Massage Therapy

Principles and Practice

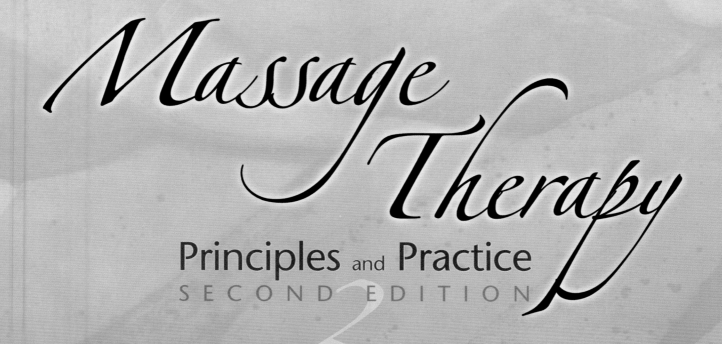

Massage Therapy

Principles and Practice

SECOND EDITION 2

SUSAN G. SALVO, BEd, LMT, NTS, CI, NCTMB

Co-owner, Co-director, and Instructor
Louisiana Institute of Massage Therapy
Lake Charles, Louisiana

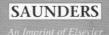

SAUNDERS

An Imprint of Elsevier

SAUNDERS
An Imprint of Elsevier

11830 Westline Industrial Drive
St. Louis, Missouri 63146

Massage Therapy: Principles and Practice

NOTICE

Massage therapy is an ever-changing field. Standard safety precautions must be followed, but as new research and clinical experience broaden our knowledge, changes in treatment and drug therapy may become necessary or appropriate. Readers are advised to check the most current product information provided by the manufacturer of each drug to be administered to verify the recommended dose, the method and duration of administration, and contraindications. It is the responsibility of the treating physician, relying on experience and knowledge of the patient, to determine dosages and the best treatment for each individual patient. Neither the Publisher nor the author assumes any liability for any injury and/or damage to persons or property arising from this publication.

Previous edition copyrighted 1999.

ISBN-13: 978–1–4160–3128–4
ISBN-10: 1–4160–3128–6

Publishing Director: Linda Duncan
Acquisitions Editor: Kellie White
Senior Developmental Editor: Kim Fons
Publishing Services Manager: Deborah Vogel
Project Manager: Kelley Barbarick
Senior Designer: Julia Dummit

Printed in China

Last digit is the print number: 9   8   7   6   5   4   3   2

To Michael; you are my love, my strength, my anchor, and my wings.

To our children, Jason, Chelsea, Christopher, Camille, Connor, Jessica, Jennifer, Justin, Juliet, and JT; you are my peace and my joy.

To my parents, Barbara and Orlando; you are my encouragement.

In memory of my grandmothers; I miss you so.

To my teachers and students; you are my inspiration.

Sandra Kauffman Anderson, BA, LMT, NCBTMB
Department Head of Anatomy and Physiology
Desert Institute of the Healing Arts
Tucson, Arizona
Member of the Exam Committee for the National
   Certification Board of Therapeutic Massage and
   Bodywork
Indications/contraindications in all body systems chapters

Michael A. Breaux, LMT
Co-owner, Director, Louisiana Institute of Massage
   Therapy
Lake Charles, Louisiana
Past Chairman, Louisiana State Board of Massage
   Therapy
Clinical Application of Massage Therapy

Alice Pilola Funk, RN, LMT
Instructor, Louisiana Institute of Massage Therapy
Lake Charles, Louisiana
Client Intake, Assessment, and Documentation

Debra C. Howard, Dipl. ABT (NCCAOM), LMT, AOBTA
   Certified Instructor
Instructor, Medical Training College, Baton Rouge,
   Louisiana; Delta College, Covington, Louisiana
President, AOBTA
Asian Bodywork Therapy: Shiatsu

Rita S. LeBleu, LMT
MA, Rhetorical and Interpersonal Communication
DeQuincy, Louisiana
Biographical Sketches

Ralph R. Stephens, BSEd, LMT, NCTMB
Owner, Ralph Stephens Seminars, LLC
Cedar Rapids, Iowa
Website: http://www.ralphstephens.com
Seated Massage

H. Micheal Tarver, PhD
Professor, Department Head of Social Sciences and
   Philosophy, Arkansas Tech University
Russellville, Arkansas
A Historical Perspective of Massage

Sandra Kauffman Anderson, BA, LMT, NCBTMB
Desert Institute of the Healing Arts
Tucson, Arizona

William L. Barry, LAc, RMT
Phoenix School of Holistic Studies
Phoenix, Arizona

JoAnn Bock, LMT, RPP
Florida School of Massage
Gainesville, Florida

Karen Brooks, NTS, LMT
New Mexico School of Natural Therapeutics
Tijeras, New Mexico

Iris Burman, LMT
Educating Hands School of Massage
Miami, Florida

Gloria Ray Carpeneto, PhD, MST, NCTMB
Villa Julie College
Baltimore, Maryland

Lauren M. Christman, MFA, LMP
Brian Utting School of Massage
Seattle, Washington

Sunny Cooper, MS, Dipl. ABT (NCCAOM)
Life Circles, Inc.
Ogden, Utah

Leopold D. Cormier, BS, DC
Austin, Texas

Don Cornwell, PhD, DOM
New Mexico School of Natural Therapeutics
Albuquerque, New Mexico

Nancy W. Dail, BA, LMT, NCTMB
Downeast School of Massage
Waldoboro, Maine

Patricia Marie Holland, BS, LMT
Desert Institute of the Healing Arts
Tucson, Arizona

Kamalapati S. Khalsa, CSMT
Phoenix Therapeutic Massage College
Phoenix, Arizona

Robert King
Chicago School of Massage Therapy
Chicago, Illinois

Glenn Manceaux, PT, DC
Flynn, Manceaux, Arcement, Chiropractic and Physical Therapy Clinic
Houma, Louisiana

Jim McKnight, BA, LMT
Delta Junction, Alabama, and Honolulu, Hawaii

Carolyn A. Nelka, BA, CMT
Catonsville Community College
Catonsville, Maryland

Therese A. Novak, MSN, RN, CS
Iowa Health Center
Iowa, Louisiana

Mary L. Puglia, MS, PhD
Phoenix Therapeutic Massage College
Phoenix, Arizona

Frank Puglia, MBA, current Arizona teaching certificate
Phoenix Therapeutic Massage College
Phoenix, Arizona

June E. Schneider, NTCMB
Baltimore School of Massage
Baltimore, Maryland

Jan Schwartz, LMT, NCTMB
Desert Institute of the Healing Arts
Tucson, Arizona

Dave Shahan
Colorado Institute of Massage Therapy
The University of Arizona Medical School
Colorado Springs, Colorado, and Tucson, Arizona

Vernon Smith, PhD, Dipl. ABT (NCCAOM), Certified Instructor (AOBTA)
Massage Therapy College of Baton Rouge
Baton Rouge, Louisiana

Sari Spieler, LMT
Seattle, Washington

Bonnie Thompson, LMT, CNMT, CFT, FT
Colorado Institute of Massage
Colorado Springs, Colorado

Dennis M. Walker, MD, FAAOS
Lake Charles Memorial Hospital
Lake Charles, Louisiana

Jerry Weinert, RN, LMT, NCTMB
Desert Institute of the Healing Arts and Southwest
  Wellness Educators
Tucson, Arizona

Pamela L. Wilson, OTR/L, NTS, LMT
Healthy Touch
Albuquerque, New Mexico

Paul Wyman, BA, CMT
Denver, Colorado

John Yates
West Coast College of Massage Therapy
Vancouver, British Columbia

Robin Zill
The Spa Center, Inc.
Hillsborough, North Carolina

A teacher's influence continues to flow outward in many directions and sometimes goes in a wide circle only to return to its source.

This is a truth for me as I write the Foreword for my former student, Susan Salvo. This is not a quote from anyone in particular but an observation from my own experience with life. I have told people many times that the best students strive to surpass the drive and wisdom of their instructors. Over twenty years have passed since Susan was in my classroom. She had the drive. She had the wisdom. And she has perfected her craft because of it. You are about to experience that craft firsthand.

Massage Therapy: Principles and Practice is the best text on massage therapy available today. Massage therapy is a newly emerging old "art form" that was practiced by those in ancient societies. It is now re-emerging, however, to take its rightful place in our present day as a "complementary medicine," working with all professions that seek to relieve human disease or suffering. Thus the book couldn't have come at a more appropriate time, given this resurgence.

As I compare the first edition with the second, I am especially impressed with the new format. Susan covers the entire scope of massage therapy, from basic setup procedures to cutting-edge therapies to client comfort and trust. The result is a polished, reader-friendly text that should be in the hands of every student, instructor, and practitioner who is serious about being up to date on the art of massage.

With this book, Susan has come full circle, extending her drive and wisdom onto the next student—you, the reader. One can also see how massage itself is following the same path, returning as a valuable form of complementary health care that started with Hippocrates, the father of modern medicine.

Sincerely,
Charles T. Brown, LMT-RMTI

Massage is multidimensional—it is simultaneously an art and a science—and through learning it, you will become a sculptor, a technician, a confidante, a musician, a teacher, an actor, and a health care professional. As a health care profession, massage therapy is one of the fastest growing career fields in the country. Massage therapy programs are emerging quickly to respond to the increasing demand, and educational standards are on the rise. With these new energies of new programs come new ideas and a revolution in the concept of massage education. This textbook was written in the spirit of this massage revolution, and it is our intention that it lead the way into the new millennium.

This textbook combines the classically accepted ideology of the past with today's new concepts. We use modern educational techniques to bridge the gap between old and new, thus creating the highest quality educational and reference materials to be found in the field of massage therapy. Our primary aim is to provide the fundamental topics that massage therapy schools must teach students to prepare them for a career in massage therapy. Through careful organization we take the reader into the world of massage. Here is how this text is organized:

Unit One–Surveying the Territory: History, Standards, Boundaries, Equipment, and Environment: A Historical Perspective of Massage; Professional Standards, Boundaries, and the Therapeutic Relationship; and Tools of the Trade and the Massage Environment

Unit Two–Benefits, Contraindications, Screening, Technique, and Special Considerations for the Massage Practitioner: Health, Hygiene, Sanitation, and Safety Standards; Massage Physiology: Effects, Indications, Contraindications, and Endangerment Sites; The Science of Body and Table Mechanics; Swedish Massage Movements and Swedish Gymnastics; Client Intake, Assessment, and Documentation; Adaptive Massage and Client Management Issues; and Putting It All Together

Unit Three–Anatomy and Physiology for the Massage Therapist: Introduction to the Human Body: Cells, Tissues, and the Body Compass; Integumentary System; Skeletal System; Skeletal Nomenclature; Muscular System; Muscular Nomenclature and Kinesiology; Nervous System; Endocrine Glands and Hormones; Circulatory System; Respiratory System; Digestive System; and Urinary System

Unit Four–A User's Guide to Complementary and Adjunctive Therapies: Hydrotherapy and Spa Applications; Clinical Application of Massage Therapy; Seated Massage; and Asian Bodywork Therapy: Shiatsu

Unit Five–Business Practices: The Business of Massage

This book is an outgrowth of the need for innovative ways to teach massage therapy. We wanted to educate the reader in a way that is at once both interesting and entertaining, easy to read, easy to use, and highly informative. This book succeeds where other texts do not; it is the only textbook that combines content (derived from the author's years of practical massage experience as a therapist and a massage school instructor) with format (learned in formal university training in the field of education). Educational techniques are used to develop an interactive approach to massage therapy instruction, which is accomplished by using a variety of formats and features, including:

Interweaving massage with the anatomical sciences. The culmination of our efforts has led to a work that, though broad in scope, successfully fuses the anatomical sciences with hands-on techniques. The anatomy and physiology chapters are written from a massage therapist's point of view. This book incorporates a general knowledge of anatomical science while focusing on the aspects that are most important to the massage practitioner. The science chapters include practical information such as specific benefits, contraindications, endangerment sites, touch research, and adaptations of massage with regard to each individual body system. Italics paragraphs highlighting massage information have been included in unit three. The massage application chapters refer back to and reinforce anatomical and physiological concepts found in the science chapters.

Emphasis on the musculoskeletal system. To thoroughly cover the topic of muscles, their origins, insertions, actions, and innervations, the skeletal and muscular systems are divided into four chapters: Two cover each system in general, and the other two highlight each system by nomenclature, listing each muscle and bone individually with illustrations and important details.

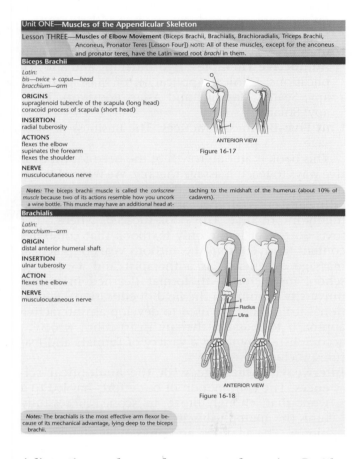

Unit ONE—Muscles of the Appendicular Skeleton

Lesson THREE—Muscles of Elbow Movement (Biceps Brachii, Brachialis, Brachioradialis, Triceps Brachii, Anconeus, Pronator Teres [Lesson Four]) NOTE: All of these muscles, except for the anconeus and pronator teres, have the Latin word root *brachi* in them.

Biceps Brachii

Latin:
bis—twice + caput—head
bracchium—arm

ORIGINS
supraglenoid tubercle of the scapula (long head)
coracoid process of scapula (short head)

INSERTION
radial tuberosity

ACTIONS
flexes the elbow
supinates the forearm
flexes the shoulder

NERVE
musculocutaneous nerve

ANTERIOR VIEW
Figure 16-17

Notes: The biceps brachii muscle is called the *corkscrew muscle* because two of its actions resemble how you uncork a wine bottle. This muscle may have an additional head attaching to the midshaft of the humerus (about 10% of cadavers).

Brachialis

Latin:
bracchium—arm

ORIGIN
distal anterior humeral shaft

INSERTION
ulnar tuberosity

ACTION
flexes the elbow

NERVE
musculocutaneous nerve

Radius
Ulna

ANTERIOR VIEW
Figure 16-18

Notes: The brachialis is the most effective arm flexor because of its mechanical advantage, lying deep to the biceps brachii.

Adjunctive and complementary therapies. Besides the base of Swedish massage techniques, this text covers such modalities as hydrotherapy, spa applications, clinical applications, seated techniques, shiatsu, and adaptations for special populations.

Key terms and glossary. Bolded in green, key terms are highlighted throughout the textbook. They can also be located in the glossary for easy access to definitions of massage terminology.

Glossary

Abdominal Anterior trunk.
Abduction Movement away from the median plane. *Horizontal abduction* refers to the direction of abduction.
Absolute contraindication Condition in which massage is inappropriate, is not advised, and may be harmful.
Absorption The processes by which the products of digestion move into the bloodstream or lymph

Active trigger points Trigger points that are noticeably painful even when there is no external physical stimulation; they can refer pain in specific patterns to other areas of the body.
Acute Refers to those conditions that last for a short time, usually a few days to a few weeks; typically these conditions have a sudden onset and run a severe course.
Adaptation A decrease in sensitivity to a pro-

Mini-labs. These short lab sessions within chapters are skill-building activities. They are designed so that left-brained and right-brained techniques reinforce each other. Direct student participation enhances the learning process by stimulating creativity and imagination. The goal is to create an interactive text that pulls the reader out of passive reading into situations in which he or she will be asked to think about, experience, and discuss topics with classmates and to write down goals and dreams.

MINI-LAB

The following exercise is designed to increase your level of sensitivity as a massage therapist and to strengthen your proprioception. Select a partner, and decide which of you is the giver and which is the receiver. Sit facing each other, and raise your hands just below shoulder level. Gently flex your fingers; allow your fingertips to touch your partner's fingertips. Both the giver and the receiver then close their eyes (Figure 10-5).

The designated giver slowly begins to move his hands in space, allowing the receiver to follow his hands while remaining connected by fingertips. This may feel awkward at first, but as the receiver expands his awareness, it begins to feel as if the two are dancing. After a minute of practice, switch roles.

After the exercise, ask yourself the following questions. How confident were you as the giver? How did you feel as the receiver? When you were the giver, did your receiver relax and follow you, or did

Biographical sketches. We have included biographies and candid interviews with many of the pioneers of massage therapy, both past and present.

ROBERT TISSERAND

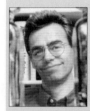

Born: November 11, 1948.

"Love what you do. Enjoy listening to people. It can be hard work, but the potential for helping people is tremendous."

Robert Tisserand, author and aromatherapist, was born in London to a father who made baskets and a mother who "did a little of this and that, but mostly raised three kids." Luckily for his "mum," the two girls were not quite as inquisitive as Tisserand, who shares his first "taste" of the aromatherapy experience.

"Curiously, I did actually drink a bottle of perfume when I was about 2 years old. My father bought it for my mother in a flea market in Paris in 1945, so the perfume would have been about 5 years old at the time. It was called *Creme de Zofali.* I survived, but the bottle has not."

Considering that it is often the smell and not the taste of foods that makes them appealing, it's easy to understand why a little boy would not think twice before turning up a bottle of slightly aged perfume. However, aromas affect more than our appetites. Odors of certain plants have been used to dedicate newborns, banish evil spirits, guide dearly departed souls to the other side, and heal all manner of ills in between. Long before frankincense and myrrh were offered to the Christ child, Egyptian physicians were using it in their practices. Greek mythology includes stories regarding the healing properties of aromatic plants, and Romans enjoyed massage with wonderfully scented, unbelievably expensive oils.

What has become a popular trend in the past few years was an academic area of study as far back as the Middle Ages. During this time, essential oils were classified according to the four elements or humors, the degree of "hotness" or "coldness" and also by the shape or color of the plant from which it was derived. For example, lungwort looks like lungs, so it was used for the respiratory system. Blue is a calming color, so plants with blue flowers were considered to have sedative properties. This way of cataloging plant essences was called the *doctrine of signatures.* Astronomy also helped play a role in organizing certain scents. Late in the sixteenth century, Nicholas Culpepper, an astrological physician, associated oils with planetary characteristics. For instance, ylang-ylang is identified as having Venus properties because it has a strong, sweet aroma and a slightly yellow tint and is considered an aphrodisiac.

The first people to dispense aromatics were the priests. They were the first perfumers, or what we would call an *aromatherapist* today. Physicians picked up the practice soon thereafter.

Although aromatherapy (the use of essential oils distilled from plants for certain conditions) has been widely used in England for some time, only recently did its climb in popularity start in the United States. Lately, massage therapists are learning more about how aromatherapy can benefit their practices. At the very least, aromatherapy adds another sensory-pleasing dimension to the pleasure of receiving a massage. However, because of the strong connection between our sense of smell and mood, it can also add other benefits. For instance, lavender is thought to be calming. On the other end of the spectrum, mints and citrus oils have an energizing effect. Mixed with oil or lotion, essential essences are considered by many to work magic on a myriad of maladies, from clogged sinuses to diarrhea. Aromatherapy can also be ingested (only by trained aromatherapists) for treatment of some ailments.

When asked which five essential oils are most important for massage therapists to always have on hand, Tisserand hesitates, pointing out that ideally, no limit should be made. However, if it is necessary to choose only five, he recommends eucalyptus, lavender, rosemary, geranium, and ylang-ylang. He also advises therapists to practice the craft in as professional a manner as

FYI (for your information), tables, charts, and checklists. Through these features, the book becomes more than an instructional text; it doubles as a practical reference guide—a welcome addition to the bookshelf of the practicing therapist. The reader can thumb through this book and take random bits of massage information.

For Your Information

The skin covers an area of about 22 square feet (ft²) and weighs approximately 9 pounds (lb), making up 7% percent of body weight. A piece of skin the size of a quarter contains more than 3 million cells, 100 sweat glands, 50 nerve endings, and 3 ft of blood vessels. The skin is thinnest over the eyelids and thickest on the soles of the feet. The fingertips have approximately 700 touch receptors on 2 square millimeters (mm²) of surface area. ⇨ □

Self-tests. We want you to pass your tests. Giving you anatomy information and teaching you massage routines is not enough if you cannot pass the licensing examinations. Self-tests are included to assist the student in self-assessment, as well as studying for and taking tests. Yes, there is a skill involved, and, if you know and understand that skill, your test-taking ability will improve. We call it becoming "test-wise." Hence, you can use this book as a study guide to prepare for and successfully pass state and/or national examinations. Other study tips include the use of mnemonic devices and an explanation of the prefixes, suffixes, and word roots of anatomical terminology.

Inspiration. Besides providing intellectual stimulation, one of our goals is to have the book inspire students emotionally and spiritually. This is accomplished through the use of insightful and thought-provoking quotations throughout the book.

"You can't turn back the clock, but you can wind it up again."

—Bonnie Prudden

Visual enhancement. For the reader's visual stimulation, we have lavishly illustrated this book with spectacular illustrations by Theodore Huff and the brilliant professional photography of Chris Salvo.

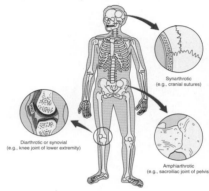

Figure 13-5 Functional classifications of joints.

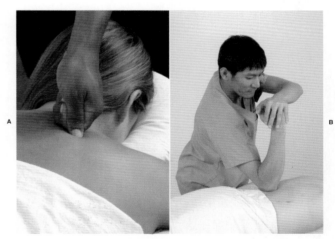

Figure 24-7 **A,** Applying ischemic compression on trigger point with thumb; **B,** using an elbow.

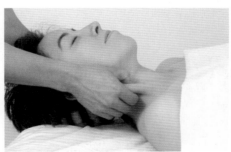

Figure 24-8 Applying ischemic compression on trigger point using a pincer grip on the sternocleidomastoid.

Unit III   Anatomy and Physiology for the Massage Therapist

314

SELF TEST

MATCHING I

List the letter of the answer next to the term or phrase that best describes it.

A. Epidermis
B. Sudoriferous glands
C. Melanocytes
D. Keratin
E. Cuticle
F. Arrector pili
G. Dermis
H. Sebaceous glands
I. Melanin
J. Nails
K. Hair follicles
L. Superficial fascia (subcutaneous layer)

____ 1. The tough ridge of skin that grows out over the nail's base

____ 2. True skin, containing adipose tissue, blood vessels, and nerve endings

____ 3. A tough, fibrous protein that provides protection by waterproofing the skin

____ 4. Tiny muscles that pull the hair upright

____ 5. Skin layer that contains melanocytes, nails, and pore openings

____ 6. Granules that gives color to the skin, hair, and the iris of the eye

____ 7. Glands whose primary functions are to regulate temperature and eliminate wastes

____ 8. Connective tissue layer that connects the dermis to underlying structures

____ 9. Specialized cells in the epidermis where skin pigment is synthesized

____ 10. Thin hard plates found on the distal ends of the fingers and toes

____ 11. Can become irritated during a massage due to allergies, hair pulling, and inadequate amount of lubricant

____ 12. Glands that secrete a fatty substance, lubricating both the hair and the epidermis

MATCHING II

List the letter of the answer next to the term or phrase that best describes it. One will be used twice.

A. Free nerve endings
B. Ruffini end organs
C. Pacinian corpuscle
D. Merkel disk
E. Meissner corpuscles
F. Krause end bulb

____ 1. Detects light pressure, adapts slowly, and is located in the dermis

____ 2. Deep pressure-sensitive receptor; shape resembles an onion slice; adapts quickly

____ 3. Responds to heat and deep, continuous pressure

____ 4. Detects light pressure, adapts slowly, and is located in the epidermis

____ 5. Pain receptors

____ 6. Receptor that is believed to respond to cold

____ 7. Also known as *nociceptors*

Web integration. Students and teachers are invited to peruse and use information published and updated on the publisher's website *http://evolve.elsevier.com/Salvo*. Expect to find links to useful websites, worksheets, and tips to enhance your massage educational experience.

Our final word of advice is to read this book three times: once during class, again as you are studying for licensing examinations, and again as a reference when situations are presented to you in your practice. Remember that this book is a very small part of your education. In fact, quality massage therapy cannot be learned solely from a book—just as you cannot learn art, music, or cooking from a book. Good role models (teachers and fellow massage therapists), a stimulating environment of classmates, curiosity, compassion, and open-mindedness are essential components of the educational process. Congratulations on beginning your education as a massage therapist. Bear in mind that your learning experience does not end with graduation from a massage school. Classroom education is simply to provide basic training and competence. Excellence is achieved by working with the body itself, where you are your own textbook, laboratory, and teacher. The body is your guide—all you need to do is listen.

SUSAN G. SALVO
susansalvo@hotmail.com
www.massagecafe.com

ACKNOWLEDGMENTS

I would like to acknowledge the following individuals who assisted me during the writing of this book: Teena Cole, H. Micheal Tarver, Alice Funk, Susie Ogg Cormier, Deborah Howard, Cathy Allen, Ralph Stephens, Michael J. Loomis, Maria and Wayne Mathias, Sandra Kaufman Anderson, Cindy Ellender, Donny Kron, Mike Breaux, Rita LeBleu, Theodore Huff, Suzanne and Chris Salvo, all the photo models (Carrie Kennedy, Amy Nicholson, Adriana Martinez, Asha Twitty, Jack DeCourcy, Eric Henson, Sally Abbott, Michael Yong, Gloria Ward, Alvaro Morales, John Choice, Diane DeGaefan, Amber Miller, Chelsea Landow, Jennifer Peters, Carol Janak, Christina Janak, Randy Perez, Layda Cabrera, Don Jewell, Nicholas Pagel, J. Randall Short, DC, Valarie Segers, Bryant Williams, Margarita Navarrete, Tom Tuma, Terrell Bearden, Jenna Cranek, Jason DeVries), Tari Dilks, Nancy Weidner, Mark Brown, Tony Dupuis, Stewart Griffith, Monica Haynes, Jeanette Ritchey, Robin Zill, John Moreno, Kathy Lea, Robin Martin, Damon Ogle, Sandy Anderson, Connie Modyelewski, Craig Parham, Stefanie Gore, Michael Kent, Dennis Walker, Belford Carver, Kevin Bernier, Marilyn Dunn, Linda Warner, Scott Weaver, Maureen Pfeifer, Christie Hart, George King, John Fanuzzi, Ann Hawkins, Belinda Hughes, Karla Hunt, Edwin Hunter, Stephanie Ecker, Cherie Sohnen-Moe, Susan Doyle, Monica Reno, Tricia Grafelman, Nina McIntosh, William Barry, Linda Mills, Brenda Roberts, Jennifer Breaux, Trish Ecker, Dennis Verrette, Angela Stevens, Todd Nicholson, Allen Breaux, Kathlene Deaville, Catherine Dupuis, Jennifer Behn, Kim Fons, Kellie White, Jennifer Paris, James Watson, Kelley Barbarick, Barbara Karkalits, Amy Perkins, and all the reviewers.

CONTENTS

UNIT FIVE   Business Practices

APPENDIXES

Massage Therapy

Principles and Practice

UNIT ONE

Surveying the Territory: History, Standards, Boundaries, Equipment, and Environment

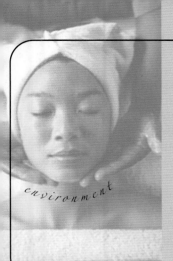

environment

A Historical Perspective of Massage

1

H. Micheal Tarver, Ph.D.

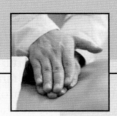

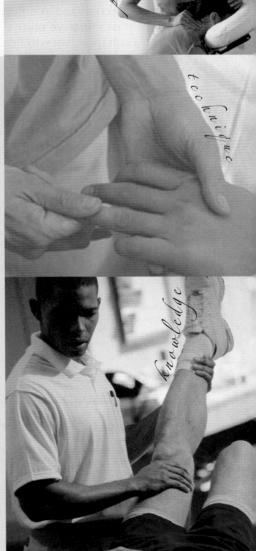

pressure

"People and places always have a past and their identity dissolves unless they recognize they have a history."

—Nathaniel Hawthorne

technique

STUDENT OBJECTIVES

After completing this chapter, the student should be able to:

- Define the term *massage*
- Name major figures in the development of medicine and specifically in massage therapy
- Discuss the ancient views and uses of massage incorporating both eastern and western cultures
- Explain the role of the European Renaissance and Enlightenment on the professionalism of massage therapy
- Distinguish the contributions of Pehr Henrik Ling from those of later physicians and therapists
- Reconstruct the development of therapeutic massage incorporating the various massage styles
- Integrate recent developments in the field of therapeutic massage into the original framework of Pehr Ling and his students

knowledge

INTRODUCTION

Massage can be defined as a systematic and scientific manipulation of the soft tissues of the body for the purpose of obtaining or maintaining health. The history of massage and healing touch is long and complex, with more than 75 different types of massage and *bodywork,* a generic term used to describe massage and its various forms. Archaeological and historical evidence seems to indicate that massage and healing touch has been practiced for thousands of years in all regions of the globe. Massage is instinctive. It is a natural response to rub our aches and pains, regardless of whether we are familiar with the medical knowledge behind those actions. In modern health care, therapeutic massage has taken on an important role. It has been shown beneficial to reduce stress, enhance blood circulation, decrease pain, promote sleep, reduce swelling, enhance relaxation, and increase oxygen capacity of the blood. Massage has also been recognized as a nondrug treatment for cancer and postoperative pain.

In this chapter, we will briefly examine the history of massage from its earliest records to the present (Figure 1-1). *The goals of this chapter are to provide the massage therapist with the information necessary to illustrate the path taken in the development of the profession and to instill in the therapist a sense of connection with those who preceded him or her.* Some names will be familiar, and others will be quite foreign. You need not memorize every name mentioned in the following pages, although some are important enough that you should know them (ask your instructor). What the names, with their different nations of origin, tell us is that the development of massage therapy was a global endeavor; people from around the world contributed to the knowledge base that transformed massage from folk remedy to scientific treatment. It should be noted that from the beginning of this chapter, the word *massage* is used to refer to *soft tissue manipulation,* even though the term did not come into use until the middle of the nineteenth century. The origin of the word *massage* is unclear, but it can be traced to numerous sources: the Hebrew word *mashesh,* the Greek roots *masso* and *massin,* the Latin root *massa,* the Arabic root *mass'h,* the Sanskrit word *makeh,* and the French word *masser.*

THE PREHISTORIC WORLD

In prehistoric times (i.e., before written records) evidence supports the position that massage was practiced by several groups around the world. Archaeologists have found artifacts that depict the use of massage in a number of world cultures. Although no direct prehistoric evidence verifies the use of massage for medical reasons, the indirect evidence clearly implies that it was used in this manner. For example, European cave paintings (c. 15,000 BC) depict what appears to be the use of healing touch. In this period, extensive pictorial records show the use of massage.

THE ANCIENT WORLD

In the ancient East a concern with illness has been documented in China for several millennia, and records have revealed that the practice of massage goes back as early as 3000 BC. However, it was in the period between the second century BC (200-101 BC)

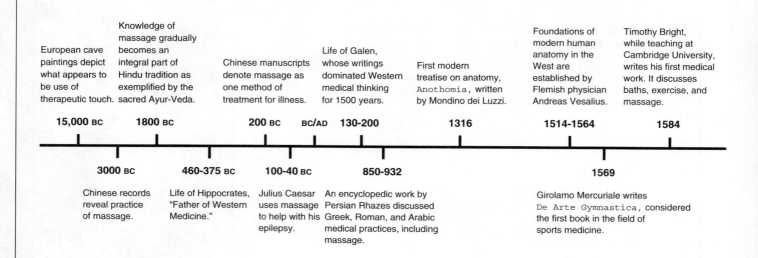

Figure 1-1   Massage time line.

and the first century AD (AD 1-100), that Chinese medicine began to take on its basic shape. Manuscripts found in China dating from the second century BC discuss massage as one of the various methods of treatment for illnesses. It should be noted, however, that acupuncture was not referred to in Chinese medical writings until 90 BC. Using their knowledge of massage and later acupuncture (Figure 1-2), the Chinese developed a style of massage that they termed *amma, amna,* or *anmo.* **Amma** is regarded as the precursor to all other therapies, manual and energetic—the grandparent of all massage techniques. The Chinese had developed the art of massage so well that they were the first to train and employ massage therapists who were blind.

As early as the first century AD, various schools of medical thought had been founded and had already begun to produce diverging ideas. These various ideas and beliefs were compiled under the name of the mythical Yellow Emperor and have become the classic scripture of traditional Chinese medicine, the *Huang-ti nei-ching.* Although the exact date of the original writing of the work is unknown, it was already in its present form by approximately the first century BC. The work, commonly known as *Nei Ching*, contained descriptions of healing touch procedures and their uses. Some debate is ongoing over the actual date of this work with some historians arguing that it was written around 2760 BC. By AD 700, a Chinese ministry of health and a public health system were established.

By the sixth century AD, the techniques and use of massage were well established in China and had found their way into Japan. In general, the Japanese

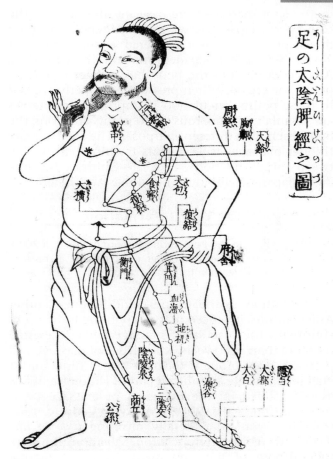

Figure 1-2 Chinese acupuncture chart. (Courtesy of the U.S. National Library of Medicine, Bethesda, Md.)

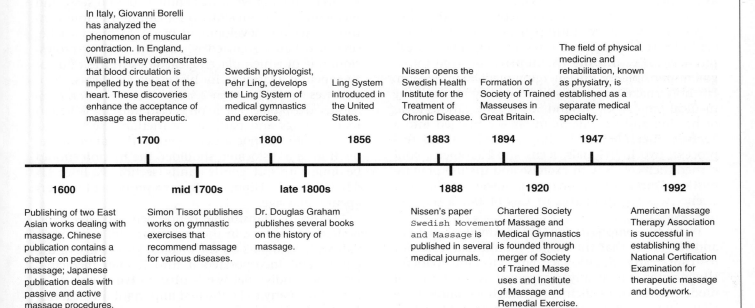

In Italy, Giovanni Borelli has analyzed the phenomenon of muscular contraction. In England, William Harvey demonstrates that blood circulation is impelled by the beat of the heart. These discoveries enhance the acceptance of massage as therapeutic.

Swedish physiologist, Pehr Ling, develops the Ling System of medical gymnastics and exercise.

Ling System introduced in the United States.

Nissen opens the Swedish Health Institute for the Treatment of Chronic Disease.

Formation of Society of Trained Masseuses in Great Britain.

The field of physical medicine and rehabilitation, known as physiatry, is established as a separate medical specialty.

1700   **1800**   **1856**   **1883**   **1894**   **1947**

1600   **mid 1700s**   **late 1800s**   **1888**   **1920**   **1992**

Publishing of two East Asian works dealing with massage. Chinese publication contains a chapter on pediatric massage; Japanese publication deals with passive and active massage procedures.

Simon Tissot publishes works on gymnastic exercises that recommend massage for various diseases.

Dr. Douglas Graham publishes several books on the history of massage.

Nissen's paper Swedish Movement and Massage is published in several medical journals.

Chartered Society of Massage and Medical Gymnastics is founded through merger of Society of Trained Masseuses and Institute of Massage and Remedial Exercise.

American Massage Therapy Association is successful in establishing the National Certification Examination for therapeutic massage and bodywork.

methods of massage were basically the same as the Chinese. In Japan, we see *shiatsu*, literally meaning finger pressure; it is considered a component of amma. *Shiatsu* is a Japanese modality based on the Asian concept that the body has a series of energy points, or **tsubo**. When pressure is properly applied to these points, circulation is improved and nerves are stimulated. Numerous tsubo points are along the body, each with different purposes. The shiatsu practitioner massages tsubo points to bring balance between mind and body. Like the Chinese, the medieval Japanese employed blind massage therapists.

For Your Information

In the Pergamon Museum in Berlin, a 2000-year-old alabaster relief depicts a massage treatment.

In addition to the Chinese and Japanese, other Asian cultures practiced massage. On the Indian subcontinent, the practice of massage has also existed for more than 3000 years. Knowledge of massage had probably been brought to India from China, and it gradually became an integral part of Hindu tradition, as exemplified by the inclusion of massage treatments in the sacred practice of **Ayur-Veda** (c. 1800 BC). The Ayur-Veda, literally meaning *code of life,* deals with rebirth, renunciation, salvation, the soul, the purpose of life, the maintenance of mental health, and the prevention and treatment of diseases. As for medicine, the most important Ayurvedic texts are the Samhitas. A later work, the ***Manav Dharma Shastra*** (c. 300 BC), also mentions massage. In addition to the above-mentioned eastern cultures, the Polynesians have also been documented as practicing therapeutic massage.

The concept of health and medicine in the West began to take shape during the seventh and sixth centuries BC. During that time, the legendary Greek physician **Æsculapius (Asclepius)** evolved into a god responsible for the emerging medical profession. His holy snake and staff still remain symbols of the medical profession. Around 500 BC, the various ideas of healing and treatments in Greece merged into a **techne iatriche**, or healing science. During this process, two individuals, Iccus and Herodicus, concerned themselves with exercise and the use of gymnastics. Among the numerous followers of this new science was **Hippocrates of Cos** (460-375 BC) (Figure 1-3).

With his emphasis on the individual patient and his belief that the healer should take care not to cause any additional harm to the patient, Hippocrates is generally recognized as the father of modern western medicine. Although we know little about him, he is reputed to have been a fine clini-

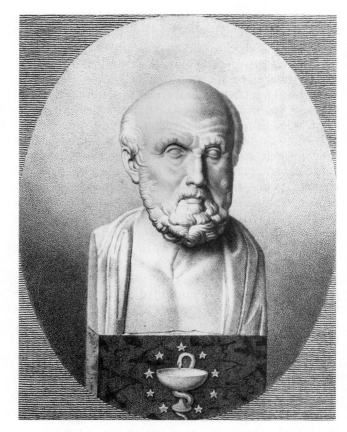

Figure 1-3   Hippocrates of Cos. (Courtesy of the U.S. National Library of Medicine, Bethesda, Md.)

cian, a founder of a medical school, and the author of numerous books, although most of the works attributed to him were written by other members of the Hippocratic school. These works are collectively known as the ***Corpus Hippocraticum***, which summarized much of what was known about disease and medicine in the ancient world. During the four centuries after the development of the techne iatriche, several debates occurred within the healing profession, one of which placed great stock in the value of therapeutic massage. In his essay *On Joints*, Hippocrates wrote, "πολλων ευπειρον σει τον ιητρον, αταρ ση και ανατριψιοξ" ("The physician must be skilled in many things and particularly friction," section IX, lines 25-26). Hippocrates also noted that after the reduction of a dislocated shoulder, the friction should be done with soft, gentle hands (section IX, lines 31-33). Obviously, Hippocrates was a proponent of therapeutic massage.

During the transitional period between Greek and Roman dominance in the ancient world, a few individuals helped pass on the medical knowledge of the Greeks and incorporated it into Roman medicine. One such individual was **Aulus Celsus**, who is regarded by many to be the first important medical historian. His ***De Medicina*** is an outstanding account of Roman medicine, and it bridges the gap between his times and those of Hippocrates. During this period, massage had gained such acceptance that Julius Caesar (c. 100-44 BC) used it to help his epilepsy.

A group of Greek physicians residing in Rome, known as the **Methodists**, supported a simplistic view of healing and restricted their treatments to bathing, diet, massage, and a few drugs. The earlier practitioners and other groups recognized the importance of touch. The founder of this school of thought was **Asclepiades**. Among his many contributions to Roman medicine was a treatise on friction (massage) and exercise. Although the work is no longer in existence, it was cited by Aulus Aurelius Cornelius Celsus (c. 25 BC-AD 50) in his writings on friction.

A later follower of Hippocratic medicine was **Galen of Pergamon** (c. AD 130-200) (Figure 1-4). Galen was a Roman physician who studied medicine in Alexandria (Egypt) and became the personal physician to the Roman emperor Marcus Aurelius. In at least 100 treatises, Galen synthesized and unified Greek knowledge of anatomy and medicine; his system continued to dominate medicine throughout the Middle Ages and until relatively recent times. Among his many works, Galen's *De Sanitate Tuenda* considers exercise, the use of baths, and massage. Following the division of the Roman Empire into eastern and western halves, the decline in learning was much more rapid and severe in the Roman West than in the Greek East (Byzantium).

Farther east of the Romans, the ancient Slavs reportedly used massage. In the Americas, the Mayas and Inca have been documented as practicing joint manipulation and massage. The Inca also used the application of heat in their treatments of joint disorders, through the use of the leaves of the chilca bush. They had a higher success rate for *trepanation,* a surgical procedure involving the removal of a segment of the skull, in 2000 BC than the Europeans did in AD 1800. In addition, records indicate that the Cherokees and Navajos used massage in their treatments of colic and to ease labor pains.

THE MIDDLE AGES

After the collapse of the Roman Empire (AD 476), western medicine experienced a period of decline. In reality, it was only because of the writing efforts of a number of western physicians (e.g., Oribasius and Alexander of Tralles) that the ancient medical knowledge of the Greeks and Romans was preserved. Among the last of the Greco-Roman writers to consider treatment by mechanical means (as opposed to drug therapy or surgery) was **Paul of Aegina** (AD 625-690), who advocated the bending, stretching, and rubbing of paralyzed limbs. As a consequence of his writings, Galen became the central medical authority in the West for centuries. After the decline of Rome, the Hippocratic-Galenic tradition survived in the Greek-speaking East. After the fall of Alexandria (AD 642), knowledge of Greek medicine spread throughout the Arabic world.

After the expansion of the Islamic world in the seventh and eighth centuries, the comprehensive body of Greco-Roman medical doctrine was adopted, together with extensive Persian and Hindu medical knowledge. One such example of this synthesis of knowledge was an encyclopedic work *(Kitabu'l Hawi Fi't-Tibb)* by the Persian physician **Rhazes** (Abu Bakr Muhammad ibn Zakariya al-Razi) (c. AD 850-932), which discussed Greek, Roman, and Arabic medical practices, including massage. Another important work was by the Persian physician Abu-Ali al-Husayn ibn-Sina (AD 980-1037), generally known as **Avicenna**. He also authored numerous medical books that remained the standard until the seventeenth century. His *Canon of Medicine* was an especially famous medical text, which compiled the theoretical and practical medical knowledge of the time. The work illustrates the tremendous influence of Galen on the medical knowledge of the era; the text makes numerous references to the use of massage. In fact, by the end of the ninth century, almost all of Galen's lengthy medical texts had been translated into Arabic. In general, it appears that the Islamic physicians of the European Middle Ages were more interested in developing and commenting on the truths learned from the Greeks and Romans than they were in discovering new knowledge. The Muslims simply incorporated

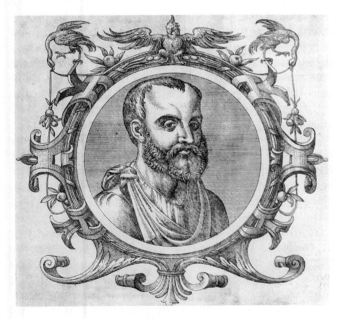

Figure 1-4   Galen of Pergamon. (Courtesy of the U.S. National Library of Medicine, Bethesda, Md.)

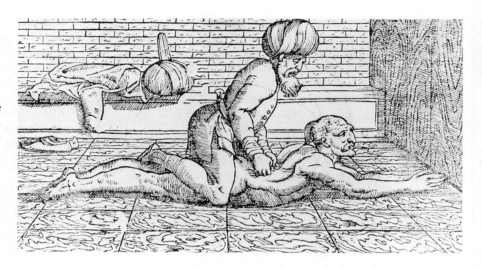

Figure 1-5 Print of woodcut of massage therapy dated 1595. (Courtesy of the U.S. National Library of Medicine, Bethesda, Md.)

Greco-Roman medical knowledge into the Islamic framework. It was through Latin translations of these Arabic authors that most of the knowledge of Greek medicine was revived in the Christian West (i.e., Europe).

For the most part, western medical practitioners of the Middle Ages abandoned massage in favor of other treatments. Massage did, however, remain an important procedure for folk healers and midwives, and its procedures were passed on as an art form. Subsequently, no early compilation of these techniques and procedures was undertaken. It is also very likely that monastic clergy used massage in their *hospitale pauperum* because they would have had copies of earlier Greco-Roman medical writings.

During the course of the later Middle Ages, the collection, preservation, and transmission of classical medical knowledge occurred (Figure 1-5). After the twelfth century, medieval medical knowledge in the West expanded, thanks in part to the existing works by the Muslims, who had earlier translated Greek and Latin medical texts into Arabic. By the thirteenth century, medical knowledge had advanced to the point that three major European centers (Montpelier, Paris, and Bologna) were offering degrees in medicine. In 1316, Mondino dei Luzzi wrote **Anothomia**, the first modern treatise on anatomy.

With the revival of classical Greek learning during the Renaissance, western medicine was revitalized by new translations of old Greek and Latin texts. Among the newly revived texts was Aulus Celsus's *De Medicina,* which came into circulation again, thanks to the newly invented printing press.

 When you steal from one author, it's plagiarism; if you steal from many, it's research.
　　　　　　　　　　　　　　—Wilson Mizner

THE EUROPEAN RENAISSANCE AND ENLIGHTENMENT

The **Renaissance** (c. 1250-1550) was an exciting period in the history of medicine and medical treatments. The word *renaissance* means rebirth, and it was during that time that the foundations of modern human anatomy (in the West) were established by the Flemish physician **Andreas Vesalius** (1514-1564). His *De Humani Corporis Fabrica* (1543) is considered one of the most important studies in the history of medicine. In addition, the foundations of chemical pharmacology, as opposed to herbal remedies, were laid by the Swiss physician Philippus von Hohenheim (1493-1541), better known as **Paracelsus**. New surgical procedures were also established, particularly those by the French military surgeon **Ambroise Paré** (c. 1510-1590) (Figure 1-6). In addition to inventing several surgical instruments, Paré was among the earliest modern physicians to discuss the therapeutic effects of massage, especially in orthopedic surgery cases. Paré even went so far as to classify various types of massage movements.

Two other notable Renaissance physicians were **Girolamo Mercuriale** (1530-1606) and **Timothy Bright** (c. 1551-1615). Mercuriale spent several years in Rome examining the manuscripts of the ancient writers. His extensive knowledge of the attitudes of the Greeks and Romans toward diet, exercise, and their effects on health and disease is evident in *De Arte Gymnastica* (1569), considered to be the first book in the field of sports medicine. The work compiled the history of gymnastics up to that time, synthesizing all that had been written on the use of exercise (for both the purpose of health and the treatment of disease).

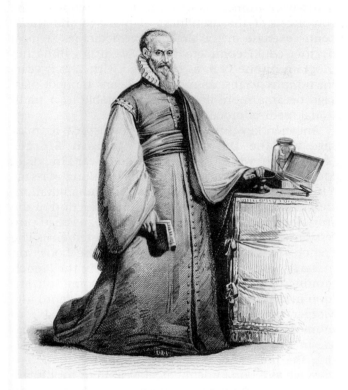

Figure 1-6   Ambroise Paré. (Courtesy of the U.S. National Library of Medicine, Bethesda, Md.)

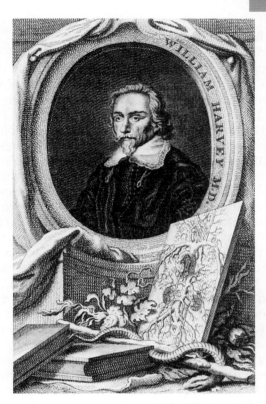

Figure 1-7   William Harvey. (Courtesy of the U.S. National Library of Medicine, Bethesda, Md.)

Bright's first medical work (c. 1584) was divided into two parts, *Hygienina on Restoring Health* and *Therapeutica on Restoring Health*. In this work, Bright discussed baths, exercise, and massage, and he began teaching his ideas to students at Cambridge University in Cambridge, England.

Around the sixteenth century, we see two important East Asian works that dealt with massage. The Chinese published ***Chen-chiu ta-ch'eng***, which contained a chapter on pediatric massage, and the Japanese published ***San-tsai-tou-hoei***, which mentioned both passive and active massage procedures.

By the end of the seventeenth century, western medicine had experienced a revolution in both ideas and knowledge. In Italy, **Giovanni Alfonso Borelli** (1608-1679) carried out extensive anatomical dissections and had analyzed the phenomenon of muscular contraction. In England, **William Harvey** (1578-1657) had demonstrated that blood circulation in animals is impelled by the beat of the heart through arteries and veins (Figure 1-7). This discovery enhanced the acceptance of massage as a therapeutic measure. Another crucial development during the seventeenth century was the realization that it was necessary to compile complete clinical descriptions of disease, generally at bedsides, and to develop specific remedies for each specific disease. In this area, the English physician **Thomas Sydenham** (1624-1689) was most prominent. At the same time these scientific advances were being made, massage was reemerging as a therapy acceptable to the medical profession and as a therapeutic practice for health and disease.

The European renaissance and enlightenment era also had an impact on western medicine. What emerged was an optimistic outlook concerning the role and benefits of the field of medicine. It was widely believed that health was a natural state to be attained and preserved. Within this new philosophy, massage came to be viewed as a popular treatment in Europe. **Simon André Tissot** (1728-1797) published several works on gymnastic exercises that recommended massage for various diseases and gave indications for its use. The eighteenth century also saw the creation of new medical systems, which incorporated the anatomical, physiological, and chemical discoveries of the previous 200 years. These comprehensive systems were necessary to provide a rationale for and guidance to clinical activities. Some believed that the gathering and dispensing of this new knowledge would add prestige to the medical profession and help weed out the "quacks."

THE MODERN ERA

The era of modern massage began in the early nineteenth century when a wide variety of authors were advocating massage and developing their own systems. The most important of these writers was **Pehr Henrik Ling** (1776-1839), a Swedish physiologist and gymnastics instructor. Through his experiences at the University of Lund and the Swedish Royal Central Institute of Gymnastics, Ling developed his own system of medical (Swedish) gymnastics and exercise, known as the *Ling System, Swedish Movements,* or *Swedish Movement Cure.* The primary focus of Ling's work was on gymnastics applied to the treatment of disease and/or injury. In this regard, Ling was a proponent of gymnastics, a subject that was promoted more than 2000 years earlier by Herodicus, the teacher of Hippocrates. According to Ling, gymnastics were a therapeutic system by which we try—by means of influencing movement—to overcome discomfort that has arisen through abnormal conditions.

Ling's system consists of three primary movements: active, passive, and duplicated. Active movements were those performed by the patient (e.g., exercise). Passive movements were movements of the patient performed by the therapist (e.g., stretching, range of motion). Duplicated movements were those performed by the patient with the cooperation of the therapist (e.g., active assistive). As part of duplicated movements, patient's movements may be opposed by the therapist (active resistive). Other terms used to describe Swedish gymnastics are *remedial gymnastics, table stretches, joint mobilizations,* and *range-of-motion exercises.*

Massage was viewed as a component of Ling's overall system and was known commonly as **Swedish massage**. Ling, the father of Swedish massage, and his followers used a system of strokes that created a very relaxing experience. In general, these followers used massage strokes in tandem with the movements described above. Its movements of the joints promoted general relaxation, improved circulation, relieved muscle tension, and improved range of motion.

From 1813 to 1839, Ling taught these techniques at the Royal Central Institute of Gymnastics in Stockholm, Sweden, which he founded with governmental support. Although Ling is also considered the father of physical therapy, actually his students would be responsible for the spreading of his ideas throughout the world. Among the more important cities with established schools teaching Ling's methods were St. Petersburg, London, Berlin, Dresden, Leipzig, Vienna, Paris, and New York. Within 12 years of his death (1839), 38 institutions in Europe were teaching the Swedish Movement System. Included in these students were numerous medical doctors who became convinced of the usefulness of massage and therapeutic exercise in the practice of medicine. Medical doctors could complete Ling's Swedish gymnastics program in one year, as compared with 2 to 3 years for nonphysicians. As more physicians trained, massage became more and more acceptable as a traditional medical procedure and practice.

Another key individual in the history of massage was the Dutch physician **Johann Mezger** (1839-1909), who was born the same year Ling died. Mezger is generally given credit for making massage a fundamental component of physical rehabilitation. He has also been credited for the introduction of the still-used French terminology into the massage profession (e.g., effleurage, pétrissage, tapotement). The French translated several of the Chinese books on massage, and this probably explains why the French terminology for the procedures has become so common in massage texts like this one. Unlike Pehr Ling, Mezger, being a physician, was much more able to promote massage using a medical and scientific basis. In this regard, Mezger was quite successful getting the medical profession to more readily accept massage as a bona fide medical treatment for disease and illness. A number of European physicians began to use massage therapy and to publish scientifically the positive results of the modality. What occurred was the inclusion of the art of massage in the science of medicine.

The Swedish Movement system was introduced into the United States in 1856 by two brothers, **George Henry Taylor** and **Charles Fayette Taylor**. The Taylors had studied the techniques in Europe and returned to the United States where they opened an orthopedic practice with a specialization in the Swedish Movements. The two physicians published a number of important works on Ling's system, including the first American textbook on the subject in 1860. A third prominent American follower of the Swedish Movement was **Douglas O. Graham**. Not only was Dr. Graham a practitioner of the system, but from 1874 to 1925, he also authored several works on the history of massage.

Another prominent practitioner in the United States was **Hartvig Nissen**, who in 1883 opened the Swedish Health Institute for the Treatment of Chronic Diseases by Swedish Movements and Massage (Washington, D.C.). Nissen presented the paper, *Swedish Movement and Massage,* in 1888, which was subsequently published in several medical journals. The result of publication was numerous letters from physicians who wanted to know more about Ling's system, and this inquiry led him to publish *Swedish Movement and Massage Treatment* in that same year. Taken together, Nissen's book and Graham's *A Treatise on Massage, Its History, Mode of Application and Effects* (1902)

PEHR HENRIK LING

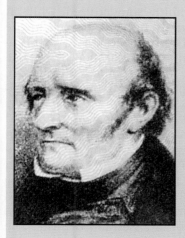

Born: 1776; died: 1839. Father of physical therapy and Swedish massage.

(Courtesy of Armand Dedrick Maanum, the last Master-Master Masseur-Teacher of the Sjuk Gymnastiken Passiva Rorelser Massage of Pehr Henrik Ling.)

Born in Smaaland, one of the southern provinces of Sweden, Pehr Henrik Ling led a very interesting life. After being expelled from school for disciplinary problems, Ling traveled through Europe and eventually returned to Sweden where he learned fencing (the art of using a sword). In 1804 he accepted a post at the University of Lund, where he taught fencing and gymnastics. At the same time, he studied anatomy and physiology. In his teaching of fencing techniques, he noted that the movements he often wanted his pupils to make were hindered by motions that the student had learned from habit. Ling therefore resolved to teach the movements of the body in a systematic manner. For Ling, this training was important for military concerns, and he viewed fencing as an important part of gymnastics. What he meant was that soldiers could be taught to use weapons and move muscles in ways that were new to them.

At the same time, Ling also developed what is referred to as *Swedish gymnastics,* through which we try—by means of influencing movements—to overcome discomfort that has arisen through abnormal conditions. These gymnastics comprised only a few stretching movements done by the student alone (active movements), performed by another pupil while the student relaxed (passive movements), or performed by the student with the cooperation of the pupil (duplicated movements such as active assistive and active resistive). In Ling's system, very little, if any, mechanical apparatus was involved.

In 1813, Ling opened the Swedish Royal Central Institute of Gymnastics where he further developed his own system of medical gymnastics and exercise, known as the *Ling system, Swedish movements,* or the *Swedish movement cure.* The primary focus of Ling's work was on gymnastics applied to the treatment of disease and/or injury. Massage was viewed as a component of Ling's overall system. Known commonly as *Swedish massage,* Ling and his followers used a system of long, smooth, slow strokes that created a very relaxing experience. The movements of the joints promote general relaxation, improve circulation, relieve muscle tension, and improve range of motion.

Ling was not a physician, and his system of Swedish gymnastics was bitterly opposed by many within the medical profession during much of his lifetime. However, many of his students were physicians, and these individuals spread his teachings and began to publish success stories of his techniques in respectable medical journals. Ling's influence was so great that by 1851, 38 schools located throughout Europe were teaching his system of gymnastics and massage.

After years of failing health, Pehr Henrik Ling died in 1839. His legacy is seen today throughout the health professions, especially in the teachings of massage therapy, physical therapy, kinesiology, and gymnastics.

are generally credited with arousing interest in the U.S. medical profession in the benefits of massage.

While the Taylor brothers, Graham, and Nissen were convincing the medical community of the benefits of massage and gymnastics, several other individuals were busy convincing the general public. Among the most famous of these was **John Harvey Kellogg** (1852-1943) of Battle Creek, Mich. He

wrote numerous articles and books on massage and published *Good Health,* a magazine that targeted the general public. Efforts by men like Kellogg helped popularize massage in the United States.

The end of the nineteenth and beginning of the twentieth centuries witnessed important changes in the use of massage, the most important of which was the development of the field of physical therapy.

Physical therapy, which developed from physical education, was responsible for the training of women to work in hospitals where they used massage and therapeutic exercise to help patients recover. These women were often trained in mechanotherapy, which is the healing of the body by means of manipulations (massage and special exercises).

World War I provided countless opportunities for the use of therapeutic massage, exercise, and other physiotherapeutic methods (electrotherapy and hydrotherapy) in efforts to rehabilitate injured soldiers. During the course of treating war casualties, the earlier ideas of **Just Lucas-Championniere** (1843-1913) were eventually recognized. Dr. Lucas-Championniere advocated the use of massage and passive motion exercises after injuries, especially fractures.

By the beginning of the twentieth century, massage had begun to be used throughout the West. Once the procedures of massage were accepted, what developed was the profession of massage. In Great Britain, *The Society of Trained Masseuses* (1894) was formed by several women who realized the need for the standardization and professionalization of their trade. The organization was successful in several key areas: establishing a massage curriculum; accrediting massage schools, which had to undergo regular inspections; requiring qualified instructors for the massage classes; and establishing a board certification program. By the end of World War I (1918), the Society had nearly 5000 members.

In 1920 the Society merged with the Institute of Massage and Remedial Exercise, and the new group became known as the *Chartered Society of Massage and Medical Gymnastics*. This new group also took some important steps at professionalism. Among the new membership requirements were the requirement for physician referrals and the issuance of certificates of competence to those who passed the required tests.

By 1939 the membership in the organization numbered approximately 12,000.

After World War I, medical organizations such as the *American Society of Physical Therapy Physicians* also formed. In the 1920s and 1930s, programs for physical therapists were becoming standardized, while at the same time physicians were being trained in the field. In 1926, **John S. Coulter** became the first full-time academic physician in physical medicine at the Northwestern University Medical School in Evanston, Ill. By 1947 the field of physical therapy and rehabilitation was established as a separate medical specialty.

Although many masseurs and masseuses frowned on the encroachment of the medical profession on their art form, the events just described can be viewed with excitement. By the early part of the twentieth century, the western medical profession had begun to realize what the Chinese and masseurs/masseuses had long preached: therapeutic massage had an important place in the treatment of illnesses and diseases. The professionalism of medical gymnastics (now called *physical therapy*) simply meant that in addition to learning the art of massage the therapist needs also to acquire the scientific background necessary to understand human anatomy and physiology. As this textbook illustrates, the authors and contributors also believe in a well-educated, well-trained massage therapist.

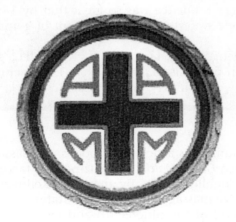

Figure 1-8 Membership pin of the American Association of Masseurs and Masseuses. (Courtesy of the American Massage Therapy Association, Evanston, Ill.)

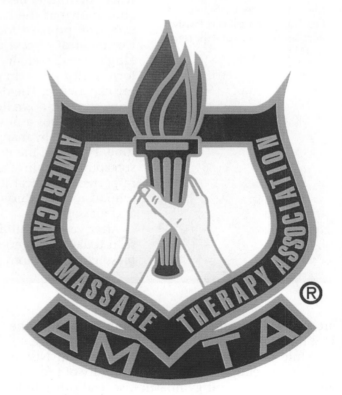

Figure 1-9 Current logo of the American Massage Therapy Association. (Courtesy of the American Massage Therapy Association, Evanston, Ill.)

As technology and medical advances caught up with the profession, a simple massage became less crucial on its own; it became one procedure in the arsenal of rehabilitation. As a consequence, the *British Chartered Society of Massage and Medical Gymnastics* changed its name to the *Chartered Society of Physiotherapy*. In 1943, postgraduates from the College of Swedish Massage in Chicago created the *American Association of Masseurs and Masseuses (AAMM)* (Figure 1-8). The AAMM changed its name to the *American Massage and Therapy Association* in 1958 and then again changed its name to the *American Massage Therapy Association (AMTA)* in 1983 (Figure 1-9). Over time the AMTA came to represent the professional masseurs and masseuses, preferably called *massage therapists*. It is the largest massage therapist organization with chapters in all 50 states and currently has more than 47,000 members in 30 countries.

> *Nature, being well-instructed, does what is needed without being taught.*
>
> —Hippocrates

NEW METHODS

To date, about 75 methods of massage therapy have been classified (Figure 1-10). Although space limitations prohibit detailed discussions of these procedures, a listing has been complied of several styles (see Figure 1-10). These styles or **modalities** (any technique, procedure, or product used to produce a positive response for the client) have been categorized according their primary approach on the human body/mind/spirit. Many of these techniques go beyond the original concepts of Swedish massage, and most were developed in the United States since 1960.

Figure 1-10 Massage family tree.

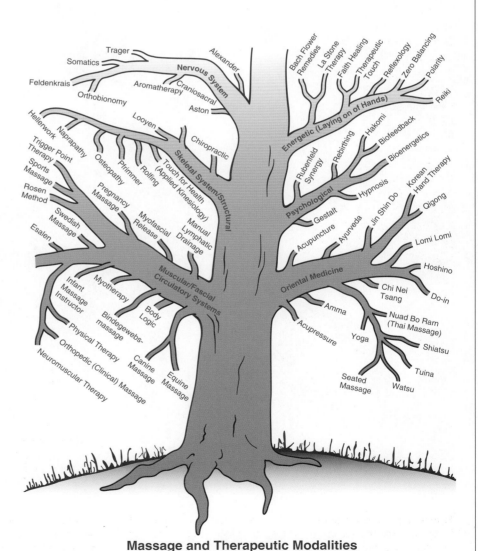

Massage and Therapeutic Modalities

SUMMARY

In the past 25 years, massage has risen in popularity in the United States. Especially important in this rise of popularity are those individuals who are looking for alternative/complementary therapies (e.g., diet, exercise, herbal remedies, acupuncture, acupressure, and massage) to supplement their medical treatments and thus help them with their lives and their health. Massage, as one method of physical therapy, has been shown to be beneficial for many people.

As a consequence of this increase in popularity, the profession has also grown during that time. In 1988 the AMTA pushed for the development of national certification, which came in 1992 with the independent National Certification Examination for Therapeutic Massage and Bodywork. As such, massage therapy has become a respected and much-used allied health care profession. According to Eisenberg et al's *Trends in Alternative Medicine Use in the United States, 1990-1997,* massage therapy was the third most prevalent type of alternative/complementary medicine used by adults in the United States in the 1990s. New uses for massage therapy are being discovered daily, with a recent (April 2001) study published in the journal *Archives of Internal Medicine* documenting the effectiveness of massage for chronic back pain. The study also noted that massage was found to be superior to both acupuncture and self-care, over both the short- and long-term.

By no means is this study of massage history complete and exhaustive. A detailed history of massage would take volumes and entail years of research. This chapter should have given you a thorough sense of how the profession developed and in what direction it appears to be headed. More than 75 different varieties of massage and bodywork are available. This chapter has given you a glimpse of how they first began.

MATCHING I

Write the letter of the best answer in the space provided.

A. Johann Mezger
B. Nei-ching
C. Ayur-Veda
D. Passive
E. Physical therapy
F. Hippocrates

G. George and
   Charles Taylor
H. China
I. Pehr H. Ling
J. Greece
K. Arte Gymnastica

L. Amma
M. Massage
N. Active
O. Tsubos
P. William Harvey

—— 1. The first written accounts of therapeutic rubbing (massage) originated in which country

—— 2. The original massage technique

—— 3. Energy points in the Japanese massage system where pressure is applied

—— 4. The application of massage was included in what sacred Indian practice

—— 5. The father of modern western medicine

—— 6. Systematic and scientific manipulation of the soft tissues of the body for the purpose of obtaining and/or maintaining health

—— 7. Western massage texts tend to use French terminology, primarily because of the efforts of this individual

—— 8. The classic scripture of traditional Chinese medicine

—— 9. The scientist that demonstrated that blood circulation is impelled by the beat of the heart through arteries and veins

—— 10. The work generally credited as being the first book in the field of sports medicine

—— 11. The father of Swedish massage and physical therapy

—— 12. Along with duplicated and active, this term is also one of the different kinds of movements used in Ling's system of medical gymnastics

—— 13. The Swedish movement system was introduced into the United States by these individuals

—— 14. Movements performed by the client

Bibliography

Basham AL: The practice of medicine in ancient and medieval India. In Leslie C, editor: *Asian medical systems,* Berkeley, Calif, 1976, University of California Press.

Buikstra JE: Diseases of the pre-Columbian Americas. In Kiple KF et al: *The Cambridge world history of human disease,* New York, 1993, Cambridge University Press.

Castiglioni A: *A history of medicine,* New York, 1947, Alfred A. Knopf (Translated by EB Krumbhaar).

Coulter J: *Physical therapy,* New York, 1932, Paul B. Hoeber.

Eisenberg D et al: Trends in alternative medicine use in the United States, 1990-1997: results of a follow-up national survey, *JAMA* 280(18):1569-1575, 1998.

Fryback P, Reinert B: Alternative therapies and control for health in cancer and AIDS, *Clin Nurse Spec* 11(2):64-69, 1997.

Goldberg J et al: The effect of therapeutic massage on H-reflex amplitude in persons with a spinal cord injury, *Phys Ther* 74(8):728-737, 1994.

Hippocates: *Hippocates, vol iii, on wounds in the head. in the surgery. on fractures. on joints. mochlicon,* Cambridge, 1928, Harvard University Press. (Transated by ET Withington.)

Liddel L: *The book of massage: the complete step-by-step guide to eastern and western techniques,* New York, 1984, Simon and Schuster.

McMillan M: *Massage and therapeutic exercise,* Philadelphia, 1921, WB Saunders.

Means PA: *Ancient civilizations of the Andes.* New York, 1931, C Scribner's Sons.

Meintz SL: Alternatives and complementary therapies: whatever became of the back rub? *RN* 58(4):49-50+, 1995.

Mulliner MR: *Mechano-therapy: a text-book for students,* Philadelphia, 1929, Lea & Febiger.

Nissen H: *Practical massage in twenty lessons,* Philadelphia, 1905, FA Davis.

Rahman F: *Health and medicine in the Islamic tradition: change and identity,* New York, 1987, Crossroad.

Salmon JW, editor: *Alternative medicine: popular and policy perspectives,* New York, 1984, Tavistock.

Solomon W: What is happening to massage? *Arch Phys Med* 31:521-523, 1950.

Unschuld PU: History of Chinese medicine. In Kiple KF et al, editor: *Cambridge world history of human disease,* New York, 1993, Cambridge University Press.

U.S. Department of Health and Human Services: *Acute pain management in adults: operative procedures—quick reference guide for clinicians,* Rockville, Md, 1992, The Department.

U.S. Department of Health and Human Services: *Management of cancer pain: adults—quick reference guide for clinicians,* Rockville, Md, 1994, The Department.

Veith I, Huang T: *Nei ching su wen,* Baltimore, 1949, Williams and Wilkins.

Wanning T: Healing and the mind/body arts: massage, acupuncture, yoga, tai chi, and Feldenkrais, *AAOHN J* 41(7):349-351, 1993.

White J: Touching with intent: therapeutic massage, *Holist Nurs Prac* 2(3):63-67, 1988.

Wide AG: *Hand-book of medical and orthopedic gymnastics,* New York, 1905, Funk and Wagnalls.

Zyzk KG: *Religious healing in the Veda, with translations and annotations of medical hymns in the Rgveda and the Atharvaveda and renderings from the corresponding ritual texts,* Philadelphia, 1985, American Philosophical Society. (Transactions of the American Philosophical Society, vol 75, p 7.)

Web Resources

The American Massage Therapy Association: *A short history: the American Massage Therapy Association,* accessed Nov 1, 2002. Available at *http://www.amtamassage.org/about/history.htm.*

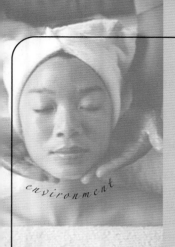

environment

Professional Standards, Boundaries, and the Therapeutic Relationship

2

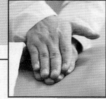

"Good fences make good neighbors."

—Robert Frost

pressure

technique

STUDENT **OBJECTIVES**

After completing this chapter, the student should be able to:

- Define the massage therapist's scope of practice
- List 15 different standards of conduct from the Code of Ethics
- List 15 different items from the Standards of Practice
- Define self-disclosure and confidentiality; give examples of confidentiality exceptions
- Define the concept of boundaries as they relate to your personal and professional life
- Write a set of personal and professional boundaries for yourself
- Create boundary management skills and procedures for handling "fire drills" and scenarios of client conflict
- Describe when it is appropriate to terminate the massage session in the event that a client violates your professional boundaries

knowledge

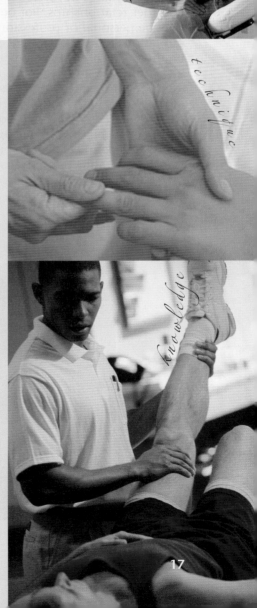

INTRODUCTION

The prevailing professional parameters for the massage therapy profession can be divided into two areas: professional standards and boundaries. *Professional standards* consist of a list of guidelines that are established by a profession itself to promote consistent professionalism and integrity. These standards apply to all massage therapists in a given jurisdiction and define how the individual therapist relates to the profession as a whole. Although geographically these standards may vary widely, they include a number of vital elements: educational requirements; professional scope of practice; a code of ethics; standards of practice; confidentiality; and regional, state, or municipal laws. It is the responsibility of the student/therapist to know the laws and standards that govern their profession and abide by these laws and adopt these standards.

The second area, *boundaries,* consists of our individual standards in interactions with our clients and all other relationships. For our purposes, boundaries may be personal or professional. As the Robert Frost quotation reminds us, fences (a type of physical boundary) can enhance our relationships with others. Boundaries in relationships impart a sense of self, a personal or professional space to grow, and a sense of protection. As we explore the topic of boundaries, we will discuss personal boundaries, professional boundaries, boundary management, issues of intimacy and conflict, client abuse and client neglect, transference and countertransference, how to handle problem situations, inappropriate behavior and its consequences, session termination procedures, and incident reports (Figure 2-1).

PROFESSIONAL STANDARDS

In general, professional standards help define and distinguish our profession from that of other health care professions. As our profession grows, more distinct borders that give our profession limitations are defined. We call these parameters our professional standards. These standards include the requirements for education and certification, testing and licensing, scope of practice, code of ethics, and standards of practice.

What's in a Word? The Educational Requirements

The terms *licensed, certified, registered,* and *nationally certified* are all adjectives used to describe educated massage therapists. Credentials and identifying titles are important parts of professional image and allow you to promote yourself as qualified and competent to the general public. These adjectives are often confusing because different agencies who issue the right to use these descriptions often have different requirements. Each region (e.g., state, county, parish, city) may have its own rules and regulations for the practice of massage therapy.

Massage therapy schools today teach certification courses that range from 100 to more than 2000

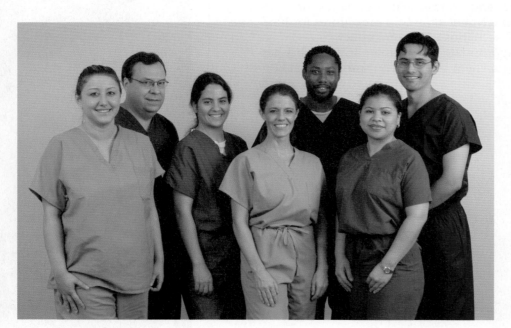

Figure 2-1 The massage therapist is a professional.

hours. At the time of this writing (2002), the national average of formal training in the United States is 500 hours. The terms *masseur* and *masseuse* were dropped in favor of massage therapist. In some areas, this was done to move from the gender-specific French terms to a title that is not gender specific. In other areas of the country, the change in terminology was made to differentiate between individuals who were apprentice trained and those who received formal classroom training in anatomy and physiology, as well as knowledge, skills, and abilities in performing massage. These educated therapists were described by a confusing variety of terms and titles because no national standard is recognized by every region. These titles included certified massage therapist (C.M.T.), registered massage therapist (R.M.T.), licensed massage therapist (L.M.T.), and simply massage therapist (M.T., Ms.T., or M.Th.).

According to *Webster's New Collegiate Dictionary,* one meaning of the word *certify* is to attest authoritatively as to the validity of something. Therefore to certify a massage therapist means to attest the training, knowledge, and skill of a practitioner. Such verification is usually made by a nongovernmental institution such as a trade school, massage school, or professional organization. Because the students choose voluntarily to take the classes in the massage field, the certification itself is only as good as the reputation and credentials of the certifying body. A massage therapy school therefore certifies that the student has completed a course in massage therapy and is granted the title of Certified Massage Therapist or C.M.T. This certification usually involves completion of a required number of hours of classroom instruction in combination with other educational requirements: apprenticeship; internship; and successful passing of examinations that cover science and applied skills. In many states, one must obtain a state license after receiving an official certificate of successful completion of a course of study to practice massage therapy legally.

The word *licensing* means that permission has been granted by a competent authority for a person to engage in an occupation that would otherwise be considered to be unlawful. It is a government body such as a state, province, or municipality that grants the license to practice massage therapy as a means of regulating the profession according to law. Licensure is a mandatory (or nonvoluntary) process because it is passed into law by a legislative body. Everyone who wants to practice massage therapy must complete the licensing process in states that require it. Once a therapist has been qualified (through certification) to take the licensing examination(s), successfully passing the examination(s) leads to a license. The massage therapist is then known as a *Licensed Massage Therapist* or

L.M.T. once this and perhaps further requirements (e.g., paying a license fee) are met.

The massage profession appears to have a broad range of usage of the word *registered*. Two definitions of register are (1) to make a record of or (2) a book or system of public records. When the state of Texas created its massage therapy law, it chose to use the designation *registered* instead of *licensed* massage therapist. According to the American Massage Therapy Association (AMTA), *registered* is generally "somewhat less restrictive than licensing," but each state varies in its use of the term.

Between 1954 and 1991 the AMTA also had a registered massage therapist program that sought to elevate standards by creating a higher tier of the profession. This program required successful completion of certain education, experience, and testing standards. AMTA's development of a membership examination, standards for massage training, and the creation of National Certification replaced the R.M.T. program, which was abolished in 1991.

In 1987, with the purpose of promoting higher standards for massage therapists, AMTA initiated the formation of a National Certification Commission consisting of representatives from AMTA, the American Oriental Bodywork Therapy Association (AOBTA), the American Polarity Therapy Association (APTA), the Rolf Institute, and the Trager Institute. The Commission organized the National Certification Board for Therapeutic Massage and Bodywork. By 1992, the National Certification Board for Therapeutic Massage and Bodywork (NCBTMB), a nonprofit organization that is governed by an elected board of directors, was established. This independent national board was accredited by the National Organization for Competency Assurance (NOCA) in 1993. The goal of the NCBTMB was to define and implement high standards for the massage therapy profession through the successful completion of a nationally recognized test.

The NCBTMB has been quite successful, and, although it has not been accepted unanimously in all states, some states with licensing laws accept the national examination in lieu of their own state written licensing examination. An NCBTMB national code of ethics, standards of practice, and a disciplinary board is available for processing grievances filed against nationally certified practitioners.

In summary, massage therapy schools certify graduates. The majority of the states license their massage therapists through a testing procedure. Some states opt to use the term *registered* to define massage therapists in their regions. National certification is a process designed to raise professional standards and create additional professional recognition for those who can complete it.

Distinguishing Between Basic and Advanced Massage Practice

Modality specialization involves additional training, possible additional certification criteria, and concentration on a select clinical area within the field and scope of massage. Changes are occurring in the health care field necessitating the need for massage therapists with specialty skills. The massage profession itself has evolved and now provides its members with the knowledge to advance their practices. Although many states require a minimum number of continuing education units (CEU) every year, additional certifications are elective. Only therapists who graduate from a basic 500-hour curriculum should be candidates for this supplementary training.

What has evolved is a two-tiered structure in massage therapy education; basic training and advanced training. This trend is not unlike what happened to the field of medicine recently. Doctors can be general practitioners or specialists. Nurses can be licensed practical or vocational nurses, registered nurses, or nurse practitioners. The massage profession is still in transition and is responding to this development in

a variety of ways. Massage schools are trying to beef up the curriculum in an attempt to satisfy the specialty trend. Another development has been the offering of workshops and seminar series. Some states have recognized this trend and developed two licenses to reflect massage therapists with different training levels; a massage therapy license offered to a therapist with the minimum required hours (500 being the national average) and a master's license for individuals who have gone beyond basic educational requirements and received an additional 200 hours or more in an area of specialization (neuromuscular massage, manual lymphatic drainage, shiatsu, myofascial release, and so on). Advanced certificates are elective and can only be obtained if primary, or basic requirements are met.

One model used for conceptualizing this tiered system of massage therapy is a practice wheel. The hub of the wheel is a basic 500-hour curriculum (for a discussion on if 500 hours is enough training, read the section on How Safe Is Massage in Chapter 5) and advanced training extends in all directions from the wheel's center (Figure 2-2). Moving toward basic and advanced massage practices will help advance the

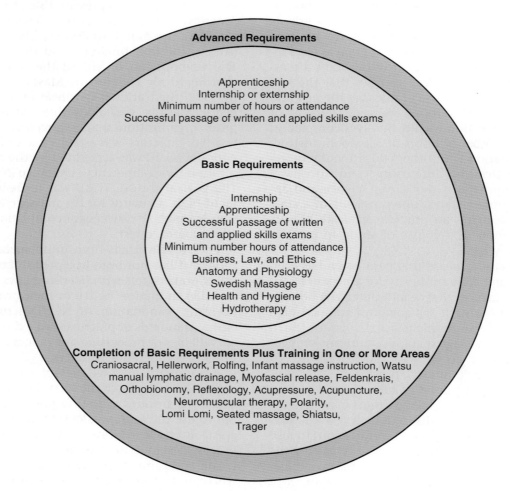

Figure 2-2 Massage practice wheel.

profession and offer options to therapists, their clients, and referring physicians.

The Scope of a Massage Therapy Practice

Scope of practice, often derived from the legal definition of massage, defines the working parameters of a particular profession, according to training, education, and licensure, and is solely a matter of state law. Scope of practice defines what services massage therapists can provide; it may also list specific practices such as ultrasound treatments that massage therapists may not offer because a separate license is required. Professional massage therapy associations and certifying bodies such as massage therapy schools, workshops, and national organizations may also have their own requirements. However, state law, where applicable, supersedes any other conflicting legal definitions and professional parameters. State law should define scope of practice as the minimum standard by which massage therapists must practice (Figure 2-3).

It is the responsibility of every therapist to obtain a copy of the state law where practicing and learn its rules, regulations, and legislated scope of practice. The scope of practice should contain a definition of massage therapy.

1. Your scope of practice may say that massage therapy is the application of any form of manual treatment of bodily soft tissues for the purposes of general relaxation, improving the health of the client, and maintaining or restoring the client to proper health. The term soft tissue denotes the various layers of the integument, muscles, tendons, ligaments, fascia, cartilage, nerves, blood vessels, viscera, and membranes of the body. The term manual treatment includes all forms of therapy whereby the soft tissues of the client's body are treated with direct or indirect contact of the massage therapist's hands, feet, elbows, knees, and forearms. Direct contact may include the application of pressure to the tissues and may introduce movement to the joints to affect surrounding tissues. *Direct* contact may also include various devices, such as mechanical vibrators or handheld pressure bars for applying static pressure or cross-fiber friction. *Indirect* contact may be energetic in nature—that is, it may not necessarily involve actual touch as much as sensitivity to and manipulation of the energy fields surrounding the body.

2. Scope of practice includes the general assessment of the client's condition by intake form, interview, palpation, and consultation with the client's other health care providers. Assessment is needed to determine treatment goals, contraindications, and the need for referral to other health care professionals. *General assessment* refers to the massage therapist's ability, based on past training and experience, to recognize specific pathologies and to formulate an appropriate treatment based on established protocol.

3. Scope of practice does not include diagnosis of illness or injury. Although it may include joint mobilizations and range of motion, it does *not* include performing spinal or joint manipulations. Prescribing or advising the use of medication, or rendering a prognosis, both of which are in the domain of medical and chiropractic physicians, are also omitted. Instead of a prognosis, massage therapists can give an estimated duration of treatment or opinion regarding the client's progress.

4. Because of the popular use of massage therapy as recreational, massage therapists have open access to the public. A doctor's prescription is *not* required for someone to see a massage therapist. However, in cases involving insurance reimbursement for treatment of illness or injury, the massage therapist must have a written diagnosis and referral from a medical or chiropractic physician.

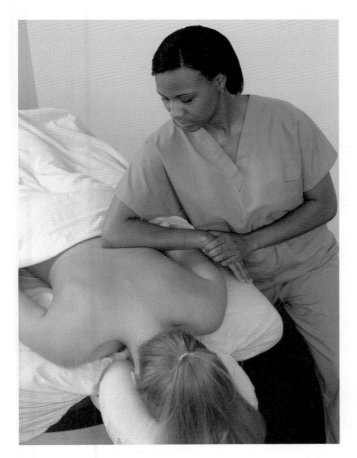

Figure 2-3 Massage therapists' scope of practice is determined by state law.

5. Scope of practice may include the use of hydrotherapy and aromatherapy. Hydrotherapy encompasses the therapeutic use of ice packs, heat packs, whirlpools, saunas, and steam baths. Aromatherapy includes the use of essential oils to heighten the relaxation effect of the therapy.

If a client requires services that are out of your scope of practice, please refer them to the proper health care provider.

Code of Ethics and Standards of Practice

When you enroll in a massage therapy school, you agree to accept certain rules and standards. Likewise, when you enter into the profession in a state that requires licensure, you also inherently accept the massage therapy laws and ethical standards practiced in that state. Typically the licensing board of your state is responsible for creating and distributing its code of ethics. Professional massage therapy organizations may have their own codes of ethics and standards of practice, which if you are a member you are expected to incorporate into your practice.

A **code of ethics** is a set of guiding moral principles that governs one's course of action (Box 2-1). Most licensed health care professions have a code of ethics that members of those professions are expected to follow when working within their scope of practice. Most codes of ethics for massage therapists include governing principles for therapeutic relationships, professional behavior, business policies, and even guidance in decision making. An ethical decision is required to solve a problem that has long-term implications. For example, most state

---

BOX 2-1

The National Certification Board for Therapeutic Massage and Bodywork Code of Ethics

The Code of Ethics of the National Certification Board for Therapeutic Massage and Bodywork (NCBTMB) specifies professional standards that allow for the proper discharge of the massage therapist's and/or bodyworker's responsibilities to those served, that protect the integrity of the profession, and that safeguard the interest of individual clients.

Those practitioners nationally certified in therapeutic massage and bodywork in the exercise of professional accountability will conduct themselves as follows:

1. Have a sincere commitment to provide the highest quality of care to those who seek their professional services.
2. Represent their qualifications honestly, including education and professional affiliations, and provide only those services that they are qualified to perform.
3. Accurately inform clients, other health care practitioners, and the public of the scope and limitations of their discipline.
4. Acknowledge the limitations of and contraindications for massage therapy and bodywork, and refer clients to appropriate health professionals.
5. Provide treatment only when there is reasonable expectation that it will be advantageous to the client.
6. Consistently maintain and improve professional knowledge and competence, striving for professional excellence through regular assessment of personal and professional strengths and weaknesses and through continued educational training.
7. Conduct their business and professional activities with honesty and integrity, and respect the inherent worth of all people.
8. Refuse to unjustly discriminate against clients or other ethical health professionals.
9. Safeguard the confidentiality of all client information, unless disclosure is required by law, court order, or absolutely necessary for the protection of the public.
10. Respect the client's right to treatment with informed and voluntary consent. The NCTMB practitioner will obtain and record the informed consent of the client, or client's advocate, before providing treatment. This consent may be written or verbal.
11. Respect the client's right to refuse, modify, or terminate treatment regardless of prior consent given.
12. Provide draping and treatment in a way that ensures the safety, comfort, and privacy of the client.
13. Exercise the right to refuse to treat any person or part of the body for just and reasonable cause.
14. Refrain, under all circumstances, from initiating or engaging in any sexual conduct, sexual activities, or sexualizing behavior involving a client, even if the client attempts to sexualize the relationship.
15. Avoid any interest, activity, or influence that might be in conflict with the practitioner's obligation to act in the best interests of the client or the profession.
16. Respect the client's boundaries with regard to privacy, disclosure, exposure, emotional expression, beliefs, and the client's reasonable expectations of professional behavior. Practitioners will respect the client's autonomy.
17. Refuse any gifts or benefits that are intended to influence a referral, decision, or treatment and that are purely for personal gain and not for the good of the client.
18. Follow all policies, procedures, guidelines, regulations, codes, and requirements promulgated by the National Certification Board for Therapeutic Massage and Bodywork.

From National Certification Board for Therapeutic Massage and Bodywork: *Code of ethics (adopted 2/17/95) and standards of practice (adopted 2/9/00)*, McLean, Va, The Board.

laws do not require therapists to post a list of fees for a given service, nor do states require that the therapist equally charge every client. No one will argue with a therapist who gives a discount to senior citizens, the disabled, or the economically disadvantaged. But how will a therapist be judged if an attorney or a doctor is charged more than the normal fee? While it may be legal to do so, it is not ethical. For more information, see the NCBTMB Code of Ethics in Box 2-1.

Most people have a personal code of ethics that governs their behavior. Many of us form our codes as a result of early interactions with family, members of our religious congregation, and members of our community. So your personal code of ethics may not be very different from your professional code of ethics. When acting unethically, you are acting in contradiction to your own personal code and a generally accepted standard of conduct set forth by your peers and/or your profession.

In addition to a code of ethics, many health professions publish a standards of practice. These standards, also published by the National Certification Board for Therapeutic Massage and Bodywork, cover the following areas: Professionalism, Legal and Ethical Requirements, Confidentiality, Business Practices, Roles and Boundaries, Prevention of Sexual Misconduct. The primary goal of the **standards of practice** is to assist you in making good decisions while your are conducting your day-to-day responsibilities within your scope of practice. Box 2-2 contains the published code of ethics and standards of practice adopted by the NCBTMB.

The Good Samaritan Law

Every state in the United States has a Good Samaritan law to protect individuals who give medical aid in emergency situations from criminal and civil liability. Within each state, the law concerning the Good Samaritan may vary slightly, but in general, if a health care professional or civilian renders help to an individual in need, such as performing cardiopulmonary resuscitation (CPR), she is not held liable for any harm to the individual as a result of her decision to help in the emergency.

Self-Disclosure and Confidentiality

Beginning at the initial contact and during the course of the therapeutic relationship, clients will reveal their thoughts and feelings to the therapist. Honest and open sharing of these emotions, ideas, and insights is known as **self-disclosure**. As time spent with the therapist progresses, and the client experiences emotional safety, more of themselves will

be revealed. This information should be closely guarded by the therapist. The safekeeping of this knowledge is called **confidentiality** and is considered nondisclosure of privileged information—that is, it may not be divulged to a third party. Both self-disclosure and confidentiality are important components of the client-therapist relationship.

The two basic exceptions to the confidentiality rule are as follows. The first exception is when clients give permission for the massage therapist to reveal their name or specific personal information to a third party. This may occur when the therapist is part of a therapy team, working in connection with a client's mental health counselor, doctor, attorney, insurance company, or other involved profession. Release of information may also involve a family member such as a parent of a minor client or the adult child of an elderly client. Other third-party involvement can include a translator for someone with a language barrier or a relative who has power of attorney for a disabled client.

The second exception occurs when keeping information confidential would cause harm to either the client or a third party. These situations might involve a client who, taking the massage therapist into his confidence, discusses plans of suicide or actions that will harm others (e.g., homicide). In these cases, the therapist should contact the client's psychotherapist, medical doctor, or the emergency contact person listed on the client intake form. Reporting the situation initiates a process, often an investigation. In some areas, the massage therapist may be required to report situations of child abuse, elder abuse, or certain criminal activities to law enforcement. Call the local district attorney's office or the massage therapy board in your state to find out which agency in your area is appropriate for each situation.

You may also be required to report cases of communicable diseases such as tuberculosis or hepatitis to your public health department to make sure that you and others are not at risk of infection. Contact your local health department and inquire what your responsibilities are as a health care provider.

How Do We Refer to Our Patrons, as Clients or Patients?

A great deal of discussion is ongoing over whether the patrons of massage therapy should be referred to as clients or patients. If your state law specifies the use of client or patient, then the language of the law supersedes any professional preference. When the law does not specify or if your state currently does not require licensure, how we refer to our patrons may be strictly situational. For example, if you are in private practice or are employed by a nonmedical establishment such

BOX 2-2

The National Certification Board for Therapeutic Massage and Bodywork Standards of Practice

Standard I: Professionalism

The certificant must provide optimal levels of professional massage and bodywork services and demonstrate excellence in practice by promoting healing and well-being through responsible, compassionate, and respectful touch. In his or her professional role the certificant shall commit to the following:

1. Adhere to the NCBTMB Code of Ethics, Standards of Practice, policies, and procedures.
2. Comply with the peer review process conducted by the NCBTMB Ethics and Standards Committee regarding any alleged violations against the NCBTMB Code of Ethics and Standards of Practice.
3. Conduct themselves in a manner in all settings meriting the respect of the public and other professionals.
4. Treat each client with respect, dignity, and worth.
5. Use professional verbal, nonverbal, and written communications.
6. Provide an environment that is safe and comfortable for the client and which, at a minimum, meets all legal requirements for health and safety.
7. Use standard precautions to ensure professional hygienic practices and maintain a level of personal hygiene appropriate for practitioners in the therapeutic setting.
8. Wear clothing that is clean, modest, and professional.
9. Obtain voluntary and informed consent from the client before initiating the session.
10. If applicable, conduct an accurate needs assessment, develop a plan of care with the client, and update the plan as needed.
11. Use appropriate draping to protect the client's physical and emotional privacy.
12. Be knowledgeable of their scope of practice and practice only within these limitations.
13. Refer to other professionals when in the best interest of the client and/or practitioner.
14. Seek other professional advice when needed.
15. Respect the traditions and practices of other professionals and foster collegial relationships.
16. Not falsely impugn the reputation of any colleague.
17. Use the initials NCTMB to designate his or her professional ability and competency to practice therapeutic massage and bodywork only.
18. Remain in good standing with and maintain NCBTMB certification.
19. Understand that the NCBTMB certificate may be displayed prominently in the certificant's principal place of practice.
20. When using the NCBTMB logo and certification number on business cards, brochures, advertisements, and stationery, do so only in a manner that is within established NCBTMB guidelines.
21. Not duplicate the NCBTMB certificate for purposes other than verification of the practitioner's credentials.
22. Immediately return the certificate to NCBTMB if it is revoked or suspended.

Standard II: Legal and Ethical Requirements

The certificant must comply with all the legal requirements in applicable jurisdictions regulating the profession of massage therapy and bodywork. In his or her professional role the certificant shall commit to the following:

1. Obey all applicable local, state, and federal laws.
2. Refrain from any behavior that results in illegal, discriminatory, or unethical actions.
3. Accept responsibility for his or her own actions.
4. Report to the proper authorities any alleged violations of the law by other certificants.
5. Maintain accurate and truthful records.
6. Report to the NCBTMB any criminal convictions regarding himself or herself and other certificants.
7. Report to NCBTMB any pending litigation and resulting resolution related to his or her professional practice and the professional practice of other certificants.
8. Respect existing publishing rights and copyright laws.

Standard III: Confidentiality

The certificant shall respect the confidentiality of client information and safeguard all records. In his or her professional role the certificant shall commit to the following:

1. Protect the client's identity in social conversations, all advertisements, and any and all other manners unless requested by the client in writing, medically necessary, or required by law.
2. Protect the interests of clients who are minors or who are unable to give voluntary consent by securing permission from an appropriate third party or guardian.
3. Solicit only information that is relevant to the professional client/therapist relationship.
4. Share pertinent information about the client with third parties when required by law.
5. Maintain the client files for a minimum period of four years.
6. Store and dispose of client files in a secure manner.

Standard IV: Business Practices

The certificant shall practice with honesty, integrity, and lawfulness in the business of massage and bodywork. In his or her professional role the certificant shall commit to the following:

1. Provide a physical setting that is safe and meets all applicable legal requirements for health and safety.
2. Maintain adequate and customary liability insurance.
3. Maintain adequate progress notes for each client session, if applicable.
4. Accurately and truthfully inform the public of services provided.
5. Honestly represent all professional qualifications and affiliations.
6. Promote his or her business with integrity and avoid potential and actual conflicts of interest.

From National Certification Board for Therapeutic Massage and Bodywork: *Code of ethics (adopted 2/17/95) and standards of practice (adopted 2/9/00)*, McLean, Va, The Board.

BOX 2-2

The National Certification Board for Therapeutic Massage and Bodywork Standards of Practice—cont'd

7. Advertise in a manner that is honest, dignified, and representative of services that can be delivered and remains consistent with the NCBTMB Code of Ethics.
8. Advertise in a manner that is not misleading to the public by, among other things, the use of sensational, sexual, or provocative language and/or pictures to promote business.
9. Comply with all laws regarding sexual harassment.
10. Not exploit the trust and dependency of others, including clients and employees or co-workers.
11. Display or discuss schedule of fees in advance of the session that are clearly understood by the client or potential client.
12. Make financial arrangements in advance that are clearly understood by and safeguard the best interests of the client or consumer.
13. Follow acceptable accounting practices.
14. File all applicable municipal, state and federal taxes.
15. Maintain accurate financial records, contracts and legal obligations, appointment records, tax reports and receipts for at least 4 years.

Standard V: Roles and Boundaries

The certificant shall adhere to ethical boundaries and perform the professional roles designed to protect the client and practitioner and safeguard the therapeutic value of the relationship. In his or her professional role the certificant shall commit to the following:

1. Recognize his or her personal limitations and practice only within these limitations.
2. Recognize his or her influential position with the client and shall not exploit the relationship for personal or other gain.
3. Recognize and limit the impact of transference and countertransference between the client and the certificant.
4. Avoid dual or multidimensional relationships that could impair professional judgment or result in exploitation of the client or employees and/or co-workers.
5. Not engage in any sexual activity with a client.
6. Acknowledge and respect the client's freedom of choice in the therapeutic session.
7. Respect the client's right to refuse the therapeutic session.

8. Refrain from practicing under the influence of alcohol, drugs, or any illegal substances (with the exception of prescribed dosage of prescription medication, which does not significantly impair the certificant).
9. Have the right to refuse and/or terminate the service to a client who is abusive or under the influence of alcohol, drugs, or any illegal substance.

Standard VI: Prevention of Sexual Misconduct

The certificant shall refrain from any behavior that sexualizes, or appears to sexualize, the client/therapist relationship. The certificant recognizes that the intimacy of the therapeutic relationship may activate practitioner and/or client needs and/or desires that weaken objectivity and may lead to sexualizing the therapeutic relationship. In his or her professional role the certificant shall commit to the following:

1. Refrain from participating in a sexual relationship or sexual conduct with the client, whether consensual or otherwise, from the beginning of the client/therapist relationship and for a minimum of 6 months after the termination of the client/therapist relationship.
2. In the event that the client initiates sexual behavior, clarify the purpose of the therapeutic session, and if such conduct does not cease, terminate or refuse the session.
3. Recognize that sexual activity with clients, students, employees, supervisors, or trainees is prohibited even if consensual.
4. Not touch the genitalia.
5. Only perform therapeutic treatments beyond the normal narrowing of the ear canal and normal narrowing of the nasal passages as indicated in the plan of care and only after receiving informed voluntary written consent.
6. Only perform therapeutic treatments in the oropharynx as indicated in the plan of care and only after receiving informed voluntary consent.
7. Only perform therapeutic treatments into the anal canal as indicated in the plan of care and only after receiving informed voluntary written consent.
8. Only provide therapeutic breast massage as indicated in the plan of care and only after receiving informed voluntary consent from the client.

From National Certification Board for Therapeutic Massage and Bodywork: *Code of ethics (adopted 2/17/95) and standards of practice (adopted 2/9/00)*, McLean, Va, The Board.

as a salon or a spa, *client* is the appropriate reference for a patron. If you work in a medical setting, such as a hospital, a physical therapy office, or a chiropractic clinic, the preferred terminology is *patient*. The major difference is that the term *patient* denotes that a patron is under the medical supervision of another health care professional.

Discrimination vs. Right of Refusal

It is the right of either the therapist or the client to decide not to engage in or maintain the therapeutic relationship. The therapist has the right to refuse any client as long as a justifiable reason is provided for the refusal of service, and the therapist should in-

MOSHE FELDENKRAIS, DSc

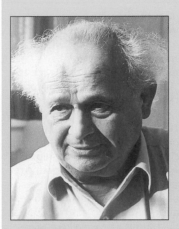

(Courtesy of Feldenkrais Institute, Tel Aviv, Isreal.)

Born: May 6, 1904; died: February 9, 1984.

"We settle for so little! As long as we can get by, we let it go at that."

Moshe Feldenkrais's father sold bits of forests, and that was the only ordinary thing about the man. Feldenkrais was reared in the Talmudic tradition and came from a long list of rabbis, some still famous today. Feldenkrais changed his nationality three times before he left home at 13—from Polish to German to Russian. In 1918 at the close of WWI, he left for Turkey, never to see his family again.

Although he would eventually obtain his doctorate in science and degrees in both mechanical and electrical engineering and proceed to work on the French atomic research program and the British antisubmarine program, he found his passion quite early in life.

As a boy of 16 in Palestine, Feldenkrais was part of a group called the *Haganah*, which means self-defense force. They learned some basic jujitsu, which did not prove successful. It was then that Feldenkrais realized that the only way to learn was to start at the beginning—with the first move.

And I built this system of defense for any sort of attack where the first movement is not what you think to do, what you decide to do, but what you actually do when you are frightened. And I said, "All right, let's see now, we will train the people so that the end of their first spontaneous movement is where we must start."

—Moshe on Moshe on the Martial Arts. From Feldenkrais Journal 12, Issue #2.

Feldenkrais published an instructional book on the subject, which gained him admission to his first judo exhibition. The Japanese minister of education, rather taken by Feldenkrais and what he had accomplished without any formal training, asked him to introduce judo to Europe. Feldenkrais refused, explaining he could not devote himself to such an enterprise and continue his university studies at the same time, but the minister was determined. Soon it was agreed that an expert would come to France and work with Feldenkrais when time would allow.

Thus Feldenkrais became the first European to hold a black belt in judo. He was also a fierce soccer player. A soccer injury flared up during the German invasion of France and prompted him to use both his martial arts experience and his engineering and mechanical background to explore the relationship between the nervous system and body function. (A 50/50 chance that surgery would correct the problem was not worth it to Feldenkrais.)

The result of his work is pure genius, but it was his philosophy that became his legacy. He believed in, and made a difference to, the potential of humankind. He helped men and women become more themselves. He saw the infinite possibilities because he, like Descartes, viewed the human being as a tabula rasa, or clean slate.

The problem is that much of what we have learned is harmful to our system because it was learned in childhood, when immediate dependence on others distorted our real needs. Long-standing habitual action feels right. Training a body to be perfect in all the possible forms and configurations of its members changes not only the strength and flexibility of the skeleton and muscles, but makes a profound and beneficial change in the self-image and quality of the direction of the self.

—From: "Mind and Body." Moshe Feldenkrais.

Feldenkrais believed that habitual patterns are imprinted in the nervous system, good or bad, but that verbally directed exercises and manipulation could help the brain and body learn movements that would free bodily limitations and instill our natural birthright, a sense of grace.

MOSHE FELDENKRAIS, DSc—cont'd

His methods led to what could be considered incredible results. People with multiple sclerosis and cerebral palsy gained a new lease on life, and athletes without any obvious physical limitations sought his therapy.

A typical session consists of an instructor leading a group in various exercises or manipulating an individual through small, repeated movements. This creates a new awareness or spatial reality, which the brain recognizes as being immediately right or better than the original impeded movement.

The sensations experienced in these sessions bring into focus the tension and stress that make our movement inefficient and prepare us to learn new patterns that permit the body to function at a level much closer to its full human potential. Feldenkrais was big on the concept of learning. He thought it was the gift of life, inextricably tied to personal growth and the key to a healthy body and mind.

My way of learning, my way of dealing with people, is to find out, for that person who wants it, what sort of accomplishment is possible for that person. People can learn to move and walk and stand differently, but they have given up because they think it's too late now, that the growth process has been completed, that they can't learn something new, that they don't have the time or ability. You don't have to go back to being a baby in order to function properly. You can, at any time of your life, rewire yourself, provided I can convince you that there is nothing permanent or compulsive in your system, except what you believe to be so.
—From: "Movement and the Mind." Moshe Feldenkrais and Will Shutz.

Practitioners worldwide are achieving dramatic results with Functional Integration and Awareness Through Movement. In North America alone, 1500 certified practitioners are listed. Training takes about 3 years, and because Feldenkrais believed the only way he could teach his work was through direct experience, graduates leave not only with a diploma and an opportunity for a promising career but also with improved posture, flexibility, coordination, and ease of movement (at any age); freedom from or reduction of pain; profound psychological and emotional growth; improved physical well-being and vitality; and the ability to understand how to learn effectively and enjoyably in any area of life.

form the client of the reason for refusal. A justifiable reason may include health-related issues such as contraindicated conditions, improper hygiene, and personal safety. The therapist may not refuse a client for reasons of race, creed, political affiliation, disability, religion, gender, marital status, national origin, ancestry, sexual orientation, or social or economic status. The massage therapist should perform her work in an unbiased, nonjudgmental, and professional manner.

Conversely, the client has the right to refuse, modify, or terminate treatment and to cancel or reschedule appointments. Clients are not required to divulge reasons; however, inquires should be made directly to the client (not to a third party). If the client exercises her right, the therapist must comply immediately.

BOUNDARIES: THE EXTENT OF OUR ROLE AS MASSAGE THERAPISTS

A *boundary* can be defined as a set of parameters that indicates a border or limit. In this section, boundaries will include not only boundaries that pertain to our profession but also personal boundaries. Violation of a boundary system can vary greatly and may range from mild issues such as inconsideration or rudeness to the more serious issues of abuse. We will also explore issues of intimacy and personal disclosure with clients, consequences of misconduct, and how to handle problematic situations.

Boundaries represent the limits we establish between ourselves and others in regard to various aspects of our lives; we thereby establish our personal space, emotional separateness, and professional distance. Let's look at various boundaries as they occur in real estate. A property line exists between two lots and is generally respected by neighbors, even though the line is typically unmarked. Repeated violations of this invisible boundary may cause feelings of anger or anxiety. The walls and doors of our homes are also boundaries that shut or open. A home with open or even unlocked doors may be considered unsafe; without an invitation such as a knock, it would be difficult to control who entered. Professional boundaries are very similar.

In her work *Exploring Boundaries,* Pat Ogden, developer of Hakomi Integrative Somatics, offers a very comprehensive description of boundaries. She states that boundaries are as follows:

> Infinitely flexible and changeable, depending, moment to moment, upon both inner and outer conditions. A healthy sense of boundaries indicates that we can connect with the experience or sense of ourselves as both separate and in unity with the world. A "holding environment" for one's own presence, a container for our individual sense of self, of who we are, is established through healthy boundaries. We are aware of our differences, yet we can sense the interconnectedness of all beings. We can maintain both differentiation and connection.
>
> Through boundaries we are able to screen input from the world, to know what input is appropriate to let in and assimilate, and what input we need to keep out. With healthy boundaries, we keep ourselves from accepting subtle or overt kinds of abuse, and we also are sensitive to and respect the rights and boundaries of others.

In this section, we will explore the concept of boundaries as they relate to our personal and professional lives. Perhaps the most important part of Ogden's description is her statement about healthy boundaries: "With healthy boundaries, we keep ourselves from accepting subtle or overt kinds of abuse. . . ." Boundaries are about self-protection.

Odgen also states, "And we also are sensitive to and respect the rights and boundaries of others." It is from this aspect of healthy boundaries that the majority of our professional boundaries as massage therapists are derived. By respecting the boundaries of others, we instill a sense of dignity and respect to our clients, our profession, and ourselves.

Imagine that you are always surrounded by a semipermeable membrane and this membrane can expand or contract depending on the person or situation you encounter. You are able to choose, either consciously or unconsciously, how physically and emotionally close to you this other person is allowed. This may be difficult if you have never been exposed to the concept of boundaries. Some relationships do not honor or respect (and therefore do not teach or reinforce) good healthy boundaries. In these cases, the therapist is encouraged to obtain as much information as possible on boundaries, putting into practice what is learned.

Personal Boundaries

Personal boundaries are boundaries that you create to protect yourself, nurture yourself, make your life less stressful, and maintain a healthy sense of your separateness from others. Many people get by without having to commit them to paper, but writing down personal boundaries is a good idea. The very act of writing these boundaries down helps anchor them in the conscious and unconscious mind. Remember that boundaries are extremely personal decisions that are unique to the individual based on their personal belief systems, needs, and environment. Examples of healthy boundaries may include the following:

- I will recognize and respect the boundaries of others. I realize that I may not be able to meet their every need, but I will be sensitive to them; meet the needs I can; and when someone says stop, I will comply.
- I will say no when I am at my limit. I realize, in some occasions, I have gone out of my way to please others. Although it's okay to do favors out of love and kindness for other people, I have overcommitted myself in the past and have become resentful. When solicited for help, time, or money, I will take 24 hours to think about it before giving the person an answer. This reduces my stress level and often prevents me from making impulsive decisions.
- If someone is being verbally abusive toward me, I can state my feelings about the situation and ask him or her to stop being verbally abusive. Although I cannot change the person, I can always remove myself from the situation by leaving.

The aforementioned boundaries were thought out and planned, but boundaries also can be innate. You may recognize some of these boundaries as things you do naturally. For example, when you get into a crowded elevator with strangers, everyone's physical boundaries are compressed. As a coping mechanism for the physical closeness, the normal reaction is to emotionally distance yourself from the other passengers. This is usually accomplished through silence and by staring at the numbers of the floors going by. Our physical boundaries are different for different people. Some people are not comfortable touching at all; others warrant a handshake; others, a hug; and some, a kiss.

Personal boundaries can surround privacy issues such as nudity, doors being closed, finances, telephone conversations, mail, journals, and diaries. Personal boundaries include personal space in a variety of situations with friends, strangers, family, or lovers, as well as people who smoke, wear too much fragrance, or who are noisy. Personal boundaries also encompass our mental, emotional, and spiritual beliefs. We may choose with whom we share our feelings, beliefs, decisions, and spirituality (self-disclosure); all these help us define who we are as individuals. Many people with unhealthy boundaries find themselves taking on the likes, dislikes, belief systems, and even the personalities of those with whom they are in a relationship. The following list contains illustrations of unhealthy boundaries. Unhealthy boundaries are usually not chosen by the individual, but occur as inappropriate behaviors of others are modeled, or they are a coping mechanism that may have worked during childhood, but is no longer valid for the individual as an adult.

- I tell my problems to anyone who will listen, even extremely personal information concerning my body, my sexuality, my finances, or my problems with my spouse and family. I make no distinction about whether I talk about these things in private or in a crowded room.
- I really don't like to go to action movies with my spouse, but I never tell him that I would rather see a romance or drama instead. Usually I just sit through it with him, resenting that I'm wasting my time and treating him coldly for the rest of the evening.

These types of behaviors often lead to feelings of self-dissatisfaction, isolation, and depression. People with poor boundary systems typically find themselves being either withdraw and vulnerable, on one end of the spectrum, or aggressive and intrusive, at the other end. With healthy boundaries come both security and the ability to give and receive in relationships.

 The best way out is always through.
—Robert Frost

Professional Boundaries

Professional boundaries relate directly to the integrity of the therapist. **Integrity** comes from the word *integer* meaning to integrate thoughts, values, intention, and actions. Integrity is the condition of being whole and undivided. *Webster's New Collegiate Dictionary* on p. 662 defines *integrity* as the "firm adherence to a code of moral or artistic values." Integrity is central to our work as massage therapists and to our relationships with clients, colleagues, and other health care professionals. In *A Year of Living Consciously*, author Gay Hedricks, Ph.D., defines some guidelines for acting with integrity. They are as follows:

- Don't deny your feelings, but don't wallow in them either.
- Communicate effectively without assigning blame.

- Tell the whole truth.
- Make commitments selectively, and keep the ones you make.
- Take responsibility for everything you do, and ask others to do the same.

The majority of the professional boundaries discussed in this chapter will be *client-focused* so that, according to Ogden, "we also are sensitive to and respect the rights and boundaries of others." In a healthy therapeutic relationship a balance exists between safety, care, and compassion (existing in a boundary) and risk-taking (stretching boundary limits). No formula is available for achieving this balance, but healthy boundaries can provide the foundation on which the therapist builds his professional relationship with the client. Boundaries are always contextual—that is, they are interpreted in the context of the relationship; boundaries will be different in intimate relationships than they are in therapeutic relationships.

Boundary Management

A boundary is a defining border. A massage therapist should know her professional boundaries, which should be linked to her scope of practice. The therapist should not only guard her boundaries but also be prepared to extend or expand it as a bridge while maintaining her integrity when in contact with individuals or groups of individuals with which she needs to collaborate.

As a boundary manager, massage therapists should know how to temporarily overlap boundaries. This technique is used when resolving conflict, participating in negotiations, or mediating between groups. However, when someone crosses her boundary, she is put on alert and prepares for communication or other actions across the borderline. Conflicts may result.

The following list contains several examples of professional boundaries. Notice that they include issues that may not be covered directly in the Code of Ethics or Standards of Practice. Each item can be used as a topic for discussion, or therapists may use the list to form their own individual professional conscience regarding their practices. The purpose of the following list is to begin examining ways to manage boundaries and to prevent situations of boundary violation, abuse, or neglect to both the client and the therapist.

- I will schedule a minimum of 30 minutes between client appointments. This will give me the flexibility of dealing with late clients, time to extend appointments from 60 to 90 minutes if requested, change linens, return phone calls, or take a break.
- I will make house calls or out-calls to hotels only with clients who have been referred by an existing client or with clients who have a history of treatment at my office.

- In my office, I will always provide a container for the client's jewelry and personal items so that valuables will not get misplaced.
- I will respect the client's physical appearance. I will not make rude or disrespectful comments about any large or unusual scars, tattoos, body piercing, birth defects, body hair, body coloring, body size, or anomalies, even if I am surprised by their appearance.
- I will not use high-pressure tactics to sell the client vitamin supplements or other merchandise or to get the client to make a commitment to long-term massage treatments.
- I will avoid hugging the client unless it is solicited by the client and only then if I feel comfortable with the situation. The client will be fully clothed and not on the massage table during hugging.

Client Abuse and Client Neglect

When any professional, whether doctor, attorney, minister, or massage therapist, does not recognize or respect the rights and boundaries of the client, the result may be client abuse or client neglect. **Client neglect** is defined as *unintentional* physical or emotional harm sustained by the client because of insensitivity or lack of knowledge on the therapist's behalf. An example of a neglectful act might be a therapist who mistakes a cyst for a trigger point, causing tissue damage through prolonged pressure. Another example might be a therapist who, rather than providing emotional support for the client, oversteps his training, slips into a counseling role, and gives unsolicited and/or untrained advice. In each case the therapist did not intend to harm the client, and yet it happened. Negligent treatment is often spawned by ignorance. Our chief tools in the prevention of negligence are (1) developing a cautious and professional attitude, (2) providing ourselves with continuing education, and (3) maintaining professional boundaries.

Client abuse is defined as physical or emotional harm sustained by the client resulting from *deliberate* acts of the therapist. An abusive therapist is one who makes a conscious decision to take advantage of a client physically, sexually, financially, or emotionally.

Although rare, physical abuse may include deliberately disregarding the client's request for lighter pressure because the therapist feels that additional pressure is better. In cases of bruising as a result of physical abuse, the therapist is liable, and the client may elect to file assault charges with the district attorney or a civil suit for damages.

Sexual abuse may be verbal or **nonverbal** (transmission of messages by means other than the spoken word), but its intent is to give or receive sexual gratification. This type of abuse is not limited to ad-

vances made while the client is receiving a massage. Contact made with the client while not performing professional activities still falls within the realm of the therapeutic relationship. If a more intimate relationship is desired, NCBTMB recommends discontinuing the client-therapist relationship for a minimum of 6 months before the new relationship is initiated. This type of restriction represents practicing good boundaries. For more information, read the section later in this chapter on Consequences of Inappropriate Behavior and Sexual Misconduct.

Financial client abuse is taking advantage of a client's resources. It can be charging more than the standard rate simply because the therapist knows the client is in a high-income bracket. Accepting expensive gifts or access to living quarters for a weekend is financially abusive. A good rule of thumb is not to accept a gift (or tip) from a client if it exceeds the cost of the massage (e.g., $50). Failing to inform new clients about prices or old clients about upcoming price increases is abusive to the client and sabotages the trust of the client-therapist relationship.

Emotional abuse is usually involved in all other types of abusive relationships where an imbalance of power is evident and when the person who wields the greater power does not recognize or respect the boundaries of the other. The therapeutic relationship between a client and the massage therapist is particularly vulnerable to this type of abuse. In relationship to the client, the massage therapist has the authoritative position. The client enters into the relationship because the massage therapist has particular skills, knowledge, and abilities. The relationship may be considered personal because it involves skin-to-skin contact. The client may feel vulnerable both physically and emotionally because she is usually lying down and draped, whereas the therapist is standing and clothed. Often when someone removes her clothing, she may feel emotionally naked and vulnerable. It is because of the vulnerability of the client that the therapist must have good professional boundaries.

Issues of Intimacy: Therapeutic Relationships vs. Multidimensional Relationships

Being friendly is good for business. No one ever lost a client or customer by smiling and by being nice and polite. The problem is that being *too* friendly can sometimes wound the therapeutic relationship. If we are attracted to some of our clients and develop friendships or dating relationships with them, we are assuming multidimensional relationships. We may become unclear about where to draw the line between clients and friends or clients and lovers.

Multidimensional relationships are relationships that exist in addition to the therapeutic relationship. Also referred to as *dual relationships,* multidimensional relationships are where the therapist assumes more than one role in the client's life. These roles can be reversed. In these complex interweaving of roles, it may be difficult, if not impossible, to maintain healthy professional boundaries. It may be difficult to treat all clients the same if some are personal friends and others are not. It is easy to see how conflicts of interest arise, boundaries become blurred, and the potential for client abuse is heightened in multidimensional relationships.

In addition to our roles as therapist, what other roles are possible? Can a therapist become friends with a client? What about a client who becomes a business partner? What if a client becomes romantically or sexually involved with the therapist? Should a therapist rent property or borrow money from a client? It's not hard to imagine how a romantic, sexual, or financial relationship might evolve from a professional client-therapist relationship. Let's explore the most common multidimensional relationship, friendship.

It is helpful to realize that the therapeutic relationship is not a friendship. In a friendship, the relationship is 50/50—a certain amount of give and take occurs between parties. In a friendship, your friend knows as much about you as you know about her. This is not the case in a therapeutic relationship; it is not an equal partnership. In a therapeutic relationship, the therapist knows much more about the client than the client knows about the therapist. The therapeutic relationship exists to benefit the client. In some ways, the therapeutic relationship can be compared with the parent-child relationship. The relationship is one-sided; the therapist having the more powerful position. Along with power comes responsibility of using the power wisely to create good and not harm. Despite this fact, friendships with clients routinely develop, and bonds of intimacy are formed. However, as we examine multidimensional relationships in the context of intimacy, we can clearly differentiate between friendship and professional relationships.

Intimacy is a sensual (meaning an experience of the senses) bond to another in which the following elements exist: choice, mutuality, reciprocity, trust, and delight. This definition of intimacy is generally true for those to whom we are closest, usually family and friends. The element of *choice* is present in that we can choose to be in the relationship; we cannot be forced into intimacy. *Mutuality* goes hand in hand with choice; both parties elect to enter and maintain intimacy. *Reciprocity* is the knowledge that if I choose to be in the relationship, over time, I will receive as much from the relationship as I give to the relationship. *Trust* is the result of continued risk taking. We can choose to trust blindly without a history of trust,

but we are more likely to get hurt. Finally, *delight* is the sensual experience that the relationship brings to us because of these first four elements: choice, mutuality, reciprocity, and trust.

The therapeutic relationship then is very similar to an intimate relationship with a few important differences. Choice and mutuality exist, or no relationship would. Trust is built from the continued risk taking of subsequent sessions. Delight may even be experienced at times by both parties. It is for these similarities that people often confuse the closeness of a love relationship with the closeness of the therapeutic relationship, but the key element missing is reciprocity. The roles are not equal. The massage therapist is getting paid to be in this relationship, and although it may be argued that what the client is receiving is worth the money exchanged, the relationship is at best one-sided. Although the massage therapist is caring and compassionate, he also keeps a therapeutic distance from personal involvement outside the therapy room with his clients (Figure 2-4).

In fact, you may soon discover is that distance makes the therapeutic relationship a safe place for the client's experience. Let us consider Chapter 11 of the *Tao Te Ching:*

> *Thirty spokes share the wheel's hub;*
> *It is the center hole that makes it useful.*
> *Shape clay into a vessel;*
> *It is the space within that makes it useful.*
> *Cut doors and windows for a room;*
> *It is the holes which make it useful.*
> *Therefore profit comes from what is there;*
> *Usefulness from what is not there.*
>
> —Lao Tsu

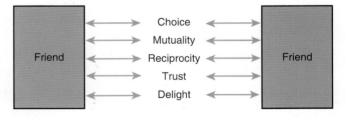

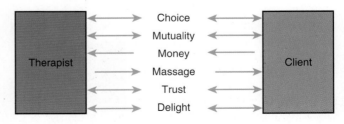

Figure 2-4 Intimate vs. therapeutic relationships.

When the space is provided for clients to relax and be themselves, healing is more likely to occur. If we fill up the space in the relationship with too much conversation or our own agendas or concerns, the client does not have the opportunity to come out from behind her wall (often in the form of muscular tension). The distance we can provide, like the pauses in a symphony, are often the places we can feel peace, sanctity, and oneness. This is a gift not often acknowledged. This is the gift of the therapeutic relationship and why it is so important to protect it by not entering into multidimensional relationships with our clients (Figure 2-5).

What about friends who become clients? For a therapeutic relationship to occur, boundaries must be established, and both parties should understand their individual position and responsibilities. The massage therapist will provide massage therapy, for which the client will pay the requested fee. It is best to keep the conversations during the massage sessions focused on the massage session.

Communication, Conflict, and Conflict Resolution

Massage therapists can be described as trilingual; we speak three languages. One is the language of *physical therapy* (clinical massage); the second is the language of *comfort* (relaxation massage); third is the language of *business* (money exchanged for services). You may be fluent in other languages, but these languages are most used in the work setting. Ambiguity and resultant conflict arise when lack of communication, a blurring of boundaries, or assuming subroles occur (see the following section on Transference and Countertransference). These conflicts may be within the therapist or health care field or between the therapist and the client.

Interpersonal conflicts may arise within the therapist when she has wonderful abilities using one language but not another. For example, she may be a great communicator, knows how to comfort a client while on and off the table, gives a great relaxation massage, but doesn't return phone calls to clients or make deposits to her business checking account. Another source of inter-conflict is not managing boundaries between personal and professional life such as working late into the day and not making time for spouse and children (see the section on Boundary Management earlier in this chapter).

Conflicts may arise interprofessionally with communication between massage colleagues or other health care providers. Some sources of conflicts between physical therapists, chiropractors, or even fellow massage therapists may occur when one professional refers to another and the professional being referred to does not reciprocate. Other potential conflicts are when one set of professionals perceives another as an economic threat or unfair competition.

Conflicts between the client and the therapist often arise when expectations are not met: the therapist is late starting a massage, problem areas stated by

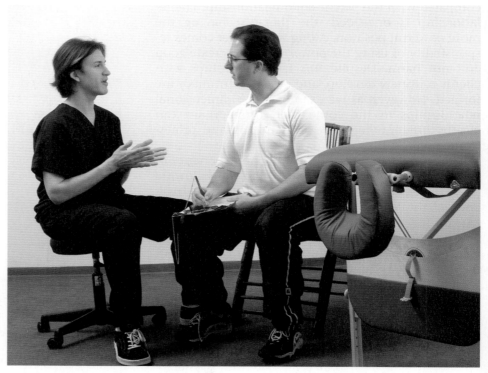

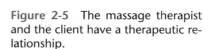

Figure 2-5 The massage therapist and the client have a therapeutic relationship.

the client are not addressed by the therapist during the massage, or the client cancels an appointment for the third time in a month.

However, negotiations and arriving at a resolution are both part of being a competent, successful businessperson and are necessary for having and maintaining healthy relationships. When conflicts arise, it is an invitation to explore resolution options. Creativity must be used because all conflicts will not be resolved using one method. Listed below are suggestions for problem solving when conflicts arise (Table 2-1).

- Identify and accept the problem.
- Communicate with *I* messages instead of *you* messages; you messages feel like blaming to the other party.
- Have healthy boundaries; this is essential to conflict resolution.
- Look for solutions that are in the best interest of the relationship.
- Be open to a variety of solutions.
- Do not take problems and differences personally.
- Let each party keep his or her respect and dignity.
- Do not deny an adversarial reaction if it is present, but do not assume one either.
- Take full responsibility for your own behavior.

- Communicate clearly about what you want and need; consistently foregoing what you want and need is not conflict resolution.
- Consider both the wants and needs of yourself and others as important.
- Separate issues from people.
- Avoid power plays.
- Pick your battles carefully, asking yourself if this issue will matter in 5 or 10 years.
- Save ultimatums for absolute nonnegotiations or late-stage negotiations.
- Do not waste time negotiating nonnegotiables.
- Take time out when angry emotions are running high; step back and look at the problem before reacting.
- Look for the gift or the lesson after the conflict is resolved.

Transference and Countertransference

In some cases, the client wishes for more of a relationship with the therapist. Psychotherapists have long been taught about a phenomenon of personalization that often takes place between counselors and their clients. These phenomena are referred to as *transference* and *countertransference*. **Transference** is

TABLE 2-1

Healthy and Unhealthy Conflict Resolution Strategies

Strategy	Action	By
Fight	Trying to impose one's preferred solution on the other party	Insisting Blaming Criticizing Accusing Shouting
Submit	Lower aspirations and settle for less than one would have liked	Giving in Giving up Agreeing just to end conflict Surrendering to what the other wants
Flee	Choose to leave the scene of the conflict	Ceasing to talk Leaving physically, cognitively, and/or emotionally Changing the topic
Freeze	Choose to wait for the other's next move	Waiting Doing nothing
Problem solve	Pursue alternatives that satisfy both sides; a win-win situation	Talking Listening Gathering information Thinking Generating options Resolving

the unconscious tendency of the client to assign to others feelings and attitudes associated with significant people in one's early life (e.g., parents). **Countertransference** is an emotional reaction of the therapist that reflects their own inner needs and conflicts. It may also be a reaction to the client's behavior of transference. The feelings that are projected in both the transference or countertransference processes may be affectionate, which results in a positive transference or countertransference, or they may be feelings of hostility or animosity, which creates a negative transference or countertransference.

Massage therapists and their clients are just as susceptible to these phenomena as are counseling professionals; massage therapists are not always trained or prepared to recognize and deal with these problems. Transference occurs when the client begins to personalize the professional relationship. This is usually because some needs that were not being met in his personal relationships are now being met in the professional relationship. These may not only be touch needs but also the human needs for attention, listening, validation, and nurturing (a list of human needs can be found in Chapter 12 in the section on Touch Research). A blurring of reality occurs. Instead of seeing that he is a client paying a therapist to perform a specific service, the perception is that the therapist is a caring friend, confidant, or possible lover.

This is not to suggest that the professional relationship should be cold and sterile. Some of the most successful massage therapists are those who are extremely personable and friendly. People like to give business to someone who truly cares about them. Simple acknowledgment that a business relationship exists needs to occur. It is the responsibility of the massage therapist to maintain this balance.

Countertransference occurs when the therapist has trouble maintaining her professional detachment from the client. Detachment is not thinking less of a client, but thinking of a client less. In countertransference, the therapist may reverse roles and try to get her needs met through the interactions with her client within the professional relationship. It may be the attention produced from the transference that may trigger the therapist into taking a personal interest in the client; becoming overly responsible for the client's recovery; thinking about the client between appointments; and in more extreme cases, possibly getting into romantic and sexual fantasizing.

If the transference-countertransference process is allowed to continue once it has been identified, these feelings may progress into sexual behavior. It is important that massage therapists be able to recognize these situations and take appropriate steps to set firm boundaries with the client who wants to personalize the relationship. If boundaries are not firmly identified, the client's behavior may be progressive. If countertransference develops unnoticed by the therapist, the result may be emotional and sexual intimacy. Ultimately, the situation damages the therapeutic relationship and removes the focus of healing from the client.

So what can a massage therapist do if he suddenly finds himself in such a situation? The first step is to tell someone about the relationship. This can be done by going to a licensed counselor, a closed support group for professionals only, or another massage therapist who can be unbiased, nonjudgmental, and supportive. The act of breaking the secret brings the situation out into the light of reality where it can be examined. The supporting counselor, support group, or colleague may then ask questions and offer feedback on handling the situation. If the relationship has progressed so far that countertransference has occurred, it is generally best to terminate the professional relationship and refer the client to another massage therapist. This prevents the dynamic from progressing to an emotional/sexual relationship, which is detrimental to both the client and the therapist.

The dynamics of the situation should be explained to the client with care. The therapist might say that a personal issue prevents him from providing the client with the best possible care. The massage therapist should then take a close look at his own needs and examine which ones are not being met. It is typical that this pattern will repeat itself with other clients as long as the therapist is not getting his own needs met. At this point, the massage therapist should consider going to a licensed counselor who can help him identify his needs and develop appropriate ways of getting them met.

 Attachment is the great fabricator of illusions; reality can be attained only by someone who is detached.

—Simone Weil

Consequences of Inappropriate Behavior and Sexual Misconduct

Part of understanding boundaries means accepting the consequences when we choose to cross them. It is therefore necessary that every massage therapist understand the consequences of inappropriate behavior, particularly sexual misconduct. Becoming sexual with a client, even if it is in a dating situation and not the massage room, is considered to be sexual abuse. This is true because the power dynamic between client and therapist does not empower the client to say "no" easily to the therapist. Therapists should gain the knowledge to look for warning signs in themselves and their colleagues and should learn how to help clients handle complaints about other therapists.

Inappropriate behavior and sexual misconduct are forms of client abuse because therapists take advantage of their more powerful positions in the therapeutic relationship to meet their own emotional or sexual needs. The professional relationship is considered a business arrangement between therapist and client, which benefits the client through healing touch and massage. When a therapist violates the boundaries of the therapeutic relationship through severe misconduct, the consequences associated with the violation are often of a corresponding severity. Possible consequences of this type of behavior include loss of income, reputation, marriage, friendships, relationship with peers and colleagues, license, membership in professional organizations, and insurance coverage, as well as lawsuits for damages, criminal charges, fines, attorney's fees, court costs, and time in jail.

Remember that the therapist is always responsible and liable for her actions, even if the client initiated the situation. Do not depend on professional liability insurance to cover any damages. Although your insurance company may well provide an attorney to assist in your defense, it typically does not cover damages resulting from sexual misconduct.

This is not to say that sexual feelings are wrong or unhealthy. We are all sexual beings. Individual sexuality is a large part of self-esteem and identity. We simply need to keep some healthy separateness between our individual sexuality, which is part of our personal life, and the profession.

At one time or another you may feel an attraction to one of your clients, and sometimes it will be sexual. Nothing is wrong with this; it is natural and healthy. When we experience sexual feelings toward a client, we can honor this feeling by acknowledging it to ourselves and to a supportive colleague (not to the client). Having done so, we then focus on the job at hand and put our minds back in professional mode. Again, it is not the attraction that is dangerous; it is acting out the attraction with inappropriate behavior that is cause for concern.

Fire Drills: Applying Conflict Resolution

When you were in elementary school, your teachers marched you in a single file down the halls and out a prescribed exit during a fire drill. Why? Because when you establish a habit by performing an action when you have time to think clearly, you will most likely react to threatening situations by repeating the ingrained habit. Had there been an actual fire,

you and your classmates would have known what to do.

Regarding massage therapy, most uncomfortable situations can be handled tactfully if we prepare for them through "fire drills"—forming a rational plan of action so that you act instead of react at a time of stress. The fire drill should consist of the situation and several possible ways of resolution. These steps should be in order from simple to complex. The simplest usually reflects the most gracious means of handling an uncomfortable situation, whereas the most complex or drastic usually focuses on protecting the therapist physically and emotionally. The therapist should use the most gracious means first and should try more drastic measures if resolution does not occur.

Fire drills are designed to act out the situation in a safe environment with a fellow classmate (under the direction of an instructor or with a colleague). You may run into a client who wants to go beyond a professional relationship. This may be someone who has an honest attraction to you as a person, or it could be someone who believes that massage therapy is related to sexual service. This violates not only your professional space but your personal space as well. Fortunately, these situations tend to be the exception rather than the rule. Clients may approach the therapist in one of two ways: *covertly* or *overtly*.

Clients acting covertly typically begin by testing your boundaries. The word *covert* suggests that their approaches will be subtle and sneaky rather than honest and direct. Clients may hint about their loneliness and failed loves. Sometimes the client may ask personal questions about you and your love life. He may "accidentally" expose himself. Or he may "accidentally" brush his hands up against you while you are working. Inform the client that you are in the business of therapeutic massage and that his behavior is unacceptable. In most cases, your directness will put an end to his subterfuge.

Overt behavior is obvious, and there is no doubt what the client has in mind. Overt violations are clear in intent and may include grabbing the therapist sexually or verbally propositioning the therapist for sex, or the client may be intentionally stimulating himself on the massage table. Do not compromise yourself under these circumstances. Every incident of overt behavior must be confronted. Some therapists think that ignoring the situation will make it go away. Silence and nonaction are typically not the best responses in cases like these; silence is often taken as permission. Even in ordinary conversation, silence is generally accepted as agreement with the speaker. Disagreement is expressed verbally and through action. If the overt behavior is not harmful, such as a client's asking you out on a date, then he needs to understand the boundaries of the therapeutic relationship. If the overt behavior is harmful physically or emotionally, then take control of the situation.

These types of situations and other conflicts can be resolved using skills and procedures learned in a fire drill activity. Let's say the topic for the fire drill is "Client makes a pass [a covert romantic overture] toward the therapist." The sample fire drill for this situation might look like this:

Situation: Client tests the boundaries of the relationship by making a pass toward the therapist; specifically, he asks the therapist if she is married.

Step 1. The therapist informs the client that she is married and tries to redirect the conversation by changing the subject. She might say, "Yes, my husband and I have been married for 5 years. We just had a wedding anniversary and went to New York to see Broadway plays. Do you like theater [or do you like to travel]?" Client responds, "I'd like anything with you. You said you're married, but are you *happily* married?"

Step 2. At this point the client has made it clear that he does not respect the boundary of marriage, and the therapist must take control of the conversation. She might say, "I'm very happy with my married relationship, but I'm not happy with the trend of this conversation. Let's keep *our* relationship on a professional level." Most clients will be uncomfortable to continue the conversation trend at this point, but this client is being a little more aggressive and presses the issue by asking the therapist out to dinner.

Step 3. The therapist informs the client that she is not interested in anything outside of their therapeutic relationship, states that she is feeling uncomfortable with the direction of the conversation, and tells the client that the massage will be terminated if the conversation continues in the direction it is heading.

With this direct response, the majority of all conflicts will be resolved. For argument's sake, let's assume that the unacceptable behavior continues and the client overtly grabs the therapist, pulling her toward him, presumably for a kiss.

Step 4. The therapist leaves the room and terminates the session according to an established plan. A session termination form is given to the client by a fellow therapist or can be slid under the door if no one is available to assist. The client is then left alone in the massage room to get dressed. An example of the session termination form is shown in Figure 2-6.

By using the fire drill approach to reestablish violated boundaries, you can protect yourself from many types of abuse. Even subtle abuse may take its toll on the body, mind, and spirit. It is important to be able to recognize abuse both personally and for our clients.

MINI-LAB

Make a list of five or more situations to create fire drills. They can be repeats of past unpleasant experiences or situations that constitute the most uncomfortable or frightening scenarios that could happen to you as a massage therapist. For example, it could be that a client goes into heart failure on the table, you accidentally undrape a client, or someone makes a pass at you.

Act out each situation with a classmate in front of the class. Once the situation is complete, ask the class and/or instructor for other options. Revise the fire drill if necessary. This activity will help you become more prepared to handle difficult situations.

Session Termination Procedure

Rarely does it happen that a massage therapist will have to terminate a session because of some inappropriate statement or action by the client, but if it does happen, the therapist must be prepared to deal with the situation by standard procedure. Usually, this involves the following three steps:

1. **Notifying the client of the session termination.** If the client commits some faux pas or inappropriate behavior that the therapist judges to be mild, subtle, or covert, the therapist has the option of providing the client with an initial verbal warning that, if the behavior is repeated, the session will be terminated. If the behavior is overt, such as sexual touching or a direct proposition, then a warning is not necessary. The therapist should terminate the session immediately. The therapist may want to vocalize the termination by using one of the following statements: "I do not believe anything therapeutic is going on, so this session is now over," or "I do not feel comfortable with your behavior, and this session needs to end." If the therapist is uncomfortable with verbalizing the termination, he or she should find a reason to leave the room. The actual termination can be accomplished by handing the client the session termination notice (see Figure 2-6) and promptly leaving the room.

2. **Have the client leave the premises, thereby reestablishing therapist safety.** Once the client has been notified of the session termination, the therapist should leave the room and take steps to ensure her own safety. Each situation will have to be judged independently. If you work with others, get a coworker to stay with you until the client has left the building. If you work alone or the client physically intimidates you, use the phone to make contact with a colleague, friend, or family member. The therapist should inform the per-

SESSION TERMINATION NOTICE

You have been handed this notice due to the use of language or behavior that the massage therapist perceives to be inappropriate.

This is to notify you that your massage session has been terminated at the therapist's discretion. You should dress and leave.

Charges for the entire session will be collected at the business office.

OR

You will receive a bill for the entire session.

The language or behavior constituting session termination is recorded on this form below and is confidential between the therapist, coordinator, and department manager.

You may request an incident review by calling (a persons name) at (phone number).

Future appointments will not be accepted without an incident review and resolution of the situation.

Date: _____ Client's Name: _____

Time: _____ Therapist's Name: _____

Location of Massage: _____

Description of Events:

Actions Taken:

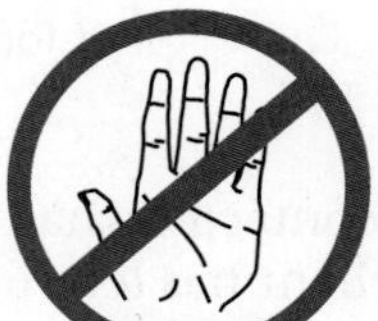

Proposed Resolutions:

Case Reviewed and Resolved:

Date: _____

Time: _____

Place: _____

Those in attendance: _____

Figure 2-6 A sample session termination notice. (Permission is hereby granted to reproduce this form in its entirety, including the copyright notice, for commercial or instructional use but not for resale.)

INCIDENT REPORT FORM

Date:_____ Client's Name: _____

Time:_____ Therapist's Name: _____

Place:_____

Therapist's Perceptions of Incident:

Actions Taken:

Proposed Resolutions:

_____   _____   _____   _____
Signature of Massage Therapist   Date   Signature of Client   Date

Reviewed and Resolved:

Date:_____   Time: _____

Place: _____

Those in attendance:

Figure 2-7 A sample incident report form. (Permission is hereby granted to reproduce this form in its entirety, including the copyright notice, for commercial or instructional use but not for resale.)

son contacted that she will call again as soon as the client has left, usually within 3 minutes. If the friend does not receive a call back, the friend is instructed to alert the proper authorities. If the therapist feels that she may be harmed physically by the client, the therapist may choose to dial 911 and have a police unit sent to the premises to escort the client out. The therapist may also want to lock herself in a room as a safety measure until the client has left. The therapist must use her discretion to distinguish the potentially threatening situations from those that are merely nuisances.

3. **Documenting the session termination in writing.** A session termination form is simply a document to record the events as they took place from the therapist's point of view. The first copy that was handed to the client should just be a brief statement of the problem. The office copy should be a total replay of the entire incident. The main purpose of this form is to have a written record

that can be used as a reference should the case go to court. It is important for the therapist to document every detail of the situation that led her to terminate the session. If it was sexual improprieties, document the statements verbatim or describe actions that gave that impression. For more information on documentation, see the following section on Client Incident Reports.

One other situation merits mention here, and that is the *house call* or *out-call*. In business arrangements, where the massage therapist makes trips to the client's home or hotel, the session termination may have to be handled differently. During a house call, you are on the client's turf with your equipment. The most straightforward response is to tell the client that the massage is over and that you will be leaving. If for any reason the client tries to intimidate you, it is best to simply leave your equipment behind and come back for it with the authorities (hotel security or the local police). It is still in your own best interest to port should be filled out and retained to document the unusual things that happen to a client, in the same way that the session termination form documents unusual things that happen to the therapist. Incident reports most often involve a client who slips and falls, who misplaces belongings, or who becomes ill during a massage session. The incident report should include the date, time, and exact location of the occurrence, who was present, and what was done to alleviate the problem. If physical injury was involved, the report should include the condition of the client when he departed from your establishment. If possible, obtain signatures from all individuals who were present during the incident (Figure 2-8). It is also helpful to have a camera handy to take photographs of actual accidents or accident scenes.

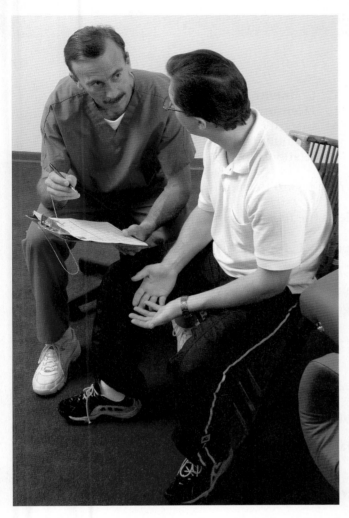

Figure 2-8 The incident report form should be reviewed with the client and then signed by both the massage therapist and the client.

record the circumstances surrounding the session termination. Hopefully, the use of session termination forms will be minimal. This form is merely another useful tool in establishing professional boundaries and preserving the therapeutic relationship.

Client Incident Reports

Incident reports are also known as *accident reports* or *unusual occurrence reports* (Figure 2-7). Regardless of how small the accident or unusual the episode, a re-

SUMMARY

The professional image and behavior of a massage therapist can be divided up into the areas of professional standards and boundaries.

Professional standards are set from within the profession itself and govern the actions of the individual practitioners. This is done by defining a certain scope of practice, educational requirements, code of ethics, and standards of practice. These may all vary slightly from state to state but share the same common belief in professional, client-centered care.

Boundaries are our personal and professional parameters that specify how we will interact with others, including our personal space, professional conduct, and emotional boundaries. Having healthy boundaries also means respecting the boundaries of others, even if their standards are different than our own. Observing boundaries prevents client abuse, reduces conflict, and limits opportunities for becoming too intimate or disclosing too much personal information to our clients. Understanding boundaries means accepting the consequences for our actions when we choose to disregard boundaries. It is therefore necessary that every massage therapist understand the consequences of inappropriate behavior and sexual misconduct. Likewise, when clients behave inappropriately, the therapist must be prepared to terminate the session.

MATCHING

Write the letter of the best answer in the space provided.

A. Standards of practice
B. Incident report
C. Scope of practice
D. Confidentiality
E. Client abuse

F. Transference
G. Intimacy
H. Code of ethics
I. Boundaries
J. Client neglect

K. Countertransference
L. Licensure
M. Integrity
N. Multidimensional
   relationship

_____ 1. Limits we establish between ourselves and others in regard to various aspects of our lives

_____ 2. An emotional reaction of the therapist that reflects the therapist's inner needs and conflicts

_____ 3. A report to document unusual things that happen to a client during a session

_____ 4. A condition of being whole and undivided

_____ 5. The unconscious tendency of the client to assign to others feelings and attitudes associated with significant people in his or her early life

_____ 6. Nondisclosure of privileged information

_____ 7. A sensual bond to another that involves choice, mutuality, reciprocity, trust, and delight

_____ 8. Relationships that exist in addition to the therapeutic relationship

_____ 9. Unintentional physical or emotional harm sustained by the client resulting from lack of knowledge or insensitivity on the therapist's behalf

_____ 10. A mandatory process to be completed to engage in an occupation that would otherwise be considered to be unlawful

_____ 11. A list of standards to assist the professional in making good decisions while conducting day-to-day responsibilities within their scope of practice

_____ 12. Set of guiding moral principles that govern one's course of action

_____ 13. The working parameters of a profession

_____ 14. Physical or emotional harm sustained by the client due to deliberate acts of the therapist

Bibliography

American Massage Therapy Association: *Credentials used for the massage therapy profession,* accessed May, 2002. Available at: *http://www.amtamassage.org.*

American Massage Therapy Association: *What are certification, licensing and accreditation?,* accessed May, 2002. Available at: *http://www.amtamassage.org.*

Baron RA: *Psychology,* ed 2, Boston, 1992, Allyn and Bacon.

Carnes P: *Out of the shadows: understanding sexual addiction,* Minneapolis, 1983, CompCare.

Fritz S, Grosenbach MJ, Paholsky K: Ethics and professionalism, *Massage Mag* Jan/Feb 1997, p 46.

Gill S: Avoid those ticking time bombs: safety or the massage professional, *Massage Bodywork: Nurture Body, Mind, Spirit,* Feb/Mar 2000, p 92.

Hamric AB, Spross JA, Hanson CM: *Advanced nursing practice: an integrative approach,* Philadelphia, 1996, WB Saunders.

Hedricks G: *A year of living consciously: 365 daily inspirations for creating a life of passion and purpose,* Harper and Row, 2000.

Ignatavicius DD, Bayne MV: *Medical-surgical nursing,* Philadelphia, 1991, WB Saunders.

Johanson G, Kurtz R: *Grace unfolding, psychotherapy in the spirit of the Tao-te Ching,* New York, 1991, Harmony Books.

Kasl CD: *Women, sex and addiction: a search for love and power,* New York, 1989, Ticknor and Fields.

Kellogg T: *Sex and sexuality: a workshop,* Dallas, 1998, Author.

Kurtz R: *Body-centered psychotherapy: the Hakomi method,* Mendocino, Calif, 1990, LifeRhythm Books.

McIntosh N: *The educated heart: professional guidelines for massage therapists, bodyworkers, and movement therapists,* Memphis, 1989, Decatur Bainbridge Press.

Miller-Keane encyclopedia and dictionary of medicine, nursing, and allied health, ed 6, Philadelphia, 1997, WB Saunders.

National Certification Board for Therapeutic Massage and Bodywork: *Code of ethics (adopted 2/17/95) and standards of practice (adopted 2/9/00),* McLean, Va, Author.

Ogden P: *Boundaries II or somatic psychology,* Boulder, Colo, 1995, Hakomi Integrative Somatics.

Roberts B: *Boundaries and the massage therapist: a workshop,* Lake Charles, La, 1999, Author.

Torres LS: *Basic medical techniques and patient care for radiologic technologists,* ed 4, Philadelphia, 1993, JB Lippincott.

Tsu L: *Tao Te Ching,* New York, 1972, Vintage Books (Translated by Gia-Fu Feng and Jane English).

Webster's new world college dictionary, Springfield, Mass, 1995, G and C Merriam.

Whitfield CL: *Boundaries and relationships: knowing, protecting and enjoying the self,* Deerfield, Fla, 1993, Health Communications.

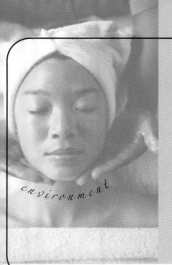

environment

Tools of the Trade and the Massage Environment

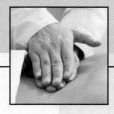

3

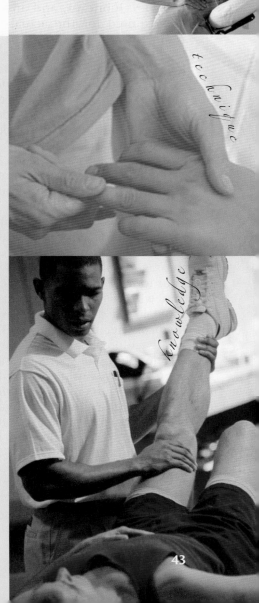

pressure

technique

knowledge

"All labor that uplifts humanity has dignity and importance and should be undertaken with painstaking excellence."

—Martin Luther King, Jr.

STUDENT OBJECTIVES

After completing this chapter, the student should be able to:

- Identify and discuss massage table features
- Choose the correct massage table for practice
- Apply fabric care to the massage tabletop and table accessories
- Discuss differences in massage media and aromatherapy
- Design a massage room

INTRODUCTION

Your career as a massage therapist not only depends on your education and skills training but also on your ability to use wisely the tools of the trade. Like any other skilled artisan, the massage therapist will use these tools to implement the massage work itself. The finished product depends both on the quality of the tools and how well the artisan uses them. The tools of the massage therapist include the massage table and related accessories, the massage lubricants, and even the room environment. In this chapter we will open the therapist's toolbox and examine each item in detail. Practical suggestions are included to assist the massage therapy student in making wise decisions when choosing equipment or designing a room.

First of all, we need to distinguish between a massage *room* and a massage *office*. A massage room is the place where the massage service itself is actually performed. This room contains the massage table, accessories, lubricant, and any other incidentals that are required for the actual massage. The massage room is often referred to as a *massage studio*. This chapter will concern itself with the massage room and the objects that may be found there.

The massage office, also known as the *paper office,* is where massage appointments are scheduled, telephone calls are placed, and records are kept. All business-related activities take place in the office. These activities are necessary for your massage practice to run smoothly and efficiently. Equipment such as the telephone, answering machine, computer, filing cabinets, files, and accounting supplies are located in the massage office.

Before you start buying furniture and equipment for your massage room, spend some time evaluating yourself and your prospective clientele. The kind of massage you want to offer will play a part in how your room looks and feels. If clinical massage is what you will be doing, your massage room may look more like a doctor's office with anatomical charts, medical references on a bookshelf, little or no music, lightly colored walls, and white massage linens.

The room of a sports massage therapist may have sports-type paintings or photographs, reference books on sports-related problems, and a single free-standing locker for clients' garments. A sports massage therapist is more likely to own a portable massage table to be used when his or her services are needed at sports events.

A massage therapist who focuses on stress-reduction massage will want to create a relaxing environment. The walls may be painted in warm colors; only natural or subdued lighting may be used, with a hint of lavender scent in the air.

THE CORRECT EQUIPMENT

Massage equipment refers to the objects or machinery used in the successful execution of massage therapy services. When considering the purchase of massage equipment, several things must be kept in mind.

First, will it ergonomically support you, the therapist, by reducing stress? **Ergonomics** is the scientific study of anatomy, physiology, and psychology relating to humans' work; adjusting the environment and equipment to support the alignment and balance of the body in its activities. If your back, neck, or wrist is in pain after performing one or more massage sessions, chances are that your equipment is *creating* stress. Use the section on Massage Table Features to help you better understand table mechanics and assist you in altering your equipment to better suit your body. If it is not the massage equipment, then you need to look at your body mechanics. See Chapter 6 for assistance in correcting any inefficient body postures you may be using.

Second, will your massage equipment add comfort to the client? Does the padding support the client's body, and are the physical dimensions of the table comfortable? For example, a table that is too narrow may not allow the client's arms to rest comfortably at his or her side. This may create a feeling of unease in the client. Use of bolsters take stress off low back, ankles, and neck.

Third, how long can you expect this piece of equipment to last? Most table manufacturers offer a 5- to 10-year warranty. However, top-quality tables last much longer, especially if you are willing to remove and replace worn padding and top fabric. Eventually, you may want to have a stationary table for your office and a lightweight, portable table for home visits. This prolongs the life of both tables. It's like rotating two pairs of shoes; both pairs last longer.

Lastly, is it a wise investment? Because your equipment, especially your massage table, is an investment in your business, resist the urge to buy impulsively. Ask veteran massage therapists which equipment they use and why. Why did they choose a particular table width or padding? Besides other therapists, contact several table companies and ask them to mail you product catalogs. If possible, go to a massage school or a massage convention where you can see and lie on tables from several different manufacturers. If you can compare, you will have a better understanding about table features. This will help you make an informed decision (Figure 3-1).

Ergonomics, client comfort, durability, and workmanship are all important factors in purchasing massage equipment. Because these four elements are so important, we will discuss these factors throughout the chapter.

MASSAGE TABLE CHECKLIST

TYPE OF MASSAGE TABLE

☐ Stationary Massage Table   ☐ Portable Massage Table

                                              ☐ Hydraulic Lift Table

MASSAGE TABLE FEATURES

Frame   ☐ Aluminum   ☐ Wood-Type: _____

Width   ☐ 26" ☐ 28" ☐ 30" ☐ 32" ☐ Custom Width: _____

Height   ☐ Standard Height   ☐ Custom Height: _____

Length   ☐ Standard Length   ☐ Custom Length: _____

PADDING

Layering   ☐ Single Layer   ☐ Multiple Layering System

Density   ☐ Light   ☐ Medium   ☐ High

Thickness   ☐ 1½"   ☐ 2"   ☐ 2½"   ☐ 3"   ☐ Other

Fabric   ☐ Vinyl   ☐ Textured Vinyl   ☐ Vinyl Suede

               ☐ Velour   ☐ Cotton Velvet   ☐ Ultra Leather

Color: _____

Other Options: _____

_____

ACCESSORIES FOR YOUR MASSAGE TABLE

Face Rest: ☐ Standard   ☐ Deluxe/Tilting

☐ Arm Shelf   ☐ Side Extenders   ☐ Foot Rest

☐ Carrying Case   ☐ Table Skates/Cart   ☐ Stool

BOLSTERS AND SUPPORTIVE DEVICES

☐ Bolster (3" × 27")   ☐ Bolster (6" × 27")

☐ Bolster (8" × 27")   ☐ Soft Neck Bolster

Figure 3-1   Massage table checklist. Use this to compare the features of several massage tables. (Permission is hereby granted to reproduce this form in its entirety, including the copyright notice, for commercial or instructional use but not for resale.)

One word of caution: some therapists resort to building their own massage tables or to having their tables made by well-meaning friends or family members. Some table companies offer table kits that you can assemble. This may not be a good idea in the long run because the only tables that can be guaranteed by a reputable table manufacturer are those that are assembled by the table manufacturer. With a homemade table or a table kit, you may be held liable if table failure occurs during a massage. Should something happen to your table, it is preferable to have a table manufacturer who can stand behind its materials and workmanship. In addition, all table companies make accessories that can be purchased to add to the comfort or transportability of their massage tables.

MASSAGE TABLES

The two most popular styles of massage tables sold to massage students and therapists are stationary and portable tables. Stationary tables are made to stay in a massage room. Portable tables are designed to be folded in half and carried, like an oversized suitcase, from one location to another.

Portable tables account for 90% to 98% of all table sales by table manufacturers with prices ranging from $200 to $600. Some advantages of portable tables are that the therapist is able to make home or office visits (going to the client), the table can be moved if the therapist is using multiple office locations, and, if the massage therapist shares office space with other therapists, he or she can easily move the portable table out of the office.

As a massage therapist, you must feel totally confident in your equipment, and your massage table is the fundamental tool of your business and will be one of your major expenditures. It is the massage therapist's responsibility to make every effort to control the factors he or she can, including purchasing professional-grade equipment for the comfort, safety, and security of clients. Purchase your table from a reputable, well-established massage product company. This will accomplish several things. First, these companies tend to provide great customer service. Second, because they are generally well known in the industry, their products will be easier to turn around, will sell quickly, and will bring a better price. Third, most established table manufacturers offer a trial period for you to try out their product and, if you are not satisfied, will refund your money once the table is returned. Last, these massage product companies offer the best warranties, usually 5 years and up.

Massage Table Features

When you are considering the purchase of a stationary or a portable massage table, most table manufacturers let you decide the specifications on features such as width, height, length, frame material, padding, and fabric (Figure 3-2). One suggestion is to purchase a massage table that fits the therapist's height and weight and buy accessories to accommodate your client's body (wide client: side extensions;

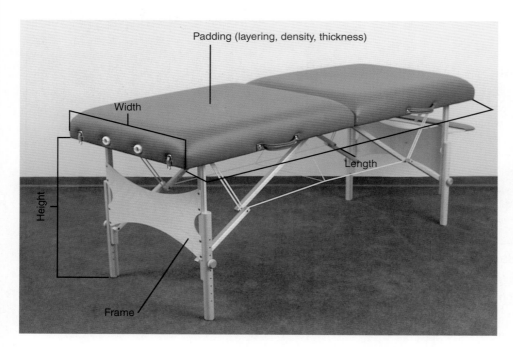

Figure 3-2 A typical portable massage table.

long client: table extender). Let us look at a few more table guidelines.

Width. Most massage tables sold are between 28 and 31 inches wide. In most cases, the width of the table depends on the height of the therapist. Shorter therapists should consider tables that are 28 and 29 inches wide because it is easier to reach across the table, safeguarding proper body mechanics. Taller therapists usually can work with a wider table (30 to 31 inches wide). Other considerations include your clients. For example, if your table is less than 28 inches wide, your large-framed clients may feel uneasy when they are lying supine because their arms tend to hang off the sides of the table (use side extension). If your table is wider than 31 inches, it may be difficult for you, as the therapist, to reach across the table and effectively apply massage strokes because of loss of leverage. Wider portable tables are taller (when folded up) and heavier, which is a consideration because they are lifted and carried from lo-

cation to location (carrying them up and down stairs can be tricky). It is helpful to massage several body styles on a range of table widths before choosing which table width to purchase.

Height. All manufactured portable and stationary tables have an adjustable height range, which is usually between 22 and 34 inches high. Adjustment is achieved, usually in half-inch increments, by lengthening or shortening the four legs of the table. The optimum working height of the massage table is determined by the height of the practitioner and his preferred style of massage.

For Swedish massage, three generally accepted methods determine the height of the tabletop. Take care to relax your shoulders fully to get an accurate measurement.

- As you stand by a massage table, arm to your side, extend your wrist in a 90-degree angle (open palm facing the floor). The proper table height is where the table rests under your palm (Figure 3-3, *A*).

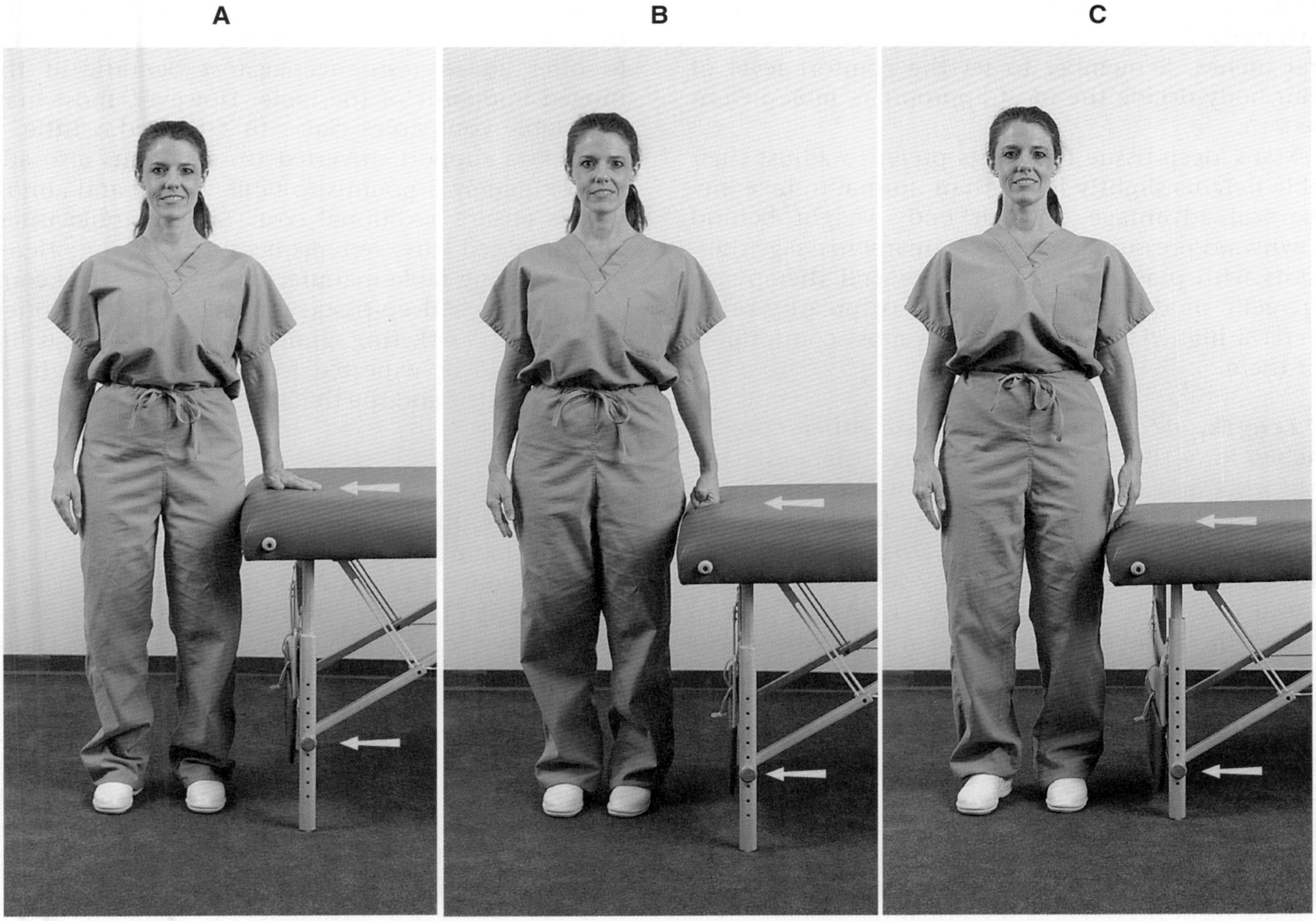

A   B   C

Figure 3-3 Three methods of determining the correct height for a massage table. **A,** Wrist extended 90 degrees with palm touching tabletop; **B,** hand in a fist touching tabletop; **C,** hand relaxed with fingertips touching tabletop.

- Alternatively, you can stand by the massage table with arms to your side and make a fist with your hand. Using this method, the table height is where the table touches your fist or set of knuckles (Figure 3-3, *B*).
- Stand by the massage table with arms to your side and wrist and fingers straight. The height of where your fingertips slightly brush against the table represents the appropriate table height for you (Figure 3-3, *C*). This method is often favored by therapists who practice deep-tissue techniques.

For several massage sessions, try all of these methods for deciding table height. Notice how your body feels. If your arms or shoulders feel achy, the table is probably too high; you could be overcompensating from not being able to use leg strength or leverage. If your lower back feels stiff after giving a massage, most likely your table is too low; you could be overcompensating and having to bend too much to apply strokes. After a massage, the therapist should feel anywhere from relaxed to energized. Raise or drop the tabletop by small increments until optimal table height is achieved. Also, take into consideration your clients' girth when deciding on the level of the table. This variable can alter how low your table is by several inches. Remember to let the comfort level of your body decide the most appropriate table height for you.

Many deep-tissue therapists prefer to adjust their table heights slightly lower than normal to take mechanical advantage of their body weight behind downward pressure. Conversely, many massage therapists who practice Trager, craniosacral therapy, or energetic modalities such as Reiki or polarity often prefer a higher table because it is most comfortable for them.

Length. Most massage tables are either 72 or 73 inches long. Because most massage therapists use face rests and bolsters, your 6-foot-plus client can have ample room. This is because a face rest adds 10 to 12 inches to your table, and a 6- or 8-inch–wide bolster will shorten the client's leg length when placed under the knees or ankles. Using bolsters to change the client's joint angles can reduce the occupied table length by 6 to 12 inches.

Frames. Table frames are made of either wood or aluminum, the most popular being wood. The major difference between wood and aluminum is that wood frames are heavier. Welded aluminum frames have a slight advantage in lateral stability over wooden frame tables, but this difference probably will not be noticed with a high-quality wooden table. Aluminum tables also have the advantage of quicker leg adjustments. Although the therapist may think they will seldom adjust the height of their massage table, client's torso girth varies enough to make leg adjustability a consideration. This is especially true when working on the fourth, fifth, or sixth client of the day. Energy conservation and proper body mechanics are paramount.

Beware of aluminum-framed massage tables that are fastened with rivets because they can become loose and are difficult to tighten. The chief reasons for buying aluminum tables are their light weight and strength. Small-framed massage therapists often purchase aluminum-frame tables because they are easier to transport. Therapists who are conscious of body energy fields avoid aluminum, citing that the metal interferes with the energy field of the body.

If the table you are thinking about purchasing has a single-knob attachment, make sure the leg extensions are attached to the table legs by a tongue-and-groove mechanism. A two-knob attachment or a tongue-and-groove system is more stable and increases the table-to-table leg integrity. Tighten up the table leg knobs at the beginning of every week. This ensures that the table is as strong and stable as possible.

Many table manufacturers also offer an inverted truss system. The theory behind this frame option is to offer added resistance against bending at the hinged midpoint of the table. However, most massage table companies claim that this adds little, if any, extra support. Inverted truss systems also add approximately 5 pounds to table weight and almost always ensure additional cost. Table manufacturers offer inverted truss systems because they are offered by competing table manufacturers. Also, some companies offer a deep-tissue upgrade, which is often more of a marketing gimmick. Any high-quality table should be expected to support the weight of both the client and the therapist during a deep-tissue session.

Padding. If you ask clients what they remember about being on your massage table, they will often mention table padding. This material adapts to and supports your client's body. When selecting a pad for your massage tabletop, decisions must be made regarding layering, foam density, and thickness. Let us examine these areas.

- **Layering.** Some tables are padded with a single layer of foam, whereas other manufacturers pad their tables with multiple (two or three) layers. In the multiple-layer system, the most dense foam is on the bottom. The lower layers of foam support the bony structure and prevent the body from bottoming out on the wood platform of the table. The upper layers are less dense to conform to the contours of the body. Multiple-foam layering usually outlasts single-foam layering and is much more comfortable to the client. Ask the table manufacturer, when purchasing your table, if the layered foam is also glued to each other layer and adhered to the plywood tabletop. If they are not, the foam tends to shift under the vinyl and, in some cases, roll up into waves.

- **Density.** Most foam pads are divided into three grades of density: light, medium, and high. High-density foams generally have better memory, which is the ability of the foam to return to its original height after its surface has been disturbed. Higher-density foams are heavier and will add weight to your massage table; they are typically not found on a table designed for light weight. High-quality tables use a medium- to high-density foam because light-density foam does not have enough memory, even when used as a top layer.

- **Thickness/loft.** Foam thickness typically ranges from 1.5 (firm) to 3 inches (plush). Deep-tissue practitioners traditionally work on tables with firm foam thickness. Using a firm padding prevents loss of the therapist's energy when downward pressure is applied. Without a firm pad, the client sinks down into the foam. If you like to work beneath the client's body, a plush foam top is best. Plush foam is preferred by stress-reduction therapists because it is more comfortable. Because of government regulations, all table manufacturers use padding that is chlorofluorocarbon-free (CFC-free). This manufacturing process does not damage our fragile ozone layer.

Table Fabric. Table fabric covers the foam padding of your massage table. The most common fabric choice is vinyl because it is long lasting and easy to clean. Other fabrics available are textured vinyl, vinyl suede, velour, cotton velvet, and ultra leather.

Vinyl fabrics also resist oil, perspiration, and makeup stains; however, they also tend to be stiff, retain the cold, and are not as comfortable as velour, cotton velvet, or ultra leather. Vinyl is sensitive to changes in environmental conditions and may become dry and brittle and may crack, especially if you leave your massage table in your car between appointments (see the following section on Vinyl Fabric Care). Vinyl fabrics can be easily punctured by keys, hairpins, jewelry, and pets. Massage linens have a tendency to slip on a slick vinyl surface.

Ultra leather is soft and resists punctures better than vinyl fabrics. All ultra leather products offered by table manufacturers are imported because the process used to make ultra leather is unsafe for the environment. If you make decisions according to how a product affects the environment, you will probably not choose ultra leather as your table fabric.

The cloth fabrics such as cotton velour, velour, and other textured fabrics are very soft and provide the utmost in client comfort. Unfortunately, they are difficult to clean and impossible to disinfect. Many state laws require therapists to use surfaces that can be disinfected such as vinyl.

MINI-LAB

If you are fortunate enough to have several manufactured tables on display at your school, try these three tests before you finalize your purchase.

1. **One-Knee Test.** Kneel down and place your weight on one-knee and see if you bottom out. This will indicate the integrity of the foam and what a client might be feeling when he or she is pressed into the table.

2. **The Bounce.** Lean your body weight against the massage table and lay your forearm on the tabletop. Gently bounce up and down. Notice how much the table flexes when you jump. The ideal table will resist you as you bounce. If the tabletop is not firm, some of the energy you use pressing into the client's muscles will be lost. This also translates into conserving the therapist's energy.

3. **Table Rock.** Rock the table back and forth to check for lateral stability. If the table wobbles, the integrity of the table should be questioned (or the joints should be tightened).

4. **Ready, Set, Go!** Fold the massage table, and close it securely. Holding it by the handles, lift the table and walk around the room. Unfold the table and set it up on its four legs, noticing the ease or difficulties you encounter.

Vinyl Fabric Care. The most important thing to know about the care of your table's vinyl fabric is to keep it clean. For daily cleaning, simply wipe down the table surface with a mild cleanser such as a solution of liquid hand or dishwashing detergent and water. Dry with a soft, lint-free towel or old but clean T-shirt. Avoid using vinyl conditioners or protectants because they are unnecessary and may damage the vinyl top coat.

The three worst substances for the vinyl surface of the table are the very things with which you might expect it to come in contact: oils, isopropyl alcohol, and chlorine bleach. Body oils or massage oils can erode the protective top coat, which is specially designed to keep the fabric soft. When the top coat is damaged by oil, the plasticizers that give the vinyl its softness, suppleness, and resilience are broken down. The other two substances, isopropyl alcohol and chlorine bleach, are often used in the disinfecting process. Use the chlorine bleach and water solution

(10 parts water to one part chlorine bleach) to disinfect the vinyl surface *only* when it comes into contact with bodily fluids. All three substances will shorten the life of the vinyl by causing it to become dry and brittle, making it susceptible to cracking or splitting.

Vinyl table fabrics are like fine wine; they do not like wide temperature ranges. This becomes a problem only if you keep your massage table outdoors or in your car. After a home or office visit, put the table back in your office or your home. If your table fabric does get cold, allow it to return to room temperature before you begin your next massage. Direct sunlight can also break down vinyl and cause it to become dry and cracked, and high temperatures can soften it; again, allow the table to return to room temperature before using it. Pressure on a hot table may cause permanent damage by leaving stretch marks in the fabric.

Avoid table fabric wear and tear by transporting your portable table in a carrying case. It is virtually impossible to keep your tabletop unblemished when you have to haul the table from your office or home, to the car, to your client's home, back to your car, back to your office or home, and so on. If you are going to own and carry a portable table, get a carrying case. Your table is certainly worth it.

When your table arrives, with it will be a packing slip that lists your table model, dimensions, color, and manufacturer's address and telephone number. Make a copy of this packing slip and attach it to the bottom of your table with a sheet of adhesive laminate. The original packing slip should be filed in your office in case the massage table is lost or stolen. Now you will always have the information at your fingertips when you want to order additional equipment or supplies such as table pads or linens.

 When the only tool you have is a hammer, every problem looks like a nail.
—Albert Einstein

Accessories for Your Massage Table

Face Rest. A face rest, or face cradle, allows clients to keep their heads and necks relatively straight while they are lying prone. The face rest extends the functional length of the table by 10 to 12 inches. It consists of two parts, a cushion and a frame (Figure 3-4). The cushion is generally attached to the frame by loop-and-pile fasteners. This enables the crescent-shaped cushion to be spread or narrowed to accommodate a wide variety of facial structures. The cushion fabric is usually the same fabric as the massage table.

The face cradle frame is attached to the massage table with support rods that insert into grommets at either or both ends of the table. Standard face rests

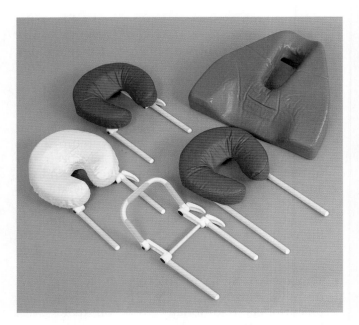

Figure 3-4   Standard and adjustable face rests and a prone pillow.

allow the head and neck to be in only one position—parallel to the tabletop. Adjustable models can be purchased that allow the neck to be flexed for client comfort and easy access of the posterior head and neck for the therapist. The more adjustments that can be made, the more positions available to the client and therapist. This feature is important when working with clients with special needs, such as elderly or large clients or clients who are physically challenged. Adjustable face rests can be folded down instead of removed from the table when not in use.

Some face rests can be removed from the table and locked into a U shape, allowing clients to lay prone on the floor with comfortable breathing space. Working on the floor may be needed when working with clients who cannot get on and off your table, such as the elderly.

Other face rest options include a face hole with plug and the prone pillow. The face hole is an oval opening in the table surface that allows the client to lie face down looking through the table. The hole can be closed with a fitted plug when the client is lying supine. The prone pillow (see Figure 3-4) is contoured foam covered with vinyl, which sits on top of the table and supports the face comfortably above the table surface.

Arm Shelf/Side Extensions. Arm shelf provides a place for the arms to rest in the prone or supine position. The arm shelf model used in the supine position looks like a pair of bolsters connected by a wide strap. Also referred to as an *arm support* or *side extension*, this option simply widens the

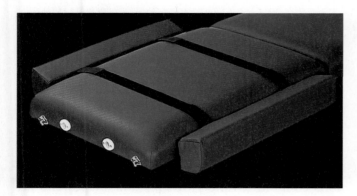

Figure 3-5 Arm support side extension. (Courtesy of Oakworks, Shrewsbury, Pa.)

table (Figure 3-5). Other models slide into grommets located in the sides of the table. Make sure you have enough room in your studio to maneuver around the table with its additional width.

Another model of arm shelf is a small platform suspended below the face cradle (Figure 3-6). This particular arm shelf is solely for use in the prone position. Arm shelves that attach to the table frame seem to be more stable than those that suspend from the face rest, but because they are permanently attached, they are usable at only one end of the table and usually cannot be adjusted in height. The arm shelf that suspends from the face rest may become unclipped or may tilt, swing, or slip, especially if the client presses down on the arm shelf when it is time to turn over. Both models come in a full range of

fabrics and colors to match your massage table. Either style is preferable to having a client's arms go numb from compression when lying prone with arms hanging off the sides of the table.

Footrest. A footrest is basically a padded platform covered with table fabric. The same width as your massage table and extending from one end, the footrest attaches to the table by either sliding rods or by a locking hinge mechanism. Using a footrest can increase the length of your massage table by 10 to 12 inches, depending on the length of the footrest. When it is not in use, it can either fold down or slide out of the grommets.

Carrying Case. A carrying case helps protect your table fabric from being damaged during transport, while adding a few handles, pockets, and padded straps, which makes the table easier to lift and carry. Many massage therapists consider a carrying case absolutely necessary if the table is placed in a vehicle's trunk. Most cases are made of tough synthetic fabrics such as Cordura nylon.

Table Skates and Carts. If you move your table often, table skates or a table cart can save your back and shoulders from ache and injury and help you conserve your energy. These devices allow your table to be rolled across the floor instead of being lifted and carried (Figure 3-7). Table skates and carts are made by using two high-quality casters mounted on a strip or two of thick plywood board or

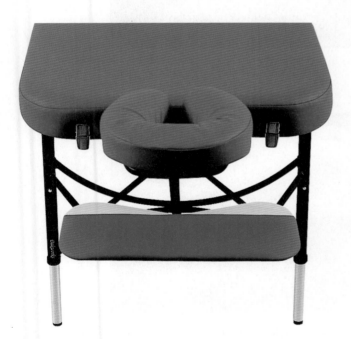

Figure 3-6 Arm shelf for use in prone position. (Courtesy of Oakworks, Shrewsbury, Pa.)

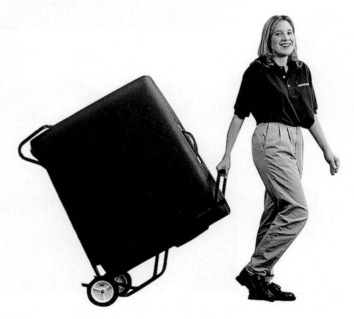

Figure 3-7 Table cart. (Courtesy of Oakworks, Shrewsbury, Pa.)

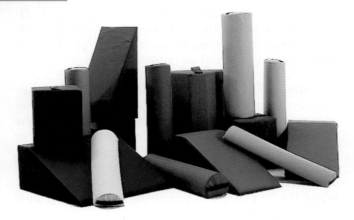

Figure 3-8 Bolsters are used to support your client on the massage table. (Courtesy of Oakworks, Shrewsbury, Pa.)

aluminum framing. The boards are attached to the folded table by means of an adjustable quick-clip strap. Once the skate or cart is attached, the table can be easily pushed or pulled. This accessory makes transporting your table much easier in some ways, but you will still need to lift the table over curbs and up stairs.

Bolsters and Supportive Devices. Bolsters and supportive devices are used to enhance relaxation of the client's muscles and spine. These cushions come in a variety of sizes and shapes and are used to support your client on the massage table (Figure 3-8). Pillow shapes include tubular, square, rectangular, and wave shaped (orthopedic); they support the neck, ankles, and knees (Figure 3-9, *A* and *B*).

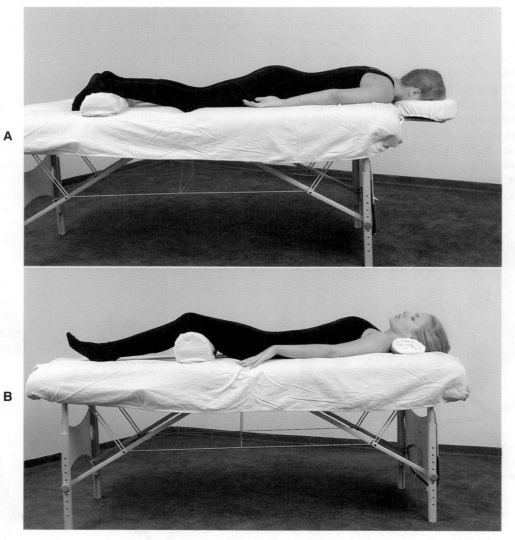

Figure 3-9 Bolsters are used to support the client's neck, ankles, and knees. **A**, Prone; **B**, supine.

These pillows can be made of foam or stuffed with feathers or seeds such as buckwheat or flaxseed.

A soft, tubular pillow is typically used for the neck while the client is in the supine position. Always cover the neck pillow with a pillowcase, which should be laundered after each use. Besides your neck pillow, it is a good idea to keep four to six regular-size bed pillows on hand, which can be used when positioning the client in a side-lying posture.

The most popular sizes of knee and ankle bolsters are 3 × 26 inches, 6 × 26 inches, and 8 × 26 inches. Flat-bottomed bolsters tend to stay in place. All knee and ankle bolsters are covered with vinyl, making them easy to clean and disinfect. Most manufacturers offer a variety of styles; full-round and half-round bolsters are available. It is recommended that a variety of sizes be available for your clientele. More elaborate cushion systems can also be purchased for your massage practice.

The fabric surfaces of body cushions, bolsters, and supportive devices must be wiped down with mild cleanser and draped with a clean cloth or paper cover before the start of each massage. Because of the damage caused by disinfecting chemicals, disinfect the fabric surfaces *only* when they come into contact with body fluids, for sanitation (client coughs and sneezes), and client comfort.

A stool can be regarded as a table accessory and is listed as such in the massage table checklist (see Figure 3-1). However, it is discussed later in this chapter in the section on Furnishing the Massage Room.

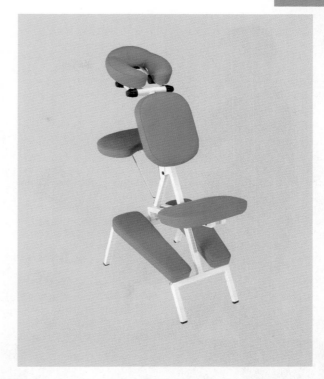

Figure 3-10   Massage chair. (Courtesy of Golden Ratio, Emigrant, Mont.)

MASSAGE CHAIRS

Introduced in the 1980s, chair massage has grown in popularity and is found in many settings from shopping malls and airports to private offices (Figure 3-10). A massage chair takes up a relatively small amount of space compared with an open massage table. Seated massage is performed on the client while the client is completely clothed. (For more information on seated massage, see chapter 25.) Many therapists purchase a massage chair after their table purchase and use it as an adjunct to their table work. However, some therapists conduct an exclusive chair practice. The cost of a massage chair is almost the same as a massage table.

Many different massage chairs are on the market today. Just as when choosing a massage table, different features appeal to different therapists. Important considerations when choosing a massage chair are that the chair is lightweight and simple to set up and take down. The chair should also be sturdy and strong because a wobbly chair makes the person sitting in it feel unsafe. Make sure all the adjustable levers and latches are enclosed completely because exposed ones can pinch therapists' fingers and catch clients' hair. A desktop model is also available (Figure 3-11).

MINI-LAB

Obtain a 3 × 26–inch bolster, a 6 × 26–inch bolster, and an 8 × 26–inch bolster. Lie on your back (supine position) and place the 3 × 26–inch bolster behind your knees for 1 minute. Next, place the 6 × 26–inch bolster behind your knees for 1 minute. Then, place the 8 × 26–inch bolster behind your knees for 1 minute. On a sheet of paper, note the differences you feel in your back, hips, knees, ankles, and feet. Repeat the procedure, but this time lie on your abdomen (prone position) and place the bolsters under your ankles for 1 minute. Again, noting the differences in specific body joints, jot down your findings on a sheet of paper. This will help you understand why bolsters are used in your massage practice and why it is preferable to include the three sizes. One will usually feel more comfortable than the other two, but this will vary from person to person. All three sizes need to be offered to the client.

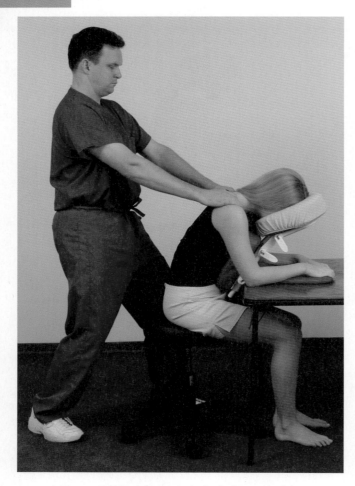

Figure 3-11   Massage chair desktop model.

CLEANING MASSAGE EQUIPMENT

Maintenance of massage equipment involves daily cleaning and periodic disinfecting. Cleaning removes dirt, body oil, and massage lubricants from the equipment surfaces. Recall that the three worst substances for vinyl are oils, isopropyl alcohol, and chlorine bleach. Disinfectants are used to kill viral, bacterial, and fungal agents. If you work in a hospital setting, your equipment must be cleaned in accordance with hospital policy and state law.

All massage equipment is draped with linens during the massage session and all draping material is laundered after each massage; therefore vinyl surfaces need only be cleaned at the start of each workday. Cleaned equipment includes face rests, arm or footrests, bolsters, and the massage tabletop. Use a mild cleanser such as liquid hand soap or dish soap.

A disinfectant will remove germs when applied to equipment surfaces. Because frequent disinfectant use will damage the vinyl, disinfect the massage equipment only when necessary. For example, if

your client has a contagious skin condition or a local or general infection or if any body fluid seeps, cleaning and disinfecting are required after the client leaves the room. Note that most situations that require immediate cleaning and disinfecting are also contraindications for massage. Many massage therapists periodically disinfect the vinyl surfaces every month and after an incidence of contact with viral, bacterial, or fungal agents.

Choose good-quality cleaning and disinfecting agents, both of which are available in either liquid or aerosol form. Using disposable towels, apply the agent to the equipment surface. Disposable or single-use towels are preferred over cloth towels because they are more sanitary and can be discarded after each use. Using a circular motion, wipe the equipment, beginning with the least soiled area, and move toward the most soiled area. This prevents the areas that are clean from being contaminated by the areas that are heavily soiled. If you are ever in doubt whether a piece of equipment or a supply is clean, do not use it until it has been properly treated.

MASSAGE LINENS

Massage linens consist of the following: a top and bottom sheet for the massage table, bolster covers, face rest covers, pillowcases, eye pillow covers, towels, armrest covers, and blankets. All linens used on massage tables or to cover equipment must be cleaned before the massage and then removed and laundered after the massage. The amount of linens needed depends on the number of clients you see per day; a two-day supply on hand is recommended. Replace the linens whenever they become stained, odorous, or threadbare. If washing and folding linens is something you do not wish to do, locate a linen service in your area.

Popular linen fabrics are flannel, cotton, cotton blends, and percale. Be cognizant of the weight and thickness of the fabric. Many inexpensive linens such as cotton-polyester blends, are too transparent to be appropriate draping material. If you find yourself in this predicament, a blanket over the top drape can remedy the problem. If you choose to use flannel sheets, you can buy sets of single-size (twin) fitted and flat sheets or purchase sheets from the manufacturer of your table. Many therapists drape with bath-size towels or bath sheets. Whichever type of drape you choose, have an alternative drape available if your client makes a request.

White, off-white, or soft pastels look great and these colors bleach well. Darker colors may show oil stains too easily. Some massage oil manufacturers sell a product that is added to the wash water to help remove the appearance and smell of oil from massage linens. If you are using oil as your primary medium, this product would be an asset.

Towels are often used as draping material. They are thicker and heavier than sheets, provide good client coverage, and provide easy access to the abdominal region when the client is supine. Other reasons massage therapists cite for using towels are that towels are easier to maneuver than sheets and oil stains are less obvious on towels than on sheets.

Have at least two cotton or woolen blankets to drape over your client on cold days, should he or she become chilled. As the body begins to relax, blood pressure is lowered, circulation returns to the core (the circulation pattern changes from the skeletal muscles to the internal organs). With this change, the body often feels cooler. Along with feeling warmer, the weight of the blanket adds a feeling of comfort and security for the client during the massage. Make sure the blankets you choose are machine washable and that they can be tossed in the dryer. Always drape a blanket over the original drape used to cover the client. The blanket does not replace the original drape.

MASSAGE MEDIA: OILS, LOTIONS, CREAMS, BUTTERS, POWDERS, AND LINIMENTS

The primary purpose of massage media is to reduce the friction between the therapist's hands and the client's skin. If not enough lubricant is used, the client may report that he or she is experiencing a burning sensation to the skin. The therapist should adjust lubricant use accordingly. Several factors must be considered when choosing a good quality lubricant. A few basic guidelines can be used when deciding what medium works best for you and your clients.

1. **Does the lubricant nourish the skin?** Ingredients such as cold-pressed vegetable, nut, and seed oils and plant essences are good for the skin, whereas ingredients like mineral oil and isopropyl alcohol can clog the pores and deplete nutrients from the skin. Even though stearyl and cetyl alcohol do not nourish the skin, they are safe and often used as emulsifiers and stiffening agents in various creams and lotions. Always read the ingredients list to ascertain the contents of a massage lubricant.

2. **How will my client's skin react to the lubricant?** Clients with certain skin types will be sensitive to some products and not to others. During the massage consultation, inquire about allergies to nuts or other products that act as ingredients in massage lubricants or allow the client to read the contents

on the lubricant container to see if she recognizes any potential problems in the ingredients. Because lubricant sensitivity cannot always be predetermined, keep a bottle of hypoallergenic cream or lotion available to use on request or when you are unsure about how a client will react to your primary lubricant. However, the word *hypoallergenic* does not mean that your client will not have an allergic reaction to the product. Hypoallergenic generally means that the product has undergone lengthy testing and that the majority of the subjects in the study did not have an allergic reaction to the product tested. Scented lubricants often increase allergic reactions. Many allergic reactions do not show up for 24 to 48 hours after the agent comes into contact with the skin. This means that most allergic reactions will not be apparent until a day or two after treatment. This is another argument in favor of hypoallergenic lubricants.

3. **Will the lubricant easily stain my massage linens?** Oil-based products are more likely to stain linens than water-based products. Creams and lotions are typically oil based. Massage linens like bolster covers and bottom sheets are more susceptible to staining and may have to be replaced more often. Conversely, top sheets are the least likely to become stained by oily products. Do not use linens that are stained. Even if clean, stained linens appear unsanitary, which may reduce client confidence.

The amount of lubricant you use will depend on (1) how emollient is the massage lubricant, (2) the dryness of the client's skin, (3) the amount of body hair, and (4) the intention of the massage. The more emollient the lubricant, the less is required. Dry skin requires more lubricant. Large amounts of body hair require more lubricant. In Swedish massage, the hands' ability to glide across the skin is important, and a fair amount of lubricant is required to accomplish this task. When performing some types of deep-tissue massage, such as myofascial release, the ability to grasp superficial layers of skin and fascia is important and therefore very little lubricant is needed. In general, excessive amounts of lubricant will prevent you from manipulating tissue, and inadequate amounts of lubricant will pull and irritate the skin. Experience will teach you how much lubricant is the right amount. Less is better; you can always add more lubricant if necessary.

When choosing a lubricant dispenser, make sure the dispenser contents do not become contaminated when applying and reapplying the lubricant to the client's skin. A pump container works best. The downside to pumps is that they break easily if dropped. The dispenser can be placed on the massage table between the knees for easy access and to prevent it from being knocked off the table during the massage. Placing the dispenser on the floor requires the therapist to continually bend over or squat in between lubricant applications and is not recommended. Lubricant holsters are also available; they allow the lubricant and dispenser to be worn around the therapist's hips.

Never apply the lubricant directly on the client's skin. Place the proper amount in your own hands, warming it by rubbing the fingers and palms together. Apply lubricant only on the area you will be massaging, never on adjacent areas. If too much lubricant is accidentally used, wipe off the excess with the back of your hand.

It is preferred to have both unscented and scented lubricant available. Ask the client to state her preference. If you discover that your client has numerous allergies, she may be sensitive to scented lubricants. If allergies are not a consideration and the client chooses the scented lubricant, place a small amount on the back of the client's hand before the massage begins so she may smell and approve or disapprove the scent.

Types of Lubricants

Oils.   Massage oils are the most traditional and most commonly used lubricant. Nut and seed oils are the best because they are the most nutritive. Healing agents such as vitamin E, may be added to the oil. Vitamin E, an antioxidant, also acts as a preservative, which is important, because natural, cold-pressed oils can become rancid. Some therapists mix their oil with a lotion in a 50/50 solution. They will separate, so blend the mixture before use by shaking the container.

The drawback of massage oils is that they not only stain massage linens but clothing as well. You may choose to inform your clients about the possibility of oil stains on their garments when they call and schedule the massage appointment so they can plan accordingly. This usually involves wearing loungewear to the session or bringing a change of clothes to be used after the massage session. Offer the client a hand towel to wipe any excess oil from the skin. A shower after the massage may remedy this problem.

Avoid mineral oil because it is a known **carcinogen** (substance that cause cancer). Mineral oil, or liquid petroleum, is not miscible in body oils and adds no nutritive value to the skin because it does not penetrate the skin. Often, mineral oils serve as a barrier that may clog the pores. Most brands of body lotions and creams contain mineral oil because it is inexpensive and has an infinite shelf life. Baby oils consist primarily of mineral oil.

Lotion.   Lotions are preferred by deep-tissue massage therapists because of the limited amount of glide they afford. When you do not want to slip and slide over the skin's surface, lotion is a good choice. This gives you more control over the lubricant because glide can be decreased by working longer. Lotion will not leave the skin feeling greasy. However, lotion does not have the staying power of oil or cream and is quickly absorbed into the skin. Therefore you will use more lotion than oil or cream, but lotion is generally less expensive than cream.

Cream.   Creams are more emollient than lotion but less greasy than oils. Because they cannot be spilled like oils or lotions, creams are less messy than any other massage medium because they are more viscous. This quality also gives them a staying power almost equal to that of massage oils. Creams are less likely to stain clothing but are typically the most expensive massage medium.

Cocoa Butter Sticks.   Cocoa butter sticks provide precise lubrication application and are often used in deep-tissue work because they allow more control and are easily absorbed by the skin. A small amount will cover a large area on the body because the client's body temperature will melt the cocoa butter. Allergic reactions to cocoa butter are rare.

Powder.   Baby powder, talc, powdered chalk, or cornstarch may be used during the massage, but it is not as efficient at friction reduction as other forms of massage media. Occasionally, you may have a client who may request powder or a client who does not want any topical agents used that will leave a residue. Powder may be used as an alternative lubricant and is the lubricant of choice for therapists who practice manual lymphatic drainage. Be careful when applying powder to the skin because the powder particles can enter the nasal passages and cause the client or therapist to sneeze or cough.

Liniments.   Liniments are alcoholic, oily, or soapy agents used in massage to create the sensation of heat. All liniments are *rubefacient,* which means they redden the skin because of the counterirritation caused by the ingredients. As the skin is irritated, the vessels become dilated, and the supply of blood increases. Liniments can also produce an analgesic effect. Avoid using liniments or liniment-type lotions on a client's hands or near mucous membranes.

AROMATHERAPY

The use of scents for therapeutic purposes is called **aromatherapy**. Aromatherapy can be used in baths, candles, candle-lit diffusers, massage lubricants, incense, and specially designed aromatherapy diffusing units or heating units. Massage and aromatherapy are often combined to enhance the therapeutic value of each other. How aromatherapy works is discussed in Chapter 20.

Essential oils are concentrated essences of aromatic plants. They have been used for thousands of years for their healing properties. For use in massage therapy, essential oils can be used to scent a room and scent the massage lubricant. Before using any of these essential oils, read the product label carefully for precautions and warnings. For example, many essential oils are not recommended for use on pregnant women or clients with certain neurological conditions such as seizure disorders, especially birch, cedar, clary sage, jasmine, juniper, marjoram, peppermint, and rosemary. Other essential oils are contraindicated for some skin conditions because of the possibility of irritation. As a rule, most fair-haired, fair-skinned people have sensitive skin. With the exception of lavender and tea tree oil, do not use oils "neat" or directly on the skin, especially cinnamon, ginger, lemon, melissa, peppermint, lemongrass, and orange. Always dilute the essential oil in a carrier oil such as almond oil. Some essential oils are photosensitive and may cause hypersensitivity in the presence of ultraviolet light or sunlight, especially bergamot and lemon. Do not use essential oils if you or your client has dermatitis or any skin allergies, especially jasmine, pine, rose, germanium, and ylang-ylang. In any case, use essential oils sparingly (only a few drops at a time). Used safely, essential oils can enhance your client's health and well-being.

According to a manufacturer of massage products and essential oils, the 12 most popular essential oils are lavender, clary sage, eucalyptus, sandalwood, rosemary, tangerine, vetiver, peppermint, lemon, juniper, chamomile, and ylang-ylang. If you wish to use aromatherapy in your massage practice, these essential oils are recommended to begin your collection. To obtain a more complete list of essential oils, ask your instructor to recommend a book on aromatherapy.

1. **Lavender.** The most widely used essential oil, it combats insomnia, calms, and balances the mind and emotions, and helps ease irritability.
2. **Clary sage.** This essential oil acts as an antidepressant. It is said to calm and balance the mind and emotions. Because of its calming effect, it is great before and during menstruation but is not recommended during pregnancy.
3. **Eucalyptus.** Highly used for respiratory congestion, eucalyptus helps bring comfort when experiencing loss and grief. This oil is also used during periods of physical and mental fatigue and exhaustion. Use sparingly because it can irritate the skin.
4. **Sandalwood.** Sandalwood promotes deep relaxation, abates depression, and quiets the mind and emotions.

5. **Rosemary.** Aiding in stimulating mental clarity, concentration, and memory, rosemary promotes cerebral activity. Rosemary also brings balance by helping detoxify the mind and body. Do not use during pregnancy or on clients with seizure disorders.
6. **Tangerine.** Tangerine is said to clear away negativity and opens up the heart by inspiring sensitivity and empathy. It also helps calm an overactive nervous system.
7. **Vetiver.** Vetiver promotes a sense of balance by activating a feeling of security and stability and by erasing worries.
8. **Peppermint.** Peppermint adds a sense of excitement and enthusiasm. It is great for a pick-me-up or after a long period of depression. This oil is used for headaches, nausea, and motion sickness. Do not use during pregnancy. If your client is taking homeopathic remedies, avoid using peppermint because it can act as an antidote.
9. **Lemon.** Lemon is used for added energy to the mind and body and a sense of clarity, which makes it useful during times of indecisiveness. Lemon essential oil may irritate the skin.
10. **Juniper.** This scent promotes a sense of strength and well-being. Juniper can ease the pain in muscles and joints. Avoid during pregnancy.
11. **Chamomile.** Chamomile helps ease depression, stress, anger, tension, and irritability. It can also restore the mind and body after a long illness.
12. **Ylang-ylang.** This oil can calm the nervous system, ease depression, and reduce frustration. Used topically, ylang-ylang can irritate the skin.

MASSAGE SUPPLIES

Massage supplies are items such as paper towels and lubricants that are bought and used often. They are needed to provide a clean, sanitary, and comfortable massage environment. Some massage supplies are not necessary for direct massage services but should be considered as minor accompaniments such as hair spray, disposable cups, and cotton balls. Use the checklist (Figure 3-12) when shopping for your massage supplies and incidentals. Extra lines have been added to the checklist for you to write in your own massage items not mentioned in this chapter.

FURNISHING THE MASSAGE ROOM

The furnishings and fixtures you choose for your massage will help you create the best setting for you and your clients. These items include a mirror, clock, water dispenser, wastebasket, supply cabinet, chairs and stools, a place for your client's clothes and per-

MASSAGE SUPPLY CHECKLIST

☐ Lubricant

☐ Liquid Soap

☐ Vinyl Gloves and Finger Cots

☐ Cleaning and Disinfectant Supplies

☐ Box of Tissues

☐ Paper Towels

☐ Toilet Paper

☐ Cotton Balls

☐ Disposable Cups

☐ Hairspray

☐ Contact Lens Solution

Facial Massage Supplies:

☐ Makeup Remover

☐ Cleansing Cream

☐ Toner/Astringent

☐ Moisturizing Cream

☐ Clay Masque

☐ Other: _____

☐ Other: _____

_____

Figure 3-12 Massage supply checklist. (Permission is hereby granted to reproduce this form in its entirety, including the copyright notice, for commercial or instructional use but not for resale.)

sonal items, and wall hangings. Window treatments, light sources, and floor and wall treatment are also important. Most furnishings are intended to increase client comfort and to provide minor conveniences. Some suggestions for your massage room can be seen in Figure 3-13, *A* and *B*.

Mirror. A mirror is an essential for massage rooms. Clients use mirrors to groom themselves after their massage to make sure they are presentable when returning to work or home. Therapists use full-length mirrors to aid in assessing body posture with clients. Mirrors are also used to reflect light and to make a room appear larger.

Clocks. Wall or desk clocks are needed to keep the therapist on schedule and to time certain treatments such as ice packs or facial masks. The two standard types of clocks are digital and analog. The digital clock displays the time numerically, whereas the analog clock has a numbered circular face with hour, minute, and sometimes second hands. The digital

clocks are more convenient if the therapist does a lot of small, timed treatments during the session. It is often easier to monitor a 3-minute treatment from 2:35 to 2:38 than it is to estimate the analog clock's hand movement from across the room. The clock should be quiet and more visible to the therapist than to the client, for whom it may be a distraction.

Water Dispenser. Clean, pure drinking water is an important element in maintaining health. Most people do not drink enough fluids. A water dispenser makes it easy to get the water your body requires. Clients will want to take advantage of a water dispenser as well. Part of your massage service can include offering each client a cup of fresh water before and after each massage.

Wastebasket. A wastebasket is needed in the massage room for used paper towels, tissue paper, disposable gloves, and other items. Most states require that the wastebasket have a closing and sealing lid. The lidded wastebaskets that open using foot

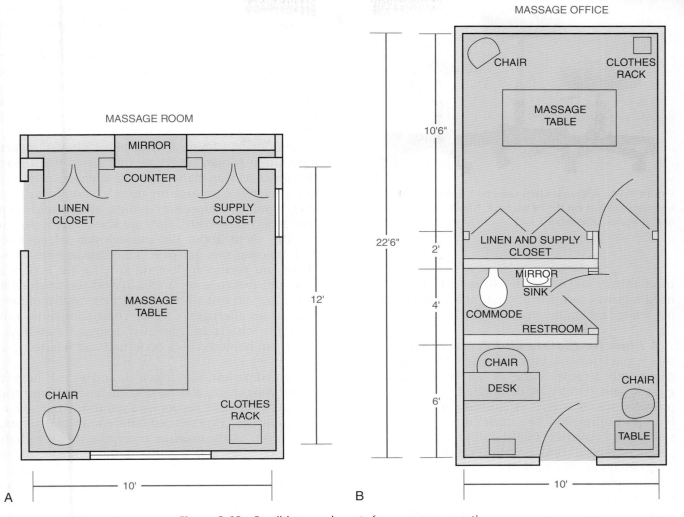

Figure 3-13 Possible room layouts for a massage practice.

pedal are preferred to ones that must be opened by lifting the lid by hand because of the possibility of cross-contamination.

Supply Cabinet. A supply cabinet with hinged doors is preferred to open shelves because supply items are kept out of sight. A supply cabinet can be used to store your massage linens. Cabinets or closets fitted with louvered doors allow linens to breathe, reducing the formation of a rancid odor. These types of doors also hide stereo speakers while still allowing sounds to move through the slats. Line the top surface of your shelves with laminate (e.g., Formica), which resists stains from lubricant dispensers and linens and is easy to clean and disinfect. Be sure to provide a place to store soiled linens separately from clean ones.

Chairs and Stools. A chair provides a place for the client to sit while removing trousers, stockings,

shoes, and socks. Depending on available space and personal taste, you may choose a simple straight-back chair; a plush, oversized chair; a chaise lounge; or an ottoman. Upholstery fabrics are available in a wide variety of textures and colors and contribute to creating the desired atmosphere.

A stool is often used by the therapist when performing massage on the head, neck, hands, or feet. Sitting on a stool takes the place of kneeling on the floor or sitting on the massage table. The best stool design is one that can be raised or lowered for the best administration of different massage techniques (Figure 3-14). Remember, all massage equipment, including furniture, should ergonomically support the therapist. All kinds of different height adjustment mechanisms are available, from hydraulic to screw type. The hydraulic type can be quietly adjusted while the therapist is sitting on the stool. The screw-type mechanisms often require the therapist to remove himself from the stool first. Some screw-type

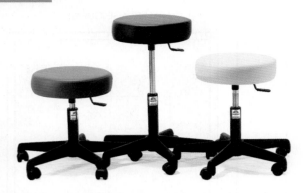

Figure 3-14 A stool is often used by the therapist when performing massage on the head, neck, hands, or feet. (Courtesy of Oakworks, Shrewsbury, Pa.)

mechanisms are noisy and time consuming if you need a great change in height. Many therapists also use a large inflatable physioball as a stool.

A Place for Clothes and Personal Items. For the application of most massage techniques, the client will remove some or all of his garments, glasses, and jewelry. A designated place should be provided for all articles of clothing, including coats, hats, and umbrellas. The most common devices are wall hooks, coat tree, free-standing locker, or valet.

Often, a small desk or table is placed next to the designated clothing removal area for the client's personal items. A small dish or basket can be provided for clients to place items such as keys, pocket change, wallet, eyeglasses, wristwatches, and jewelry. In this way, clients can easily take their personal property with them if they move from one location to another. Make sure these items are safe and secure and are not accidentally misplaced.

Wall Hangings. Most massage therapists use wall hangings in their massage studios for four reasons. First, wall hangings can add ambiance to the room. Second, wall hangings can be used to inform and educate the client. Third, some wall hangings provide acoustical properties to help achieve a quieter room. Fourth, certain wall decor will add a sense of professionalism to the room.

When choosing a wall hanging for ambiance, consider color and content. Warm or soft colors such as peach and beige are calming and tranquil. Bright, intense colors such as red and yellow stimulate our nervous system and typically do not provide a relaxing environment.

In selecting art such as paintings or prints, nature scenes of waterfalls and open meadows help provide a relaxing environment. Save your battle scene pictures of the American Civil War for your living room.

A picture or painting of an ocean or sunset adds a serene, tranquil feeling to your massage atmosphere. Visual art is music for your eyes. Keep it simple; if it is too busy, it may distract the client from the massage experience. You want your art to make a statement, not an exclamation. Before you make an art purchase, it's a good idea to obtain feedback from at least three other individuals; this helps to ensure objectivity.

Anatomical charts, trigger point charts, or acupuncture meridian charts are often used by massage therapists as wall hangings. These charts provide a quick reference for locating muscles, bony markings, trigger points, acupressure points, and other important areas of the body. They are also used for educating the client about her musculoskeletal anatomy and mechanisms of pain and discomfort. These charts are perfect if you are striving for a clinical look and feel to your studio. If you use anatomical charts but do not want to use them wall mounted, there is an alternative. Many chart companies now offer flip charts in specially designed notebooks. These can be stored on a bookshelf and referred to as needed.

Framed diplomas, certificates, and awards help instill in your clients a sense of confidence in your abilities. Achievement papers are a reminder that you are accomplished, experienced, and committed to your profession. Many massage therapists prefer to hang their diplomas and awards in their offices and to keep the studio atmosphere artistic and relaxing; the studio space belongs to your clients. Other professional documents to display include a photographic collage of you working on clients, receiving awards, or giving lectures.

Window Treatments. Windows treatments include vertical and horizontal blinds, shades, and an assortment of drapes. Window treatments have four main functions; (1) they provide wall decoration; (2) they insulate from sound and outside temperature variations; (3) they block or filter light; and (4) they provide privacy for clients.

Window treatments can be simple or can be an addition to your wall ornamentation. When choosing window treatments as a form of decoration, the material (wood, textile, or metal), color, and shade of the walls and floor must be taken into consideration. For example, window treatment fabrics with a pattern usually do not look good with a printed wallpaper. Ask someone who has talent or training in interior decorating to assist you in this selection.

For privacy, all windows that provide a view *into* the studio should be covered by a window treatment. Heavy drapes absorb more sound than shades or blinds; a combination of blinds, drapes, and shades is often used to create the right effect. Massage therapists prefer window treatments that are light blocking over those that are light filtering because it is easier to add more light than to try to reduce it. Fabric-covered blinds are more attractive than the vinyl and aluminum versions but are also more expensive. Window treatments come in a wide variety of styles, weights, and colors, but all may be stained by being touched by oily hands.

Flooring and Walls. Carpet is the best choice for flooring in your massage room. As an insulator, carpet provides warmth and absorbs sound. Carpeted floors also provide safety for clients; oily feet can pose a liability risk on slick flooring. If your massage room has vinyl or hardwood flooring, a thick throw rug that takes up the majority of the room will suffice.

To reduce further unwanted sounds from outside the massage room, interior walls can be insulated, or sound-absorbing panels can be placed in the room. Textured wallpaper, hanging pictures, and other large decorations on the walls will minimize the echoing sounds. Hollow-core doors can be replaced with solid-core doors to reduce further undesired sound.

 Where the spirit does not work with the hand, there is no art.
—Leonardo da Vinci

The Massage Room Environment

Beyond your professional appearance, one of the most important factors for client appeal is the atmosphere of your massage studio. The surroundings of the room set the tone for the massage session. Ideally, you want a place that is quiet, private, easy to heat or cool, and draft free. The room must also be free of tobacco odor, pet dander, and the smell of cleaning solutions. All supplies such as bolsters, blankets, lubricants, and pillows should all be within easy reach. Convenient access to a bathroom is desirable. However, local ordinances may dictate part of the massage environment; check with the proper authorities.

The importance of atmosphere cannot be overemphasized. The symbol for space in Chinese is the symbol for gates in Japanese. Open the gates to relaxation and healing by creating a space for this to occur. If possible, atmosphere should begin when the client drives up to your office and should be maintained all the way to your treatment room. Atmospheric considerations include lighting, music, temperature, and room color. The examples here are given to stimulate your imagination and to help you set your goals.

The dining-room metaphor is one way of explaining why the massage room ambiance is so essential.

When you are serving a specially prepared meal, adjustments are made to make the dining experience extraordinary. The table is set using attractive linens, plates, cups, flatware, and flowers. Soft music is playing in the background, and the lights are dimmed. Give your massage clients the same kind of care and consideration. Let them feel, through the environment you create, that they are honored guests in your establishment. The food makes the meal, but the setting can greatly enhance the experience.

MINI-LAB

If possible, receive massages from a variety of therapists. After the experience, write a summary on how you felt about the massage environment. Use this information when deciding not only the type of equipment you will use but also the décor. This mini-lab can be expanded to include the therapist's interviewing skills and the massage technique used.

Light Sources and Lighting. Lighting serves several purposes in a massage setting. First, you must provide adequate lighting so your clients can read, remove garments, maneuver around the room, get on the massage table, get off the massage table, redress, and exit the office. This same lighting can be used for the therapist visually to assess the condition of the skin before and during a massage. Second, most massage therapists lower the lights during the massage to assist the client in achieving relaxation.

The best light source is sunlight. Natural light coming in a window can be controlled through your window treatments. If you live in a predominantly sunny climate, you can also tint exterior windows of your massage room to create the best lighting for massage therapy.

Even if you use sunlight as your main light source, other forms of light will have to be used on overcast days or after sunset. Indirect lighting is best. Indirect lighting means that the bulbs are obscured from view by means of opaque shades or baffles. A similar effect can be achieved by placing floor lamps in the corners of the room or by using recessed ceiling lights at the corners of the rooms.

After natural light, incandescent bulb lighting is the next best choice, and they can be used in a variety of lamps and fixtures. The higher the wattage of the bulb, the more light it will emit. However, many lamps require a medium- to low-wattage incandescent bulb. The intensity of many lamps and light fixtures can be adjusted by using a special switch known as a *rheostat* or *dimmer*. Your lighting needs will vary from time to time, depending on if you are assessing the client or performing a stress-reduction massage. Offer several lighting possibilities.

STEVEN HALPERN, PhD

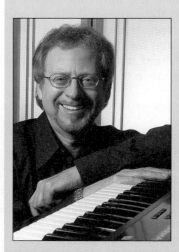

Born: April 18, 1947.

"Mother Nature gave us eyelids. She didn't give us ear-lids or body-lids."

As the true pioneer in the field of relaxation music, Steven Halpern is far from being simply a gifted musician. His eternal thirst for knowledge has benefited the field of massage therapy, and any therapist who has used any of his music can attest to this undeniable fact. His extensive research has taken music to a scientific level and beyond.

His interest in music actually began as a toddler growing up in Long Island, N.Y. Surprisingly, his parents never played music in the home. In fact, it wasn't uncommon for him to crawl down the hallway of his apartment building to the doors of neighbors playing music. This allowed him to follow his heart and listen to music that he truly enjoyed at a very young age. A short while after starting in the school music program, he found himself becoming bored with just playing "little black dots written by dead white composers." This led to his involvement in jazz, which allows a great deal of improvisation.

While in college in the late 1960s his curiosity about music led to his revolutionary research on the effects of certain rhythms on the human body. At the time it was practically a virgin field. Few schools would allow such research, but fortunately he was introduced to the University of California at Sonoma. Here he had access to biofeedback equipment and conducted investigations on the effects of music using subtle rhythms, gentle tones, and non-traditional harmonics. The result has been the hallmark of his approach to composition. "One of the most fundamental responses of the human organism is that it is easily rhythm entrained to an external rhythmic stimulus," he says. "In other words, if there is a steady beat, your heart and pulse will naturally synchronize to that rhythm." This explains why it is impossible to relax to music that has a beat faster than a resting heartbeat.

This theory instantly made Halpern's music popular with massage therapists and clients. After hearing this new type of music, people actually hired him to play live as they were receiving massages. Many massage professionals claimed that as a result of listening to his music, clients were actually relaxing before they even placed a hand on them. Thus therapists received much less resistance from clients, which in turn resulted in making their work much easier.

Although music is important, Halpern reminds us not to forget about other forms of sound. Having a great deal of control over her environment, a therapist needs to be aware of the noises that are often taken for granted. He says he is amazed at how many therapists have a loud ticking clock or a noisy air conditioner. These factors should be taken care of before music can even be considered. Many of us have conditioned ourselves to block out certain sounds. Halpern states, "Mother Nature gave us eyelids. She didn't give us ear-lids or body-lids." Whether we are consciously aware of it, our entire body is picking up and responding to all sounds.

Halpern notes that "while listening to true relaxation music, an altered state can be entered . . . whereas dancers say they become one with the music, a massage therapist can become one with the massage. This state allows therapists to consciously lose track of the exact strokes they are going to do next, yet they always seem to do exactly the right ones." He claims that some of the best massage professionals he has talked with say that such music has helped them reach the zone in which the realm of massage lives and a wonderful healing energy can be tapped. He admits that this phenomenon has yet

STEVEN HALPERN, PhD—cont'd

to be scientifically documented, but after hearing it from so many people, he feels that it must be true. He invites all massage professionals to keep their awareness and hearts open to this because it can be of great service and benefit to their clients. "Music is much more powerful, and the effects of music are much more pronounced than most people realize," says Halpern. "In the past 25 or 30 years, people have forgotten how to listen in a lot of respects, but I now start to see people come back."

The two other forms of light bulbs used are halogen and fluorescent lights. Even though both types of bulbs use very little energy, a few problems should be noted. A few incidents of exploding halogen bulbs have been reported. Fluorescent lights often emit a humming noise and a bluish color, which may contribute to the onset of headaches and annoy clients with attention deficit disorder (ADD) or attention deficit with hyperactivity disorder (ADHD) by aggravating their symptoms. If your office already has fluorescent lighting, you may want to leave it off and use table or floor lamps or replace the fluorescent bulbs with a full-spectrum bulb. The full-spectrum bulb will take care of the color problem but will not take care of the humming problem.

Still other mood lighting suggestions can be accomplished rather inexpensively. Line a window, corner, or beam with strings of clear Christmas lights that do not flash. Try placing a nightlight behind a large object such as an oversized vase. Many massage therapists include the use of candlelight in their practice. Although candles are unbeatable for creating a relaxing ambiance, they are also a fire hazard. Regardless of how careful you are, candle wax spills and soot deposits occur on shelves and walls. However, you may decide the benefits are worth the risks.

Music. Because "music soothes the savage beast," it is reasonable to include it in creating an environment conducive to massage therapy. Music is art for the ears, and most massage therapists will tell you that it makes a difference in how clients relax (if the music is soft and slow). It also helps the therapist in keeping a rhythm with massage movements.

Music systems can range from a transportable box style with a handle to a multicomponent system. The most convenient feature on a cassette player is an auto reverse or a repeat button on a compact disc player. This allows uninterrupted massage time because your time will not be spent turning the tape

over or restarting it. It is helpful to listen to the mechanical sounds of the music system during its operation. Many units are quite noisy when the tape is reversing direction or may pause too long when changing discs.

If you have detachable speakers, place them at your client's ear level when he or she is lying down on your massage table. Small, hidden speakers are preferred to overly large speakers that look like furniture. Thanks to technology, small, high-quality speakers are available. Most music systems can accommodate as many as four to six speakers.

Have a variety of cassette tapes or compact discs available for your client's (and your own) listening pleasure. Some therapists encourage clients to bring their own music selections to the session. Although music, like room decor, is a matter of taste, most therapists prefer a slow, even melody. Most classical selections are not appropriate because of an ebb and flow of crescendos and decrescendos. Be careful of New Age music, because most selections have jumpy melodies and are too stimulating. Music companies are now subdividing New Age music including a category called *minimalism,* which is suitable for massage. Nature sounds such as waves breaking on the shore, whale songs, and thunderstorms, combined with orchestral music, are also a good choice. Beware of trickling water sounds; they may induce some clients to request a visit to the bathroom during the massage.

MINI-LAB

Lie on your massage table in the prone and the supine positions. Get the client's perspective. Notice what the major issues are: visual stimuli, odor, sound, and so on. Do what you can to maximize the positive effects and minimize the negative effects.

Temperature of the Massage Room. The temperature range for your massage room is between 72° and 75° F. Clients may have difficulty relaxing if the room temperature is not comfortable. As the massage progresses, pulse rate, respiration rate, and blood pressure decrease. This is why clients often become chilled during the massage, even though they felt comfortable at the beginning of the massage. Always ask the client if he is warm enough halfway through the massage session.

Once your room temperature is set, there are several ways to keep your client warm as her body physiology changes. A small portable heater can be placed in the room if additional warmth is needed. Make sure that no one is in danger of touching the heating element on the unit. In winter months, a heating blanket can be added to the massage tabletop. Blankets can be placed on top of the client for warmth as well. Many clients express that the room temperature is fine, but their feet feel cold. Clients may elect to bring and wear socks while on the massage table, or an extra blanket can be draped over their feet for added warmth. If you have a ceiling fan in your room, you may want to set it at the lowest speed blowing up. This will create a circulation effect for moving the warm air collected near the ceiling out to the sides of the room and down the walls. The room maintains a more constant air temperature without directing a draft toward the client. Conversely, clients who are warm-natured or pregnant may actually request that the ceiling fan be set to blow on them to cool them down in warmer seasons.

The massage therapist may become warm during the massage because of physical exertion. If you become overheated easily, try wearing clothes made of natural fibers that fit loosely to allow air to evaporate perspiration. A small oscillating fan can be placed on the floor and the airflow directed at the therapist's feet. No matter where the therapist is standing, the air will reach him as the fan turns. The fan should not interfere with keeping the client warm. Make sure the fan or fan cord is not in a location to create a safety hazard. If the room has vertical blinds, ensure they are not in the path of the fan, otherwise the breeze will disturb them, creating an audible distraction.

Color. Colors used for your massage room can be divided into two categories, warm and cool. Warm colors naturally bring a feeling of warmth but also stimulation; cool colors can make a room feel cool, but they are also relaxing. The shade of a particular color has an impact on what you are trying to achieve.

Warm colors are reds, browns, yellows, and oranges; cool colors are blues, violets, and greens. White is the absence of color, and black is the combination of all colors. You can choose what you like; if you do not have a strong preference, go with the color most of your clients like. Color can also open up a small room or make a large room appear smaller and cozier.

The most important color considerations in your massage room are the walls, floor, window treatments, and linens. Choose colors that contrast well, such as tan walls and sage green linens, or green walls and beige linens. Neutral colors work best because they do not overwhelm the client's nervous system.

MINI-LAB

Using all the elements discussed in this chapter, design your massage room.

SUMMARY

Career success depends not only on knowledge, skills, and abilities but also on your capacity to use wisely the tools of the trade. Tools or massage equipment includes the massage table, face rests, arm shelves, carrying cases, table carts, linens, bolsters, and massage lubricants. Equipment should be chosen with consideration to ergonomics, client comfort, longevity, and wise investment.

Your massage table is your most important tool. When purchasing a stationary or a portable massage table, most table manufacturers let you decide the specifications of features such as width, height, length, frame, padding, and fabric.

It is essential that the therapist understand the procedures and frequency of simple cleaning and disinfecting each piece of equipment.

Massage linens include towels, sheets, blankets, pillowcases, bolster and face rest covers, and so on. Popular linen fabrics are flannel, cotton, cotton blends, and percale.

Massage media or lubricants include oils, creams, lotions, powders, and liniments. Good lubricants should nourish the skin. They should not cause allergic reactions or stain clothing and linens.

Finally, the massage room environment ties everything together. Considerations should be made for temperature, lighting, color, music, decorations, and client comfort.

Using these recommendations can produce a great savings of time and money and improve the quality of the therapist's work.

SHORT ANSWER

Complete the questions with an appropriate response.

1. In choosing the right kind of massage equipment, what are important considerations?

2. What are some important features of massage tables?

3. Massage tables that are too wide make it difficult for the therapist. Explain.

4. Massage tables that are too high make it difficult for the therapist. Explain.

5. What are the three *worst* substances for your table and accessory vinyl?

6. List some accessories you might want to purchase for your massage table.

7. How often is your massage vinyl cleaned and with which type of cleanser?

8. When is the massage table vinyl disinfected?

9. How does the therapist determine the amount of massage lubricant used?

10. Why is keeping your client warm during the massage important?

Bibliography

Clark S: *Essential chemistry for safe aromatherapy,* New York, 2002, Churchill Livingstone.

McClure VS: *Infant massage instructor handbook,* 1997 (self-published manuscript).

Price S, Price L: *Aromatherapy for health professionals,* ed 2, New York, 1999, Churchill Livingstone.

Tisserard R: *The art of aromatherapy handbook,* Boulder, Colo, 1977, Healing Arts Press.

UNIT TWO

Benefits, Contraindications, Screening, Technique, and Special Considerations for the Massage Practitioner

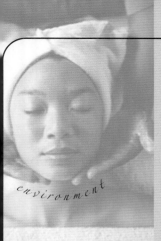

environment

Health, Hygiene, Sanitation, and Safety Standards

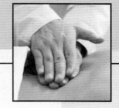

4

"The pessimist sees difficulty in every opportunity. The optimist sees the opportunity in every difficultly."

—Winston Churchill

pressure

STUDENT OBJECTIVES

After completing this chapter, the student should be able to:

- List and give examples of pathogens
- Explain basic rules and procedures of sanitation and how they are used to control transmission of pathogens
- Discuss universal precautions and how they are applicable to the practice of massage therapy
- Determine when gloves are needed for massage therapy
- Demonstrate proper handwashing techniques
- List five hygiene tips
- Recommend three health tips to your clients and colleagues
- Design a massage facility using basic rules of safety and accessibility

technique

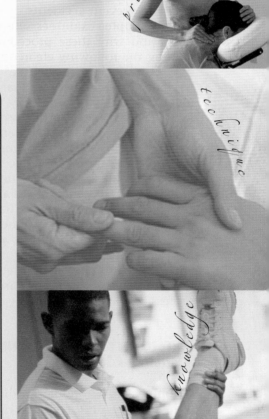

knowledge

INTRODUCTION

Massage therapy is one of the safest, least intrusive, and yet most effective treatment modalities in the health care field today. However, the client is susceptible to harm in certain areas of our practice. These areas may be obscure, such as incidental exposure to disease-causing agents or an accidental injury. Contagious or communicable diseases may be transferred to clients by unclean hands and nails and by unsanitary equipment and supplies. The therapist must adopt a policy of impeccable cleanliness before coming into contact with a client. Hippocrates, the father of Western medicine, declared that physicians should "do no harm." All medical professionals practice high standards of sanitation. Every precaution must be taken to protect clients and therapists through personal and professional procedures and clinic modifications that minimize disease transmission and prevent accidents.

This chapter examines safety and hygiene procedures and why these procedures are necessary, including the following elements: basic pathophysiology as it relates to disease transmission, proper hygiene and sanitation, and safety standards for your massage facility. Familiarity with these facets of health will support you in providing the best environment possible for your clients. The pathophysiology section includes pathogenic agents and their related diseases, how to reduce the transmission of disease-causing microorganisms, and the handling of biohazardous material (blood and other body fluids). Health and hygiene covers basic sanitation procedures and techniques for handwashing and gloving and health tips for therapists and clients. The safety module provides standards for the physical facility and information on client safety. These standards for health, hygiene, sanitation, and safety are a part of professional massage conduct across the country.

PATHOPHYSIOLOGY AND DISEASE AWARENESS

To build a better understanding of disease and its transmission, a fundamental overview of *pathophysiology,* the study of biological and physical manifestation of disease, is required. A **pathogen** is a biological agent capable of causing disease. Pathogen comes from the Greek words, *pathos,* meaning disease, and *gen,* meaning to produce. Examples of pathogens are bacteria, fungi, protozoa, and viruses. One way to develop a disease is to be exposed to a pathogen. Effective exposure results in contamination. **Contamination** occurs when an infectious, or pathogenic, agent resides in or on an organism.

Pathogens can be airborne or fluid-borne, or they can infect through direct contact.

Once the organism is contaminated, the next phase is infection. Infection elicits response from the body's defenses. Inanimate objects, or **fomites**, can also become contaminated. The body's natural defense mechanisms against exposure are (1) physical and chemical barriers such as the skin, mucosa, cilia, digestive enzymes, perspiration, and vaginal secretions; (2) inflammation; and (3) the body's immunological responses. The following section examines pathogens in more detail. Once the mechanism of transmission is identified, ways to stop its transmission become apparent.

The Host/Pathogen Relationship

When a pathogen first penetrates a target organism, a relationship between the pathogen and the host is initiated. The host's reacts to fight the pathogen, and the pathogen tries to overcome the host's reactions. As a pathogen enters the body, the immune system is put on alert and a complex series of reactions begins. This includes the secretion of chemicals such as enzymes and acids of the gastrointestinal tract. Reflexes like coughing and vomiting may occur in a physical attempt to remove the infectious agent. White blood cells (WBCs), part of the body's immune system, begin to mobilize to destroy the invader.

The susceptibility of the host to infection is dependent on factors such as age, genetics, nutrition, state of health, and immune response, along with factors that have not yet been identified. The success of the pathogen depends on various factors including the portion or number of organisms that gain access, which areas are attacked, the pathogen's ability to spread and replicate itself, and its resistance to host defenses. Thus a weak host with a strong pathogen results in disease, whereas a strong host with a weak pathogen overcomes the introduction of disease.

However, if the immune system is depressed by chronic stress, malnutrition, radiation, some medications, or a preexisting illness such as acquired immune deficiency syndrome (AIDS), the organism is then more susceptible to diseases caused by pathogens. It is for this reason that the human immunodeficiency virus (HIV) is so deadly; it weakens the host by crippling its immune response so that a second infection, which would normally be contained or suppressed by the immune system, becomes fatal.

Types of Diseases

To understand how to reduce the likelihood of transmitting disease, disease itself must be examined. This section explores the types of diseases, both pathogenic and nonpathogenic. As you may recall, the presence of a pathogen does not ensure that a disease will develop. The body's immune system often declares biological war on the pathogen and destroys it before disease can manifest itself. Some signs and symptoms that may show us the organism is trying to defeat a pathogen are fever, mild nausea, altered metabolism, cardiovascular changes, anemia, leukocytosis (elevated WBC count), and a general feeling of low energy.

The types of diseases are *infectious, deficiency, metabolic, genetic, cancerous,* and *autoimmune.*

1. **Infectious diseases** are caused by a biological agent such as a virus or a bacterium and are highly contagious. Also known as *communicable diseases,* infectious diseases can be transmitted to a person by another person, an animal, or a fomite; either by direct or indirect contact. Examples of infectious disease are pneumonia, measles, and tuberculosis.
2. **Deficiency diseases,** caused by a lack of an essential vitamin or nutrient, typically interfere with the body's growth and development. This may help establish metabolic diseases. Types of deficiency diseases are scurvy (deficiency of ascorbic acid or vitamin C), rickets (deficiency of vitamin D), and beriberi (deficiency of thiamine or B_1). Deficiency diseases are not contagious.
3. **Metabolic diseases** involve abnormal activities of cells and/or tissues such as Cushing's disease, diabetes, cardiovascular conditions, and jaundice. Metabolic diseases are not contagious but may have originated from a contagious disease such as hepatitis, which can lead to jaundice or vice versa.
4. **Genetic diseases** are caused by an imperfect genetic code in the chromosomes. Chromosomes, the body's genetic material, are structures found in the nucleus of cells. Examples of genetic diseases are Down syndrome, cystic fibrosis, sickle cell anemia, and hemophilia. These genetic disorders are not contagious but may be passed down from generation to generation.
5. **Cancerous diseases** are characterized by the uncontrollable growth of abnormal cells that invade surrounding tissue and metastasize. **Metastasis** is the process of cancerous cells spreading to distant parts of the body, usually through the bloodstream or the lymphatic circulation. The definite cause of cancer is undetermined, but many potential causes are recognized. More than 80% of cancer cases are attributed to exposure to **carcinogenic** (cancer-causing) chemicals, tobacco, ionizing radiation, and ultraviolet rays. Stress tends to promote cancer growth. Cancer is not contagious, but it can metastasize and spread internally. Some cancers are **benign** (not life threatening), and some are **malignant** (condition that worsens and causes death if not treated).
6. **Autoimmune diseases** are part of a large group of diseases marked by an inappropriate or excessive response of the body's immune functions. These disorders result from an attack by the body's own immune system. The body mistakenly identifies one or more tissues as invading organisms and attacks that tissue. Examples of autoimmune diseases are rheumatoid arthritis, lupus, and multiple sclerosis.

Agents of Disease

Four basic pathogenic agents promote disease in the body: *bacteria, fungi, protozoa,* and *viruses* (Table 4-1).

1. **Bacteria.** Most bacteria are not pathogenic and do not require living tissue for survival. Some bacteria are important for plant growth, such as nitrogen-fixing bacteria in the soil. Others are used for processing certain foods such as bread, cheese, yogurt, and wine. "Good" bacteria also occur as natural flora in the body (mouth, intestines) and aid digestive processes. Harmful bacteria are transmitted directly from person to person or animal to person or through a fomite. Bacteria may enter the body through ingestion and lead to diseases like botulism and salmonella. Improper food handling, such as chopping vegetables or fruits after handling raw meat or chopping on unclean surfaces, can contaminate food. Another common method of obtaining bacteria is by not washing the hands after using the toilet then touching the nose or mouth. Some diseases that are caused by bacteria are boils (staph), tuberculosis, strep throat, and tetanus.
2. **Fungi.** Fungal agents include molds and yeast, and their growth is promoted by warm, moist environments. Only a few fungal varieties are pathogenic. When an individual has a fungal infection, it is typically superficial, tenacious, and difficult to eradicate. Generally, fungal spores are transmitted by a fomite; for example, athlete's foot fungus may be picked up off a locker room floor. However, some fungal infections can infect the body internally such as thrush, which is a yeast infection of the tissues of the mouth. In hosts with severely suppressed immune function, fungi can become systemic and may be life threatening. Moreover, fungi can be transmitted directly from person to person. *Candida albicans* normally grows in the mucous membranes of the mouth and vagina, can be found in the axilla and under the breast, and can be transmitted to a new host through touch. Another fungal infestation is ringworm, which manifests on the skin.

TABLE 4-1

Pathogenic Agents, Reservoir, and Infection or Disease

Organism/Pathogen	Reservoir	Infection/Disease
Bacteria		
Escherichia coli	Colon, manure	Food poisoning, diarrhea, enteritis
Staphylococcus aureus	Skin, hair, nose	Cellulitis, pneumonia, impetigo, acne, boil
Streptococcus pneumoniae	Throat, skin, lungs	Pneumonia
Streptococcus pyogenes	Throat, skin	Strep throat, scarlet fever, rheumatic fever
Mycobacterium tuberculosis	Lungs	Tuberculosis
Neisseria gonorrhoeae	Genitalia, rectum, mouth	Gonorrhea
Rickettsia rickettsii	Tick	Rocky Mountain spotted fever
Borrelia burgdorferi	Tick	Lyme disease
Clostridium botulinum	Food (improperly handled)	Botulism, food poisoning, gastroenteritis
Salmonella enteritidis	Food (improperly handled)	Salmonella, food poisoning, gastroenteritis
Clostridium tetani	Intestines, feces	Tetanus
Helicobacter pylori	Duodenum, stomach, saliva	Ulcers
Chlamydia trachomatis	Urinogenital tract, eye	Chlamydia, pelvic inflammatory disease, urethritis, trachoma, lymphogranuloma venereum
Fungi		
Candida albicans	Mouth, skin, genitalia, intestines	Candidiasis, thrush, dermatitis
Epidermophyton floccosum	Fomite, skin	Athletes foot, ringworm, jock itch, onychomycosis
Protozoa		
Plasmodium falciparum	Mosquito	Malaria
Trichomonas vaginalis	Urinogenital tract	Trichomoniasis
Trypanosoma brucei rhodesiense	Tsetse fly	African sleeping sickness
Entamoeba histolytica	Water, food, feces	Amebic dysentery
Viral		
Human immunodeficiency virus	Body fluids	AIDS
Influenzavirus type A, B, C	Droplets, lung	Influenza
Paramyxovirus	Droplets	Measles, mumps, respiratory infections
Human papillomavirus	Skin	Warts
Rhabdovirus	Saliva, brain tissue	Rabies
Herpesvirus type 1 and 2	Mucous membrane, genitalia, rectum, blisters	Herpes simplex, genital herpes

3. **Protozoa**. These single-celled organisms are considered the simplest form of animal life; pathogenic protozoa can only survive in a living subject and are commonly transmitted through contact with feces or contaminated food and water. Protozoa are responsible for diseases such as trichomoniasis, amebic dysentery, African sleeping sickness, and malaria.

4. **Viruses**. Viruses are considered to be nonliving entities because they do not carry out independent metabolic activities. They can only replicate themselves within the cell of a living plant or animal host. Because viruses easily mutate, antibiotics are relatively ineffective. Viruses are usually transmitted from person to person or animal to person. Viral diseases include the common cold, influenza, AIDS, measles, mumps, rabies, herpes simplex, viral hepatitis, and Ebola.

Premassage consultations should query the client regarding illness. In general, massage therapists are exposed to no more viruses and bacteria than the average person, with one major difference: we are touching an unclothed person. Massage therapists who are hospital-based or who work with hospice or nursing homes may be at a higher risk of infection. The pathogen that the massage therapist is most likely to contact is fungi (yeast). Massage therapists may not only contract the fungi, but the fungi also can be spread to other parts of their client's body. Contamination can occur in both directions: from therapist to client and from client to therapist.

Paths of Infection

For infection to pass successfully from an infected agent to a living organism (or host), a mode of transmission is required. The infected agent is often referred to as a *reservoir*, which can be living or inanimate. By understanding the various modes of transmission, this information can be used to protect therapists and clients from disease.

1. **Direct physical contact.** Pathogens can enter a host through direct contact with *mucous membranes* or *intact* or *broken skin.*
   - **Mucous membranes.** This includes the touching of an infected mucous membrane to an uninfected mucous membrane (e.g., nose, mouth, and genitals) and the exchange of bodily fluids and secretions by kissing or by oral, genital, or rectal sexual activity (the latter are also known as *sexually transmitted diseases* [STDs]).
   - **Intact skin.** This method of transmission includes contact with someone who is infected with agents or pathogens such as fleas, scabies, lice, ticks, fungi, poison oak, poison ivy, and poison sumac. Inoculation through intact skin can occur when an infected insect or animal stings or bites a host, causing a break in the skin. Malaria and rabies are two examples of diseases caused by inoculation.
   - **Broken skin.** This type of transmission can also include pathogen entry through breaks in the skin. The reason for the skin break does not matter; it could be accidental, a surgical intrusion, a dog or mosquito bite, skin eruptions from a prior infection, a hangnail, or a self-inflicted wound (e.g., intravenous [IV] drug use). Most parasites gain entry to the body through breaks in the skin of the feet.
2. **Indirect physical contact.** Pathogens can enter a host by indirect contact through *ingestion* or *inhalation.*
   - **Ingestion.** This includes the consumption of contaminated water, undercooked meats, or food that has not been properly handled, stored, or refrigerated. (NOTE: Refrigerators should be set at 40° F.)
   - **Inhalation.** This mode of transmission includes infectious agents that are inhaled and absorbed through the respiratory mucosa. Although no

direct contact is made with infected mucous membranes, contamination occurs when the host comes into contact with airborne droplets of fluid arising from the respiratory tract and salivary glands of the reservoir, primarily through coughing, sneezing, massaging, or talking within a 3-foot distance. Most respiratory diseases are spread by this method.

 A musician must make music, an artist must paint, a poet must write, if he is to be ultimately at peace with himself.
—Abraham Maslow

Controlling Transmission of Pathogens in a Massage Practice

The best thing a massage therapist can do to control transmission of pathogenic organisms is to practice good hygiene and sanitation. Handwashing and using only clean linens and equipment are common-sense measures. The therapist should bandage breaks in the skin and avoid those of the clients. Many sanitation practices are routinely performed, and others are performed only when stricter standards are needed, such as gloving up to reduce the likelihood of cross contamination. Other ways in which you, as a massage therapist, can control the spread of pathogenic microorganisms in your practice are by disinfecting equipment if contaminated, using a closed dispenser for massage lubricant, and not working when you are ill.

These safeguards will be explained in detail later in the chapter. Discuss these methods for controlling the transmission of infectious disease with other massage therapists. You may decide to incorporate other methods of sanitation in your practice. Remember that all the rules for sanitation are to prevent the spread of infectious agents in any direction: from therapist to client, client to therapist, and one part of the client's body to another.

Universal and Selective Precautions

In December 1991, the Occupational Safety and Health Administration (OSHA) supported and helped pass federal legislation that now requires all health care providers to prescribe to a plan that prevents the exposure to and spreading of blood- and fluid-borne pathogens. Body fluids that can carry harmful microorganisms are semen; vaginal secretions; blood; saliva; breast milk; urine; feces; and cerebrospinal, synovial, pleural, peritoneal, and pericardial fluids. From this legislation, the Centers for Disease Control and Prevention (CDC) established **universal**

precautions to reduce the transmission of communicable disease. These precautions protect the client *and* the health care provider.

Universal precautions include mandatory handwashing, use of gloves, protective eyewear, nose/ face masks, protective clothing, laundering linens and uniforms, cleaning or disinfecting equipment, and observing proper methods for disposing of used medical supplies and biological material. Universal precautions are required when performing invasive

TIFFANY FIELD, PhD

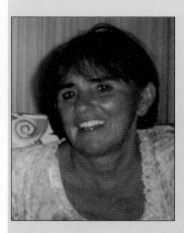

"The best pioneers are the ones actually out there doing massage. They get devotees just from having put their hands on them. That's what keeps the field alive and moving."

Tiffany Field has always been a woman on the move. As the daughter of an insurance executive and teacher, she lived in 12 different places when she was growing up, but now she's found her home and her life's calling—on the beach in Hollywood, Fla.

She is not a massage therapist, and she has not developed any particular massage modality; however, her work has dramatically affected the credibility of the profession. Tiffany Field is a professor of pediatrics, psychology, and psychiatry, and she is the director of the University of Miami School of Medicine's Touch Research Institute (TRI). TRI was established in 1992 and is the only center in the world devoted solely to the study of touch and its applications in science and medicine.

According to a recent article in *Massage Therapy Journal* by Mirka Knaster, Field holds a doctorate in developmental psychology and has 25 years of research experience, with numerous publishing credits, awards, and research grants. She has written for 50 professional journals and retains membership in more than a dozen professional organizations.

TRI evolved after her team's research findings supported touch as a factor that increased birthweight in premature infants. Premature infants who receive massage put on weight faster and leave the hospital earlier. With 470,000 premature births in the United States each year, that could add up to $7.05 billion in annual savings.

The potential for Field's research and the cost-cutting measures earned the grant money to explore touch therapy further. Currently, her group is studying the effects of massage on all ages, from cocaine-exposed newborns to arthritic geriatric patients. *Massage Therapy Reduces Anxiety and Enhances EEG Pattern of Alertness and Math Computations* is one of the most recent studies being conducted.

Some of the work being examined at TRI is particularly groundbreaking. Still considered by many a contraindication for massage, an ongoing breast cancer study shows an increase in natural killer cells (cells that kill cancer cells) and other pathologies after massage. In a society that values scientific proof, such findings could eventually make massage therapy a component of mainstream medicine.

Field has a hectic schedule that involves lots of travel for fund-raising, overseeing projects, and writing grant proposals. To unwind, she swims daily; practices yoga, ballet, and tai chi when she has spare time; and of course she gets a massage whenever she can.

For over a decade, Field has probably been one of the most instrumental individuals in helping gain respect for massage therapy and advises new massage therapists to "join a group practice to learn the ropes of operating a business."

medical procedures or when handling body fluids. Invasive medical procedures involve puncturing or penetrating body tissues or entering a body cavity.

How involved do massage therapists have to become with these medical precautions? The answer to this question varies according to your practice. Although massage therapists are not involved with surgical procedures, we do occasionally enter a body cavity such as the mouth for temporomandibular joint (TMJ) massage (where legal). A therapist who works in a medical clinic or hospital has a greater exposure risk than the therapist who works in a private practice. In a clinical setting, the therapist may be required to perform rehabilitative therapy on patients who have pins, wires, stitches, staples, or open wounds near the treated area.

Contact with body fluids seldom occurs in a private massage therapy practice. A small blemish may break, lesions or minute scabs on recently shaved legs may drain, a client may cough or sneeze mucus, or a nauseated client may vomit. These and similar situations must be handled according to an aseptic protocol, which involves the use of methods to eliminate the presence and/or spread of pathogens and are outlined later in the chapter.

Glove Use in Massage Therapy

The use of intact gloves ensures client and therapist protection from transmission of disease. Massage therapists working with people who are HIV positive, or who have a condition where the immune system is compromised, must be particularly careful not to infect their clients with something that could prove fatal in their weakened state. For more information on massage, gloves, and the human immunodeficiency virus (HIV), see Chapter 9.

If you must wear gloves during a massage, make sure they fit your hands well. Be aware that glove use may reduce your palpatory abilities. Performing massage with gloved hands also creates more friction, especially in thick body hair, and this may be uncomfortable for the client. How to reduce the additional friction depends on the type of glove used. The two most popular gloves used in the health care industry are latex and vinyl. Each has its assets and liabilities.

1. **Latex gloves** are very thin, very strong, and tend to conform like a second skin to the therapist's hands. They are readily available in a variety of sizes and are affordably priced. Most massage lubricants are oil-based; these break down latex glove material. If latex gloves are used, a water-based lubricant is needed. Many people have latex allergies or are latex-sensitive.

When Should the Massage Therapist Use Gloves?

1. When handling any form of blood or other body fluid or secretions (this includes removing these linens from the table or removing trash that may be contaminated).
2. Anytime the therapist has a break in the skin or an infectious skin disease on one or both hands. If the injury or infection is only on the end of the finger, a finger cot may be worn.
3. For reasons of hygiene, such as internal TMJ massage.
4. Whenever the client requests that the therapist wear gloves.
5. Whenever the therapist does not feel comfortable without them.
6. If several of these conditions are present, then the therapist may decide that the risk factor is high enough to warrant double gloving or rescheduling the massage until the conditions change.

2. **Vinyl gloves** may be used with oil-based lubricants and are fine for clients with latex allergies. Vinyl gloves are thicker and may reduce tactile sensitivity of the therapist. They do not have the stretch capability of latex and so do not conform to the contours of the hands as readily. Vinyl gloves are also rarely available in stores and are a little more expensive.

Inform the client about the use of gloves for safety and protection (e.g., open cuts). Some clients may be offended that you are donning gloves before the massage and ask you not to use gloves. You may refuse to perform the massage on the client if this occurs. Conversely, the client may refuse the massage if he suspects you have an open wound or an infection (e.g., cold or influenza). Before gloving up, wash your hands and dry them thoroughly. Glove up discreetly and quietly. If a glove is torn or damaged during a procedure, it must be removed, the hands rewashed, and a new glove replaced immediately.

Once the decision has been made to use gloves, care must be taken when removing and disposing of them to restrict possible contamination from the glove surface. One safe method of glove removal is to peel the first glove from the cuff to fingers so that it is inside out (Figure 4-1, *A*). Then, place the removed glove into the palm of the other hand (Figure 4-1, *B*) so that when you peel off the second glove, the first will be contained inside (Figure 4-1, *C*). Dispose of the removed gloves in a closed container (Figure 4-1, *D*). Even though you have been careful in removing and discarding the used gloves, wash your hands immediately.

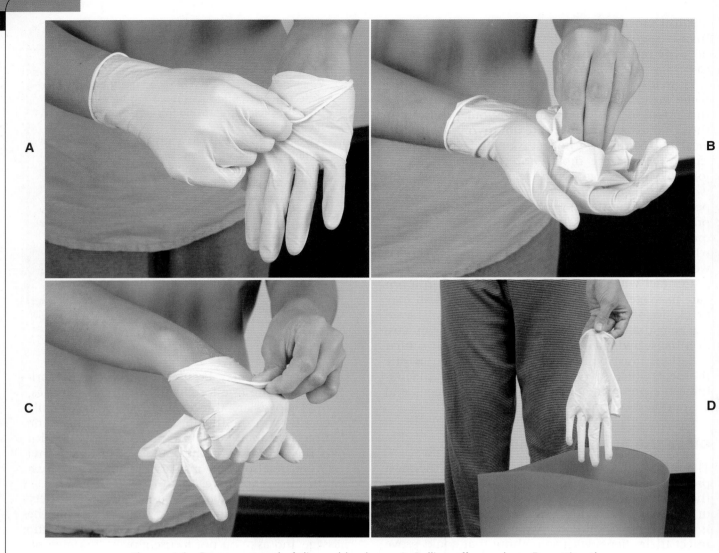

Figure 4-1   Proper removal of disposable gloves. **A,** Pulling off one glove; **B,** putting the removed glove in the palm of the gloved hand; **C,** removing the other glove with the first removed glove inside; **D,** disposal of the used gloves.

SANITARY PROCEDURES FOR THE MASSAGE THERAPIST

One of the best things we can do for our clients is to follow basic rules of sanitation. **Sanitation** involves the application of measures to promote a healthful, disease-free environment. This includes laundering the massage linens after each use, following a handwashing procedure, and cleaning and disinfecting massage equipment and supplies used for the client (Box 4-1).

Handwashing removes or destroys pathogens from the forearms, hands, and nails. Other aseptic handwashing techniques include the use of special hand-cleaning solutions that are designed to be used without water. These high-alcohol content gels are designed for field use in sporting events and on-site chair massage appointments where handwashing may not be convenient or even possible. Be sure to follow the directions listed on the container. Because it is more difficult to remove microorganisms from small cracks and crevices found in ornate jewelry, wearing rings, bracelets, or wristwatches while performing massage therapy is not advisable. Long nails or cracked nail polish also provides hiding places for microorganisms and is not in keeping with sanitary standards. Long nails and jewelry can also potentially injure the client or break the protective barrier of gloves.

The garments you wear as you perform the massage, including your laboratory coat (if you wear

BOX 4-1

Handwashing Procedure

1. Approach the sink. Turn on the valve (Figure 4-2, *A*). Adjust the water valve until the water is a comfortable temperature and is not splashing in the sink.
2. Wet your hands, forearms, and elbows. Keep your hands lower than your elbows, or water, soil, and microorganisms will run up your arms and onto your garments (Figure 4-2, *B*). Using a nailbrush or orange stick, clean underneath the nails (Figure 4-2, *C*). A single-use nailbrush or orange stick is preferred. Nails must be cleaned before hands.
3. Using soap, generate lather in your hands and rub the soap up the forearms using a firm, circular motion. Massage your soapy hands and forearms for 30 seconds. If you have broken skin on your fingers, hands, forearms, or elbows or come into contact with body fluids such as blood, mother's milk, or semen, *increase the handwashing time to 2 minutes.*
   - The friction created by rubbing your hands together is essential to emulsify the oils on the skin and to lift microorganisms and dirt from the skin's surface. These unwanted impurities become suspended in the lather, which will be rinsed away.
   - When washing, include the areas between your fingers (Figure 4-2, *D*).
   - Liquid soap in a pump dispenser is preferred over bar soap because liquid soap does not become contaminated by direct contact and is therefore more sanitary. If you are using bar soap, rinse the bar before and after use.
   - Liquid dishwashing soap can be used as an alternative to liquid hand soap.
4. Rinse the hands and forearms thoroughly, using tap water until all lather is removed. Allow the water to run from the fingers to the elbows. This rinsing technique ensures that the hands will be the most sanitary area. Do not skimp on this step. Leaving soap residue on the skin may result in chapped or dry skin.
5. Using paper towels, dry your hands and forearms well (Figure 4-2, *E*). Using the same paper towels, turn off the water valves (Figure 4-2, *F*). Continue to use the same paper towels to open door handles until you reach the room in which you will perform massage. Discard the paper towels.

one), must be laundered after being worn each workday. Machine wash and dry your uniforms in hot water with detergent. If you suspect any exposure to contaminated fluids/droplets or a communicable disease, add ¼ cup of chlorine bleach with the detergent during the wash cycle; machine dry afterward. Do not wear your massage uniform for other purposes. Short sleeves are more sanitary than long sleeves because they do not touch the client's skin.

Do not confuse disinfection with sterilization. **Disinfection** is the removal of pathogens or their toxins from surfaces by a chemical and/or mechanical agent. This often does not remove *spores* (the reproductive unit). Disinfection includes the use of antiseptics, which remove pathogenic organisms from fomites or tissues of the skin's surface and mucosa without damaging or destroying these tissues. **Sterilization** destroys microorganisms using heat, water, chemicals, and/or gases. Disinfection or sterilization of surfaces is required by law in most states when a surface comes into contact with body fluids; you can lose your license if you do not uphold these standards for clients.

In some circumstances, state law or employers require the massage therapist to be immunized against diseases such as hepatitis B, rubella, rubeola, poliomyelitis, diphtheria, and tuberculosis. Some employers of massage therapists, such as hospitals, may

highly recommend vaccination, but it is not mandatory. However, you should understand that it is accepted practice that all nonimmunized employees are sent home for the duration of any outbreak. This will vary with the microorganism in question. The following rules for sanitation will guide you in using aseptic protocol to ensure the highest quality of health care possible (Box 4-2).

Handwashing

The premiere source of microorganism cross-contamination is by contact with human hands. It seems reasonable that the best measure to prevent the spread of infection would be handwashing. Massage therapists must wash their hands before and after each massage; using gloves for massage therapy does not preclude handwashing. The handwashing procedure shown in Figure 4-2 and described in Box 4-1 is recommended for health care professionals to ensure that appropriate steps have been taken to protect them and their clients.

For Your Information

In 1843, Semmelweis, a Hungarian physician, reintroduced handwashing between patients to prevent the spread of disease.

BOX 4-2

Rules of Sanitation for Massage Therapists

1. Using an approved handwashing procedure, wash and dry your hands thoroughly before and after performing massage therapy. One example is provided in Box 4-1.
2. Use only clean linens for each massage session and launder all massage linens (i.e., sheets, towels, bolster covers, and face rest covers) after each session. If blood or tissue fluid seepage is evident from any superficial wounds, remove the linens with gloved hands. According to the CDC, machine wash and dry contaminated linens separately in hot water, using laundry detergent and ¼ cup chlorine bleach. Once contaminated linens have been removed from the massage table, clean the table with a solution of water and chlorine bleach in a 10:1 solution. Finally, wash your hands.
3. Wear a clean uniform each day. Avoid contact between used linens and your uniform. If your uniform becomes contaminated with body fluids or secretions, machine wash and dry clothing separately in hot water, detergent, and ¼ cup chlorine bleach.
4. To prevent lubricant contamination, use only closed dispenser-type containers. Jar containers run the risk of cross-contamination because the therapist must remove the lubricant from the jar, place it on the client's skin, and reach back into the jar for additional lubricant after touching the client. The lubricant in the container is then used for another massage. **Cross-contamination** (the passing of microorganisms from one person to another) can occur if the lubricant becomes contaminated. If a jar container is used, use a clean spatula or tongue depressor and remove enough lubricant for single-client use, placing it on a disposable palette or in a separate sanitary container.
5. Disposable gloves are to be worn anytime the therapist has a cut or open wound on the hands, when handling contaminated linens, or cleaning massage equipment that contains body fluids. A finger cot may be used over a bandage to keep the edges smooth or in place of a glove if the area of broken skin is relegated to only one finger.
6. Provide an operative toilet and lavatory with hot and cold running water in a private restroom setting. Each restroom shall be equipped with toilet tissue, soap dispenser with soap or other hand-cleaning material, sanitary towels or other hand-drying device such as a wall-mounted electric hand drier, and waste receptacle. Massage establishments located in buildings housing multiple businesses under one roof such as a shopping mall or in hotels may substitute a centralized restroom. Facilities and fixtures shall be kept clean, well lit, and adequately ventilated to remove offensive odors.
7. Maintain clean shower facilities and other equipment used to enhance the massage or for client use, such as a whirlpool bath, sauna, steam cabinet, or steam room.
8. Do not perform massage therapy while you are ill or have coldlike symptoms such as sneezing, coughing, fever, or a runny nose. In these cases, it is preferred to cancel your clients or arrange for an associate to substitute, rather than to wear a surgical mask to prevent the spread of airborne pathogenic microorganisms.
9. Avoid massaging clients who are ill.
10. Remove all trash from the premises daily.
11. Exterminate all insects, termites, and rodents on the premises and maintain a pest-free facility.

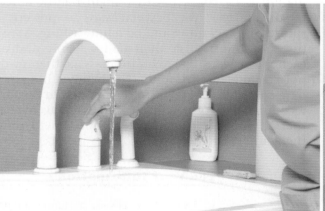
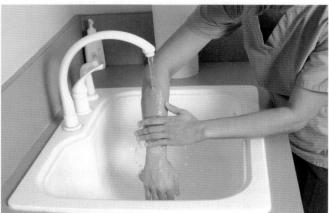

A **B**

Figure 4-2 **A,** Turning on the water; **B,** wetting hands, forearms, and elbows.

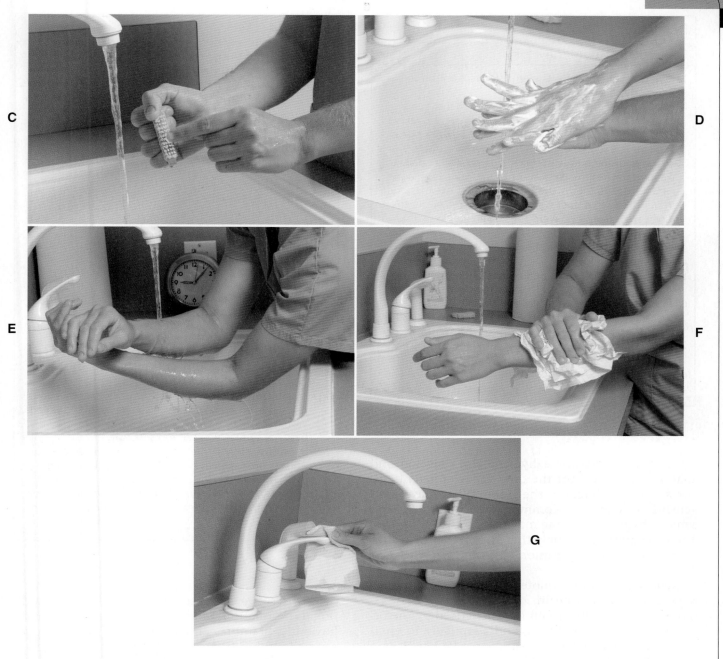

Figure 4-2—cont'd   C, cleaning underneath fingernails; **D,** soaping the hands; **E,** rinsing; **F,** drying the hands; **G,** turning off the water.

HYGIENE AND HEALTH FOR THE MASSAGE THERAPIST

Hygiene is defined as the collective principles of health preservation. In states requiring licensure of massage therapists, good grooming and hygiene are required by law. This is because proper hygiene habits not only preserve health but also help protect the public from the transmission of microorganisms. A list of tips has been compiled to aid you in practicing a recommended hygiene regimen (Box 4-3).

These hygiene tips will enable you to be more effective health care providers. As such, you are making the statement that you care about health—that is, your health and the health of your clients.

BOX 4-3

Professional Hygiene Tips

1. Bathe or shower daily. Use an antiperspirant or deodorant if necessary.
2. Wash your hair often. Choose a hairstyle that keeps hair out of your way during a massage; secure hair so that it does not touch the client. Because of its porosity, hair is a source of harmful microorganisms.
3. Brush your teeth at least twice a day and floss daily to keep gums healthy. Regular brushing removes plaque and reduces the growth of bacteria. Because massage requires close contact with clients, you may elect to use a mouthwash or avoid food that can cause an offensive odor on workdays.
4. Shave often or keep facial hair neat, trimmed, and well groomed.
5. Keep nails clean, short, and neatly trimmed. Long nails can injure the client and hide bacteria.
6. If you perspire heavily while performing a massage, wear sweatbands at the wrists and forehead to ensure that perspiration does not drip onto the client's skin.
7. Avoid perfumes, colognes, or scented lotions. Respect the client's allergies and hypersensitivities.
8. Wash your hands thoroughly after using the toilet and before and after each massage session.

BOX 4-4

Health Tips to Keep Fit for Massage and Model a Healthy Lifestyle

1. Exercise at least three times a week for 30 minutes for cardiovascular fitness.
2. Lift weights three times a week (see a fitness trainer for personal program).
3. Stretch or practice yoga to keep yourself flexible.
4. Drink water daily—at least $1/2$ ounce per 1 pound of body weight per day.
5. Eat low-fat, high-fiber foods and maintain a balanced diet for your energy needs.
6. Limit your intake of salt, sugar, caffeine, and alcohol.
7. Avoid all forms of tobacco use.
8. Schedule "stress breaks" of at least 15 minutes to relax, especially on crowded days. Breathe slowly and deeply while allowing your body and mind to rest in a comfortable position. Start the day with morning meditation or "quiet time" to avoid a stressful day.
9. Remember to schedule regular massage therapy for yourself.
10. Honor your emotions by expressing them appropriately. Keep a journal, see a counselor, or join a support group.
11. Laugh. Surround yourself with positive, happy people. Go to a comedy club. Tell stories with old friends. Watch a Monty Python or Marx Brothers movie. It is best not to take yourself too seriously.
12. Stimulate yourself intellectually, spiritually, and emotionally on a regular basis. Go to art galleries, museums, worship services, and concerts. Read a book, write poetry, or see a foreign film. Talk about religion and politics with someone who has differing philosophies.

As you observe these hygiene tips, develop and maintain a respect for the diversity of different cultures found throughout the globe. What may be offensive to some are commonplace to others, and what is hygienic to some may be offensive to others. Each therapist must apply these tips to her own situation with her own common sense and knowledge of local customs.

René Dubos, often quoted in nursing education, says, "The states of health or disease are the expressions of the success or failure experienced by the organism in its efforts to respond adaptively to environmental challenges." In other words, health is a reflection of how well our bodies adapt to our environment. Health can be broken down into three primary elements—*nutrition, exercise,* and *relaxation.* The health tips described in Box 4-4 touch on all three elements. Each day, the massage therapist takes time to attend to himself or herself with health-promoting activities; you and your clients will reap the benefits.

The simple fact is that we cannot give away what we do not have. The best gift we can give to our clients is by giving to ourselves first. *Charity begins at home* means that self-care is not being "selfish" but being self-nurturing in a way that allows us to pass along our gifts to others. The health tips described in Box 4-4 can be used to achieve good health in our own lives so we can become better care givers. Additional information on activities to increase strength, flexibility, stamina, and hand-developing exercises can be found in Chapter 6.

SAFETY PROCEDURES FOR THE MASSAGE THERAPIST

Safety procedures provide an environment that is hazard free and barrier free. Safety has two aspects for the massage therapist: (1) safety of the physical space or massage facility and (2) safety of the procedure itself. A safe facility is accessible to all patrons, even the elderly or those who are physically challenged. For the massage therapist to provide a safe procedure, knowledge of endangerment sites, human physiology and pathophysiology, first aid, artificial respiration, and cardiopulmonary resuscitation (CPR) must be

BOX 4-5

Rules for Facility and Procedural Safety

Facility Safety

1. Comply with all state and municipal building fire and safety codes.
2. Establish and maintain current liability insurance coverage. The original or copy of this policy must be kept on the premises at all times and be available for inspection.
3. Maintain an operative fire extinguisher and heat or smoke detectors on the premises. Fire extinguishers must be located at eye level and in clear view (ratings specified by the city ordinance).
4. Have a fire escape route posted in the office and clearly mark all building exits.
5. Provide safe and unobstructed human passage in the public areas. Safe passage includes level flooring. Omit area rugs because they can be a slipping or tripping hazard.
6. Choose only nonslip flooring, especially in bathrooms and wet areas.
7. Bathrooms should be accessible to the physically challenged and should include a wheelchair-height lavatory with lever-style faucets. Grab bars should be located near the toilet for clients who need assistance transferring to and from the toilet seat.
8. Lever-style door handles are required for physically challenged people.
9. Have a designated handicap-accessible parking space. Slopes, not steps, between the parking space and the building, should be available for use. The space should be marked with the international symbol for accessibility. Exterior ramps should be designed so that they drain easily and do not hold water.
10. Public telephones should have an adjustable volume control.
11. Maintain a list of all emergency phone numbers by the telephone: the local fire station, police department, sheriff's department, local hospital, and ambulance.
12. The street address should be outside the building in clear view. This will make it easier for emergency assistance to locate your business.
13. Maintain all equipment used to perform massage services in safe condition. This includes checking and tightening your massage table hinges, knobs, and locks on your massage table and other equipment before each business day.

Procedural Safety

1. Obtain and maintain training or certification for first aid and CPR.
2. Keep a first-aid kit on the premises in a location known by all personnel.
3. After each massage, wipe the client's feet to remove the massage lubricant with a paper towel to decrease the likelihood of the client falling. You may wish to spray isopropyl alcohol on the client's feet and wipe it off with a paper towel to more effectively remove the lubricant. However, do not use alcohol on client's feet if the skin is broken or if athlete's foot is present.
4. Be able to identify endangerment sites and contraindications of massage therapy. Use this information in your massage therapy practice (see Chapter 5).
5. Do not perform massage therapy under the influence of alcohol or other recreational drugs.

included in massage training. Skill training and knowledge of the human body helps ensure that the massage therapist is safe and competent.

The safety rules described in Box 4-5 will assist you in providing a safe, barrier-free environment for the practice of massage therapy. Once these safety rules have been followed, you and your client may proceed with the massage therapy. Check with state and local officials to be certain that you are within the standards set forth by these legal systems.

SUMMARY

As health care professionals, we seek to improve the health and well-being of our clients through massage therapy and to ensure that no accidental injuries nor transmission of disease in our offices from client to client or from therapist to client occur. Protecting the client has many facets, some of which include understanding basic pathophysiology, practicing proper health and hygiene, and meeting safety standards for the massage facility.

Pathophysiology includes knowing causative agents of disease: bacteria, fungi, protozoa, and viruses. The six types of disease are infectious, deficiency, metabolic, genetic, cancerous, and autoimmune. Infectious diseases are directly related to pathogens, which can be transmitted through several different modes. Disease can be prevented by interrupting these modes of transmission. Transmission interruption is accomplished by following the basic rules of health, hygiene, safety, and sanitation, including handwashing, and using gloves. Additional responsibilities are to provide equal access to your business and to prevent accidental injury to your clients by compliance with local building safety codes. The goal of health, hygiene, sanitation, and safety standards is to protect the client and the therapist by causing no harm.

MATCHING

Write the letter of the best answer in the space provided.

A. Infectious disease
B. Universal precautions
C. Cancerous disease
D. Carcinogen

E. Sanitation
F. Pathogen
G. Fomite
H. Cross-contamination

I. Handwashing
J. Hygiene
K. Disinfection
L. Autoimmune disease

_____ 1. Disease marked by an inappropriate or excessive response of the body's immune functions

_____ 2. A biological agent capable of causing disease

_____ 3. Removal of pathogens from surfaces by a chemical and/or mechanical agent

_____ 4. Disease characterized by uncontrollable growth and metastasis of abnormal cells

_____ 5. An inanimate object

_____ 6. Passing of microorganisms from one person to another

_____ 7. Highly contagious disease caused by a biological agent

_____ 8. The application of measures to promote a healthful, disease-free environment

_____ 9. Cancer-causing agent

_____ 10. The best thing a massage therapist can do to control transmission of diseases

_____ 11. Established by the Centers for Disease Control and Prevention to reduce the transmission of communicable diseases

_____ 12. Collective principles of health preservation

Bibliography

Applegate EJ: *The anatomy and physiology learning system,* ed 2, Philadelphia, 2000, WB Saunders.

Damjanov I: *Pathophysiology for the health-related professions,* Philadelphia, 1996, WB Saunders.

Frazier MS, Drzymkowski JW: *Essentials of human diseases and conditions,* ed 2, Philadelphia, 2000, WB Saunders.

Gould BE: *Pathophysiology for the health-related professionals,* Philadelphia, 1997, WB Saunders.

Jacob S, Francone C: *Elements of anatomy and physiology,* Philadelphia, 1989, WB Saunders.

Larson E, Mayur T, Laughon BA: Influence of two hand washing frequencies on reduction in colonizing flora with three products used by health care personnel, *Am J Infect Control* 23:17, 1989.

Louisiana State Department of Social Services: *Uniform federal accessibility standards accessibility checklist,* Baton Rouge, La, 1995, United States Architectural and Transportation Barriers Compliance Board.

Ogg S: Personal communication, Lafayette, La, 1997, Lafayette General Hospital.

Thibodeau G, Patton K: *Structure and function of the body,* ed 11, St Louis, 2000, Mosby.

Torres LS: *Basic medical techniques and patient care for radiologic technologies,* Philadelphia, 1993, JB Lippincott.

Tortora GJ: *Introduction to the human body: the essentials of anatomy and physiology,* ed 3, New York, 1994, Harper-Collins.

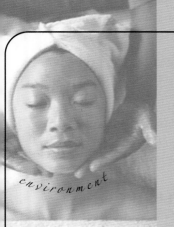

Massage Physiology: Effects, Indications, Contraindications, and Endangerment Sites

5

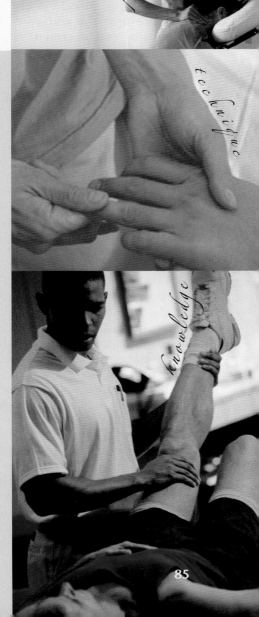

"He who feels it knows it more."

—Bob Marley

STUDENT **OBJECTIVES**

After completing this chapter, the student should be able to:

- Compare mechanical and reflexive responses of massage
- Discuss the effects of massage in various body systems and body tissues
- Using the gate theory, discuss how massage relieves pain
- Identify indications for massage therapy
- Identify local and absolute contraindications of massage therapy
- Recognize and modify treatment over endangerment sites

INTRODUCTION

Massage is a very popular form of therapy. In the United States alone, almost 50% of adults used at least one form of alternative/complementary therapy in 1997 and the popularity continues to increase. Most people visit massage therapists for **chronic** conditions such as back pain, anxiety, depression, and headaches. Current research helps us to understand how massage benefits clients and to identify conditions improved with massage.

Although massage is effective for many bodily ailments, a few conditions are evident for which massage is *contraindicated*. If massage therapy is to be administered safely, the prudent professional will screen clients for these conditions.

Various anatomical landmarks are also evident for which caution is recommended or where pressure should be avoided. These topographical regions known as *endangerment sites,* are regions in the body where nerves, blood vessels, and other fragile structures lie near the surface of the skin. Locations of the major endangerment sites are included in this chapter.

HOW SAFE IS MASSAGE?

Most massage therapists must go to school and become licensed before starting a practice and seeing clients. Much of class hours are devoted to learning massage strokes, routines, and how to design a treatment plan. Many hours are also spent learning anatomy, physiology, and pathology, with special emphasis on musculoskeletal systems. Anatomical, physiological, and pathological knowledge is essential to understanding effects and contraindications and locating endangerment sites. Ultimately, you will be expected to conduct a client intake, perform a massage treatment that will address the client's needs, and "do no harm."

But how safe is massage? Can a client become injured? Massage is one of the safest modalities of complimentary medicine and physical therapy. Although it is possible for a client to become injured, it is highly improbable when a therapist respects boundaries, contraindications, endangerment sites, and client's request regarding pressure. In an article published in the *Journal of the American Medical Association,* liability claims against massage therapists were compiled and analyzed. The percentage of claims filed against massage therapists was less than one tenth of 1% (1990-1996). Most claims were related to minor injures such as bruising and other soft-tissue damage. A significant portion of claims filed were related to sexual misconduct. Because 500 hours represents the national average of training required in the current 27 states that mandate massage, the low rate of filed claims clearly indicate that these 500 hours are adequate to train a safe, competent massage therapist. Areas of specialization are available for additional training.

MECHANICAL AND REFLEXIVE RESPONSES TO MASSAGE

The body responds to pressure in one of two ways. One is a *mechanical response,* and the other is a *reflexive response.* A **mechanical response** occurs as a result of pressure, force, or range of motion. Tissues are pulled, lifted, rubbed, compressed, and manipulated. Examples of the mechanical responses of pressure are increased blood circulation, reduced swelling, and the reduced formation of scar tissue.

To create a **reflexive response** in the body, nerves are stimulated which in turn, activate a reflex arc. Examples of reflexive responses are decreased arousal of the sympathetic nervous system (general relaxation), triggering of stretch receptors (e.g., muscle spindles), increased diameter of blood vessels, and reduced blood pressure. Massage responses can be primarily mechanical or reflexive in nature, but both responses are closely related and often occur simultaneously.

EFFECTS OF MASSAGE

Both mechanical and reflexive responses are linked to massage techniques that deliver moderate to deep pressure, which stimulate pressure receptors. This type of massage is often referred to as *Swedish massage* or *therapeutic massage.* Some of the benefits outlined in this chapter are related to touch, but most are linked to Swedish massage. One study in particular implemented deep Swedish massage or deep tissue massage. In this study, massage using light pressure generally produced adverse results. In fact, it was criticized because it stated that massage did not have any effect on circulation but, after closer examination, it was discovered that only light pressure was used for the experimental (massaged) group.

In a study conducted by Cherkin et al, speculation was offered to explain why massage was effective in the treatment of low back pain. As you would expect, effects on soft tissues were noted. Other factors attributed to massage effectiveness were the client spending 1 hour in a relaxed environment, receiving ongoing attention from the therapist, being touched in a therapeutic context, and increased body awareness during and after the massage. Education about exercise and other positive lifestyle changes was another benefit clients received as part of their massage.

Do the effects of massage last? Most benefits cease shortly after the massage treatments are terminated, but this is also true of other health-related treatments such as diet, exercise, and meditation. The key to long-term effects is the education clients receive concerning lifestyle habits and changes. These changes can be a more healthy diet, frequent walks, and increased fluid intake. Clients are also taught other methods of self-care such as how to breathe for relaxation, a basic self-massage routine, or the stretching of muscle groups. Massage does have long-lasting effects on some specific injuries or pathologies. These effects include reducing scar tissue formation, decreasing edema, loosening lung phlegm, and relieving constipation. Chronic conditions often require ongoing massage treatments.

Massage therapy and the response it creates within the body can affect the cardiovascular system, lymphatic/immune systems, skin and related structures, nervous and endocrine systems, muscles, connective tissues, respiratory system, digestive system, and urinary system. Also noted are miscellaneous effects and indications for specific conditions and individuals. Although most claims made about the benefits of massage therapy are the result of scientific experiments, a few are from empirical clinical observations and speculation based on physiological principles. By examining the effects of massage on each body system, we can understand the scientific application of massage therapy and how it benefits clients.

Effects of Massage on the Cardiovascular System

- **Dilates blood vessels.** The body responds to massage by reflexively dilating the blood vessels. This, in turn, aids in improving blood circulation and lowering blood pressure (see the following).
- **Improves blood circulation.** Deep stroking improves blood circulation by mechanically assisting venous blood flow back to the heart. The increase of blood flow is comparable to that of exercise. It has been documented that during a massage local circulation increases up to 3 times more than circulation at rest.
- **Decreases blood pressure.** Blood pressure is decreased by dilation of blood vessels. Both diastolic and systolic readings decline and last approximately 40 minutes after the massage session.
- **Creates hyperemia.** Increased blood flow creates a hyperemic effect, which is often visible on the surface of the skin.

- **Stimulates release of acetylcholine and histamine for sustained vasodilation.** These two substances are released due to vasomotor activity, helping prolong vasodilation.
- **Replenishes nutritive materials.** Another benefit of increased circulation, products such as nutrients and oxygen are transported to the cells and tissues more efficiently.
- **Promotes rapid removal of waste products.** Not only are nutrients brought to cells and to tissues, but metabolic waste products are removed more rapidly through massage. It is often said that massage "dilutes the poisons."
- **Reduces ischemia.** Massage reduces ischemia and ischemic-related pain. Ischemia is also related to trigger point formation and associated pain referral patterns.
- **Reduces heart rate.** Massage decreases heart rate through activation of the relaxation response.
- **Lowers pulse rate.** As one would expect, a reduced heart rate would lower the pulse rate.
- **Increases stroke volume.** Stroke volume is the amount of blood ejected from the left ventricle during each contraction. As the heart rate decreases, more time is available for the cardiac ventricles to fill with blood. The result is a larger volume of blood pushed through the heart with each ventricular contraction, thereby increasing stroke volume.
- **Increases red blood cell (RBC) count.** The number of functioning RBCs and their oxygen-carrying capacity are increased. It is speculated that this effect is achieved by (1) promoting the spleen's discharge of RBCs; (2) recruiting excess blood from engorged internal organs into general circulation; (3) stimulating stagnant capillary beds and returning this blood into general circulation. All three events increase RBC count.
- **Increases oxygen saturation in blood.** When RBC count rises, a greater oxygen saturation occurs in the blood.
- **Increases white blood cell (WBC) count.** The presence of WBCs increases after massage. The body may perceive massage as a mild stressor (an event to which the body must adapt) and recruits additional WBCs. The increase in WBC count enables the body to more effectively protect itself against disease.
- **Enhances the adhesion of migrating WBCs.** The surfaces of WBCs become more "sticky" following a massage, increasing their adhesive quality and therefore their effectiveness.
- **Increases platelet count.** Gentle but firm massage strokes increase the number of platelets in the blood.

MINI-LAB

You have two uninflated balloons—a small one and another twice the size of your first. Place a cup of water in each balloon. Which balloon has the lesser amount of pressure, the smaller or the larger? The larger one has the lesser pressure. This illustrates how massage can lower blood pressure through reflex action and increasing the parasympathetic response. By increasing the diameter of the vessel, the pressure inside the vessel decreases (Figure 5-1).

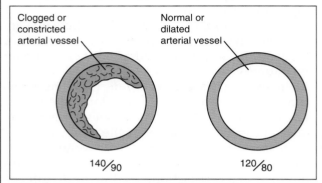

Figure 5-1   Blood pressure and blood vessel diameter.

Effects of Massage on the Lymphatic/Immune Systems

- **Promotes lymph circulation.** Lymph is a fluid that moves slowly within its own system of vessels. Lymphatic circulation depends entirely on pressure: from muscle contraction, pressure changes in the thorax and abdomen during breathing, or applied pressure from a massage.
- **Reduces lymphedema.** Massage reduces lymphedema (swelling) by promoting lymph circulation, which helps remove waste from the system more effectively than either passive range of motion or electrical muscle stimulation.
- **Decreases the circumference of an area affected with lymphedema.** When an area swells, the diameter increases. When the swelling subsides, circumference decreases.
- **Decreases weight in patients with lymphedema.** Fluid retention adds weight to a patient. When lymphedema is addressed with massage, weight is consequently reduced.
- **Increases lymphocyte count.** Lymphocytes are types of WBCs. This effect indicates that massage supports immune functions.
- **Increases the number and function (or cytotoxicity) of natural killer cells.** Natural killer cells are also types of WBCs. This further suggests that massage strengthens immune functions and might help individuals with immune disorders.

Effects of Massage on the Skin and Related Structures

- **Increases skin temperature.** Warming of the skin indicates a reduction of stress and other benefits outlined below.
- **Improves skin condition.** As superficial blood vessels dilate and circulation increases, the skin appears hyperemic. This brings added nutrients to the skin, improving the skin's condition, texture, and tone. Clinical observations have determined that massage also improves the appearance (i.e., color and texture) of the skin.
- **Stimulates sebaceous glands.** Stimulation of the sebaceous (oil) glands causes an increase in sebum production. This added sebum improves the skin's condition and reduces skin dryness.
- **Stimulates sudoriferous glands.** Sudoriferous (sweat) gland stimulation increases insensible perspiration. Insensible perspiration is the constant evaporative cooling that occurs as microscopic beads of perspiration evaporate from the skin's surface.
- **Improves skin pathologies.** Unless a condition contraindicates massage, skin pathologies may improve by decreasing redness, reducing thickening/hardening of the skin, increasing healing of skin abrasions, and reducing itching.
- **Reduces superficial keloid formation.** Massage applied to scar tissue helps reduce the formation of superficial keloids in the skin and excessive scar formation in the soft tissues beneath the site of massage application.

Effects of Massage on the Nervous and Endocrine Systems

- **Reduces stress.** Stress is reduced by activation of the parasympathetic nervous system.
- **Reduces anxiety.** Interestingly, a reduction in anxiety is noted in both the person who received the massage and the person who gave the massage.
- **Promotes relaxation.** General relaxation is promoted through activation of the relaxation response. Relaxation also has a diminishing effect on pain.
- **Decreases beta wave activity.** Associated with relaxation, a decrease in beta brainwave activity occurred during and after the massage (confirmed by electroencephalogram [EEG]).
- **Increases delta wave activity.** Increases in delta brainwave activity are linked to sleep and to relaxation; both are promoted with massage (confirmed by EEG).
- **Increase in alpha waves.** An increase in alpha brainwave during massage indicates relaxation (confirmed by EEG).

- **Increases dopamine levels.** Increased levels of dopamine are linked to decreased stress levels and reduced depression.
- **Increases serotonin levels.** Increased levels of serotonin suggest a reduction of both stress and depression. It is believed that serotonin inhibits transmission of noxious signals to the brain, indicating that increased levels of serotonin may also reduce pain.
- **Reduces cortisol levels.** Massage reduces cortisol levels by activating the relaxation response. Elevated levels of cortisol not only represent heightened stress but also inhibit immune functions.
- **Reduces norepinephrine levels.** Massage has been proven to reduce norepinephrine, a stress hormone; reduced norepinephrine levels are linked to the relaxation response.
- **Reduces epinephrine levels.** Epinephrine, another stress hormone, is reduced with massage.
- **Reduces feelings of depression.** Both chemical and electrophysiological changes from a negative to a positive mood were noted and may underline the decrease in depression after massage therapy.
- **Decreases pain.** Massage relieves local and referred pain caused by hypersensitive trigger points, presumably by increasing circulation, thereby reducing ischemia. Massage also stimulates the release of endorphins (endogenous morphine), enkephalins, and other pain-reducing neurochemicals. General relaxation brought on by massage therapy also has a diminishing effect on pain. The pressure of a massage interferes with pain information entering the spinal cord by stimulating pressure receptors, further reducing pain (gate theory, Figure 5-2). Massage interrupts the pain cycle by relieving muscular spasms, increasing circulation, and promoting rapid disposal of waste products (Figure 5-3). Massage also improves sleep patterns. During deep sleep, a substance called somatostatin is normally released. Without this substance, pain is experienced.
- **Reduces analgesic use.** Because pain is reduced with massage, so is the need for excessive use of pain medication.
- **Activates sensory receptors.** Depending on factors such as stroke choice, direction, speed, and pressure, massage can stimulate different sensory receptors, affecting the massage outcome. For example, cross-fiber tapotement stimulates muscle spindles, which activates muscular contraction, while a slow passive stretch and deep effleurage activate Golgi tendon organs, which inhibits muscular contraction. Activation of sensory pressure receptors reduces pain (see Figure 5-2).
- **Faster and more elaborate development of the hippocampal region of the brain.** Part of the limbic system, development of the hippocampal region is related to superior memory performance.
- **Increases vagal activity.** Increased activity of the vagal nerve lowers physiological arousal and stress hormones. A decrease in stress hormones leads to enhanced immune functions. One of the branches

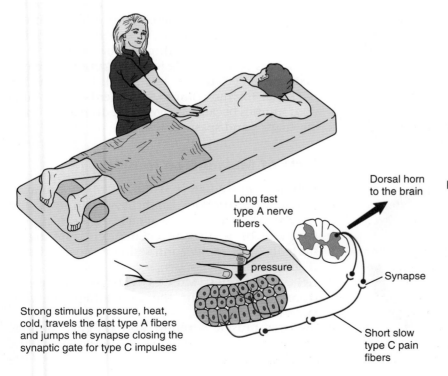

Strong stimulus pressure, heat, cold, travels the fast type A fibers and jumps the synapse closing the synaptic gate for type C impulses

Long fast type A nerve fibers

pressure

Dorsal horn to the brain

Synapse

Short slow type C pain fibers

Figure 5-2 The gate theory.

The Gate Theory

In 1965, Wall and Melzack postulated the gate theory of pain relief, which explains why massage, ice, and heat are effective in the treatment of pain. The *gate theory* refers to the exclusion of certain nerve impulses when multiple impulses are competing for the same synaptic "gate" or entry into the central nervous system. To understand this, we will examine the two types of nerve fibers: Type A and Type C.

The sensory transmitters for pressure, temperature, and sharp acute pain lie close together in large concentrations near the body's surface. These sensory nerve pathways are composed of long, fast type A nerve fibers, which are important for protecting the body from external harm. Strong stimuli to these surface transmitters generate a quick sensory input to the cord segment, where a reflex-motor impulse is generated to move the affected body part out of harm's way. Touching a needle or a hot pan elicits this type of immediate reflex response.

The sensory transmitters for deep aching pain such as myofascial pain originate in the deeper tissues. These nerve pathways are composed of short, slow type C nerve fibers, which tend to transmit pain that has been present for some time and requires no immediate protective action (i.e., headache or muscular pain). These nerves transmit stimuli that are of lesser importance and lesser consequence to the body. The purpose of type C nerve pathways is to make the conscious mind aware that a problem exists, which can be used to prevent overuse or dependence on an injured body part.

Suppose that an Olympic gymnast is having her performance compromised by pain in her right Achilles tendon. This pain originates from the deeper, slower type C nerve network. When a pressure stimulus such as massage is applied to the calf, the new sensory input travels along the faster, longer type A nerve network and bridges the synaptic gap ahead of the type C sensory input. The synaptic gate is closed, thus excluding the pain information from entry to the spinal cord. The body experiences the pressure of the massage stroke as interruption of pain (see Figure 5-2).

Massage therapists can use the gate mechanism a number of ways including in the application of cold, heat, pressure, vibration, percussion, and superficial rubbing or light stimulation of cutaneous tissue. Any of these applications has the potential to interfere or interrupt pain signals.

For Your Information

The pain-cycle is initiated when painful stimuli result in reflex muscle contraction and localized muscle splinting or guarding. The localized muscle guarding restricts movement and decreases local circulation, which restricts the amount of oxygen available to the tissues and the removal of metabolic wastes. The subsequent swelling creates more pain. From this point, muscle splinting is intensified and the cycle repeats itself. A more generalized secondary pain results that outlasts or exceeds the original discomfort. Massage interrupts the pain cycle on all levels.

of the vagus nerve is known as the "smart branch." Stimulation of this nerve branch increases facial expression and vocalization, which reduces feelings of depression.

- **Right frontal EEG activation shifted to left frontal EEG activation.** Right frontal EEG activation is associated with a sad affect and left frontal EEG activation is associated with a happy affect. This implies that the client experienced an improvement of mood during the massage.
- **Decreases H-amplitude levels during massage.** A decrease of 60% to 80% was noted. This reduction is crucial for the comfort of patients with spinal cord injuries because it signifies a decrease of muscle cramps and spasm activity.

Effects of Massage on Muscles

- **Relieves muscular tension.** Massage relieves muscular restrictions, tightness, stiffness, and spasms. These effects are achieved by direct pressure and by increasing circulation, resulting in more flexible, supple, and resilient muscle tissues (Figure 5-4).
- **Relaxes muscles.** Muscles relax as massage reduces excitability in the sympathetic nervous system.
- **Reduces muscle soreness and fatigue.** Massage enhances blood circulation, thus increasing the amount of oxygen and nutrients available to the

THE PAIN CYCLE

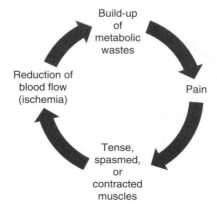

Figure 5-3 Massage interrupts the pain cycle.

muscles. Increased oxygen and nutrients reduce muscle fatigue and postexercise soreness. Massage promotes rapid disposal of waste products, further reducing muscle fatigue and soreness (see Figure 5-3). A fatigued muscle recuperates 20% after 5 minutes of rest and 100% after 5 minutes of massage. A reduction in postexercise recovery time was indicated by a decline in pulse rate and an increase muscle "work" capacity.

- **Reduces trigger point formation.** Trigger point formation is greatly reduced by the pressure applied during a massage, affecting trigger points in both muscle and fascia.
- **Manually separates muscle fibers.** Compressive strokes and cross-fiber friction strokes separate muscle fibers, reducing muscle spasms.
- **Increases range of motion.** When muscular tension is reduced, range of motion is improved. The freedom of the joints is dictated by the freedom of the muscles.
- **Improves performance (balance and posture).** Many postural distortions are removed when trigger points are released and when muscle tension is reduced. Range of motion increases, gait becomes more efficient, the posture is more aligned and balanced, and improved performance is the net result.
- **Improves motor skills.** Not surprisingly, if a massage was found to improve performance, balance, and posture, motor skills are also enhanced.
- **Lengthens muscles.** Massage mechanically stretches and broadens tissue, especially when combined with Swedish gymnastics (joint mobilization and stretches). These changes are detected by Golgi tendon organs, which inhibit contraction signals, further lengthening muscles. Massage retrains the tissue from a contracted state to an elongated state, increasing resting length. This is one of the principles behind neuromuscular reeducation.
- **Increases flexibility.** By lengthening muscles and promoting muscular relaxation, massage has also been shown to increase muscle flexibility.
- **Tones weak muscles.** Muscle spindle activity is increased during massage strokes (e.g., tapotement, vibration). An increase in muscle spindle activity creates muscle contractions, helping tone weak muscles. This effect is particularly beneficial in cases of prolonged bed rest, flaccidity, and atrophy.
- **Reduces creatine kinase activity in the blood.** Creatine kinase is an enzyme that helps ensure enough adenosine triphosphate (ATP) is available for muscle contraction. By reducing the activity of creatine kinase in the blood, massage indirectly helps decrease muscle contraction and therefore increase muscle relaxation.

- **Improves muscular nutrition.** As a result of an increase in blood-transported nutrients, massage improves muscular nutrition. This hastens muscle recovery and enables muscles to function at maximum capacity after recovery.
- **Decreases electromyography (EMG) readings.** This signifies a decrease in neuromuscular activity and reduction of neuromuscular complaints.

MINI-LAB

Sit in a chair with your feet flat on the floor. Moving only your head and neck, look over your left shoulder, and notice how far you can comfortably move. Do the same, looking to the right. Take your right hand and grab the top of your right shoulder. As you apply pressure, slowly move the shoulder up and down ten times. Maintain the pressure, and roll your shoulder back ten times, then forward ten times. Do this same movement with the left shoulder. Squeeze the back of your neck. Without releasing the pressure, turn your head (as if saying no), nod your head (as if saying yes), and circle your nose clockwise and counterclockwise 10 times each. After the "squeeze and move" activity, look over your right and left shoulders again. Notice how much farther you can go. This increase is the result of self-administered massage.

Effects of Massage on Connective Tissues

- **Reduces keloid formation.** Massage applied to scar tissue helps reduce keloid formation in scar tissue.
- **Reduces excessive scar formation.** Deep massage reduces excessive scar formation, helping create an appropriate scar that is strong yet does not interfere with the muscle's ability to broaden as it contracts.
- **Decreases adhesion formation.** The displacement of scar tissue during massage helps reduce formation of adhesions. This, in turn, facilitates normal, pain-free motion of the affected muscles and joints.
- **Releases fascial restrictions.** Pressure and the heat it produces converts fascia from a gel-state to a sol-state (thixotropy), reducing hyperplasia. Fascia loosens and melts, becoming more flexible and elastic. Softening of the fascia surrounding muscles allows them to be stretched to their fullest resting length, increasing joint range of motion, and freeing the body of restricted movements.
- **Increases mineral retention in bone.** Massage increases the retention of nutrients such as nitrogen, sulfur, and phosphorus in bones.
- **Promotes fracture healing.** When a bone is fractured, the body forms a network of new blood vessels at the break site. Massage increases circulation around the fracture, promoting fracture healing.

Increased circulation around a fracture leads to increased deposition of callus to the bone. Callus is formed between and around the broken ends of a fractured bone during healing, and is ultimately replaced by compact bone.

- **Improves connective tissue healing.** Occurring only with deep pressure massage, proliferation and activation of fibroblasts was noted. Fibroblasts generate connective tissue matrix, which promotes tissue healing by increasing collagen production and increasing the tensile strength of healed tissue.
- **Reduces surface dimpling of cellulite.** Massage flattens out adipose globules located under the skin and makes the skin seem smoother. Cellulite, a type of adipose tissue, appears as groups of small dimples or depressions under the skin, caused by an uneven separation of fat globules below the skin's surface, which are displaced by manual manipulation. Massage does not reduce the amount of cellulite below the skin; instead, it temporarily alters the shape and appearance of cellulite.

Effects of Massage on the Respiratory System

- **Reduces respiration rate.** Massage slows down the rate of respiration because of activation of the relaxation response.
- **Strengthens respiratory muscles.** The muscles of respiration have a greater capacity to contract, helping improve pulmonary functions.
- **Decreases the sensation of dyspnea.** Dyspnea is shortness of breath or difficult breathing, and is lessened as a result of massage.
- **Decreases asthma attacks.** Through increased relaxation and improved pulmonary functions, the client experiences fewer asthma attacks.
- **Reduces laryngeal tension.** Laryngeal tension may occur from excessive public speaking or singing. Massage reduces the stress on the larynx and tension on the muscles of the throat.
- **Increases fluid discharge from the lungs.** The mechanical loosening and discharge of phlegm in the respiratory tract increases with rhythmic alternating pressures. Tapotement (cupping) and vibration on the rib cage are often used to enhance this effect. Phlegm loosening and discharge is further enhanced when combined with postural drainage (promoting fluid drainage of the respiratory tract through certain body positions) and when the client is encouraged to cough.
- **Improves pulmonary functions.** Relaxation plays a big role in how massage improves pulmonary function, but massage also loosens tight respiratory muscles and fascia. The affected pulmonary functions are as follows:
  - **Increased vital capacity.** This is the amount of air that can be expelled at the normal rate of exhalation after a maximum inhalation, representing the greatest possible breathing capacity.
  - **Increased forced vital capacity.** This is the amount of air that can be forcibly expelled after a forced inhalation.
  - **Increased forced expiratory volume.** This is the volume of air that can be forcibly expelled after a full exhalation.
  - **Increased forced expiratory flow.** This is the volume of air that can be forcibly expelled after a full inhalation.
  - **Improved peak expiratory flow.** This is the greatest rate of airflow that can be achieved during forced expiration beginning with the lungs fully inflated.

Effects of Massage on the Digestive System

- **Promotes evacuation of the colon.** By increasing peristaltic activity in the colon through massage, bowel contents move toward the anus for elimination.
- **Relieves constipation.** Because evacuation of the colon is promoted, constipation is relieved.
- **Relieves colic and intestinal gas.** Increased peristaltic activity also helps relieve colic and the expulsion of intestinal gas.

Figure 5-4 Muscle tension's relationship to blood flow.

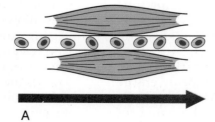

A

Capillaries running between two relaxed muscle fibers; round forms are red blood cells.

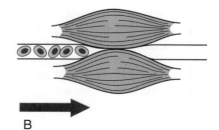

B

Capillary is compressed —squeezed— by the shortened thickened fibers of contracted muscle.

- **Stimulates digestion.** Massage also promotes activation of the parasympathetic nervous system, which stimulates digestion.

Effects of Massage on the Urinary System

- **Increases urine output.** Massage activates dormant capillary beds and recovers lymphatic fluids for filtration by the kidney. This in turn increases the frequency of urination and amount of urine produced. Massage is also relaxing. This promotes general homeostasis and increases urine output.
- **Promotes the excretion of nitrogen, inorganic phosphorus, and sodium chloride in urine.** Levels of these metabolic wastes are elevated in urine after massage.

Miscellaneous Effects of Massage

- **Reduces fatigue and increases vigor.** Many clients experienced a sense of renewed energy after massage by taking a break from the stresses of the day.
- **Improves sleep patterns.** When clients went to sleep, they reported a deeper sleep and felt more rested upon waking.
- **Reduces job related and posttraumatic stress.** Massage reduces many types of stress. In particular, job related stress and posttraumatic stress decreased after massage.
- **Improves mood.** The mental health status and mood improved in the subjects of the experimental (massaged) group.
- **Decreases feelings of anger.** Clients reported a decrease in aggression and feelings of anger with massage.
- **Improves body image.** Massage improved body image in clients who stated having a poor body image prior to the massage session.
- **Improves self-esteem.** Individuals who received and who gave massages reported enhanced self-esteem.
- **Promotes communication and expression.** Individuals who received and gave massages reported an increase in the quantity and quality of their social interactions. They talked more freely and openly and enjoyed themselves more during these social interactions. Massage can also assist the ease of emotional expression through relaxation.
- **Improves lifestyle habits.** Following massage, clients reported improved lifestyle habits such as increased activities of daily living (ADLs), fewer cups of coffee, fewer somatic symptoms, fewer doctor visits, and increased levels of exercising (walking).
- **Increases physical well being.** Massage enhances well-being through stress reduction and subsequent relaxation.

- **Reduces touch aversion and touch sensitivity.** Massage given to victims of rape and spousal abuse reported a reduction in touch aversion. Hypersensitivity to touch reduced in other individuals.
- **Increases academic performance.** A decrease in math computation time and an increase in math accuracy was noted in massage studies.
- **Increases mental alertness.** Massage increases mental alertness by relaxing the body/mind and by removing unwanted stress.
- **Satisfies emotional needs.** Clients reported using the therapeutic relationship to satisfy their emotional needs for attention, acceptance, caring, and nurturing touch, which were not being met through their other relationships.

 You can be born with a talent. But you have to acquire a craft to know how to use that talent.

—Sid Caesar

INDICATIONS OF MASSAGE FOR SPECIFIC CONDITIONS AND SPECIFIC INDIVIDUALS

Massage is a relatively low risk form of therapy. Massage is contraindicated for several conditions, and these are listed later in the chapter. In general, massage is beneficial for just about every other condition that does not fall into the contraindication category. It would be almost impossible to list all the conditions for which massage is in indicated. This section focuses on a few conditions that have been scientifically documented to benefit from massage. For further reading, please see the bibliography at the end of the chapter.

- **Alzheimer's disease.** Massage decreased physical expressions of agitation (i.e., pacing, wandering) and improved sleep patterns.
- **Anemia.** An increase in RBCs and an increase in oxygen saturation in the blood suggests that massage is beneficial for individuals with anemia.
- **Asthma.** It was found that massage improved pulmonary functions, and reduced the occurrence of asthma attacks.
- **Attention deficit hyperactivity disorder (ADHD).** Individuals diagnosed with ADHD who receive massage were observed to be less fidgety and hyperactive, and spent more time completing assigned tasks.
- **Autism.** Massaged autistic children spent less time in solitary play and had an increase in attention to sounds and their social relatedness to their teachers. Autistic behavior such as touch aversion was reduced.
- **Burn victims.** Burn victims who were massaged experienced a decrease in pain and itching and reduced anxiety before débridement. Massage also lowered feelings of depression and anger.

- **Cancer.** Lymphedema, pain, anxiety, and feelings of anger and depression were reduced when cancer patients had routine massages. Massage also increased lymphocyte and natural killer cell counts.
- **Cerebral palsy (CP).** Massage promotes circulation of blood and lymph and relieves muscular tension in individuals with CP. Increases in flexibility were also reported.
- **Chronic fatigue syndrome (CFS).** Clients with CFS experience reduced feelings of depression and anxiety and fewer somatic symptoms such as fatigue. CFS affects muscle strength; improved grip strength was also documented for clients receiving massages.
- **Constipation.** Elimination problems were relieved through massage.
- **Diabetes.** Blood glucose levels, anxiety, and depression were reduced with massage. An increase in dietary compliance was also reported.
- **Eating disorders.** Anorexia nervosa and bulimia nervosa patients stated a reduction of depression and anxiety. These individuals stated that they experienced an improvement in eating habits and an increase in positive body image with regular massage treatments.
- **Fibromyalgia.** Not only were stress, anxiety and feelings of depression reduced with massage, but decreases in pain, stiffness, fatigue, and insomnia were documented in individuals with fibromyalgia. Massage was rated more effective than standard physical therapy or prescriptive drugs.
- **Headaches.** Most headaches (muscular, cluster, eye strain, mental fatigue, sinus) were relieved with massage. Subjects also reported more headache-free days and less analgesic use as a result of pain reduction.
- **High blood pressure.** Massage decreased blood pressure (both systolic and diastolic readings) and helped promote healthy lifestyle habits in patients with hypertension.
- **Individuals infected with the human immunodeficiency virus (HIV).** The number of natural killer cells and their ability to fight pathogens increased after massage. Massage also helped individuals infected with HIV to relax.
- **Hospitalized and hospice patients.** Postoperative pain was reduced and patients had a decline in heart rate and blood pressure, indicating decreased stress and anxiety. Hospice patients experienced the same effects.
- **Infants.** Preterm, cocaine-exposed, HIV-exposed, and full-term infants experienced less colic, less repetitive crying, improved feeding habits, and gained more weight than nonmassaged infants in the same categories. Massage was found more effective than rocking for inducing infant sleep.
- **Injuries.** Massage speeds the healing of overuse injuries, sprains, and strains.
- **Insomnia.** Insomnia is alleviated by inducing relaxation.
- **Low back pain.** Low back pain is decreased by addressing trigger points. Medical costs were reduced by about 40% along with reduced analgesic use. Massage increased range of motion and promoted relaxation. Patients reported that massage made them feel cared for, happy, physically relaxed, less anxious, calm, restful, and gave them a feeling of closeness with the individuals who gave massages. Massage was rated more effective than standard physical therapy or prescriptive drugs.
- **Lung disease.** For clients with chronic obstructive pulmonary disease (COPD), massage strengthened respiratory muscles, reduced heart rate, increased oxygen saturation in blood, decreased shortness of breath, and improved pulmonary functions. Respiratory drainage is encouraged through cupping tapotement and vibration. Clients with cystic fibrosis further reported decreased anxiety and improved mood with massage treatments.
- **Lymphedema.** Swelling resulting from lymphedema was reduced with massage if it was not a result of inflammation or disease. Edema resulting from traumatic inflammation may be aided with techniques such as light centripetally applied effleurage.
- **Multiple sclerosis (MS).** Individuals with MS who received massages experienced reduced anxiety and depression, improved self-esteem and positive body image, and implemented changes to their lifestyle that promoted health such as exercising and stretching.
- **Nerve entrapment.** Conditions of nerve entrapment that occur when soft tissues constrict the nerve, such as carpal tunnel syndrome, thoracic outlet syndrome, and sciatica, were relieved by release of the myofascial component.
- **Poor circulation.** Massage improved blood circulation.
- **Pregnancy and postpartum.** Massaged pregnant women reported fewer obstetric and postpartum complications, reduced prematurity rates, shorter and less painful labors, and fewer days in hospital after labor and delivery. When nurses, midwives, or spouses massaged the pregnant or laboring women's perineal area, injury such as tearing during fetal delivery was reduced. Feelings of postpartum depression declined with massage. Depressed adolescent mothers reported less stress, anxiety, and depression. These were supported by a reduction of stress hormones in the blood.

JOHN F. BARNES, PT

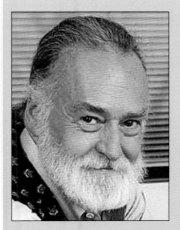

Born: February 3, 1939.

"The master therapist is real, calm, nonjudgmental, intelligent, sensitive, strong yet flexible, supportive, compassionate, empathic, and joyful."

One of the major differences between myofascial release and many other forms of bodywork is that, at its best, it allows the therapist to bring more to the table. It is systematic, physiologically grounded, and intuitive without apology. Its founder, John Barnes, is a physical therapist and teacher who values a wide range of modalities such as the work of Ida Rolf, Milton Trager, John Upledger, and Paul St. John.

Barnes's father died when he was 3, and he was raised by his mother. He remembers enjoying being alone in the forest and learning to be so quiet that the wildlife would venture out. He studied karate and, as a result, learned about the role of Qi. As a junior in high school, he knew he wanted to be a physical therapist.

With warm eyes, a burly build, and a full beard, he looks like the type to live in a log cabin and love nature—and he does. He's been called an old soul and doesn't scoff at the label. He doesn't believe in assembly-line quick fixes. How could he? He knows how insidious pain can be.

As a teen, Barnes was weightlifting and couldn't get out of a dead squat, so he turned a backflip and landed on his tailbone with an extra 300 pounds to boot. It wasn't long afterward that his back locked up just as he was about to kiss a girl he was crazy about. Nevertheless, he didn't pay much attention to his condition. He had youth on his side and charged on, until a skiing accident left him in worse condition. Surgery made a big difference, but the pain left an indelible scar.

Robert Calvert of *Massage Magazine* quotes Barnes as saying, "I don't really mean this should happen, but in a way, every physician or therapist should be severely injured, and not just hurt for a week or two or a month, but a couple years. It's a whole different story when you are a prisoner in your own body. I felt broken, and I was broken. It was a horrible, horrible experience."

Yet another injury led him to explore the advantage of alternative therapies that hadn't been offered in his traditional physical therapist training. He began to blend experience with principles from different disciplines and discovered how fascia and energy flow are connected. Basically, myofascial release is based on understanding the role of fascia, a web of interconnected tissue that travels the body without interruption. It surrounds individual cells, organs, systems, and then wraps it all up in one huge package, head to toe. This network also serves as the communication medium from cell to cell and organ to organ. Trauma, posture, or inflammation can change the consistency of the web, solidifying and shortening fibers and blocking the flow of messages that are necessary for homeostasis. This web, if pulled too tightly in one place, can leave other areas restricted, creating pressure on nerves, muscles, organs, and bones.

As a physical therapist, Barnes's style had always been focused, slow, and rhythmic. Sometimes his touch was light. Sometimes the tissue beneath his hands granted him deeper access. He didn't know he was practicing *myofascial release*, per se, until he attended a physicians' course on connective tissue. Afterward, he began to see and treat the interrelationship of the whole body (including the mind or spirit) rather than the isolated sore neck, bum knee, or other body part. This shift in thinking enhanced the results of his work, but stirred up emotions that demanded his attention. As his work evolved, so did Barnes. (The goal of myofascial release is not necessarily to incite emotional response, but considering the pervasive nature of myofascial system

Continued

JOHN F. BARNES, PT—cont'd

and the complex nature of humans, many forms of bodywork are considered and may eventually be proven to be therapeutic for emotional and physical trauma.)

Barnes started teaching others his form of bodywork in the mid-1970s. His task begins by reawakening the therapist's ability to "feel" what is happening with the body. Then he teaches the techniques to evaluate and release restricted areas in a systematic way. In his opinion, a comprehensive program should also include exercise and flexibility programs, movement awareness facilitation techniques, instruction in body mechanics, mobilization and muscle energy techniques, nutritional advice, biofeedback, and psychological counseling.

Even with such a systematic and comprehensive approach, Barnes is realistic about results. Therapists do not "fix" clients. We can offer tools for change not only in the form of bodywork but also in "mindwork." When it gets right down to the nitty gritty, we can't help our clients unless they are ready to help themselves. That's a humbling thought, yet being proficient and humble is a good starting point.

Barnes's advice for beginning massage therapists is to continue learning advanced methods after graduating from the typical 500-hour program. Just reading about a bodywork concept or simply being introduced to a modality isn't sufficient to practice it successfully and in some cases may lead to learning bad habits or faulty techniques. Barnes suggests learning as many forms of bodywork as possible in order to adapt to the wide range of client needs.

- **Premenstrual syndrome.** Massage reduced swelling, pain, and anxiety and improved the mood of women experiencing premenstrual syndrome.
- **Psychiatric patients.** Child, adolescent, and adult psychiatric patients were observed to be better adapted to a group and the medical staff reported better clinical progress with massage treatments. A decrease in depression and anxiety was noted with reduced cortisol levels and norepinephrine blood levels and increased in dopamine levels. In many individuals, a decreased self-destructive behavior was reported and the mental health status in the subjects of the massaged group. A decrease in the episodes of dysfunctional behavior was found in patients with dementia.
- **Rheumatoid arthritis (RA).** Massage reduced trigger point formation, pain, anxiety, and morning stiffness in individuals with adult and juvenile RA.
- **Skin conditions.** Skin problems such as mild dryness and itching were alleviated by massage because of the increase of sebum production and blood circulation.
- **Stress and anxiety.** Stress and anxiety are reduced by activation of the parasympathetic nervous system and promotion of the relaxation response.

- **Temporomandibular joint (TMJ) dysfunction.** The muscular component of TMJ dysfunction was addressed with massage and reduced pain and dysfunction was the result.

Once the benefits and indications of massage are known, an understanding of contraindications and endangerment sites becomes clear. For instance, by increasing lymph circulation, massage affects the tissue and fluids of the body; because massage increases the circulation of blood, thrombosis must be a contraindication.

CONTRAINDICATIONS FOR MASSAGE THERAPY

This section considers pathologies and symptoms that may contraindicate massage. The professional therapist exercises caution under certain conditions. During the intake process before treatment begins, the therapist conducts a consultation with the client to establish goals, note precautions, and determine any preexisting conditions that might affect treatment. It is the duty and obligation of the therapist to rule out the presence of any conditions in which massage may have harmful effects. However, if the client refuses to disclose his medical history, the therapist has the right to refuse treatment.

It is highly recommended that the massage therapist postpone treatment with anyone under the influence of prescription or over-the-counter (OTC) drugs that reduce pain, alcoholic beverages, or any other substance that would inhibit or distort the client's response or ability to give feedback regarding discomfort or pain during treatment.

The two categories of contraindications are *absolute* and *local*. Conditions in which massage is inappropriate, is not advised, and may be harmful to the client are known as **absolute contraindications**. It is rare that a physician would order massage under these conditions, but some exceptions occur. Note that absolute contraindications are typically contagious viral or bacterial pathologies or chronic aliments in which massage would better serve the client if the ailment were in remission. A physician's clearance is advised. Some of these conditions are so severe that the patient may be hospitalized.

A few contraindications for massage that have been followed by massage therapists for decades are controversial, such as varicose veins and cancer. Physician research refutes the need for contraindications of these two pathologies. No research currently links massage to increasing varicosities. In fact, massage helps empty veins, aiding circulation. No reported cases in which massage has worsened the status of cancer patients is evident. Research proves that massage decreases lymphedema, increases natural killer cell count, and promotes relaxation, which is important because stress impairs immune responses. More research is needed with regard to contraindications. A pathology book may need to be consulted because many conditions have both a common name, such as *boil,* and a medical name, such as *furuncle.*

Many pathologies are **local contraindications** in which massage can be administered while avoiding the infected area or area in question. These conditions or situations merit caution and adaptive measures to ensure that the massage is safely administered. Each situation must be assessed before a decision is made to either avoid the area or postpone the massage. If a mutual decision has been made to continue with the massage, the therapist should be fastidious about using a closed dispenser of lubricant to prevent cross contamination. Many pathologies listed below can be spread if they are accidentally touched during the massage. For additional information, see the pathology index in the appendix, the anatomy chapter of the system affected by the condition (chapters 12 through 15 and 17 through 22), or books and articles listed in the bibliography at the end of this chapter.

For many conditions massage is fine, but a physician must be consulted. Obtain the physician's "okay" and ask if there are any modifications that can be applied to the client's treatment. Much will depend on the client's vitality. Box 5-1 contains a list of pathologies grouped into three categories: conditions that require a physician's clearance before treatment, local contraindications, and absolute contraindications.

Some conditions just require adaptive measures to position the client comfortably, reduce pressure, shorten the length of treatment, or increase the frequency of treatments. Examples of adaptive massage are working with pregnant clients or with clients who are chronically ill. These and many other conditions requiring adaptive measures are presented in Chapter 9.

Exercise good judgment and use common sense when identifying these situations. After determining contraindications, you may decide to refer your client to his personal physician for further evaluation and treatment recommendations. As a rule, the therapist should be conservative. If any doubt about a specific condition or injury is evident, ask the client to obtain written medical clearance from his personal physician.

During the massage, monitor the client's response continuously. If the client reports that his pain has increased either during or after the massage session, modify or discontinue the massage treatments until further evaluation. If the client becomes ill or nauseated, discontinue treatment immediately.

 It is the heart that understands and the hand that soothes.

—Martha Rogers

ENDANGERMENT SITES

Endangerment sites are areas of the body that contain superficial delicate anatomical structures that are relatively unprotected and are therefore prone to injury. These sites merit caution during treatment. Often, the therapist simply adjusts pressure or avoids sustained pressure. Endangerment sites include such structures as nerves, blood vessels, organs, small or prominent bony projections, and any abnormalities such as cysts. These areas may be treated during a massage session, and often are, but caution must be exercised, working slowly, lightly, and carefully when in or around these sites. Exceptions to this rule would be energy work and techniques with which little or no pressure is used, such as therapeutic touch.

This section examines types of endangerment sites and why caution is warranted. In the next section,

BOX 5-1

Pathologies and Massage Contraindications

Conditions That Require Physician Clearance
- Acromegaly
- Aneurysm
- Atherosclerosis
- Burns
- Cancer
- Cerebrovascular accident
- Chronic obstructive pulmonary disease
- Congestive heart failure
- Coronary artery disease
- Hemophilia
- Hodgkin's disease
- Kidney stones
- Leukemia
- Myasthenia gravis
- Nephrosis
- Peritonitis
- Polycystic kidney disease
- Uremia

Conditions With Local Contraindications
- Abdominal diastasis (avoid abdomen)
- Abnormal lumps (avoid area)
- Acne vulgaris (avoid infected area)
- Athlete's foot (avoid infected area)
- Blister (avoid area)
- Bruise (avoid bruised area if less than 72 hours old)
- Carpal tunnel syndrome (avoid inflamed area)
- Colitis (avoid abdomen)
- Cretinism (avoid throat area)
- Crohn's disease (avoid abdomen)
- Cystitis (avoid cysts Baker's ganglion, sebaceous)
- Decubitus ulcers (avoid ulcerated area)
- Diverticular diseases (avoid abdomen)
- Folliculitis (avoid infected area)
- Foreign objects embedded in the skin such as glass, pencil lead, and metal (avoid area)
- Furuncle/carbuncle (avoid infected area)
- Goiter (avoid throat area)
- Gouty arthritis (avoid infected area)
- Graves' disease (avoid throat region and any enlarged lymph nodes)
- Hernia such as hiatal, femoral, inguinal, and umbilical (avoid herniated area)
- Hyperthyroidism (avoid throat area)
- Hypothyroidism (avoid throat area)
- Irritable bowel syndrome (avoid abdomen)
- Local inflammation (avoid inflamed area)
- Onychomycosis (avoid infected area)
- Open wounds (avoid wounded area)
- Paronychia (avoid infected area)
- Phlebitis (lightly over affected area)
- Polyps (avoid abdomen)
- Poison ivy, poison oak, poison sumac (unless affected area is widespread, in which case this is an absolute contraindication)

- Seborrhea keratosis (avoid infected area)
- Shingles (avoid infected area)*
- Spina bifida (avoid lumbosacral area)
- Swollen lymph glands (avoid swollen area)
- Thrombophlebitis (lightly over affected area; avoid inner thigh region)
- Ulcers (avoid abdomen)
- Unhealed burns and wounds (avoid injured area)
- Urinary incontinence (avoid abdomen)
- Urinary tract infection (avoid abdomen)
- Varicose veins (lightly over affected area)
- Wart (avoid infected area)

Conditions With Absolute Contraindications
- Appendicitis
- Autoimmune diseases or acute inflammatory processes during exacerbation period (or flare-up)
- Cardiac arrest
- Chickenpox
- Cholecystitis (during flare-up)
- Cirrhosis of the liver (if due to viral agent)
- Contact dermatitis (if widespread area is involved)
- Diarrhea (if due to infection)
- Embolism
- Encephalitis
- Fever
- Gallstones (if during a gallbladder attack)
- German measles
- Gout (during acute phase)
- Hemorrhage
- Hepatitis (during acute phase)
- Herpes simplex (avoid infected area)
- Hives (during acute phase)
- Hypertension (if not controlled by diet, exercise, and/or medication)
- Impetigo (avoid infected area)
- Infectious diseases (many are contained in this list)
- Influenza
- Intestinal obstruction
- Jaundice
- Laryngitis (if caused by infectious agent)
- Lice
- Lupus (during a flare-up)
- Measles
- Meningitis
- Migraine headache (during the migraine headache episode)
- Mononucleosis
- Multiple sclerosis (during flare-up)
- Mumps
- Pancreatitis (if acute pancreatitis)
- Pericarditis
- Pharyngitis (if due to infection)
- Pleurisy (if caused by infectious agent)
- Pneumonia (during acute phase)

BOX 5-1

Pathologies and Massage Contraindications—cont'd

- Preeclampsia
- Psychiatric diagnoses of manic depressive psychosis, schizophrenic psychosis, and paranoid conditions
- Pulmonary embolism
- Pyelonephritis
- Rabies
- Recent injury (wait 72 hours or until medical clearance is given)
- Recent surgery (until medical clearance is given)
- Respiratory distress syndrome

- Rheumatoid arthritis (during flare-up)
- Ringworm
- Scabies
- Scarlet fever
- Scleroderma (during flare-up)
- Severe, acute pain
- Sickle cell disease (during flare-up)
- Tonsillitis
- Tuberculosis

*If you, the therapist, have not had the chicken pox, do not massage; it is a contraindication for you.

areas of the body where most endangerment sites exist will be identified.

- **Nerves.** When nerves are compressed during massage, the client may experience numbness, tingling, burning, or shooting pain. It is doubtful that this will damage the nerve, but it may alarm your client or make her feel uncomfortable. If the pressure is prolonged, the client may experience a temporary loss of motor control.
- **Blood vessels.** Pressure applied to superficial blood vessels may cause a temporary reduction in blood flow and may possibly affect blood pressure. When massaging an area where a known or suspected superficial artery is present, apply light pressure and feel for a pulse. If a pulse is felt, avoid prolonged pressure on the specific pulse location. Veins are generally superficially located. Apply gliding movements such as effleurage centripetally (toward the center) to promote venous blood flow.

    Caution areas for arteries also include the neighboring veins of the same name with the exception of the aorta, the carotid artery, the great saphenous vein, and the jugular vein. Arteries and veins lie in proximity to each other, and caution of one generally reflects caution of the other. Note that many of these endangerment sites are common pulse point locations (see Figure 19-6).
- **Bony structures.** Compression of certain small, fragile, or prominent bony areas may cause pain, bruising of surface tissues and, in some cases, fracture of the bony projection.
- **Organs/glands.** Pressure or striking movements such as tapotement to the kidney or eye area may cause bruising, sharp pain, nausea, or temporary dysfunction. Swollen lymph nodes are also endangerment sites.
- **Abnormal findings.** Any abnormal findings such as suspicious lumps, masses, or moles are endangerment sites.

The following specific locations of each type of endangerment site can be located on the endangerment site map (Figure 5-5, *A* and *B*). All endangerment sites are bilaterally symmetrical with the exception of those located on the midline of the body. Remember, you can and should work these areas, but be mindful of the following anatomical structures:

- **Abdomen.** The structures to be aware of regarding pressure in the abdomen include the abdominal and descending aorta, liver, linea alba (connective tissue band running down the abdominal wall; it can herniate), lumbar plexus, vagus nerve, and xiphoid process.
- **Axilla.** The axillary region contains several nerves and blood vessels that can become compressed during massage, such as the axillary and brachial arteries; axillary, median, musculocutaneous, radial, and ulnar nerves; and brachial plexus.
- **Elbow.** The areas of endangerment of the elbow are the brachial, radial, and ulnar (antecubital) arteries; median (antecubital), radial (lateral epicondyles of the humerus), and ulnar (medial epicondyles of the humerus-ulnar notch) nerves, and cubital veins (antecubital).
- **Face.** Avoid direct pressure on the eyeball, facial arteries (alongside the upper and lower jaw), and transverse facial arteries (anterior to the ear).
- **Femoral triangle/medial thigh.** The borders of the femoral triangle are the gracilis, sartorius, and inguinal ligament. This area contains the femoral arteries and nerves, great saphenous veins, and obturator nerves.
- **Low back.** Do not get carried away with the striking tapotement or the electrical massager on the low back. Two structures to watch out for here are the floating ribs and kidneys (located retroperitoneally).
- **Popliteal.** Located behind the knee are the common peroneal and tibial nerves and the popliteal arteries.

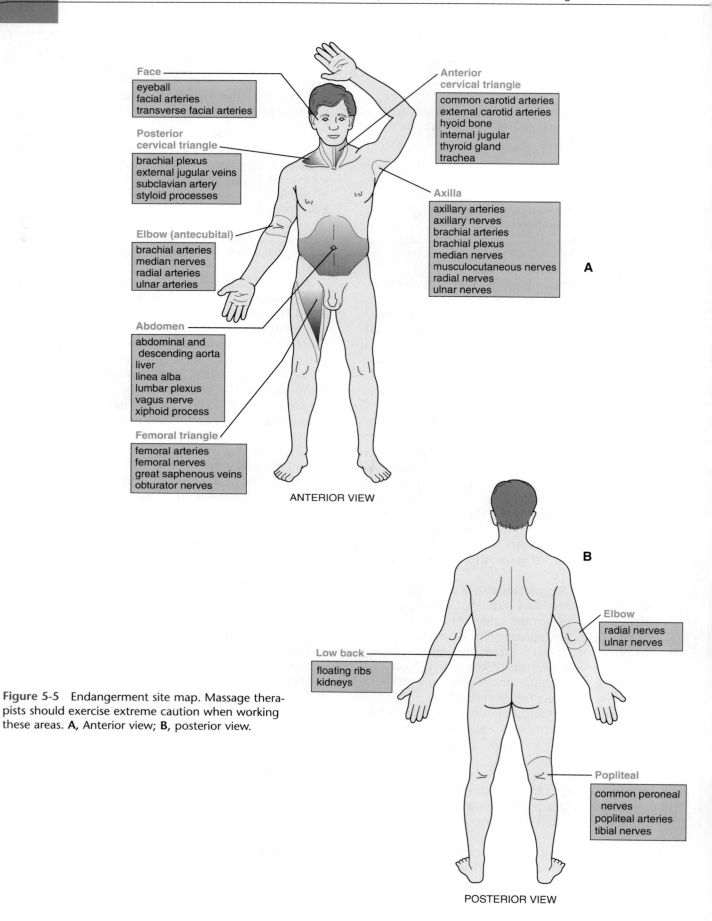

Face
eyeball
facial arteries
transverse facial arteries

Posterior cervical triangle
brachial plexus
external jugular veins
subclavian artery
styloid processes

Elbow (antecubital)
brachial arteries
median nerves
radial arteries
ulnar arteries

Abdomen
abdominal and
 descending aorta
liver
linea alba
lumbar plexus
vagus nerve
xiphoid process

Femoral triangle
femoral arteries
femoral nerves
great saphenous veins
obturator nerves

Anterior cervical triangle
common carotid arteries
external carotid arteries
hyoid bone
internal jugular
thyroid gland
trachea

Axilla
axillary arteries
axillary nerves
brachial arteries
brachial plexus
median nerves
musculocutaneous nerves
radial nerves
ulnar nerves

A

ANTERIOR VIEW

B

Elbow
radial nerves
ulnar nerves

Low back
floating ribs
kidneys

Popliteal
common peroneal
 nerves
popliteal arteries
tibial nerves

POSTERIOR VIEW

Figure 5-5 Endangerment site map. Massage therapists should exercise extreme caution when working these areas. **A**, Anterior view; **B**, posterior view.

- **Throat.** The throat region contains two triangular regions, the anterior and posterior cervical triangles. The *anterior cervical triangle,* whose defining borders are the trachea, base of the mandible, and sternocleidomastoid, contains seven endangerment sites, which are the common carotid arteries, external carotid arteries, hyoid bone, internal jugular veins, thyroid gland, trachea, and vagus nerves. The *posterior cervical triangle,* which uses the clavicle, sternocleidomastoid, and trapezius as its defining borders, possesses the following endangerment sites: brachial plexus, external jugular veins, facial nerve (just posterior to the mandibular ramus), subclavian artery, and styloid processes of the temporal bone (located anterior to insertion of the sternocleidomastoid and posterior to the mandibular angle).

SUMMARY

Massage has a powerful impact on the health and functioning of the body and has beneficial effects on virtually every body system. Yet it is not the preeminent answer for all problems and ills. The massage therapist who has studied and learned the indications and contraindications inspires confidence in his clients by demonstrating a strong grasp of anatomy, physiology, and pathology. This includes the science of how massage provides pain relief through such mechanisms as the gate theory. No greater gift can be given to a client than the attention to and caution against contraindicated conditions and vascular, nervous, osseous, and other miscellaneous endangerment sites. In this way the therapist also demonstrates an appreciation for his own abilities, an awareness of his own limitations, and an unflagging reputation for acting in the best interest of his clients.

For Your Information

When in doubt, don't.

MATCHING

List the letter of the answer next to the term or phrase that best describes it.

A. Reduces swelling
B. Retroperitoneal
C. Common peroneal nerve
D. Mechanical response
E. Local contraindication

F. Fever, lice, pleurisy
G. Reflexive response
H. Endangerment sites
I. Herpes simplex, warts, seborrhea

J. Absolute contraindication
K. Reduction of ischemia
L. Decreases excessive scar and adhesion formation

G   1. A physiological response to pressure as nerves are stimulated, activating a reflex arc

F   2. Examples of absolute contraindications

E   3. Condition in which massage can be administered while avoiding an infected area or area in question

L   4. A massage effect on connective tissues

D   5. A physiological response that occurs as a result of pressure, force, or range of motion

K   6. Which is a massage effect on the cardiovascular system

B   7. A term describing the location of the kidneys

A   8. An effect of massage on the lymphatic/immune systems

C   9. The structure located in the popliteal space

H   10. Areas of the body containing superficial delicate anatomical structures that are relatively unprotected and prone to injury; these sites merit caution during treatment

I   11. Examples of local contraindications

J   12. Condition in which massage is inappropriate, is not advised, and may be harmful to the client

Bibliography

Applegate EJ: *The anatomy and physiology learning system,* ed 2, Philadelphia, 2000, WB Saunders.

Barr JS, Taslitz N: Influence of back massage on autonomic functions, *Phys Ther* 50(12):1679-1691, 1970.

Beeken JE et al: The effectiveness of neuromuscular release massage therapy in five individuals with chronic obstructive lung disease, *Clin Nurs Res* 7(3):309-325, 1998.

Bell AJ: Massage and the physiotherapist, *Physiotherapy JCSP* 1964.

Bernal GR: How to calm children through massage, *Childhood Educ* 74:(1), 1997.

Bodian M: Use of massage following lid surgery, *Eye Ear Nose Throat Mon* 48(9):542-547, 1969.

Bonica JJ: The management of myofascial pain syndromes, *Phys Ther Rev* 39(6), 1959.

Cady SH, Jones GR: Massage therapy as a workplace intervention for reduction of stress, *Percept Motor Skills* 84:157-158, 1997.

Cherkin DC et al: Randomized trial comparing traditional Chinese medical acupuncture, therapeutic massage, and self-care education for chronic low back pain, *Arch Int Med* 161:1081-1088, 2001.

Consumer Reports Magazine: *The mainstreaming of alternative medicine,* May 2000.

Coward DD: Lymphedema prevention and management knowledge in women treated for breast cancer, *Oncol Nurs Forum* 26(6):1047-1053, 1999.

Cuthbertson DP: Effects of massage on metabolism: a survey, *Glasgow Med J* vol 131, 1933.

Cyriax J: Treatment by manipulation, massage, and injection. In *Textbook of orthopedic medicine,* vol 2, ed 11, London, 1984, Bailliere-Tindall.

De Domenico G, Wood E: *Beard's massage,* Philadelphia, 1987, WB Saunders.

Dennis W, Pergrouhi N: Infant development under environmental handicap, *Psychol Monogr: Gen Appl* 71(7), 1957.

Despard LL: *Textbook of massage and remedial gymnastics,* ed 3, New York, 1932, Oxford University Press.

Eisenberg DM et al: Trends in alternative medicine use in the United States, 1990-1997: results of a follow-up national survey, *JAMA* 280(18):1569-1575, 1998.

Evans P: The healing process at a cellular level: a review, *Physiotherapy JCSP* issue 66, 1980.

Fassbender HG: *Pathology of rheumatic diseases,* New York, 1975, Springer-Verlag.

Ferell-Torry AT, Glick OJ: The use of therapeutic massage as a nursing intervention to modify anxiety and the perception of cancer pain, *Cancer Nurs* 16(2):93-101, 1993.

Field T: *Touch in early development,* Hillsdale, NJ, 1995, Lawrence Erlbaum Associates.

Field T: Chronic fatigue syndrome: massage therapy effects on depression and somatic symptoms in chronic fatigue, *J Chron Fatigue Syndr* 3:43-51, 1997.

Field T: Sexual abuse effects are lessened by massage therapy, *J Bodywork Movement Ther* 1:65-69, 1997.

Field T: Children with asthma have improved pulmonary functions after massage therapy, *J Pediatr* 132(5), 1998.

Field T, Hernandez-Reif M, Seligman S: Juvenile rheumatoid arthritis: benefits from massage therapy, *J Pediatr Psychol* 22:607-617, 1997.

Field T, Seligman S, Scafidi F: Alleviating posttraumatic stress in children following hurricane Andrew, *J Appl Dev Psychol* 17:37-50, 1996.

Field T et al: Massage reduces anxiety in child and adolescent psychiatric patients, *J Am Acad Child Adolesc Psychiatry* 31(1):125-131, 1992.

Field T et al: Massage and relaxation therapies' effects on depressed adolescent mothers, *Adolescence* 31(124):903-911, 1996.

Field T et al: Massage therapy for infants of depressed mothers, *Infant Behav Dev* 19(124), 1996.

Field T et al: Massage therapy reduces anxiety and enhances EEG pattern of alertness and math computations. *Internat J Neurosci* 86:197-205, 1996.

Field T et al: Autistic children's attentiveness and responsively improved after touch therapy, *J Autism Dev Disord* 27:333-338, 1997.

Field T et al: Burn injuries benefit from massage therapy, *J Burn Care Rehabil* 19:241-244, 1997.

Field T et al: Job stress reduction therapies, *Alternat Ther Health Med* 3:54-56, 1997.

Field T et al: Labor pain is reduced by massage therapy, *J Psychosom Obstetr Gynecol* 18:286-291, 1997.

Field T et al: Massage therapy lowers glucose levels in children with diabetes mellitus, *Diabet Spectr* 10:237-239, 1997.

Field T et al: Adolescents with attention deficit hyperactivity disorder benefit from massage therapy, *Adolescence* 33(129):103-108, 1998.

Field T et al: Bulimic adolescents benefit from massage therapy, *Adolescence* 33(131):555-563, 1998.

Field T et al: Elder retired volunteers benefit from giving massage therapy to infants, *J Appl Gerontol* 17(2), 1998.

Field T et al: Pregnant women benefit from massage therapy, *J Psychosom Obstet Gynaecol* 19:31-38, 1999.

Fraser J, Kerr JR: Psychophysiological effects of back massage on elderly institutionalized patients, *J Adv Nurs* 18:238-245, 1993.

Garner DM, Olmsted MP, Polivy J: *Anorexia nervosa: recent developments in research,* New York, 1983, Alan R. Liss.

Gehlsen GM, Ganion LR, Helfst R: Fibroblast responses to variation in soft tissue mobilization pressure, *Med Sci Sports Exerc* 31(4):531-535, 1999.

Goldberg J, Seaborne D, Sullivan S: The effects of therapeutic massage on H-reflex amplitude in persons with a spinal cord injury, *Phys Ther* 74(8):728-737, 1994.

Grafelman T: *Graf's anatomy and physiology guide for the massage therapist,* Aurora, Colo, 1998, DG Publishing.

Hammer WI: The use of transverse friction massage in the management chronic bursitis of the hip or shoulder, *J Manipulative Physiol Ther* 16(2):107-111, 1993.

Herandez-Reif M: Multiple sclerosis patients benefit from massage therapy, *J Bodywork Movement Ther* 2:168-174, 1998.

Herandez-Reif M et al: Migraine headaches are reduced by massage therapy, *Int J Neurosci* 96:1-11, 1998.

Hernandez-Reif M et al: Cystic fibrosis symptoms are reduced with massage therapy intervention, *J Pediatr Psychol* 24:183-199, 1999.

Hillard D: Massage for the seriously mentally ill, *J Psychosoc Nurs Ment Health Serv* 33(7), 1995.

Holland B, Pokorny M: Slow stroke back massage: its effect on patients in a rehabilitation setting, *Rehabil Nurs* 26(5):182-186, 2001.

Hovind H, Nielsen SL: Effect of massage on blood flow in skeletal muscle, *Scand J Rehabil Med* 6(2):74-77, 1974.

Hulme JH, Waterman V, Hillier F: The effect of foot massage on patients' perception of care following laparoscopic sterilization as day case patients, *J Adv Nurs* 30(2):460-468, 1999.

Ironson G et al: Massage therapy is associated with enhancement of the immune system's cytotoxic capacity, *Int J Neurosci* 84:205-218, 1996.

Jacob S, Francone C: *Elements of anatomy and physiology,* Philadelphia, 1989, WB Saunders.

Jacobs M: Massage for the relief of pain: anatomical and physiological considerations, *Phys Ther Rev* 40(2), 1960.

Jancin B: Massage effective in treating chronic low back pain, *Fam Pract News* 29(22), 1999.

Johanson R: Perineal massage for the prevention of perineal trauma in childbirth, *Lancet* 355(9200):250-251, 2000.

Jones NA, Field T: Massage and music therapies attenuate frontal EEG asymmetry in depressed adolescents, *Adolescence* 34(135):529-534, 1999.

Juhan D: *Job's body, a handbook for bodyworkers,* Barrington, NY, 1987, Station Hill Press.

Kim EJ, Buschmann MT: The effect of expressive physical touch on patients with dementia, *Int J Nurs Stud* 36(3):235-243, 1999.

Kresge CA: Massage and sports. In *Sports medicine, fitness, training, injuries,* Baltimore, 1987, Urban and Schwarzenberg.

Krieger D: Therapeutic touch: the imprimatur of nursing, *Am J Nurs* 75(5):784-787, 1975.

Krusen FH: *Physical medicine,* Philadelphia, 1941, WB Saunders.

Leivadi S, Hernandez-Reif M, Field T: Massage therapy and relaxation effects on university dance students, *J Dance Sci* 3:108-112, 1999.

Lindrea KB, Stainton MC: A case study of infant massage outcomes, *MCN Am J Matern Child Nurs* 25(2):95-99, 2000.

Little L, Porche DJ: Manual lymph drainage, *J Assoc Nurses AIDS Care* 9(1):78-81, 1998.

Lucia SP, Richard JF: Effects of massage on blood platelet production, *Proc Soc Exp Biol Med* 1933.

Lundeberg T: Long-term results of vibratory stimulation as a pain relieving measure for chronic pain, *Pain* 20:13-23 1984.

Lundeberg T et al: Vibratory stimulation compared to placebo in alleviation of pain, *Scand J Rehabil Med* 19:153-158, 1987.

Lundeberg T et al: Effect of vibratory stimulation on experimental and clinical pain, *Scand J Rehabil Med* 19:153-158, 1988.

McKechnie A et al: Anxiety states: a preliminary report on the value of connective tissue massage, *J Psychosom Res* 27:125-129, 1983.

Meek S: Effects of slow stroke back massage on relaxation in hospice clients, *Image J Nurs Sch* 25(1):17-21, 1993.

Melzack R, Wall PD: Pain mechanisms: a new theory, *Science* 150(699):971-979, 1965.

Mennell JB: *Physical treatment,* ed 5, Philadelphia, 1945, Blakiston.

Merck manual, ed 17, Whitehouse Station, NJ, 1998, Merck and Company.

Mitchell JK: *Massage and exercise in system of physiological therapeutics,* Philadelphia, 1984, Blakiston.

Mock HE: Massage in surgical cases. In *AMA handbook of physical medicine,* Chicago, 1945, Council of Physical Medicine.

Modi N, Glover J: *Massage therapy for preterm infants,* research paper presented at the Touch Research Symposium, April 1995.

Morelli M, Seaborne DE, Sullivan J: Changes in H-reflex amplitude during massage of triceps surae in healthy subjects, *J Orthop Sports Phys Ther* 12:55-59, 1990.

Morelli M, Seaborne DE, Sullivan J: H-reflex modulation during manual muscle massage of human triceps surae, *Arch Phys Med Rehabil* 72:915-919, 1991.

Mosby's Medical, Nursing, and Allied Health Dictionary, ed 4, St Louis, 1994, Mosby.

Myers TW: *Anatomy trains: myofascial meridians for manual and movement therapists,* New York, 2001, Churchill Livingstone.

Nixon N et al: Expanding the nursing repertory: the effective of massage in postoperative pain, *Aust J Adv Nurs* 14:21-26, 1997.

Nordschow M, Bierman W: Influence of manual massage on muscle relaxation: effects on trunk flexion, *Phys Ther* 42:653-657, 1962.

Ottoson D, Ekblom AT, Hansson P: Vibratory stimulation for the relief of pain of dental origin, *Pain* 10:37-45, 1981.

Pemberton R: Physiology of massage. In *American Medical Association handbook of physical therapy,* ed 3, Chicago, 1939, Council of Physical Therapy.

Premkumar K: *Pathology A to Z, a handbook for massage therapists,* Calgary, Alberta, Canada, 1996, VanPub Books.

Preyde M: Effectiveness of massage therapy for subacute low-back pain: a randomized controlled trial, *CMAJ* 162(13):1815-1820, 2000.

Prudden B: *Pain erasure,* New York, 1980, Random House, Ballantine Books.

Puustjarvi K, Pontinen PJ: The effects of massage in patients with chronic tension headaches, *Acupunct Electrother Res* 15(2):159-162, 1990.

Reed B, Held JM: Effects of sequential connective tissue massage on autonomic nervous system of middle-aged elderly adults, *Phys Ther* 68(8):1231-1234, 1988.

Rich GJ: *Massage therapy: the evidence for practice,* St Louis, 2002, Mosby.

Richards A: Hands on help, *Nurs Times* 94(32):69-72, 1998.

Rodenburg JB et al: Warm-up, stretching, and massage diminish harmful effects of eccentric exercise, *Int J Sports Med* 15:414-419, 1994.

Rogeness GA, Javors MA, Pliszka SR: Neurochemistry and child and adolescent psychiatry, *J Am Acad Child Adolesc Psychiatry* 31(5):765-781, 1992.

Rowe M, Alfred D: The effectiveness of slow-stroke massage in diffusing agitated behaviors in individuals with Alzheimer's disease, *J Gerontol Nurs* 25(6):22-34, 1999.

St. John P: *St. John neuromuscular therapy seminars, manual I,* Largo, Fla, 1995, Author.

Salvo SG: *Pathology: a guide for massage therapists,* St Louis, 2004, Mosby.

Samples P: Does sports massage have a role in sports medicine? *Physician Sportsmed* 15(3), 1987.

Sansone P, Schmitt L: Providing tender touch massage to elderly nursing home residents: a demonstration project, *Geriatr Nurs* 21(6):303-308, 2000.

Schachner L et al: Atopic dermatitis symptoms decrease in children following massage therapy, *Pediatr Dermatol* 15:390-395, 1998.

Schanberg S: Genetic basis for touch effects. In Field T, editor: *Touch in early development,* Hillsdale, NJ, 1984, Lawrence Erlbaum Associates.

Scull CW: Massage: physiological basis, *Arch Phys Med* pp 159-167, 1945.

Smith L et al: The effects of athletic massage on delayed onset muscle soreness, creatine kinase, and neutrophil count: a preliminary report, *J Orthop Sports Phys Ther* 19(2):93-99, 1994.

Stewart K: Massage for children with cerebral palsy promotes tactile stimulation, *Nurs Times* 2(50), 2000.

Sullivan SJ: Does massage decrease laryngeal tension in a subject with complete tetraplegia? *Percept Mot Skills* 84:169-170, 1997.

Sullivan SJ et al: Effects of massage on alpha motoneuron excitability, *Phys Ther* 71(8):555-560, 1991.

Sunshine W et al: Fibromyalgia benefits from massage therapy and transcutaneous electrical stimulation, *J Clin Rheumatol* 2:18-22, 1997.

Taber's cyclopedic medical dictionary, ed 13, Philadelphia, 1977, FA Davis.

Tappan FM: *Healing massage technique, holistic, classical and emerging methods,* Norwalk, Conn, 1988, Appleton and Lange.

Thibodeau G, Patton K: *Structure and function of the body,* ed 11, St Louis, 2000, Mosby.

Tortora GJ: *Introduction to the human body: the essentials of anatomy and physiology,* ed 3, New York, 1994, Harper-Collins.

Tortora GJ, Grabowksi SR: *Principles of anatomy and physiology,* ed 9, New York, 1994, John Wiley and Sons.

Travell J: Referred pain from skeletal muscles, *NY State J Med* 55:2, 1955.

Travell JG, Simons D: *Myofasical pain and dysfunction, the trigger point manual,* Baltimore, 1983, Williams & Wilkins.

Van Der Riet P: Effects of therapeutic massage on preoperative anxiety in a rural hospital: part 1 and part 2, *Aust J Rural Health* 1(4), 1993.

Vickers A, Zollman C: Massage therapies, *BMJ* 319:7219, 1999.

Voss DE, Ionta MK, Myers BJ: *Proprioceptive neuromuscular facilitation,* Philadelphia, 1985, Harper and Row.

Wakim KG: *Manipulation, traction and massage,* New York, 1976, Robert E. Krieger.

Wakim KG et al: The effects of massage on the circulation in normal and paralyzed extremities, *Arch Phys Med* 30:135-144, 1949.

Weeks VD, Travell J: Postural vertigo due to trigger areas in the sternocleidomastoid muscle, *J Pediatr* 47(162), 1955.

Williams RE: *The road to radiant health,* College Place, Wash, 1977, Color Press.

Zeitlin D et al: Immunological effects of massage therapy during academic stress, *Psychosom Med* 62(1):83-84, 2000.

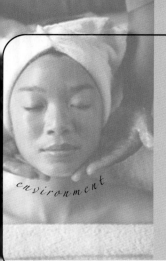

environment

The Science of Body and Table Mechanics

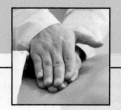

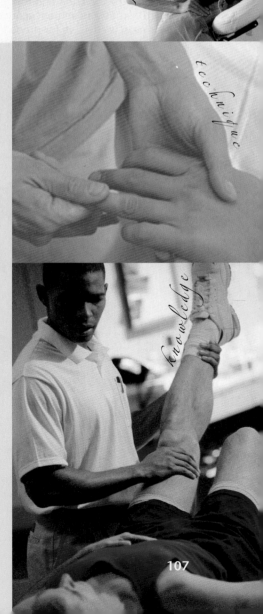

pressure

technique

knowledge

"Hands are the heart's landscape."

—Pope John Paul II

STUDENT OBJECTIVES

After completing this chapter, the student should be able to:

- Discuss ways to reduce the risk of repetitive motion injuries
- Implement the concepts of health that relate to the practice of body mechanics
- Identify basic foot stances
- Explain guidelines for proper body mechanics
- Use appropriate positioning equipment and bolstering devices and position the client in the prone, supine, side-lying, and seated positions
- Properly drape the client with sheets and towels
- Maintain appropriate draping while the client rolls over
- Assist the client on and off the massage table while maintaining the appropriate drape

INTRODUCTION

To ensure a successful long-term career in massage, the massage therapist must maintain her own physical condition and avoid the pitfalls associated with repetitive motion injuries.

To accomplish this goal, we examine some of the causes of repetitive motion injuries and two impor-tant aspects of massage therapy: *body mechanics* and *table mechanics*.

Body mechanics includes the principles of strength, stamina, breathing, stability, balance, and groundedness/centeredness. It also encompasses the practice of foot stances, body postures, and leverage techniques to decrease the likelihood of injury. **Table mechanics** addresses the practical issues of setting the table height and positioning, bolstering,

Preparing for the Massage

The following exercises are designed to assist the therapist in preparing her shoulders, elbows and hands for the physical exertion involved in massage therapy.

- **Warm-up.** Begin by rubbing your palms and fingers to-gether, creating friction and warmth; then vigorously rub the backs of your hands and arms. Shake your hands and fingers at the wrists and then drop your hands to your sides and roll your shoulders forward for 10 repetitions. Reverse the direction and rotate your shoulders back-ward. Do this movement sequence 10 times. This quick warm-up is effective for preparing the hands right before a massage or before other hand-developing exercises. Remember to breathe as you move.

- **Hand swishing.** Press your palms and fingers together at chest level with fingertips pointing up to your chin. Quickly rotate your fingers forward until they are point-ing downward toward the toes and then reverse back to the starting position. This motion should be playful, quick, and vigorous. NOTE: The elbows and shoulders re-main fixed while the wrists rotate together.

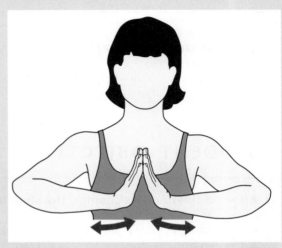

Digit stretch.

- **Wrist circles.** Begin with your arms at your sides. Flex the elbows while lifting your hands in front of you to chest level. With your fingers extended, circle both wrists in one direction for 10 revolutions and then reverse the direction for 10 revolutions. Repeat the wrist circles in both directions, but this time, close your hands into a fist. Do 10 revolutions in both directions.

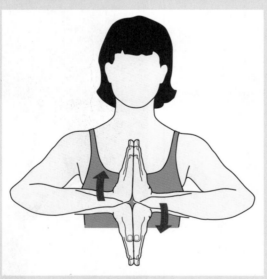

Hand swishing.

- **Digit stretch.** Press your fingertips together as you keep your wrists apart about 6 to 8 inches. Release this pres-sure while maintaining contact. Repeat the fingertip press-and-release sequence 10 times.

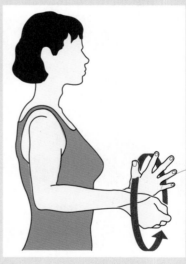

Wrist circles.

and draping your client in a manner that is professional, ethical, and efficient. Assisting the client on and off the table will also be addressed as it involves both body and table mechanics.

REPETITIVE MOTION INJURIES

The number one reason why massage therapists decide to leave the industry is not professional burnout or missed employment opportunities; it is because of injuries resulting from repetitive motions and cumulative trauma to the wrist and fingers. Our bodies were designed to be in motion. We begin to have problems when we stop moving or start moving the

same joints repetitively. Even with the use of proper body mechanics, body tissues react negatively when the same motion is repeated excessively. Because this type of injury can shorten your career, let us examine repetitive motion injuries in detail.

Repetitive motion injuries, also known as repetitive strain injuries (RSIs), are basically self-inflicted injuries related to inefficient biomechanics including general posture, sporting movements, and work habits. A repetitive or constant motion, combined with compressive forces or joint hyperextension, causes injury to soft tissues. Usually the resulting injury is cumulative in nature, having built up from self-abuse over an extended period. This injury type encompasses a broad spectrum of injuries. The

---

Preparing for the Massage—cont'd

- **Grab and stretch.** Start with your open palms at your sides. Pull your hands up to chest height, closing the palms into fists. Without stopping, continue the upward thrust of your hands over your head, stretching your fingertips out and inhaling simultaneously. Reverse the direction, bringing your arms back down. Close your hands as you pass your chest and reopen them as they reach your sides, exhaling forcefully. Keep your pace slow and your movements graceful. Repeat the sequence five times. Stop immediately if you become lightheaded.

- **Ball squeeze.** Place a tennis ball or a racquet ball in the palm of your hand and wrap your fingers around it. Squeeze the ball as hard as you can for 10 seconds. Repeat 10 times. Switch hands and repeat the sequence.

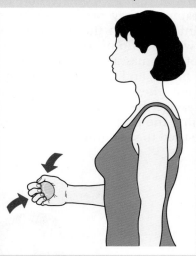

Ball squeeze.

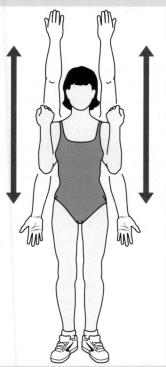

Grab and stretch.

most common types of repetitive motion injuries are carpal tunnel syndrome, thoracic outlet syndrome, tennis elbow, and rotator cuff problems. The symptoms and damage are progressive, unless the inefficient biomechanics or repetitive strain is altered. The general symptoms of RSI are related to the inflammation response: pain, redness, heat, swelling, limited range of motion (ROM). Initial symptoms are usually limited to the soft tissues. The progression of injury typically goes from muscle soreness, to increased tonus, to the formation of multiple trigger points, and in some cases to nerve entrapment. Chronic RSIs may result in neuropathy; subluxation; deterioration or trauma to the joints including bursitis; arthritis; and even stress fractures of involved bones.

The muscles of the therapist's anterior forearm quickly become large and tight because of repeated finger flexing. Over time, the flexor retinaculum begins to compress against the tendons and nerves supplying the hand. You may begin to feel a numbness or weakness in the forearm, wrist, or hand. The digits most likely involved are the middle and ring fingers and the thumb. Compression damage and nerve entrapment may occur because of excessive trigger point work with the tips of the fingers and thumb or with the tip of the elbow. If you begin to have symptoms, massage the entire arm, pectoralis major and minor, and the neck musculature.

To prevent these injuries from occurring, frequently massage the anterior forearm muscles while strengthening the posterior forearm muscles. A barbell can be used to strengthening these muscles (Figure 6-1).

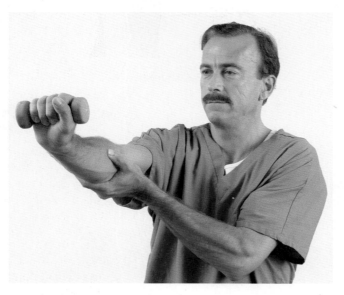

Figure 6-1   Therapist doing wrist extension curls for prevention of repetitive motion injuries.

For our clients, improper work habits are probably the leading cause of these types of injuries, and they are 100% preventable. All it takes is a little education. Initially, the client has to be made aware of the potential damage being done to his body, the warning signs and symptoms, and the consequences of that damage. The client can then implement a new work habit. This again involves education of proper body mechanics such as lifting and keyboarding. The only way to break an old bad habit is to replace it with a new good one. The worst thing about repetitive motion injuries is that they take time to occur. By the time they are symptomatic, we are already in the habit of doing an activity improperly.

An example of a job-related RSI is the office worker who holds the phone to his ear with his shoulder to free his hands to do other things. Years of this behavior, especially if he favors one shoulder, may lead to headaches, muscular tension, and eventually degenerative disk disease or herniation. This may sound like an exaggeration, but it is not. How can the seemingly innocuous act of holding the phone to the ear with the shoulder lead to degenerative disk disease? It simply happens through the mechanisms of muscular imbalance and postural distortion.

Muscular imbalances are common in the body. They occur when the strength of one muscle or muscle group is greater than the opposing muscle(s). Quadriceps muscle imbalances are a common cause of hamstring tears in sprinters and hurtlers. So what does this have to do with the telephone? Holding the phone by using the right side of the head, neck, and shoulders contracts muscles such as the right trapezius, right scalenes, and right levator scapulae. This daily activity occurring over a period of several years develops these muscles; they become stronger, enlarged, and tighter. With this type of muscular imbalance, postural distortions come into play. The stronger right neck muscles begin to compress the cervical vertebrae together. The weaker muscles on the left have less pressure across the cervical joints. Over time, the action of right lateral flexion and rotation actually disrupts the integrity of the disks between the vertebrae. If the disk migrates (bulges) toward the left because of the increased vertebral compression on the right, the disk may press against the left nerve root, causing an impingement or pinched nerve. Often, the pattern appears as neck pain on one side of the body and arm numbness or pain on the opposite side. The preventive measure is simple enough; an earphone with wraparound pencil microphone or even a simple speakerphone allows him to perform a task without the muscular imbalance and ensuing pain.

As you can see, these types of injuries will not only affect your work as a therapist, but clients will present these types of injuries to you. Pain is the great equalizer. It eventually gets everyone's attention, so pay attention to your body, or your client's body, when it is speaking to you.

The best ways for you to reduce the likelihood of RSI affecting you, are to (1) use a variety of strokes, (2) rest your hands by spacing your clients, (3) stretch between sessions, (4) adjust the height of the massage table, (5) avoid sustained pressure or delayed compression, (6) keep your body physically fit using weight and flexibility training, (7) use proper body mechanics, and (8) get massages.

BODY MECHANICS FOR THE PRACTITIONER OF MASSAGE THERAPY

Body mechanics is defined as the proper use of postural techniques to deliver massage therapy with the utmost efficiency and with minimum trauma to the practitioner. Also known as *biomechanics,* proper body mechanics influences the execution of the massage, decreases fatigue and discomfort during and after the massage session, and helps prevent repetitive motion injuries. The key to a long healthy career as a massage therapist is the ability to provide treatment without incurring injury. Proper body mechanics is as critical to a successful practice as anatomical knowledge, manual skills, and business acumen. Few occupations use upper-body strength at the force or frequency as massage. Upper-body stress is all too common in the massage field. Incorrect working posture and poorly executed hand techniques can increase stress on the joints, creating RSIs.

Bonnie Prudden, in her book *Pain Erasure: The Bonnie Prudden Way* (1980), classifies occupations into five categories, according to the degree of physical activity required to perform the job. These categories are (1) *sitting,* (2) *standing,* (3) *walking,* (4) *active,* and (5) *strenuous occupations.* She lists massage therapy in the strenuous category because of the expenditure of physical energy and the use of torque (twisting and turning motions that occur in the torso). She also states that strenuous occupations often result in back pain (Box 6-1). An important part of body mechanics lies in taking steps to prepare our bodies for the massage. A personal fitness program can help us do just that.

It is significant to note that most members of western cultures focus on strength and stamina as the primary goal of a fitness regimen. Eastern cultures focus on building balance and the ability to become grounded and centered as the foundations of health; strength and stamina comes with discipline. Both viewpoints have merit. The concepts discussed below combine several key principles of both eastern and western cultures. All fitness activities help you explore the body's landscapes and build its natural bioenergy. Of course, anyone with health problems should consult a personal physician before initiating any fitness program, but generally, if a person is healthy enough to do massage, then she is healthy enough to exercise. Massage is a physically demanding profession. To minimize such stress and damage, health-promoting principles should be practiced.

The elements of body mechanics and the *kata* in martial arts are similar in nature. To help us better understand these systems of movement, the ancient practices of kendo and aikido need to be examined. Students of these martial arts are required to follow four basic principles: (1) *eyes first* (for focus and attention), (2) *footwork next* (foot position for weight transference), (3) *courage third* (assessing timing, space, your opponent, and how you are going to initiate your movements), and (4) *strength last* (body moves into action, or weight effort). It is important to note that strength and weight effort come last in the list. If we apply these principles to massage therapy, focus, foot stance, and assessment come before the massage strokes.

MINI-LAB

Using a full-length mirror in your massage room, occasionally observe your body mechanics during a massage. Adjust your stance when needed.

PRINCIPLES OF BODY MECHANICS

In Chapter 4, the concept of health is examined in the context of nutrition, exercise, and relaxation. However, this chapter explores some related concepts to these three areas of health, which are vital to the principles and practice of massage therapy. These principles are (1) strength, (2) stamina, (3) breathing, (4) stability, (5) balance, and (6) groundedness/centeredness.

Strength

Massage requires physical strength. If you do not possess adequate strength through exercise and proper diet, you not only fatigue faster, you are also more prone to injury. You may be asked to assist your client on and off the table or lift and move a client who is elderly or physically challenged. The best activities to add muscle strength to your body are floor exercises such as sit-ups, push-ups, and weight/resistance training. Muscles only become stronger when they are challenged. Because massage involves the entire body, all major muscle groups should be addressed during strength training.

BOX 6-1

Occupations and Related Pain Hazards

Occupations Classified by Kind or Degree of Physical Activity Required

Sitting	Standing	Walking	Active	Strenuous
Accountant	Bank teller	Detective	Carpenter	Athlete
Administrator	Barber	Flight attendant	Carpet layer	Construction worker
Anesthetist	Bartender	Floorwalker	Dairy worker	Dancer
Architect	Beautician	Librarian	Electrician	Diver
Artist	Blacksmith	Nurse	Farmer	Heavy equipment operator
Astronaut	Butcher	Orderly	Fireman	Linesman
Author	Cafeteria server	Postal carrier	Forester	Longshoreman
Bookkeeper	Clerk	Real estate agent	Maintenance	Martial arts instructor
Broadcaster	Cook	Restaurant wait staff	Mason	Massage therapist
Bus driver	Dental hygienist	Service station attendant	Mechanic	Miner
Cab driver	Dentist	Train conductor	Painter	Steel worker
Chauffeur	Doctor	Usher	Photographer	Wood worker
Computer programmer	Electrologist	Watchman	Plumber	
Crane operator	Elevator Operator		Police officer	
Dispatcher	File clerk		Sailor	
Draftsman	Hairdresser		Ski instructor	
Editor	Machinist		Soldier	
Educator	Sales clerk		Sports coach	
Electronics repairer	Sculptor		Tree remover	
Engineer	Surgeon			
Executive	Teacher			
Glass blower	Veterinarian			
Jeweler				
Keypunch operator				
Lawyer				
Pilot				
Psychiatrist				
School bus driver				
Secretary				
Student				
Telephone operator				
Truck driver				
Weaver				

Sitting

Sitting occupations often put trigger points in the upper and lower back. Because the body is constantly bent, the groin may be involved. If circulation is impaired by overweight, the legs and buttocks, which are constantly compressed against chairs, become involved.

Standing

Occupations requiring long hours of standing in one place contribute to the risk of low back pain. The upper back is also in danger, as are the arms and the shoulders and neck. Swelling may also occur in the feet and ankles.

Walking

Occupations requiring ordinary walking are not at risk. However, when the walking includes carrying (postal carrier or restaurant wait staff), the back is in danger.

Active

Active occupational all entail danger. For example, carpenters damage their elbows and experience tennis elbow, the plumber working with pipe threaders and large wrenches puts trigger points in the chest muscles, the mason strains the back, and the dancer damages the legs and lower back.

Strenuous

Strenuous occupations often result in back pain, and the injuries often involve torque, such as the ladder that gets away, the barrel that rolls the wrong way, or anything that pulls the torso with a twisting motion.

Modified from Prudden B: *Pain erasure: the Bonnie Prudden way*, New York, 1980, Ballantine Books.

Stamina

Most massage sessions last at least 1 hour. The therapist must possess enough stamina and endurance for all her clients all day long. This usually means including some cardiovascular training in your fitness program. Thirty minutes three times a week is the minimum time to spend to enhance your health and influence stamina. Additional complex carbohydrates added to a balanced diet are the best fuel food for keeping your energy level high. Make sure you get plenty of rest. Good body mechanics suffer when a therapist is tired. Fatigue can also be reduced by proper breathing technique.

Breathing

The use of proper breathing will help keep the therapist relaxed, pace massage movements, and fuel the muscles. Proper breathing technique enhances our mental and physical health, thus positively affecting the quality of massage. According to William Barry, author and instructor of massage therapy, correct

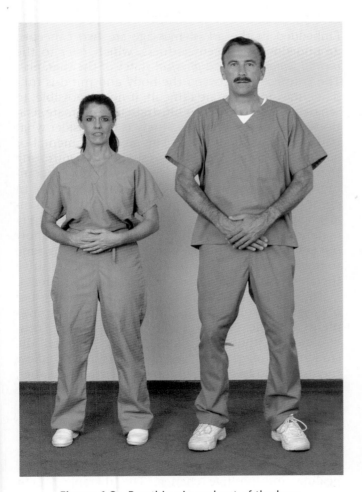

Figure 6-2   Breathing in and out of the hara.

breathing is often referred to as the *foundation of massage*. Try combining volitional breathing and massage therapy. As you massage, the strokes that require the therapist to reach may be accompanied by an exhalation, and the return strokes may be accompanied by an inhalation. Some deep breathing modifications such as sighing and yawning may be indicators that the body needs more oxygen. If this occurs, take a few slow deep breaths. This is also a great way to release tension. Encourage your clients to sigh or yawn before, during, and after the massage. By placing your tongue on the roof of your mouth, nasal breathing is encouraged.

Aikido masters often use breathing to guide the student to shrink their focus to a space about the size of a quarter, 2 inches below and behind the navel. This ancient center of gravity is called the **hara** (Japanese term) or the **dantien** (Chinese term). This is a topographical *and* meditative point of reference, known for thousands of years in many cultures as the center of physical and spiritual balance. A simple way to experience the power of this dynamic center is to allow your breath to move into and out of the hara (Figure 6-2). On exhalation, the therapist should contract the muscles of the pelvic floor to lower the center of gravity and splint the lower back muscles to help maintain a straight back. Additionally, this form of abdominal breathing helps lower the center of gravity and contributes to stability.

Stability

Effective massage therapy is dependent on the therapist moving from a stable base. The lower portion of your body is capable of providing about two and a half times more power and greater stability than your upper body, just as walking is easier than doing push-ups. Proper body mechanics transmit force from the therapist to the client by using lower body stability. The upper body becomes a flexible conduit of energy while the therapist remains free of injury. With both feet firmly planted, force is transmitted to a stable base shared by both legs and diffused to the floor (Figure 6-3).

The greater the number of points of contact, the more stable the object becomes. Compare the relative stability of a pogo stick, ironing board, tripod, and chair. The tripod and chair are very stable, but the pogo stick is not. Techniques requiring the therapist to stand with most or all of his weight on one leg constitute extremely poor body mechanics. Precise articulations from the upper extremity are not possible while continually leaning on the client. Furthermore, the center of gravity is much higher, further reducing stability. The therapist needs a stable base of support. Ironically, when the therapist works

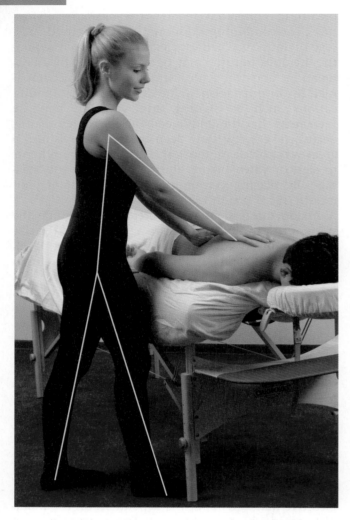

Figure 6-3   Both feet flat on the floor provides a stable base.

from a stable body stance, he is more responsive to the client. Stability is the prerequisite to balance.

Balance

Proper body mechanics are a direct result of balanced posture which respects the laws of gravity. Gravity is the mutual attraction of two objects toward each other, such as your body and the earth. When you are balanced, less energy is expended during the massage. The center of gravity, the point at which the body is balanced, is generally between the fourth and fifth lumbar vertebrae on the front of the spine, or an inch or two below and behind your navel (hara). The principle of balance can be expanded to an emotional/spiritual awareness or energetic experience of ourselves in relation to our surroundings. This sensation of peaceful energy is often experienced in the same place as our center of gravity. Exercises that encourage balance include yoga and martial art

disciplines such as tai chi and aikido, which can also be used for meditation or grounding.

MINI-LAB

Choose a partner. Have her stand with her feet 24 inches apart. Ask your partner to concentrate on her head. After a moment, gently and gradually begin pushing against her shoulder. Question her about how her body responds to the change. Next, ask your partner to concentrate on an area between the fourth and fifth lumbar vertebrae on the front of the spine or about 1 to 2 inches below and behind your navel. After allowing time for concentration, give another gentle push. Have your partner report on the difference she felt during each push. Which area of concentration felt more stable? Switch roles and allow your partner to gently push you. Compare experiences, noting similarities or differences. The area that felt more stable is the area from which you initiate your massage movements.

Groundedness/Centeredness

Embedded in the art of massage are two concepts, groundedness and centeredness, which refer to the *mental, emotional,* and *physical* states of the therapist. The connection between the body and mind is fundamental, and they are difficult, if not impossible, to separate. The best way to illustrate this intimate relationship between mind and body is to consider what happens to the body when you are under mental or emotional stress. The body responds by mirroring that state of mind; headaches and insomnia are common. Conversely, when people are physically ill or in chronic pain, it affects them mentally and emotionally, which is often expressed by their attitude. Many common tasks become difficult, and we either show our emotions too easily or not at all. Thus taking time to prepare our minds helps us become more sensitive therapists, so we then have more to offer our clients.

The martial art aikido is helpful for guiding the massage therapist into useful application of movement principles. When teaching the concept of centeredness to students of aikido, masters often tell the students to place their weight underside and allow themselves to feel light on top. As mentioned earlier, abdominal breathing from the hara helps ground the therapist.

When you are grounded, you may feel the presence of God, nature, or your higher power, in addition to the company of your client. You become part of a larger whole and recognize that you are just a vessel for healing and positive change. The therapist might imagine that all his tensions are draining from his body, and he connects to the ubiquitous energy and power that brings peace and serenity (Box 6-2). Using the vessel as a psychological and spiritual reference point, the stress, tension, and excess energy that are released by the client during a massage are not absorbed by the therapist but are effectively channeled to the grounding source itself. Being both grounded and centered makes a difference in how you deliver the massage; it will help you stay focused on what is at hand. By clearing your mind and experiencing the moment, your body mechanics will be greatly enhanced.

FOOT STANCES RELATED TO BODY MECHANICS

We do not just massage with our hands; the whole body plays a role in how the massage is delivered. The placement of the feet influences the type and direction of the massage stroke, while providing a stable base. Remember, the lower extremities have two and a half times more available strength than the upper extremities, so it makes sense to use the body's natural strength to deliver massage. Foot placement, which is the source of your stable base, has a profound effect on body mechanics and body alignment.

The massage therapist typically uses one of two basic foot stances when applying massage strokes: the *bow* and *warrior stances*. Both the bow and warrior stances provide a stable foundation and balanced body posture. The foot stance used most often depends on the style of massage you perform and the type of strokes you use most often. When in a bow or warrior stance, each foot makes contact with the earth at three points (Figure 6-4; see Chapter 14 for more information). Two feet represent six points of contact. This double-tripod structure provides a stable foundation for movement. While practicing movement from

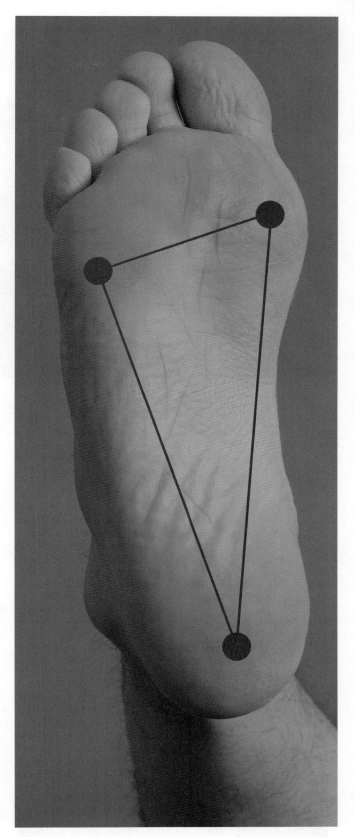

Figure 6-4 The foot forms a base of support with three points of contact.

BOX 6-2

Serenity Prayer

God, grant me
the serenity to accept the things I cannot change,
the courage to change the things I can,
and the wisdom to know the difference.
Living one day at a time;
enjoying one moment at a time;
accepting hardships as the pathway to peace.
Taking, as He did, this sinful world as it is, not as I would have it.
Trusting that He will make all things right if I surrender to His will.
That I may be reasonably happy in this life and supremely happy with Him forever in the next.
Amen.

—Rev. Reinhold Niebuhr

A   **B**   **C**

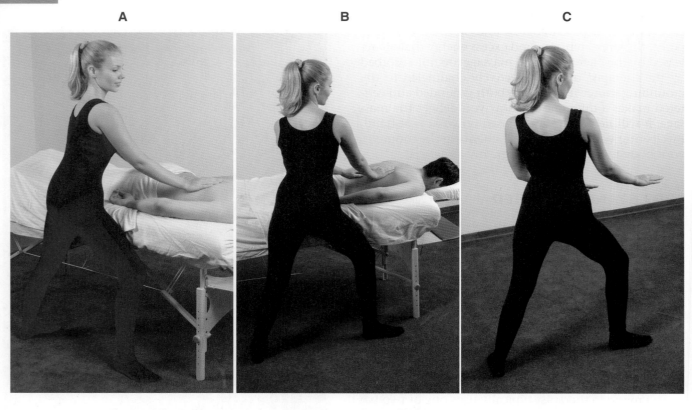

Figure 6-5   **A,** Therapist in bow stance from side angle. **B,** Therapist in bow stance from back angle. **C,** Therapist in bow stance from back angle without table and client.

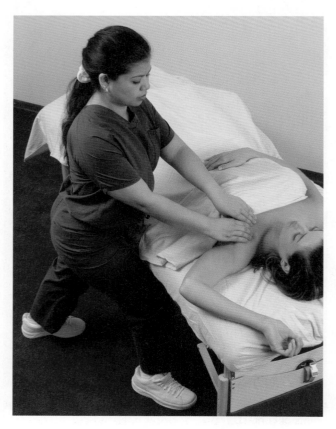

Figure 6-6   Get behind your work.

both the bow and warrior stances, let movement be initiated from your stable base (feet planted firmly on the floor) up to the center of balance (*hara* or *dantien*) and then through the arms and hands (see Figure 6-3).

The Bow Stance

Also known as the *archer stance* or *lunge position,* the **bow stance** is often used when applying effleurage, or any stroke where the therapist proceeds from one point to the next along the client's body. The feet are placed on the floor in a 30- to 50-degree angle, one pointing straight forward (lead foot) and one pointing off toward the side (trailing foot). The lead foot is pointing in the direction of movement (Figure 6-5, *A*). The distance between the two feet will vary.

To apply massage along a limb or the trunk, keep the rear leg planted on the floor and shift the weight, while flexing the knee, onto the forward leg up to about 60% (beyond this, balance may be lost). Avoid movements that bring the knee beyond the placement of the foot. For longer stroking or to advance along the table, place the trailing foot behind the lead foot, then step forward with the lead foot (Fig 6-5, *B* and *C*). With the bow stance, you will shift your body weight and return to your original position, without bending over or losing contact with

A   B   C

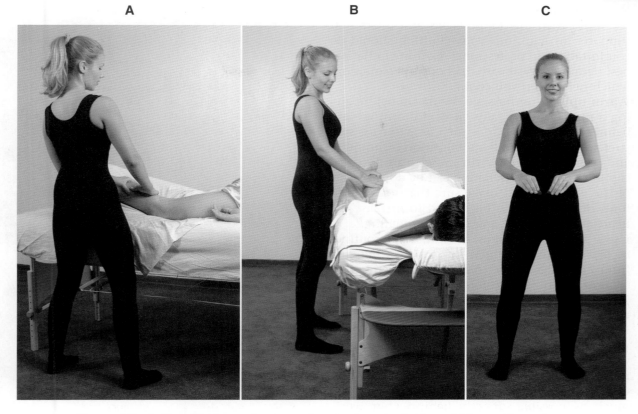

Figure 6-7   A, Therapist in warrior stance from back angle. **B,** Therapist from side angle. **C,** Therapist from front angle.

your client and while maintaining a constant flow. Keep the upper and lower torso in as straight a line as possible during the massage. Never bend at the waist while advancing over the client. Whenever possible, get behind your hands while working in the bow stance (Figure 6-6).

The Warrior Stance

Also known as the *horse stance*, the **warrior stance** is used to perform massage strokes that traverse relatively short distances, such as pétrissage and certain friction strokes, and reaching over to the far side of the body. Both feet are placed on the floor, toes pointing forward a little more than hip distance apart (Figure 6-7, *A* through *C*). The actual distance between both feet depends on your hip size and height. Shorter people have a lower center of gravity and their feet tend to be closer together. Taller people, who have a higher center of gravity, place their feet farther apart. You may find that women, who have wider hips, place their feet farther apart.

If you are having difficulty maintaining balance, readjust your foot distance until maintaining the warrior stance feels effortless. Once the proper foot distance is located, soften your knees by allowing them to flex slightly. Keep your hips pointed forward and

your back straight. Your shoulders should be relaxed while your hands and arms perform the work, transfering the load through the torso to the legs and feet. As long as both feet are on the floor, you may lean against the table with your thighs. Shift your weight from one foot to the other as your hands move across the client's skin and muscles. This stance works particularly well for a two-handed alternating pétrissage. If a lifting or lowering action is required to apply a massage stroke, raise or lower your body by bending your knees and keeping your back straight.

GUIDELINES FOR PROPER BODY MECHANICS

1. **Check table height.** If you are working on a table that is not yours or if someone else has borrowed your table, check the table height before beginning the massage to make sure it is appropriate for you. A proper table height allows you to use your weight rather than your strength to develop pressure. Position the table accessories (e.g., head rest, arm shelf, and bolsters) to fit the client's body proportions to give you optimum access to the various body parts with a minimum of strain. For further discussion, see Chapter 3.

2. **Wear comfortable attire.** Wear sensible supportive shoes with low or no heels and good arch supports. In addition, your clothing should be comfortable and professional. Cotton clothes are best because they absorb the body's perspiration, which helps keep you cool.

3. **Warm up before massage.** Warm up before giving a massage, especially on cold mornings and before strenuous routines such as active assisted stretching, Trager, body mobilization techniques, and sports massage. Warm muscles are less susceptible to injury. Stretching can be done as part of the warm-up, but make sure that some other form of warm-up has been used to increase the heart rate and blood flow before stretching.

4. **Use a variety of strokes.** Most massage routines incorporate an assortment of strokes. Changing from effleurage to pétrissage to tapotement to friction uses different muscle groups, thus reducing fatigue and repetitive motion injuries. As the therapist, you must also listen to your own body. If the right forearm is fatiguing, use the left arm more; if compressive movements are irritating wrist and knuckle joints, change to a lifting move such as pétrissage.

5. **Get behind your work.** Position yourself, as much as possible, directly behind your work. Both arms and legs should face the direction in which pressure is applied. If pushing a heavy object, you would not stand beside it; you would stand directly behind (see Figure 6-6).

6. **Check in with hips, knees, and feet.** Hips should be level and knees slightly bent. Never lock the knees straight or back. Keep your feet planted firmly on the ground while standing. Shift weight from one foot to another to reflect what your hands are doing.

7. **Position shoulders, arms, wrists, and fingers.** Place your shoulders comfortably on top of your rib cage. Keep your upper arm perpendicular to your upper body and your forearm parallel to the ground whenever possible. When your arms are far away from your body, they tend to fatigue faster. Avoid reaching across the table because this can strain your back. Your shoulders and upper back should be relaxed to help you keep your wrist and fingers in proper alignment. Avoid raising your shoulders toward your ears.

The hand and wrist are designed for articulation and dexterity, not weight bearing, so it is important that you perform exercises to stretch and strengthen these muscles and practice moderation when applying strokes.

Keep the wrists as straight as possible (Figure 6-8). At times, it will be necessary to flex and extend the wrist, but remember that the greater the pressure, the straighter the wrist should be. Hyperextending the wrist while applying pressure

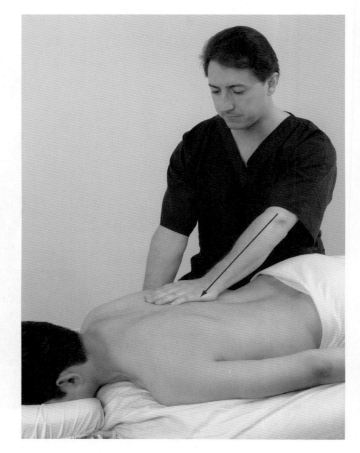

Figure 6-8   Correct wrist posture.

can produce overuse injuries such as tendonitis and carpal tunnel syndrome. When not being used, keep wrists and fingers relaxed.

Do not let the digits become hyperextended while applying direct pressure. Use braced finger and thumb techniques to avoid joint hyperextension (Figure 6-9, *A* and *B*).

8. **Lean or sit.** Lean, sit, or brace yourself against the table when needed. Most Swedish moves require that the therapist be in motion, but some modalities require the therapist to lean on the client, brace themselves against the table, or sit on the table for a short time. Leaning into the client can be used for ischemic compression requiring deep static pressure. Make sure both feet are on the floor, and you are not overly contracting your arm and shoulder muscles to produce downward force. Avoid staying on your feet the entire day. A stool can be used while performing foot, neck, or facial routines (Figure 6-10, *A* and *B*). Keep both feet flat on the floor with the back straight while seated. This maintains a stable base and reduces strain on the upper body.

9. **Body aligned.** Keep your back straight by tilting your pelvis backward (posterior tilt), which flattens out the low back and reduces an exaggerated

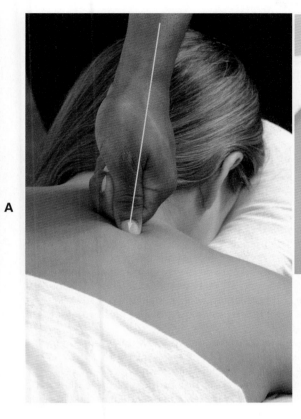

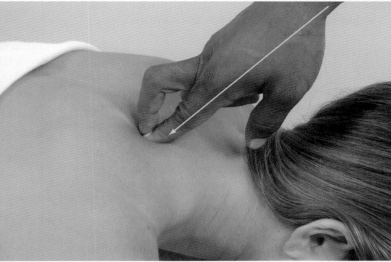

Figure 6-9 **A,** Braced thumb techniques; **B,** braced finger technique.

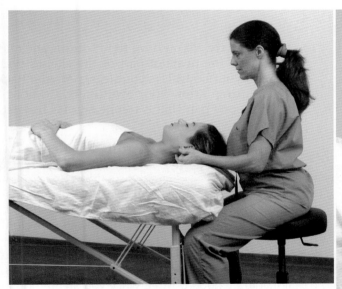

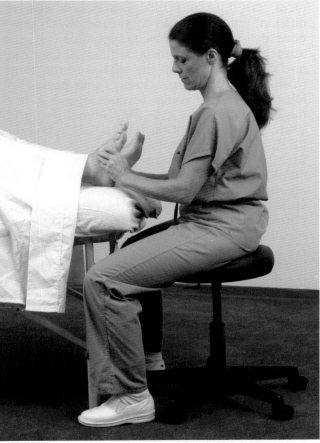

Figure 6-10 Therapist using stool. **A,** Neck work; **B,** foot work.

lumbar curve. Use the penny-pinching technique (see the Mini-Lab for instructions).

MINI-LAB

To experience a posterior-tilted pelvis, try the penny-pinching technique. While standing, imagine that you have a penny between your buttocks. To keep the penny from falling to the ground, contract your gluteal muscles and "pinch" the penny. This simple exercise straightens your back muscles, pulls in your abdominal muscles and tilts your pelvis backward.

Keep your body in correct alignment by maintaining your head over your neck and shoulders. Avoid a forward head posture. When working on a muscle or group of muscles, keep your eyes forward, your neck straight, and your head erect. If you spend a great amount of time looking down, your neck may become stiff. If you must observe your work, lower yourself to the level of your hands by kneeling down on the floor or sitting on a stool. Look up, out the window, or at the corners of the ceiling occasionally to stretch the anterior neck musculature. Another way to reduce the strain on your neck is to turn your head away from the direction of the massage stroke. Experiment with different head and neck positions for different massage strokes to discover which positions are more comfortable for you (Box 6-3).

10. **Stretch.** Take stretch breaks while walking from one side of the table to the other. Use this time to shake out your arms, stretch your neck, and relax. Between massage sessions spend a few minutes doing exercises to strengthen and stretch the muscles of the hands. See the box on pp. 108-109 for suggestions.

11. **Breathe.** During the massage, use deep, full abdominal breathing. This will aid you in self-relaxation and helps keep a steady pace with your massage strokes. Apply the pressure stroke during the exhale and the return stroke while inhaling. While you breathe, be aware of facial expression; keep your jaw unlocked, your forehead relaxed, and your tongue on the roof of the mouth.

12. **Move smoothly.** Find your *own* rhythm and then move *with* it. For example, pétrissage can be done more efficiently in the warrior stance with a side-to-side rocking motion. The rocking motion itself can be learned from an instructor, but the rate or rhythm is an internal component that originates within the therapist. Keep your movements smooth and flowing. What is jerky and rough for you is jerky and rough for your client too.

BOX 6-3

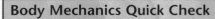

Body Mechanics Quick Check

The following is a list of questions for determining correct body mechanics during the massage:
1. Is your massage table the correct height for you?
2. Are you warming up before your first massage of the day and stretching between massage sessions?
3. Are your knees slightly bent?
4. Are your feet firmly planted on the ground?
5. Are you shifting your weight as you move, working with your whole body?
6. Are your forearms parallel to the ground?
7. Are your wrists straight?
8. Are your thumbs and fingers supported while applying direct pressure?
9. Is your back straight and your pelvis posteriorly tilted?
10. Is your head centered over your neck and shoulders?
11. Are you using a variety of strokes in your massage? Are you positioning yourself behind your strokes?
12. Is a stool nearby to be used during facial and foot massages?
13. Is your face relaxed and your jaw unlocked during the massage?
14. Are you using proper lifting techniques?

If you answered no to one or more of these questions, you may be at risk for stress, strain, and injury due to poor body mechanics.

13. **Lift correctly.** If you have to lift during the massage, keep the heaviest part of the client's body close to your body. Use your legs, not your back, when lifting. Know your own limits. Do not try to lift a body part that is too heavy. Ask for assistance.

MINI-LAB

Stand in front of a full-length mirror. Place one foot 18 inches in front of the other and place your hands on your hips. Lunge forward, shifting your weight from the back leg to the front leg. As you move forward and backward, keep your shoulders and hips level. Look in the mirror to check your progress. Maintaining a good posture while you are in motion promotes good working posture while performing massage therapy.

 The moment you commit and quit holding back, all sorts of unforeseen incidences, meetings, and material assistance will rise up to help you. The simple act of commitment is a powerful magnet for help.

—Napoleon Hill

PAUL ST. JOHN, LMT

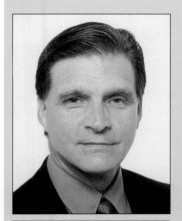

Born: July 27, 1945.

"Where all the growth is in this profession and in life is the line of most resistance. Oftentimes we resist so much of what life wants to teach us and why we're here."

The St. John method of neuromuscular therapy is a comprehensive program of soft-tissue manipulation techniques that balance the central nervous system with the structure and form of the musculoskeletal system. On a more basic level it is the study of how form affects function. The St. John method can free the body to move, stand, and simply "be" the way it was created to be from a structural and biochemical model.

Unlike some therapies that relax individuals and relieve minor pain, deep neuromuscular work zeroes in on both the problem and effect. According to St. John, the five principles of neuromuscular therapy are biomechanics, postural distortion, trigger points, nerve entrapment/nerve compression, and ischemia, all of which upset homeostasis.

Much of the charisma and commitment of Paul St. John, the man behind the method, was captured by Robert Calvert in an interview for *Massage Magazine*. St. John was 3 years old when his father, an illegal alien, was deported. Young St. John was a street kid and an average student who later discovered a learning disability. Playing high school football, he suffered a broken back, his first injury. This lead him to taking an Army recruiter's aptitude test. After doing exceptionally well, however, St. John still was not quite ready to join. Instead, his mother's battle with cancer motivated him into a career in radiology. While practicing radiology, he was drafted into Vietnam War. When his plane was shot down, two Chinese doctors accomplished in minutes what the hospital who managed his earlier leg injury in high school had not been able to do in weeks.

After returning home, his family hounded him to get a job. He hitchhiked to Florida and worked as a garbage collector until his third injury. With debilitating pain and mounting health bills, he experienced no improvement. A friend in chiropractic care then introduced St. John to the work of Dr. Raymond Nimmo, responsible for a technique known as *receptor tonus*. St. John studied this technique and soon began helping friends cope with pain. He then began massage therapy school and is now a teacher and practitioner who never wants to lose touch with clients. His own encounters with pain and those living with pain fuel his desire to do even more. He considers himself a perpetual student.

Today, he is changing the quality of lives with his methods, giving hope to people who have not found relief through conventional means. "Medicine has unconsciously become totally function oriented," explains St. John. "It ignores form, but if you have someone with a collapsed diaphragmatic posture, peristaltic action and nutrient absorption is affected. The stomach collapses and loses tone. The medical community might suggest a laxative. You've got to treat the cause and not the effect. America spent over $4 billion for analgesics, medicines to suppress symptoms, this past year [1997]."

St. John shares the results of one of his latest cases. "A young woman who was about to have a surgery to correct her scoliosis spent some time at my clinic. Doctors were going to put a rod in her back. We corrected her curvature 27%, and we have the x-rays to prove it."

He goes on to share other relationships between structure and disease. "Parkinson's patients almost all have a distortion in their cranium. In many stroke victims a forward-head posture of 6 to 8 inches is seen. This traps the arteries. Patients with cardiac problems usually have a slumping shoulder pos-

PAUL ST. JOHN, LMT—cont'd

ture. An abdominal posture affects the diaphragm, aorta, vena cava, and esophagus. That's why so many of these people develop hiatal hernias.

"Neuromuscular therapy is the best value for the money. If your carburetor needs fixing, you get it fixed, right? But we let our bodies stay broken down."

After treatment, St. John's clients ask, "Why hasn't my doctor done this? It makes so much sense!" Still, skeptics abound. A man with a bad knee who had practically been dragged to the clinic told St. John, "I know what's wrong with my knee. I'm 72 years old." St. John then pointed to the patient's good knee and said, "Oh yeah, so how old is that knee?

"He had a belief," explains St. John, "a belief in permanence creating a state of mind called *inertia*. So I created doubt by asking him about his good knee. Doubt is energy in itself. Once I created doubt in the permanence of his condition, it opened the door for me to point out that his right shoulder and pelvis were inferior, the knee was twisted and compressed, the left shoulder and pelvis were elevated."

St. John has many success stories, but because of his commitment to his work, he has little time to recount them all. He has patients waiting. The interview is over with these words of advice for the beginning therapist, "Take personal responsibility. Specialize in a certain area if you really want to make a living. Techniques that work best conform to the laws of the universe. One third medicine is intellectual; two thirds is art."

In an earlier interview, St. John offers direction for anyone seeking success. "People who accomplish great things are ordinary people who have great dreams. It's not that they are more gifted and God has smiled upon them. People who become great have great work ethics and they put a lot of sweat equity into it. They aren't lucky people, you know; they work hard, and they're committed."

TABLE MECHANICS FOR THE MASSAGE PRACTITIONER

The science of **table mechanics** involves a variety of practical considerations concerning the placement of the client on the table during treatment. These considerations include (1) client positioning (prone, supine, side-lying, or seated), (2) positioning equipment (bolsters and pillows), and (3) draping, using towels or sheets. The following table mechanic techniques are not only professional and effective; but they are designed to be time efficient and low stress to reduce workload on the therapist.

Client Positioning

Once you have interviewed your client, and directed her to the massage table, you must determine how to position her while she receives the massage. Client positioning promotes client comfort through positional release, promotes relaxation through proper body alignment, and addresses health conditions such as swelling or recent surgeries. Consider the following questions:

In which position would you like the client to lie: prone, supine, side-lying, or seated position?

How do you position the client's joints during the massage (e.g., head/neck, knees, and ankles)?

Does the client have any health condition or physical limitations that would require an adjustment to the table or additional bolstering?

The last question addresses the client who has a condition which time on the table could make worse. For example, some clients may have sinus problems that limit time spent in the prone position. A swollen ankle may need additional support and elevation. A client with severe lordosis may need a cushion under her abdomen while in the supine position.

Regardless of which positions you and the client decide, it is a good idea to ask your client, "How can you become even more comfortable?" This process allows you to fine-tune the client's position and address her comfort needs.

How to Begin?

Prone? Supine? How do you decide? What are the pros and cons of beginning prone or supine? Some therapists prefer to start their clients prone and end the massage with their clients supine or vice versa, whereas other therapists let the clients decide. The following sections detail the possibilities.

Beginning Prone, Ending Supine

Most clients complain of back-related pain. Beginning the client in the prone position allows you to massage this essential area first. Ending supine allows your client's sinuses to drain, otherwise she may leave your office with a stuffy head from laying prone last. Beginning prone also allows the genital region of the body to be underneath the client's body (an emotionally vulnerable area) and allows time for trust between the client and therapist to develop. Even with the best face rest, the client's neck may become stiff while lying prone. Beginning prone and ending supine allows the neck to be worked in the last half of the session to reduce or eliminate any neck stiffness that may have occurred from lying prone. Many therapists wrap their client up in the bottom sheet like a human cocoon. Ending supine allows this type of treatment conclusion.

Beginning Supine, Ending Prone

Clients often enjoy conversing with their therapists but also enjoy silence during the massage. When you begin the massage with the client in the supine position, eye contact between client and therapist is easy. Conversation may flow easily from the client. When the client rolls onto her abdomen, this often signals a time of quiet rest. Ending prone also allows the back to be worked last, which is often the primary area of complaint.

After these considerations, weigh the pros and cons, and decide which position sequence you or your client prefers. No matter how you begin, you may decide to finish the massage with the client in the side-lying position, allowing her to rest before getting up off the table. The side-lying position also facilitates stretching of the client's back, especially if you ask her to pull both knees to her chest into a fetal position.

Positioning Equipment

To provide greater client comfort and proper body mechanics in the prone, supine, or side-lying position, use positioning equipment and bolstering devices. These cushions support the client's individual joints, which in turn more fully relaxes the muscles (Figure 6-11). The most commonly bolstered areas are the *face/head, neck, ankles,* and *knees.* Special placement of bolsters for clients in the side-lying position is discussed in the draping section of this chapter. In the absence of commercially manufactured bolsters, a rolled-up towel, blanket, or pillow may be used.

Many therapists store bolsters under the table, on a low shelf, or on the floor. The therapist may bend down to get these bolsters, replacing them in their storage areas before the client rolls over, and before the client gets up when the massage is finished. Typically, three bolsters are used per session. If you see six clients per day, you will be bending about 36 times per day just for bolsters. Avoid bending over because this action alone may cause low back strain. Instead, squat down to get bolsters, stand the bolsters on their end in a convenient corner, or place them on a shelf at chest level for easy frequent access.

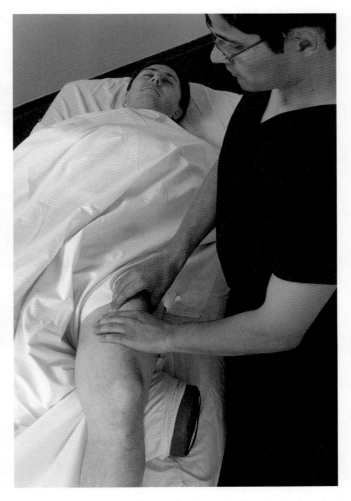

Figure 6-11 Supine client using knee bolster to help relax back musculature.

Position the seam running lengthwise on the bolster away from the client's body. This prevents any uncomfortable sensations or compression marks left on the client's skin. Always drape the bolster or pillow with a protective covering such as a towel, pillowcase, or specially designed bolster cover. These covers are washed after each client use. The bolster may also be placed between the bottom sheet and the table surface. Remove the bolster before your client gets up off the massage table to dress. When needed, clean your bolster with a mild detergent such as dish soap. See Chapter 3 for more discussion on bolsters.

Prone Position

The most commonly supported areas when the client is in the prone position are anterior ankles and the head/neck complex. If possible, use a face rest or specially designed prone pillow. This allows your client to keep her neck straight while lying face down. Some tables possess a wide slit for the face, allowing the client to lie prone without a face rest. If a face rest is not available, one or two standard-size pillows may be used, placing them either horizontally or diago-

nally under the forehead and shoulders. Large-chested women may need additional pillow support under the breasts or lengthwise along the sternum.

A vinyl-covered 3- or 6-inch diameter bolster under the anterior ankles allows the hips, legs, and ankles to relax fully during the massage. Try both sizes to see which one works best for each client. If the client complains of his low back feeling strained by lying prone, a pillow or soft cushion placed under the abdomen or pelvis reduces the anterior curve, which may reduce the strained feeling. For added shoulder and arm relaxation, an arm shelf or linen-draped stool placed under the face rest can be used for a forearm rest (Figure 6-12, *A* and *B*).

Supine Position

When the client is in the supine position, the most commonly supported areas are the posterior cervical region and the posterior knees. Use of a knee bolster helps relax the low back. A soft cloth-covered cervical pillow is best; place it at the lower cervical region, not the occipital region (Figure 6-13). A rolled-up bath-size towel can be used as a cervical pillow; fold both long sides toward the middle, leaving a 1-inch

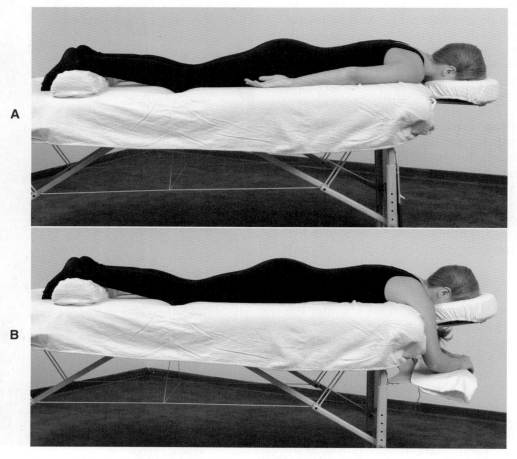

Figure 6-12   A, Prone client with bolsters and face rest; **B,** with the addition of an arm rest (see Figure 3-8, *A*).

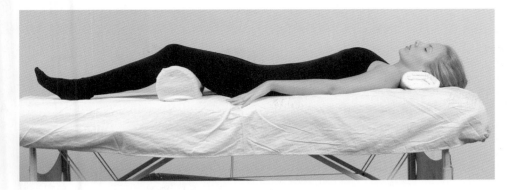

Figure 6-13 Supine client with bolsters (see Figure 3-8, *B*).

space down the middle before rolling the towel (Figure 6-14). If you are working on a narrow table and have a large client, consider providing a side extension accessory, giving additional width to the table and support for your client's arms.

While you are massaging the feet in the supine position, place a large pillow under the feet to elevate them; this provides easier access to the feet and facilitates proper body mechanics for you (Figure 6-15). This added foot support also assists dependent drainage in cases of lymphedema. You may sit on the massage table or on a stool while massaging the client's feet. Avoid permitting the client to raise her own feet simultaneously because this may strain her low back. Instead, ask her to place one foot on the pillow at a time or lift her feet for her onto the pillow.

If needed, the therapist can use a modified supine position for pregnant clients, clients with respiratory problems, or any client who is more comfortable in this position. The modified supine position has the client's upper body elevated about 30 degrees. See Figures 9-10 and 20-5 in this text.

Side-Lying Position
The side-lying position is preferred for pregnancy, some older adults, and for various other conditions. The client may lie in either a right lateral or a left lateral recumbent position. Ask the client to lay on the

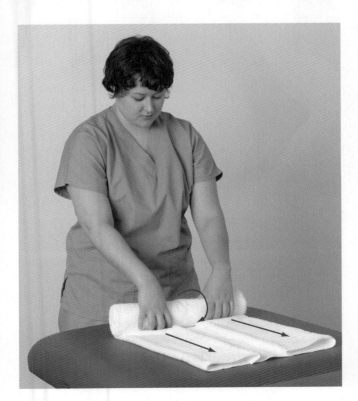

Figure 6-14   Rolling up a bath-size towel for a cervical pillow

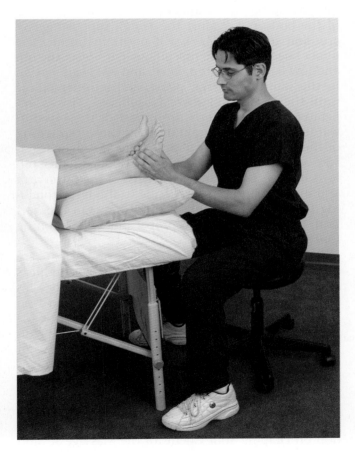

Figure 6-15   Therapist sitting on a stool, massaging a clients foot placed on a pillow.

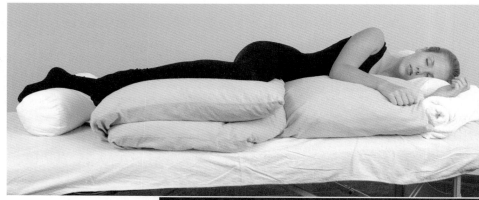

Figure 6-16 **A,** Side-lying client with bolsters and pillows.
B, Overview of side-lying position.

A

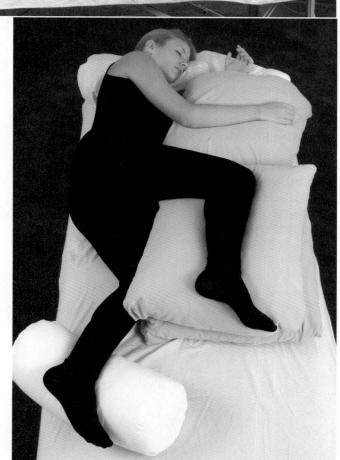

B

side on which she feels most comfortable, but you may dictate the direction. The client will spend most of the treatment time on the first side, as much of the body can be accessed from this position.

Ask the side-lying client to slide back so her backside is near the edge of the table (approximately 4 inches). This not only will make it easier for the therapist to work the client's back, but it also provides additional table space in front of the client for pillows to be placed. Use three or four pillows; place the first pillow underneath her head. The next pillow should be placed under the upper arm (the side of the body not against the table), supporting her arm and shoulder. The last is positioned under the upper knee and ankle; this pillow helps relax the hip and low back. If the hip, knee, and ankle are not all in the same horizontal plane, add another pillow until the proper alignment is achieved. This is imperative; if the ankle is unsupported, the hip outwardly rotates. This rotation may cause tightening of the outward rotator musculature and may aggravate sciatic conditions. Two additional smaller pillows may be added under the wrist of the lower arm and under the lower ankle (side of the body touching the table). See Figure 6-16, *A* and *B* in this section, which demonstrates proper pillow positioning for the side-lying position.

Because the back, parts of the legs, and feet are approached from a side position, the therapist adjusts his body position for the best leverage. This may include using a stool, squatting, or kneeling down on the floor.

Roll the client over and complete the massage on the second side-lying position; treatment time spent should be considerably shorter. Before your client changes positions, or before she gets up from the massage table after the session, remove all pillows and bolsters to reduce obstacles that may impede a smooth recumbent-to-upright transition. See the section on Draping Your Client for the Massage Session for more information on draping the side-lying client.

MINI-LAB

Acquire approximately six pillows of various sizes, a massage table, and a partner. Ask your partner to lie on the massage table in the supine position, and use the pillows to create a variety of comfortable positions. Once all possibilities are explored, remove the pillows from the massage table and ask your partner to turn over and lie on his side. Reuse the pillows to position your partner's arms, legs, and so on. Repeat the activity in the prone position. This method will help you discover new and creative ways to work with pillows as positioning equipment.

Seated Position

The seated position is a massage given while the client is seated. The client may be sitting in an ordinary chair or a specially designed massage chair. Devices are also available that sit or clip onto a tabletop that accommodate the client leaning forward. When an ordinary chair is used, the client may lean forward and rest her head on a cushion placed on the top of a nearby table (Figure 6-17, *A* through *C*). The seated position may be preferable in one of the following situations:

- The client prefers a seated massage.
- A massage table is not available.
- Adequate physical space is not available to set up a massage table or to use proper body mechanics during the massage.
- The client has a condition (e.g., handicap, pain, mobility problem, or medical condition) that makes it difficult to get on or off a massage table.
- The client is in a wheelchair. NOTE: It may not be feasible for the client to transfer to a massage table or chair. Work with him in the wheelchair. Simply roll the chair up to the side of the massage table so that his legs are underneath. Lock the wheels in position, lean the client forward on a cushion, and proceed with the massage. See Chapter 9 for more details.
- The client has reservations about removing clothing for the massage.

If you have determined that the seated position is best for serving your client, refer to Chapter 25 for specific details on how to position your client for comfort and accessibility.

Draping Your Client for the Massage Session

Draping is essentially covering the body with cloth. The purpose of using a drape during massage therapy is to (1) provide a professional atmosphere, (2) support the client's need for emotional privacy (modesty), (3) offer warmth, and (4) provide access to individual parts of the client's body. Covering up the body with cloth allows the client to be undressed while receiving the massage.

The primary comfort consideration is warmth. As the massage session progresses, the client becomes relaxed and shifts into a parasympathetic state. When this occurs, a drop in basal body temperature and blood pressure occurs. The client may become chilled and have difficulty relaxing. Always ask the client if he is comfortably warm at least twice during the session—once before you start the massage and halfway through. If he indicates that he is chilled, additional draping may be added by placing a blanket across the top sheet. On the flip side of the issue, your client may become too warm due to pregnancy or being peri- or postmenopausal. If this occurs, expose more body surface area, provided the following areas remain draped: the genital region on both men and women, the gluteal cleft, and in some regions, breast area on females.

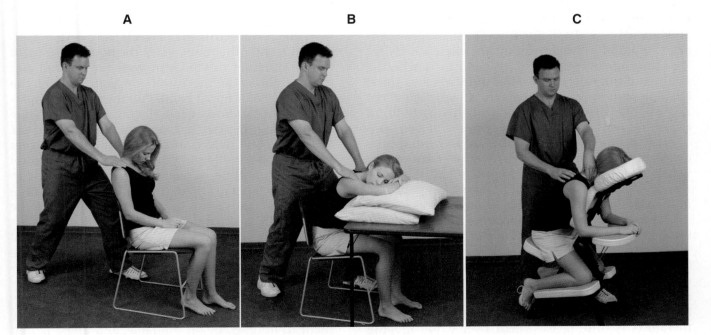

A   **B**   **C**

Figure 6-17   **A** and **B,** Client receiving seated massage in ordinary chair. **C,** Client receiving seated massage in a massage chair.

The drape not only constitutes the therapist's professional and ethical boundaries, but it also represents the client's modesty boundary. In regard to modesty of either the therapist or client, three basic rules apply. The *first rule* is the state or local laws regarding draping. This is your minimum draping standard, and you cannot drape with less than the law requires without endangering your license. The *second rule* is to honor the client's individual request for draping. As long as it does not conflict with your state laws, you may add extra draping or remove superfluous draping. The *third rule* is that the massage therapist also has to be comfortable with the level of draping. For example, a female client may schedule a massage from a therapist in a state that has no massage therapy legislation. The female client may be perfectly comfortable with no top drape, but the therapist may be uncomfortable with this situation. In this case, the therapist discusses the situation with the client. The resolution may range from the massage performed with a top drape or the client locating a different therapist. For more information regarding draping and ethics, see Chapter 2.

A general rule is to expose only the body areas being massaged. For example, if you are massaging the back, both legs should be draped. If you are working on the posterior aspect of the left leg, the back *and* the right leg should be draped. By exposing only the areas that are being massaged, all areas of concern are addressed—that is, warmth, privacy, professionalism, and easy access.

It is improper to lift, fluff, or move the sheet in such a way as to make the fabric leave the client's body. The sudden feeling of "air space" may violate the client's feelings of warmth, security, relaxation, and privacy, thus detracting from the massage experience. Avoid lifting the sheet off the client's body for the turning over process. When an anchoring method of turning (described in the Sheet and Towel Draping sections of this chapter) is used, the client can feel the drape in contact with his body at all times and feel secure about his privacy. If you accidentally expose the client, look away and redrape the exposed area. It is generally better to acknowledge your error with a simple pardoning of yourself while remaining composed. A look of horror on your face only makes the uncomfortable situation worse.

The two main types of drapes are sheets and towels. Become proficient at using *both* types of drapes because you may find yourself in a situation requiring the use of the one you do not normally use. Be patient with yourself while learning draping techniques; it takes time and practice and is considered an art in itself. A challenge for most new massage therapists is turning the client over while keeping the draping securely in place. It is in turning the client that most accidental exposures occur.

Work like everything depends on you and pray like everything depends on God.
—Thomas Aquinas

MINI-LAB

One way to practice draping is to put on a pair of bright undergarments OVER your regular attire. Lay on a table with the drape over you. Have a classmate practice turning you over while NOT exposing your bright undergarments.

Towel Draping

Towels are often used as draping materials. They are thicker, heavier, more opaque than sheets, smaller, and easier to use when accessing treatment areas such as the abdomen. However, towel draping is more difficult to master. Typically, one towel is used for draping male clients, and two towels are used to drape female clients, but do provide more drape if a client requests it. A flat or fitted sheet is used as a table cover beneath the client with towel(s) draped over the client.

When using towel draping, fold the towel back or under to reveal the area to be massaged. In most circumstances, the towel stays where it is folded, but it may be tucked underneath the body to provide a more secure drape. Avoid using towels when a client is in a side-lying position; they typically do not provide enough coverage.

Towel Draping Male Clients. Instruct the client to undress, lie on the table, and drape himself with one towel across the pelvis (Figure 6-18, *A*). After you reenter the room, grasp the bottom corner of the towel closet to you with your lower hand and the top corner of the towel (opposite side of the table) with your upper hand. Pull these corners apart until slight traction is felt (Figure 6-18, *B*). While maintaining traction and keeping the center of the towel over the pelvis, rotate the towel 90 degrees with the top hand pulling the far corner of the towel across the midline of the clients body to the hip nearest the therapist. At the same time, with the same speed, move the lower hand away until the corner held is on the opposite side of the clients body (Figure 6-18, *C*). The towel is now draped down the legs (Figure 6-18, *D*). The towel will be turned back in its original position before the client is turned over.

Towel Draping Female Clients. Instruct the client to undress, lie on the table, and drape herself crossways with the two towels—one across her torso and the other across her pelvis (Figure 6-19, *A*). The

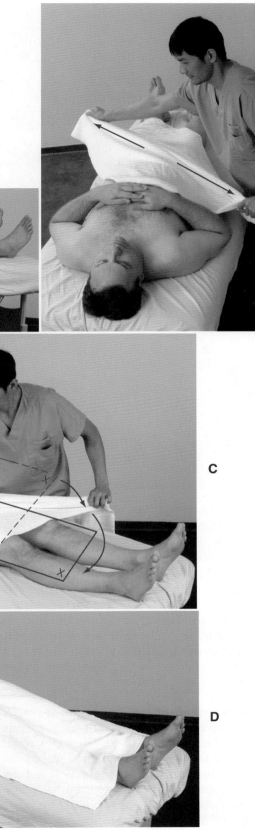

Figure 6-18 **A,** Male client on table with towel draped across pelvis. **B,** Therapist holding towel at opposite corners with traction, ready to rotate. **C,** Therapist rotating towel 90 degrees. **D,** Client on table with towel draped down legs.

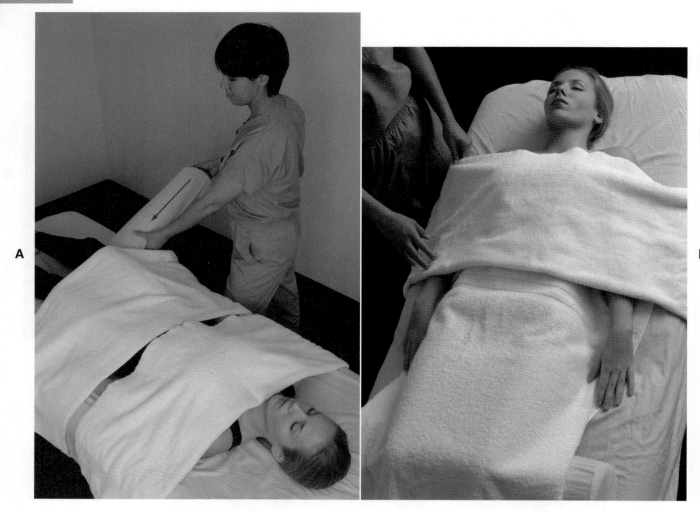

Figure 6-19   A, Supine female client on table with two towels draped across torso and pelvis. **B,** Client on table with towels in T formation.

two towels should be parallel to each other but perpendicular to the client's body, like an equal sign (=). After you reenter the room, use the technique detailed previously to rotate the bottom towel 90 degrees. When towel rotation is complete, the bottom towel will be parallel to the body, creating a T where it meets the top towel (Figure 6-19, *B*). The towels will be returned to the equals sign formation before the client is turned over.

Accessing the Abdominal Area on Female Clients.   Towel draping is convenient for accessing the abdomen in the supine position. The top towel is pulled down until the top edge is at the level of the clavicles. The bottom corners of the top towel are lifted with both hands and the towel is fanfolded on itself across the breasts to act as a bikini top. Care must be taken to keep the female breasts covered while the abdomen is being exposed (Figure 6-20, *A*). To redrape the client's abdomen, simply anchor the top edge of the towel with one hand at the sternum and pull the center of the towel down toward the

lower towel, unfolding the fanfolds as you go (Figure 6-20, *B*).

Turning the Client Prone to Supine.   NOTE: This discussion assumes the therapist is using two towels. Modify the instructions for a single towel. When turning the client from prone to supine, it is necessary that the direction of rotation be *toward the therapist.* This prevents undraping the client accidentally. First, remove all positioning equipment from the table before turning the client over. Instruct the client to scoot down until her head is resting on the table and off the face rest, guiding the towels down with her for proper coverage. Rotate the lower towel back to the equal sign position if the towel placement is still in the T formation (Figure 6-21, *A*).

Grasp the top corner of the top towel with your upper hand and the lower corner of the top towel and upper corner of the bottom towel with your lower hand. Anchor the towel edges nearest you by leaning on them, thus securing them to the table. Instruct the client to turn to face you and continue

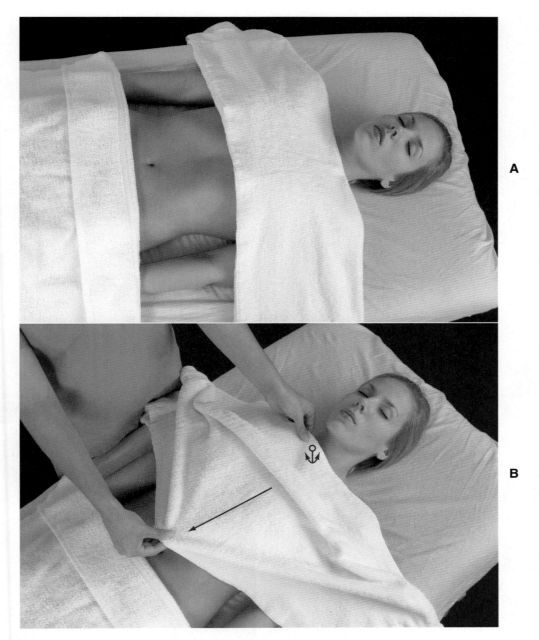

Figure 6-20 **A,** Supine female client on table with towel draping, abdomen exposed.
B, Therapist holding top of towel while unfolding the fanfolds with other hand.

turning (Figure 6-21, *B*) until she is all the way over onto her back (180 degrees) (Figure 6-21, *C*). Use verbal instructions and hand gestures such as tapping the table to direct the client which way to turn. Return the bottom towel to the T formation before proceeding with the massage (Figure 6-21, *D*). Place bolsters under the client's neck and behind the knees (see Figure 6-19, *A*).

Turning the Client Supine to Prone. NOTE: This discussion assumes the therapist is using one towel on a male client. If needed, modify the instructions for two towels. When turning the client from supine to prone, it is necessary that the direction of

rotation be *away from the therapist.* This prevents undraping the client accidentally. First, remove all positioning equipment from the table and rotate the towel until it is perpendicular to the body. Anchor the towel against the table with your body (Figure 6-22, *A*). Instruct the client to turn to face away from you and continue all the way over until he is on his abdomen (Figure 6-22, *B*). Use verbal instructions and hand gestures such as tapping the table to direct the client which way to turn. The client may scoot up and make use of the face rest. Rotate the towel 90 degrees until the towel is parallel to the client's body, draping him from the waist to the ankles (Figure 6-22, *C*). Place a bolster under his ankles (Figure 6-22, *D*).

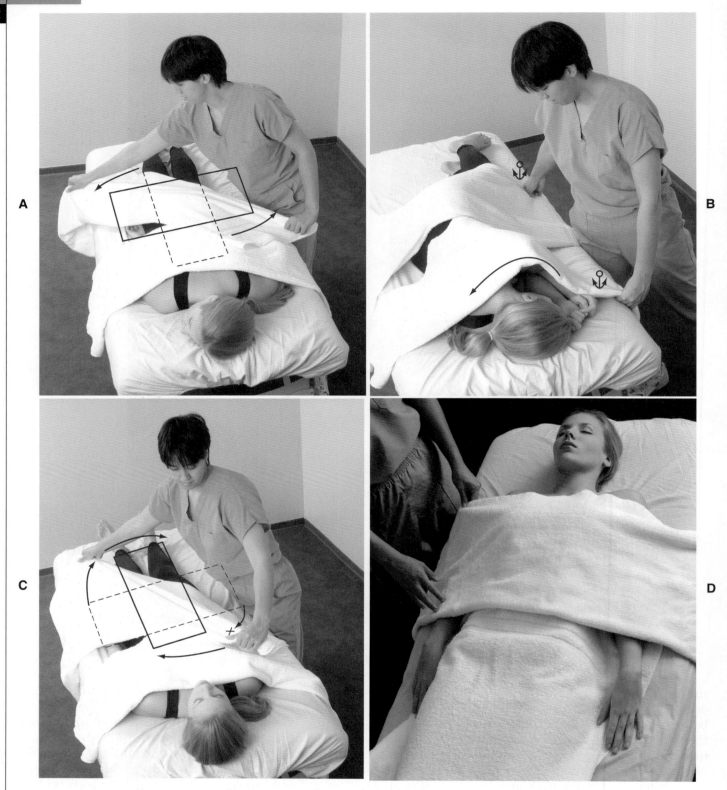

Figure 6-21   A, Therapist rotating lower towel back parallel on prone female client. **B,** Client rolling over while therapist maintains holds and anchors towels. **C,** Therapist rotating lower towel back to T formation. **D,** Supine client draped with towels in T formation.

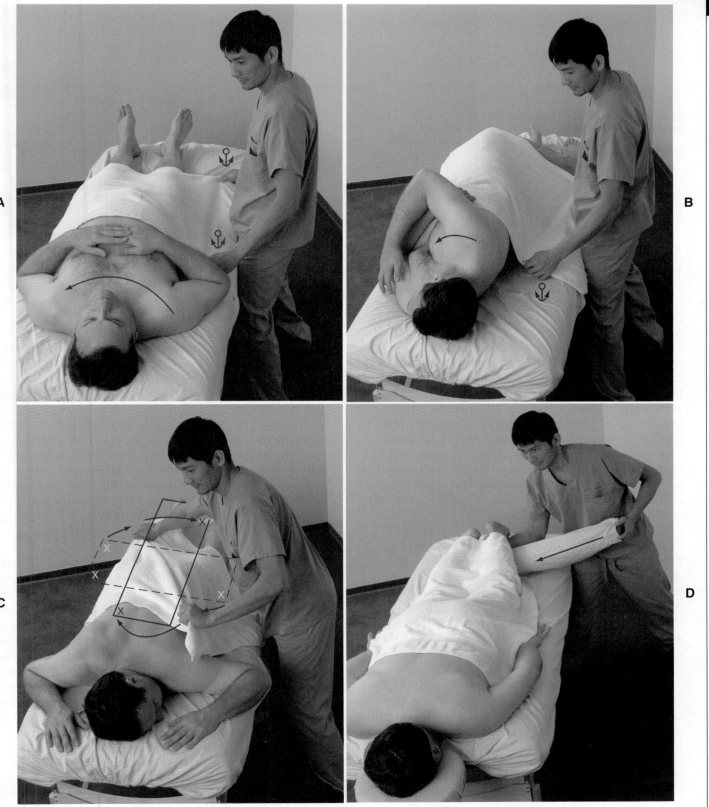

Figure 6-22 **A,** Therapist holding towel and client ready to turn. **B,** Client rolling over while therapist anchors and holds towel. **C,** Therapist rotating towel. **D,** Client draped with towel down legs.

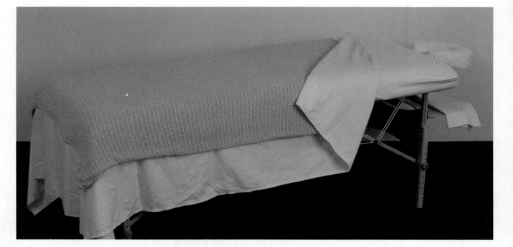

Figure 6-23 Sheet arrangement on table without client.

Sheet Draping

Two sheets are required for each client: one sheet draped over the client and one sheet covering the massage table. Clients and therapists may prefer using sheets because they are already familiar with this arrangement; it is how beds are made. Twin-size sheet sets are preferred (fitted sheet for the table drape and flat sheet for the client drape), but a double-size flat sheet folded in half may be used as the table drape. Arrange the top flat sheet neatly on the bottom sheet, folding down the top corner edge to reveal the bottom sheet. This gives the draped massage table an inviting appearance (Figure 6-23). As you undrape specific areas of the body for massage, tuck the ends of the fabric underneath the client's body. Untuck the sheet, and re-drape when moving to a different area for massage.

Accessing the Abdominal Area on Female Clients. Two different methods of sheet draping can be employed to work the abdominal region on a female. First, the lower edge of the sheet can be pulled up to waist level, which creates a surplus of material around the midsection. The sheet is then arranged in a C-shaped window to expose the abdominal area while keeping the pelvic and breast regions covered (Figure 6-24, *A*).

The second method of accessing the abdominal area requires the use of a towel or pillowcase. A towel is draped on top of the sheet, across the breasts, and perpendicular to the body. The top center edge of the towel is held at the level of the clavicles with one hand. The other hand pulls the sheet out from under the towel without moving the towel from its location. Once the sheet is clear of the towel, the sheet is folded back to expose the abdomen, with the towel acting as a bikini top (Figure 6-24, *B*).

Turning the Client Prone to Supine. When turning the client from prone to supine, it is necessary that the direction of rotation be *toward the therapist.*

This prevents undraping the client accidentally. Remove all positioning equipment from the table. Uncover the feet because they may become entangled in the sheet while the client is turning over. Instruct her to scoot down until her head is resting on the table and not on the face rest. Grasp the sheet along the opposite edge of the table, while anchoring the sheet with your thighs on the side of the table closest to you (Figure 6-25, *A*). The therapist's hands are holding the sheet at the level of the client's shoulder and pelvis. Instruct the client to turn and face you and to continue turning until she is all the way onto her back (180 degrees) (Figure 6-25, *B*). Sometimes it helps to pull a little extra top sheet material toward the therapist before beginning to turn the client (Figure 6-25, *C*). It may be helpful to reinforce your instructions to the client by the use of hand gestures such as tapping the table to direct the client which way to turn.

Turning the Client Supine to Prone. When turning the client from supine to prone, it is necessary that the direction of rotation be *away from the therapist.* This prevents undraping the client accidentally. Remove all positioning equipment from the table and uncover the feet to prevent getting entangled in the sheet while the client is turning over. Hold the sheet along the opposite edge of the table, while anchoring the edge of the top sheet on the side of the table closest to you (Figure 6-26, *A*). Instruct the client to turn away from you (Figure 6-26, *B*) and to continue all the way over until he is on his abdomen (Figure 6-26, *C*). Ask him to center himself on the table and to move up and make use of the face rest (if any). Place a bolster under the ankles. Again, it may be helpful to reinforce your instructions to the client by the use of hand gestures such as tapping the table to direct the client which way to turn.

Side-Lying Draping Technique Using Sheet Draping. Drape the side-lying client with a sheet. Proceed with the massage as usual, exposing one area

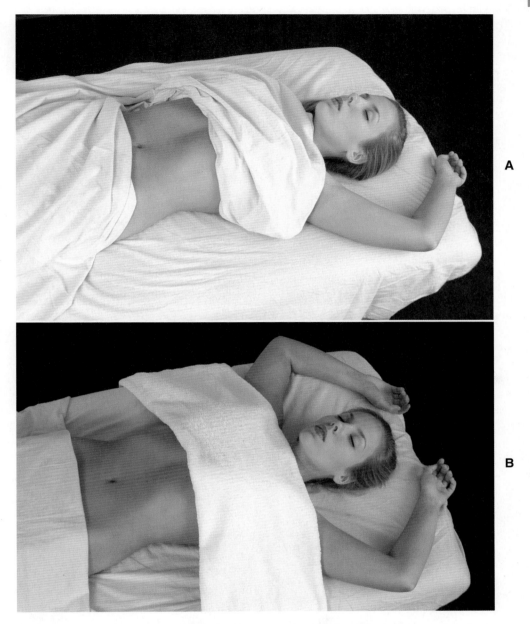

Figure 6-24 A, Female client using sheet draping to create a window to access the abdomen. **B,** Using a sheet and towel to access the abdomen.

at a time. When the back, and neck are uncovered, use a towel folded in half lengthwise, draping it over the client's side to secure the sheet drape (Figure 6-27, *A*). The arm is worked from the front while the client is draped from the chest down (Figure 6-27, *B*). For the bottom leg, drape as you would if the client were lying prone or supine (Figure 6-27, *C*). For the top leg, undrape and tuck the sheet back around under the leg (Figure 6-27, *D*). The back can be worked while the therapist is seated in a stool or chair (Figure 6-27, *E*).

Turning the Client Supine to Side-Lying or from Side-Lying to Opposite Side. Remove all

positioning equipment from the table, except the head pillow. With the client in the supine position, grasp the sheet along the opposite edge of the table, while anchoring the sheet with your thighs on the side of the table closest to you (Figure 6-28, *A*). Ask her to turn and lay on the side that she feels most comfortable. She will roll 90 degrees or a quarter turn either toward or away from you (Figure 6-28, *B*). Use the bolstering recommendations located in the Positioning Equipment section earlier in this chapter (Figure 6-28, *C*). Typically, the massage time is shorter on the second side because the back and neck were already addressed.

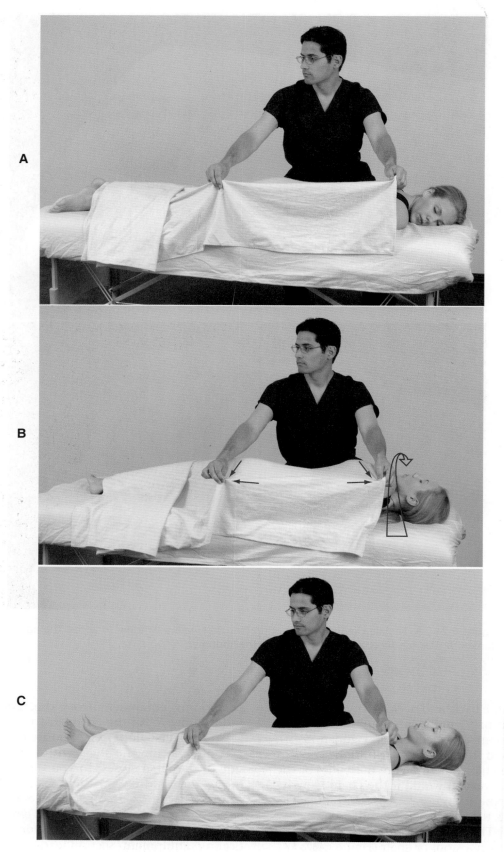

Figure 6-25 **A**, Prone female client with feet uncovered ready to turn while therapist holds sheet in place. **B**, Client in mid-turn while therapist holds sheet in place. **C**, Client now in supine position.

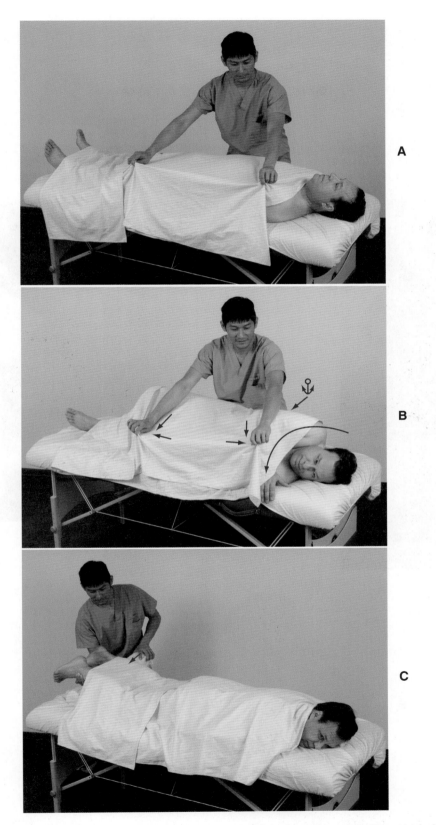

Figure 6-26 **A,** Supine male client with feet uncovered ready to turn while therapist holds sheet in place. **B,** Client in mid-turn while therapist holds sheet in place. **C,** Client now in prone position.

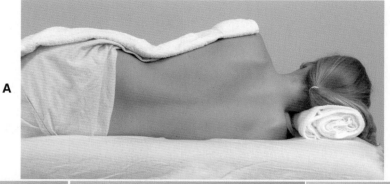

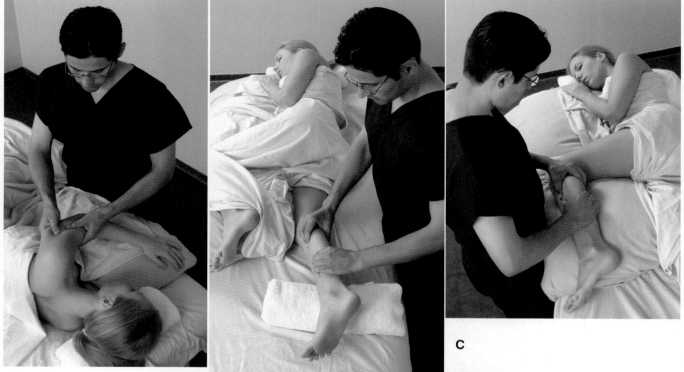

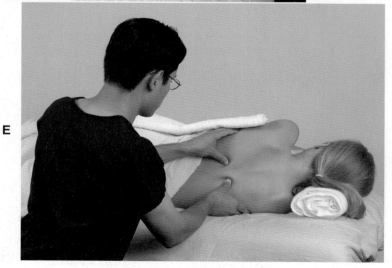

Figure 6-27   **A,** Female side-lying client with exposed back and neck while a towel holds sheet in place. **B,** Therapist massaging client's arm. **C,** Side-lying client with bottom leg exposed. **D,** Side-lying client with top leg exposed. **E,** Massaging back of side-lying client.

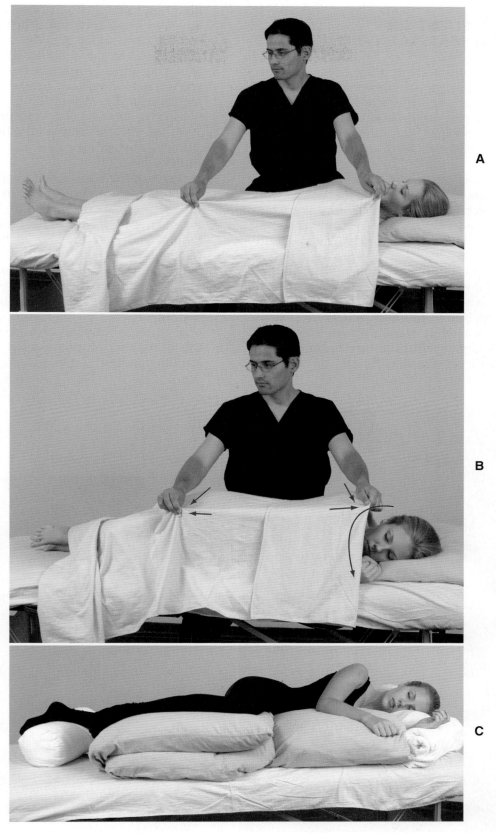

Figure 6-28   **A,** Supine female client with head pillow ready to turn while therapist holds sheet in place. **B,** Side-lying client rolling over. **C,** Client on other side with bolsters and pillows in place.

ASSISTING A CLIENT ON AND OFF THE MASSAGE TABLE

From time to time, a client may need assistance getting on the table or sitting up and getting off the massage table once the massage is complete. Geriatric clients may use a stool when getting on the table. The therapist may offer her forearm as a brace for the client to lean on while getting on or off the table.

A variety of methods assist the client getting off the table, while keeping the client comfortably draped and protecting the therapist's back against injury. This method assumes the therapist is using sheets as the drape; however, towels may be substituted.

Remove all positioning equipment used during the massage and explain the procedure to the client. The client needs to be in the supine position, so you may have to ask him to roll over. Follow these steps:

1. Face the client while standing with the side of your hip or thigh against the massage table at the client's waist level (Figure 6-29, *A*).

2. Place your closest arm under the client's closest arm and grasp under and behind her shoulder. Ask the client to reach under your arm and grasp your closest arm or shoulder (Figure 6-29, *B*).

3. Slide your other arm under the client's back until you are supporting the opposite shoulder from behind. Grasp the edge of the top drape while supporting the shoulder with your arm (Figure 6-29, *C*).

4. With the client assisting, raise her to a seated position. Use your legs, not your back, to assist in lifting.

5. Pull the sheet loosely about her neck and shoulders while continuing to secure the top edge of the drape (Figure 6-29, *D*).

6. Reach over the client's knees and cup your palm around and over the side of her opposite knee (Figure 6-29, *E*).

7. While supporting the client's back with your upper arm, pull her knees toward you in a swivel so that her lower legs dangle off the table edge (Figure 6-29, *F*).

8. Maintaining your upper arm around her shoulders, use your other arm to support the client into a standing position (Figure 6-29, *G*). Do not let go of

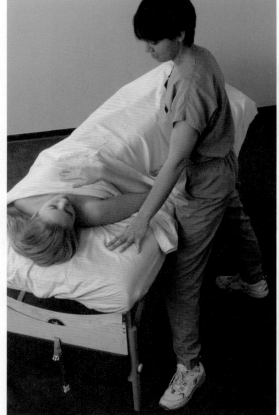
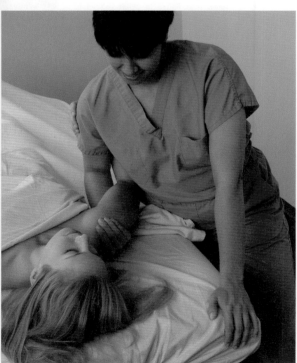

Figure 6-29   A, Therapist's body prior to assisting client, highlighting stance. **B,** Therapist grasping behind client's near shoulder and client grasping therapist's shoulder.

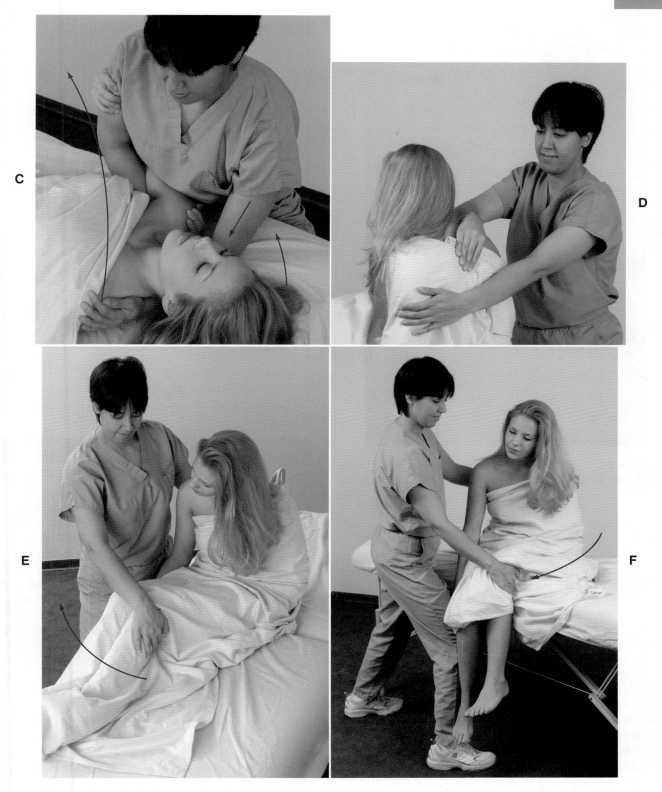

Figure 6-29, cont'd   C, Therapist sliding other hand under client to opposite shoulder. **D,** Therapist adjusting and securing drape once client is in seated position. **E,** Therapist reaching over both client knees. **F,** Therapist rotating client till feet dangle off table edge.

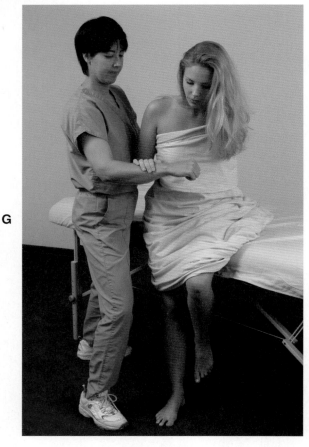

G

Figure 6-29, cont'd   **G,** Therapist maintaining drape while client gets off table, using therapist's other arm for support.

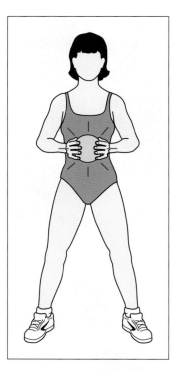

Figure 6-30   Bioenergy exercise.

the top edge of the drape until your client has it securely in her hand and drapes herself appropriately.

MINI-LAB

To generate bioenergy, begin by rubbing your hands together vigorously for 1 minute. Separate them about 5 inches, and be receptive to a light sensation between your hands. It may feel like the attraction or resistance of two magnets. Experiment by moving your hands very slightly closer together and then farther apart. Let your right hand move in a small circle while your left hand is still. Reverse. Imagine a ball of energy between your hands. Move your hands back and forth, and imagine the ball becoming malleable. Breathe in and out slowly as your hands move. Imagine the ball growing as you separate your hands and compressing as you move your hands together (Figure 6-30). Finally, separate your hands as far as possible, and turn the palms outward, allowing the ball of energy to dissipate.

SUMMARY

As a precursor to giving the massage, we have explored two subjects that must be taken into consideration regarding both the client and the therapist. One topic is *body mechanics,* which refers to personal health care and the proper use of postural techniques to deliver massage therapy with the utmost efficiency and with minimum trauma to the practitioner. Body mechanics reduce the physical toll taken on the therapist's body both on a daily basis and cumulatively over a long career. Specifically, body mechanics includes the use of foot stances, body postures, and leverage techniques based on the principle elements of strength, stamina, proper breathing, stability, balance, and being grounded or centered. Each of these elements is essential to the success of the massage. Use self-care techniques to prevent or treat minor aches and pains that arise from working too hard or too long (Figure 6-31). The other main topic is the study of table mechanics, which comprises setting the table height, positioning, bolstering, and draping the client. Table mechanics ensure that every step has been taken to provide a physically secure and emotionally comfortable space for the client in a way that is time and energy efficient to the therapist.

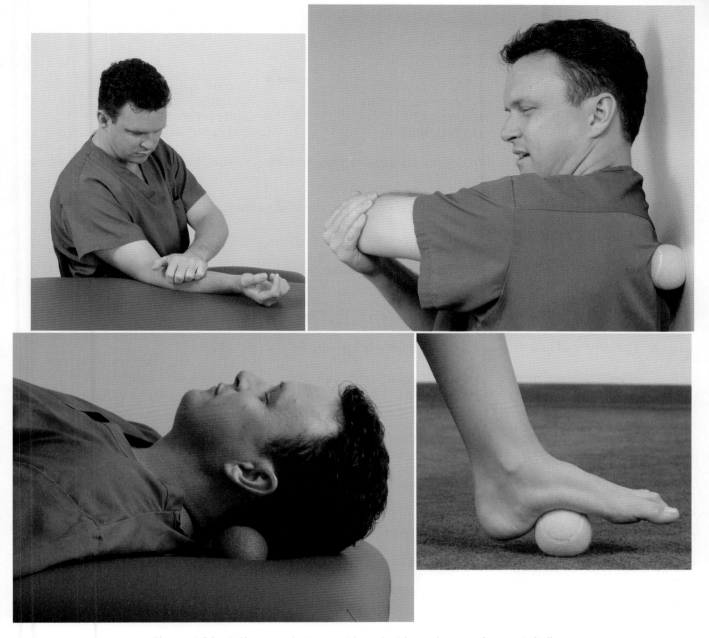

Figure 6-31   Self-care techniques with and without the use of a tennis ball.

MATCHING

List the letter of the answer next to the term or phrase that best describes it.

A. Bow stance
B. Side-lying position
C. Repetitive motion injuries
D. Prone

E. Warrior stance
F. Hara or dantien
G. Warmth
H. Breathing

I. Supine
J. Draping
K. Body mechanics
L. Strenuous occupation

_____ 1. Postural techniques used to deliver massage therapy with the utmost efficiency and with minimum trauma to the practitioner

_____ 2. According to Bonnie Prudden, how the profession of massage therapy is classified

_____ 3. The position of a client when lying on his abdomen

_____ 4. Covering the body with a cloth for professionalism, client's emotional privacy, and warmth, while accessing the client's body for massage

_____ 5. According to William Barry, the foundation of massage

_____ 6. The center of gravity located 1 to 2 inches below and behind the navel

_____ 7. The foot stance most often used when applying effleurage, or any stroke where the therapist proceeds from one point to the next along the client's body; one foot pointing in the direction of movement

_____ 8. The foot stance used to perform massage strokes that traverse relatively short distances; both feet are placed on the floor with toes pointing forward at a little more than hip distance apart

_____ 9. Injuries related to inefficient biomechanics; a constant motion, combined with compressive forces, causing injury to soft tissues

_____ 10. Position preferred for pregnancy, some older adults, and various other conditions

_____ 11. In the art of draping, the primary comfort consideration

_____ 12. The position of a client when lying on his back

Bibliography

Barry W: Massage body mechanics, *Massage Magazine* vol 60, 1996.

Barry W: *Personal communication,* 2001.

Beck MF: *Theory and practice of therapeutic massage,* ed 3, Albany, NY, 1999, Milady.

Coughlin P: *Principles and practice of manual therapeutics,* New York, 2002, Churchill Livingstone.

Grafelman T: *Graf's anatomy and physiology guide for the massage therapist,* Aurora, Colo, 1998, DG Publishing.

Prudden B: *Pain erasure,* New York, 1980, M Evans and Co.

Torres LS: *Basic medical techniques and patient care for radiologic technologies,* Philadelphia, 1993, JB Lippincott.

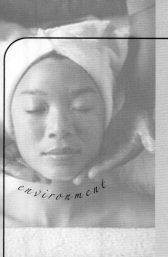

environment

Swedish Massage Movements and Swedish Gymnastics

7

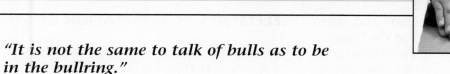

pressure

"It is not the same to talk of bulls as to be in the bullring."

—Spanish Proverb

STUDENT OBJECTIVES

After completing this chapter, the student should be able to:

- Describe and implement the following basic elements used in applying Swedish massage strokes: intention, touch, pressure, depth, excursion, speed, rhythm, continuity, duration, and sequence
- Describe and perform the five basic Swedish massage strokes and their variations: effleurage, pétrissage, friction, tapotement, and vibration
- Perform Swedish gymnastics (stretches and joint mobilizations) on articulated body segments

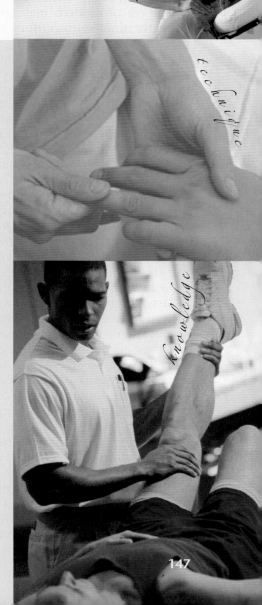

technique

knowledge

INTRODUCTION

Massage has been around for millennia, probably since early man hit his head on the roof of the cave and instinctively began to rub it to reduce the pain. Massage in Asian countries developed according to eastern philosophy, spirituality, theories of energy movement, and clinical practice. Massage in western society was originally based on early religious and medical ideas and has evolved under the influence of modern medicine, biology, and sports models. This chapter concentrates primarily on a western style of massage, Swedish massage.

Swedish massage is the systematic and scientific manipulation of the soft tissues of the body for the purpose of establishing or maintaining good health. One writer defined massage as organized, intentional touch. Massage is used for a variety of reasons: to bring a client to a deeper level of relaxation, to rehabilitate, to prevent an injury, or to slow the progression of an illness.

The era of modern massage began to develop in the early nineteenth century, when a wide variety of practitioners were advocating massage and developing their own systems. The most important of these writers was Pehr Henrik Ling (1776-1839), a Swedish physiologist and gymnastics instructor. Because of his nationality, Ling's system became commonly known as *Swedish massage,* and he became known as both the father of Swedish massage *and* physical therapy.

The most widely used system of massage therapy in North America is the Swedish system. The five basic massage strokes or movements used to administer Swedish massage are effleurage, pétrissage, friction, tapotement, and vibration. Dutch physician Johann Mezger promoted Swedish massage using the western medical model and is given credit for introducing and popularizing the use of French terminology into the profession (see Chapter 1.)

Swedish gymnastics, part of the Ling system, is also discussed in this chapter. The primary movements used in Swedish Gymnastics, which include stretches and joint mobilizations, can be performed actively and passively. Furthermore, the therapist can assist or resist active movements.

Understanding the effects of these movements on the body is an essential prerequisite for the *scientific application* of massage. *Masterful application* requires the addition of one basic ingredient—practice, practice, and more practice. Recall any distinguished musical composer or performer; a musician practices scales before advancing to symphonies.

A master of massage, like a martial arts master or professional dancer, no longer has to think about the moves; she has totally integrated science and art—the physical, emotional, intellectual, and spiritual aspects of movement—into her own body. The massage therapist uses her whole being when practicing her craft. This includes using all of her sensory facilities, spatial awareness, and client receptiveness for meticulous execution of massage strokes. Your skills of massage will evolve and mature as you evolve and mature as a therapist.

 It's not the age; it's the mileage.
—Harrison Ford as Indiana Jones
in Raiders of the Lost Ark

ELEMENTS IN APPLICATION OF STROKES

During your study of massage therapy, you quickly discover that applying massage movements is much more than placing your hands on the body and manipulating skin, muscle, and fascia. Skillful application of massage strokes is a blend of the hand movements themselves, and your body mechanics, as well as pressure and depth, excursion, rhythm and continuity, speed, duration, and sequence. These elements affect not only the body's response to massage therapy but also the intensity of the response.

A client seeks massage therapy services for many reasons, but what a client may yearn for are the three Ts—touch, talk, and time. In our advanced, technological society, many people feel distant and out of touch. The time your client spends on your table or chair has many benefits that cannot be scientifically measured. Massage is an art *and* a science.

As you begin your study of massage, your initial struggle is just to remember the names and order of the strokes. As you practice, your strokes integrate certain qualities (intention, touch, depth, pressure, excursion, speed, rhythm, continuity, duration, and sequence) which vary within a session and from client to client. Let us examine these concepts to deepen your understanding and then use them as you evaluate your own progress and digest the critiques of others.

Intention

Based on a plan of action, **intention** is a consciously sought out goal or a desired end. All other elements in the application of massage are dependent on intention. The massage therapist begins to formulate her intention when the client states her current and long-term needs. As the therapist begins to palpate the tissues and administer the massage, objective findings are taken into account, helping her further establish the massage treatment's intention. An example of a current need may be to reduce tension in the upper shoulders. A long-term goal may be to circumvent the build up of stress and tension. This process is ongoing and changes as massage is integrated into your client's experiences.

Touch

Touch is the medium of massage and a powerful therapeutic tool. In this context, touch is not casual but full of meaning and intention. In some methods, touch is a modality in and of itself (e.g., in therapeutic touch and healing touch). Touching the client on the head, feet, or back is one of the best ways to begin and end the massage session (Figure 7-1). Often, a moment of quietness accompanies the initial contact with your client, giving him the opportunity to become accustomed to you without distracting conversation.

Pressure and Depth

Pressure is the application of force applied to a surface (the client's body). Usually the therapist uses her own hands, elbows, or forearms when applying pressure; however, handheld tools can be used. Most massage tools are made of wood, rubber, glass, or stone. If a tool is used to apply pressure, disinfect it between sessions. Pressure may also be applied with the knees or feet when integrating the use of Eastern techniques.

Achieved through the application of pressure, **depth** is the distance traveled into the body's tissues. The therapist can control the amount of pressure exerted on the tissues, but the client often influences depth during treatment. A tense, contracted muscle prevents the therapist from going deep into the tissues

(guarding). A relaxed muscle will yield and allow the therapist to push deep into the tissues. Hence, the depth achieved is a combination of the calculated depth and the muscle receptivity or resistance.

Initially, the pressure should be light to moderate, gradually adding more pressure until the desired effect is achieved. More pressure may be applied simply by changing your body position to put more (or less) of your own body weight into the stroke or by lowering (or raising) your massage table. Avoid applying pressure past the client's pain threshold. Pressure tolerance is best known by asking the client. The amount of applied pressure is ultimately determined by the intention of the massage and client tolerance. Pressure to affect lymph flow is different than pressure to reduce the hypersensitivity of a trigger point. After tissue release has occurred or the desired results have been accomplished, gradually release the pressure.

The amount of pressure that the therapist uses depends on the following:
- Purpose or intent of the massage stroke
- Condition of the tissue before the application of a massage stroke
- Massage stroke the therapist is using
- Area on the body where the pressure is being applied
- Response of the client (i.e., reaching the client's pain threshold) during the application of pressure

If too much pressure is used, the client guards by tensing the muscle, decreasing the stroke's effectiveness so that little depth is achieved. Too much pressure irritates tissues, causing soreness and/or bruising. Avoid heavy pressure on delicate or thin-tissued areas such as the face, dorsum of the hand, and anterior throat. Thick muscular areas such as the back,

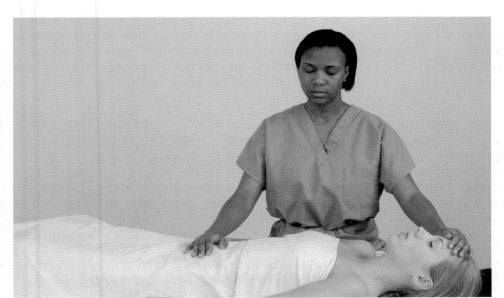

Figure 7-1 Supine client with therapist touching the client's forehead and abdomen in a quiet focus.

legs, or hips can withstand greater pressure. Sufficient pressure is needed to create positive tissue changes as evidenced by hyperemia, softening of tight bands, and deactivation of trigger points. With appropriate training, practice, and common sense, you can make good pressure judgments.

As pressure is being applied, observe the client's facial expressions or changes in breathing patterns. Distorted facial features or an alteration in the client's breathing (e.g., shallow breathing, holding the breath) often indicates pressure that is too great. The client may lift a limb or lift the head up off the table to indicate discomfort. Often, the therapist simply increases the surface area contacting the client's skin without reducing pressure. For example, if you are using a fingertip to apply pressure, change to the palm of your hand.

Keep your pressure consistent as your hands move over the client's skin, releasing pressure while maintaining contact. The use of even pressure and anticipated motion helps build trust with your client. It is easier for relaxation to take place when the client feels safe. If each long movement feels like a rollercoaster ride, the client will always be braced for the next unpredictable push.

Excursion

Excursion is the distance traversed during the length of one massage stroke. Once the therapist has applied the desired pressure of a stroke, the next consideration is how far across the skin the movement should go. The therapist decides if the massage movement will cover the length of the muscle, the area of tissue restriction, or a topographical region such as the lower leg or the lateral border of the scapula.

Excursion has a relationship with body stance and foot placement. Longer strokes are best achieved while standing in the bow stance; shorter strokes are done in the warrior stance. Proper foot stance is vital to ensure a smooth continuum of the excursion without a change in pressure or a break in flow.

Speed

Speed refers to the change of your hand position over time or how fast (or slow) a massage movement is being executed. The therapist determines the stroke speed, but the following general rules apply:
- Rapid massage movements tend to be stimulatory.
- Slower massage movements tend to be relaxing.
- The client should be able to track the movements across his skin.
- Quick delivery of massage movements may alarm the client, causing a tensing reaction.
- Fast massage movements have a tendency to fatigue the client.

- The therapist cannot palpate and assess the soft tissues if the hand speed is too fast or too slow.

Rhythm and Continuity

The repetition or regularity of massage movements is its **rhythm**. Massage therapy is delivered using both strong and soft elements. A distinct connection exists between pressure, speed, and rhythm. Alter the rhythm of the massage to fit the intent of the session; a slower technique is ideal for stress reduction, whereas a faster tempo is more stimulatory and is ideal for pre-event sports massage.

The concept of **continuity** in massage refers to the uninterrupted flow of strokes and to the unbroken transition from one stroke to the next. It is more difficult for the client to relax when the massage lacks smooth rhythm and fluid continuity. During the massage, the therapist should keep his hands relaxed and flexible, which allows them to be lifted, without losing contact, around the bony regions and contours of the body. Rhythm and continuity come not only from what the hands are doing, but also from what the rest of the therapist's body is doing (e.g., foot placement, distance between the client and the therapist) and the height of the table.

Duration

Duration refers to the length of time spent on an area, which may be difficult to determine. Working an area too long is setting the stage for disaster. The desire to help may be overwhelming because you really want to help and, well, more massage is better, right? Wrong. More massage, especially deep pressure massage, may create inflammation and make clients sore, doing more harm than good. In this arena, experience is the best teacher. Learn to work effectively by using a variety of strokes and use ice packs posttreatment if you suspect the client may become sore. Massage soreness is like exercise soreness or even overexposure to the sun. You really do not know you have overdone it until later and often not until the next day.

Sequence

A sequence is the arrangement of massage strokes. The therapist combines massage strokes in a series of movements based on the client's plan of care. Typically, effleurage is applied initially to evaluate and warm up the tissues. Pétrissage often follows effleurage to work on tissues more deeply. Friction is used to address specific areas. Vibration and percussion may be used when the therapist deems them necessary. A series of ending effleurages often flushes out the area. Using a sequence also helps prevent repetitive motion injury to the therapist.

The Routine

The union of these aforementioned elements results in a routine. In the classroom and under the supervision of a caring and experienced instructor, you will learn several routines. Learning a routine from a book is difficult, at best. By its very nature, routines are dynamic. Each time you begin a massage, your routine will change. As you evolve as a therapist, your routine will change. With each postgraduate seminar you attend, your routine will change. With each massage you receive, your routine will change. Stay in tune with the client during the routine. A conscientious therapist continually listens to the client and the client's body, modifying her original protocol as needed. See Chapter 24 for clinical massage techniques (e.g., ischemic compression) that may be used during the routine when localized pain is found.

CLASSIFICATION OF SWEDISH MASSAGE MOVEMENTS

The five basic Swedish massage strokes have been categorized into groups according to their application. These groups are *effleurage, pétrissage, friction, tapotement,* and *vibration.* Each of these strokes are described, technically discussed, and photographically represented. Also included are stroke variations. At times, it may seem as if the description of these moves is like describing a kitten; you have a better chance of understanding them through sight and touch. Hence, learning these strokes takes more than a book. Rely on your experienced instructor(s) to demonstrate properly each move, to model technique as you go, and to guide your practice. Use the self-assessment guide to help you evaluate your progress (Box 7-1).

Hybrid strokes exist in Swedish massage, as they do in most systems. Some pétrissage variations such as ocean waves combine lifting and squeezing followed by a downward compression often seen in effleurage strokes. Pincement tapotement is a hybrid of pétrissage and tapotement as it has elements of both. The classifications presented below are one view based on tradition, research, observation, and experience (Table 7-1). Feel free to reinterpret the definitions and regroup the variations.

Effleurage (Gliding Strokes)

Description

The most commonly employed Swedish stroke is effleurage (ef-flur-ahzh). The term comes from the French word *effleurer,* which means *to flow or glide.* **Effleurage** is the application of unbroken gliding

BOX 7-1

Massage Therapist's Self-Assessment Guide

- Are the movements smooth and easy for you to do? Are the movements jarred, rough, or abrupt?
- Are your transitions smooth?
- Is your own body as fluid, easy, and open as the movement qualities you want to give to the client?
- Do you pause enough? Do you leave time for the client to respond?
- Do you know how far a stroke needs to go? Are your excursions long enough or are they too long?
- Is there depth without invasion or intrusion?
- Do you know when to stop so as not to overwork part of the body?
- Do you use your body well (positioning, stance, leverage, and wrist angle)? Are your body mechanics complementing your massage movements?
- Are you working within an appropriate amount of time?
- Is the session feeling whole and integrated?
- Does your client feel honored and invited?

movements that are repeated and follow the contour of the client's body. This stroke may be applied with the therapist's hands (palm, knuckles, fingertips), or forearm; the pressure may be either superficial (gentle) or deep. Variations are *one-handed, two-handed,* by *alternate hand,* and *nerve stroke.*

Effleurage is used to introduce touch and for applying lubricant. It is excellent for assessing and exploring surface and underlying tissues. It is also the stroke used to begin and end a massage because it is so proficient at moving blood and lymph. Effleurage can be used to prepare tissue for deeper massage and to flush out the tissue after using other strokes. Oftentimes, it is the only stroke needed to eliminate discomfort in a painful area. Effleurage can be used on virtually every type of body surface, making it the preferred transition stroke to use between other strokes.

Technique

The hand placement used in most effleurage variations is shaped like the letter L (Figure 7-2, *A* and *B*). Effleurage is, in effect, a *pushing* of the tissue both downward and away from the therapist and is delivered using a *lean-and-drag* technique. When working on the extremities, apply pressure **centripetally**, or toward the heart (or center), to promote venous blood flow. Once the excursion is complete, drag your hands back using no added pressure and only the weight of your hands. Remember to maintain contact during each repetition. Additionally, a deeper effleurage is more effectively delivered by going more slowly.

When working the extremities, work the area most proximally first, proceeding distally, stroking in

TABLE 7-1

Massage Strokes and Their Variations

Massage Stroke	Variations
Effleurage *(gliding)*	One-handed *(raking, ironing, circular)*
	Two-handed *(heart, circular)*
	Alternate hand *(raking, circular)*
	Nerve stroke
Pétrissage *(kneading)*	One-handed
	Two-handed *(praying hands, ocean waves)*
	Alternate hand
	Fulling
	Skin rolling
Friction	Superficial warming *(sawing)*
	Rolling
	Wringing
	Cross fiber
	Chucking
	Circular
Tapotement *(percussion)*	Tapping *(punctuation, pulsing, raindrops)*
	Pincement
	Hacking *(quacking)*
	Cupping
	Pounding *(rapping)*
	Clapping
	Diffused
Vibration *(shaking)*	Fine
	Jostling
	Rocking

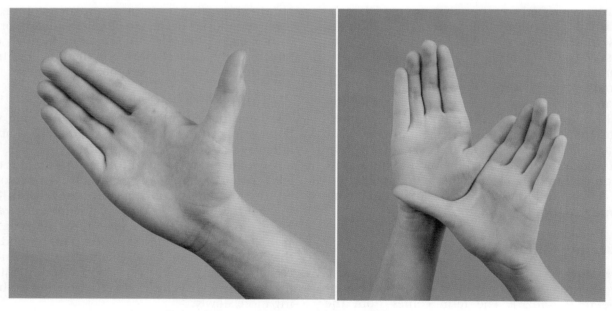

Figure 7-2   Hand(s) in L formation used in effleurage.

the direction of the heart. For example, the posterior thigh is massaged from the knee to the hip first and then the calf from the ankle to the knee. If a stroke has several phases or progressions up the leg or arm, apply more pressure when gliding from distal to proximal. When applying effleurage on the back, centripetal application does not apply because the heart is centrally located.

Avoid hyperextension of the wrist by keeping the angle between 100 and 180 degrees. This reduces repetitive motion injuries such as carpal tunnel syndrome. The therapist's hands, arms, shoulders, back, and legs should all be aligned along path of movement in order to reduce injuries and increase the ease of stroke application (Figure 7-3).

The hands should be relaxed and the movement even. Mold your hands to the contours of the client's body. Gradually increase the pressure with each repetition. Effleurage is often repeated six times on an area or until the desired effect is achieved (e.g., hyperemia, release of taut bands of tissue). Remember to apply pressure in only one direction, or you may induce friction.

Variations

One-Handed Effleurage. This variation implies that one hand or one thumb is used to apply gliding pressure and is used for small areas such as in between the metacarpals or metatarsals (Figure 7-4) or in the neck and shoulder area (Figure 7-5). Fingertips together or apart moving in one direction is called *raking*. A deep one-handed effleurage is often referred to as *ironing effleurage* and is often done with the forearm (Figure 7-6), fist, or palm of hand. The deeper the glide, the slower the move. *Circular* one-handed effleurage can be performed around the shoulder, hip, and knee and also on the abdomen (Figure 7-7).

Two-Handed Effleurage. Two-handed effleurage is executed using both hands gliding on the skin simultaneously. The hands may glide together or move apart. This variation works well up or down the back in a heart shape or *heart effleurage* (Figure 7-8), up the leg (Figure 7-9), or up the arm (Figure 7-10). One hand may be placed next to or on top of the other hand to perform the *circular two-handed effleurage* (Figure 7-11).

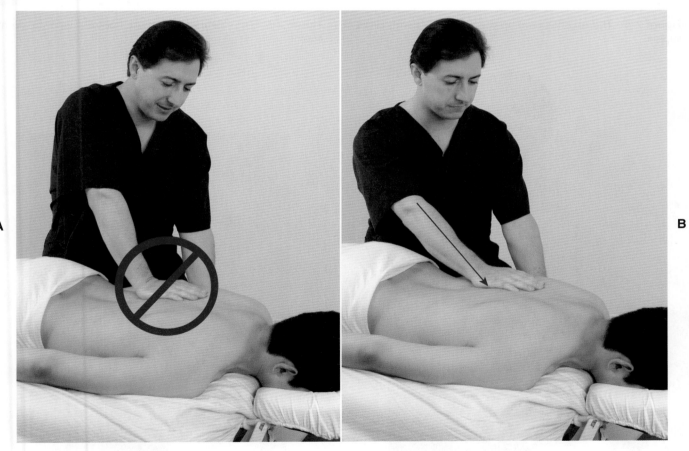

A   **B**

Figure 7-3   Incorrect **(A)** and correct **(B)** wrist alignment (see Figure 6-8).

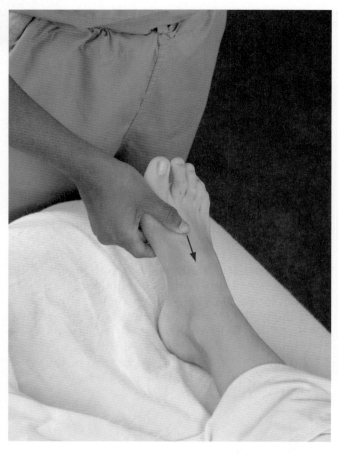

Figure 7-4 Thumb effleurage up the metatarsals with client supine.

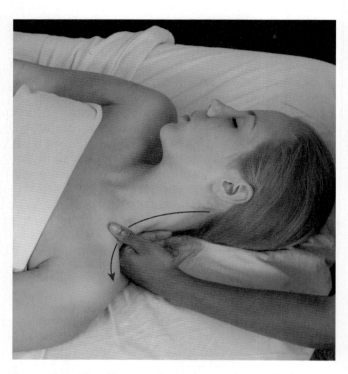

Figure 7-5 Fist effleurage down the trapezius with the client supine.

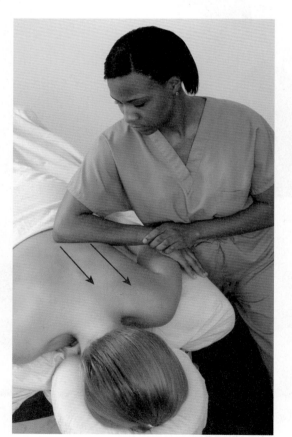

Figure 7-6 Forearm iron effleurage on the back with client prone.

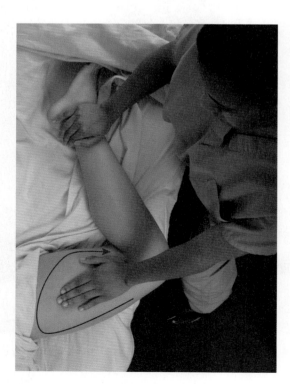

Figure 7-7 Palmar circular effleurage on a prone client's iliotibial band with knee flexed and hip outwardly rotated.

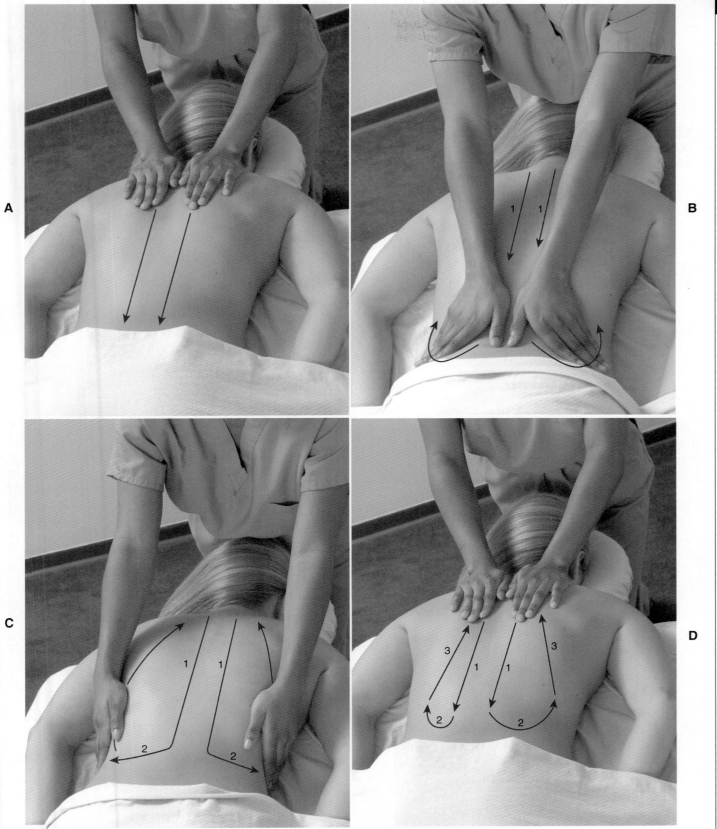

Figure 7-8   Heart effleurage with client prone.

Figure 7-9 Two-handed effleurage up the leg on client supine.

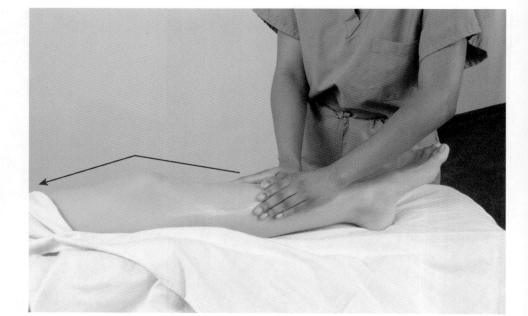

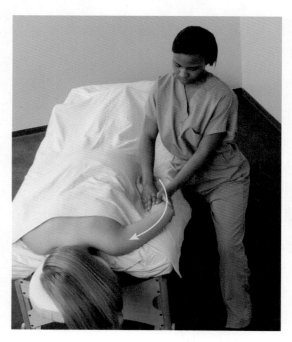

Figure 7-10 Two handed effleurage up arm with client prone.

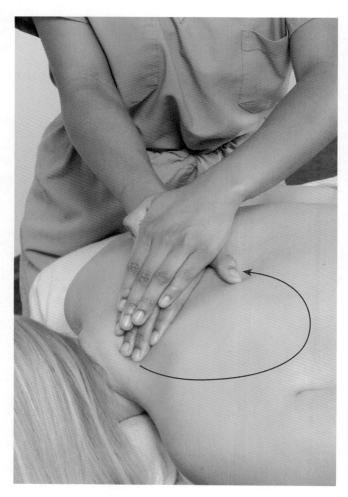

Figure 7-11 Two handed circular effleurage on shoulder with client prone.

Alternate Hand Effleurage. To perform alternate hand effleurage, glide one hand or thumb across the skin, lifting it up as the other hand or thumb follows behind in succession (Figure 7-12). Done properly, the sequence resembles a paddlewheel (Figure 7-13). The index and middle finger forming the letter V may be placed on either side of the spine. This variation, known as *alternate finger raking,* is used to move from one side of the table to the other without losing contact with the client (Figure 7-14). *Alternate hand circular effleurage* can be performed as one hand circles a region and the other hand moves behind the first hand in a half circle or a crescent shape (Figure 7-15). Because of the full- and half-circle sequence, this variation is also known as *sun-moon.* Move both hands in the same direction in all variations.

Nerve Stroke. Considered a light effleurage, nerve stroke is feather-light finger tracing over the skin. This is used as a finishing stroke in massage therapy and is typically done at the end of massaging a body segment and at the completion of the massage. Avoid pressure that is too light because it may be perceived as ticklish or produce goose bumps. The stroke may be applied to bare skin or clothed clients (sports or seated massage) or through the massage drape. The direction of nerve strokes is superior to inferior or proximal to distal because downward movements are more relaxing (Figure 7-16). Many therapists consider nerve stroking as "icing on the cake."

Benefits

Effleurage has the capacity to do the following:
- Warm bodily tissues, making them more extensible
- Relax the client and prepare an area for deeper strokes
- Soothe an area after deep work
- Soothe places too painful for deep work
- Calm the nervous system when done slowly
- Stimulate the nervous system when done quickly

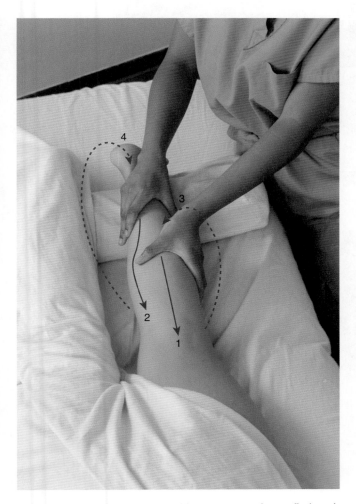

Figure 7-12 Alternate hand effleurage using butterfly hands on prone client's leg.

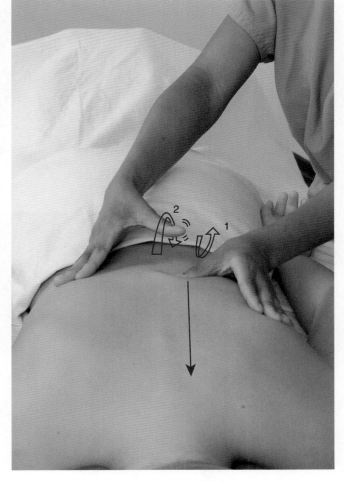

Figure 7-13 Alternate hand (thumb) effleurage up one side of the paraspinals.

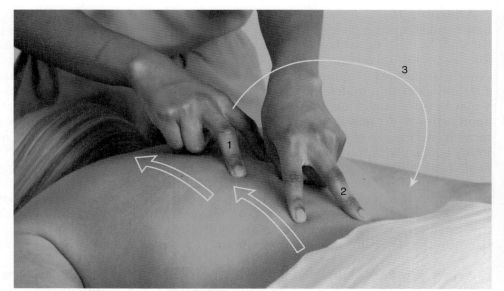

Figure 7-14 Raking up the paraspinals.

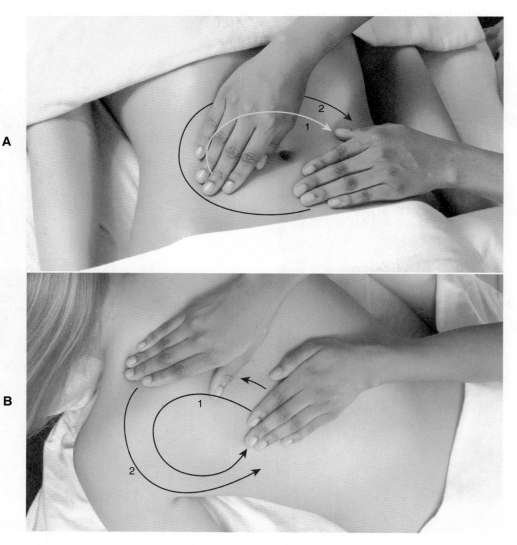

Figure 7-15 **A,** Alternate hand circular effleurage on abdomen with client supine. **B,** Alternate hand circle effleurage on shoulder.

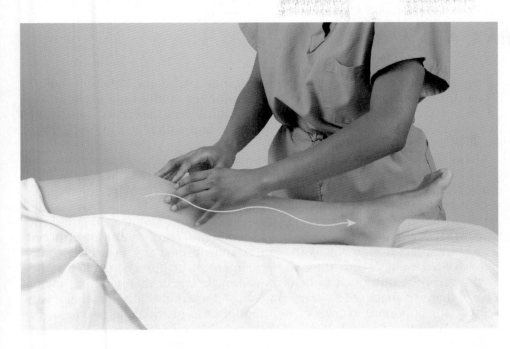

Figure 7-16 Nerve stroke down the leg while client is supine.

- Aid in the moving of wastes out of congested areas (also known as flushing)
- Create length in a muscle, if applied with fiber direction
- Increase blood and lymph circulation
- Soothe tired, achy muscles
- Relieve insomnia

Pétrissage (Kneading Strokes)

Description

The term *pétrissage* (peh-tre-sahzh) comes from the French word *petrir* meaning *to mash or to knead.* In a Swedish massage routine, pétrissage typically follows effleurage strokes. The application of **pétrissage** consists of a cycle of rhythmic lifting, squeezing, and releasing of tissue. Pétrissage is the stroke of choice to "milk" the tissue of metabolic wastes and draw new blood and oxygen into the tissues. This technique also stretches and broadens the tissue. It is important to repeat the effleurage stroke after pétrissage to flush the stirred-up waste from the area and back into the circulatory system. Pétrissage strokes can also be followed with friction, then with effleurage strokes. Several variations of pétrissage are *one-handed, two-handed, alternate hand, fulling,* and *skin rolling.*

Technique

Grasp the skin or muscle with the hand in a C formation (Figure 7-17). Lift up the skin and the underlying muscle tissue and firmly knead, wring, or squeeze. This movement should raise the muscle from its usual position, away from the bone. As you relax the grasp, repeat the first move with the opposite hand (Figure 7-18). Repeat the lifting, compressing, and releasing using one or both hands intermittently. Work in one area using several repetitions before proceeding to another area. It helps imagine that the palm of your hand is a suction cup and that you are "slurping" up the tissue. The focus is on lifting the tissue and moving it vertically or horizontally rather than just pinching it.

In general, pressure should be applied in a rhythmic circular pattern to achieve alternate compression and relaxation of the muscle. On large muscular areas such as the back, use as much of the hands as possible. Enough pressure must be used to engage

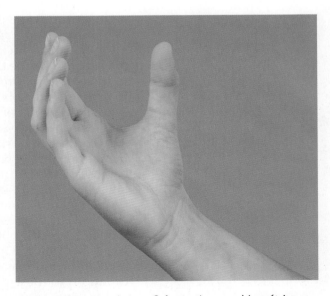

Figure 7-17   Hands in a C formation used in pétrissage.

JAMES HENRY CYRIAX, MD, MRCP

Born: 1904; died: June 17, 1985. Physician. Father of orthopedic medicine.

"He could often be seen walking backwards along Lambeth Palace Road round to the bus stop on Westminster Bridge so as to keep an eye on the oncoming buses."

James Cyriax was born in London to Edgar and Annyuta (Kellgren) Cyriax, both of whom studied medicine. His mother's family used exercise and manipulation in the treatment of musculoskeletal disorders, something that was not in common practice at the time, and which became very influential in Cyriax's medical career.

Young James was educated at University College School (Gonville) and Caius College (Cambridge) before finally graduating from St. Thomas's Hospital Medical School (London). Soon after passing his qualifying medical examinations, Cyriax became affiliated with St. Thomas's Hospital in the department of orthopedic surgery. He is generally given credit for coining the term *orthopedic medicine* and was probably one of Great Britain's most noted orthopedic practitioners. In 1938, Cyriax transformed the massage department at St. Thomas's into the first department of orthopedic medicine. His new department did much to help transform the art of manipulation into a science that was practiced by trained medical doctors and physical therapists.

Especially important in Cyriax's contributions was his system of soft tissue diagnosis. According to his *Textbook of Orthopedic Medicine* (1982 edition), Cyriax had a four-step process for determining problems of soft tissues: (1) active motion (to assess the patient's range of motion, strength, and willingness to move the affected area); (2) passive motion (to assess the degree of motion available and the direction of limitation, the use of palpable sensation at the end of passive motion that Cyriax called *end-feel,* and the determination of resistance felt by the practitioner during the end-feel testing; (3) resisted contractions (to determine the reaction of the muscle, tendon, and bony attachments to contraction); and (4) palpation (to confirm involvement of the structures suggested by the preceding three steps in the diagnostic procedure (Hayes et al, 1994).

In efforts to determine the exact location of a soft tissue lesion, Cyriax's work is extremely important (although not without numerous critics) in that it helps therapists identify the tissues causing the pain and, consequently, select the best methods of treatment to diminish the pain. In general, Cyriax advocated the use of manipulation, deep friction massage (without the use of creams or oils), and the injection of selected drugs in the treatment of soft-tissue lesions. Even though Cyriax's ideas were (and remain) controversial, he provided the first systematic diagnostic approach to determine the cause of a patient's soft-tissue disorder.

It is important to note that Cyriax was a firm believer in deep-tissue massage (deep transverse friction), either alone or in conjunction with passive or active movements, for the treatment of muscular, ligamentous, and tendinous lesions. In his *Textbook of Orthopedic Medicine* (1982 edition), he wrote, "Deep transverse friction restores mobility to muscle in the same way a manipulation frees a joint. Indeed, the action of deep transverse friction may be summed up as affording a mobilization that passive stretching or active exercises cannot achieve."

According to Cyriax's obituary in the *British Medical Journal* (July 1, 1985), he was apparently *persona non grata* within the British medical establishment because of his nontraditional views and consequently was never elected a fellow of the British Royal College of Physicians. His work continues to be scrutinized, as an examination of the various journals within the physical medicine profession attest. He was an individual who brought out the extremes in individuals, with both his supporters and critics being adamant about their views. Regardless, Cyriax was instrumental in advancing the concepts of manipulation and massage in the medical profession, making incalculable contributions to those professions.

A key indicator of the importance of James H. Cyriax's contributions is the fact that his *Textbook of Orthopedic Medicine* is presently in its ninth edition.

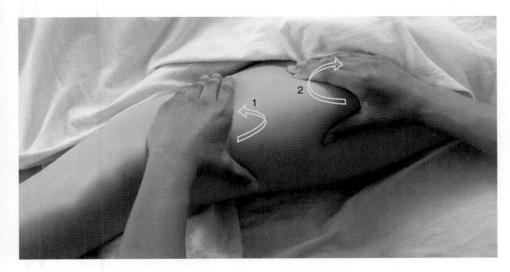

Figure 7-18 Alternate hand pétrissage on quadriceps.

the muscle, but not so much that you cause pain. If your client has a lot of body hair, a circular pétrissage may matte and pull the hair. As an alternative, use the back and forth pattern (as with ocean waves described later) instead of a circular pattern or perform the pétrissage movement on top of the sheet. Do not lose contact with the skin while you are switching hands.

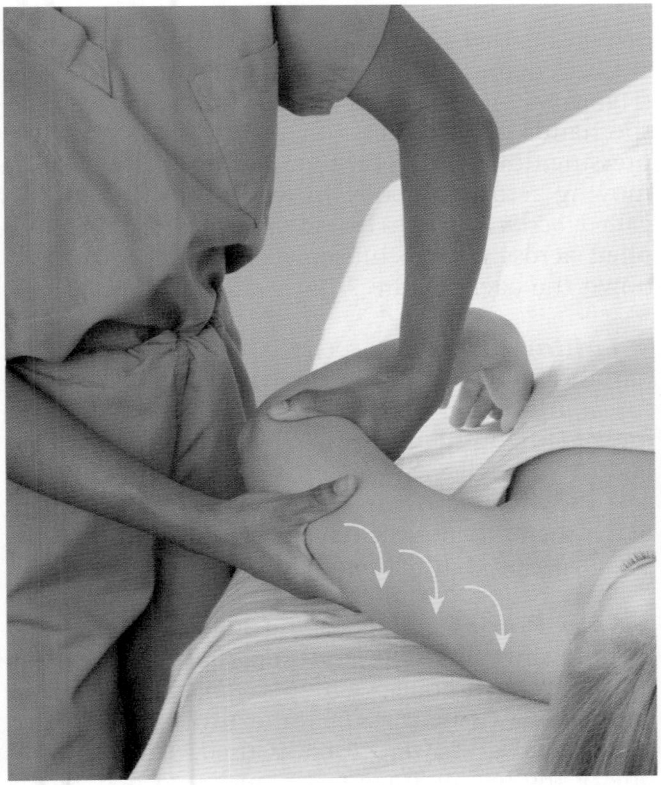

Variations

One-Handed Pétrissage. As much as the entire hand or as little as the pads of the fingers and thumb can be used to lift the tissue (Figure 7-19). This variation is well suited for smaller muscular areas such as the arms, top of the trapezius (Figure 7-20), or the arms and legs of a child.

Alternate Hand Pétrissage. Lift the skin and the underlying tissue with one hand and compress.

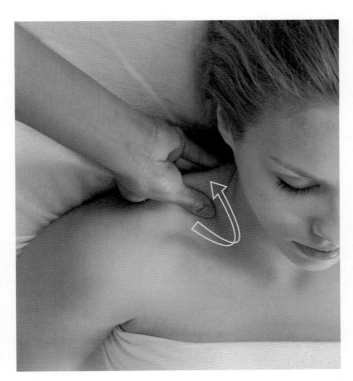

Figure 7-19 One-handed pétrissage of triceps with inwardly rotated shoulder and elbow flexed on supine client.

Figure 7-20 One-handed pétrissage using pads of fingers and thumb on trapezius with client supine.

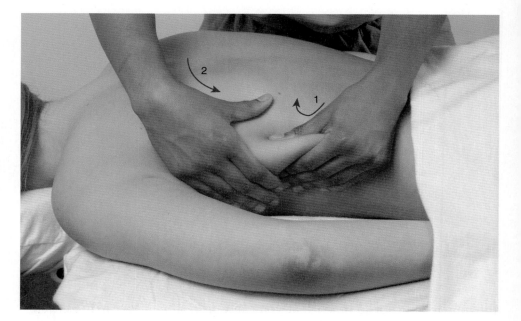

Figure 7-21   Alternate hand pétrissage on the axillary portion of the latissimus dorsi muscle with client prone.

Next, lighten the grip enough to allow the muscle tissue to be released while still remaining contact with the skin (Figure 7-21). Repeat the first move with the opposite hand. Duplicate the sequence alternating both hands (see Figure 7-18).

Two-Handed Pétrissage.   The technique for two-handed pétrissage is the same as for one-handed pétrissage, except both hands are lifting, compressing, and releasing the tissue simultaneously. Two hands are often used to address larger muscular areas such as the back. One variation uses the heels of both hands on the sides of a muscle, lifting it up before releasing it. To help maintain proper position, the fingers are interlaced in a *praying hands* position (Figure 7-22). Another variation of two-handed pétrissage adds compression to the stroke, covering both the top and sides of an area (Figure 7-23). Use a back and forth movement while the hands oppose each other, lifting the sides and pressing down while on top. Because the hands are moving across the body in waves, this variation is called *ocean waves*. This variation is typically applied across a large muscular area or horizontally down the back (Figure 7-24).

Fulling Pétrissage.   Grasp the tissue with both hands; lift it up and away from the bone while spreading it out laterally (Figure 7-25). Repeat the movements until the tissues feel warm and elastic. Fulling pétrissage is effective for broadening muscles and their related tissues and mimics the movement of a muscle when it contracts. Because of this, fulling pétrissage is often referred to as *broadening*.

Skin Rolling.   Skin rolling involves lifting and compressing the skin and superficial fascia. Skin rolling is a technique essential to *Bindegewebsmassage* (connective tissue massage) and myofascial release. Because no downward force is used, skin rolling is one of the few massage techniques that may be applied over bony areas. It may be initially uncomfortable for the client, so move gently and respect the

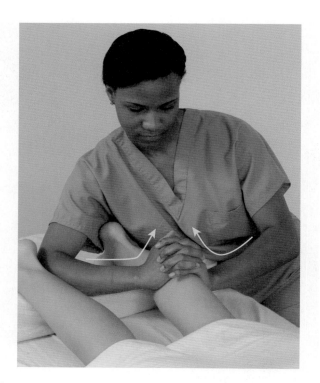

Figure 7-22   Praying hands two-handed pétrissage on prone client's calf.

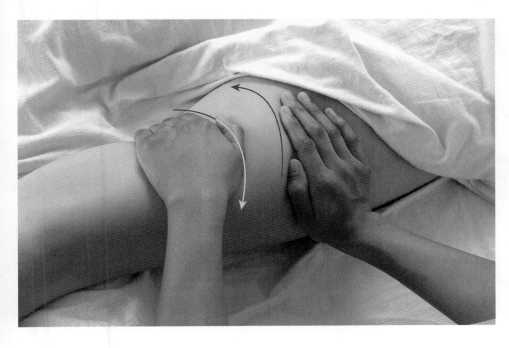

Figure 7-23 Ocean waves pétrissage on the quadriceps.

client's pain threshold. These areas are vascular and sensitive, so overworking an area may leave the client bruised and sore.

Remove any excess lubricant. Hot packs may be used to prepare the skin and fascia. Grasp and lift the skin between the fingers and thumbs, compressing the tissue. Roll the skin as though you were rolling a pencil, using your fingers to scoop up the skin as you move across the area (Figure 7-26). Continue the rolling technique until the designated area has been treated. Tissue may be lifted using the sides of two hands (Figure 7-27). The skin may also be lifted between the thumb web of one hand and the fingers of the other hand (Figure 7-28). Because the superficial fascia lies in several planes, lift and roll the skin in several directions. If the skin is not lifting, do not force the tissue into this position. It is recommended that you address the area two or three times in a session, allowing time between each application.

Benefits
Pétrissage affects physiology by doing the following:
- Increasing blood flow
- Working out metabolic wastes
- Reducing local swelling
- Relieving general fatigue
- Improving cellular nutrition
- Mechanically relaxes and lengthens the muscle
- Addressing tension *under* the surface
- Reducing muscle soreness and stiffness
- Stimulating the nervous system
- Softening superficial fascia
- Producing analgesia by stimulating the release of pain-relieving substances such as endorphins (skin rolling)

Friction

Description
The term *friction* comes from the Latin word *frictio*, meaning *to rub*. Friction typically follows pétrissage in the sequential order of massage strokes. **Friction** massage is performed by compressing tissues in several directions. Because this stroke increases circulation, it is often used for areas that have little or no

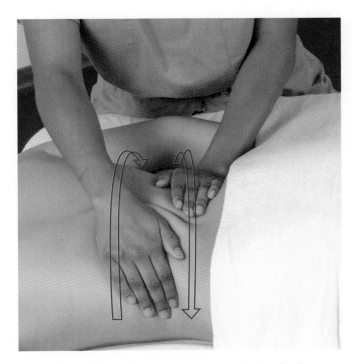

Figure 7-24 Ocean waves across the low back.

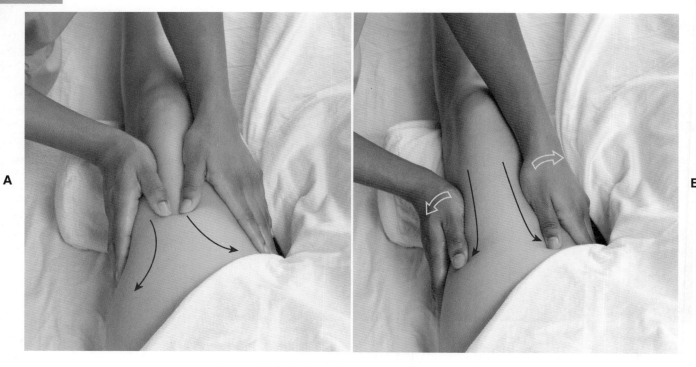

A   **B**

Figure 7-25   Fulling pétrissage on the quadriceps.

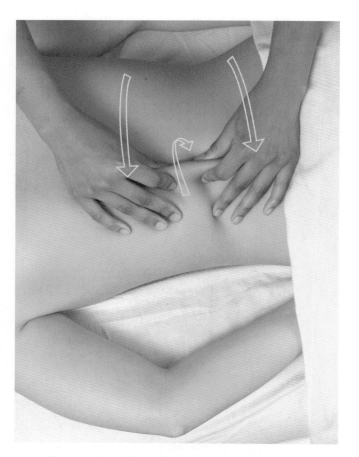

Figure 7-26   Skin rolling pétrissage on the back.

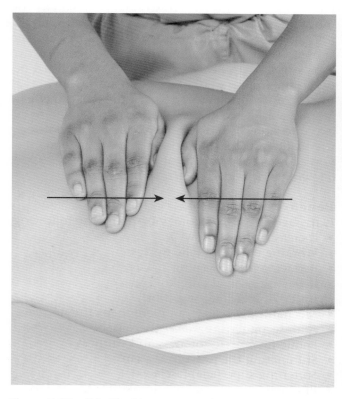

Figure 7-27   Skin lifted between two hands while they lie flat over the clients back.

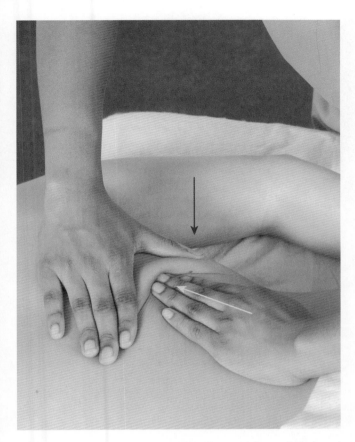

Figure 7-28 Skin lifted between fingers of one hand and thumb web of the other.

blood supply, such as ligaments and tendons. Varieties of friction range from general techniques such as *superficial warming, rolling,* and *wringing* to deep, specific techniques such as *cross-fiber, chucking,* and *circular.* General friction is used to address large areas such as the back or the arm. Deep friction is well suited for areas that lack muscle bulk such as the ankle, the sides of the head, or the suboccipital region. Friction may be applied with the palm of one or two hands, or specific work may be done with the tips of the thumb, fingers, or elbow. The variation depends on the intent of the massage and the size of the surface area to be treated.

Technique

Friction may be delivered superficially by sliding the therapist's hands, palms, finger, or knuckles back and forth over the client's skin or to deeper tissue layers. To access these deeper layers, the therapist's hands do not slide over the skin but moves the skin (and sometimes the superficial fascia) across the deeper tissue layers. Friction may be applied either by pressing down or around an area or with circular or linear reciprocating movements. Deep frictioning techniques are typically done dry, using little or no lubricant.

Variations

Superficial Warming Friction. Also known as a *heat rub,* superficial warming friction generates heat by creating resistance to motion. Place both hands palm down on the client's skin. The fingers of each hand should be together firmly. Move the hands briskly and simultaneously in opposite directions, moving one toward you and one away from you (Figure 7-29). The hands should pass each other in midstroke and continue to alternate like pistons. Begin to pick up speed to build resistance and create heat. The muscles of the shoulder and upper arm are used to propel the hands, reducing the stress on the therapist's hands. The fingertips, knuckles, or ulnar surface of one or both hands may be used if the surface area treated is small (Figure 7-30). The latter variation is called *sawing* (Figure 7-31). Superficial warming friction may also be done with a towel, rubbing it quickly on the client's skin.

Rolling Friction. Rolling is best suited for the extremities. Compress the tissue firmly with open palms and extended fingers of both hands. Roll the skin, muscle, and surrounding tissues around the bone, moving both hands in opposite directions. As you roll the tissue around an extremity, use a back

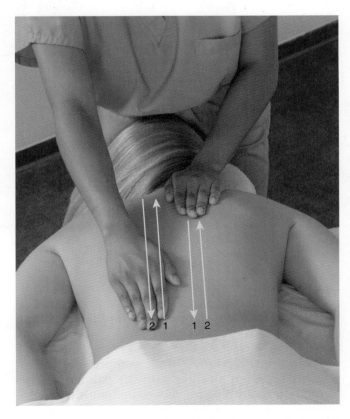

Figure 7-29 Alternate hand superficial friction on the back of prone client.

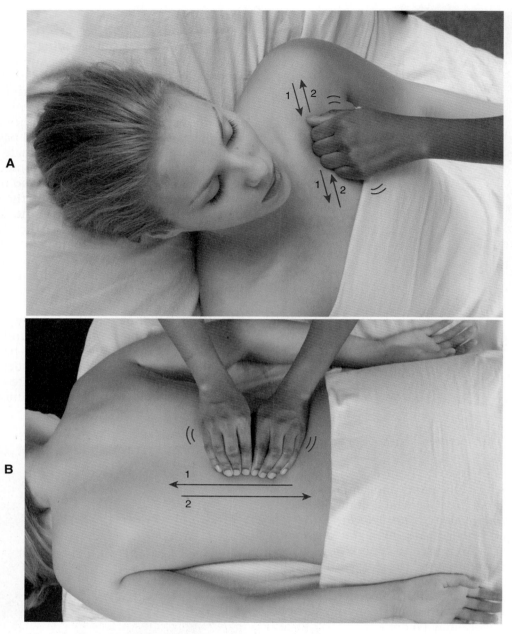

Figure 7-30 **A,** Superficial warming friction using knuckles of one hand on pectoralis major below clavicle with client supine. **B,** Superficial warming friction using fingertips up and down the paraspinals.

and forth movement (Figure 7-32) while you compress the tissue and slide your hands from distal to proximal. The client may assist by holding the limb still.

Wringing Friction. While compressing the lubricated tissue on all sides with the palmar surfaces of the hands and fingers, move the hands in opposing directions. Slide the hands toward the trunk of the body during the massage movement (distal to proximal). Wringing friction is performed vigorously,

like wringing water out of a cloth (Figure 7-33). This movement is best suited for arms, legs, and fingers. To wring the fingers and other small body areas, modify your technique; compress the tissue using only the fingers rather than your entire hand.

Cross-Fiber Friction. Also known as *deep transverse friction,* cross-fiber friction is a very precise and penetrating form of friction popularized by Dr. James Cyriax of London (see p. 160). The direction of movement should be across and perpendicular to the

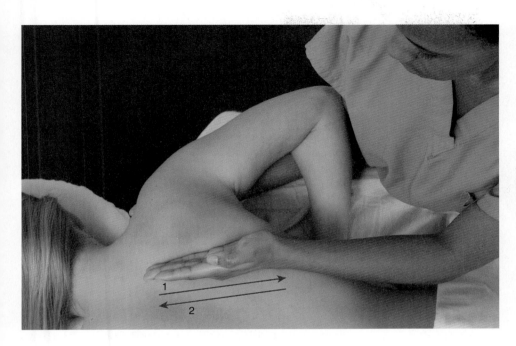

Figure 7-31 Sawing superficial friction using the ulnar sides of the hands on the rhomboids with client prone.

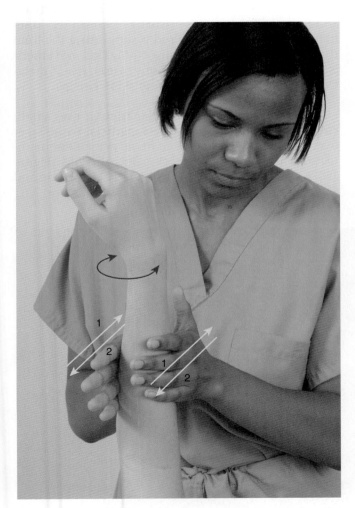

Figure 7-32 Rolling friction on extended arm with client supine.

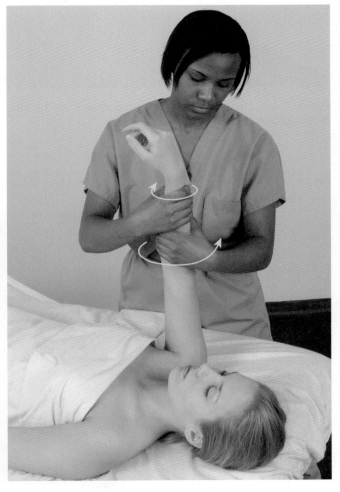

Figure 7-33 Wringing friction on extended arm with client supine.

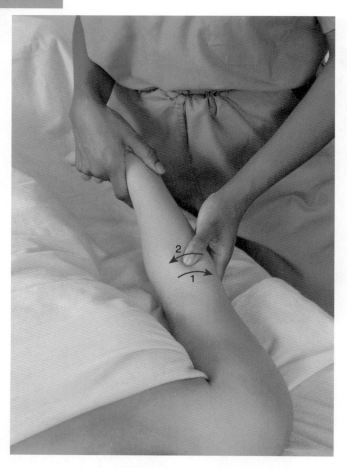

Figure 7-34 One thumb cross-fiber technique on the forearm musculature.

Figure 7-35 Cross-fiber friction of the paraspinals using the tips of several fingers.

pattern of muscle fibers. Success of this method depends on the therapist's ability to identify contracted or injured tissue by palpation and then apply the technique. The therapist must have a good knowledge of muscular fiber patterns.

One or more fingers are placed on the skin at the exact site of a pain or injury. Applying firm, consistent pressure in one or both directions, move the fingers in a back-and-forth motion (Figure 7-34). The fingers and skin must move as one unit, or a blister may form. Apply moderate to heavy pressure, according to the client's tolerance, for up to 1 minute. Repeat if needed. This massage movement is a rehabilitative stroke and is remarkably effective in treating most muscular, tendinous, or ligamentous injuries, especially when adhesions and fibrosis are involved (Figure 7-35).

Chucking Friction. Chucking or *parallel friction* refers to deep friction applied in the same direction as muscle, tendon, or ligamentous fibers. The therapist uses his thumb or fingers to rub back and forth, moving the superficial tissue over the underlying structure. Chucking is usually performed one-handed, while the other hand is supporting the limb that is being massaged (Figure 7-36). This movement is often applied between bony areas (e.g., metacarpals, metatarsals, forearms, and lower legs).

Circular Friction. Circular friction uses small, circular movements that glide superficial tissue layer over underlying tissue layer in several different directions using the fingers or palm of hand (Figure 7-37). This movement is particularly useful around joints and in bony areas (Figure 7-38).

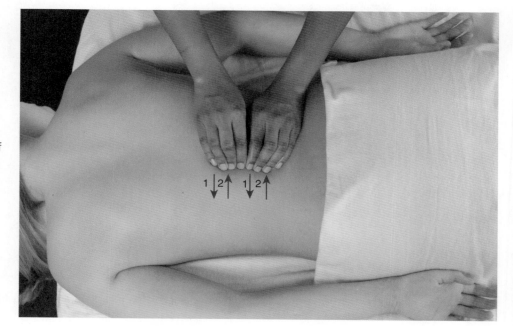

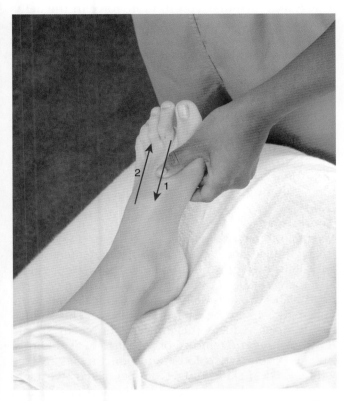

Figure 7-36 Chucking friction on metatarsals with client supine.

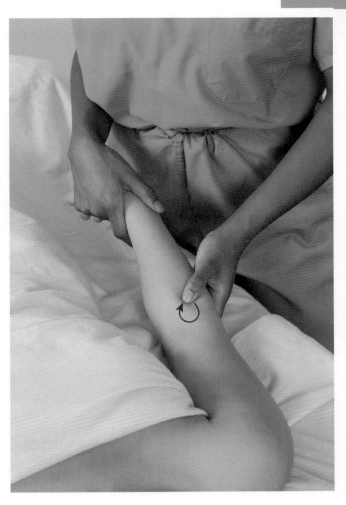

Figure 7-37 Circular friction on the forearm musculature.

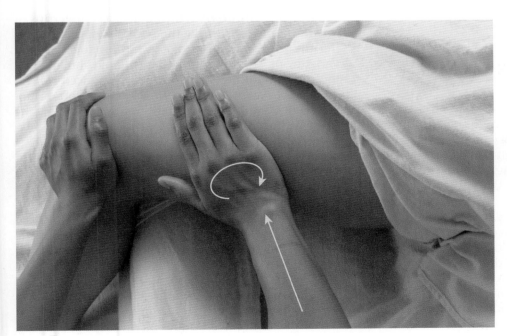

Figure 7-38 Palmar circular friction on the iliotibial band.

Benefits

Friction can benefit the client through the following:

- Generating heat
- Dilating the capillaries
- Increasing circulation
- Promoting venous blood flow
- Loosening stiffness in joints
- Relaxing muscles
- Improving the glandular action of the skin
- Promoting proper scar formation by reorganizing collagen, creating a more biofunctional pattern (This is accomplished by *stressing* the scar formation at the injury site, using mild, controlled pressure in a specific direction. *Stress,* in this instance, is defined as a physical factor that requires a physical response.)
- Breaking down and freeing adhesions
- Softening hyperplasia
- Mimicking muscle broadening and stretching that occurs in normal muscle movement
- Reducing trigger and tender point formation
- Reducing trigger and tender point activity

MINI-LAB

To illustrate how cross-fiber friction can have an effect on scar tissue repatterning, do the following activity. Place 50 toothpicks in a haphazard formation under a thick towel. Lay your hand, palm down, on the towel and begin moving your hand using a back and forth motion. Continue doing this for several minutes and notice what happens to the toothpick arrangement. Do they remain haphazard or do they line up straight? How does this relate to applying cross-fiber friction on restricted fascia or a scar? Write down your conclusion and share it with your class.

Tapotement (Percussion Strokes)

Description

Tapotement involves repetitive staccato striking movements of the hands, moving either simultaneously or alternately. This stroke may be delivered with the ulnar surface of the hand, tips of the fingers, open palm, cupped palm, or back or ulnar surface of a loosely closed fist. Performed skillfully, tapotement has a pleasant, stimulating effect. The word *tapotement* (tap-ot-mon) is a French derivation of an Old French term *taper* that means *a light blow,* which in turn was derived from the Anglo-Saxon term *taeppa,* meaning to *tap,* in the sense of draining fluid from a cavity. At first, this may seem like a strange etiology, but interestingly enough, the mechanical impact of the tapotement techniques is still used by respiratory therapists and nurses to loosen phlegm congestion in the lungs. The synonym *percussion* comes from *percussio,* which means *a striking.*

The technique variations are *tapping, pincement, hacking, cupping, pounding,* and *clapping.* The style of the percussion depends on the location where it is employed and the desired effect. Muscular areas such as legs and hips may absorb more force in the delivery, and thin-tissued or delicate areas such as the face require a smaller, lighter tap. Most therapists use tapotement to finish an area or end the massage (like nerve stroking). Avoid the application of tapotement immediately after exercise because this stroke can activate muscle spindles and stimulate cramping. Heavy tapotement over the kidneys in the low back area is not advised because they are not adequately protected by bodily tissues. You may want to warn the client about the loud noise that often accompanies some tapotement varieties (e.g., quacking, cupping, clapping).

Technique

Percussion may be applied directly to the skin or through the drape. When applying tapotement, begin with light pressure and moderate strike speed, gradually increase speed, and finally diminish speed and depth. The stroke is delivered rhythmically, allowing your hands to spring back after contact. This sudden bounce-back reduces the impact. The client should feel the onset and removal of pressure. To avoid bruising, keep your wrists loose and your fingers relaxed while making skin contact. Proper percussive techniques should be learned under the supervision of a qualified instructor because percussion delivered with too much force can bruise a client.

Variations

Tapping Tapotement.   Using your fingertips of one or both hands, strike the body's surface. Modifying the time and speed of the tap produces several varieties of tapping tapotement. Rapid, but consistent delivery of pressure and speed produced *punctuation tapotement* (Figure 7-39). A hard version of tapping punctuation tapotement is excellent for the soles of the feet. *Pulsing tapotement* is performed one-handed, with an alternate deep and light tap. The deep tap is comparable to a full note, and the light tap is comparable to a half note. The sound produced by the soft and hard tap reverberates like the sound or feel of a beating heart (lubb-dubb, lubb-dubb). Commonly used on the face or scalp, *raindrops tapotement* feels like light rain—each fingertip of the hand strikes the skin lightly at a different time (Figure 7-40).

Pincement Tapotement.   Pincement, or *plucking,* tapotement lifts the skin much the same way as the skin rolling technique mentioned previously.

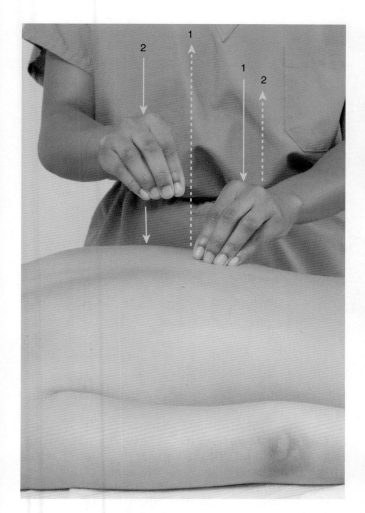

Figure 7-39   Tapping tapotement applied to the back.

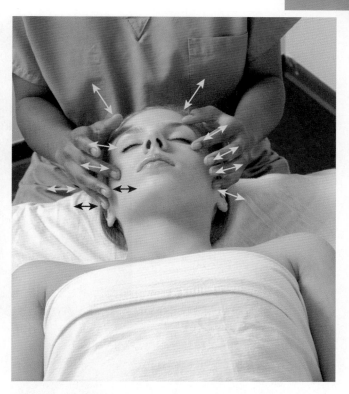

Figure 7-40   Raindrops tapotement on the face of a supine client.

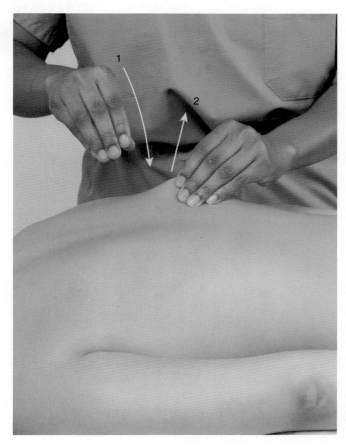

Figure 7-41   Pincement tapotement on the back.

The skin is grasped using a quickly delivered striking motion, lifted, and released while the fingers of the opposite hand follow suit (Figure 7-41). This action is classified as a tapotement but resembles pétrissage because of its distinct lifting effect.

Hacking Tapotement.   Using the ulnar edge of one hand or both hands alternately, strike the surface of the client's skin. The hands should be held loosely with the finger slightly spread. On contact, the momentum of the stroke causes each finger to contact the one below it. This produces a slight vibratory action coupled with the percussive action. Hacking *along* muscle fibers, with the fingers parallel, produces relaxation in the muscle (Figure 7-42).

Hacking applied *across* large muscles, with the fingers perpendicular (across the grain), stimulates muscle spindle activity (Figure 7-43). Minute contractions of the muscle are the result. A variation of hacking, *quacking,* places the palms of both hands together. The skin is struck using only the sides of the third, fourth, and fifth finger. The air moving out of

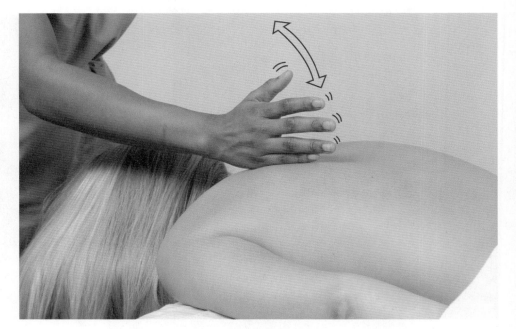

Figure 7-42   One-handed hacking along the back parallel to the paraspinals with client prone.

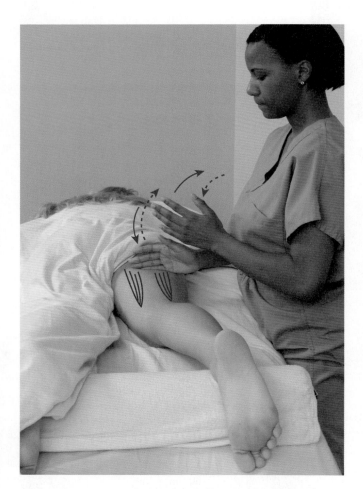

Figure 7-43   Alternate hand hacking perpendicular to the hamstrings with client prone.

the hands during the strike make a quacking sound (Figure 7-44).

Cupping Tapotement.   Curve the palmar surface of the hand into a cup, as if holding water. Strike the client's skin with the edges of a cupped hand, making a muffled horse-hoof sound (Figure 7-45). A vacuum is created when lifting the palm from the skin's surface, hence, the hollow sound of suction. This is the stroke of choice for loosening mucus and phlegm in the chest cavity. Additionally, it is a very vigorous stroke and may induce coughing. Therapists using this type of stroke therapeutically should interrupt the technique to allow for coughing and have plenty of tissues on hand for the client. It often helps to orient the client with the head lower than the chest by using pillow bolsters under the abdomen and chest to induce positional drainage. Make sure you end this section with several soothing strokes. This type of tapotement may not be considered a pleasant experience, so make sure that you thoroughly explain the procedure before treatment.

Pounding Tapotement.   Pounding tapotement is performed with the sides of one or both loose fists, contacting the skin alternately. These blows are delivered rhythmically using moderate pressure (Figure 7-46). Pounding tapotement, or *loose fist beating,* is used on large, muscular areas such as the posterior legs and the hips. The loose fists may be placed palm down, striking the skin's surface like the therapist is

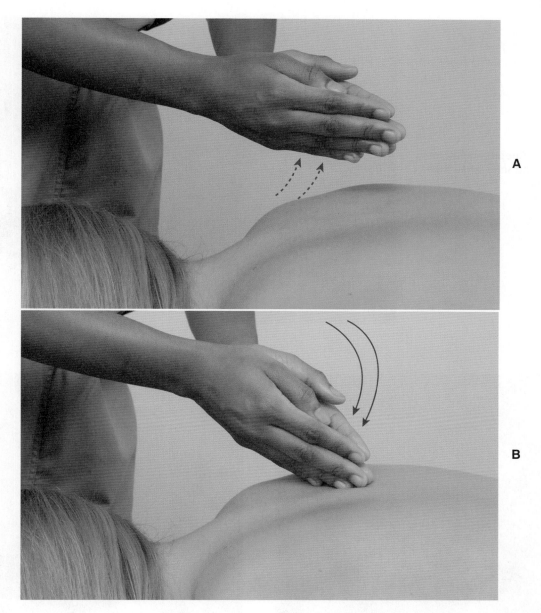

Figure 7-44 Quacking tapotement on the rhomboids with client prone.

knocking on a door (Figure 7-47). This variation is called *rapping*.

Clapping Tapotement. Clapping, or *slapping,* tapotement is performed with the palmar surface of the hands and fingers, striking the skin with alternate strokes (Figure 7-48). The fingers are held together. A loud smacking sound is heard if done correctly. A light upward slapping may be done on the sides of the face. Although it is often an invigorating stroke, clapping tapotement is not recommended for use on clients who are known to be survivors of abuse as it may trigger painful past episodes of abuse.

Diffused Tapotement. Lay the palmar surface of one hand on the client's skin. Using a relaxed fist, strike the dorsal surface of your open hand to diffuse the force (Figure 7-49). Diffused tapotement is commonly used over the abdominal region. Drag the open hand across the skin as you move across the skin's surface.

Benefits
The massage therapist may use tapotement to do the following:
- Stimulate nerve endings initially, becoming more sedative if continued

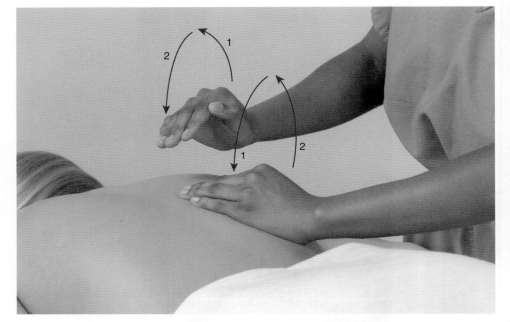

Figure 7-45 Cupping tapotement on the back and sides while the client is prone.

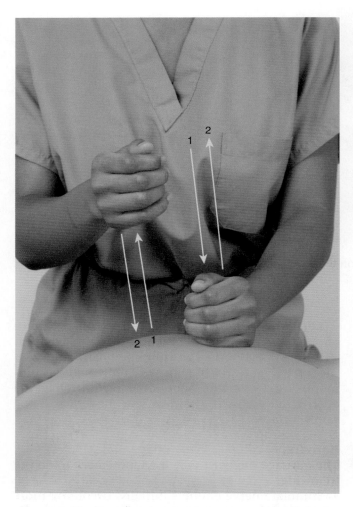

Figure 7-46 Pounding tapotement on prone client's back.

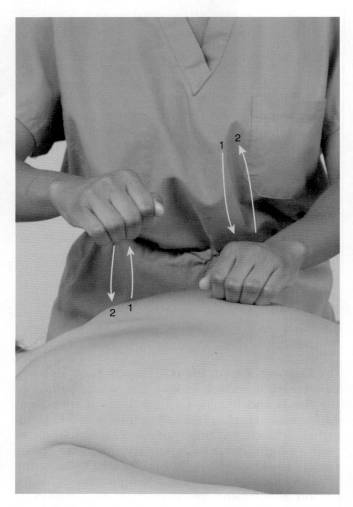

Figure 7-47 Rapping tapotement on prone client's back.

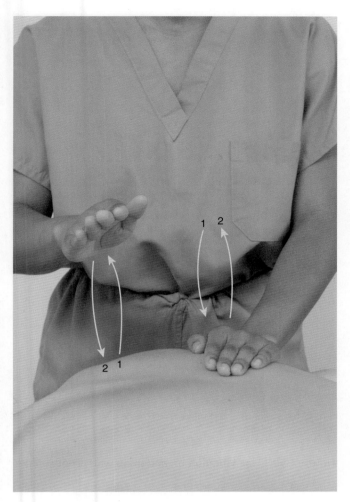

Figure 7-48 Slapping tapotement on the back with client prone.

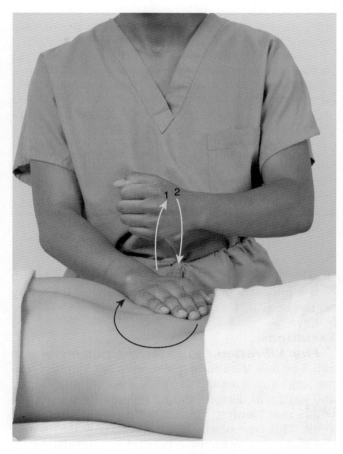

Figure 7-49 Diffused tapotement on supine client's abdomen.

- Aid in decongesting the lungs by loosening and mobilizing phlegm in the respiratory tract
- Tone atrophied muscles
- Increase local blood flow
- Access deeper structures such as hip rotators
- Create an ultrasound effect manually
- Relieve pain (perhaps due to the gate theory)
- Desensitize a hypersensitive area after a few minutes of tapotement stimulation

Vibration

Description

The term **vibration** comes from the Latin term for *a shaker*. Vibration is rapid shaking, quivering, trembling, or rocking movements applied with the fingertips, full hand, or an appliance. Done properly, you will be able to observe the tissue moving near the area of contact. As in tapotement, the client should feel the onset and removal of pressure.

However, vibration differs from tapotement in that the hands do not break contact with the client's skin. Performing vibration correctly requires coordination and practice. The three categories of vibration are *fine, coarse,* and *rocking.* Vibration is the most physically demanding massage stroke (Box 7-2). Many therapists use an electrical device to apply vibration. A discussion on the use of such appliances is included in this section.

Technique

Each variety of vibration requires a slightly different delivery. Fine vibration uses the fingertips or hands to tremble the skin. When applying coarse vibration, the therapist grasps the muscle or limb with one or both hands and shakes or pulls it vigorously. Rocking involves pushing the client's body with one hand or tossing the body back and forth on the table between two hands. The therapist will notice that each body has its own type of movement pattern, depending on

---

BOX 7-2

Ultrasound

Ultrasound is acoustic mechanical vibration of high frequency that produces thermal and nonthermal effects. Therapeutic ultrasound is unique because it falls within the acoustic spectrum and not the electromagnetic spectrum. Physical and physiotherapists use an ultrasound machine to project microwaves beyond human hearing. While ultrasound therapy is outside the scope of massage therapy sonic (sound) energy can be transmitted into the body during tapotement delivery. Therapeutic ultrasound is known for its thermal effects, but its acoustic pressure changes are the most important. Therapeutic ultrasound is referred to as *micromassage.* It is also interesting that lower frequencies of sound penetrate farther into the tissue.

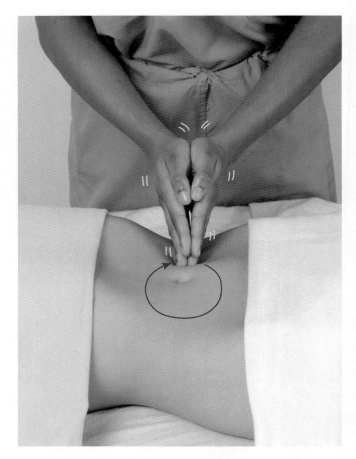

Figure 7-50   Fine vibration on abdomen with client supine.

---

the size of the body, density of the tissues, and health of the joints. Avoid imposing an unnatural rhythm on the body.

Variations

Fine Vibration.   Place the fingertips on the skin and begin a trembling movement by rapidly contracting and relaxing the arm, keeping the fingers and wrist stiff. Fingers should be moving side to side while maintaining contact with the skin (Figure 7-50). This type of vibration is especially useful over the abdomen to increase peristalsis, stimulating digestion and elimination. The therapist's hand may remain in one location or glide down or around an area, such as the back, legs, or arms, while applying the quivering movement (Figure 7-51).

Another way to apply fine vibration is to compress and lift the tissue into your hands (Figure 7-52). Done properly, the stroke feels as if you are slurping up the tissue in your hands. Once this is done, begin trembling the hand that is in direct contact with the tissue.

Jostling.   Jostling, or *coarse,* vibration can be used on a muscle belly or limb. When applying it to muscle, grasp the muscle belly or bellies and shake vigorously, but rhythmically, back and forth. This may feel like rolling friction. Shortening the muscle by moving the attachments closer together creates slack in the muscle before applying vibration. If applied to a limb, use one or both hands to grab the limb securely (Figure 7-53). The most proximal joint (e.g., shoulder or hip) is preferred. Add a small degree of traction by leaning back, shaking the limb (Figure 7-54). As in fine vibration, you can slide down the limb, supporting it from behind, thumping it on the table (Figure 7-55). Coarse vibration

can loosen up muscles surrounding a joint and is the principle stroke used in the Trager technique.

Rocking .   Rocking vibration requires a pitch-and-catch motion. Push, or "pitch," the body with one or both hands, retrieving, or "catching," it as the body swings back toward you (Figure 7-56). Pitch and catch the body until it begins to move easily or fluidly. You can also pitch and catch the body using one hand on each side of the body (Figure 7-57). A wonderful bodily sensation for the client, rocking is often physically taxing to the therapist, who should closely monitor her own personal exertion for setting the duration of the stroke. Not unlike pushing someone on a swing, timing of this stroke is everything. Some bodies have a quicker "rattle," whereas others have a slow, full rock. Support the client's own movement pattern, whether it is a rattle or a rock. The gentle rocking in a mother's womb or in a parent's arms is probably the first motion your body experiences. Even as adults, we find comfort in this sensation.

Use of Mechanical Vibration.   Place a towel on the client's skin for a more comfortable delivery of mechanical vibration. The cord must be long

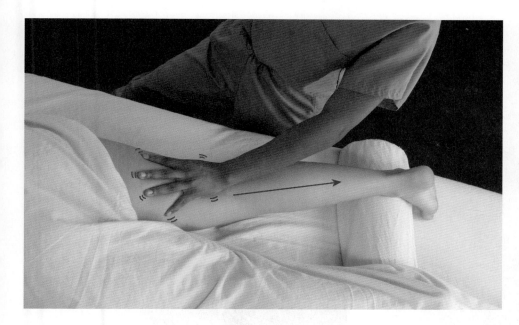

Figure 7-51 Fine vibration sliding down the leg with client prone.

enough to reach the area of treatment from an electrical outlet. Make sure the cord does not touch the client. If the cord is long enough, drape it over your shoulder while holding the appliance (Figure 7-58). Never leave the appliance on the floor or the cord stretched out for someone to trip over. Check the cord often for wear, and replace it immediately if it is frayed.

The use of handheld vibrators or electric vibrators that strap to the back of your hand should be kept to a minimum. Prolonged use of these appliances has a harmful effect on the nervous system of the

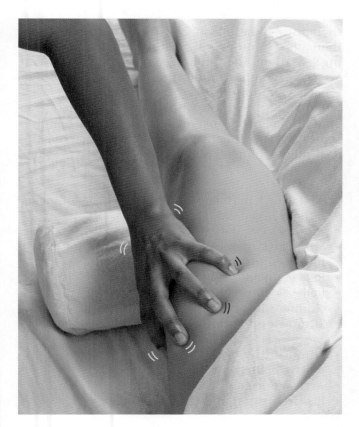

Figure 7-52 Fine vibration slurping up the tissue on the quadriceps with client supine.

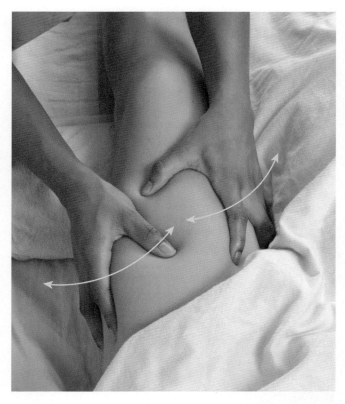

Figure 7-53 Jostling on the quadriceps with client supine.

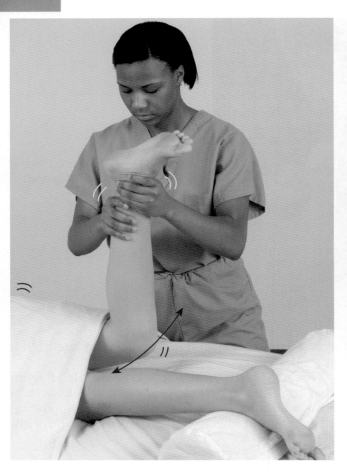

Figure 7-54   Hip joint jostling vibration with client prone.

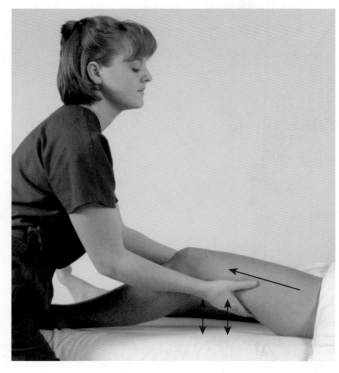

Figure 7-55   Sliding down the back of the leg while coarsely vibrating with client supine.

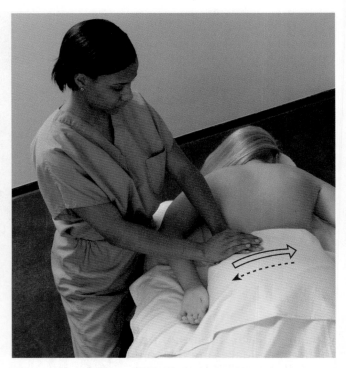

Figure 7-56   Rocking vibration using hand-over-hand with client prone.

therapist. Vibration applied on one area for more than a few minutes will create an unpleasant numbing sensation. After prolonged mechanical vibration, a rash may appear, indicating tissue irritation. Prolonged vibration also can breakdown collagen. Often, massage therapists who use handheld electric vibrators experience nerve damage of the hand. In some cases, nerve damage was so severe that opening a jar lid was difficult and painful.

Benefits
Used during a massage, vibration does the following:
• Enhances general relaxation
• Increases circulation
• Stimulates muscle spindles, thus creating minute muscle contractions
• Relieves pain
• Relieves upper respiratory tract congestion, including sinus congestion
• Stimulates peristalsis of the large intestine
• Moves gas in the lower gastrointestinal tract
• Stimulates synovial fluid production in joints when applied with traction
• Accesses deeper structures such as hip rotators
• Reduces trigger and tender point activity

 Often the hands will solve a mystery that the intellect has struggled with in vain.
—C.G. Jung

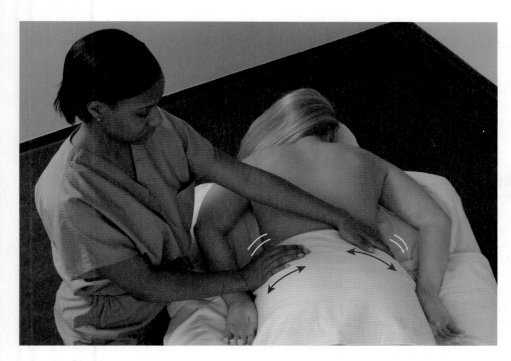

Figure 7-57 Rocking vibration with two hands on either side of the hips with client prone.

MINI-LAB

To demonstrate the ability to relax the body during vibration, do the following activity. With a partner, decide who will be the giver and who will be the receiver. Stand about 18 to 24 inches apart. The giver grasps the receiver's wrist and pull, using moderate force. Note the response of the receiver's body. Let go and again grasp the receiver's wrist. Pull, using moderate force, only this time rock or shake the arm as you do so. Note the response of the receiver's body. Ask the receiver to share his experience with both techniques. Do the exercise again, reversing roles. Is it more difficult to tense up and resist the forward movement while your body is being rocked? Could the rocking movement also be providing a distracting element, interfering with the body's tendency to stiffen?

SWEDISH GYMNASTICS

During the massage, the therapist takes special care to address the client's needs with massage strokes, applying pressure up to the client's tolerance on tender areas. To further assist the client in restoration of healthy tissue and pain-free movements, the therapist may use another method of the Swedish system called **Swedish gymnastics**. These are movements to reduce pain, restore mobility, and maintain health. These movements provide a variety of treatment options, add a kinesthetic element to the session, and can easily be applied before, during, or

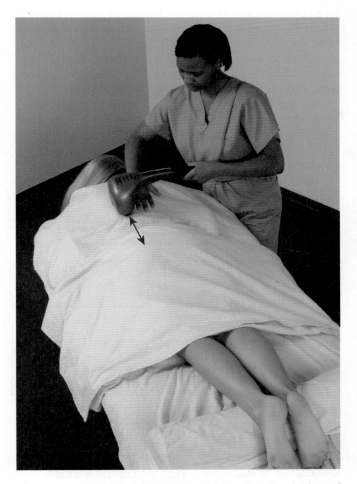

Figure 7-58 Mechanical vibration on prone client's draped back with cord over therapist's shoulder.

after the massage. If the latter two are used, you may need to wipe off any excess lubricant. Ideally, the therapist uses Swedish gymnastics to mobilize and/or stretch articulated segments of the client's body. Also referred to as *therapeutic exercise,* much of Swedish gymnastics can be used by the client at home to extend the benefits received during the massage.

Description

The movements used in Swedish gymnastics can be classified into two primary categories, *passive* and *active.* **Passive movements** are applied by the therapist while the client remains relaxed (or passive) and are commonly used during the massage treatment. **Active movements** involve the therapist describing or demonstrating the movement while the client actively performs the movement. Active stretching has two variations: *active assisted* and *active resisted.* **Active assisted movements** are performed by the client while the therapist assists throughout the range of motion or stretch. **Active resisted movements** involve the therapist applying gentle resistance while the client is actively engaged in the movement (Figure 7-59). When active assisted or active resisted movements are performed at home, the client may use a wall, towel, or other object to provide the assistance or resistance. Active movements are vital to health. Passive movements do not dynamically engage the muscle and therefore do not tone muscles or prevent muscle atrophy.

The most commonly used movements are *stretches* and *joint mobilizations.* In the practice of massage, stretching and joint mobilizations go hand in hand.

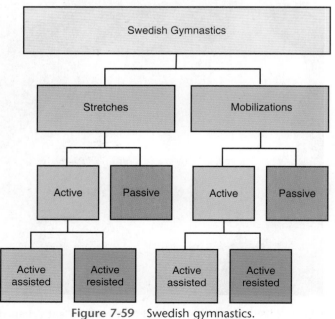

Figure 7-59   Swedish gymnastics.

The therapist may mobilize the joint, performing a stretch by changing the joint position to lengthen a specific muscle. How far a muscle can be stretched or how well a joint can be mobilized depends on numerous factors, including the client's flexibility, genetic limitations, the health of the involved joint, fascial restrictions, muscle tension, muscle guarding, past injuries, and past surgeries. *Flexibility* is the ability of muscles and other soft tissues to lengthen and shorten through the range of motion for which they are intended. Although these factors may reduce a person's ability to move, we can use massage therapy and Swedish gymnastics to increase flexibility, reduce pain, and restore function.

MINI-LAB

Place your hand, palm down, on your anterior thigh. Keeping your hand flat, raise up your index finger and notice how high it can go. Now raise your index finger again, but this time, use your other hand to lift your finger to its fullest extent. Notice how much farther your index finger can go with active assistance.

Stretching routines are not joint mobilizations. **Joint mobilizations** involve moving a joint through its normal range of motion. **Stretching** involves a single muscle (and its synergist) being drawn out to its fullest length. Be familiar with the type of joint with which you are working and the movements possible at that joint (muscles causing the movement). The information found in Chapters 13, 14, 15, and 16 will prove invaluable. Furthermore, use proper body mechanics when applying stretching or joint mobilizations because they are physically demanding on the therapist, particularly when the client is large. Avoid stretching or mobilization if swelling is present around the area.

The purpose of this section is to give the beginning massage therapist a basic understanding of both stretching and joint mobilizations and to foster a desire for further learning. Books and workshops are available to assist the student in this task. Additionally, massage therapists should check their state's definition of scope of practice for the inclusion or exclusion of Swedish gymnastics (stretching modalities and joint mobilizations).

Technique

Use caution if any abnormality is present, such as a surgical replacement, pins, or wires, and any conditions where movement must be limited or avoided, such as edema, inflammation, osteoporosis, rheumatoid or osteoarthritis, dislocations, scoliosis, spondylolisthesis, spondylosis, or hypermobililty. It is important that the body is warmed up before applying stretches or joint mobilizations. If the movements are performed before the massage, the therapist may use rocking vibration or superficial warming friction. If the movements are performed by the client at home, light activity should be done before the stretches or mobilizations. The principle is simple; like clay, warm tissues are pliable and can move and stretch without tearing. Cold tissues tend to be rigid and less malleable, making them more susceptible to injury.

Avoid fast, bouncy, or *ballistic* movements because they can cause the muscle to contract, limiting the effectiveness of the movement. A succession of ballistic movements can cause irritation or even tear the muscle, fascia, tendons, and ligaments (Box 7-3). The lengthening and sweeping motions should be gentle and not induce pain. Avoid over-extending or over treating; use a *static* stretch. It is helpful for the client to relax and inhale at the beginning of the movement and exhale during the stretch or mobilization. Take the joint through three range-of-motion exercises or a muscle through three stretch repetitions. **Range of motion** is a measure of possible joint movement from the least

to the greatest by a particular joint. Hold the stretched muscle for up to 30 seconds, release, and then take up the slack and hold again for the second repetition. Repeat for the third and final repetition. Try to sense movement drag and endfeel. These offer vital feedback as to the condition of the tissues and the limitations of motion.

The techniques presented in the following section are basic passive movements. A brief description of the movement is presented with pictorial representation. Both mobilization and stretches are addressed in the prone and supine positions. Practice these Swedish movements many times with an instructor or an experienced therapist.

Neck
Movements of the neck include flexion, extension, lateral flexion, and rotation. These movements, performed while the client is in the supine position, include *neck circles, neck lateral flexion, neck lateral flexion with rotation,* and *neck forward flexion* (Table 7-2). Apply these movements using gentle to moderate pressure.

Wrist/Hand
The four movements of the wrist are abduction, adduction, flexion, and extension. Do not apply excessive pressure while moving the wrist and hand. Swedish gymnastics used for this area, which can be done while the client is lying prone or supine, are *flip wrist, interlace fingers during movements, metacarpal scissors, circumduct fingers,* and *pull fingers* (Table 7-3).

Shoulder/Elbow
The movements of the shoulder are adduction, abduction, medial and lateral rotation, and circumduction. Flexion and extension are permitted at both the shoulder and the elbow. Most of the basic gymnastic movements are best applied while the client is supine but can be adapted for the prone client. The basic movements are *pull arm down side, pull abducted arm, push adducted arm, pull arm overhead, big shoulder circles,* and *little shoulder circles* (Table 7-4).

Chest
The Swedish gymnastics movements for the chest area use simple pulling and compressing of the ribcage while the client is supine. Hence these movements are called *lift ribcage* and *compress ribcage* (Table 7-5).

Back
The Swedish gymnastics movement for the spine use a lengthening and twisting motion on the supine-lying client and is called *spinal twist* (Table 7-6). The upper or lower portion of the spine may be isolated with a simple modification.

BOX 7-3

Stretch Reflexes

The two types of reflexes associated with stretching are the *myotatic stretch reflex* and *inverse stretch reflex.* Each reflex is associated with a corresponding sensory nerve initiating the reflex. Both reflexes are safeguards activated by extremes in movement. The myotatic stretch reflex is initiated when a muscle is pulled suddenly, initiating contraction. The receptor detecting the abrupt stretch, the *muscle spindle,* is located within the muscle belly. An impulse is sent to the spinal cord, triggering a motor response of contraction. This reaction is designed to protect the joint from further movement in that direction and the muscle from overstretching by causing the muscle to contract. The force of the muscle contraction is somewhat related to the force and speed of the stretch that triggers it.

The second stretch reflex, the inverse stretch reflex, is mediated by the *Golgi tendon organs.* These receptors measure changes in distance or degree of tensile force between the fibers of the muscle/tendon junction. When Golgi tendon organs are stimulated by slow, low-force stretches, they inhibit regular muscle contraction, relaxing the entire muscle, allowing maximum stretching.

In summary, myotatic stretch reflex stimulates muscle spindles, which initiates muscle contraction; inverse stretch reflex stimulates Golgi tendon organs, which inhibits muscle contraction.

TABLE **7-2**				
Neck Gymnastics				
Movement	Figure Number	Stretch or Mobilization	Prone or Supine	Description
Neck circles	7-60	Mobilization	Supine	Place one hand on the client's forehead, rocking head back and forth while your other hand intermittently pulls the tissue in lamina groove on the opposite side up and toward the therapist.
Neck lateral flexion	7-61	Stretch	Supine	With one hand, pull the client's head toward the near shoulder while your hand stabilizes the client's far shoulder.
Neck lateral flexion with rotation	7-62	Stretch	Supine	With one hand hold and pull the client's head (that is rotated toward the near shoulder) toward the near shoulder while your other hand stabilizes the client's far shoulder. Repeat with client's head rotated toward far shoulders.
Neck forward flexion	7-63	Stretch	Supine	With one or both hands, hold the client's shoulders while your crisscrossed forearms support the client's posterior head and neck as the head is lifted toward the chest.

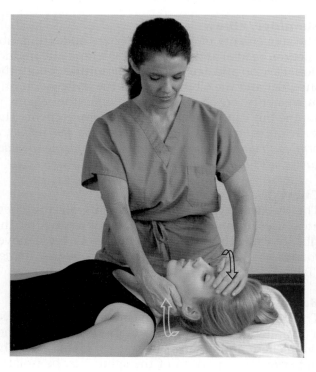

Figure 7-60   Neck circles.

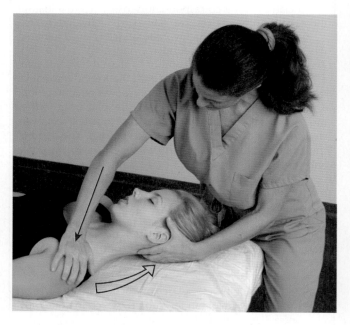

Figure 7-61   Neck lateral flexion.

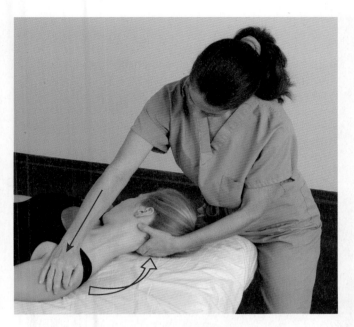

Figure 7-62   Neck lateral flexion with rotation.

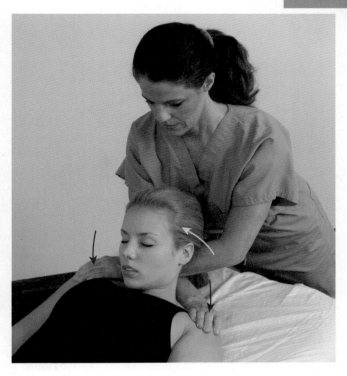

Figure 7-63   Neck forward flexion.

TABLE 7-3

Wrist and Hand Gymnastics

Movement	Figure Number	Stretch or Mobilization	Prone or Supine	Description
Flip wrist	7-64	Mobilization	Prone or supine	Use your fingers below the client's wrist to flip it while your thumbs stabilize the top of the client's wrist.
Interlace fingers during movements	7-65	Mobilization	Prone or supine	Interlace your fingers with the client's fingers while moving the wrist into flexion, extension, abduction, and adduction as your other hand stabilizes the client's flexed arm above the wrist.
Metacarpal scissors	7-66	Mobilization	Prone or supine	While holding the client's metacarpals, alternately move them up and down.
Circumduct fingers	7-67	Mobilization	Prone or supine	With one hand, hold the client's hand while your other hand circumducts each finger and thumb with mild traction.
Pull fingers	7-68	Stretch	Prone or supine	With one hand, hold the client's hand while your other hand pulls each of the client's fingers and thumb.

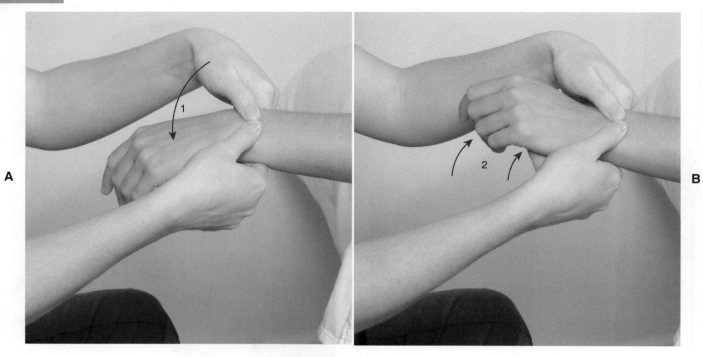

A   B

Figure 7-64   Flip wrist.

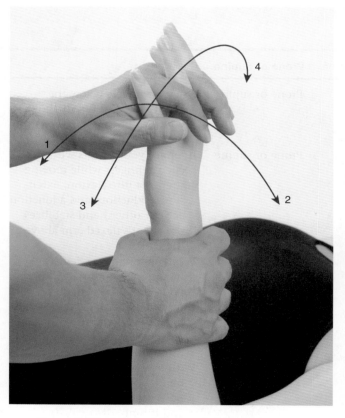

Figure 7-65   Interlace fingers during movements.

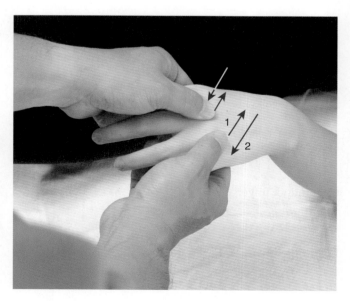

Figure 7-66   Metacarpal scissors.

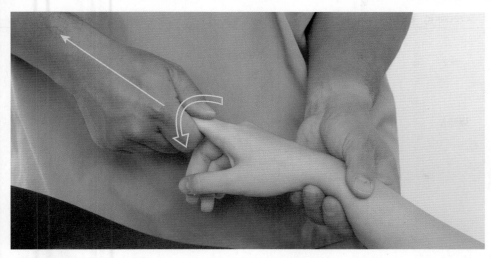

Figure 7-67 Circumduct fingers.

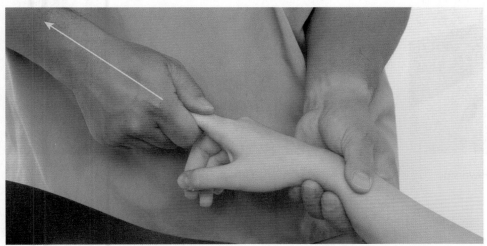

Figure 7-68 Pull fingers.

TABLE 7-4

Shoulder and Elbow Gymnastics

Movement	Figure Number	Stretch or Mobilization	Prone or Supine	Description
Pull arm down side	7-69	Stretch	Prone or supine	While standing tableside, grasp the client's wrist and pull firmly several times.
Pull abducted arm	7-70	Stretch	Prone or supine	While standing several feet away from the table's side, grasp the client's wrist and pull firmly several times.
Push adducted arm	7-71	Stretch	Supine	Push the client's shoulder horizontally across the table.
Pull arm overhead	7-72	Stretch	Supine	While standing at the head of the table, grasp the client's wrist and pull firmly several times.
Big shoulder circles	7-73	Mobilization	Supine	Beginning with the client's arm at their side, pull arm up over the head, then down to side by bending the elbow while maintaining traction during the movement.
Little shoulder circles	7-74	Mobilization	Prone or supine	Grasp above and below the client's shoulder, moving it in a circular direction.

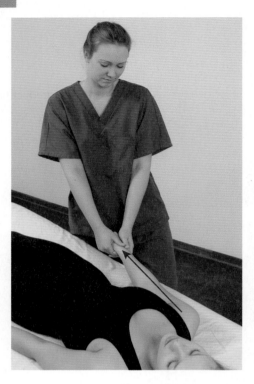

Figure 7-69 Pull arm down side.

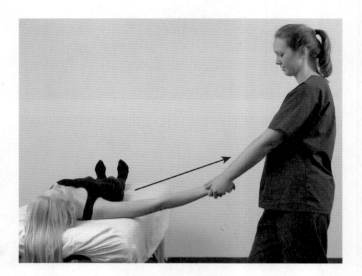

Figure 7-70 Pull abducted arm.

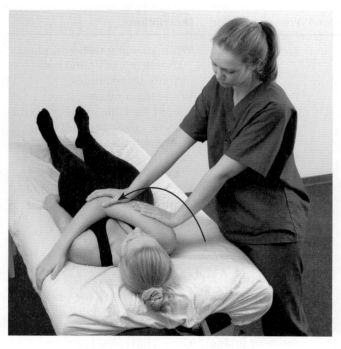

Figure 7-71 Push adducted arm.

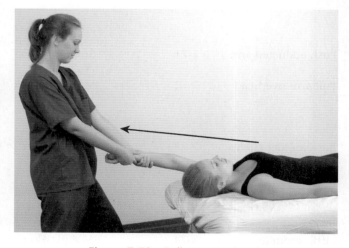

Figure 7-72 Pull arm overhead.

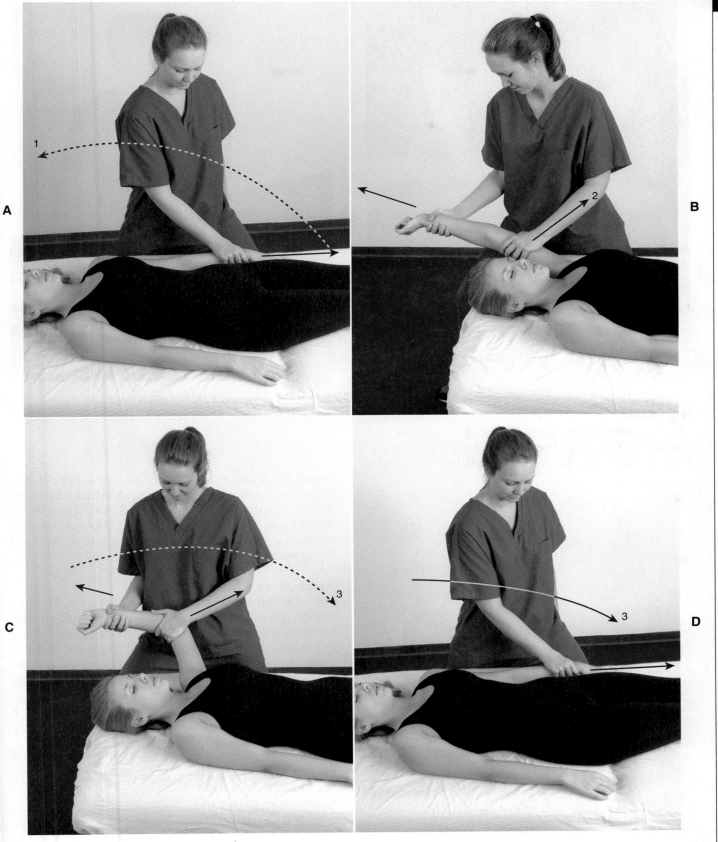

Figure 7-73 Big shoulder circles.

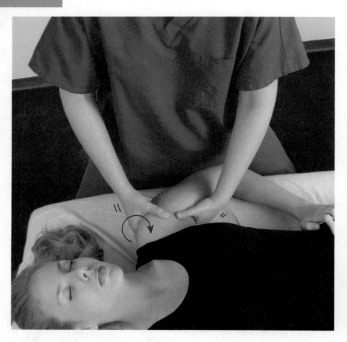

Figure 7-74   Little shoulder circles.

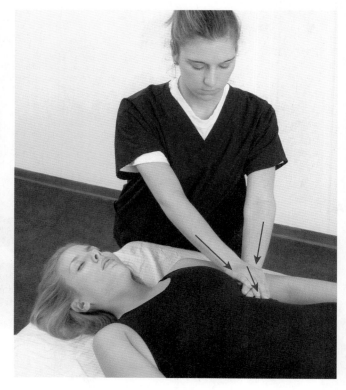

Figure 7-76   Compress ribcage.

Hip/Knee

The hip movements are adduction, abduction and circumduction. Both the hip and knee can flex, extend, medially and laterally rotate. When the knee is

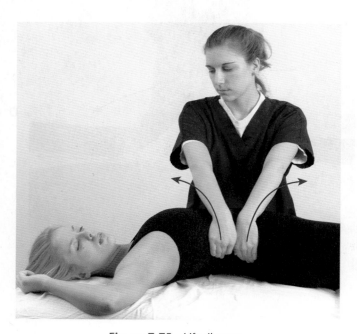

Figure 7-75   Lift ribcage.

flexed, the thigh may be flexed so that it rests on the abdomen. Most of the Swedish gymnastics can be applied while the client is prone or supine. These basic movements are the *leg pull, leg rock, hip clock stretch, hip circles, groin stretch, hip rotations, heel to hip,* and *hip hyperextension* (Table 7-7).

Ankle/Feet

The ankle and foot movements, which include dorsiflexion, plantar flexion, inversion, and eversion, can be applied while the client is prone or supine. These gymnastics movements are *plantar flex ankle, dorsiflex ankle, leg rotations* (using the foot to mobilize the hip), *metatarsal scissors, circumduct toes,* and *pull toes* (Table 7-8).

Benefits

Benefits of Swedish Gymnastics include the following:

- Promotes relaxation
- Decreases pain
- Increases circulation
- Relieves muscle soreness
- Aids in rehabilitation

TABLE 7-5

Chest Gymnastics

Movement	Figure Number	Stretch or Mobilization	Prone or Supine	Description
Lift ribcage	7-75	Stretch	Supine	While reaching across table, grasp the back of the ribcage, pulling up and toward you. Release and repeat.
Compress ribcage	7-76	Mobilization	Supine	Using one or two hands, gently compress rib cage down several times. Release after each compression.

TABLE 7-6

Back Gymnastics

Movement	Figure Number	Stretch or Mobilization	Prone or Supine	Description
Spinal twist	7-77	Stretch	Supine	With the client's near leg bent and the foot placed on the lateral side of the far knee, push the bent knee away from you while pulling the far shoulder toward you.

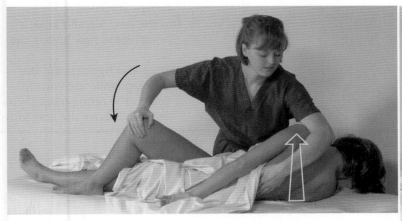

A

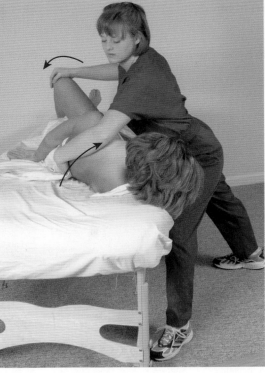

B

Figure 7-77   Spinal twist.

TABLE 7-7

Hip and Knee Gymnastics

Movement	Figure Number	Stretch or Mobilization	Prone or Supine	Description
Leg pull	7-78	Stretch	Prone or supine	While standing at the foot of the table, grasp the client's ankle and pull firmly several times.
Leg rock	7-79	Mobilization	Supine	While standing tableside, place your hands above and below the client's knee and rock back and forth.
Hip clock stretch	7-80	Stretch	Supine	Flex the client's hip and knee while supporting both the knee and heel; imagining the client's lower leg the hour hand of a clock, push and stretch the hip in a 10 o'clock, 12 o'clock, and 2 o'clock stretch.
Hip circles	7-81	Mobilization	Supine	Move the flexed hip and knee in a circular direction. Reverse direction
Groin stretch	7-82	Stretch	Prone or supine	Place the flexed far leg on the table with the foot by the straight near knee; stretch by gently compressing the far knee.
Hip rotations	7-83	Mobilization	Prone or supine	Picking up the near leg above and below the knee, rotate the hip by pushing the leg in, to the side, and out several times. Reverse direction.
Heel to hip	7-84	Stretch	Prone	Flex the near hip and knee, bringing the heel toward the hip.
Hip hyper-extension	7-85	Stretch	Prone	Pick up and hyperextend the near hip while the knee is flexed. The lifting hand should be placed above the near knee.

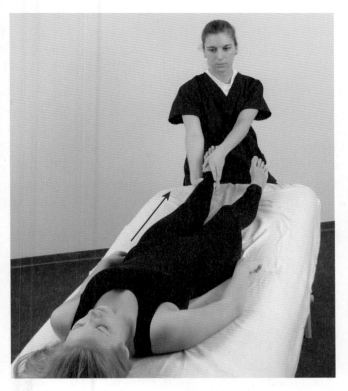

Figure 7-78   Leg pull.

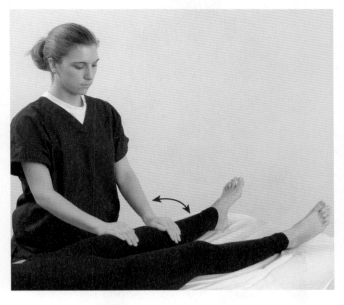

Figure 7-79   Leg rock.

A   B   C

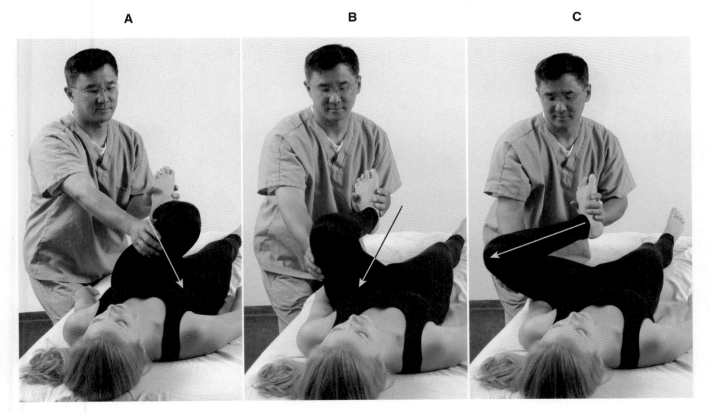

Figure 7-80   Hip clock stretch.

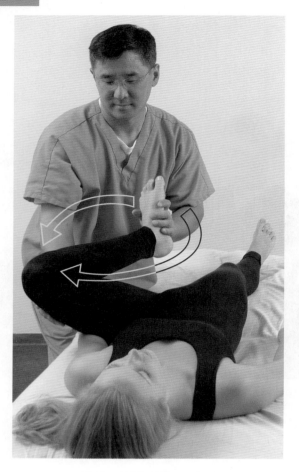

Figure 7-81   Hip circles.

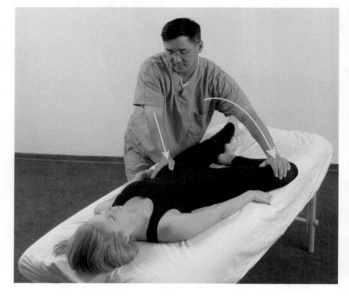

Figure 7-82   Groin stretch.

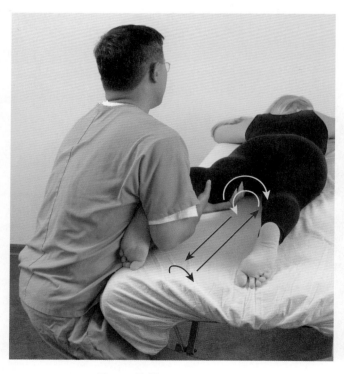

Figure 7-83   Hip rotations.

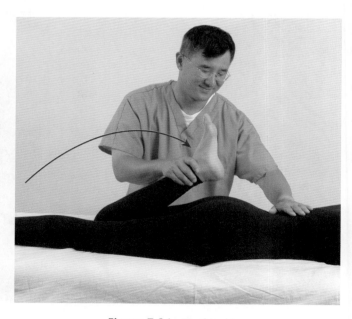

Figure 7-84   Heel to hip.

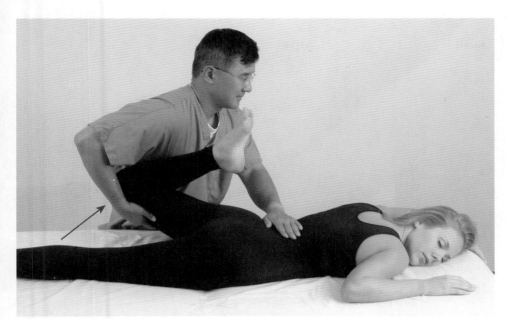

Figure 7-85   Hip hyperextension.

TABLE 7-8

Ankle and Foot Gymnastics

Movement	Figure Number	Stretch or Mobilization	Prone or Supine	Description
Plantar flex ankle	7-86	Stretch	Prone or supine	While holding the client's heel with one hand, push down on the top of the foot with the other hand.
Dorsiflex ankle	7-87	Stretch	Prone or supine	Hold the client's heel with one hand, while pushing the ball of the foot toward the knee with the other hand.
Leg rotations	7-88	Mobilization	Supine	Rotate the hip by circumducting the toes as you hold the client's heel. Reverse direction.
Metatarsal scissors	7-89	Mobilization	Prone or supine	While holding the client's metatarsals, move them up and down.
Circumduct toes	7-90	Mobilization	Prone or supine	Support the client's foot with one hand while the other hand circumducts each toe with mild traction.
Pull toes	7-91	Stretch	Prone or supine	With one hand, hold the client's foot while your other hand pulls each of the client's toes.

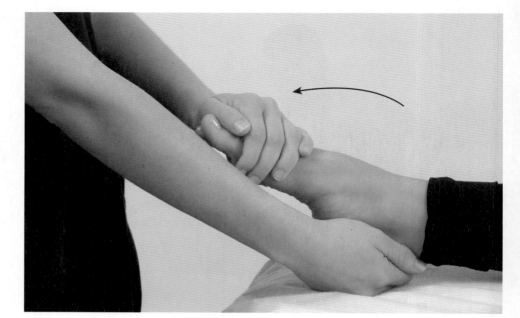

Figure 7-86   Plantar flex ankle.

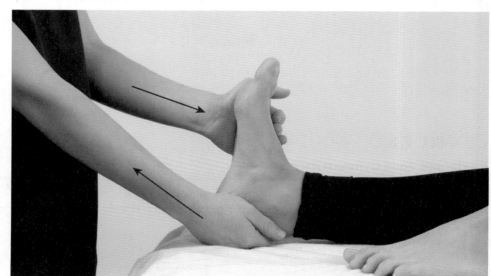

Figure 7-87   Dorsiflex ankle.

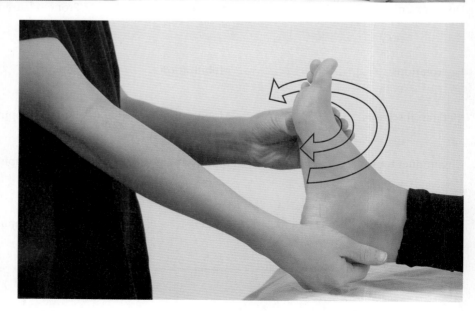

Figure 7-88   Leg rotations, using ankle as fulcrum.

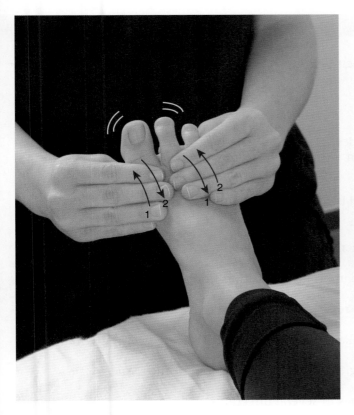

Figure 7-89   Metatarsal scissors.

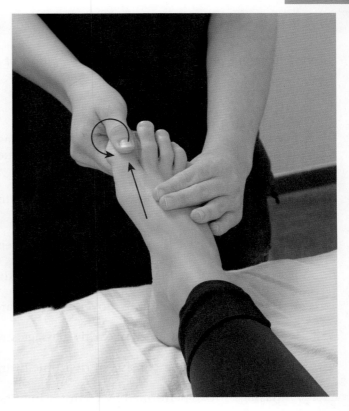

Figure 7-90   Circumduct toes.

- Increases and maintains flexibility and range of motion
- Reduces muscle guarding
- Resets the muscular tone around a joint, increasing joint mobility
- Stimulates synovial fluid production
- Increases kinesthetic awareness
- Improves body alignment and posture
- Assists the therapist in assessing tissues

SUMMARY

Massage may be used to relax the body or to rehabilitate an injury. Swedish massage is the grandparent of most western forms of massage therapy. It uses the following five main strokes: effleurage, pétrissage, friction, tapotement, and vibration. Execution of these strokes can be measured by several qualities, including intention, touch, depth, pressure, excursion, speed, rhythm, continuity, duration, and sequence.

Swedish gymnastics, performed on articulated body segments, includes stretches and joint mobilizations and can be performed actively and passively. Active movements can be assisted or resisted.

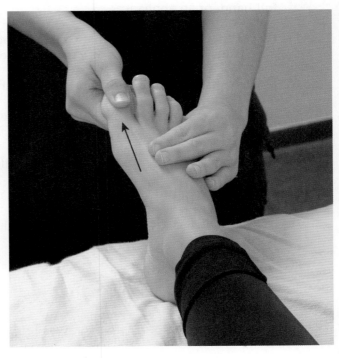

Figure 7-91   Pull toes.

MATCHING

List the letter of the answer next to the term or phrase that best describes it.

A. Active movements
B. Tapotement
C. Cross-fiber friction
D. Active assisted movements
E. Vibration
F. Passive movements

G. Stretching
H. Effleurage
I. Pétrissage
J. Swedish gymnastics
K. Joint mobilization

L. Rhythm
M. Nerve stroke
N. Continuity
O. Active resisted movements
P. Friction

_____ 1. Movements that are described or demonstrated by the therapist while the client actively performs the movements

_____ 2. The repetition or regularity of massage movements

_____ 3. The uninterrupted flow of massage strokes; the unbroken transition from one stroke to the next

_____ 4. The application of gliding movements that are repeated and follow the contour of the client's body

_____ 5. Considered a light effleurage, this massage stroke is feather-light finger tracing over the skin

_____ 6. Massage stroke that consists of rhythmic lifting, squeezing, and releasing of the tissue

_____ 7. Massage stroke performed by compressing tissues in several directions

_____ 8. A very precise and penetrating form of friction, popularized by Dr. James Cyriax of London, in which the direction of movement is across and perpendicular to the tissue fibers

_____ 9. Repetitive staccato striking movements of the therapist hands on the client's skin

_____ 10. Rapid shaking, quivering, trembling, or rocking massage movements applied with the fingertips, a full hand, or an appliance

_____ 11. Part of the Swedish system that consists of active and passive stretches and joint mobilizations to reduce pain, restore mobility, and maintain health

_____ 12. Movements applied by the therapist while the client remains relaxed (or passive)

_____ 13. Active movements performed by the client while the therapist assists throughout the range of motion

_____ 14. The therapist applies a gentle resistance while the client is actively engaged in a movement

_____ 15. Moving a joint through its normal range of motion

_____ 16. Drawing out a single muscle (and its synergist) to its fullest length

Bibliography

Anderson B: *Stretching,* Bolinas, Calif, 1980, Shelter Publications.

Beck MF: *Theory and practice of therapeutic massage,* ed 3, Albany, NY, 1999, Milady Publishing.

Chaitow L: *Modern neuromuscular techniques,* New York, 1996, Churchill Livingstone.

Coughlin P: *Principles and practice of manual therapeutics,* New York, 2002, Churchill Livingstone.

Drez D: *Therapeutic modalities for sports injuries,* St Louis, 1989, Mosby.

Hayes KW et al: An examination of Cyriax's passive motion tests with patients having osteoarthritis of the knee, *Phys Ther* 74(8):697-708, 1994.

Juhan D: *Job's body, a handbook for bodyworkers,* Barrington, NY, 1987, Station Hill Press.

Kendall F, McCreary E: *Muscles: testing and function,* Baltimore, 1983, Williams and Wilkins.

Krieger D: Therapeutic touch: the imprimatur of nursing, *AJN* 75(5):784-787, 1975.

Mattes A: *Active isolated stretching,* self-published by Aaron Mattes, 1995.

Mennell JB: *Physical treatment,* ed 5, Philadelphia, 1945, Blakiston.

Moore KL: *Clinically oriented anatomy,* ed 2, Baltimore, 1985, Williams and Wilkins.

Platzer W: *Color atlas and textbook of human anatomy: locomotor system, vol 1,* ed 3, New York, 1984, Thieme.

Prudden B: *Pain erasure,* New York, 1980, M Evans.

Reed B, Held JM: Effects of sequential connective tissue massage on autonomic nervous system of middle-aged and elderly adults, *Phys Ther* 68(8):1231-1234, 1988.

St. John P: *St. John neuromuscular therapy seminars: manual I,* Largo, Fla, 1995, Author.

Taber's cyclopedic medical dictionary, ed 13, Philadelphia, 1977, FA Davis.

Tappan FM, Benjamin PJ: *Tappan's handbook of healing massage techniques; classic holistic, and emerging methods,* Stamford, Conn, 1998, Appleton and Lange.

Thompson C: Oil on troubled waters? *Nurs Times* 97(15):74-77, 2001.

Travell JG, Simons DG: *Myofascial pain and dysfunction: the trigger point manual,* Baltimore, 1983, Williams and Wilkins.

Voss DE, Ionta MK, Myers BJ: *Proprioceptive neuromuscular facilitation,* Philadelphia, 1985, Harper and Row.

Williams RE: *The road to radiant health,* College Place, Wash, 1977, Color Press.

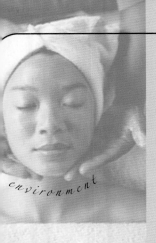

environment

Client Intake, Assessment, and Documentation

8

Alice Pilola Funk, RN

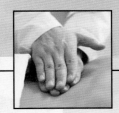

"The body tells the story. It is, in fact, a living autobiography."

—Elaine Mayland

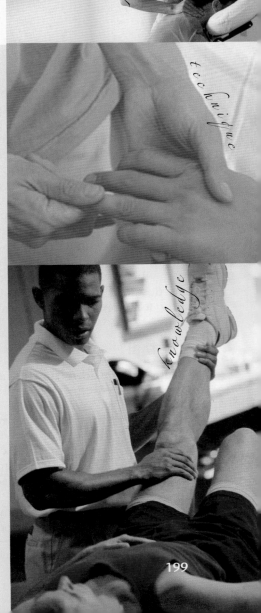

pressure

technique

knowledge

STUDENT OBJECTIVES

After completing this chapter, the student should be able to:

- Develop a health intake form
- Identify the stages of client care
- Describe the components and focuses of the initial and investigative stages
- Explain the components and focuses in the collection of data stage
- Using the categories listed in the chapter, complete a treatment record
- Using collected data, formulate massage therapy goals, including short-term and long-term goals
- Apply supportive documentation relative to case scenarios
- Use medical abbreviations in documentation and decipher prescriptions

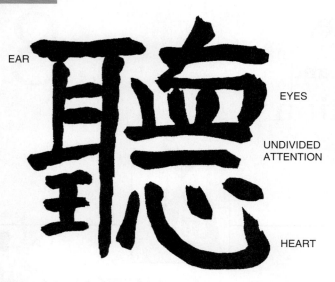

EAR
EYES
UNDIVIDED ATTENTION
HEART

Figure 8-1 Calligraphy depicting communication. (From LOOKING OUT/LOOKING IN 7E 7th edition by ADLER. ©1993. Reprinted with permission of Wadsworth, a division of Thomson Learning: www.thomsonrights.com. Fax 800 730-2215.)

INTRODUCTION

This chapter examines the collection of client information, assessment, and applying a method of documentation. Documentation, professional communication, and respecting boundaries safeguard the therapist and protect the client. As a massage therapist begins her journey into practice, she must be aware of and employ all the types of communication techniques, including verbal, nonverbal, and written (Figure 8-1). A prudent therapist uses patience, skills, knowledge, and a positive frame of mind. All of these affect the outcome of a massage session. The therapist moves the client through four distinct stages of care when performing massage therapy. These stages are designed to provide quality service and opportunity for client assessment and proper documenta-

tion. As we move forward through specific stages and their components, practice, practice, practice, along with continued education, builds confidence in the therapist and positive outcomes for the client. The four stages include *initial, investigative, charting,* and *supportive documentation* (Table 8-1), but first, we need to design and adopt a health intake form.

Today, clients are choosing a variety of massage modalities for specific health benefits. The focus is on the whole person—body, mind, and spirit. Clients are also choosing to be educated partners in their own healing processes.

DESIGNING THE HEALTH INTAKE FORM

Information gathered and documented on a health intake form varies between questionnaires (Figure 8-2). To keep from overlooking and forgetting vital information, a well-tailored health intake form is essential. The form should encompass a variety of information such as the client's personal and contact information, health and medical history, and client consent. Design the intake form to be user-friendly so the client can circle or check off items quickly. The type on the intake form must be readable, logically organized, appropriate to massage, and confined to a single one-sided page. The more education and higher certificates a person holds, the more the therapist can do within her scope of practice. Let us examine, section by section, the information that may be required on the client intake form.

Personal and Contact Information

- Name
- Street address
- City, state, and ZIP code
- Contact telephone numbers (home, work, mobile, and pager numbers)
- Occupation
- Date of birth

TABLE 8-1

Stages, Related Activities, and Focuses of Assessment of Documentation

Stage	Activity	Focus
Initial	Meeting clients, obtaining health history, consent, referrals, consults	Gather appropriate data and clarify necessary information ("find out")
Investigative	Use visual and palpation skills	Perform assessment and treat ("hands on")
Charting	Document activities performed and collected in APIE	Identify what was done and is to be done ("write out")
Supportive documentation	Release forms Progress report	Other documents necessary ("back-up")

APIE, Assessment, plan (of care), implementation, and evaluation.

Client Intake Form

Date: ___-___-___ Name: _____ DOB: ___-___-___ Job: _____
Address: _____
Phone number: ____-_____-_____ Referred by: _____
Healthcare Provider: _____ Insurance: _____
* *

Health Data
Allergies: _____ Reason for visit: _____
Areas that need attention today? _____
Any injuries or surgeries within the past 72 hours? ___Yes ___ No   Explain: _____
_____
First massage ___Yes ___ No   If yes, for _____
Medical-surgical history (any complications) _____
_____
Medications (ASA, steroids, blood thinner) _____
_____
Do you take medications as ordered? ___Yes ___ No
Check all that apply:
Fire Element (heart/small intestine)

___ dry scalp
___ bitter taste
___ facial redness
___ hot hands/feet
___ acne

___ tonsillitis
___ dislikes heat
___ itching/burning skin
___ uterine bleeding
___ gum problems

Earth Element (stomach/spleen)

___ indigestion
___ food allergy
___ halitosis
___ gas
___ anemia

___ diarrhea
___ weakness
___ heartburn
___ sores in mouth

Metal Element (lung/large intestine)

___ constipation
___ shallow breathing
___ hay fever
___ bronchitis/asthma

___ dry skin
___ pneumonia
___ sinus infections
___ coughs

Water Element (kidney/bladder)

___ heart palpitation
___ fatigue
___ hearing loss
___ sciatic/nerve pain
___ headaches
___ emotional instability
___ premature aging
___ hair thinning/loss
___ bladder infections

___ shoulder/neck tension
___ ear infections
___ joint pain
___ lower backache
___ muscle spasms
___ dislikes cold
___ cold hands/feet
___ change in sexual energy
___ rapid weight gain

Wood Element (liver/gallbladder)

___ migraines   ___ poor eyesight
___ dry eyes   ___ skin eruptions
___ shingles   ___ rashes
___ nervous   ___ twitching
___ jaundice   ___ hepatitis
___ cold sores   ___ ulcer
___ chest discomfort
___ irregular menses

___ eye infections
___ eczema
___ warts
___ seizures
___ hemorrhoids
___ herpes
___ loss of appetite

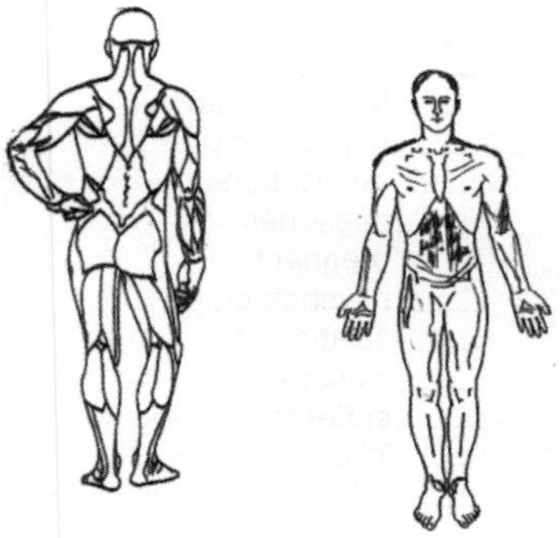

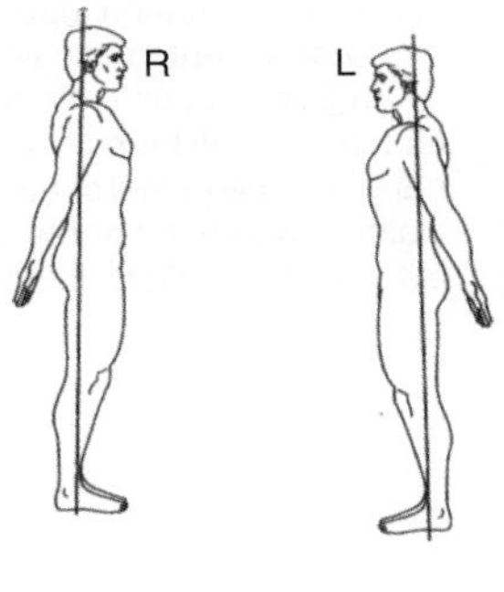

Figure 8-2   Sample client intake forms.   *Continued*

- Insurance information (if applicable)
- Social security number (if applicable)
- Emergency contact person (name, relation to client, and phone number)
- Name of person referring to your office

Health and Medical History

- Current reason for seeking massage services
- Allergies
- Use of orthotics

- Water consumption
- Sleeping habits or sleeping positions
- Type of stress breaks used
- Recent illnesses, injuries, accidents, or surgeries, including cosmetic surgeries (within the last 12 months)
- Any serious illnesses, injuries, accidents, or surgeries
- Current medications (prescription and over-the-counter [OTC])
- Name and telephone number of primary physician

Client Intake Form

Date: ___/___/_____ Name: _____ Date of Birth: ___/___/_____
Mailing address: _____
Employer: _____ Occupation: _____
Contact numbers: Home: (_____)_____-_____ Work: (_____)_____-_____
Fax: (_____)_____-_____ Voice mail: (_____)_____-_____ E-mail: _____
Emergency name and phone number: _____

Health Data

Allergies: _____ Reason for visit: _____
Have you had a massage before? ___ Yes ___ No   If yes, what kind of massage? _____
Any injuries within the past 72 hours? ___ Yes ___ No   Explain _____
_____

Check all that apply:
_____ breathing problems (lung)
_____ bruise easily
_____ carpal tunnel
_____ contact lenses
_____ diabetes
_____ exercise
_____ heart problems
_____ high blood pressure
_____ medications
_____ migraines
_____ pregnant
_____ psychotherapy
_____ sciatica
_____ sinuses
_____ suffer from stress
_____ TMJ (jaw pain)
_____ last consumption of alcohol _____

Mark appropriate stress zones:

Informed consent: The above information is accurate to the best of my knowledge and I freely give my permission to be massaged. I agree to inform the therapist of any experience of pain during the session. I understand this does not deter me from seeking medical treatment for medical conditions. I understand that no inappropriate comments or conduct will be tolerated. Any indication of such behavior will automatically end the session.

   I agree to update the massage therapist in regard to changes in my health and understand that there shall be no liability on the therapist's part should I forget to do so. I agree to hold harmless the establishment, all management, including volunteers, from and against any and all claims. I agree to handle suit at its sole expense and agree to bear all costs related even if claims, etc., are groundless, false, and fraudulent.

_____   _____
Signature   Date

Figure 8-2, cont'd

- A checklist of information and various conditions that may help the therapist screen for contraindications or use adaptive measures during treatment, including:
  - Arthritis
  - Autoimmune disorder
  - Bruise easily
  - Cancer
  - Carpal tunnel syndrome (wrist pain)
  - Contact lenses
  - Depression
- Diabetes
- Epilepsy
- Foot problems, including bunions, corns, plantar warts, calluses, and improper fitting shoes
- Headaches or migraines
- Heart condition
- Low back pain
- Numbness, tingling, or pins-and-needles sensations
- Phlebitis
- Pregnant

J. Michael Brown & Associates
Licensed Massage Therapists

403 West 18th Street
Lake City, LA 70601

(504) 555-1212 phone
(504) 555-1211 fax

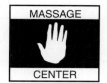

MASSAGE

CENTER

Personal Data

Today's date: _____   Date of birth: _____

Name: _____   Home phone: _____

Mailing address: _____   Pager #: _____

City, state, ZIP: _____   Fax #: _____

Occupation: _____   Work phone: _____

Whom may we thank for your referral? _____

Health Data

Reason for initial visit: _____

Serious illnesses, injuries, or surgeries: _____

_____

Name of regular doctor: _____

Emergency contact: _____   Phone: _____

Please check the appropriate boxes:

Suffer from stress	❏ Yes	❏ No	Pregnant	❏ Yes	❏ No
Contact lenses	❏ Yes	❏ No	Diabetes	❏ Yes	❏ No
Bruise easily	❏ Yes	❏ No	Epilepsy	❏ Yes	❏ No
Carpal tunnel (wrists)	❏ Yes	❏ No	TMJ (jaws)	❏ Yes	❏ No
High blood pressure	❏ Yes	❏ No	Sciatica (hips)	❏ Yes	❏ No
Cardiac problems	❏ Yes	❏ No	Migraines	❏ Yes	❏ No
Psychotherapy	❏ Yes	❏ No	Exercise	❏ Yes	❏ No
Chiropractic	❏ Yes	❏ No	Medication	❏ Yes	❏ No

Informed consent: Please take a moment to carefully read the following and sign where indicated.
The above information is accurate to the best of my knowledge and I freely give my permission to be
massaged. Since massage is contraindicated for some serious medical conditions, it may be necessary
to obtain a doctor's release or prescription before beginning therapy. I agree to inform the therapist of any
experience of pain during the session. I understand that massage therapy should not be construed as a
substitute for medical examination, diagnosis, and treatment, and that I should see a medical or
chiropractic physician or other healthcare specialist. I agree to update the massage therapist in regard to
changes in my health and understand that there shall be no liability on the therapist's part should I forget
to do so. Should I have to cancel an appointment for any reason, I agree to give the therapist a 24-hour
notice.

Patient signature: _____   Date: _____

Figure 8-2, cont'd   *Continued*

- Rotator cuff injury (shoulder pain)
- Sciatica (buttock, thigh, lower leg, or foot pain)
- Scoliosis
- Sensitivity to cold, heat, or pressure
- Skin conditions
- Sports or exercise habits
- Stress (divorce, finances, teenagers, or work)
- Thoracic outlet syndrome (arm pain)
- Temporomandibular joint (TMJ) disorder, including clenching or grinding

- Trauma or motor vehicle accident
- Varicose veins
- Vertebral disc problems (bulging or ruptured)
- Vitamin or mineral usage (megadoses of vitamin E can increase bruising; lack of minerals may cause spasms)
- Whiplash (neck pain)

On the back of the form, areas for assessments, proposed treatments, and progress notes for initial and subsequent sessions may also need to be completed.

Client Health Record

Name: _____ Telephone: (____) _____ Date of Birth: _____

Address: _____ City: _____ State: _____ Zip: _____

Referred by: _____ Telephone: (___) _____

In case of emergency: _____ Telephone: (___) _____

General & Medical Information

Occupation: _____ Height: _____ Weight: _____ ❏ Male ❏ Female

Are you basically in good health? ❏ Yes ❏ No

Has there been any change to your health in the past year? ❏ Yes ❏ No

   If so, please explain: _____

Physician: _____ Telephone: (___) _____

If you answer "yes" to any of the following questions, please explain as clearly as possible.

Do you suffer from acne? ❏ Yes ❏ No	Do you wear dentures? ❏ Yes ❏ No

Do you suffer from acne? ❏ Yes ❏ No   Do you wear dentures? ❏ Yes ❏ No

Do you have allergies? ❏ Yes ❏ No   Do you have a pacemaker? ❏ Yes ❏ No
Specify:

     Are you currently being treated by a
     physician for any condition? ❏ Yes ❏ No
Do you have arthritis? ❏ Yes ❏ No   Please explain:

Do you have high blood pressure? ❏ Yes ❏ No   _____
If yes, what medication are you taking?

_____   Do you have any other medical condition I should know about?

Do you suffer from epilepsy or seizures? ❏ Yes ❏ No   _____

Do you suffer from claustrophobia? ❏ Yes ❏ No   Are you taking any medications (*including non-prescription drugs*)

Do you have varicose veins or distended   ❏ Birth Control Pills   ❏ Diuretics
capillaries? ❏ Yes ❏ No   ❏ Accutane   ❏ Vitamins/Supplements
       ❏ Hormone Therapy   ❏ Antibiotics
Do you have any contagious diseases? ❏ Yes ❏ No   ❏ Aspirin/Ibuprofen/Acetaminophen
       ❏ Vitamin A (topical or internal)
Do you have heart disease? ❏ Yes ❏ No
     Are you using any of the following products?
Do you have diabetes? ❏ Yes ❏ No
       ❏ Renova   ❏ Benzoyl Peroxide
Do you have asthma? ❏ Yes ❏ No   ❏ Glycolic Acid   ❏ Retin-A

Have you ever had or are you being   How much water do you drink a day? _____ glasses
treated now for cancer? ❏ Yes ❏ No
Please explain: Do you exercise regularly? ❏ Yes ❏ No

_____   How would you describe your overall level of stress?
       ❏ Low   ❏ Medium   ❏ High
Do you suffer from any blood disorder? ❏ Yes ❏ No

Do you have seborrhea? ❏ Yes ❏ No   Comments: _____

Have you ever had surgery? ❏ Yes ❏ No   _____
Please explain:

_____   _____

Are you pregnant or nursing? ❏ Yes ❏ No   _____

Do you wear contact lenses? ❏ Yes ❏ No

Please take a moment to carefully read the information you have provided and sign where indicated. If you have a specific medical condition or specific symptoms, certain esthetic treatments may be contraindicated. A referral from your primary care provider may be required prior to service being rendered.

Client Signature: _____ Date: _____

Figure 8-2, cont'd

Intake Questionnaire and Assessment Worksheet

PERSONAL DATA AND LIFESTYLE:

Client _____ Phone _____ Date _____

Address _____ Date of Birth _____

Occupation _____ Interests _____

Posture assumed most of day _____ Previous professional bodywork/massage? _____

How often do you exercise? _____ Type of exercise? _____

With whom do you live? _____ Pets? _____

Are you happy with your general energy level? _____

Do you have much stress in your life? _____ What are the primary stressors? (circle)

   job   family   finances   school   relationships   health   other _____

What is your goal or concern for today's session? _____

Is there an area where you seem to hold more tension? _____

MEDICAL HISTORY:

1. Have you experienced any illnesses, injuries, or surgical procedures? Please give date, nature of injury or surgery, and any remaining aftereffects or pain syndrome _____

   _____

2. Are you currently under medical supervision? _____ Condition _____

3. Are you currently taking any medications? _____ What? _____

4. Do you wear contact lenses? _____ dentures? _____ hearing aid? _____ pacemaker? _____
   transdermal patch medication? _____ surgical pins, plates, artificial joints? _____

5. Do you have any chronic conditions? Examples: allergies, headaches, asthma, diabetes, high blood pressure, epilepsy, arthritis, fibroid tumors, cancer, arteriosclerosis, PMS or menopausal symptoms, depression, anxiety, insomnia, digestive problems, etc. _____

   _____

6. Do you have any chronic or frequent pain problems? _____

DIET, HABITS, AND PREFERENCES:

1. Are you happy with your diet? _____ What would you change? _____

2. Are you happy with your body? _____ What would you change? _____

3. Are you happy with your sleep/rest? _____ What would you change? _____

4. Are you happy with your activity level? _____ What would you change? _____

5. Are you happy with your emotions? _____ What would you change? _____

6. Which activity do you prefer? (circle): walking, sitting, lying down, standing, reading

7. What is your best time of day? _____ Worst time of day? _____

8. Are there any flavors you crave often? (circle): salty, sweet, spicy, sour, bitter

9. Do you use any of the following regularly? (circle): tobacco, alcohol, soft drinks, caffeine, fried food, artificial sweetener, drugs or medication, (prescription or otherwise)

Figure 8-2, cont'd

MINI-LAB

Collect a variety of intake forms from other professionals including massage therapists, physicians, chiropractic care professionals, dentists, physical therapists, and counselors. Use them to create your own health intake form. Ask your instructor or a massage therapist to critique it for advantages and disadvantages. Continue revising it until it is comprehensive and satisfactory.

INITIAL STAGE

During the initial stage, the therapist meets the client and conducts the massage consultation. The client completes a client intake form, or the therapist updates the form used previously. The therapist explains the session and obtains consent. If the massage services were requested by a physician, important forms such as a prescription or referral form must be obtained.

Massage Consultation

The massage consultation is a two-part process. First, the client completes the intake form, reads and signs the consent form, and gives the therapist any prescriptions or referral forms. Both processes are needed; the written intake form begins the process, but the client's answering of questions builds rapport and gives the therapist greater insight into the client's condition.

Thus begins the first record keeping. While the client is completing the form, the therapist should be available for questions. The health intake data may be obtained by the client completing the form or through the therapist's interview and the recording of the client's responses on the intake form (Figure 8-3). If the latter is chosen, the form should be given to the client to read before signing.

The interview process follows, in which the therapist evaluates the information offered by the client, asking the client for clarification or additional information. If the client completes the form, the therapist should read over it once it is returned. Make sure that all relevant information is complete, dated, and signed. Look for problem-prone areas or contraindications for massage therapy. The therapist needs to review the information before doing the APIE documentation discussed later in this chapter. If this is not the initial appointment, the therapist then reviews the client intake form, updating information as needed. This information is necessary to formulate a massage treatment plan.

A comfortable place for the consultation to take place should be provided—that is, a place free of distractions such as pagers, mobile telephones, television, pets, and people. Poor planning with a lack of organization in collecting data weakens the credibility of the therapist and hampers the outcome of a session.

During the interview portion of the consultation, the therapist should face the client. This, along with nodding while the client is speaking, lets her know that she is being heard and that the therapist is interested in helping her. While being interviewed, the client may use nonverbal communication when speaking. Nonverbal communication, known as *body language,* includes body gestures, facial expression, and changes in posture. The therapist observes the client's body language to gain clues about the client's feelings. Reciprocal observation is made by the client, so the therapist should be aware of his own body language. A genuine caring professional image should be exhibited, strengthening the weight a therapist's words carry. Generally, the strongest message the listener receives and remembers is the unspoken one, perceived to be the most honest.

A successful consultation produces satisfied clients. A working, therapeutic relationship and a thoughtful therapist who is well-prepared for the consultation establishes this success and resultant satisfaction. Proper preparation includes the following list of topics to discuss with the client:

- What is the chief complaint? (If you could only correct one thing with today's session, what would it be?)
- When did it start?
- How often does it occur? Is it constant or periodic?
- What are the symptoms?
- Describe the pain using the following pain scale: 0-1 = minimal, 2-3 = moderate, and 4-5 = severe.
- What activities make the symptoms worse? How much worse?
- What activities make the symptoms disappear?
- Do you administer any self-treatment? What are the results of that self-treatment?
- Does referral pain accompany the symptoms? (Client should state location and sensation described.)
- Are you experiencing any problems with activities of daily living (ADLs)?
- What other professionals have been seen? What were the results of those visits?
- If applicable, what are your impressions of the previous session?
  - How long was relief experienced from previous massage sessions?
  - Which areas feel better?
  - Which areas still need attention?
  - Where have you experienced any adverse effects such as soreness or bruising?

Once the consultation is complete, a therapist may realize that the client requires services that are

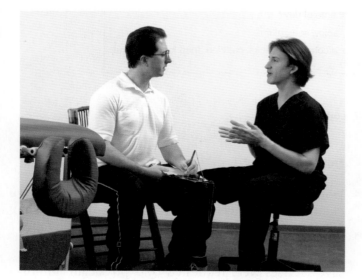

Figure 8-3   Therapist and client sharing information.

Consent for Therapy

I understand that

- The relationship between the client and the massage therapist is a confidential one and that all information provided to the therapist are to be kept confidential.

- My body will be properly draped at all times for comfort, security, and warmth.

- The massage is solely for the purpose of therapeutic massage and that the massage therapist also has the right to be free from any unwanted, harmful, offensive, and/or physical contact or behavior.

- I have the right to request and require that any procedure or technique be modified, changed, stopped, or simply not performed.

- The information given is accurate and agree to update the therapist of health changes at future appointments as appropriate.

- It may be necessary to obtain permission from my healthcare provider, to receive or continue therapy.

- I will inform the therapist of any discomfort, so that the application of pressure or strokes may be adjusted to my level of comfort.

- The benefits of massage and discomfort that I may feel have been explained.

- The therapeutic massage is ancillary treatment, not primary medical treatment.

- The therapist is state-licensed.

- By signing this form, I also give consent for future sessions. I have read this form and hereby freely give my permission to be massaged.

As a minor, I have been informed in the presence of my guardian

_____   _____
(Print name)   (Signature)

_____   _____
(Date)   (Therapist's signature)

Should I have to cancel an appointment for any reason, I agree to give the therapist a 24-hour notice.

Figure 8-4   Sample consent for therapy.

---

out of the scope of her practice. If this occurs, the therapist should be prepared to refer the client to the proper health care provider for further evaluation and treatment.

Informed Consent

The initial interview process includes obtaining consent for treatment. The consent may be written or verbal. **Informed consent** is a client's authorization for professional services based on adequate information provided by the attending therapist. This information includes modalities used, expectations, potential benefits, possible undesirable effects, and professional and ethical responsibility. An informed client can make an educated decision to participate in his care. The consent may be on a separate form or combined on the health intake form (Figure 8-4). The consent should be reviewed verbally with the

client, giving him an opportunity to ask questions and receive answers. A signature should be obtained from the client. If the therapy is provided to a minor, a parent or guardian may sign the consent.

Client consent should include any or all of the following features:

- *The above information is true to the best of my knowledge.*
- *I freely give my permission to receive massage therapy treatment.*
- *I understand that massage is contraindicated for some medical conditions and that it may be necessary to obtain a physician's clearance, release, or prescription before beginning treatment.*
- *I agree to inform the therapist of any experience of pain during the session.*
- *I understand that I have the right to refuse any treatment or ask that it be modified in regard to pressure or modality.*

- *I understand that I will be draped during treatment in accordance with state laws and that I may request additional draping if desired.*
- *During future sessions, I agree to update the therapist in regard to changes in my health and medical history and understand that there shall be no liability on the therapist's part if I should neglect to do so.*
- *I understand that massage therapy should not be construed as a substitute for medical examination, diagnosis, and treatment, and that I should see a medical or chiropractic physician or other health care specialist to address concerns that are outside the scope of a massage therapist.*
- Patient signature
- Date of signature

Prescriptions and Referral Forms

Massage therapists have direct access to the public, meaning that no physician prescription or referral is needed to receive treatment. However, most insurance companies require documentation of referral or prescription when insurance is billed for massage services. In these cases, one of two forms must be completed by a physician, chiropractic care professional, or nurse practitioner. The two forms are a prescription or a referral.

A **prescription**, which literally means *take thou this,* is a written order by a physician or nurse practitioner authorizing massage therapy treatment. These orders are usually written on the physician's own personalized prescription pad like a prescription for antibiotics or exercise. The prescription must specify massage therapy, not physical therapy. The simplest form of prescription is when the physician writes the order "to evaluate and treat" and leaves the specifics up to the discretion of the therapist. Parts of a prescription include the following:

- Date of the order
- Client's name
- Diagnosis and diagnosis code (**diagnosis** is identifying a disease or illness by scientific evaluation from a qualified health care practitioner)
- Treatment order
- Frequency of treatments
- Duration of treatments
- Referring physician's name, signature, and contact information

A prescription may order a specific modality and adjunctive therapy, such as the use of ice or heat (Figure 8-5). A **modality** is a general term used to denote any technique, procedure, or product that produces a positive response for the client (e.g., soft-tissue mobilization, manual lymphatic drainage). *Frequency* specifies the number of sessions per week, and duration refers to *total calendar treatment period* (e.g., 3× wk for 6 wk). Sometimes other information is written on the prescription pad. The massage therapist must be able

to decipher any medical jargon. If understanding the order is troublesome, the physician's nurse or assistant should be contacted to verify the order.

The second kind of form is the referral form. **Referral forms** are generally produced by the provider (therapist) and completed by a physician or nurse practitioner authorizing massage therapy treatment. These forms may be personalized with the massage therapist's logo, name, address, telephone, fax number, and other contact information. The form should have room for the patient's name, diagnosis, treatment choices (preferably with check boxes), and blanks for frequency and duration. At the bottom is a space for a signature and office address stamp. These referral forms can be given one at a time to a specific client seeking massage therapy services. She can then take it to her physician for completion. Alternatively, the therapist can drop a tablet of these forms off at the offices of physicians who support massage therapy for their clients. It is irrelevant on whose form the order is written. If one physician gives an order for massage therapy treatment for a client, and that order is written on another practitioner's referral form, the client can still bring the form to a therapist for service. This is much like the choices of pharmacies available to health consumers; they also have a choice of therapists for massage treatment. However, note that as with prescriptions, an order for physical therapy cannot be treated with massage therapy by a massage therapist.

The date or orders on a prescription or referral form should *never* be changed. If the frequency and duration need modification to suit the client or therapist's schedule, the physician or her nurse or assistant should be contacted for a confirmation of changes (Figure 8-6).

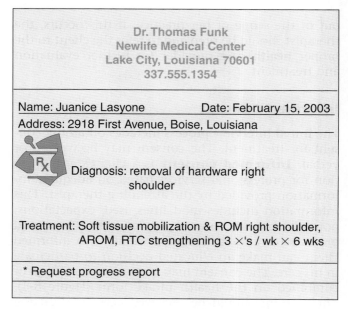

Dr. Thomas Funk
Newlife Medical Center
Lake City, Louisiana 70601
337.555.1354

Name: Juanice Lasyone   Date: February 15, 2003
Address: 2918 First Avenue, Boise, Louisiana

Diagnosis: removal of hardware right
shoulder

Treatment: Soft tissue mobilization & ROM right shoulder, AROM, RTC strengthening 3 ×'s / wk × 6 wks

* Request progress report

Figure 8-5   Sample prescription.

Massage Referral

Tranquil Moments Massage Centre
2918 Fifth Avenue
Lake City, Louisiana 70601

To Whom It May Concern:

I began treatment on _____ on _____ for the
                      (Client's name)   (Date)

condition of _____. The client's medical history is as follows:
_____
_____
_____

The scheduled treatments are as follows:

COMPLAINT	OBSERVATION	APPLICATION	OUTCOME

At this time I am asking for further assistance in treatments and procedures that will offer
_____ a quicker recovery.
(Client's name)

Thank you for your assistance. If I can assist in any way, contact me by phone at 337-555-1354 or
by fax at 337-555-1543.

Yours in health,

_____
(Massage therapist)

I hereby grant _____ permission to release information to the referring
agency to assist in the continuity of care. I am also granting permission of the referring agency to send
back to _____
_____
recommendations and reports on any and all of the treatments performed on

_____   _____   _____
(Print client's name)   (Client's signature)   (Date)

Figure 8-6 Sample physician referral forms.

INVESTIGATION STAGE

> *The body never lies.*
>
> —Martha Graham

The investigative stage begins when the therapist assimilates the subjective information on the intake form and begins to assess the client. The main goal of the investigation stage is to gather objective information about the client. The focus of these assessments are the skin; soft tissues such as muscle and fascia; and structure, posture, and movement patterns. Assessing the client is a multisensory experience, but the primary assessment tools are observation and palpation, which are used before, during, and after the actual massage session (Figure 8-7). Some conditions can be assessed both visually and by touch, such as edema.

Observation

Visual observations begin when the client walks in the door. The attentive therapist observes how the client stands and moves, noting any deviations from normal. During the consultation, the therapist may observe abnormalities in the tissues, such as swelling

Physician's Referral

Physician's Name: _____

Physician's Address: _____

Physician's Telephone: (_____) _____

I have been treating this patient since _____ for the following condition(s):
                                              date

_____

_____

_____

I have prescribed (specific massage therapy or bodywork treatment) for this patient's condition as follows:

_____

_____

Rx:_____ times per week for a period of _____ weeks.

Please note that the following considerations/medications warrant special concern:

_____

_____

Should you notice anything unusual or suspicious in the treatment or progress of this patient, please notify my office immediately.

Physician's Signature_____ Date _____

Please return completed form to:

MEMBER
ABMP

Figure 8-6, cont'd

or signs of trauma. Visual clues in body language, movement, and posture may help the therapist form ideas about cause and effect. A high right shoulder may be from carrying a heavy purse. Chronic ankle and knee pain may be from a pronated gait pattern resulting from fallen arches. This information is used in therapy sessions to relieve pain, restore health to the tissues, correct faulty posture patterns, and empathize with the client emotionally.

During visual assessment, the following observations can be made:

- **Skin color.** Color is normal for client's race and skin tone and not ashen, gray, or pale (ischemic); yellow (jaundiced); pink or red (inflamed, burned); or stretched and shiny (edematous). Note any bruising.

- **Circulation of nail beds.** The nail should be pressed firmly and released; normal refill is less than 2 seconds.
- **Skin condition.** Skin is moist; evidence of edema, lesions, and skin pathologies should be checked. All birthmarks, moles, and body hair should appear normal, and all scars are properly healed and accounted for on the intake form.
- **Structure.** Bone structure appears symmetrical bilaterally with no noticeable distortions along the horizontal or vertical axes.
- **Breathing.** Smooth, even movements should be heard during breathing.
- **Gait.** Client walks using a normal cross pattern and does not list or lean; arms swing freely at the sides, and toes point forward.

J. Michael Brown & Associates

403 W. 18th Street
Lake City, LA 70601

Lic # LA0034
(337) 555-1212

Physician's Referral and Prescription Form

Date: _____

Patient name: _____

Diagnosis: _____

ICD9 Code: _____

Contraindications: _____

It is my recommendation that this patient undergo the following procedure(s) ancillary and adjunctive to my treatment for the diagnosis listed above.

Procedure:

❑ Soft-tissue mobilization

❑ Neuromuscular re-education

❑ Manual lymphatic drainage

❑ Ice/heat packs

❑ Other _____
       (*please specify*)

Scheduling:

❑ 3 times per week for _____ weeks

❑ 2 times per week for _____ weeks

❑ 1 time per week for _____ weeks

❑ PRN for _____ weeks

Follow-up:

Patient will be re-evaluated on the _____ day of _____ , 20_____ , at which time the patient will be released or further orders for treatment will be authorized.

Physician's signature: _____

Please stamp
with your office ⟶
return address

Figure 8-6, cont'd

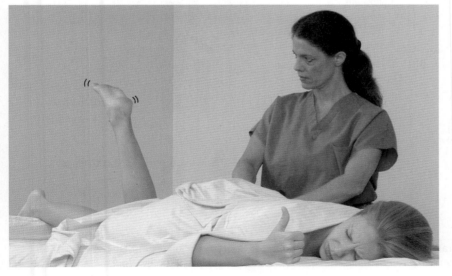

Figure 8-7 Therapist standing using visual and palpatory skills.

- **Body language.** Body language is monitored for changes in facial expression and other signs indicating discomfort and change in emotions.

Palpation

Palpation is defined as assessment through touching with purpose and intent. Palpatory assessment begins as the therapist runs his fingers over the client's main areas of complaint to note tissue health and abnormalities. Palpatory examination is easier when a small amount of lubricant is used, allowing for easier recognition of tissues below the surface. When palpating, light to moderate pressure should be used. This information is needed to determine which massage techniques to use during treatment.

During palpatory assessment, the following specifics may be noted:

- **Skin temperature.** Skin is not overly warm or hot, suggesting inflammation, or cool, indicating ischemia.
- **Skin condition.** Skin is not overly dry, suggesting excessive stress (sympathetic nervous system over activation).
- **Superficial fascia.** The skin should glide easily when moved over the underlying structures; difficult movement indicates adhesions of superficial fascia.

- **Muscle spasms.** The underlying musculature houses localized or general tension.
- **Local twitch response.** This is an involuntary firing or twitching in a muscle (a reflex motor output) in response to the sensory stimulation (pressure) on a trigger point.
- **Muscle atrophy.** Muscle lacks tone and feels flaccid to the touch.
- **Endfeel.** During functional assessment, endfeel is what is felt at the end of a passive range of motion (ROM). Hard endfeel has an abrupt stop of motion; soft endfeel has springy, spongy end of motion
- **Tenderness.** Pressing the area produces pain or discomfort.
- **Edema.** The area feels swollen, mushy, and congested; **pitting edema** (prolonged existence of pits produced by applying pressure) should be assessed.
- **Swollen lymph nodes.** This may denote possible local or systemic infection.
- **Anomalies.** Superficial and deep masses such as lipomas and other irregularities.

MINI-LAB

With the help of a classmate, use palpation to find and note the differences between a bone, muscle, lymph nodes, veins or arteries, and hair.

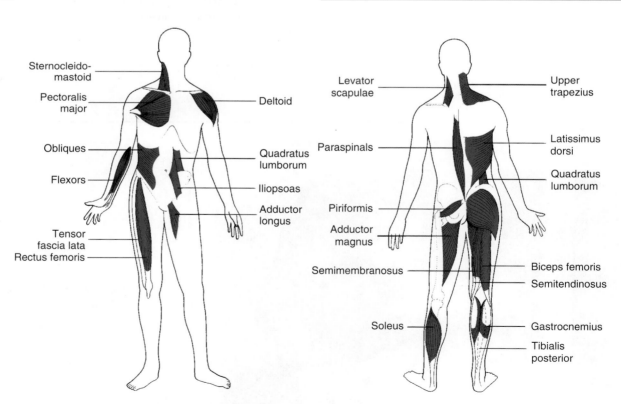

Figure 8-8   Major postural muscles, anterior and posterior views. (From Chiatow L, Delaney JW: *Clinical application of neuromuscular techniques V: vol 1—the upper body,* New York, 2001, Churchill Livingstone.)

Skin Assessment

During the consultation, a general survey of the skin can be made by observing and palpating any areas not covered with clothing. When the client is on the massage table, the areas not checked during the consultation should be quickly assessed. The above information can be used under observation and palpation to inspect the skin for skin color, temperature, and condition.

Postural (Structural) Assessment

Posture is the position of the body in space, such as standing, sitting, and lying down. Standing is considered the baseline measure of balance and alignment because standing posture is maintained through strength and tone of the muscles against gravitational forces (Figure 8-8). The human body maintains balance while standing and in motion. Structural misalignment is often the source of chronic pain. Disruption in the normal balance of the vertebrae can lead to degenerative disc disease, chronic myofascial pain, and further misalignment or compensation. Forward head posture creates excessive strain on neck muscles, throwing the entire body out of alignment in an attempt to compensate. Because of compressive forces in the chest cavity as a result of abnormal posture, lung capacity may be affected.

With age, a person's posture changes and height may decrease. The abdominal muscles often weaken and a redistribution of fat to the hips and the lower abdomen may cause the lower abdomen to protrude. Any spinal curvatures, such as lordosis, kyphosis, Dowager's hump, and scoliosis, require bolstering to increase client comfort while on the massage table. Chronic diseases of the lung, abnormal shape of the ribcage, or a barrel chest may rotate the shoulders forward. Women with large breasts and who wear improperly fitting brassieres may experience neck and shoulder pain resulting from an anterior pull or bra strap that may compress the trapezius and/or the brachial plexus. Use modalities to restore postural support and alignment. Client education should include stretching and strengthening techniques.

Major postural signs of imbalance should be observed. The therapist must visually observe the structure by taking a baseline measurement in several planes of the body to find deviations. Ways to assess the client's structure are to use the following landmarks (Figure 8-9):
- **Horizontal landmarks.** These should be symmetrical on both sides of the body and equidistant from the ground.
  Anterior
  - Ears
  - Eyes
  - Top of the acromioclavicular joints
  - Anterior superior iliac spines

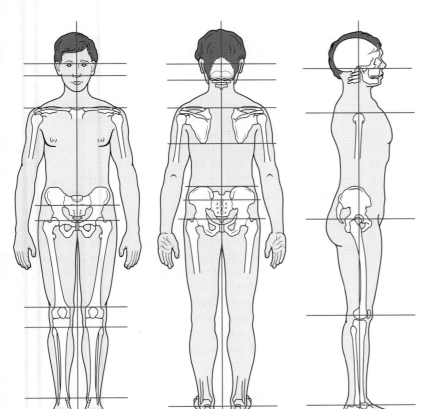

Figure 8-9   Horizontal and vertical landmarks.

- Top of the greater trochanters
- Top of the patellas
- Top of the fibular heads
- Top of the medial malleoli

Posterior
- Ears
- Occiput
- Scapulas
- Posterior superior iliac spines
- Top of the greater trochanters
- Calcaneus

- **Vertical landmarks.** These should be in a vertical line perpendicular to the ground.

Midsagittal Plane
- Nasal septum
- Manubrium
- Umbilicus
- Pubic symphysis

Coronal Plane
- External auditory meatus
- Humeral head
- Femoral head
- Lateral epicondyle of femur
- Lateral malleolus

Functional Assessment

Structure relates to function, posture relates to gait, and flexibility relates to posture and range of motion (ROM), so the body must be regarded as a unit. To move freely and without discomfort, each structure must play its part. Alterations in structure such as dysfunctional knees, spinal curvatures, high/low hip, long/short leg (Figure 8-10), and forward head posture produces distortions in body function and movement. When assessing for function, excess tension or atrophy in major muscle groups can be compared bilaterally. Muscular imbalances between anterior musculature and posterior musculature should be assessed. According to osteopath Andrew Taylor Still the human body structure governs function, so tension in muscles and misaligned bones causes unnecessary strain on the body as a whole. This theory, proposed in 1874, still holds true today.

Gait Assessment

Gait refers to a person's walking pattern. A normal gait pattern is smooth, coordinated, and rhythmic. During an efficient gait pattern, the body is erect, eyes are looking forward, arms are extended at the sides and swinging forward in opposition to the legs (Figure 8-11). The thumb and forefinger of the hand should face forward and not toward the backs of the hands. The toes point forward with the feet positioned slightly apart. Common abnormalities in gait result from muscle weakness, postural imbalance, pain, and connective tissue restriction; abnormalities may be acute or chronic. The longer the abnormali-

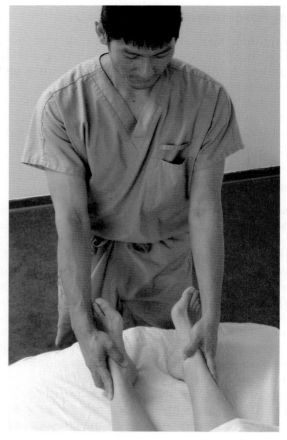

Figure 8-10 Therapist checking supine client's leg length using thumbs on medial malleoli.

ties in gait persist, the more soft-tissue compensations are involved. If an internal rotation of the knees, shoulders, hips, or feet occurs, the body cannot efficiently dissipate momentum, and trigger points can develop. Waddling gait patterns can contribute to lumbar disc deterioration. Neurological disorders or musculoskeletal injuries can often be detected while observing gait patterns.

The two phases to a gait pattern are the stance phase and the swing phase. The stance phase occurs when one leg and one foot bears most of the client's weight. When one leg is in the swing phase, the opposite leg is in the stance phase. The swing phase refers to the period during which the leg is actually moving: from the time it leaves the ground to the time it touches down again. The stance phase refers to the period during which the leg is bearing weight. Most gait abnormalities occur in the stance phase. The swing phase is the actual walking stage, when one foot is up and the opposite leg and foot bear the entire client's weight. The following are points to remember when assessing gait:

- **Slow gait.** Pain may be age-related or resulting from a neurological disorder.
- **Balance and grace.** Balance may altered because of pain in the shoulders, neck, weak upper extremity, poor posture, brain disorders, or use of prosthesis.

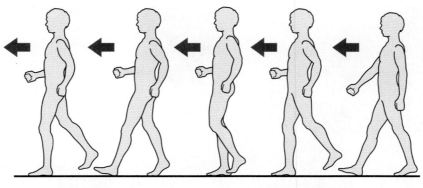

Left leg stance phase
Right leg swing phase

Right leg stance phase
Left leg swing phase

Figure 8-11   Stance and swing phases.

- **Short, shuffling steps.** Weak quadriceps or a neurological disorder such as Parkinson's may cause short steps.
- **Torquing or listing movements in the torso.** Arms or legs approach or cross the midline during stride.
- **Dragging feet.** This is indicator of weakness in the ankle dorsiflexors (drop-foot).
- **Waddling.** This may be the result of pain in the lower back, hip, knees, ankles. Generalized leg pain or use of prosthesis or orthotics may also cause waddling.
- **Limping.** This may occur as a result of a muscle cramp, bone spur, recent injury, neurological disorder, or a chronic condition such as sciatica.

MINI-LAB

Split the class into two groups; one group will observe while the other classmates walk. The observers assess posture and gait. Hold a group discussion to identify structures and the muscle groups used.
Then, check for balance and coordination:

1. To test foot extensor and flexor muscles, instruct a classmate to walk several feet on his heels and then turn around and walk toward the instructor on his toes.
2. To test proximal and distal muscle strength in the legs, instruct a classmate to hop in place for 10 seconds.
3. To check proximal muscles and hip extensors, instruct a classmate to stand up from a sitting position without using her arms. NOTE: This activity should be avoided by classmates with disabilities and severe illnesses.

Range of Motion

Assessing muscle and joint function is valuable in determining the location and level of dysfunction. Furthermore, evaluating ROM pre- and postmassage

demonstrate to the client treatment progress and effectiveness. ROM is an objective test that is measurable and can be recorded as such. A goniometer (Figure 8-12) can be used to measure degrees of movement. When documenting, name the action (e.g., flexion, extension, circumduction) and identify the type of movement (e.g., active, active assisted, active resisted, or passive). Note any joint deformity, tenderness, swelling, or crepitus. The following is a method for testing actively, which can be adapted for other movements:

1. **Explain why.** Explain to the client that you will be examining movement of a particular joint and that this will give information about its condition.
2. **Therapist demonstration.** Demonstrate the exact movement; the client will have less apprehension, knowing what to expect.
3. **Move the unaffected side first.** Assist the client in performing the movement correctly on the unaffected side if the condition is not bilateral. This establishes a baseline for the client's "normal" range.
4. **Move the affected joint.** Ask the client to move the affected joint and stop at the point of discomfort. Emphasize not to move the joint if discomfort is evident when initiating movement. Note when the client encounters pain by watching for facial grimaces, muscle guarding, apprehension, or the use of accessory muscles.

For example, if the client complains of neck pain, the therapist should ask him to demonstrate (or describe if the pain is severe) the movement in which the pain is experienced and to stop when he feels pain. After working the muscles involved, the therapist should then ask the client to repeat the movement.

Active ROM measures the client's movement using voluntary muscles. Passive ROM measures movement while the client relaxes voluntarily. In general, active movements are preferred to passive for assessment, especially for muscles, tendons, and tendon

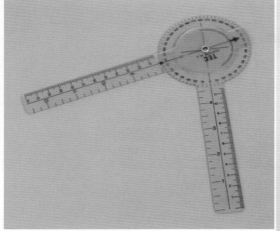

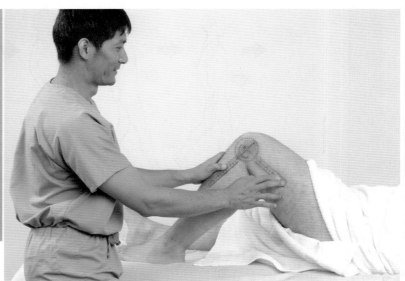

A   **B**

Figure 8-12 **A**, Goniometer; **B**, goniometer use.

sheaths. Passive ROM and stretching can test for ligaments, joint capsules, and some tendons.

Based on advice from the *Expert 10-Minute Physical Examination,* use the following key to grade and document muscle strength/weakness and range of motion.

0	**Complete paralysis.** No visible or palpable muscle contraction or movement of the extremity (severe decrease in normal range).
1	**Very severe weakness.** Weak muscle contraction is visible, but the extremity does not move (severe decrease in normal range).
2	**Severe weakness.** Client can roll the extremity but cannot lift it. Client can perform full ROM but not against gravity (severe decrease in normal range).
3	**Moderate weakness.** Client can perform full ROM against gravity but not against resistance (moderate decrease in normal range).
4	**Slight weakness.** Client can perform full ROM against gravity and slight resistance (mild decrease in normal range).
5	**Normal muscle strength.** Client can perform full ROM against gravity and resistance (normal range).

The most common error massage therapists make in charting functional assessment is to state that conducting massage improved ROM without recording pre- and postmassage measurements and observations. Making no note of what joint improved or what particular movement improved is also a mistake. By assessing and documenting pre- and post-

therapy, a clearer picture emerges of the client's improvement. Methods for accessing whether a client has full and painless ROM are as follows:

- Check if ROM is full and painless in the neck, shoulders, wrists, hips, knees, and ankle joints.
- During passive movements, the therapist moves the joint slowly and gently until a slight resistance is felt or the full range is accomplished.
- During active, active assisted, and active resisted movements, the therapist should confirm a contraction of the muscle during palpation to identify weak muscles or if the client is using accessory muscles to perform the movement.

CHARTING STAGE

Documentation is a record of client care. One way to organize client data obtained during the initial and investigative stages is by use of the APIE format, defined later in this section. The client's **treatment record** is the documentation obtained by using the APIE format. Massage therapy is a part of the health care system, and it is through written record that therapists can confirm their educated assessment, choice of massage, and the evaluation of the client's progress. With written documentation, the therapist can reread information to aid in recall and review. The effectiveness of the treatment is hard to determine when not documented. Memory is a poor method of record keeping. Charting is also a vital tool for communicating with other health care providers. Documentation and client records are legal evidence; this serves to protect the therapist by establishing professional accountability and showing that the care given met the client's expectations and needs. Adequate and accurate documentation also

MILTON TRAGER, MD

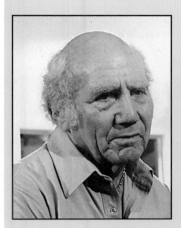

Photo courtesy of the Trager Institute, Mill Valley, Calif.

Born: April 20, 1908; died: January 20, 1997.

"Not until we experience it is it more than just words. After we experience it, there is no need for words."

It is the roaring '20s in sunny Miami. But for a high school dropout who lied about his age to get the $.65-an-hour post office job, it's all work. He barely has time to breathe—until today. Today, the posted health tip instructs him to do so and to sign his name indicating that he has done so.

Back then, Milton Trager probably had no idea that he possessed a talent that would develop, without outside influence, into a revolutionary method of bodywork. He inhaled and then exhaled, and that one deep breath put Trager in touch with his body for the very first time. "It was the beginning of me," he recalls. Soon he started working out at the beach, doing acrobatics, developing his muscles, and listening to the waves as he swayed to their ebb and flow.

Fascinated by the movements of boxers in the ring, he took up the sport. One day he offered to "turn the table" and massage his trainer. The trainer was stunned at his ability. He then worked on his father, who had severe sciatic pain. After just four sessions, his father's pain was gone, never to return again.

At age 19, Trager helped a child walk who had been unable to for 4 years. The proverbial 90-pound weakling had grown into a strong, agile young man whose acrobatic antics along his mail route captured the attention of the Hollywood studios. However, his unique mode of hands-on therapy went virtually unnoticed.

He enlisted with the Navy medical corps. After his release, he decided it was time to get the credentials that would make the medical field take notice of his work, but the only medical school that would accept a 42 year old was in Guadalajara, Mexico. So he headed south with his wife and embarked on the arduous task of earning a medical degree in a Spanish-speaking country.

Establishing a medical practice was difficult for someone with his background, but Trager finally settled in Honolulu. Sadly, the medical community remained disinterested in his work, but he did not feel the need for its blessing to feel secure in his knowledge. His method of holding, listening to, rocking, and freeing the body continued to evolve.

A well-known psychologist experienced Trager's methods and convinced him to demonstrate at Esalen, a workshop and meeting place for developing human potential. Jack Liskin, Trager's biographer, writes, "And so it was that an aging and unusual doctor with an unusual talent, unattached to any movement, New Age or conventional, came face-to-face with the California counterculture."*

The Trager Approach uses nonintrusive movements to lull the body into a better, more mobile, lighter state of being by releasing deep-seated physical and mental patterns.

Essential to Trager work is the term *hook-up,* which means that the practitioner becomes so totally focused that she achieves a hypersensitivity to body cues. It is as though the practitioner's mind/body communicates without using words. Additionally, what is being said to the receiver is, although he may have hidden them from his consciousness, that he holds the keys to unlock patterns that are holding him physically and mentally hostage. The therapist is just there to give his body the cues to gently remind him of his own potential—nothing more.

A Trager session does not end with tablework. Mentastics reinforces the results. *Mentastics* is Trager's term for *mental gymnastics,* the gentle, mindful

*From Liskin J: *Moving medicine: the life and work of Milton Trager, M.D.,* Barrytown, NY, 1996, Station Hill Press.

MILTON TRAGER, MD—cont'd

movement exercises that help the body recall positive physical or mental changes that occurred on the table and reinforce these changes.

Although Trager never cared for explaining his work, those who experienced, practiced, and witnessed its results have filled in the gaps.

"The practitioner uses the vast sensory capacities of the skin and deeper tissue to transmit messages. Using wavelike, moving rhythms that are at the core of all forms and matter of life, it communicates its messages thousands of times during a session to break habitual patterns," writes Liskin.

Trager never cared to be referred to as a genius, guru, or healer, claiming instead to have a talent. His talent did touch lives and change minds about what was possible. For example, Betty Fuller, a frequent seminar leader at Esalen, was prepared to live the rest of her days in chronic pain. When Trager reached out to examine her, she practically shrieked, "No one touches my neck." Yet he persisted in his gentle but unyielding manner. Soon, she was pain free and became Trager's first instructor. In Trager, she saw the same deep reverence for the mind's ability to heal the body that she had experienced as a student of Moshe Feldenkrais. It was to Fuller that Trager turned to protect his name and his work, and in 1980, the Trager Institute was founded.† Today, practitioners worldwide are using the Trager Approach and Mentastics Movement Education to ease headaches, back pain, and the debilitating effects of Parkinson's, cerebral palsy, polio, and multiple sclerosis.

†From What could be lighter? the work of Milton Trager, *Massage Mag* 67:56-63, 1997.

helps in justifying reimbursement, improving the quality of care, and demonstrating to the public that the therapist follows the accepted standards of care mandated by law, the profession, and the health care facility. When documenting, it is important to use accepted abbreviations common to the medical profession (Table 8-2).

Computerized charting is increasing in popularity. Fewer errors are made because the formats are standardized, legibility is improved over handwriting, and it requires less time and expense to record electronically.

For written documentation, corrections of any errors should be done on a single line, marked void, and initialed by the therapist. Scribbling and the use of correction fluid introduce doubt about the care provided and suggest the hiding of information. This is not acceptable documentation. The same color ink should be used consistently throughout the entire period of treatment. One entry in a different color may look like it was added later as a correction. Blue ink is the recommended color for intake forms and all handwritten documentation. Photocopy technology has advanced to the point that it may be difficult to tell an original in black pen from a photocopy. A

blue-ink original lends more credibility to the document.

One of the most valuable skills a therapist can have is being an effective listener and communicator. The goal is to help the client reach her highest functional level with minimal risks and problems. A problem-solving process is needed to direct the care in a systematic approach. This can be achieved using the APIE format, defined as follows:

- **Assessment:** Subjective data and objective data
- **Plan (of care):** What should be done today and in the near future
- **Implementation:** Modalities applied during today's session
- **Evaluation:** Therapist's determination of treatment outcome to date

Obtaining this information in these categories helps the therapist write appropriate documentation and guides the therapist with a feasible plan. The sum of the information gathered in the subjective/objective data, the plan and implementation of care, and evaluation of treatment are like spokes of a wheel. Each spoke shares in carrying the weight and helps maintain strength, mobility, and integrity of the wheel. A weak spoke such as improper collection

TABLE 8-2

Common Abbreviations, Symbols, Prescriptive Directions, Medical Terminology, Pathologies, Modalities, and Findings

Abbreviations/Symbols	Meaning	Abbreviations/Symbols	Meaning
General		INF	inferior
p; post	after	stat	immediately
ANT	anterior	INT	internal
≈	approximately	LAT	lateral, left anterior thigh
ASAP	as soon as possible	L	left
PRN	as needed	<	less than, minus, negative, absent
@	at		
hs	at bedtime	LTG	long-term goal
a; pre	before	#	number
BIL	bilateral	qwk	once a week
CAUD	caudal	OTC	over-the-counter prescription
CEPH	cephalic	pt	patient
℅	complains of	+	positive, plus, present, and
CSTx	continue same treatment	Rx	prescription, drug, or medication
CNT	could not test		
CSR	craniosacral rhythm	Px	prognosis, physical examination
DOB	date of birth		
DOI	date of injury	PROX	proximal
↓	decrease, below	O—<	recumbent
Dx	diagnosis	R	right
DNK	did not keep	2°	secondary, due to, as a result of
dist.	distal		
Eval	evaluate	STG	short-term goal
qd	every day	×	times, time
qod	every other day	per, /	through, or by
ft	foot	Tx	treatment, therapy
>	greater than	b.i.d.	twice a day
Hx	history	c; w	with
↑	increase, above	s; w/o	without
Symptoms		INFLAM	inflammation
Abr	abrasion	kyph	kyphosis
ASP	abnormal spine posture	max	maximum
AI	accidental injury	min	minimum
Adh	adhesion, fibrosis	MAEW	moves all extremities well
AOB	alcohol on breath	P & B	pain and burning
BA	backache	POM	pain on motion
CON	congested	SFLE	stress from life experience
crep	crepitus	SOB	shortness of breath
Flat	flatulence	SOBOE	shortness of breath on exercise
FOOSH	fell on outstretched hand		
HA	headache	st	stiffness
HOH	hard of hearing	STI	soft-tissue injury
HT	hypertonus, tension, tight muscles	SP	spasm
		TP	trigger point
Pathologies		DDD	degenerative disk disease
CTS	carpal tunnel syndrome	DJD	degenerative joint disease
CVA	cerebral vascular accident	DEV	deviation
CHF	congested heart failure	ed	edema
CFS	chronic fatigue syndrome		

Continued

TABLE 8-2

Common Abbreviations, Symbols, Prescriptive Directions, Medical Terminology, Pathologies, Modalities, and Findings—cont'd

Abbreviations/Symbols	Meaning	Abbreviations/Symbols	Meaning
Pathologies—cont'd			
Fl up	flare up	RTC	rotator cuff
FT	fibrous tissue	TeP	tender point
FX	fracture	TP	trigger point
HBP	high blood pressure	TMD	temporomandibular joint dysfunction
HTR	hypertrophy		
LBP	low back pain	TOS	thoracic outlet syndrome
lord	lordosis	spr.	sprain
OA	osteoarthritis	str.	strain
PTSD	posttraumatic stress disorder	VV	varicose vein
RA	rheumatoid arthritis		
Massage Techniques and Modalities			
AAS	active assisted stretching	MFW	myofascial web, continuous fascial planes
Abd/ABD	abduction		
Add/ADD	adduction	NMT	neuromuscular therapy
AROM	active ROM	PB	paraffin bath
aroma	aromatherapy	PAROM	passive-assisted ROM
CST	craniosacral therapy	Pas Ex	passive exercise
XFF	cross-fiber friction	PNF	proprioceptive neuro-muscular facilitation
DP	direct pressure		
EXT	external, extension	PROM	passive ROM
ext. rot.	external rotation	PT	physical therapy
ever	eversion	ROM	range of motion
FLEX	flexion	ROS	review of symptoms/systems
int. rot.	internal rotation	SFT	soft-tissue mobilization
inver	inversion	SCS	strain, counterstrain
MLD	manual lymphatic drainage	SUP	superior, supination
M	massage	SwM	Swedish massage
Ms	muscle, musculoskeletal	Ther-X	therapeutic exercise or procedure
MET	muscle energy technique		
MFR	myofascial release	WNL	within normal limits
Muscles and Landmarks			
abs	abdominal	LEV	levator scapulae
AC	acromioclavicular	LB	low back
ACL	anterior cruciate ligament	L1->5	lumbar vertebrae, spine
ASIS	anterior superior iliac spine	LN	lymph node
bi	biceps	Mm	major, minor
C1->7	cervical vertebrae, spine	pecs	pectoralis
DH	dominant hand	QL	quadratus lumborum
E	energy	SI	sacroiliac
ES	erector spinae group	S1->5	sacral vertebrae, sacrum
gastroc	gastrocnemius	SCM	sternocleidomastoid
IF	iliofemoral	TFL	tensor fascia latae
ITB	iliotibial band	traps	trapezius
IP	iliopsoas	TMJ	temporal mandibular joint
IT	ischial tuberosity	T1-12	thoracic vertebrae, spine
lats	latissimus dorsi		

of data damages the entire structure of the wheel, jeopardizing the success of the entire therapy session.

Assessment

Attainment of assessment data is a two-fold process. First, information is obtained through the client's perspective (subjective data). Second, the therapist collects information through objective assessment methods. The combination of these builds a foundation for the other three components (plan, implementation, and evaluation) to take place.

Subjective data are any information you gain from the client. It is considered subjective because the client cannot present the information to the therapist without personal bias; he is the one experiencing the pain. Subjective information includes all written disclosure given on the intake form and all the information gathered through questioning during the interview process of the consultation. Of special note are the client's chief concern or complaint and his explanations of various symptoms. A **symptom** may be anything he subjectively notices as unusual or uncomfortable. The therapist can explore symptoms by asking the client to describe the pain (i.e., sharp, dull, burning, or aching) or identify its onset. When asking a client about pain, it is important to be consistent by using the same pain scales for each session and with each client (Figure 8-13). This information is recorded on section *S* of the APIE notes on the client's intake form (Figure 8-14, *S* on APIE record).

Objective data are the recordings of the therapist's assessments gathered during the investigation stage described earlier. **Objective data** are measurable and quantitative, such as the size and shape of a mole, whether the right shoulder is higher than the left, or if the left knee is swollen (larger) and by how many centimeters more than the right. It may be a comparison of ROM as measured by a goniometer before and after treatment.

Use of a record assessment protocol (RAP) such as the one presented below ensures consistency in assessment. Note how this list is derived from observable and palpable data provided in earlier sections. This protocol is a checklist of assessment criteria that helps prevent errors of omission. It is not necessary to waste time and space charting normal conditions, chart only the deviations from the norm. Assessment speed comes with practice and experience. Use of critical thinking, learning to think beyond the problem, and developing "thinking fingers" along with an "inquiring mind" are all pertinent to this process. Use of medical abbreviations is required to record findings in section *O* of the APIE notes on the client's treatment record in an abbreviated summary style (see Figure 8-14, *O* on APIE record).

Record Assessment Protocol

The following is an example of a RAP:

- Skin color
- Skin temperature
- Skin condition
- Swollen lymph nodes
- Anomalies
- Superficial fascia
- Localized or generalized tenderness
- Muscle tension, tone, spasms, and atrophy
- Horizontal structural landmarks
- Vertical structural landmarks
- Breathing
- Gait
- Range of motion

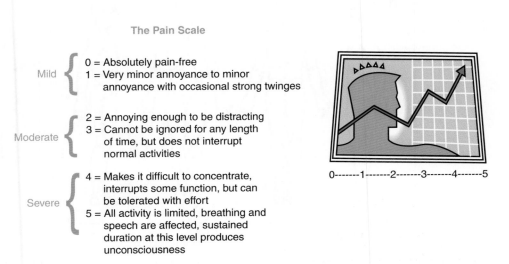

The Pain Scale

Mild {
0 = Absolutely pain-free
1 = Very minor annoyance to minor annoyance with occasional strong twinges

Moderate {
2 = Annoying enough to be distracting
3 = Cannot be ignored for any length of time, but does not interrupt normal activities

Severe {
4 = Makes it difficult to concentrate, interrupts some function, but can be tolerated with effort
5 = All activity is limited, breathing and speech are affected, sustained duration at this level produces unconsciousness

0-------1-------2-------3-------4-------5

Figure 8-13   Pain scale and illustration.

APIE Treatment Record   Date_____ Page _____ of _____

Name: Wanda Victorian   DOB: 11/18/50   PH 555-2918

Job: Special Needs school bus aid, works at the Hanger—clothing store

Notes: previously seen for neck, posterior shoulder pain, left hip pain with referral pattern down lateral side of leg. Requests relaxation massage with extra work for neck & shoulders.

A: subjective/objective data

S: c/o's of neck pain worse × 2 wks, reports being tense between the shoulders—"those nasty muscles", hurts and c/o's soreness left hip to the knee on the side. This past week mom, 80, pulled dislocated hip and fell fracturing her good hip, father with dementia and incontinence of bowel and bladder—wears diapers, she has been helping.

O: tenderness noted posterior cervicals with taut bands, mild dowanger's hump. hypertonus rhomboids Mm, tenderness and congested L. outerglutes with referral pain pattern down L-ITB

P: STG: neck, shoulder, hip pain by the end session. LTG: bring tennis ball on bus routes to trigger between shoulder, and trigger hip also can carry cold gel packs on bus route to use. Homework: cont. with salt and soda baths. ↑ water intake, will contact a sitters registry, cont. with neck, shoulder exercises, wear shoe lift. Requests to set up 30 minute sessions weekly × 2 for neck and shoulder discomfort, then a full body on 3rd week. Client to perform/mirror neck and shoulder exercises.

I: Jacuzzi × 10 minutes with cool compress to upper neck. TP to posterior neck & shoulders, XFF to upper anterior ribcage, myofascial stretch–w/Sw Gymnastic to upper torso. Sw Massage, cool compress under neck while lying supine before completion of session. PNF–L hip. Ended with thoracic stretch.

E: Feels very frustrated trying to handle 2 jobs with parents both sick. Reports she has to work in order to pay bills, allowed client to vent, likes the change in the neck routine "seems like my neck is finally releasing.", would like to keep the neck routine as part of future massage sessions. The use of cold compress while in the Jacuzzi was very soothing. Encourage client to continue to wear Rx. heel lift

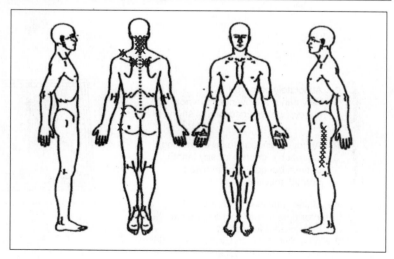

Figure 8-14   APIE sample treatment record.

Plan

The *P* in APIE is for plan or plan of care. After the completion of the session, the short-term goals (STGs) and long-term goals (LTGs) are set, along with treatment strategies for future sessions. Client education and suggestions of lifestyle modifications can assist the client in reaching her goals. Success of treatment is proportionate to the effort that goes into the plan; establishing confidence in the treatments and aiding the body's healing processes. Careful planning helps set priorities in the massage sessions.

STGs involve using specific modalities to decrease discomfort in a specific area by the end of the session. The STG for a specific session may be applying ischemic compression to active trigger points in the client's right shoulder. Subsequent treatments may focus on deeper musculature; passive ROM; and finally, active ROM. Each of these sessions may include client education and various homework assignments when appropriate such as ROM exercises, stretching, and strength building. Each of these STGs are the increments of progress that assist in reaching the LTG.

Client education empowers the client to take control of their health. Keep health-related information on hand that is easy to understand. Areas of education include ergonomics, musculoskeletal self-care activities, exercises, and postural adjustments. If handout literature includes exercises or stretches, demonstrating them prior to issuing them to clients is helpful. Alternatively, the client can be asked to mirror the exercise so that she may do it properly and not injure herself. The client needs to understand all the factors that can play a part in her healing process.

LTGs focus on restoration of normal function. The goal is generally to return to the same level of health enjoyed before an accident. For example, a muscle spasm that is relieved in a session is short-term; the ability to return to work, pain free, without the use of a brace is long term. These goals should be recorded in section *P* of the APIE notes on the client's treatment record (see Figure 8-14, *P* on APIE record).

When establishing goals, they should be kept simple and realistic. The client needs continued success to keep him motivated and maintain healthy habits. Finding ways to support and encourage him is important. For example, if the client is not an avid water drinker, design creative ways to help him increase his water consumption. The benefits of water can be explained—how water intake improves the metabo-lism of the body and affects the aging process and how water assists to metabolize fat. Relevant articles should be available, providing a schedule on how to "sneak" water into the diet. Teaching a client a skill lasts longer than willpower.

If a physician or physical therapist is assigning exercise, it would be inappropriate to add more or different activities. Professional boundaries should be obtained; commenting negatively on the assignments from another practitioner is discouraged. Networking directly with other health care providers is sometimes necessary. The therapist should explain to the client that her health care provider is being contacted. A signed release form should be obtained from the client while she is in your office (Figure 8-15).

Implementation

The *I* in APIE is for implementation, or techniques used during therapy. The choice of therapy depends on the assessments (subjective and objective data) during the initial and investigative stages and the knowledge base of the therapist. Numerous modalities can be used to give the client maximum benefit from the session. Documentation of the types of modalities used help the therapist recall what worked for the client, if the client reports receiving benefit. If a local contraindication exists, this influences the massage application. Documentation of this information protects the therapist and decreases liability risks. The documentation should include the use of any adjunctive therapies such as aromatherapy, hydrotherapy, or support/bolstering devices that are out of the ordinary. Also, whether the client needed assistance should be documented. Findings made during the treatment can be recorded in the in section *I* of the APIE notes on the client's treatment record (see Figure 8-14, *I* on APIE record).

Evaluation

The *E* in APIE stands for evaluation. The outcome of a session should be recorded to evaluate the effectiveness, problems, or concerns of that session. **Outcome** is the client's response to therapy and progress toward STGs and LTGs. The client may have made comments during the session, so the therapist should use this area to make reminders for future sessions. Any revisions to the previous plan should be documented,

Release of Information

Client name:_____ Medical record no:_____

Address:_____

Phone: (____)_____ DOB:_____ ZIP code:_____

Releasing facility:_____

Address:_____

City, state, ZIP code:_____

Fax: (____)_____ Phone: (____)_____

Send or fax information to:

Receiving facility:_____

Address:_____

City, state, ZIP code:_____

Fax: (____)_____ Phone: (____)_____

I hereby grant permission to release health information regarding my care for the dates:

_____ to _____. This release expires on _____.

_____   _____
(Patient signature)   (Date)

Figure 8-15   Sample release form.

with record made of evaluations in section *E* of the APIE notes on the client's treatment record (see Figure 8-14, *E* on APIE record). Evaluation is an ongoing process that occurs every time a client visits. Documentation with clear statements demonstrates progress toward attaining goals. Realize that a 100% return of function and complete freedom from pain are not possible in all cases. Sometimes 50% improvement is tremendous achievement for the client.

For Your Information

Evaluation addresses posttreatment conclusion.

SUPPORTIVE DOCUMENTATION STAGE

APIE notes are important client and treatment documents. Additional paperwork may be necessary to supplement information or support the care provided in a session. Quality assurance is necessary to update files and improve services. Other supportive documentation includes a *release form* or *progress notes*.

Release Form

To send out any information about the client, the client must release the information because of its confidential nature. The release form gives the therapist

authorization to release certain information from the client to specific parties. The form should have the client name, the institution and address maintaining the client records, and the institution and address of the receiving institution. The client should sign and date the release form, and a signature from a witness should be obtained. The release of information should have an expiration period. If the client is a juvenile, a parent/guardian must sign (see Figure 8-15).

Progress Notes

Progress notes or progress reports are addenda to previous APIE notes used in follow-up visits. This form indicates the improvement the client has made with appropriate data gleaned from previous sessions. The information should be kept chronological, with the self-care capabilities, initial dates of sessions, and the response made by the client included. Previous visits can be referred back to by dates with a brief synopsis. STGs and/or LTGs can be examined at this time (Figure 8-16).

For Your Information

The therapist must keep important records for an established period. The National Certification Board of Therapeutic Massage and Bodyworkers (NCBTMB) recommends 4 years, but it varies from state to state.

Progress Note

Name: _____ Dx: _____

Date: _____ Last visit: __/__/__ for _____

Changes in health ___ yes ___ no

Assessment (subjective/objective data) _____

_____

_____

Objective: see body map for changes from visit: __/__/__

Problem	Plan	Implementation

***pain scale: _____   ***pain scale: _____

pain scale: 0-1 = mild 2-3 = moderate 4-5 = severe

Other: _____

Plan:

___ ↑ water intake   ___ cold compress   ___ warm compress

___ stretching ex.   ___ salt & soda soaks   ___ referred

Other: _____

Evaluation: _____

Illustration key: X = adhesion @ = trigger point 0 = pain → = refers to

---

Progress Note

Name: _Wanda Victorian_ Dx: _____

Date: _03/28/02_ Last visit: _03/15/02_ for _Relaxation_

Changes in health ___ yes ✓ no

Assessment (subjective/objective data) _Since last session. Neck_

L shoulder. L hip pain much improved. Wearing shoe lift and started

walking exercise in the mall. Focus today — neck — back of neck

also c/o's of HA

Objective: see body map for changes from visit: _03/15/02_

Problem - assessed	Plan	Implementation
neck—post cervical	STG - ↓ neck,	
thick, taut bands	shoulder pain	
Bil. traps (↑) upper		See gymnastics
congested		for neck, shoulder (L)
	LTG - Minimize	Hip - L
Rhomboids L > R	pain and increase	
w/tenderness	mobility of upper	TP (L) lateral
L-/ITB—tenderness	torso - neck -	1T Band.
	shoulders	

***pain scale: _4_   ***pain scale: _1_

pain scale: 0-1 = mild 2-3 = moderate 4-5 = severe

Other: _____

Plan:

✓ ↑ water intake   ✓ cold compress   ✓ warm compress

✓ stretching ex.   ✓ salt & soda soaks   ___ referred

Other: _Instructed to try cold compress @ post. base_

of neck, warm compress on feet × 10 min in

a quiet room w/relaxed music for HA

Evaluation: _Today's session lasted 1 hour — 40 min_

spent on neck routine — 20 min for the rest

of session. Met goal. Pain level 2.

Illustration key: X = adhesion @ = trigger point 0 = pain → = refers to

Figure 8-16 Sample progress notes.

SUMMARY

Navigating through the sea of information obtained in the initial and investigative stages can tailor the appropriate therapy for the client. The knowledge gained in the previous chapters can guide a therapist into developing a plan of care for enhancing the client's health and wellness.

Using the charting format of APIE is the documentation backbone to the massage therapy service (Table 8-3). APIE documentation helps categorize information from the client to develop and evaluate the care provided. Assessment data of subjective and objective information is critical information to develop a therapeutic session. The subjective data allow the client to share information from their understanding and what they perceive is their problem. The objective data allows the therapist to determine those problems shared by the client. Plan is the client's map of health maintenance. Implementation of therapy and the array of knowledge a massage therapist has enable the therapist to administer her "healing hands" to the client. Not only is it a quality assurance check, it also helps the therapist determine whether she would have done anything differently if she were starting over with that client. Therefore the evaluation phase is the check and double-check role.

Supportive documentation is the supplemental information that accommodates the charting and gives aid to the therapist for her documentation of services. A variety of forms can assist documentation.

Success in using professional behavior, appropriate treatments, and documentation results in an open door for massage therapists, acknowledging them as important members of the health care teams in medicine.

TABLE 8-3

Stages of Assessment and Documentation

Stage	Activity	Focus
Initial	Completion of health intake form	Clarification of information
	Sign consents, reviews past intake and notes	
	Provide referrals/consultation	
Investigative	Assimilates subjective/objective data	Assessment of client
Charting	Complete treatment	Notes on subjective/objective assessments, plan, implementation, application of modalities, and evaluation
	record by categories	
Supportive documentation	Integrates other forms to communicate care	Helpful forms to provide, continue, or promote care

MATCHING I

List the letter of the answer next to the term or phrase that best describes it.

A. Outcome
B. Subjective data
C. Pitting edema
D. Diagnosis
E. Palpation

F. Palliative
G. Gait
H. Posture
I. Informed consent
J. Symptom

K. Treatment record
L. Objective data
M. Modality
N. Prescription

_____ 1. The documentation obtained using the APIE format

_____ 2. A technique, procedure, or product that produces a positive response for the client

_____ 3. Type of care that eases or reduces pain

_____ 4. Any information gained from the client

_____ 5. Client's authorization for professional services based on adequate information provided by the attending therapist

_____ 6. A written order by a physician or nurse-practitioner authorizing massage therapy treatment

_____ 7. Assessment through touching with purpose and intent

_____ 8. A person's walking pattern

_____ 9. Anything that is subjectively noticed as unusual or uncomfortable

_____ 10. Identifying a disease or illness by scientific evaluation from a qualified health care practitioner

_____ 11. The recordings of the therapist's assessments; it is measurable and quantitative

_____ 12. Position of the body in space, such as standing, sitting, and lying down

_____ 13. The client's response to therapy and progress toward STGs and LTGs

_____ 14. The prolonged existence of pits produced by applying pressure

MATCHING II

Mark the following statements as S, subjective; O, objective; I, implementation; P, plan; and E, evaluation.

_____ 1. Complains of lower back pain (LBP)

_____ 2. Hamstring stretch 4 × daily

_____ 3. Guarding right shoulder

_____ 4. Hypertonus/thickening of rhomboids

_____ 5. "My back hurts, so I bought slip-on shoes because I can't bend over to tie shoes"

MATCHING II—cont'd

___ 6. "Ouch, that feels like a *10!*"

___ 7. During the follow-up consult, the client reports the lumbar work enabled him to stand upright with minimal pain

___ 8. Trigger point work to upper and middle trapezius muscles

___ 9. Return for follow-up in 2 weeks

___ 10. Client "walks like a duck"

___ 11. During intake, client reports generalized feelings of tension

___ 12. Right posterior shoulder presents with a mole that is dark with an irregular border and cauliflower appearance

___ 13. Guarding with piriformis stretch during assessment

___ 14. Client increases water intake and takes stress breaks at work

___ 15. Swedish gymnastics, Swedish massage this session

Bibliography

Abdenour J: *TN Magazine: the professional magazine with the personal touch,* Mountvale, NJ, 1999, Medical Economics.

American Massage Therapy Association: *Code of ethics,* Evanston, Ill, 1994, The Association.

Associated Bodywork and Massage Professionals: *Successful business handbook,* Evergreen, Colo, 2001, The Associated.

Boltn R: *People skills,* New York, 1979, Simon and Schuster.

Burley-Allen M: *Listening: the forgotten skill,* New York, 1995, John Wiley.

Chaitow L: *Palpation skills: assessment and diagnosis through touch,* New York, 2000, Churchill Livingstone.

D'Ambrogio KJ, Roth GB: *Positional release therapy: assessment and treatment of musculoskeletal dysfunction,* Philadelphia, 1997, Mosby.

Davis NM: *Medical abbreviations: 7000 conveniences at the expense of communications and safety,* ed 5, Huntington Valley, Pa, 1990, Neil M. Davis Associates.

Dolan DW: *Objective structural findings in massage therapy: key to insurance reimbursement and special physician referrals,* Jacksonville, Fla, 1995, Advanced Therapeutics America.

Expert 10-minute physical examination, St Louis, 1997, Mosby.

Ignatavicius DD, Bayne MV: *Medical-surgical nursing: a nursing process approach,* Philadelphia, 1991, WB Saunders.

Loving J: *Massage therapy: theory and practice,* Stamford, Conn, 1998, Appleton and Lange.

Lowe WW: *Functional assessment in massage therapy,* Corvallis, Ore, 1995, Pacific Orthopedic Massage.

Mackey B: Massage therapy and reflexology awareness, *Nurs Clin North Am* 36(1):159-170, 2001.

McKay M, Davis M, Fanning P: *Messages: the communication skills book,* Oakland, Calif, 1987, New Harbinger.

National Association of Nurse Massage Therapists: *Standards of practice,* Jupiter, Fla, 1992, The Association.

National Certification Board of Massage Therapy: *Code of ethics,* McLean, Va, 1995, The Board.

Reese NB: *Muscle and sensory testing,* Philadelphia, 1999, WB Saunders.

Rubino J: *Been there done that,* Charlottesville, Va, 1997, Upline Press.

St. John P: *St. John neuromuscular therapy seminars, manual I,* Largo, Fla, 1995, Author.

Salvo SG: *Massage therapy principles and practice,* ed 1, Lake Charles, La, 1999, WB Saunders.

Shealy NC: *Alternative medicine: the complete family guide,* Versailles, Ky, 1996, Rand McNally.

Sohen-Moe C: Taking care of business: the ultimate client interview, *Massage Ther J* pp 133-136, 1996.

Springhouse Corporation: *Charting made incredibly easy!* Springhouse, Pa, 1998, Springhouse.

Starlanyl D, Copeland ME: *Fibromyalgia and chronic myofascial pain: a survival manual,* ed 2, Oakland, Calif, 2001, New Harbinger.

Strong J et al: *Pain: a textbook for therapists,* New York, 2002, Churchill Livingstone.

Thompson DL: Hands heal: *Documentation for massage therapy,* ed 2, Seattle, 2001, Lippincott Williams and Wilkins.

Torres LS: *Basic medical techniques and patient care for radiologic technologies,* Philadelphia, 1993, JB Lippincott.

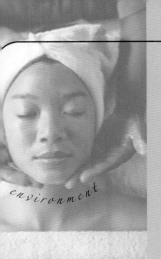

environment

Adaptive Massage and Client Management Issues

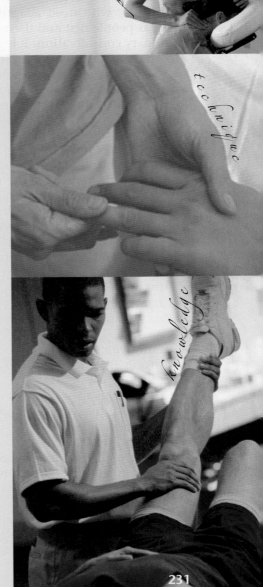

pressure

technique

knowledge

"It is only with the heart that one can see rightly. What is essential is invisible to the eye."

—Antoine de Saint-Exupéry

STUDENT OBJECTIVES

After completing this chapter, the student should be able to:

- Learn modifications for the client's position on the massage table when someone requires variation from the norm
- Adjust massage techniques to suit the client's various conditions
- Adapt massage therapy for pregnant clients
- Accommodate clients who have visual, auditory, or speech impairments
- Adjust massage to accommodate someone who is physically challenged or in a wheelchair
- Discuss emotional releases and describe ways they can be appropriately handled

INTRODUCTION

The standard massage routine is designed to suit the needs of the average client, who may represent the majority of your clientele. However, you will encounter individuals who have unique situations that include physical, emotional, and health-related challenges. You will need to accommodate these individuals and modify or adapt massage therapy to fit their special needs. The client's needs may range from relatively simple ones such as bolstering for breast implants or pregnancy; to communication needs for those with speech, vision, or hearing impairments; to moderate needs such as working around central venous catheters, colostomies, and pacemakers; to emotional needs for those who have been sexually abused or have chemical dependencies; and to those living with illnesses such as cancer and human immunodeficiency virus (HIV).

The most important way in which you can assist individuals who need adaptive massage is to view them as people first and their special needs only as a secondary consideration. It is generally best to regard all injuries and conditions with the attitudes of gentleness, kindness, and acceptance. Many clients who have special needs may be touch-deprived, and massage can go a long way to provide safe touch and meet psychosocial and physiological needs. Adopting this attitude sets the stage for a therapeutic relationship that can be fulfilling to both of you.

When adapting your massage for special populations, keep in mind that the massage strokes themselves may not change. The alterations come in how you modify the pressure, speed, duration, and frequency of the massage; how you position your client on the massage table; and other safety precautions you must take. Adaptations to consider include the following:

- Amputations
- Clients who are athletes
- Breast implants or large breasts
- Cancer
- Central venous catheter
- Chronic illness
- Colostomy or ileostomy
- Contact lens users
- End-of-life massage
- Geriatric clients
- Hearing impaired clients
- Clients with HIV or who are living with acquired immune deficiency syndrome (AIDS)
- Infants
- Large clients
- Menstruation
- Pacemaker users
- Paraplegia, quadriplegia, and hemiplegia
- Pediatric clients
- Postoperative clients and scar tissue
- Pregnant clients
- Sexual abuse
- Speech difficulties
- Spinal abnormalities such as kyphosis, lordosis, and scoliosis
- Substance abuse and drug addiction issues
- Visually impaired clients
- Clients in wheelchairs

The client may make you aware of her special need when she calls to get information about your services or to set up an appointment. If so, spend a few minutes looking up the condition in this textbook, a pathophysiology book, or a medical dictionary before the scheduled appointment. The best way to obtain information about her special need is to ask her directly during the premassage interview. Each situation will be different, and you must be willing to be open-minded, patient, tolerant, and flexible. Each client will teach you, if you are willing to listen and learn. Although each client will have different needs in the delivery of the massage, the therapist's boundaries should always be consistent. See Chapter 2 for an in-depth discussion of personal and professional boundaries and confidentiality issues for the massage therapist.

The following sections can help you make the necessary accommodations.

Amputations

If your client has an amputation, obtain consent to massage the stump during the premassage interview. Also, inquire about the actual surgical procedure; most clients know about their particular situation. For instance, if a midhumeral amputation has a smooth stump with no protruding bone, it helps to know if the triceps or biceps was used to wrap the stump end. This helps you locate trigger points. While massaging the stump, ask the client if it is sensitive or numb. Use light tapotement, towel friction, or mechanical vibration to desensitize any hypersensitive areas. Many practitioners of energy work such as polarity and Reiki treat the energy field of the missing limb as if it were still present.

Approximately 70% of all people with amputations experience *phantom limb sensation* (feeling pain and other sensations in all or part of an amputated limb). The onset of pain is generally within the first week but may occur several months or years after the amputation. One possible explanation of this phenomenon is that a *neuroma* (tumor found in nervous tissue) forms on the severed nerve ends of the amputated limb. Another theory states that abnormal sensory input along the afferent nerve in the amputated area enters the higher centers of the brain, resulting in pain. Another postulation is that the nerves in the central nervous system still send out signals to the length of the missing limb. Clearly phantom limb sensation is complex and does involve both the peripheral and the central nervous systems. However, the calming effects of massage generally have a positive outcome on phantom limb pain regardless of the cause.

Amputations may not be obvious because of prosthetic appliances. Some clients may not want to remove the prosthetic because of the time factors, whereas others are glad to be free of them for awhile. Look out for chafing or friction wounds where the prosthetic limb fits to the stump. Avoid any inflamed areas broken skin, or open wounds. Clients with leg amputations may walk using leg prosthetics and at other times may be on crutches or in a wheelchair (see the section Clients in Wheelchairs).

Athletes

An athlete is anyone who possesses a natural or acquired ability such as the strength, endurance, and agility required for participating in a sport. To properly massage an athlete, ask questions regarding his training schedule and areas of soreness or tenderness. Address these areas during treatment and use your palpatory skills to locate and reduce the discomfort of tender areas, using hydrotherapy as needed. Unless you are working at a sports event, you are essentially providing your athletic client with a maintenance massage, which ranges from addressing general soreness to specific work.

Athletic massage, or sports massage is divided into two main types, depending on when or how it is administered: *event* and *maintenance massage*. Event massage can be further divided into *pre-event, postevent,* and *inter-event*. Pre-event sports massage leaves the athlete relaxed and ready for the event. Inter-event massage keeps the athlete tuned up between events. Postevent massage flushes out metabolic wastes and reduces muscle spasms and soreness. Maintenance sports massage encompasses both *injury prevention* and *rehabilitative care*.

Breast Implants or Large Breasts

When massaging a woman with breast implants or large breasts, several options are available to make her more comfortable while she is lying prone. You may offer the client a rolled-up towel or cylindrical pillow to be placed under, above, or between her breasts, whichever is most comfortable. Many clients prefer a supportive device both above *and* below the breasts (Figure 9-1, *A*). Use a face rest that can be adjusted above the level of the table (Figure 9-1, *B*). Several commercial bolsters provide sternal support (Figure 9-

2). Additionally, several massage table manufacturers now carry tables fitted with breast recesses that allow the client to lie prone more comfortably. This table option includes two small, round cushions that can be inserted to fill the breast recess spaces when not use.

In the supine position, it is sometimes difficult to access muscles in the chest area of full-figured women. If massage is needed in the pectoral region, the serratus anterior, or in the walls of the axilla, you may ask the client to use the back side of her hand to cup the breast tissue and retract it medially (Figure 9-3). This technique establishes a safe physical boundary between client and therapist. You may decide to work on this area in a side-lying position with the client holding her top arm above the elbow with her bottom hand (Figure 9-4). These modifications are also useful to a postpartum or nursing mother.

Cancer

At one time, cancer was seen as a terminal illness, so a cancer patient's most common question to his physician was, "How long do I have to live?" With advanced technologies and medications, cancer is now often viewed as a chronic condition, and the focus, as survival rates continue to rise, is on the cancer patient's quality of life. Inactivity and social withdrawal are often coping mechanisms for a patient who is besieged with pain, but when pain is effectively managed, cancer patients remain active, having more energy and fewer physical problems than those who simply give in to their disabilities. Massage is now one viable option used to help cancer patients lead a more active, pain-free life after this life-changing diagnosis.

The American Cancer Society advocates massage to comfort and help improve the quality of life for cancer patients, although not to specifically treat cancer. Cancer may be a reason to begin, continue, or increase the frequency of massage treatments. Besides the benefits of relaxation, improved sleep, pain reduction, and increased blood flow, massage also bolsters immune functions, reduces or prevents lymphedema, decreases nausea, improves the quality and survival of skin during radiation therapy (perhaps as a result of the quality moisturizers in massage lubricants). Massage also reduces fatigue, which affects 72% to 95% of all cancer patients.

Massage is as safe as activities of daily living (ADLs), mild exercise, or a hot bath, all of which increase circulation.

Cancer is treated through *surgery, chemotherapy,* or *radiation therapy.* Surgery removes the cancerous tumors or organs and often neighboring lymph nodes. After surgery, the patient may experience lymphedema. If no inflammation is involved, the massage

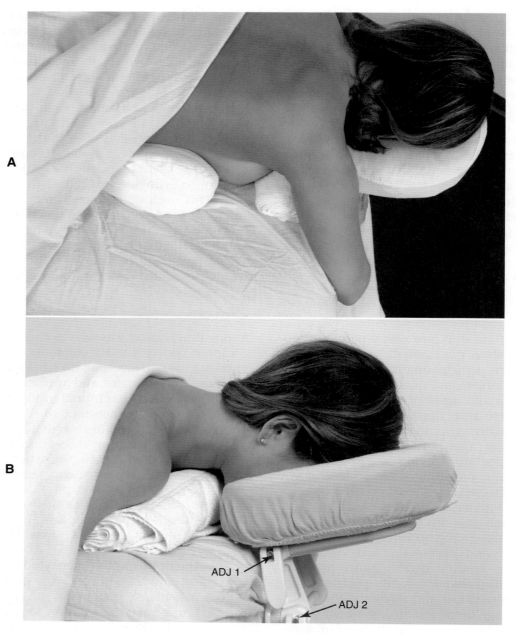

A

B

ADJ 1

ADJ 2

Figure 9-1 **A,** Prone large-breasted woman with cylindrical pillows above and below breast. **B,** Face rest adjusted properly, above the level of the table.

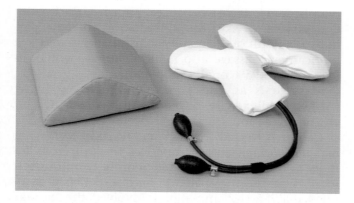

Figure 9-2 Sternal pad and breast comfort pillow.

therapist should use techniques to promote lymph flow (special training in manual lymphatic drainage is recommended) and elevate the swollen area during treatment.

Radiation therapy uses radiation to eradicate cancer cells. Common side effects from radiation include skin that appears sunburned, hair loss, reduced white blood cells (WBCs) and platelets, blood vessel fragility, fatigue, loss of appetite, and weight loss. A gentle massage is indicated, avoiding lubricant on the treatment area (usually marked with ink) because massage lubricant may interfere with cancer treatment. However, a cool towel can be placed on areas that burn or itch from radiation treatment.

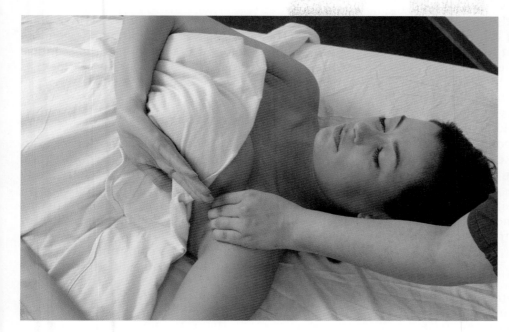

Figure 9-3 Woman retracting her breast tissue using the back of her hand.

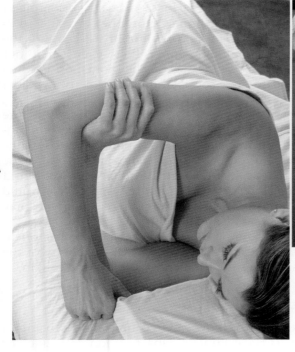

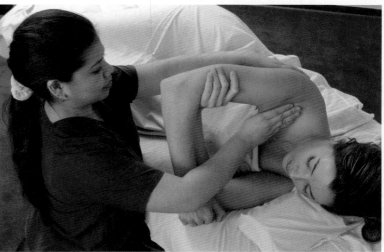

A   B

Figure 9-4 **A,** Side-lying large-breasted woman holding her upper arm away from her body. **B,** Therapist applying massage therapy.

Chemotherapy consists of a regimen of drugs given to slow or stop the growth of cancer cells. Common side effects of chemotherapy include nausea, vomiting, diarrhea or constipation, reduced WBCs and platelets, blood vessel fragility, fatigue, weight loss or gain, fever, and hair loss. Fatigue may be so severe that the client may need assistance on and off the massage table and when he changes positions. Again, a cool towel can be placed on areas that itch or burn.

Following are important guidelines for massage therapists:
- Obtain medical consent first.
- Be attentive about pressure, client position and comfort, and the areas to avoid. Use only gentle pressure or switch to modalities that use little or no pressure such as therapeutic touch, polarity, Reiki, or craniosacral therapy. The massage intent is to comfort, not to stir up and release toxins. Gentle pressure is especially important if the cancer pa-

tient is undergoing chemotherapy or radiation therapy because both tend to reduce platelet count, which causes the client to bruise easily.

- Each subsequent appointment, inquire about client health (just as you would other clients).
- Use a side-lying position if the client cannot lay prone because of central lines on the upper chest wall, radiation burns, or surgical wounds.
- If cancer has spread to the bones, bone integrity may be affected so, again, be cautious of pressure, traction, and range-of-motion (ROM) activities.
- Avoid intravenous (IV) lines, catheters, surgical wounds over known cancer sites, radiation burns, or known tumors sites. For more information, see the following section on central venous catheters.

Central Venous Catheter

A *central venous catheter,* or central line, is a flexible tube inserted and sewn into a large vein (usually the right subclavian vein in the upper chest) and then left in place for an extended period. This type of catheter is used to keep a vein open for dialysis, blood withdrawal, chemotherapy, and frequent administration of medications, which must be taken regularly but cannot be taken orally. The three common types of central venous catheters are *Hickman, Quinton,* and *Groshong* catheters. Another style of central venous catheter inserted under the skin of the chest wall, a port-a-cath, does not have an external opening.

The use of these catheters makes it difficult or impossible for the client to comfortably lie prone. Use bolsters, pillows, or other positional modifications such as a side-lying position for the client's comfort. Sometimes a small towel or washcloth over the area is all that is needed. The catheter is usually sutured to fascia and muscle. During the massage, the massage therapist should take precautions not to dislodge the catheter by exerting tension or excessive movement on nearby skin tissues. Do not allow the massage lubricant to come into contact with the catheter dressing or sutures. If a catheter is placed in the arm, do not massage the area below the catheter. Massage work above the catheter in these extremities should be gentle.

Chronic Illness

A **chronic illness** is a condition of the body for which no cure is known, such as multiple sclerosis, chronic fatigue syndrome, fibromyalgia, Parkinson's disease, lupus, and rheumatoid arthritis. When a client has a chronic illness, massage therapy can reduce his suffering and increase his personal comfort. Clients who are chronically ill may experience good days and bad days. For the chronically ill, not getting

any worse is considered an improvement. Obtain medical clearance, and administer the massage more gently, more frequently, and for shorter periods. Constantly monitor these clients during treatment as massage therapy can be tiring for them.

Colostomy or Ileostomy

A *colostomy* is an incision in the colon for the purpose of making an opening between the bowel and abdominal wall. A bag is attached outside the body to gather fecal material that passes through the opening. Colostomies are sometimes temporary bypass methods, which are used in conjunction with surgeries.

An *ileostomy* is similar to a colostomy except the ileostomy connects the small intestine to the external abdominal wall. Clients who have lower colostomies can regulate their bowels. The bowel material of upper colostomies and ileostomies is too loose to afford the client the ability to control bowel movements.

When clients who have a colostomy or ileostomy make an appointment for a massage, recommend that they not eat 2 hours before they arrive. This 2-hour delay decreases bowel motility. Because of the anterior abdominal opening, these clients may not be able to receive massage in the prone position. Accommodate these special individuals by using a side-lying position.

Suggest to a client that he empty his bag before the massage begins. A bag can burst or become unclipped during the session, spilling its contents. Should this occur, remain calm and reassure the client that accidents like this do happen. Ask him if he would prefer to clean himself up or if he would like your assistance. If he has a spinal injury, he may require your assistance.

Do not apply lubricant on or near the bag opening. Oily substances interfere with the ability of the adhesive or cement to anchor the bag to the skin.

Contact Lens Users

Many clients remove their contact lenses before a massage. Have contact lens solution available for lens storage after removal. If contact lens users do not remove them, show the client how to adjust the face rest cover to reduce eye compression while lying prone (Figure 9-5). While the client is supine, avoid massage that is near or directly over the eyes.

End-of-Life Massage

Massage can be used at the end of life to reduce suffering and increase feelings of comfort. The massage pressure should be gentle, and treatments should be more

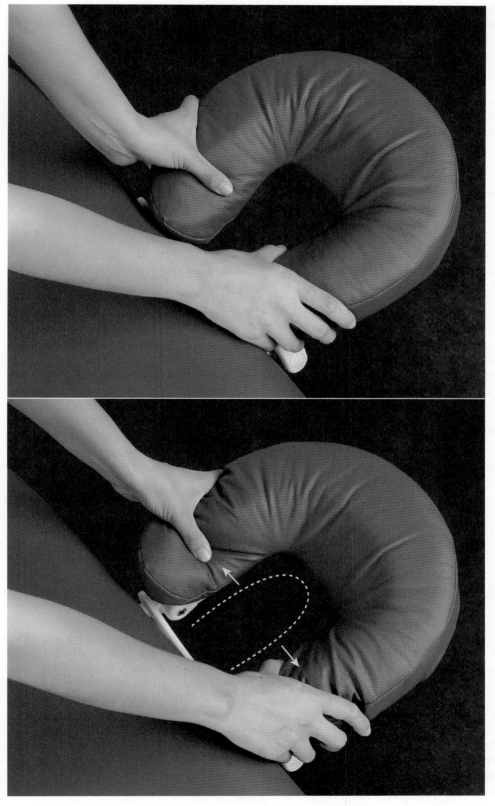

Figure 9-5 Moving the face cushion to the side of the frame to reduce eye compression of contact lens users.

frequent, but treatment time should be shorter. If working with hospice or doing a house call, the client may prefer to be massaged in her bed. Even a gentle hand and foot massage is a welcomed experience.

If you are giving the massage in the hospital, check with the doctor or nurse about additional information needed to serve the client most effectively. Work carefully around tubes, catheters, needles, monitors, and other medical equipment but limit your time spent. A 1-hour massage is rarely appropriate.

When massaging someone who is near the end of life, it is helpful to address your own feelings about death and dying. You may attend workshops that are part of a local hospice program and read books on the subject. Several authors who have written books on the subject are Elisabeth Kübler-Ross, Stephen Levine, and Bernie Siegel. These may be helpful in working with people near the end of their life as they and their support people face grief issues.

Before you decide to work with a client who is dying or terminally ill, make a personal commitment to stay with him until death because abandonment is very difficult to face at this time. Know that you will probably become attached to the client, cry when death comes, mourn the loss, grieve with his family, and grow from this experience.

Geriatric Clients

Geriatric clients represent the fastest growing populations in the massage industry. **Geriatric** refers to someone who is 70 years of age or older. The health and physical condition of the elderly decline with age, but this varies from person to person. As we age, the following changes occur to the body:

- Nerve and reflex reaction time is shorter, so more time is typically needed to perform tasks such as the intake and premassage interviews.
- Because of the effect of the nervous system, a loss or increased sensitivity to pain may occur.
- Typically a loss in hearing and vision, especially near-sighted vision, occurs that must be taken into consideration.
- A decrease in strength and muscle tone is often noted.
- Bones are neither as strong nor as flexible. Joints begin to wear down; osteoarthritis and osteoporosis are common. A mild kyphosis may be noted (Dowager's hump).
- The skin appears pale and wrinkled and becomes thinner, looser, and frailer. Age spots may appear on the skin as a result of blood leaking from damaged and weak capillaries. Liver spots may be seen on the skin of older people, especially those who have been exposed to excessive sun.
- In the case of inactivity, circulation may not be efficient. Atherosclerosis is fairly common among the elderly.

- An increase in incontinence may result from loss of muscle tone in the urinary and gastrointestinal tracts.

During the premassage interview, assess the geriatric client's condition and provide adaptations to ensure her comfort and safety. Establish rapport by acclimating her to her surroundings to help her feel safe and secure. Use a soft, clear voice, facing the client when speaking. When explaining procedures, tell her what parts of the body you will be massaging using simple, nonanatomical terms. Be sure your client understands what is being said, and allow time for asking and answering questions. Guard against chilling by using blankets over the client's body and, if appropriate, an external heat source such as a portable heating unit.

Many elderly clients live or feel alone because their spouses have passed away or because family members are busy raising their own families. If your client is living with family or friends or residing in a nursing home, knock on the door of his room before entering, make sure you put objects back in their places if disturbed, and be patient if he needs extra time to dress. It may be important that you provide an opportunity for elderly clients to talk and share their thoughts with you. Depression may also affect the elderly client. Be attentive and sensitive to the client's emotional needs. Many massage therapists offer discounts to elderly clients because most are living on fixed incomes.

When massaging an elderly person, deep work should be avoided unless ordered by her physician. Because elderly people may tire easily, massage for shorter periods. Because of decreased reaction time, possible insensitivity to pain, and thinning of the blood vessels and skin, it is easy to damage the skin or cause bruising. This can be avoided by reducing both treatment time and pressure. Avoid extreme neck mobilizations, which may harm the client because of loss of bone integrity.

Many elderly people experience a sudden drop in blood pressure when they move from a recumbent position to an upright position. The massage therapist should assist the geriatric client into a sitting posture on the table (see Chapter 6), allowing time for the client to adjust to the change in position. You may choose to spend this time massaging her neck and shoulder region while she is seated on the massage table. Help her to her feet if needed; otherwise, she may become dizzy while transferring off the table, lose her balance, and fall.

Hearing Impaired Clients

It is important to remember that hearing impaired clients communicate perfectly well; they just receive and interpret sounds differently from those of us whose hearing is intact. Be aware that even a small hearing impairment can hamper a person's ability to understand what you say.

Allow more time for the premassage interview. When initiating conversation with a client with hearing impairment, get his attention before you begin to speak. Eye contact is considered a sign of attention. It is perfectly acceptable to tap a person lightly on the shoulder or arm or to wave a hand in the person's direction to gain his attention. This is especially important when the client is lying face down in the face cradle and cannot see the therapist. Find out immediately if your client is a lip-reader and use the information in the next paragraph during the interview process. Rephrase any sentence that the client with hearing impairment does not understand; do not just repeat the same words over and over in the same sequence. Allow time for him to respond. If you have a regular client who is hearing impaired, it may be a good investment to attend a class on sign language to be used during the interview process.

The following ideas help the therapist communicate better with a client who reads lips. Face the client and maintain eye contact through the conversation. Enunciate clearly and normally but do not exaggerate your lip movements. Use facial expressions and body language to clarify your message. Do not be embarrassed to be expressive. If she has a sign language interpreter, do not direct your conversation to the interpreter; make eye contact and talk directly with the person with the hearing impairment. Stand close and do not let any object obstruct the person's view of you. Do not eat, smoke, chew gum, or hold your hands in front of your mouth while you talk. Stand in a well-lighted place. Avoid standing with your back to a light source such as a lamp or window because this throws your face into a shadow and makes it difficult for lip movements to be clearly seen.

Many people try to compensate for their hearing loss through the use of hearing aids. Do not assume that a hearing aid corrects hearing loss; it may just improve it slightly. If your client is wearing a hearing aid while she is on the massage table, avoid moving your hands close to her ears. Proximity to the hearing aid generates feedback, producing an uncomfortable squeak in her ear. Some clients may remove it before or during the session.

Remember that those clients who lost their hearing early in life may often have speech difficulties. When the cause of the speech difficulty is hearing loss, the client may pronounce words incorrectly. Many people make the mistake of assuming that someone with a speech problem is mentally handicapped. It helps to remember that the client is only hearing impaired, not unintelligent. Talking very slowly or using exaggerated lip movements only serves to frustrate the client. Give her the dignity you would afford any hearing adult in normal conversation.

Many medical establishments use a flash card system for communicating with clients with hearing or speech impairment. The system consists of a single card listing a set of simple questions. The answer area of the card has a *yes* and *no* block. The client responds by pointing to the appropriate answer. This principle can be used to create a pain tolerance level flash card for massage clients.

Clients Who Have Human Immunodeficiency Virus or are Living With Acquired Immune Deficiency Syndrome

Considered a chronic illness, AIDS is a disease caused by HIV. People with the virus are said to be HIV positive; people with AIDS have three or more opportunistic viruses, and/or a T-cell count below 200. To become infected by HIV, the following three elements must occur simultaneously:

- The virus must be in a *proper environment* to survive. The virus may be found in blood, semen, vaginal secretions, and breast milk. It has also been found in tears, sweat, and saliva.
- HIV must be in *sufficient quantity* when entering the body. The only body fluids that contain high concentrations of the virus are blood, semen, vaginal secretions, and breast milk. Tears, sweat, and saliva do not appear to contain enough of the virus to cause infection because no known cases of transmission by these body fluids have been reported. It has been speculated that it would take 6 to 10 gallons of saliva to have enough concentration for the virus to be transmitted.
- The virus must have a *port of entry*. It can enter the human body of an uninfected person through unprotected intercourse or blood-to-blood contact with an infected person. HIV cannot be transmitted by simple contact with an infected person. Intact skin is adequate protection from the virus.

The massage for a client with HIV is not that different from any other client. Inquire about the areas that need to be avoided, including the most recent site of bloodwork. If the HIV-infected client has Kaposi's sarcoma (Figure 9-6), deep massage is contraindicated because it can cause internal bleeding. Even light massage may be contraindicated around lesions, which can be extremely painful.

When massaging a client with AIDS, the therapist must take into consideration the client's general vitality and any secondary conditions that limit any Swedish gymnastics and other ROM exercises. If the client is bedridden or is inactive, bone density is reduced. If you are giving the massage in the hospital, check with the doctor or nurse about additional information needed to serve the client most effectively. Work carefully around tubes, catheters, needles, monitors, and other medical equipment. Under these circumstances, even a massage that lasts less than 1 hour can bring comfort to a client with AIDS.

If any spillage of body fluids occurs while the client is on the massage table, wash the contaminated linens separately in hot water with detergent and one quarter cup of chlorine bleach. Machine dry linens. Your massage tables and related equipment should then be wiped down with a solution of 1 part chlorine bleach to 10 parts water. Disposable linens may be used, depending on your preference. Because it is not always possible to tell if linens have come in contact with body fluids, some therapists tend to treat all sheets as "hot" or a possible exposure hazard. If you accidentally come into contact with body fluids, immediately wash the area of contact with hand soap for 2 minutes (see Chapter 4).

No known cases of a massage therapist contracting HIV from a client while performing massage has been reported. If you believe you have been exposed to HIV, contact your local HIV/AIDS foundation for testing, information, and free counseling.

Sanitation and cleanliness are important for the client and the massage therapist. Because the immune system of the client with HIV is not fully functional, he is more susceptible to contacting infections through simple exposure. If and when secondary complications occur, assess it as a separate and individual condition. You are a greater health hazard to the client with HIV than he is to you.

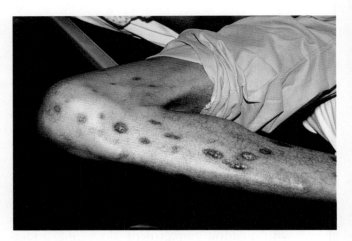

Figure 9-6   Kaposi's sarcoma. (From Damjanov I: *Pathology for the health-related professions,* ed 2, Philadelphia, 2000, WB Saunders.)

MINI-LAB

AIDS is a socially and emotionally charged issue today. Discuss with your classmates how you feel about this subject. Begin by stating how you define the problem, how it affects you as a massage therapist, and what precautions you will take in your practice.

Should massage therapists be routinely tested for HIV? Examine the legal, ethical, and medical ramifications, as well as personal and professional risk factors. What if you, as a massage therapist, discover that you are HIV positive? Should it restrict you from performing or receiving a massage?

 A baby is born with a need to be loved—and never outgrows it.

—Frank A. Clark

Infants

Infant massage is an approach of tender, loving touch that parents of many cultures have been using for centuries. It became popular in North America in 1979 with the publishing of *Infant Massage: a Handbook for Loving Parents* by Vimala Schneider McClure.

Since then, many instructors of infant massage have taught this loving method to parents and caregivers. Scientific research has identified many benefits, which include (1) encouraging parent-infant bonding; (2) relieving discomfort from teething, congestion, gas, and colic; (3) increasing relaxation and promoting sleep; (4) improving blood flow and muscle tone; and (5) increasing vocalization, thus assisting in speech and language development.

Parents also benefit from massaging their infants. A list of parental benefits include (1) promoting self-confidence and self-esteem in their parenting roles; (2) reducing stress of working parents by reinstating the connection with their infant; (3) providing parents a time to relax with their infant; (4) stimulating the release of the pituitary hormone prolactin in both mothers and fathers (in females, prolactin is involved in milk production and may help to foster maternal feelings; in males, it is believed that prolactin stimulates the desire to protect and nurture the infant); and (5) encouraging communication between the parent and infant.

Infant massage is not a technique in which a qualified therapist massages the baby. Instead, infant massage is taught by the infant massage instructor to the parents, family, or caregivers of the baby (parents, grandparents, aunts, uncles, siblings). When an infant massage instructor, acting as a parent advocate, supports and empowers the parent or caregiver, these continual life-giving experiences of interaction are more likely to occur. This is precisely why infant massage instructors are encouraged not to massage the baby; it may lower the parent's self-esteem in the process (because parents may feel they do not have the skills to do as well as the instructors).

Parents and caregivers who have continued success massaging their baby are more likely to include infant massage as a family tradition, which serves as ongoing physical and emotional nourishment for their baby. An infant massage instructor becomes a parent advocate when helping parents become increasingly more competent and eventually outgrow their need for the instructor's expertise. The instructor's obsolescence is the optimum side effect of this process.

Large Clients

When massaging the client who is large (i.e., obese or the somatotype known as an *endomorph*) or who has generous amounts of fragile subcutaneous tissue, two areas require special consideration. The first consideration is psychological and requires approaching the client with an attitude that is compassionate, caring, and nonjudgmental as large clients typically have a history of verbal abuse from society in general and health care providers in particular. Never badger a client about his weight or blame excessive size or weight on lack of morality or self-control. No one has a body that is perfect in all aspects. Make the accommodations necessary for his comfort and proceed with the session.

The second consideration is physiological in which pressure must be applied carefully to areas that contain high quantities of adipose tissue, thus reducing possible tissue damage. Adipose tissue is extremely vascular, with each pound of tissue containing approximately 1 mile of capillaries, the most fragile of vessels, making adipose tissue extremely susceptible to bruising. Avoid deep stroking of adipose tissue because it can damage and break these vessels. He may have large amounts of soft subcutaneous adipose tissue and yet may still have tense back and shoulder muscles that have become overdeveloped to support the extra weight. The back, neck, shoulders, hips, and sometimes legs of many larger clients may require extra massage work.

Palpation must be used to discern the difference between muscle and adipose tissue. If muscle fiber cannot be felt with gentle pressure, avoid working deeply into the tissue. You can ask the client to contract a specific muscle or muscle group to help you decipher the difference. If the tissue does not respond with an increase in tone, it is probably adipose tissue, and deep work should be avoided. Sometimes it is possible to gently retract adipose tissue to access muscle tissue underneath. Clients who have had recent weight loss may have areas that tend to hang in folds until the skin tightens. These areas should never be worked deeply or pinched; folds can be moved to the side while working on adjacent muscle and may be flattened out against the area to be worked so that the therapist can work through it while remaining attentive to pressure.

Inquire about the client's activity level. Just because someone is large does not necessarily mean that she is sedentary. For those who are inactive, watch for signs of edema.

Another area of consideration when working with larger clients is the therapist's body mechanics and efficiency. It may help to either lower the table height before the client's visit or have a small platform to stand on to gain height and leverage. Most table manufacturers offer electric lift or hydraulic tables that can be raised or lowered to a comfortable height.

Use a sheet or an extra-large towel as a top drape to provide adequate coverage. A client who is obese or excessively large may feel awkward or unsafe getting on and off the massage table. Have a foot stool available, and be willing to offer assistance. If you have an electric or hydraulic lift massage table, set it in the lowest position while the client is getting on and off. If the client does not feel comfortable on your massage table, she may need to receive her massage on the floor. Provide a comfortable floor mat for such an instance.

Menstruation

When a female client is menstruating, she often feels physically and emotionally uncomfortable. Because she will be wearing some kind of feminine protection (e.g., pads or tampons), it is not uncommon for undergarments to be left on. Keep feminine protection items on display in your restroom in case your female clients require them. Should any breakthrough bleeding occur while she is on the massage table, wash the linens separately in hot water with detergent and one quarter cup of chlorine bleach after the massage. Machine dry the linens. Your massage tables and related equipment should then be wiped down with a solution of 1 part chlorine bleach to 10 parts water.

Many clients cancel previously made appointments during this time of month. If they do keep their appointment, forgo deep abdominal work, particularly if they are having cramps. A moist hot pack placed on the abdomen when the client is supine or placed on the low back while the client is prone can help soothe the achy feeling associated with menses. Some extra time spent massaging her low back may offer some pain relief.

Endometriosis is a gynecological condition characterized by painful cramping before and during menstruation. It is caused by build-up of endometrial tissue that, for some unknown reason, does not slough off during menstruation. Fragments of the endometrium may be regurgitated during menstruation, moving backward through the fallopian tubes into the peritoneal cavity, where they can attach and grow.

Massage is indicated and may help relax the female client with endometriosis. However, she may be too uncomfortable to receive a massage.

Pacemaker Users

A pacemaker sends out a small electrical current to stimulate the heartbeat. Artificial pacemakers are inserted near the pectoralis major muscle with wires going directly to the heart. The newer ones are activity adjusted and automatically speed up the heartbeat during exercise. The primary concern is to make sure the incision from the surgery has completely healed before applying gentle effleurage over the area. Avoid vigorous massage on the pectoral region. While the client is prone, offer a soft pillow to be placed under the chest. This provides added comfort for the client during the massage.

Often the leads (wires) going from the pacemaker to the heart travel up over the clavicle and down into the chest cavity. For this reason, avoid moving the arm over the head when mobilizing the shoulder joint because it may disturb the lead connections.

Paraplegia, Quadriplegia, and Hemiplegia

Loss of muscle function (motor paralysis) or loss of sensation (sensory paralysis) can be the result of disease or trauma such as spinal cord injury. The massage for clients with paraplegia (paralysis of the lower extremities and trunk), quadriplegia (paralysis of the arms and legs), and hemiplegia (unilateral paralysis) (Figure 9-7) is tailored to the type of paralysis and the needs of the client.

Of primary concern with spinal cord injuries is that the client generally has large areas of numbness from the severed nerves. When working legs or arms that have no feeling, the therapist must use a pressure that is light, just enough to increase circulation, but not enough to cause any bruising or discomfort that cannot be discerned by the client. It is important to remember that being paralyzed does not always mean that the client cannot detect pressure and vibration. Sometimes only motor nerves have been damaged, leaving the client immobile but with feeling. Other clients who have had sensory nerve or total spinal cord separation may be paralyzed and sensory impaired but may be able to feel vibrations in other parts of their bodies that still have sensation. Ask the client directly for valuable feedback regarding pressure, body warmth, and how he feels positioned on the table.

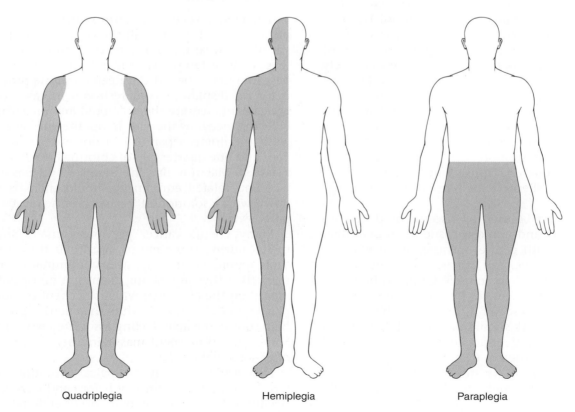

Quadriplegia   Hemiplegia   Paraplegia

Figure 9-7 Illustration of quadriplegia, hemiplegia, and paraplegia.

VIMALA SCHNEIDER MCCLURE

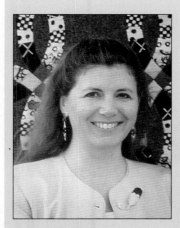

Born: June 7, 1952.

"Do all the good you can in all the ways you can, for all the people you can for long as ever you can."

—P.R. Sarkar

Vimala Schneider McClure, the pioneer of infant massage in the United States, always had the feeling that she was put here to fulfill a specific purpose. At age 21, the starry-eyed humanitarian sold everything she had and took off for India. "I was terrified," she confided, "but my sense of purpose was so strong it was worth putting myself in harm's way."

In India, she studied with Yogi Master P.R. Sarkar until a bout with malaria cut her trip short and landed her in a New York hospital for a couple of weeks.

She had recurrences for years afterward, and her health has never been perfect. McClure is a diethylstilbestrol (DES) (a drug given to prevent miscarriages now proved to have adverse effects) daughter. As a child she had open-heart surgery. She had 11 operations and has lost "every expendable organ." Today, she experiences severe fibromyalgia.

Somewhat recovered from the malaria, she returned to India and worked in an orphanage. It was there that she learned the art of infant massage from an assistant. Out of necessity, the nun who ran the orphanage spent much of her time begging for money for its support, so McClure was left to care for the children along with two Indian girls. "They couldn't speak my language, and I couldn't speak theirs," she remembers. In the evenings, when the courtyard cooled off to 90° F, she learned traditional Indian baby massage.

"They've done it in India for 10,000 years or more," she explains. Mothers massage their infants and pass along the skill to their daughters. "I began to see how relaxed these children were. . . how different [they were] from American children. They were easier with each other and less aggressive. Boys and girls alike walk around with their arms around each other. Then it began to click. I began to see massage as something that could change lives. A good analogy is that we're like a cup, and the more love that goes into that cup, until it is overflowing, the more you can give. If your cup didn't get filled as a child, then you're always looking for someone to fill it up."

McClure points out that every mammal species licks their young, which is not just for cleaning. It is a bonding process that stimulates the whole system. Without this stage, mothers kill their offspring, or offspring are affected down the road in the same way that abused children may perpetuate abuse.

McClure returned to the United States and in 1976 and became pregnant with her first of two children. In addition to everything about massage and yoga she had learned in India, she asked friends to teach her some Swedish massage techniques to develop a routine for her newborn. In *Infant Massage: a Handbook for Loving Parents*, she writes: "This joyful blend provided my son with a wonderful balance of outgoing and incoming energy, of tension release, and stimulation. Additionally, it seemed to relieve the painful gas he had been experiencing that first month."

McClure began to keep copious notes. Eventually, she invited mothers over to show them what she was doing. During these sessions she distributed a small hand-made flyer.

One of McClure's tiny flyers fell into the right hands, and she was invited to speak at a childbirth education conference. It was there that she met the owner of a baby products company who asked, "Have you ever thought about writing a book? Write one, and I'll publish it."

She had already done so, and *Infant Massage: a Handbook for Loving Parents* became, and still is, the definitive work on infant massage. Pressed by others

Continued

VIMALA SCHNEIDER MCCLURE—cont'd

to begin an organization, she founded the International Association of Infant Massage, which is a worldwide operation now, but she receives no money for her pioneering training except for royalties from the book. "I was zero percent motivated by money at the time. I didn't think about how much profit I could make. I didn't think of my work as a business venture. At this point in my life, I'm not so sure how smart that was," she confesses.

Her advice to beginning massage therapists regarding infant massage is to start with a very different mindset because what happens between parent and child is different from what happens during a therapeutic massage. McClure says, "It's the act of bonding and impacting a lifetime. That's why I trained instructors to train parents rather than training massage therapists to massage infants. As an instructor, you have to allow parents to develop their own style. Even if they don't apply strokes in an expert manner, the message comes through. You have to empower parents and not allow them to turn over their power to the instructor as the expert."

McClure considers the rearing of her two children her main mission in life. Asked how she would respond if her daughter said she was off to some Third World country to find her purpose, McClure admits, "I'd try to talk her out of it. I'm too much a mom. But if it was something she positively had to do, I'd give her my blessing." She continues to write and to help parents develop closer, more meaningful relationships with their children. Her other works include *The Tao of Motherhood, A Woman's Guide to Tantric Yoga,* and her current book, *The Path of Parenting: Twelve Principles to Guide Your Journey.*

Generally speaking, the longer the client has been inactive, the weaker the bones. Limit all ROM exercises, especially on the neck, spinal column, and hip joints. Avoid the use of electrical vibrators. Assist the client on and off the table. Most clients with these conditions are in a wheelchair (see the section on Clients in Wheelchairs).

Pediatric Clients

Children, or **pediatric** clients, are defined as young people between 3 and 18 years of age. They are often accompanied by anxious parents because most pediatric massage addresses specific tissue problems from injury or illness, resulting in pain to the client. During the premassage interview, explain the procedure to both the parents and the child, but informed consent must be obtained from the parents or legal guardians. In some states, a parent must also supervise while the massage is in progress (Figure 9-8). If the child is between the ages of 16 and 18, parental permission is not necessary; however, it is sometimes prudent to keep the parent in the room while massaging a child of the opposite gender. This is especially true, for example, when working in a sensitive area such as a pulled adductor injury in a young athlete.

Use special caution when working with adolescent boys. The reflexive sexual erection response is often very sensitive; peripheral stimulation (i.e., massage) on the thighs and belly can trigger this reflex. It is helpful to keep the top drape bunched up in the groin area to disguise any physical response to the massage. Stopping the massage for a brief period and stepping out of the room (perhaps for reason of getting a drink of water) often reduces the neurological response.

In younger children, the massage session may last only 30 to 45 minutes because of the child's smaller stature, short attention span, short neural reflex, and increased metabolism. Use the extra time to establish a rapport with the client.

Postoperative Clients and Scar Tissue

Following surgical procedures, massage can be used to promote healing and relaxation for the client or to reduce keloids or adhered scar tissue. Avoid massage therapy in the affected area until the client receives

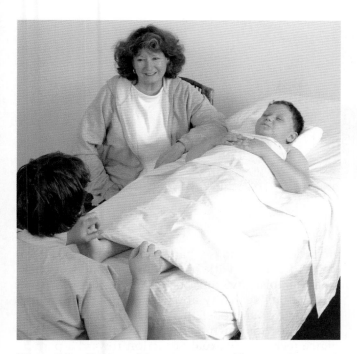

Figure 9-8   Child receiving a massage with a parent present.

medical clearance from his attending physician. During the premassage interview, ask the client why the surgery took place and obtain the physician's and patient's opinion of the success of the surgery. This helps you make good decisions on how to proceed. For example, if the reason was to remove a cancerous tumor, avoid the area over the known tumor site. Ask the client about internal staples, screens, and supports after thoracic and abdominal surgery. Omit deep abdominal moves such as massage on the psoas muscle when these are present. Use lighter pressure when massaging clients using anticoagulants because they tend to bruise easier. Obtain a verbal update on medication at every massage for up to 6 months following surgery.

Even with medical clearance, avoid massaging scar tissue within a 2-inch diameter for 6 to 8 weeks and then only if all stitches and staples have been removed. Avoid any areas that are bright red, moist, or oozing or scar tissue that is not completely healed and is scabbed over. When massaging scar tissue, use a lubricant that contains any of the following: natural oils, cocoa butter, vitamin E, aloe vera, and arnica. Work the thoroughly healed scar using skin rolling and deep friction techniques (cross-fiber, chucking, and circular). Stay within the client's pain tolerance.

Regardless of the type of surgery involved, the deep frictioning techniques can significantly reduce keloid formation and break up the uneven lumps or knots that are sometimes associated with stitches. Layers of adhered tissue can be separated by using myofascial release techniques.

Pregnant Clients

During the premassage interview, inquire about the female client's current and past pregnancies, breasts soreness, and nausea. If a history of spontaneous abortion (miscarriage) is stated, avoid massage in the first trimester because everything, including massage, is suspected should she miscarry. If she is currently experiencing eclampsia (toxemia), massage is contraindicated unless ordered by her physician. If your pregnant client reports that she is healthy with no past complications, proceed with the massage. In the first trimester, the client's position on the table is not a concern unless she is uncomfortable lying in a specific position. Avoid deep abdominal massage during the entire pregnancy and for 3 months after childbirth. If the client has breast soreness or is nursing, make modifications to her position while prone (see the section on Breast Implants and Large-Breasted Women). If the pregnant client is experiencing nausea, reduce or omit rocking from your routine.

Because of intraabdominal pressure exerted during low back massage, and the added strain on the supporting ligament and muscles when in a face-down position, prone positioning is contraindicated after the eighteenth week of pregnancy. This is not a client preference; it is up to the therapist to provide a safe and knowledgeable pregnancy massage.

Expectant mothers in their second and third trimesters should receive a massage in modified supine and side-lying positions. Typically, the modified supine and side-lying positions are the most comfortable (Figure 9-9). The modified supine position has the client's upper body elevated about 30 degrees. Because of the pressure exerted on the abdominal blood vessels by the growing fetus, massage is contraindicated in the supine position where the client is lying flat, or 180 degrees. Ask her on which side she feels more comfortable lying and allow her to spend most of the time during the session in that particular position. Side-lying position is covered in Chapter 6.

Because of the decreased clot-dissolving property of the blood during pregnancy, a client is at a higher risk for blood clots. Use only gentle pressure in the medial thigh region and restrict your techniques to the use of an open, flat hand. Pregnant women tend to urinate often because of the growing fetus pressing on the urinary bladder. Suggest to your pregnant client that she visit the restroom before getting on the massage table. Most pregnant women are also sensitive to stuffy rooms and high temperatures; avoid heating blankets and hot packs. She may be more comfortable if you keep a fan blowing in a corner of the room during the massage. If the pregnant woman has swollen ankles, elevate her knees and feet using a bolster and pillows while she is in the modified supine position; place the feet higher than the knees.

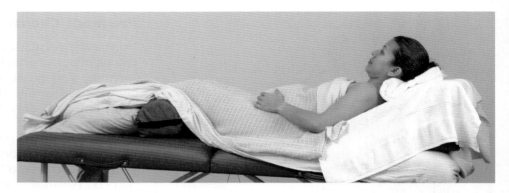

Figure 9-9 Pregnancy client in a modified supine position with wedge angling client to 30 degrees.

Sexual Abuse

It is likely that you will meet clients who are survivors of sexual abuse. Abuse crosses all population barriers, with both perpetrators and survivors being male or female, straight or gay, old or young, poor or wealthy. The majority of these incidents tend to be perpetrated by family members, extended family members, friends of family members, or friends of the survivor (e.g., date rape). Many survivors require special consideration during massage therapy, and in some cases, massage may even be contraindicated. This is generally up to the client, but she may need an extended period to build rapport with the therapist before any massage work actually begins. In any case, treatment can best be provided by a massage therapist who has an understanding of the dynamics of abuse and the steps for making massage therapy emotionally and physically safe.

One of the reasons that sexual abuse is so traumatic is because sex is such a powerful experience. It has the potential of being the ultimate expression of intimacy or one of the worst bodily assaults possible. Many survivors become people of extremes, often developing compulsive eating habits. These survivors may overeat to a point of obesity, cocooning themselves from others emotionally and physically by hiding inside excess body weight. Other survivors may relate to their bodies as the source of self-esteem and become compulsive about exercise and diet. Some survivors become anorexic or bulimic. To anesthetize the pain of the abuse, many develop alcohol, nicotine, caffeine, and narcotic dependencies. It is often depression or chemical addictions that get most survivors of sexual abuse involved in counseling. As the survivor begins to peel back different layers of various issues, she discovers incidences of abuse underneath, or she may have always been aware of the abuse.

The "extreme" behaviors may also involve sexual inappropriateness. Many survivors may fear or encourage sexual interactions; they may have difficulty understanding appropriate sexual boundaries. For a victim of sexual abuse, part of the healing process is to be in contact with positive role models. As massage therapists, we must be aware of our own issues surrounding sexuality and possess good boundaries so we can role model this behavior. If you are not clear about your own boundary issues or if you experience feelings of sexual attraction toward a particular client, refer her to another therapist.

If a client confides in you that he has an abusive history, take extra precautions to ensure a nurturing, safe, and healing environment. Some suggestions are to close window blinds, turn off the telephone, and reduce noises that may trigger a startled response. *Ask the client if he knows what his triggers are.* Common triggers are perfume, certain body positions, touch in a particular area, lightning, a specific color, and certain kinds of music. Allow the client to set the boundaries from one massage to the next and reassure him that he has control of the session. Examples of boundaries are draping issues, areas on which to work, speed and depth of massage, and length of time an area is to be worked. Often massage itself may act as a trigger mechanism for old abuse issues.

Occasionally, a client's physical body may "remember" a past traumatic event while receiving a massage. These repressed memories come to the conscious mind by a mechanism called **state-dependent memory**, which is triggered by duplicating the original position of a client, location or amount of pressure, body movements, emotions, and nervous system activation at the time the experience occurred. When your body assumes a particular position or a certain set of circumstances, it may recall the past experience, for example, when climbing on a bicycle for the first time in 20 years.

Some survivors of abuse cope with the original trauma by "leaving the body," to not feel, or to believe that the abuse was happening to someone else. This coping mechanism is called **disassociation**. Clients may relive abuse memories during a massage and repeat the disassociation. Signs of disassociation are the client becoming unresponsive, a distant look in the eyes, shaking, disorientation, loss of clarity between the present and the past, and a shift in breathing pattern.

It is not our job to change the coping mechanism by reminding the client to remain aware of her body. Neither is it our job to remove a coping skill or to use guilt for the coping skill. It takes time to learn to cope differently, and we must honor the ways in which the client has learned to survive. We must also honor her need for emotional release. Do not massage when it has just retriggered the client because further dissociative touch can be traumatizing.

 All feelings, both positive and unpleasant, come out of the same faucet. To turn down the faucet on pain is to slow the flow of pleasant feelings as well.

—Gay and Kathlyn Hendricks

Emotional Release During Treatment

Occasionally, survivors of abuse release physical or emotional tension during a massage session. These releases can manifest themselves as a deep sigh, a stream of tears, laughter, shaking, uncontrollable muscle twitching, or in rare cases, a thrashing temper tantrum. These emotional expressions may be an indication of pain, sadness, anger, or even rage. The causes of these releases may be suppressed emotions that are locked in the muscles and released through massage therapy. Muscle twitching may be a physical manifestation of body memories that are trauma induced during the time of the abuse and may occur at any time, not just during a massage. Some clients let down their defenses and release emotions during massage because of the high level of intimacy and safety they experience with their therapists.

If the client is in counseling, her emotions are typically closer to the surface, and she is more likely to experience emotional releases. The most common form of emotional release is tears or crying. Chances are that the tears are not about physical pain. Here are some tips on handling your client's tears. If the client is aware that she is likely to experience a release during the session, it is better to orient her by explaining the following process in advance:

- Approach the emotional expression with the attitude of total acceptance. Do not interfere with questions.
- Discontinue the massage and make touch contact in an area that is neutral to the abuse (e.g., shoulders, arms, feet). This should be determined before the massage begins. Most clients prefer to stop the massage because their bodies have another job now—crying. Avoid leaving the massage room unless instructed to do so by the client. Leaving the room may be interpreted as abandonment. Help provide a safe place for your client to experience

and release these emotions without explanation or judgment.
- Do not be quick to offer facial tissues. Drying someone's tears or offering the tissue too fast can be taken as disapproval of crying and of the feelings beneath it.
- When appropriate, remind your client that the tears, shaking, or fear is all right and that she is in a safe place. Ask the client if she would like to take a short break, offer a comfort measure (e.g., stroking her hair, opening a window for fresh air), or end the massage session. However, it is important not to offer too many choices all at once; keep it simple.
- Regardless of which option she chooses, be calm and accepting of the response and never encourage or repress the response.
- Get in touch with your own feelings about others expressing emotions. You must be willing to witness another person's pain without interrupting him. We may either feel empathic or uncomfortable with the client's tears, but we need to give him the time and place to experience the emotion without interruption.
- We are not counselors, but we can support the client emotionally. You can be supportive with comments such as, "It's all right to cry; in fact it's good to cry," or "Tears are part of the natural cleansing process of the body."
- In most instances, it is best to continue the massage. This allows the body to integrate the information. Clients may ask that the massage continue but to a less emotionally charged area such as the hands or feet.

Responding to Your Client After the Emotional Release

- If the client asks for an explanation of what happened, mirror back to her what you observed. Do not offer your personal interpretation or analysis; offer your understanding of state-dependent memory.
- Disassociation typically leaves the client in an emotional void. Many clients will be self-conscious. They may want to leave before they are ready to go back to the "real world." Provide a safe, private space for them to do some integrating of the experience, whether with you, by themselves, or on the telephone with their counselor. Avoid asking the client to leave while she is in a raw, open, wounded, or disassociated state.
- When appropriate, refer the client to a qualified mental health counselor.

If you are truly uncomfortable with the client's emotional release, be honest with yourself. Support her through the experience you best can while she is on the table. Later, share your feelings of apprehension with a counselor, fellow therapist, or a peer support group. Process your feelings and see if you can get past your apprehension.

If you choose not to work with survivors of sexual abuse, discuss your limitations with your client during a consultation. It is inappropriate to discuss how uncomfortable you are while she is on the massage table or immediately after the emotional release when she may feel vulnerable. Simply communicate only that you cannot provide the care the client needs. Make sure that you take ownership of the limitation or boundary, then refer the client to a massage therapist who is trained and comfortable in dealing with these issues.

Working with survivors of sexual abuse requires special skills and much empathy. If you are planning on working specifically with survivors, familiarize yourself with these issues through reading (e.g., *The Courage to Heal and Allies in Healing* by Ellen Bass and Laura Davis), attending seminars, or taking an introductory class at a university. Another resource is a support group called *Survivors of Incest Anonymous*. Although many support programs are available, there is no substitute for a qualified psychotherapist who specializes in sexual trauma. Obtain recommendations for ones in your area and refer clients to them when appropriate.

As is true with all of your clients, always remember that confidentiality is a sacred trust. Everyone has painful psychological issues at some point in their lives. Protect the anonymity of your clients. It is their right alone to divulge personal information.

Speech Difficulties

If your client has difficulty articulating speech, or enunciating words, ask him to repeat anything that is unclear or that you do not understand. It is helpful to repeat what you heard to the client and give him an opportunity to give you clarification or further instructions.

During the premassage interview, inquire about any accommodations that can be made in his behalf. Be direct and inquire about the speech difficulty. It may be the result of a physical abnormality such as cleft palate, aphasia (abnormal neurologic condition causing difficult speech and verbal comprehension) resulting from a stroke or head injury, a regional dialect or accent, dementia resulting from drug usage or illness, or inadequate pronunciation due to deafness (see the section on the Client With Hearing Impairment). If a client speaks a foreign language that you do not understand, ask of it is possible for him to bring a support person to act as an interpreter.

Spinal Abnormalities: Kyphosis, Lordosis, and Scoliosis

When massaging a client who has spinal abnormalities, positioning or table mechanics provide a way in which the client can relax in a recumbent position. Clients who have a spinal condition called *kyphosis*, or humpback condition, may be uncomfortable lying in the prone position. Place a cushion or supportive device under the clavicles and offer a standard-size pillow or a face rest for his head when your client is in the prone position (Figure 9-10). If possible, adjust the face rest higher than the table height. In this way, your client can further relax and enjoy the massage.

Lordosis, or swayback, is common in clients who are overweight or who have flaccid abdominal muscles. A pillow under the anterior superior iliac spine (ASIS) while the client is in the prone position may relieve low back discomfort (Figure 9-11). Additionally, a bolster under the ankles and using pillows to correct externally rotated femurs may help to release the hips. A 6- to 8-inch bolster behind the knees

Figure 9-10 Client with kyphosis lying prone with cushion under clavicles and face rest raised above table height.

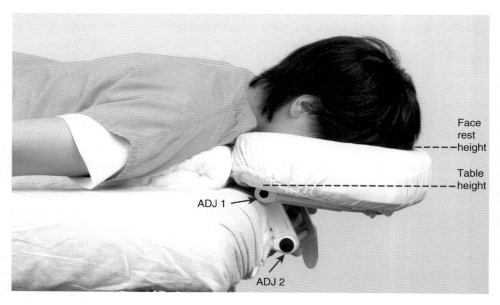

Face rest height

Table height

ADJ 1

ADJ 2

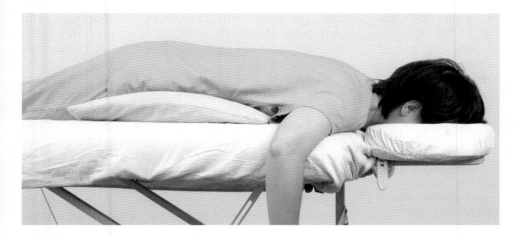

Figure 9-11 Client with lordosis with a cushion under the abdomen

while the client is lying supine may also relieve pain associated with lordosis.

Scoliosis is a lateral spinal distortion that occurs mostly in females (60% to 80%). Because the abnormal curve is in the thoracic region, the ribs and hips have distorted positions. Different degrees of spinal distortion exist, so offer your client with scoliosis several pillows and suggest that she position them until she feels supported and comfortable.

More information on spinal abnormalities can be found in Chapter 14. If any of these atypical spinal positions are present in your client or if comfort cannot be found using supportive devices, you may elect to forgo massaging in the prone position.

Substance Abuse and Drug Addiction Issues

Addictive or compulsive disorders develop when the individual starts using a mood-altering chemical as a temporary chemical escape from unpleasant emotions. Some of these uncomfortable feelings are pain, inadequacy, sadness, loneliness, anger, and fear. The behavior continues to escalate until the consequences of the addiction exceed the pain of the uncomfortable emotions that lead to the substance use in the first place, trapping the person with the disorder in a cycle of pain and escape. Examples of chemical dependency disorders range from nicotine and caffeine addiction to alcohol and narcotic abuse.

Massage therapy may be part of the recovery process for clients with addictions because it is effective for relieving stress during periods of chemical withdrawals, which often produce anxiety. Deep work should be avoided during the early stages of withdrawal because it may intensify the release of toxins into the system, which may already be overburdened during the detoxification process. During episodes of **recidivism** (relapse into a previous condition such as substance abuse), massage can be used for its psychological and physiological benefits.

Although massage can assist the recovering addict through relaxation and increased body awareness, education and support are probably the best tools for overcoming this disorder. Most massage therapists are not licensed to provide counseling services but can offer these special clients acceptance and moral support as a part of their recovery. If the client is participating in a recovery program, encourage him to continue. If not, recommend a program that deals with his particular addiction issues or refer him to a professional counselor.

Visually Impaired Clients

Massage helps people with visual impairment because of their need for tactile stimulation; touch is one of the most important ways they define their world. During the initial consultation, allow extra time to give and receive information. The best source of information when adapting your massage for a client with visual impairment is the client himself. Ask your client to explain his impairment and what assistance, if any, is needed. Do not feel offended if he declines your offer for help; this is true for any client who is physically challenged.

Keep your facilities as barrier-free as possible; the floor in your office, hallway, bathroom, and massage room should be free from clutter.

Announce your presence when you step into the room, speaking in a normal tone of voice. Begin by addressing the client by name and then state your name. When transferring a client with visual impairment from one area to another, stand just in front or to his left. He may choose to touch your right elbow and follow you. Be a gentle guide and give useful, meaningful directions. It may be helpful to describe the surroundings, using the face of a clock as a reference. Instead of saying, "There is a table in front of you," say, "There is a table at two o'clock." Go into detail about what you are going to do and what you would like him to do. Never begin a massage on a client with visually impairment until he knows that you are in the room and maintain contact throughout the massage as much as possible.

If your client has a service dog, do not feed, pet, or interact with the dog without permission from the client. This kind of interaction distracts the dog, making his important task more difficult.

MINI-LAB

Gather a blindfold (scarf or king-size pillowcase) and a dollar bill. Locate a partner. You are the "explorer." Take the dollar bill and stick it in your pocket. Your partner is the "attendant." Ask your partner to blindfold you.

The attendant guides the blindfolded explorer, on foot and in silence, to a nearby store to make a refreshment purchase. After you walk back blindfolded, remove the blindfold and reverse roles. You are now the attendant, and your partner is the explorer. Return to your starting point by a different route.

Share your experiences with each other. This activity is designed to experience what it is like to be without sight. You may notice a heightened sense of awareness in your other senses such as hearing and skin sensations.

If a store is not a convenient destination, allow the students to walk a few blocks from the school and back. This activity can be done with ear plugs and blindfolds.

Clients in Wheelchairs

The first consideration when working with a client in a wheelchair is how he will enter your massage establishment. Most municipalities require businesses to be barrier-free, but if yours is not, schedule a home visit and perform the massage off-site.

When you speak to a client who is in a wheelchair, sit down in a chair or a stool, or kneel down on the floor to be able to speak to him at his eye level. Inquire about his particular limitations. Avoid making assumptions; just because your client is in a wheelchair does not necessarily mean that he is paralyzed. People use wheelchairs for many reasons. The client may be experiencing any of the following:

- Amputation
- Spinal cord injury
- Obesity or inactivity
- Depression
- Inability to walk long distances
- Recovery from surgery
- Short-term injury (e.g., broken leg or foot)

Ask the client the reason for his wheelchair use. Spinal cord injuries must be treated differently than other conditions because of the loss of sensory input

(see the section on Paraplegia, Quadriplegia, and Hemiplegia). Clients with amputations may have special needs that must be addressed (see the section on Amputations).

Depending on time factors, reasons for impairment, and ability of the client to undress and transfer to and from the chair, some clients may elect to be massaged in the wheelchair. Often this simply involves positioning the wheelchair at the side of the massage table and placing some pillows onto which the client can lean. A desktop model massage chair may be used (Figure 9-12). Occasionally, the height of the table may have to be adjusted to accommodate the wheelchair. Make sure that the wheelchair wheels are locked in place with the brakes before starting this type of chair massage. Clients with greater mobility usually elect to use the table.

During the massage, it is important to ask the client directly for valuable feedback regarding pressure, body warmth, and how he feels in regard to positioning. Modify your massage techniques and body mechanics as needed. Trigger points may be located in the shoulders and chest area from moving about in the chair. ROM exercises can be administered to active joints.

Observe wheelchair etiquette. Never push a wheelchair without permission from the person in the chair. When moving the client from the chair to the table, he can give you the best instructions on how to proceed. Usually the person in the wheelchair has learned how to transfer, or move, himself in and out of the chair. Never assume these clients are helpless; many of them have been trained to right themselves even after falling out of the chair.

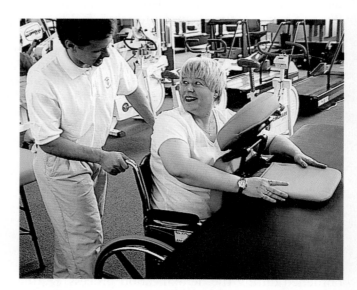

Figure 9-12 Therapist massaging client in a wheelchair using a desk topper. (Courtesy of Oakworks, Shrewsbury, Pa.)

SUMMARY

Massage is an adaptable medium of therapy; the diversity of routines is so significant that variations are endless. By applying specific combinations of these variations, we can reach out to assist those individuals with special needs who fall outside the average treatment session, including physical, emotional, and health challenges. These can be met by using adaptive massage techniques and basic client management to ensure client safety and eliminate restrictive barriers.

Client respect is the primary focus of adaptive massage. Regardless of whether you understand the client's condition, respect for him is essential before a therapeutic relationship can be established. The patients themselves are almost always the most valuable source of information. Once respect and communication have been firmly established, adaptive massage techniques can be used to heal and enrich the lives of your special clients. Working in this type of practice requires commitment, patience, discipline, and flexibility. It can also be one of the most gratifying areas of the profession.

MATCHING

Write the letter of the best answer in the space provided.

A. Chemotherapy
B. Central venous catheter
C. Athlete
D. Recidivism
E. Colostomy ·

F. Modified supine and/or
    side-lying position
G. Paraplegia
H. Quadriplegia
I. Geriatric

J. Disassociation
K. Maintenance massage
L. Phantom limb pain
M. Radiation therapy
N. Pediatric

_____ 1. Feeling pain and other sensations in all or part of an amputated limb

_____ 2. Type of sports massage that encompasses both injury prevention and rehabilitative care

_____ 3. Cancer treatment that uses radiation to eradicate cancer cells

_____ 4. Cancer treatment that consists of a regimen of drugs to slow or stop the growth of cancer cells

_____ 5. Anyone who possesses a natural or acquired ability required for participating in a sport

_____ 6. A flexible tube sewn into a large vein to keep a vein open for dialysis, blood withdrawal, chemotherapy, or frequent administration of medications

_____ 7. An incision in the colon to create an opening between the bowel and the abdominal wall with a bag attached outside the body to gather fecal material

_____ 8. Term to refer to someone who is age 70 or older

_____ 9. Paralysis of the lower extremities and trunk

_____ 10. Paralysis of the arms and legs

_____ 11. Term to refer to someone between 3 and 18 years of age

_____ 12. Expectant mothers in their second and third trimesters should receive a massage in this position(s).

_____ 13. A coping mechanism in which the client "leaves her body" or believes her own past abuse has happened to someone else

_____ 14. A relapse into a previous condition

Bibliography

Applegate EJ: *The anatomy and physiology learning system,* ed 2, Philadelphia, 2000, WB Saunders.

Barstow C: *Tending body and spirit: massage and counseling with elders,* Boulder, Colo, 1985, Author.

Bass E, Davis L: *The courage to heal,* Philadelphia, 1988, Harper and Row.

Curties D: Massage therapy and cancer, Moncton, New Brunswick, Canada, 1999, Curties-Overzet.

Falconer J: Being of service, *Massage Bodywork: Nurture Body, Mind, Spirit* Feb/Mar pp 132-137, 2002.

Fritz S: *Fundamentals of therapeutic massage,* St Louis, 1995, Mosby.

Gould BE: *Pathophysiology for the health-related professions,* Philadelphia, 1997, WB Saunders.

Ignatavicius D, Bayne MV: *Medical-surgical nursing: a nursing process approach,* Philadelphia, 1991, WB Saunders.

MacDonald G: Easing the chemotherapy experience with massage, *Massage Mag* 84:85-91, 2000.

MacDonald G: *Medicine hands: massage therapy for people with cancer,* Tallahassee, 1999, Findhorn Press.

Mathias M: *Personal communication,* 1998.

McConnellogue K: The courage to touch: massage and cancer, *Massage Bodywork: Nurture Body, Mind, Spirit* Dec/Jan pp 12-20, 2000.

McKay M, Davis M, Fanning P: *Messages: the communication skills book,* Oakland, Calif, 1987, New Harbinger.

Meek S: Effects of slow stroke back massage on relaxation in hospice clients, *Image J Nurs Sch* 25(1):17-21, 1993.

Rich GJ: *Massage therapy: the evidence for practice,* St Louis, 2002, Mosby.

Rounseville C: Phantom limb pain: the ghost that haunts the amputee, *Orthop Nurs* 11(2):67-71, 1992.

Scott D et al: The antiemetic effect of clinical relaxation: report of an exploratory pilot study, *J Psychosoc Oncol* 1(1):71-83, 1983.

Tortora GJ: Introduction to the human body: the essentials of anatomy and physiology, ed 3, New York, 1994, HarperCollins.

Weidner N: *Personal communication,* 2002.

Williams D: Touching cancer patients, *Massage Mag* 84: 74-79, 2000.

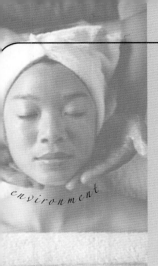

environment

Putting It All Together

10

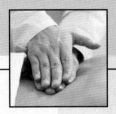

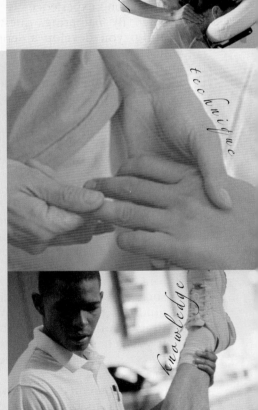

pressure

technique

knowledge

"The notes I handle no better than many pianist. But the pauses between the notes—ah, that is where art resides."

—Artur Schnabel

STUDENT **OBJECTIVES**

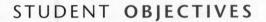

After completing this chapter, the student should be able to:

- Use proper phone etiquette for business related calls
- Prepare the studio before the client arrives
- Demonstrate how to greet a client and prepare him for the massage
- Get ready for the massage session with movement and breath work
- Address client care and comfort needs and demonstrate how communication will be handled during the massage
- Give a massage using the elements discussed in this textbook
- Design or locate follow-up information, to be dispensed to the client after the massage

INTRODUCTION

This chapter examines the massage routine in its various segments and discusses the therapist's responsibilities during each segment. The sections of the massage are (1) telephone communication, (2) before the client arrives, (3) when the client arrives, (4) before the massage session, (5) during the massage session, and (6) after the massage session.

Massage is not a rigid process. Rather, massage is a dynamic process, and the massage routine is simply a road map to help you learn your way around. As we discuss a massage routine, keep in mind that there is room, and even a need, for creativity. You can invent massage strokes. For instance, you can massage the palm of the hand and the sole of the foot at the same time. You could try massaging around the scapula and up the neck simultaneously creating a unique massage stroke. Your session will indeed be unique as long as you keep the client as the central focus of the massage.

Hands-on experience is your best and final teacher. By palpating, questioning, listening, and treating, you develop a sense of what is familiar, which, in turn, breeds knowledge, enhances skill, and promotes confidence. You will learn that mastery comes not only in the doing but also in the deciding. Many small decisions are made in the course of a workday. Good decisions are more easily made if you develop some professional awareness.

As a therapist, it is your responsibility to gain four kinds of professional awareness when practicing massage:
1. **Self awareness.** The therapist is professional in appearance and is knowledgeable, skilled, focused, calm, confident, and prepared.
2. **Client awareness.** The therapist is familiar with the client because of a thorough intake.
3. **Surrounding awareness.** Surroundings are tailored by the therapist to suit the client's needs, such as room temperature, music selection and volume, choice of lubricant, and table dressing.
4. **Precaution awareness.** The therapist determines if your client has open lesions, skin pathologies, scars that may indicate recent injuries or surgeries, or infections.

If a medical emergency arises before, during, or after the massage, contact emergency medical services (EMS) immediately. Provide the location and condition of the client.

TELEPHONE COMMUNICATION

The telephone is the second contact between the client and the therapist. The first is promotional advertising such as a business card, brochure, or word of mouth. Because of the importance of telephone communication, it makes good sense to spend time learning how to manage incoming calls and telephone communications. This is known as telephone etiquette—the behavior observed and used by people on the telephone when communicating for social or professional activities. The following tips are for communicating with your current and prospective clients by phone:
- Always answer between the second and third ring.
- Begin with "Good morning," "Good afternoon," or "Good evening," followed by your name, the name of your establishment, and an inquiry. For example, "Good afternoon. This is Jane Smith at the Nest. How may I help you?"
- Use a pleasant, expressive tone of voice; smile at the caller.
- Find out the caller's name, and use it as you speak to him.
- Give the caller your undivided attention.
- Be a good listener; find out what the caller wants first.
- Say "please," "thank you," and "you're welcome."
- If you must place the caller on hold, ask permission and wait for a reply. For example, "May I put you on hold?" If he concurs, do not leave the caller on hold for more than 1 minute. If it appears that the caller will be on hold longer than that, offer to return the call. Always thank the caller for holding.
- Be accurate and thorough when taking messages. Write down the date, time the call was received, who called, why the person called, and a return phone number and extension. Repeat all the information to the caller and check for accuracy before hanging up.
- Let the caller end the conversation, allowing him to hang up first.
- Keep your promises and follow up.
- Return calls within 24 hours; this is known as the *sundown rule.*

Inform the caller of available services and fees. If the caller schedules an appointment, recommend that she not eat or eat only lightly 1 hour before the scheduled session. If she comes directly from her work, suggest that she bring alternate clothing to wear home afterward. If you require that the client bring special items such as shorts, a swimsuit, or a towel, inform her now. Some first-time clients may be limited on time, coming to you on the lunch hour or between business appointments. If this is the case, begin the client's file by doing a telephone screening using a health intake form or mail the intake form and ask the client to bring it with her on the day of her scheduled appointment. Additionally, let the client know to schedule "downtime," or time to relax, after the session. If you have a cancellation or

DEANE JUHAN, MA

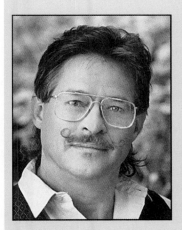

(Copyright © Karen Zurlinden Photography.)

Born: April 18, 1945.

"The principle is elegantly simple. We learn to love by being loved, we learn gentleness by being gentle, we learn to be graceful by experiencing the feeling of grace."

Deane Juhan is a bodyworker, one of the first Trager-trained instructors, an anatomy teacher/lecturer for the Trager Institute, and author of *Job's Body: a Handbook for Bodyworkers*. As the title suggests, the book offers an answer to the age-old question of "why" regarding the Old Testament book of Job . . . but that's just for starters. The book explores "the various ways through which intuitive and informed touch can positively affect a wide variety of symptoms and help to change people's lives for the better." The book was 9 years in the making, which is surprising, considering the manner in which Juhan's words easily flow during casual conversation.

Born to a woman who had "poor taste in men" and a soldier who did not hang around to become a father, Juhan was later adopted, growing up as an only child in Glenwood Springs, Colo. His father worked for the state and never drew a large salary, but his parents were wise about using resources and were determined that their only child's education would receive top priority in their lives.

Juhan describes himself as an underachiever in high school. The University of Colorado introduced him to a whole new way of living and he admits to being caught up in the novelty of its hip, liberal atmosphere until his junior year, when "his rudder finally bit the water," he says. It was then that he became interested in the aspects of art, science, and civilization.

He learned about Esalen, a workshop and meeting place for developing human potential in Big Sur, Calif., while working on his dissertation in literature. He actually managed to sneak in and start doing massage. He was so good at it. His first experience in anatomy was developing slides and lectures for Structural Integration for Rolfing lectures, but when he witnessed Milton Trager, he was hooked and abandoned all other methods to learn the Trager Approach.

"It was love at first sight," says Juhan. "I was attracted to his quality of being. It was his rich avuncular benevolence without all the preliminary folderol that made me want to learn to do what he did, so I threw myself into it and gave it my all."

It didn't come easy though for this hard-pushing 6-footer. His strength had always been, well, his strength. Nonetheless, he broke down and cried when he saw his first Trager demonstration. Then, as he clumsily applied himself to unlearning everything he ever thought he knew about bodywork, Trager reduced his ego to ashes, hollering at him during training, slapping his hand away and taking over, always admonishing him to work lighter and softer and to quit trying so hard to get the job done.

Juhan points out that Trager's use of inducing a transcendental meditation state during a session, which has been called *hook-up* is one of the things that sets Trager apart and makes the work so effective. It is during this hook-up that messages are communicated that have nothing to do with verbal and nonverbal interaction as we know it, and it is this exchange that is the key to long-term change.

For the bodywork session, the goal is to connect with the client's sensory information, process what the practitioner helps the client discover or rediscover, then help the client "wake up" to the possibility for long-term change through movement. The practitioner lays down new patterns by repeating a movement message again and again. The feeling finally becomes etched on the client's awareness, creating an experience of length, relaxation, and pain-free movement.

DEANE JUHAN, MA—cont'd

Before this can be achieved, however, the bodyworker needs to understand how the body works and what this "preverbal" language is all about. Juhan also argues for bodywork to "redress some of the underdevelopment and dysfunction we find associated with various pathological conditions." Most importantly, he wants to change the way we think about our bodies.

In short, Juhan asserts, we have stopped "listening to the only reliable source of self-regulation and preservation we have available. It is the direct result of century-long programming that has debased our subjective awareness." When we are in pain or simply feeling bad, instead of confronting what is at the root of our problem, we seek help outside the wisdom of our own bodies. We run to the doctor, shrink, psychic, minister, and self-help section of the nearest bookstore. Nothing is wrong with any of these things, of course, but Juhan reminds us that the only thing we truly know about the world is the way the body responds to it, and no one can know how our bodies are responding to stimuli the way we each individually can. In short, we are, to a very great degree, responsible for our own well-being.

Juhan writes in *Job's Body: a Handbook for Bodyworkers:* "For Job this was revelation—the perception that God was in his very flesh, in the throbbing of his heart, in the singing of his nerves, in the coiling of his muscles, to be touched and felt more intimately than an embrace."

As a beginning massage therapist, you are probably not seeking a revelation so much as you are a direction. You can probably guess that Juhan's advice is to look within. Choose the modality that will, according to Juhan, "flower in your psyche or experience. Look for what turns you on, look for what you love, not what the market says is hot."

---

late policy, let her know about it now and verify that the appointment time is appropriate for her schedule. Give her directions to your establishment and any other information that you deem necessary. Finally ask if she has any questions.

 Every artist was an amateur.
—Ralph Waldo Emerson

BEFORE THE CLIENT ARRIVES

This section is concerned with the time frame beginning when you report to work until the client arrives. If possible, arrive at least 30 to 60 minutes before your first appointment. Check your answering machine or answering service and take care of any calls. You may want to call each person the day before the scheduled massage to verify the appointment. This reduces any confusion and minimizes absenteeism. Look over your schedule; pull and review client intake forms and past notes for any clients scheduled that day. If you are expecting a first-time client, have a blank intake form and pertinent literature ready.

Check the table for safety and security. Are the knobs that connect the table legs to the tabletop loose? If so, tighten them. If you massage on a portable table, make sure the latches that keep the table closed are now flat and not protruding. Check and correct the extension of the table legs and make sure any table cords are straight and taut.

Dress the treatment table and ready the massage room. If you have prepared your massage room the day before, inspect the room for any unexpected items (e.g., dead insects). When your client enters the massage room, have the music playing, the lighting dim and indirect, and the room warm. It is a mark of professionalism to have the massage area visually appealing and ready to go (i.e., bolsters, linens, lubricant). If you do not allow enough time between massages for this preparation, have a place (e.g., waiting room, office) where your client can wait while you prepare the massage room.

Using a mirror, critique your own appearance. Is your hair in place? Are your nails trimmed, neat, and clean? Are your pockets empty of keys and change? Have you removed your jewelry and watch?

MINI-LAB

Visit a massage therapist's office. What is the initial impression you have approaching the door? List the words that describe how you feel. Is the mood serene, businesslike, busy, chaotic, impersonal, or cluttered? What do you hear or smell?

WHEN THE CLIENT ARRIVES: ROOM ORIENTATION AND PREPARATION FOR MASSAGE

This is the time frame between the client's arrival and when she undresses for the massage. Greet your client with a smile, making eye contact and calling her by name whenever possible. Introduce yourself (if this is your first time as her therapist) and escort her to the area where the massage consultation will take place. Be calm, confident, friendly, and courteous while in the presence of your client. The therapeutic relationship, which is an ongoing process, is built on a foundation of trust, good communication skills, and rapport. To show respect for the client and the relationship, avoid the use of tobacco in any form while in the company of a client. The smell of tobacco is often offensive to nonsmoking clients. Although many smoking therapists are unaware of their tobacco odor, it can be detected on their clothes, hair, and linens.

Ask the client to fill out an intake form (see Chapter 8) and review the informed consent section with her. If this is a previous client, go over the health history information and record any changes. Perform any assessments related to treatment and prioritize the client's needs based on the consultation. Explain to the client what will be done during the session and why. Ask the client if she has any questions and answer them to the best of your ability.

If any special considerations need to be addressed, discuss how the massage will be adapted to suit the client's special needs (see Chapter 9). The client may be overwhelmed by all the information that is needed to prepare for a safe and well-tailored massage session. It may be helpful to ask the client to show up 15 minutes early for her first appointment, or you may want to mail out in advance all the forms that you require (e.g., initial intake, consent, and brochure of your practice or policy and procedures). This packet may be titled *What to Expect* or *What a Massage is Like*. The purpose of this procedure is to decrease the client's stress and anxiety and to save you time.

You may wish to direct your client to the music selection, telling her what is currently playing, and asking her to make a selection if she prefers a different kind of music. Next, direct her to your massage lubricant selection and ask her to make a choice. Point out the most popular lubricant to make the selection process easier. Take into consideration any skin sensitivities and allergies. You may need to get an ingredient list in large type so the client can read the ingredients. The use of aromatherapy can also help the client to unwind (see Chapter 3).

Even though draping is discussed in the premassage consultation, often many emotions are associated with disrobing and touch that distorts the new client's perspective, making directions and instructions difficult to hear. Simple and concise instructions assist the client in the transition from the mental focus of the consultation to the physical and emotional focus of a massage session. Be sure to allow the client time to settle into the space provided for him before giving directions on the use of linens, positioning himself on the table, indicating when you will return to begin the massage. Every precaution should be taken to ensure the client's comfort, physical and emotional safety, and privacy (see Chapter 2).

Before you exit the room, address any comfort needs your client may have. Offer the client a glass of water and suggest a trip to the restroom. Show her where to place her clothes and personal items, and explain to her any special procedures you use to handle these items. Tell the client how to lie on the table (either to get underneath the top sheet or to drape towels over her body). Tell her that you are going to leave the room so she may disrobe in privacy and that, when you reenter the room, you will knock before you open the door. This alleviates any apprehension she may have about your unannounced return.

Client empathy is one of the reasons it is so important that you, as the therapist, receive massages from other therapists. By getting back in touch with what it is like to be a client, you will be a more attentive and sensitive therapist.

Clients often wear a watch or jewelry and may bring a purse, wallet, or other valuables to the massage office. Because most jewelry and watches are removed before the massage begins, care must be taken to safeguard these items. Large articles, such as purses, should not leave the client's sight. For smaller items, use a large envelope, small basket, or

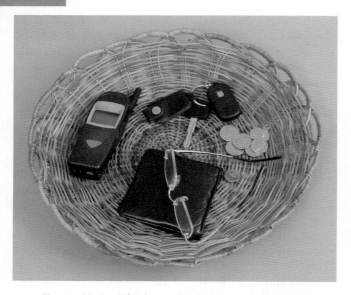

Figure 10-1   A basket or bowl for personal items.

small bowl to accommodate the client's belongings (Figure 10-1). A portable container allows these items to remain with the client if she must move from one room to another. A locker or locked box may also be used to store these items safely during the massage.

MINI-LAB

Once you have learned a basic massage routine, perform a massage blindfolded. The recipient on the table may have to assist with the draping and turning aspects of the massage because these may be too difficult for you without your sense of sight. This activity will help you get out of your head and intellect and into your hands and feeling skills.

BEFORE THE MASSAGE SESSION

This section deals with when you leave the massage room until you return to begin the massage. Wash and dry your hands and forearms (see Chapter 4). Because your hands may become cool from the handwashing, warm them by rubbing them together before the massage begins; this helps warm the massage lubricant too.

You have spent much time and energy learning a craft and preparing your massage room; spend a little time preparing your mind, body, and spirit. Grounding and centering yourself before the massage is an integral part of your therapy session. If you feel distracted and not present with your client, you will not be able to give the best massage possible.

Learning how to clear your thoughts, how to prepare your body, and how to ground and center yourself will help you be a more skilled and sensitive therapist (see Chapter 6).

Breathing and body movements are some techniques you can use to prepare yourself before the massage begins. No matter what style of massage you practice, you will expend energy. Before you enter the massage room, move and stretch your body while practicing deep breathing. If all you have is a few seconds, simply squat down to stretch your low back (only if your knees can do this comfortably) and stand up to shake out your entire body. Stretch your upper body (Figure 10-2). Relaxation allows a calm to exist. A therapist who is calm will easily project professionalism, confidence, and peace to the client with her presence and touch. If you have a minute, you might want to try the 60-Second Energy Snack in Box 10-1. It contains no calories, and it is loaded with energy.

Some massage therapists choose to incorporate elements of their own spirituality into the massage. Some therapists choose to turn their skills and the

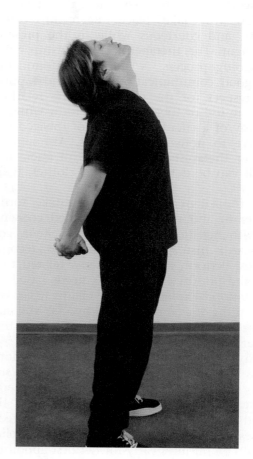

Figure 10-2   Massage therapist stretching before entering the massage room.

BOX 10-1

The 60-Second Energy Snack

1. Slap the palms of your outstretched hands together, and rub them rapidly for 5 seconds (out of earshot of clients).
2. Hold your warmed palms over your cheeks and eyes for 5 seconds.
3. Make your hands into claws and apply vigorous tapping tapotement to the scalp for 5 seconds.
4. Apply loose-fist tapotement up and down each arm for 10 seconds.
5. Gently grasp the hyoid bone and mobilize it from side to side to stimulate the thyroid gland.
6. With your right hand, cup your palm around the back of your neck and squeeze firmly about 10 times.
7. Repeat step 6 with the left hand while nodding the head at the same time.
8. Repeat step 6 with the left hand while shaking the head at the same time.
9. With the right hand reach across the midline of your body and grasp the top of your left trapezius and squeeze firmly about 10 times.
10. Repeat step 9 to the right trapezius with the left hand.
11. Do three sets of shoulder rolls forward and three backward.
12. Pincer-grip the thumb web of each hand and hold for 3 seconds (omit this step if you are pregnant).
13. Shake the hands out.
14. Stomp the feet several times.

You are now energized and ready to go!

direction of the massage over to the care of God (or a higher power). A simple prayer, verbal or silent, of gratitude for the opportunity to work with this client helps create the atmosphere for healing to occur (most massage therapists prefer to pray in silence). If you decide to pray in the massage room, ask permission from the client. Some clients will be fine with prayer; others will consider it too personal an issue and may be uncomfortable.

 No one is useless in this world who lightens the burdens of another.
—Charles Dickens

Many clients will ask you how many massages you have done today and if you are tired, or after noting the physical nature of our work, they will ask if your hands become tired. What they may really be asking is: "Do you have enough energy for me?" Assure them that you have stamina and endurance built up from frequently doing massage and that when your

hands do feel tired, you massage them back to happiness. At this point, they seem to be less fearful and greatly relieved.

MINI-LAB

When feasible, get a massage from a therapist you do not know. During the massage intake, do not reveal to the therapist that you are a massage therapist or student of massage therapy. In this way, you will get the full experience of what it is like to be a client. Along with helping you learn what to do and what not to do, this activity will also reinforce the things you are doing that work well for the client. Role reversal can be an eye-opening experience.

DURING THE MASSAGE SESSION

This section of the chapter addresses the time frame that begins when the massage therapist reenters the room and ends when the massage therapist leaves the room after the massage is complete.

Before you begin the massage, address the client's care and comfort needs one more time. Ask your client if the room temperature is comfortable. It is difficult to relax while you feel chilled. Encourage your client's proper body alignment with the placement of bolsters or pillows underneath the areas of the body that require support (e.g., neck, knees, ankles). Remind the client about the importance of being relaxed and offering feedback during the massage. If he is uncomfortable in any way, he may not become or stay engaged with the massage. Note any bruises you identify directly to the client so that you are not blamed for them.

Begin by making physical contact with the client, perhaps with quiet, motionless touch (Figure 10-3). Help your client relax by asking her to take a few deep breaths. Once you and the client are ready, proceed with the massage routine. The dozens of methods for massaging the body, each effective in its own way, are best learned in the classroom under a skilled and caring instructor.

The length of treatment is offered by the therapist but determined by the client. The client schedules the session, often in 30- to 90-minute increments. If the client is undecided about the length of her session, tell her that you will schedule a half-hour session but will block out a full hour. When 30 minutes is up, let her know, and she can then decide if she would like the massage to continue.

Focus on the client's areas of complaint during the session while working out areas that you find during the massage through palpation. Although the

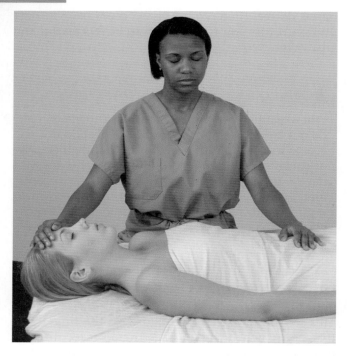

Figure 10-3   Touching your client before massage.

therapist is confined to a specific length of time, try not to let the massage feel hurried. Address the client's concerns first (e.g., back, neck, shoulder) so as to not accidentally run out of time.

Sometimes as you massage, the client's body may tense. Silently, you may decide to respond by changing your pressure or rhythm. If the client remains tense, ask for feedback. Reiterate how important communication is during the massage. You may discover that the client is ticklish or is in pain and is therefore splinting, or contracting, his muscles. He may also have to use the restroom. Address his needs and then continue with the massage. Be patient and caring; enhance your client's ability to relax.

Regarding conversation during the massage, take your cues from the client. If she is there for stress reduction, avoid becoming too talkative because this may distract from her overall relaxation. One guideline is to talk only when answering the client's questions and when addressing the client's comfort needs. Otherwise, stay silent and follow the client's lead. If one of your clients falls asleep during the massage, avoid deep work as you may either startle the client. It is also difficult to obtain feedback regarding pressure from a sleeping client.

Designing and tailoring the session to the client's individual needs are the hallmarks of a proficient massage therapist. Everybody responds differently to massage. The more you learn and practice, the greater the number of massage styles you can offer your clients. Know all your options and honor your limits. As your experience increases, you can incorporate

new moves into your routine. Like any art, mastery is a lifelong process.

The following are a few general guidelines to be considered as you are applying massage:

- Practice good hygiene with handwashing before and after each massage.
- Protect yourself by using good body mechanics.
- Promote client comfort through a restful environment and bolstering devices.
- Screen your client for local and absolute contraindications.
- Stroke lightly over bony prominences and endangerment sites.
- Address client needs regarding work on a specific area
- Be thorough and complete. Always connect body parts to themselves and to one another.
- Work deeply enough to contact and release tension but not so deep that you cause tension and pain.
- Stay relaxed and present; be focused and respect the client.

 Fish will be the last to discover water.
                                        —Albert Einstein

Providing communication and direction during the massage is a little different from normal conversation because eye contact is infrequent. When a client is lying prone, the head is to one side or in a face cradle; when a client is supine, either the eyes are closed, or a client must strain her neck muscles to obtain eye contact. Establish a method of communication in the premassage consultation, and reinforce your instructions during the session when needed. The most important feedback a massage therapist needs is how the client is receiving the massage. More specifically, the therapist must know if the massage causes any pain or discomfort. The following is an abbreviated system of communication developed by massage therapist Ralph Stephens. This system is also featured in Chapter 25; it is particularly helpful in establishing and maintaining communication and in building rapport with your client during the session.

When It Hurts or If the Pressure Is Too Hard

Tell the client, "Be sure to tell me whenever I find a tender area. Will you do that for me?" or "If at any time I am working too hard, be sure and tell me right away. Will you do that?" Quantitative measuring scales you can use are as follows:

- Ask the client to simply raise a hand if pain is felt.
- Use the 1-to-5 scale: 1 represents "no pain" and 5 represents "excruciating pain." You will know, by

the number vocalized or the number of fingers raised, how she is responding to the pressure. A 1-to-5 scale is necessary to allow easy one-handed response.

- Establish a thumbs up/thumbs down/okay gesture system. Thumbs up means that more pressure is needed (Figure 10-4). Thumbs down means that less pressure is requested. An okay symbol (index finger touching thumb with other fingers extended) means the pressure is perfect.

When It Gets Better

Tell the client, "When I find these tender places, I will stop and maintain the pressure. This sustained pressure will cause the nervous system to respond by relaxing the tender area. It may feel to you like I am letting up on the pressure or that it is beginning to feel better. Will you let me know when it gets better?"

If It Refers

Tell the client, "When I am examining or maintaining pressure on an area of tissue, you may experience some sensation somewhere else. It could be a pain, tingling, numbness, aching, or some other sensation; somewhere besides right where I am massaging. These may be trigger points that also need to be

massaged. Will you tell me if you feel anything other than pressure where I am working?"

Regardless of which system of feedback you use for assessing pain and pressure, use your peripheral vision and look for physical signs of discomfort. Some clients do not volunteer feedback about pain. They may be accustomed to denying pain and discomfort, or they may have a different sensation and perception assigned to pain. However, the body rarely lies. Body gestures that may indicate you are working too hard include (1) the client pulling away from you or contracting muscles to limit your access into the tissues; (2) general squirming; (3) raising eyebrows or frowning; (4) holding the breath; (5) white knuckles; and (6) raising the head or foot up off the table.

Another helpful tool to use when giving directions is to use tactile cues and gestures. For example, as you ask the client to scoot over to the edge of the table, gently touch her shoulder or tap the tabletop on the side you want her to move toward. This method can be used when you need the client to move up or down the table and also when to turn the head to one side or another. When asking a client to turn over, if eye contact is possible, supinate or pronate your hand to indicate the direction she should roll. When giving directions in which a client should place her arms or other body part a certain way, demonstrate it too. If you need the client to raise her head, feet, or knees to accommodate a bolster, use a gentle lifting motion with your hand. Your client may be so relaxed that verbal directions are processed slowly. Kinetic cues help the client understand what you need her to do.

When you are finished with the massage, avoid hurrying the client off the massage table. In fact, invite her to rest a few minutes. Because the client has been in one position for an extended period, it is often helpful to ask her to roll over on her side and bend her knees to her chest. Place a soft pillow under her head, and ask her to lie in this position for a few minutes before she gets up to dress. If she is afraid of falling asleep and losing track of time, tell her that you will be back in 10 minutes to remind her to get up. This short rest period allows the client some quiet time devoid of stimuli to integrate the physical and emotional aspects of the massage. It also allows transition time to move from internal focus to external focus before rescheduling an appointment, leaving your facility, and driving away. Before you leave the room, remove the bolsters and wipe off any excess lubricant from the soles of your client's feet.

You may find it necessary to instruct the client on how to get up off the table. Once lying on her side, suggest that the client allow her lower legs to fall off the edge of the table. She can then use the arm that is not lying against the massage table to push her

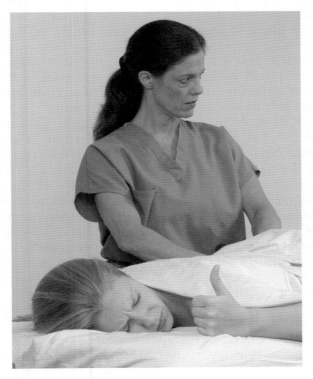

Figure 10-4   Prone client giving "thumbs up" for pressure during a massage.

upper body up into a seated position. Avoid letting the client sit straight up from a supine position because she may strain her back or neck. Remind the client that the best way for getting up off the massage table is also the best way to get out of bed in the morning. If your client requires assistance getting off the table, refer to Chapter 6.

A small portion of the population (about 10%) finds it difficult to stand up after lying down for an extended period. This is the result of insufficient cerebral circulation and a sudden drop in blood pressure that often occurs when moving into an upright position. Symptoms of this condition may include dizziness, impaired vision, and buzzing in the ears. In more severe cases, fainting may occur. With this in mind, it is helpful to do one of the following after the massage: remind your client to sit up for a few moments before standing or assist her into a standing position, pausing for a few moments to make sure she is oriented in the upright position.

If you remove a client's eyeglasses while she is on the massage table or if a client gives you her eyeglasses before the massage, hand them back to the client before she gets off the massage table and before you leave the massage room to allow her time to redress. If you neglect this important procedure, you may be liable if your client trips or falls in your massage room and incurs injuries because she was unable to see clearly.

As you leave the massage room, let the client know if she is to wait in the room for you to return or if she needs to exit the room to find you in another area.

MINI-LAB

The following exercise is designed to increase your level of sensitivity as a massage therapist and to strengthen your proprioception. Select a partner, and decide which of you is the giver and which is the receiver. Sit facing each other, and raise your hands just below shoulder level. Gently flex your fingers; allow your fingertips to touch your partner's fingertips. Both the giver and the receiver then close their eyes (Figure 10-5).

The designated giver slowly begins to move his hands in space, allowing the receiver to follow his hands while remaining connected by fingertips. This may feel awkward at first, but as the receiver expands his awareness, it begins to feel as if the two are dancing. After a minute of practice, switch roles.

After the exercise, ask yourself the following questions. How confident were you as the giver? How did you feel as the receiver? When you were the giver, did your receiver relax and follow you, or did

he tense up? Sometimes, people have a tendency to follow by anticipating the moves instead of experiencing the moves. The more sensitive the receiver becomes, then the easier it is to follow the giver. How can this type of sensitivity apply to massage therapy?

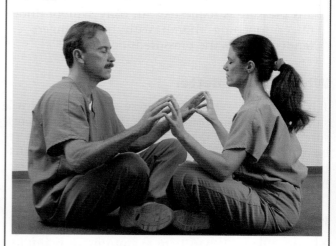

Figure 10-5 Demonstration of the position needed for push hands.

AFTER THE MASSAGE SESSION

This last section concerns the therapist's activities from the time he exits the massage room after the massage until the client leaves the premises. While your client is dressing, wash your hands and write any case notes. Make sure the lighting in the post-massage area is not too bright or too noisy because this type of environment is not very relaxing. Provide a transitional space. Take a few deep breaths, and prepare to greet the client with a smile.

Have ready any parting information that you wish to give the client. Information sheets can be anything from tips on how to use ice, self-massage, relaxation techniques, and theories about muscle soreness, to how to preserve and prolong the effects of the massage (Box 10-2). Without the educational element of massage therapy, the massage session may be no more than an expensive aspirin or bandage. Avoid just putting out fires; show clients how to prevent them. Clients really appreciate this added service of information on items such as how to alter sleeping positions to reduce muscle strain or how to sit in a chair more comfortably. Be familiar with your scope of practice to make sure "client education" is legal for a massage therapist in your state.

If the therapist removes jewelry or wristwatches for the client, it is the therapist's responsibility to make sure the client leaves with these items. The

Ten Daily Steps for Preserving and Prolonging the Effects of Your Massage

- Drink at least 0.5 oz of fresh water per 1 lb of body weight (for soft-tissue irrigation).
- Maintain a neutral sleeping posture by using pillows to bolster the extremities to keep the spine straight.
- Stretch.
- Apply ice packs on painful areas (20 minutes).
- Be aware of your posture during the day.
- Decrease the intake of caffeine and sugar as much as possible (these neurostimulants can increase pain perception and dehydrate the body).
- Breathe slowly, extending the exhale.
- Develop a positive attitude.
- Simplify/prioritize and take stress breaks.
- Love yourself.

therapist may simply indicate where the items have been placed before leaving the room for the client to dress. In the case of a client who is physically unable to put the jewelry back on herself, the therapist should offer to assist.

A client may be disoriented after a massage and may accidentally forget some of their belongings. If you do discover personal articles in a room after a massage, place them inside an envelope and seal it. Write the date, the item, and the owner of the item. If you do not know who owns the item, call the clients who were there that day and ask them if they left anything in your studio. It is generally best to let them tell you what they are missing and give a complete description before returning the item.

Some clients report becoming "sore" after a massage. Some reasons for this are the amount of pressure used during the massage, the length of time spent massaging an area, the health of the client's tissues, lack of client hydration, client inactivity, exposure to environmental toxins, and lack of post-massage care. If you worked an area deeply or for an extended period or if you suspect a client may be sore, recommend that the client drink lots of fresh water (at least 0.5 oz of water per 1 lb of body weight) and ice the area for 20 minutes.

How often a client schedules a massage can be influenced by the therapist, but, once again, is determined by the client. Massage rarely can resolve everything that has been bothering the client for years in one session. Typically, clients schedule (1) once a week, (2) once a month, (3) only when they are in a crisis, such as a headache or stiff shoulder. A client who is in the crisis management category may become a regular client if she begins to experience that massage is keeping crises from occurring. If a client asks you to decide when you think she should come back, politely tell her that only when everything you have shown her (e.g., stretching, self-massage, cold and hot packs) fails to work. This approach builds trust and confidence between the client and therapist by empowering the client.

Collect fees if you have not already done so and ask the client if he would like to reschedule. Offer the client another glass of water before he departs. After the client has gone, ready your room for your next client, take a few deep breaths, and stretch out your muscles.

Some clients may want to stay and talk after the massage. If the conversation is related to the massage and the client's health and progress, the therapist should make some time to address the client's concerns. If, on the other hand, the conversation is just a friendly chat, the therapist may have other priorities. Often the massage therapist may need to tend to phone messages, wash linens, ready the massage room for the next client, or break for lunch. Usually, simply walking the client to the door, perhaps even stepping outside with him, saying thank you and good-bye, and walking back in the office is enough (Figure 10-6). You may have to say something such as, "I really enjoy talking with you, but I have a few things to take care of." Setting a boundary is necessary to take care of yourself and to serve the other clients you have scheduled for the rest of the day.

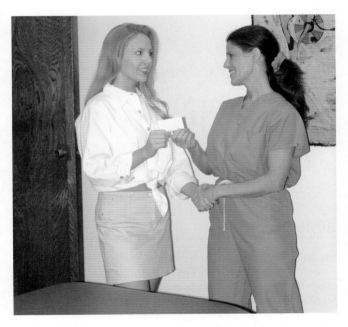

Figure 10-6 Telling a client good-bye while standing by the door.

SUMMARY

This chapter divides the massage routine into basic components and defines responsibilities for each time frame. Before the client arrives, the massage therapist should take care of room preparation, paperwork, and personal appearance. When the client arrives, the therapist should introduce herself, gather initial intake information or get an update, explain the procedures, and answer questions. Before the massage, the therapist should wash her hands and prepare herself emotionally, mentally, and physically. During the massage, the therapist continually addresses the client's needs by initiating contact, responding to muscular tension, and following the client's lead. The most important part of the massage process is establishing and maintaining a comfortable level of rapport with the client. After the massage, the therapist should again wash her hands, prepare the outside environment as a transition for the client, prepare any handouts for the client to take home, collect fees, and offer to schedule another appointment. Following these protocols enables the therapist to provide optimum care for the client (Figure 10-7).

Throughout the process, the massage therapist should cultivate and maintain an attitude of respect and courtesy toward her client.

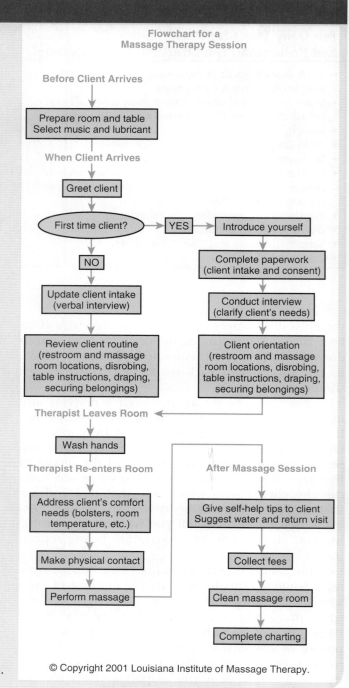

Figure 10-7 Flowchart for a massage therapy session.

© Copyright 2001 Louisiana Institute of Massage Therapy.

Bibliography

Mackey B: Massage therapy and reflexology awareness, *Nurs Clin North Am* 36(1):159-170, 2001.

Ogg-Cormier S: *Personal communication*, 1998.

Stephens R: *Personal communication*, 2002.

UNIT THREE

Anatomy and Physiology for the Massage Therapist

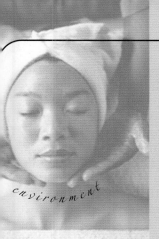

Introduction to the Human Body: Cells, Tissues, and the Body Compass

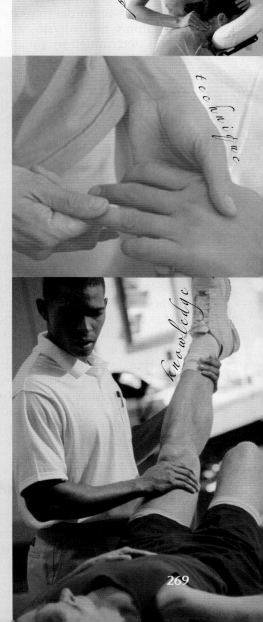

11

"The map is not the territory."

—Alfred Korzbyski

STUDENT OBJECTIVES

After completing this chapter, the student should be able to:

- Define anatomy, physiology, homeostasis, and metabolism
- Identify the parts of a cell and discuss their functions
- Describe passive and active cell processes
- Discuss the four basic tissue types and give examples of each
- Explain the three types of membranes
- State the 10 main body systems and discuss their basic functions
- Indicate the planes of the body
- Differentiate among the main body cavities and the organs contained within them
- Name the directional terminology used in anatomy and physiology; use it to locate structures of the body
- Identify body landmarks by name, location, and description

INTRODUCTION

You are about to embark on an unforgettable journey—a new path of self-discovery—into your own interiors. But first you have to learn some new language and definitions. Basic anatomical terminology is crucial to your understanding of the anatomy and physiology that follows, and to be an effective massage therapist a thorough knowledge of this material is essential.

A clear visual picture of the many possible arrangements of cells and tissues will help you truly feel what is beneath your hands. As massage therapists, you will be manipulating and comparing many types of tissues. You will be compressing and stretching fascia (connective tissue), kneading gluteus maximus (muscle tissue), chucking metacarpals (connective tissue), and feathering the epidermis (epithelial and nervous tissues). Remember, all these terms will be reinforced many times during your studies. This is only the beginning—an initial step through the door.

Anatomy and physiology are inseparable. Structure is determined by function and function is carried out through structure. Another way of looking at this concept is that form follows function. For example, consider the form (or structure) of the lungs, a pair of thin-tissued organs. Lung tissue is best suited for gas exchange. What organ (structure), with its thick, muscular walls, is suited for pumping fluids (function)? The heart, of course!

Our bodies are all physiological masterpieces. As you read this, your heart is pumping blood, your lungs are moving air, your pupils are adjusting to reading conditions, and your nerves are monitoring both the internal and external environments. These processes occur within us at every moment. During your study of anatomy and physiology, many wonders will be revealed. The philosopher Plato once noted that the "acquiring of knowledge is just a form of recollection." Learning anatomy and physiology is just becoming aware of who you are already.

This chapter is designed to serve as a reference as you continue your studies in anatomy and physiology. Here, you will learn about cells, tissues, and their membranes, and you are introduced to the organ systems. Also, you will learn terms used to navigate your way around the body. The reference for directional terminology, structural landmarks, and body cavities is known as the *body compass*.

INTRODUCTION TO ANATOMY AND PHYSIOLOGY

The two ways to approach the study of the human body are regionally and systemically. The *regional approach* is typically used in medical schools, especially in laboratory classes. In the cadaver laboratory, the student learns the regional structures of the body such as the arm, leg, and chest and the skin's many underlying structures. The most common approach for anatomy and physiology study in a lecture setting is the *systemic approach*, in which each body system is explored individually. This approach is used in the following chapters to explore nine of the 10 body systems. The reproductive system is not addressed in this text because it is irrelevant to massage. In a different manner, the regional approach is used in chapters covering skeletal and muscular nomenclature. A laboratory class format is the best way to approach the information presented in these two chapters. Both approaches are valid, and although we can look at each system individually or by region, it is important to remember that the body functions as an interrelated whole and that all the systems balance and support one another.

Almost everyone has some understanding of basic anatomy and physiology, if not from prior education classes then from practical experience of one's own body. As we begin our study, it is important to get a good definition of anatomical terms based on the medical model so that everyone speaks a common language. **Anatomy** is the study of the structures of the human body and their positional relationship to one another (the head bone is connected to the neck bone and so on). The two divisions of human anatomy are gross and microscopic.

Gross anatomy is the study of larger body structures such as bones, muscle, nerves, blood vessels, organs, and glands. *Microscopic anatomy* is the study of the smaller structures of the body, such as cells and tissues, which make up the larger structures and can best be seen through a microscope. **Physiology** is the study of how the body and its individual parts function in normal body processes.

To better understand the relationship between anatomy and physiology, a theater metaphor may be helpful. The stage, props, and cast of characters are the structures of the play (anatomy). How the characters relate to one another and the plot of the play is its function (physiology).

Homeostasis is a relatively stable condition of the body's internal environment within a very limited range. Even when the outside conditions change, the body's internal environment is relatively constant. Homeostasis is maintained by adjusting the metabolism of the body. **Metabolism** is the total of all the physical and chemical processes that occur in an organism (i.e., those that are considered to be signs of life). To maintain homeostasis the body adjusts many different metabolic functions, including heart rate, blood pressure, respiratory rate, body temperature, hormone production, glandular secretions, energy generation and consumption, the digestion and absorption of food, and the elimination of wastes.

The human body can be thought of as a universe, made up of very small parts organized to function as a unit. These follow a hierarchy based on their levels of complexity. The levels are chemical, cellular, tissue, organ, organ system, and organism levels. The chemical level encompasses the biochemistry of our body (e.g., water, hormones, deoxyribonucleic acid [DNA], oxygen, iron, or compounds). The cellular level deals primarily with cells. Cells are composed of chemicals from the chemical level and can perform all the functions vital to life. The tissue level is composed of groups of cells possessing its own unique

Biological Prefixes and Suffixes

Prefix	Meaning	Example	Prefix	Meaning	Example
a-, an-	lacking, without, not	asymptomatic	hyster-	uterus, womb	hysterectomy
ab-	away from, absent, decrease	abduct	infra-	under, below, beneath	infraspinatus
ad-	toward, near to, increase	adduct	inter-	between, together, midst	intercostals
ante-	front, before, toward	anterior	intra-	within	intravenous
anti-	against; opposed	antifungal	meso-	middle	mesentery
auto-	self	autoimmune	meta-	beyond, after, change	metacarpals
bi-, di-	twice, double, two	biceps, diencephalon	mono-	one, single	mononuclear
bio-	life	biology	multi-	many	multifidus
cephal-	head	cephalitis	narco-	sleep, numbness, stupor	narcolepsy
circum-	around	circumduction			
contra-	opposite, against	contraindication	necro-	death	necrosis
cryo-	extreme cold	cryotherapy	ophthalmo-	eye	ophthalmologist
cyto-	cell	cytoplasm	ot-	ear	otitis
de-	separate, away from, down	decapitate	para-	alongside, beside	parasympathetic
			patho-	disease	pathophysiology
			ped-	foot	pedicure
dia-	through	diaphragm	peri-	around, about	periosteum
dis-	apart, away	dislocation	post-	rear, after, behind	posterior
dors-	back	dorsiflexion	pre-, pro-	before, front	prenatal, protuberance
dys-	difficult, bad, labored	dysfunction			
ecto-, exo-, ex-	on the outer side	ectoderm	quad-	four	quadriceps
			re-	again, back	realign
endo-, em-, en-	within, inside	endometrium	recto-	straight	rectum
			retro-	backward	retroperitoneal
epi-	upon, over, in addition to	epicondyle	sub-	under, beneath, below	subscapular
			super-, supra-	above, over	superficial, supraspinatus
eu-	good, well, normal	euphoria	syn-, sym-	together, with, joined	synarthrotic, symbiotic
extend-	straighten	extension			
flex-	bend	flexibility	therm-	heat	thermotherapy
glu-, gly-	sugar, sweet	glucose	thixis-	to touch	thixotropy
histo-	tissue	histology	trans-	across, over, beyond, through	transverse
homeo-, homo-	like, same	homeopathy			
hydro-	water or hydrogen	hydromassage	tri-	three	triceps
hyper-	over, above, excessive	hyperextension	uni-	one	unilateral
hypo-	under, below, deficient	hypodermic			

Suffix	Meaning	Example	Suffix	Meaning	Example
-algia	pain	fibromyalgia	-itis	inflammation	arthritis
-ate	use, action	articulate	-oid	shaped	rhomboid
-cyte	cell	hemocyte	-ology	study of	urology
-ectomy	excision or to cut out	tonsillectomy	-oma	tumor	neuroma
-emia	blood condition	hyperemia	-osis	condition	lordosis
-gen	produce	carcinogen	-otomy	incision or to cut into	colostomy
-gram	to record	electrocardiogram	-scopy	to view or examine	orthoscopy
-ia, osis, ism	state or condition	anemia, cyanosis, embolism	-stasis	control, stopping	homeostasis
			-trophy	nourish, grow, develop	hypertrophy
-iatry	healing	psychiatry	-tropy	turning	thixotropy

TABLE 11-1

Levels of Organization

Level	Description	Examples
Chemical	Biochemistry of our bodies	Atoms, molecules, compounds, water, hormones, DNA, oxygen, iron
Cellular	Basic unit of life	Bone cell, muscle cell, nerve cell
Tissue	Groups of cells which share a similar structure and function	Epithelial, connective, muscular, nervous
Organ	Complex structures of two or more tissue types performing a specific function	Heart, kidney, brain, lung
Organ system	Related organs with complimentary functions that perform certain tasks	Circulatory, urinary, nervous, respiratory
Organism	Living entities composed of several organ systems; most complex level	Homo sapiens, fish, frog, butterfly

DNA, Deoxyribonucleic acid.

properties performing a specific function. The organ level is composed of two or more specialized groups of tissue carrying on specific functions (e.g., stomach, liver, brain). Related organs with complementary functions arrange themselves into organ systems that can perform certain necessary tasks such as respiration and digestion. The organism level is the highest level of organization, representing living entities comprised of several organ systems. All of our organ systems work together to promote life. The total of all structures and functions is a living individual (Table 11-1).

Think of these levels like the building materials of a house. The cells are similar to the individual parts such as nails, studs, tiles, bricks, and mortar. These materials are put together to make walls, floors, and ceilings, which correspond to the tissues of the body. Then put tissues together, and you get a room, which is similar to an organ. Several rooms may function as an organ system; the bedrooms might constitute one organ system, whereas the bathrooms and kitchen constitute another. These systems are all linked together into one home, which is akin to the organism level. To understand the body, the smallest components are examined first, then we proceed up to the organism level. Let us take a look at our cellular level.

MINI-LAB

In small groups or as a class, discuss the concept of being *alive*. Use a board or overhead projector to list all the ideas that accumulate. As you will discover, the concept of being alive is a very complex set of ideas.

THE CELL

In the late 1600s, Robert Hooke was examining plant tissue samples through a primitive microscope. He identified structures that reminded him of the long rows of cell rooms in a monastery. He named these cubelike biological structures cells. The **cell** is the fundamental unit of all living organisms and is the simplest form of life that can exist as a self-sustaining unit. Cells are the building blocks of the human body (Figure 11-1).

Scientists estimate that between 75 and 100 trillion active, living cells are in the body. Cells consist of four elements: carbon, oxygen, hydrogen, and nitrogen, plus trace elements such as iron, sodium, and potassium. These trace elements are very important for certain cellular functions: calcium is needed for blood clotting (among other things); iron is necessary to make hemoglobin, which carries oxygen in the blood; and iodine is needed to make a thyroid hormone, which controls metabolism. Besides the four primary elements, water makes up about 60% to 80% of all cells.

The cell contains three basic parts: (1) cell membrane; (2) cytoplasm; and (3) organelles. The organelles include the nucleus, mitochondria, ribosomes, endoplasmic reticulum, Golgi apparatus, and lysosomes (Table 11-2). The specialized nature of body tissues reflects the specialized function of their cellular makeup.

Cell Membrane

The **cell (plasma) membrane** separates the cytoplasm from the surrounding external environment. The membrane creates a semipermeable (some

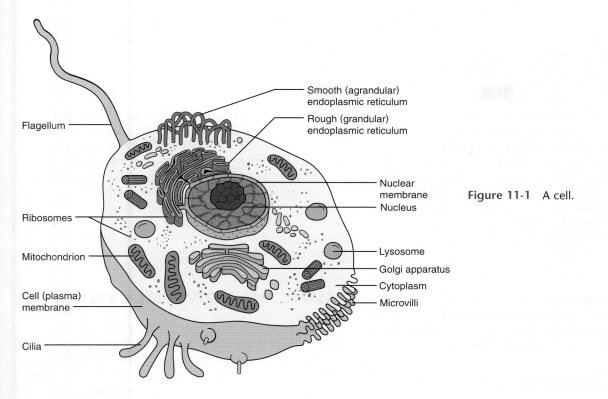

Figure 11-1   A cell.

Flagellum

Smooth (agrandular) endoplasmic reticulum

Rough (grandular) endoplasmic reticulum

Nuclear membrane

Nucleus

Ribosomes

Mitochondrion

Lysosome

Golgi apparatus

Cytoplasm

Cell (plasma) membrane

Microvilli

Cilia

materials can freely pass and others cannot) boundary that governs exchange of nutrients and waste materials. It also responds to stimulation. Movement of molecules takes place by active and passive processes, which are discussed in the next section. The cellular membrane often contains projections such as *microvilli*, *cilia*, or *flagella*, which help protect the cell and aid in its mobility.

Cytoplasm

Consisting primarily of water, **cytoplasm** (cytosol) is the gel-like intracellular fluid within the cell membrane. Within the cytoplasm are many small cellular structures called *organelles*, which provide special functions. Functions of cytoplasm are to provide cellular nutrition and to support the organelles.

Organelles

Within the cell are cytoplasmic **organelles**, (little organs), which are necessary for metabolism. Each organelle possesses a distinct structure and function within the cell. Some function in reproduction, some store materials, and some metabolize nutrients. Types of organelles are the *nucleus, ribosomes, endoplasmic reticulum, Golgi apparatus, mitochondria,* and *lysosomes.*

TABLE 11-2

Cell Structures and Functions

Cell membrane	Governs exchange of nutrients and waste materials
Cytoplasm	Provides cellular nutrition and supports organelles
Organelle:	Control center of the cell, directing nearly all metabolic activities
Nucleus	Contains DNA and RNA
Ribosomes	Synthesizes protein
Endoplasmic reticulum	Synthesizes proteins and lipids; assists the transportation of these materials
Golgi apparatus	Packing and shipping plant of the cell; alters proteins and lipids, packs and stores them till needed
Mitochondria	Power plant of the cell, responsible for cellular respiration; provides most of the cell's ATP
Lysosomes	Engulfs and digests bacteria, cellular debris, and other organelles

DNA, Deoxyribonucleic acid; *RNA,* ribonucleic acid; *ATP,* adenosine triphosphate.

Nucleus

The **nucleus**, the largest organelle in the cytoplasm, is the control center of the cell, directing nearly all metabolic activities. All cells have at least one nucleus at some time in their existence. Red blood cells lose their nuclei (enucleate) as they mature, and skeletal muscle cells possess many nuclei (multinucleate). The shape of the nucleus is usually spherical, and it is enclosed in a double-layer nuclear membrane. Each nucleus contains clusters of proteins, ribonucleic acid (RNA), and deoxyribonucleic acid (DNA), which make up chromosomes (our genetic code). Humans possess 23 pairs of chromosomes, although abnormalities can exist.

Ribosomes

Ribosomes are small granules of RNA and protein in the cytoplasm. They function to synthesize protein for use within the cell and also produce other proteins that are exported outside the cell.

Endoplasmic Reticulum

A complex network of membranous channels within the cytoplasm is the **endoplasmic reticulum**. This structure often extends from the cell membrane to the nuclear membrane and may extend to certain organelles. The endoplasmic reticulum functions in the synthesis of protein and lipids and assists the transportation of these materials from one part of the cell to another. Endoplasmic reticula are classified as rough or granular (ribosomes attached to the surface) or as smooth or agranular (ribosomes are absent).

Golgi Apparatus

The **Golgi apparatus (Golgi complex)** is a series of four to six horizontal membranous sacs. Referred to as the packing and shipping plant of the cell, the Golgi apparatus is associated with altering proteins and lipids, packing and storing them until needed. Once this process is complete, they are wrapped in a piece of Golgi apparatus membrane and jettisoned to the desired area, often out of the cell.

Mitochondria

An oval organelle, the **mitochondrion** is considered the cell's power plant because it is a site for cellular respiration, providing most of a cell's adenosine triphosphate (ATP), which is the body's energy molecule. Mitochondria consist of an inner and outer membrane; the outer shell is smooth and the inner, convoluted membrane contains many projections

called *cristae*. These inner chambers increase the surface area to enhance the mitochondrion's metabolic properties.

Lysosomes

Membrane-bound organelles containing digestive enzymes are the **lysosomes**. Lysosomes can engulf pathogens, cellular debris, and other organelles and digest them, after which any reusable matter is returned to the cytoplasm for reuse. The lysosome can also cause self-digestion of the cell when the reduction of cells in an organ is needed, such as reduction in the size of the uterus after childbirth. Lysosomes also release their digestive enzymes at injury sites to help dispose of cellular debris.

PASSIVE AND ACTIVE CELL PROCESSES

For a cell to survive, it must be able to carry on a variety of functions. In a majority of these processes, substances are exchanged across the cell membrane, which allows for the assimilation of oxygen, nutrients, and water, the elimination of pathogens, and the excretion of waste products. These processes can be classified as passive or active processes. The passive processes occur naturally by means of gradients of temperature, pressure, or concentration. It is the gradient or difference in levels of temperature, pressure, or concentration that drives the exchange of particles or fluid through the membrane. Involving no active expending of energy by the cells, passive cell processes include diffusion, filtration, and osmosis.

Active processes are those that require an expenditure of energy (ATP) by the cell itself to transport the products across the membrane. Active processes include active transport and endocytosis.

Passive Processes

Diffusion

Diffusion is the movement of molecules, or other particles, from an area of high concentration to a area of low concentration. This action continues until the distribution of particulate is equal in all areas (Figure 11-2).

Diffusion can be easily demonstrated by filling a long baking pan with cool water and setting it somewhere where no vibration or movement can disturb the pan. Open a packet of colored soft drink mix (i.e., Kool-Aid) and gently sprinkle the powder in one corner of the pan. Even though no true currents are in the pan, the colored powder diffuses across the pan. When kinetic energy, or speed, of the particles is increased (e.g., by raising the temperature), the rate of

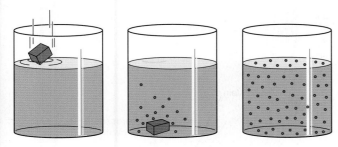

Figure 11-2   Diffusion.

the diffusion process also increases. The greater is the energy, the higher is the gradient, and the faster is the rate of diffusion. Try the Kool-Aid experiment with a pan of hot water or by gently shaking the pan and see how the rate of the diffusion process increases.

Facilitated diffusion is a special type of diffusion that uses a carrier molecule of protein to facilitate the diffusion process. Carrier molecules are contained in the cell membrane. Sometimes molecules in solution are too large to cross the cell membrane. When the solution outside the cell membrane has a high concentration of large molecules, the carrier molecules contained in the cell membrane assist the large molecules in crossing the membrane. Facilitated diffusion is limited by the number of available carrier molecules. Many of the nutrients in our digestive tract enter our bloodstream through diffusion or facilitated diffusion.

Filtration
Filtration is the movement of particles across the cellular membrane due to pressure. A pressure gradient across a cell membrane is the force that drives the filtration process. The air filter on your furnace or central air unit is a good example. The vacuum created by the suction of the fan lowers the pressure behind the filter. The atmospheric pressure in the room is then greater than that behind the filter. The air flows through the pores of the filter, which is selective and traps the larger particles of dust, pet hair, and smoke. An example of filtration is the kidney's filtering of wastes out of the body across a special membrane.

Osmosis
Similar to diffusion, **osmosis** is the movement of a pure solvent such as water from an area of low concentration (most dilute) to an area of high concentration (least dilute). This action continues until the two concentrations equalize.

Unlike filtration, osmotic movement does not depend on pressure but rather on the concentration of dissolved elements that lie in the solutions on each side of a cell membrane or vessel wall. When the solutions contain particles that are too large to cross the membrane, diffusion cannot occur. Even though

a cell membrane does not permit the particles to pass through its walls, the solvent fluid is still able to permeate the membrane. When your fingers are wrinkled from being in water too long, it is because water has been moved by osmosis from your body toward the particles in the water in which your hands have been.

Active Processes

Active Transport
Active transport moves important atoms and molecules such as ions against the concentration gradient from low levels to high levels to maintain such vital processes as nerve conduction. The mechanisms of active transport are both chemical and physical. The chemical part of the mechanism involves the breakdown of ATP within the cell. Scientists estimate that at least 40% of the ATP in the human body is used solely for active transport.

An ion is attracted to a protein molecule, which is part of the cellular membrane. The outside wall of the protein molecule opens like a clamshell, and the ion is drawn inside and binds to it. The binding causes the chemical breakdown of ATP, which again transforms the shape of a protein molecule. The clamshell closes; then the opposite side of the protein molecule opens again to release the ion to the inside of the cell membrane. This process is much like an air lock, in that only one door can be open at a time.

Endocytosis
Endocytosis is a process that moves large particles across the cell membrane into the cell. The two main types of endocytosis are phagocytosis and pinocytosis, both of which are vital to the immune defense systems of the body.

Phagocytosis, or *cell eating,* is the process by which specialized cells ingest harmful microorganisms and cellular debris, break them down, and expel the harmless remains back into the body. Phagocytosis is chiefly characteristic of leukocytes found in the blood. The process has several steps. First, the leukocyte is chemically attracted toward the microbe targeted for destruction. Second, the leukocyte adheres itself to the microbe. Next, the leukocyte forms extensions, surrounds, and ingests the microbe much like an amoeba engulfs its food. Fourth, the leukocyte produces enzymes that destroy and digest the microbe. Finally, the tiny remains are encapsulated, recycled, or expelled (Figure 11-3).

Pinocytosis, or *cell drinking,* is almost identical to phagocytosis except that the targeted object is liquid. In this process, the cell develops a saccular indention, drawing the molecule inside and then enclosing it. Pinocytic cells are more common than phagocytic cells.

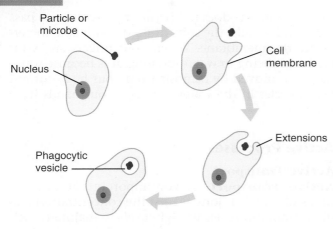

Figure 11-3   Phagocytosis.

TABLE 11-3

Cell Layers and Structures that Develop from Cell Layers

Ectoderm	Nervous system
	Special senses
	Mucosa of the mouth and anus
	Epidermis
	Fingernails
	Hair
	Skin glands
Mesoderm	Muscles
	Fascia
	Tendons
	Retinaculum
	Ligaments
	Cartilage
	Bone
	Mesenteries
	Dermis
	Hypodermis
	Blood and vessels
	Lymph and vessels
	Pleura
	Pericardium
	Peritoneum
Endoderm	Lining of the alimentary canal
	Lining of the respiratory passages
	All tissues of organs
	All tissues of glands

EMBRYONIC CELL LAYERS: ECTODERM, MESODERM, AND ENDODERM

All tissues of the body develop from one single cell. This single cell quickly becomes three individual cell (germ) layers, forming one of the first events of embryonic development. From superficial to deep, these

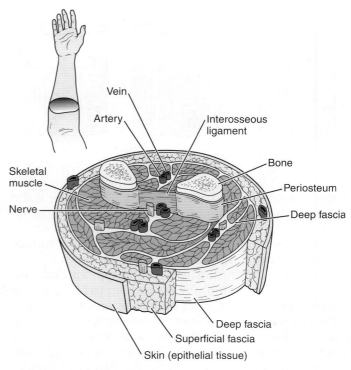

Figure 11-4   Cross-section of limb denoting tissues types.

cell layers are ectoderm, mesoderm, and endoderm (Table 11-3). As the embryo develops, these layers begin to specialize to form the four main types of tissues, from which all organs and glands are derived.

The outermost of the three cell layers is the **ectoderm**, which gives rise to the structures of the nervous system, including the special senses (e.g., ears, eyes), the mucosa of the mouth and anus, the epidermis of the skin and epidermal tissues such as fingernails, hair, and skin glands.

The middle layer is the **mesoderm**; the muscles and connective tissues of the body such as fascia, tendons, retinaculum, ligaments, cartilage, bone, mesenteries, dermis, and hypodermis arise from this embryonic cell layer. Blood; lymph and related vessels; and the pleurae of the lungs, pericardium, and peritoneum are all derived from the mesoderm.

The innermost cell layer is the **endoderm**. From this embryonic cell layer arise the lining of the alimentary canal, the lining of the respiratory passages, and all tissues of the organs and glands (e.g., lungs, urinary bladder, pancreas). Thus the endoderm comprises the lining of the body's passages and the covering for most of the internal organs.

BODY TISSUES

Tissues are defined as a group of similar cells that act together to perform a specific function. The study of tissues is known as histology (Figure 11-4). Only four major types of tissues are in the human body: epithelial, connective, muscle, and nervous.

Tissues organize themselves into organs. *Organs* are defined as a group of two or more tissue types that act together to perform a specific common function and have a consistently recognizable shape. To understand better the structure and functions of our body's organs, it is beneficial first to study the tissues that comprise the organs.

Epithelial Tissue or Epithelium

Epithelial tissue lines or covers the internal and the external (skin) organs of the body, lines blood vessels and body cavities, and lines the digestive, respiratory, urinary, and reproductive tracts (Figure 11-5). The functions of this tissue include protection, absorption, filtration, secretion, excretion, and diffusion. Epithelial tissue is typically avascular and

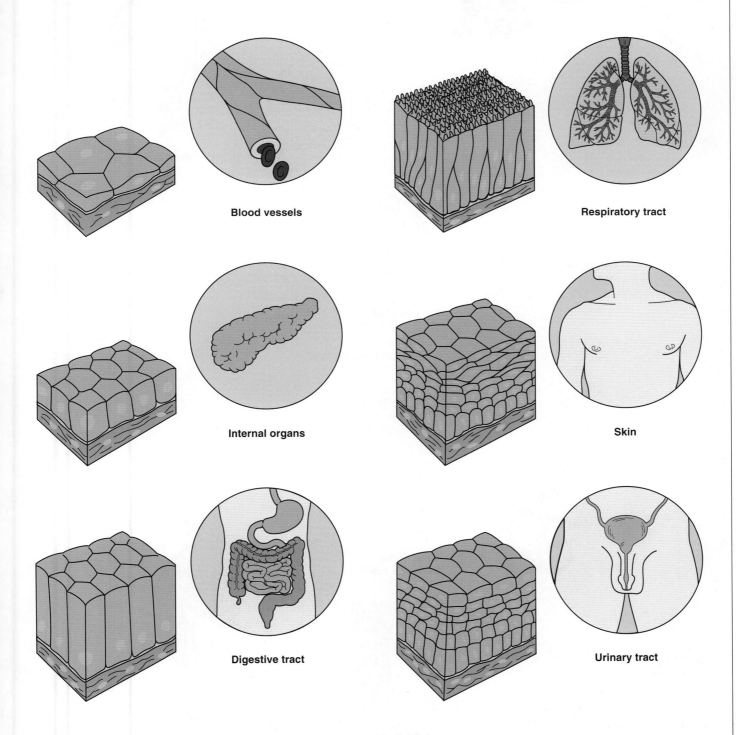

Blood vessels

Respiratory tract

Internal organs

Skin

Digestive tract

Urinary tract

Figure 11-5   Epithelial linings.

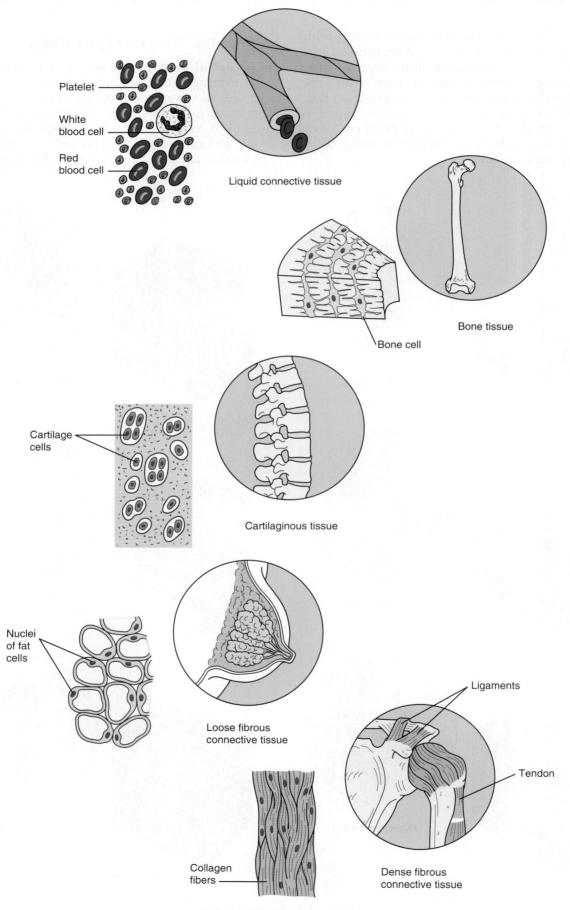

Figure 11-6 Types of connective tissue.

receives nutrition by diffusion from blood vessels in underlying connective tissues. Epithelium reproduces and regenerates quickly.

Connective Tissue

Connective tissue is the most abundant and ubiquitous tissue of the body. This tissue serves a wide variety of functions. Some connective tissue types serve as nutrient transport systems, some defend the body against disease, some possess clotting mechanisms, and others act as a supportive framework and provide protection for vital organs (Figure 11-6).

Connective tissue is highly vascularized, providing nutrition and oxygen to itself and nearby tissues (i.e., skin and muscle), with the exception of cartilage.

All connective tissue is composed of connective tissue cells scattered in a matrix. The matrix itself is a gelatinous liquid that is primarily composed of ground substance and protein. The ground substance is mostly water with some suspended solids such as carbohydrates, giving it viscosity. Within the ground substance are precursor cells called *fibroblasts*, which give rise to other connective tissue cells during tissue healing. The second component of matrix is long protein strands of collagen.

The arrangement of the fibers and the ratio of collagen to ground substance is the primary factor for determining the different types of connective tissues. Blood and lymph are dilute and have high amounts of ground substance. Bone has a very high ratio of collagen arranged to trap the mineral salts that give it density and firmness. The ligaments and fascia have a ratio of collagen to ground substance that is somewhere in the middle, giving it both durability and elasticity.

The five different classifications of connective tissue, some of which contain more than one type of tissue are (1) liquid connective tissue (blood), (2) bone or osseous tissue, (3) cartilaginous tissue, (4) loose connective tissue, and (5) dense connective tissue (Table 11-4).

TABLE 11-4

Connective Tissue Types

Type	Properties and Examples
Liquid Connective Tissue	
Blood	Fluid medium (plasma) containing three formed elements (erythrocytes, leukocytes, and platelets)
Lymph	Fluid of the lymphvascular system
Interstitial	Fluid bathing cells and tissues
Osseous Connective Tissue	
Bone	Consists of compact tissue, a spongy cancellous tissue, collagenous fibers, and mineral salts
Cartilage	
Hyaline	Most common type; elastic, rubbery, and smooth, covering ends of bones; part of the larynx and nose; forms the C-shaped rings of the trachea
Elastic	Soft and pliable, giving shape to the external nose and ears, and the epiglottis and auditory tubes
Fibrocartilage	Greatest tensile strength of all cartilage types; found in intervertebral disks, meniscus of the knee, and between the pubic bones
Loose Connective Tissue	
Areolar	Most widely distributed; forms the superficial fascia
Adipose	Specialized for fat storage; insulates the body against heat loss; provides fuel reserves for energy; provides cushion around structures
Reticular	Forms the framework for organs
Dense Connective Tissue	
Dense regular	Offers great strength and can resist pulling forces in one direction such as ligaments, tendons, retinacula, and aponeuroses
Dense irregular	Resists pulling forces in several different directions (e.g., irregular connective tissue are deep fascia, deep epidermis, and periosteum)
Elastic	Can be stretched and restored to its natural shape; found in true vocal cords, ligaments connecting adjacent vertebrae, trachea, and bronchi

Liquid Connective Tissue

Also known as *vascular tissue,* **liquid connective tissue** consists of blood, lymph, and interstitial fluid. Blood contains three formed elements, two of which are cells (erythrocytes and leukocytes) and one of which are cell fragments (platelets). The fluid medium in which these elements exist is called *plasma.* Lymph and interstitial fluid are the same substance, differing only in where they are located. Lymph resides in the lymphvascular system and interstitial fluid bathes the cells and tissues. Both lymph and interstitial fluid are chemically similar to blood plasma.

Osseous Tissue

The hardest and most solid of all connective tissue, **bone** (osseous tissue) consists of compact bone, spongy bone, collagenous fibers (for strength), and mineral salts (for hardness). Bone tissue is addressed in the skeletal system chapter.

Cartilaginous Tissue

Cartilage is an avascular, tough, protective tissue capable of withstanding repeated stress and is found in the thorax, joints, and certain rigid tubes of the body (e.g., trachea). Cartilaginous tissue can be divided into three subcategories: hyaline cartilage, fibrocartilage, and elastic cartilage.

Hyaline cartilage (gristle) is an elastic, rubbery, smooth type of cartilage that covers the ends of bones, connects the ribs to the sternum, is part of the larynx and the nose, and forms the C-shaped rings of the trachea. The skeleton of a fetus is mostly hyaline cartilage, which is replaced by osseous tissue by the time an infant is born (except for the fontanel, or soft spot, on an infant's head). This is the most common type of cartilage.

Elastic cartilage is soft and pliable (elastic) and gives shape to the external nose and ears and internal structures such as the epiglottis and the auditory tubes.

Fibrocartilage has the greatest tensile strength of all three cartilage types. It is found in the intervertebral disks, in the meniscus of the knee joint, and between the pubic bones (pubic symphysis).

Loose Connective Tissue

Loose connective tissue is regarded as the packing material of the body. It attaches the skin to underlying structures, serves to wrap and support the body cells, fills in the spaces between structures (e.g., organs, muscles), and helps keep them in their proper places. The three types of loose connective tissue are areolar, adipose, and reticular.

Areolar connective tissue is one of the most widely distributed. Along with adipose tissue, areolar connective tissue forms the subcutaneous layer of the skin (superficial fascia). This layer of tissue attaches the skin to its underlying tissues and structures.

Adipose tissue is specialized for fat storage. This connective tissue, which includes yellow bone marrow, also insulates the body against heat loss, provides fuel reserves for energy, and provides a cushion around certain structures (e.g., heart, kidneys, and some joints).

Reticular connective tissue forms the framework of certain organs such as the liver and spleen.

Dense Connective Tissue

The three types of **dense connective tissue** are dense regular, dense irregular, and elastic.

Dense regular connective tissue offers great strength and can resist pulling forces, generally in two directions; examples are ligaments, tendons, retinacula, and aponeuroses. **Dense irregular connective tissue** resists pulling forces in several different directions; examples of dense irregular connective tissue are deep fascia, deep epidermis, and periosteum. **Elastic connective tissue** can be stretched and restored to its natural shape. It is found in true vocal cords, in the ligaments connecting adjacent vertebrae, in the trachea, and bronchi.

One type of connective tissue, **fascia**, deserves more discussion, because it relates directly to your work as massage therapists. The two types of fascia are (1) superficial fascia, which is immediately under the skin, and (2) deep fascia, which surrounds muscles, holding them together and separating them into functioning groups. One may note that superficial fascia is an areolar connective tissue type and deep fascia is a type of dense irregular connective tissue.

The ground substance in fascia possesses two physical states: a relatively thin fluid (sol-state), and a thicker, more gelatinous fluid (gel-state). Fascia in its sol-state has a fluid quality and is more pliant and elastic, offering less restrictive movements. Fascia in the gel-state is tougher, more inflexible, and can restrict the body's movements.

Fascia's property of **thixotropism** refers to its ability to change the ground substance in the matrix from one state to the other. The word *thixotropy* comes from the Greek root words meaning *to touch* and *turning*. It refers to the affect of touch/friction *to change* or *turn* the state of the ground substance in the matrix from a gel- to a sol-state or vice versa.

When the body is not in efficient posture, as in forward head posture, the spine no longer adequately supports the head in space. The muscles and fascia become the supportive tissue, adapting to the situation by becoming firmer. The fascia in the neck can turn from liquid (sol-)

to solid (gel-) to help hold the head in this physically stressful position. The stiffness that the client feels is often fascia in a gel-state. This restricted fascia must be addressed during the massage.

As we apply pressure and heat, either by friction or local and general application, thixotropy occurs, converting the gel-state to the sol-state. The fascia loosens and melts, becoming more flexible and elastic. This softening of the fascia that surrounds the muscles allows the muscle to be manipulated to its fullest resting length, increasing joint range of motion and freeing the body from restrictions of movement. Thixotropism also occurs when the body is warmed by physical work, exercise, and stretching.

For Your Information

Effective conversion of fascia, from a gel-state to sol-state, will not occur easily unless the body is well hydrated; conversely, the change may not occur if the body is dehydrated. Remember to encourage your clients to consume water on a daily basis (i.e., 0.5 ounces [oz] for every 1 pound [lb] of body weight). A 140-lb person should consume 70 oz of pure water each day.

Muscle Tissue

Extremely elastic, **muscle tissue** is very vascular and has the unique ability to shorten (contract) and elongate (stretch) to produce movement. Muscle tissues are made up of muscle fibers and are usually arranged in bundles surrounded by fascia. The three types of muscle tissue are skeletal, smooth, and cardiac (Figure 11-7). Generally speaking, smooth muscle causes the contents of a tube to move, skeletal muscle causes bones to articulate, and cardiac muscle causes the heart to contract, forcing blood to move.

Smooth muscle (involuntary/visceral) forms the walls of hollow organs and tubes such as the stomach, bladder, uterus, and blood vessels. Consuming little energy, these muscle cells are adapted for long, sustained contractions. The muscle cells are spindle-shaped (pointed at both ends), and each contains one oval-shaped nucleus.

Skeletal muscle (voluntary/striated) fibers are cigar-shaped and are multinucleated; many nuclei are located near the periphery of the cell. Each skeletal muscle fiber contains bands of red and white material, causing it to appear striped or striated under a microscope.

Cardiac muscle (involuntary/striated) is located in the heart wall and is Y- or H-shaped. These shapes allow the cells to fit together like clasped fingers and help create the spherical shape of the heart. Between

each cardiac muscle cell is a structure known as the *intercalated disk*. These disks assist in the transmission of a nervous stimulus from a cardiac muscle cell to another cardiac muscle cell.

Nervous Tissue

Nervous tissue consists of oddly shaped cells called *neurons,* which can detect and transmit electrical signals by converting stimuli into nerve impulses. Located in the brain, spinal cord, and peripheral nerves, nervous tissue possesses characteristics of excitability and conductibility. Neurons detect changes both inside and outside the body, interpret the perceived information to provide a response (e.g., muscular contractions or glandular secretions), and are involved in higher mental functioning and emotional responsiveness.

The three principal parts of a neuron are the cell body, which contains the nucleus and other standard cell machinery; the dendrites, which transmit impulses to the cell body, and the axon, which transmits impulses away from the cell body (Figure 11-8).

When health is absent. . .
Wisdom cannot reveal itself
Art cannot become manifest
Strength cannot be exerted
Wealth is useless and
Reason is powerless. . . .
—Heraphilies, 300 BC

Tissue Healing: Replacement and Repair

The four different tissue types of the body have varying rates of healing. The cells of epithelial tissue, which make up the skin, are constantly being renewed by cell division. At the opposite end of the spectrum, nervous tissue regenerates very slowly, if at all. Connective tissue and muscle tissue heal at different rates because of their blood supply. Bone tissue and adipose connective tissue are highly vascular and heal quickly. Muscle tissue takes a little longer to replace, and the less vascular forms of connective tissue such as ligaments and tendons are even slower. Cartilage, a relatively avascular tissue, is among the slowest to heal.

The body's need to regain tissue integrity stimulates a healing process. Damaged tissue is replaced or repaired by several different methods. These processes are resolution, regeneration, fibrosis, and remodeling. The process activated is dependent on the degree of trauma experienced by the tissues involved. At the mild end of the trauma range, a cell reaches its natural death (tissue cells are no longer efficient) and are replaced. At the other end of the trauma range is injury, in which tissues must be

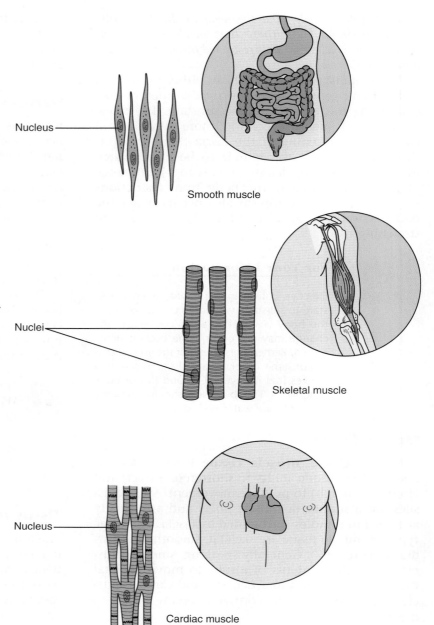

Nucleus

Smooth muscle

Nuclei

Skeletal muscle

Figure 11-7   Types of muscle tissue.

Nucleus

Cardiac muscle

repaired. Replacement of dead or mildly injured tissues occurs by a process known as *resolution*. Repair of injured tissue occurs by the process of *regeneration*. As the trauma or injury becomes larger and more severe, the bodily reaction to it is also proportional. Severe injuries are repaired by the creation of scar tissue in a process known as *fibrosis,* and the scar is modified in a phase of scar tissue maturation known as *remodeling*. However, all tissue healing begins with the same initial response—inflammation.

Inflammation, one of the body's reactions to cellular death or injury, is a protective mechanism. Its purpose is to stabilize the area, contain infection, and prepare the damaged tissue for repair. Inflammation occurs in response to events such as burns, chemical irritation, cuts, tears, and invasion by viruses and bacteria. The intensity of the inflammation is directly proportional to the extent of the trauma to the tissue. The symptoms of inflammation are local heat, redness, swelling, pain, and loss of function (Figure 11-9). Inflammation begins with vasodilation and the migration of white blood cells. When tissue trauma occurs, the tissues respond by releasing histamines and kinins. These chemicals cause sustained vasodilation at the site of the trauma and increase the permeability of the capillary walls. Vasodilation increases local blood circulation; thus an increase in heat and redness occurs. The changes in the capillary walls al-

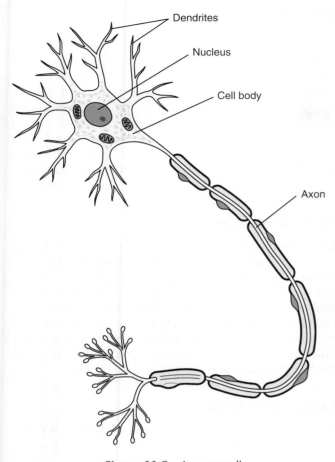

Figure 11-8   A nerve cell.

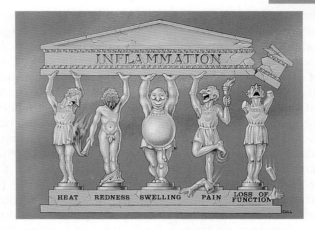

Figure 11-9 Cardinal signs of inflammation. (From Damjanov I: *Pathology for the health-related professions,* ed 2, Philadelphia, 2000, WB Saunders.)

low blood plasma to cross into the interstitial spaces; this excess fluid results in swelling. As the tissue pressure increases, the nerve receptors are stimulated, resulting in pain. The sensation of pain, combined with the swelling and muscle splinting, limits the range of motion.

As the plasma fills the tissue, several things happen. Phagocytes and white blood cells are attracted to the trauma site. The phagocytes engulf cellular debris (from cell death or damage), foreign objects, and any hostile invaders. The plasma cleanses the area and dilutes any toxic materials in the trauma site. Clotting proteins located in the blood construct a clot that seals any break in vessels or in the skin and form walls within torn tissues to isolate the wound. Once the inflammatory process is progressing, another level of tissue healing begins: resolution, regeneration, fibrosis, and/or remodeling.

Resolution
The primary method of tissue replacement is resolution. An example of resolution is the replacement of mildly damaged skin after a mild sunburn. As long as cellular membranes are intact and nuclear contents are present, tissues are repaired. Many epithelial

cells, including the digestive linings, undergo daily replacement of old dead cells that are either sloughed off externally or deteriorate to be engulfed and removed internally. When damage to the tissue is severe and tissues must be repaired, the body uses other, more drastic steps of tissue healing.

Regeneration
Regeneration is the process by which moderately traumatized tissue is repaired. Regeneration occurs when damaged tissue is replaced with new tissue of the same type. Enough undamaged tissue must be in the area so that it can reproduce itself; however, damage can be more severe, such as with a skinned knee. The open wound becomes sealed with a scab, and the healthy cells underneath the scab divide until the skin has been reproduced completely; then the scab is sloughed off. When not enough healthy cells are left to replicate, the body then enters the most extreme type of tissue healing—fibrosis.

Fibrosis
The tissue repair most often associated with moderate to severe injuries is fibrosis (scar formation), which replaces the original tissue type with a different kind of tissue. Specialized cells, known as *fibroblasts,* are mobilized to the site of injury to create scar tissue. This happens in response to the inflammatory process. As the heat level at the injury site increases, the ground substance in the matrix of the connective tissues is converted from gel-state to sol-state. As this matrix becomes more liquefied, the fibroblasts become more mobile and can migrate to the site of injury. Here they secrete collagen fiber strands to bind up the wounded tissue. Complete repair is marked by the disappearance of fibroblasts in the area.

Skeletal muscle, cardiac muscle, and central nervous system tissues do not readily regenerate and thus are generally repaired by fibrosis. The scar tissue formed by fibrosis is usually stronger than the original tissue; scarring is, in a sense, a patch. Because scar formation is not the original tissue, usually some loss of function occurs, such as elasticity. Also, remember that the word *scar* applies not only to a visible mark on the skin but to any place beneath the skin where torn soft tissues have been woven back together. This includes tears in the surface of the muscular tissues, which although not visible on the surface of the skin, may be experienced by palpation as knots; fibrous bands; and hard, crunchy striations. Fibrosis is often the last healing stage for many soft tissues, but just as often, the elastic tissues of muscle, tendon, and ligament undergo a final phase of healing following fibrosis.

Remodeling. The collagen fibers laid down in the fibrosis process are formed randomly and are consequently poorly organized. The resulting scar, although strong, may be either bulky and soft or fibrous and tough. In either case, fibrosed scar tissue in muscle, tendon, or ligament causes a loss of the tissue's natural elasticity. So after fibrosis occurs, some changes must occur within the scar tissue if it is to become pliable and function efficiently after healing. This process is called *remodeling* or *scar maturation phase*. During remodeling, the body is continually restructuring the scar tissue by a simultaneous destruction and creation of collagen fibers. This mainly occurs in response to skeletal muscle elongation and contraction. The old cross pattern patchwork of collagen fibers that was formed by fibrosis is broken down, and the new collagen fibers reorganize themselves in parallel arrangement to the muscle fibers.

What this means to massage therapists is that mobilization of a joint, contraction and relaxation of the affected muscle, exercise, myofascial release, and cross-fiber friction applied to the scar can aid in the remodeling process. Without any intervention, the tissue will heal fully, but mobility of the muscle may be impaired. Using these massage techniques increases scar pliability and strength while reducing bulk and breaking adhesions to surrounding tissue, including keloid scars.

Often during fibrosis and remodeling, excessive amounts of collagen are produced. The result can be an irregular, thick, elevated scar generally found on the surface of the skin but sometimes extending down into deeper layers of tissue. These excessive scar formations are referred to as *keloids*. Because much of the tissue healing process is dictated by genetics, the tendency of an individual to develop keloid scars is directly influenced by heredity factors.

Massage techniques such as cross-fiber friction can greatly reduce the size and appearance of keloids, often in just a few sessions.

BODY MEMBRANES

Membranes are thin, soft, pliable sheets of tissue that cover the body, line tubes or body cavities, cover organs, and separate one part of a cavity from another. Using this definition, the skin itself can be considered a membrane known as *cutaneous membrane*. Chapter 12 has been devoted to the skin.

The three basic types of membranes in the body are mucous, serous, and synovial. Mucous and serous membranes are classified as epithelial membranes; synovial is considered a connective tissue membrane.

Mucous Membrane

Membranes that line openings to the outside of the body are called **mucous membranes**, or **mucosae**. This type of membrane is found in the respiratory, digestive, reproductive, and urinary tracts. Mucous membranes secrete a viscous, slippery fluid called mucous. Many of these mucous membranes provide protection for underlying structures. The mucous membrane lining the digestive tract also aids in the processes of digestion and absorption.

Serous Membrane

Serous membranes line closed body cavities that do not open to the outside of the body. These membranes consist of two layers: a parietal layer, which lines the wall of body cavities, often adhering to it, and a visceral layer, which provides a peripheral covering to organs in closed body cavities. Examples of serous membranes are the pericardium, pleural membranes, peritoneum, and mesenteries. Serous membranes secrete a thin, serous fluid between the parietal and visceral layers. This fluid lubricates organs and reduces friction between the organs.

Synovial Membrane

Lining the joint cavities of freely moving joints (e.g., shoulder, hip, and knee) are the **synovial membranes**. These membranes secrete synovial fluid, a viscous liquid that provides nutrition and lubrication to the joint so it can move freely without undue friction. This fluid can also be contained in bursa sacs located around the joint cavity or between tendons and bones, where friction is present, and in synovial sheaths surrounding a tendon of a muscle.

BODY SYSTEM OVERVIEW

Ten body systems make up the organism discussed in this section; all are interrelated and interdependent (Table 11-5). Each system, except the

TABLE 11-5

Body Systems, Anatomical Structures, and Related Physiology

Body System	Anatomical Structures	Related Physiology
Circulatory system	Heart Blood and blood vessels Lymph Lymph vessels and glands	Transports and distributes gases, nutrients, antibodies, waste materials, and hormones; protects the body from disease; prevents hemorrhage by clotting mechanisms
Skeletal system	Bones Cartilage Ligaments Joints	Supports the body through a bony framework; protects the body's vital organs; gives leverage through muscle attachment; houses the mechanism of blood cell formation; stores fats and minerals
Integumentary system	Skin Hair Nails Oil glands Sweat glands	Protects the organism; absorbs substances such as fats, fat-soluble vitamins, oxygen, carbon dioxide, steroids, resins of certain plants, organic solvents, and salts of heavy metals; receives stimuli; regulates body temperature; eliminates wastes; converts ultraviolet rays to vitamin D
Respiratory system	Nose and nasal cavity Pharynx Larynx Trachea Bronchi and bronchioles Alveoli Lungs Diaphragm	Exchanges gases; detects smell; produces speech; regulates body pH
Reproductive system	Gonads (ovaries in females and testes in males) Ducts (fallopian tubes in females and spermatic duct in males) Gametes (ova in females and spermatozoa in males) Uterus and vagina in females Penis, prostate, and urethra in males	Produces offspring and propagates the species
Muscular system	Skeletal muscles and related fascia Tendons	Creates movement; produces heat; maintains posture
Endocrine system	Pituitary Pineal Thyroid Parathyroids Thymus Adrenals Pancreas Gonads Hormones	Produces and secretes hormones; regulates body activities; maintains the body during times of stress; contributes to the reproductive process

Continued

TABLE 11-5

Body Systems, Anatomical Structures, and Related Physiology—cont'd

Body System	Anatomical Structures	Related Physiology
Nervous system	Brain Spinal cord Meninges Cerebrospinal fluid Cranial nerves Spinal nerves Special sense organs	Receives sensory input; interprets and integrates all stimuli; initiates motor output; houses mental processes and emotional responses
Urinary system	Kidneys Ureters and urethra Urinary bladder and urine	Eliminates metabolic wastes; regulates blood pH and its chemical composition; regulate blood volume and fluid balance; monitors and helps maintain blood pressure; maintains homeostasis
Digestive system	Teeth Tongue Alimentary canal (tube from mouth to anus) Accessory glands (liver, gallbladder, pancreas, salivary)	Ingestion; digestion; absorption; defecation

reproductive system, is discussed in its own chapter. Immune functions are briefly discussed in the circulatory system (see the lymphvascular section in Chapter 19).

 The body's life is the life of sensation and emotions. The body feels real hunger, real thirst, real joy in the sun or snow, real pleasure in the smell of roses or the look of a lilac bush; real anger, real sorrow, real tenderness, real warmth, real passion, real hate, real grief. All these emotions belong to the body and are only recognized by the mind.

—D.H. Lawrence

THE BODY COMPASS

Every good travel map always has a compass drawing to indicate which way is north, south, east, and west. The map also has some distance reference such as a scale of miles per a specific measure. Any map without these items is of little or no use. Imagine trying to read a map if you cannot understand the definitions of the words *south, 5 miles, 1 block,* or *by the lake.* Think of the anatomical drawings as your map and consider this section of the book your body compass. You will learn new terms that constitute directional terminology to help you find your way around the body. These terms include names for planes of the body, locations that are relative to the body

planes, regional and directional terms for different aspects of the body, and the body cavities.

To avoid confusion when discussing anatomical directions, all parts of the body are described in relation to other body parts using a standard body position, called the **anatomical position** (Figure 11-10). In this position, the body is erect and facing forward, the arms are at the side, the palms are facing forward with the thumbs to the side, and feet are about hip distance apart with toes pointing forward.

Planes of the Body

We live in a three-dimensional structure; our height, depth, and width help describe volume in space. It is easy to think of ourselves as flat; mirrors and photographs give us the illusion that we are two dimensional, but we have sculpted fullness, curves, and angles. Because the body is three dimensional, we can refer to three planes or sections that lie at right angles to each other (Figure 11-11).

The **midsagittal** or **median plane** runs longitudinally or vertically down the body, anterior to posterior, dividing the body into right and left sections. When a plane passes through the body parallel to the median plane, we have the **sagittal plane.** The **frontal** or **coronal plane** passing through the body side-to-side to create anterior and posterior sections. The **transverse** or **horizontal plane** passes through the body and creates superior and inferior sections.

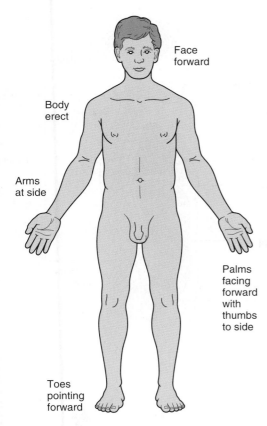

Figure 11-10   Anatomical position.

Body Cavities

The body contains organs and other structures in closed spaces called *cavities;* the two main cavities are the dorsal and the ventral. The **dorsal cavity**, located on the back or posterior aspect of the body, is further divided into the cranial cavity (containing the brain) and the spinal or vertebral cavity (containing the spinal cord). The larger **ventral cavity**, located anteriorly to the dorsal cavity, is further divided by the diaphragm into the thoracic cavity and abdominopelvic cavity. The thoracic cavity contains the right and left pleural cavities (lungs) and the mediastinum (containing the pericardium, heart, great vessels such as aorta and vena cava, esophagus, and trachea).

The abdominopelvic cavity is further divided into the abdominal cavity and the pelvic cavity. The abdominal cavity contains the digestive system and its accessory organs. The pelvic cavity contains the organs of the reproductive and urinary systems and the rectum of the digestive system (Figure 11-12).

Directional Terminology

This section defines the following directional terminology (Figure 11-13):

Prone: lying face down or belly down in a horizontal, recumbent position

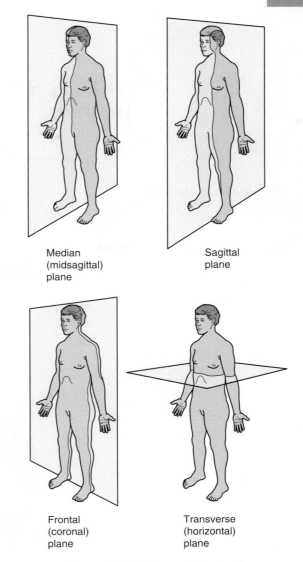

Figure 11-11   Planes of the body.

Supine: lying face up or belly up in a horizontal, recumbent position

Anterior or **ventral**: pertaining to the front side of a structure; the navel is anterior to the vertebral column

Posterior or **dorsal**: pertaining to the back of a structure; the vertebral column is posterior to the lungs

Superior, **cranial**, or **cephalic**: situated above or toward the head end; the jaw is superior to the navel

Inferior or **caudal**: situated below or toward the tail end; the sacrum is inferior to the skull

Medial: oriented toward or near the midline of the body; the nose is medial to the ears

Lateral: oriented farther away from the midline of the body; the ribs are lateral to the vertebral column

Homolateral (ipsilateral): related to the same side of the body; the right hand is homolateral to the right elbow

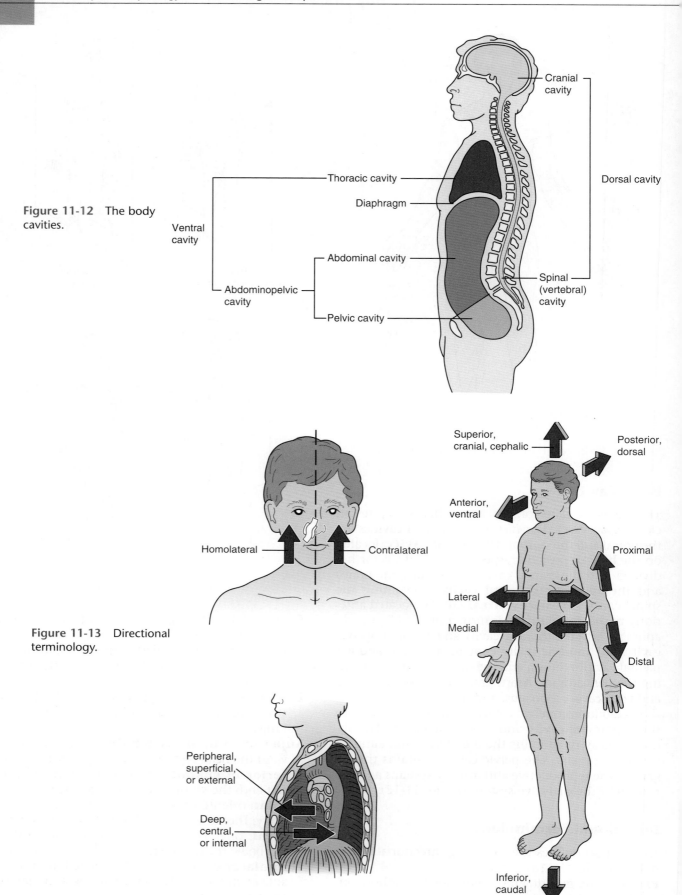

Figure 11-12   The body cavities.

Figure 11-13   Directional terminology.

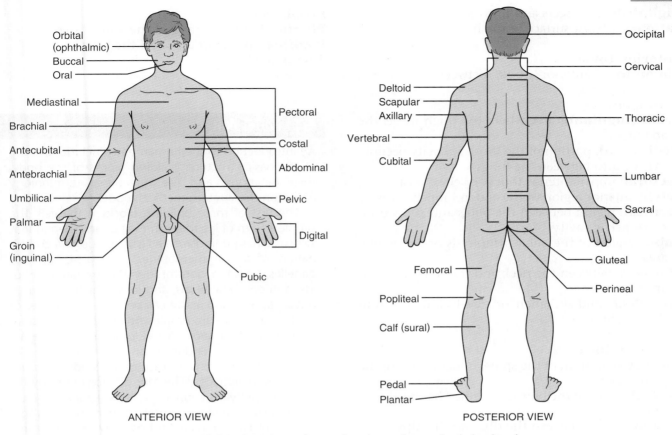

Figure 11-14   Anterior and posterior views of many body landmarks.

Contralateral: related to opposite sides of the body; the right foot is contralateral to the left foot

Proximal: nearer to the point of reference, usually toward the trunk of the body; the hip is proximal to the knee (used only on the extremities)

Distal: farther from the point of reference, usually away from the midline; the foot is distal to the hip (used only on the extremities)

Central: pertaining to or situated at a center of the body; often referred to as *deep*; the heart is centrally located, and the heart is deep to the rib cage

Peripheral: pertaining to the outside surface, periphery, or surrounding external area of a structure; often referred to as *superficial*; the skin is superficial (peripherally located) to the bones

Internal: nearest the inside (within) of a body cavity; the stomach is an internally located organ

External: nearest the outside of a body cavity; the skin is located on the external surface of the body

Regional Terms

This section identifies regions associated with body areas such as the head/neck, upper and lower extremities, and anterior and posterior torso (Figure 11-14).

Head/Neck
Buccal: cheek area
Cervical: neck area
Cranial: head end
Facial: face area
Frontal: forehead
Mandibular: lower jaw
Nasal: nose region
Nuchal: posterior neck
Occipital: posterior and inferior surface of the head
Oral: mouth region
Orbital (ophthalmic): eye area

Upper Extremity
Acromial: top of shoulder
Antebrachial: forearm; between wrist and elbow
Antecubital: space in front of elbow or at the bend of the elbow
Axillary: armpit region
Brachial: upper arm; between the shoulder and the elbow
Carpal: wrist area
Cubital: elbow
Deltoid: curve of the shoulder and upper arm formed by the deltoid muscle

Digital: digits; fingers and/or toes
Palmar: anterior surface of the hand

Anterior Torso
Abdominal: anterior trunk; between the thorax and the pelvis
Costal: ribs
Groin (inguinal): area where the thigh meets the abdomen
Mediastinal: portion of the thoracic cavity occupying the area between the lungs
Pectoral: upper anterior thorax or chest area
Pelvic: inferior region of the abdominopelvic cavity
Perineal: region between the pubis and coccyx; inferior pelvic cavity
Pubic: region of the pubic symphysis or the genital area
Thoracic: between the neck and the respiratory diaphragm
Umbilical: mid-abdomen or navel (scar left from the umbilical cord)

Posterior Torso
Coccygeal: bottom of the spine; upper region of the gluteal cleft
Gluteal: curve of the buttocks formed by the gluteal muscles
Lumbar: back; between the ribs and the hips
Sacral: sacrum of the spinal column
Sacroiliac: between the sacrum and the pelvic bone
Scapular: the shoulder blade area
Vertebral: vertebrae of the spinal column

Lower Extremity
Calf (sural): calf area of the lower leg
Coxal: hip region
Crural: entire leg
Dorsum: top of foot
Femoral: femur or the thigh area; between the hip and the knee
Patellar: knee cap

Pedal: foot/feet
Plantar: bottom surface of the foot or sole
Popliteal: posterior aspect of the knee
Tarsal: ankle

SUMMARY

An introduction to the human body includes a study of the basic structural building blocks of the body, their functions, and the directional terminology based on the western medical model.

The first of these building blocks is the cell, the simplest form of life that can exist as an independent self-sustaining unit. Each cell is made up of a combination of a cell membrane, cytoplasm, and organelles. Cells function through the exchange of fluids, nutrients, chemicals, and ions, which are carried out by passive and active cell processes. Examples of passive processes are simple and facilitated diffusion, osmosis, and filtration. Active processes include active transport and endocytosis.

Cells organize to form tissues; the study of tissues is known as *histology*. The four divisions of body tissues are epithelial, connective, muscle, and nervous. Some tissues present themselves as membranes that protect organs or separate body cavities. The three types of bodily membranes are mucous, serous, and synovial.

Tissues organize to form organs, which are classified according to organ systems. The 10 organ systems of the body are the circulatory, skeletal, integumentary, respiratory, reproductive, muscular, endocrine, nervous, urinary, and digestive.

To negotiate these body systems, it is necessary to learn the language of the body itself. Our map consists of anatomical directional terminology, planes of the body, body cavities, and regional body landmarks.

MATCHING I

Write the letter of the best answer in the space provided.

A. Cell   C. Homeostasis   E. Physiology
B. Anatomy   D. Tissue   F. Metabolism

_____ 1. The study of the structures of the human body and their positional relationships to one another

_____ 2. The human body's internal environment, remaining relatively constant within a limited range

_____ 3. The sum total of all physical and chemical processes that occur in an organism

_____ 4. How the body functions in normal body processes

_____ 5. The simplest form of life, existing as an independent self-sustaining unit

_____ 6. A group of similar cells that act together to perform a specific function

MATCHING II

Write the letter of the best answer in the space provided.

A. Diffusion   E. Filtration   I. Pinocytosis
B. Nucleus   F. Cell membrane   J. Mitochondria
C. Phagocytosis   G. Golgi apparatus
D. Lysosomes   H. Cytoplasm

_____ 1. The membrane separating the cytoplasm from the external environment

_____ 2. Gel-like fluid within the cell membrane

_____ 3. The cell's control center, directing nearly all metabolic activities; contains DNA and RNA

_____ 4. Alters, packs, and stores proteins and lipids till needed by the cell

_____ 5. Site of cellular respiration

_____ 6. Organelles containing digestive enzymes that engulf and digest bacteria and cellular debris

_____ 7. Movement of dissolved substances from a region of higher concentration to a region of lower concentration

_____ 8. Movement of particles across a cellular membrane involving pressure

_____ 9. Process by which specialized cells ingest, breakdown, and expel harmful microorganisms

_____ 10. Process by which specialized cells enclose, engulf, and expel harmful microorganisms

MATCHING III

Write the letter of the best answer in the space provided.

A. Hyaline cartilage	E. Epithelial tissue	I. Adipose tissue
B. Connective tissue	F. Osseous tissue	J. Areolar tissue
C. Dense regular tissue	G. Mucous membrane	K. Nervous tissue
D. Muscular tissue	H. Fibrocartilage cartilage	L. Synovial membrane

_____ 1. Tissue that lines or covers the blood vessels and body cavities and the digestive, respiratory, urinary, and reproductive tracts

_____ 2. The most abundant tissue type of the body, which serves as nutrient transport, disease defense, blood clotting, or support and protection for vital organs

_____ 3. The hardest and most solid of all connective tissues

_____ 4. An elastic, rubbery, smooth type of cartilage that covers the ends of bones, connects the ribs to the sternum, is part of the larynx and the nose, and forms the C-shaped rings of the trachea

_____ 5. Has the greatest tensile strength of all cartilage types and is found in the intervertebral disks, the meniscus of the knee joint, and between the pubic bones

_____ 6. The most widely distributed connective tissue type, forming the subcutaneous layer of the skin, attaching it to underlying structures

_____ 7. Connective tissue type specialized for fat and fuel storage and insulation, providing a cushion around certain structures

_____ 8. Connective tissue that offers great strength and resistance when pulled such as ligaments, tendons, retinaculum, and aponeurosis

_____ 9. This type of tissue is elastic and very vascular and has the unique ability to shorten (contract) and to elongate (stretch) to produce movement

_____ 10. This oddly shaped tissue can detect and transmit electrical signals and possesses characteristics of excitability and conductibility

_____ 11. Membrane that lines openings to the outside of the body and produces mucous

_____ 12. Membrane that lines joint cavities of freely moving joints and produces synovial fluid

MATCHING IV

Write the letter of the best answer in the space provided.

A. Distal	E. Supine	I. Medial
B. Anterior	F. Posterior	J. Proximal
C. Homolateral	G. Prone	K. Contralateral
D. Inferior	H. Superior	L. Lateral

_____ 1. Lying face down or belly down in a horizontal, recumbent position

_____ 2. Lying face up or belly up in a horizontal, recumbent position

_____ 3. Pertaining to the front side of a structure

_____ 4. Pertaining to the back of a structure

_____ 5. Situated above or toward the head end

_____ 6. Situated below or toward the tail end

_____ 7. Oriented toward or near the midline of the body

_____ 8. Oriented farther away from the midline of the body

_____ 9. Related to the same side of the body

_____ 10. Related to opposite sides of the body

_____ 11. Nearer to the point of reference, usually toward the trunk of the body

_____ 12. Farther from the point of reference, usually away from the midline

MATCHING V

Write the letter of the best answer in the space provided.

A. Antecubital	E. Antebrachial	I. Mediastinal
B. Digital	F. Popliteal	J. Costal
C. Axillary	G. Plantar	K. Cervical
D. Buccal	H. Cubital	L. Brachial

_____ 1. Cheek area

_____ 2. Neck area

_____ 3. Forearm area

_____ 4. Space in front of elbow or at the bend of the elbow

_____ 5. Armpit region

_____ 6. Upper arm region

_____ 7. Elbow area

_____ 8. Digits; both the fingers and/or toes

_____ 9. Rib area

_____ 10. Portion of the thoracic cavity between the lungs

_____ 11. Bottom surface of the foot

_____ 12. Posterior aspect of the knee

Bibliography

Applegate EJ: *The anatomy and physiology learning system,* ed 2, Philadelphia, 2000, WB Saunders.

Crawley J, Van De Graaff KM: *A photographic atlas for anatomy and physiology,* Englewood, Colo, 2002, Morton.

Goldberg S: *Clinical anatomy made ridiculously simple,* Miami, 1984, Medmaster.

Grafelman T: *Graf's anatomy and physiology guide for the massage therapist,* Aurora, Colo, 1998, DG Publishing.

Gray HT, Pickering P, Howden R: *Gray's anatomy,* ed 29, Philadelphia, 1974, Running Press.

Haubrich WS: *Medical meanings: a glossary of word origins,* New York, 1984, Harcourt Brace Jovanovich.

Jacob S, Francone C: *Elements of anatomy and physiology,* Philadelphia, 1989, WB Saunders.

Juhan D: *Job's body: a handbook for bodyworkers,* Barrington, NY, 1987, Station Hill Press.

Kapit W, Elson LM: *The anatomy coloring book,* ed 3, New York, 2002, Benjamin Cummings.

Kapit W, Macey R, Meisami E: *The physiology coloring book,* New York, 1987, HarperCollins.

Lauderstein D: *Putting the soul back in the body: a manual of imaginative anatomy for massage therapists,* Chicago, 1985, self-published manual.

Marieb EN: *Essentials of human anatomy and physiology,* ed 4, New York, 1994, Benjamin/Cummings.

Myers TW: *Anatomy trains: myofascial meridians for manual and movement therapists,* New York, 2001, Churchill Livingstone.

Spitz R: Hospitalism: an inquiry into the genesis of psychiatric conditions of early childhood, *Psychoanal Study Child* 2:53-74, 1945.

Taber's cyclopedic medical dictionary, ed 13, Philadelphia, 1977, FA Davis.

Thibodeau G, Patton K: *Structure and function of the body,* ed 11, St Louis, 2000, Mosby.

Tortora GJ: *Introduction to the human body: the essentials of anatomy and physiology,* ed 3, New York, 1994, HarperCollins.

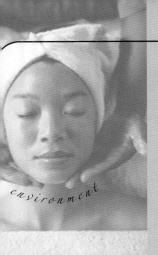

Integumentary System

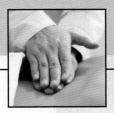

12

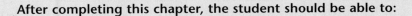

"The skin is no more separate from the brain than the surface of a lake is separate from its depths. They are two different locations in a continuous medium. To touch the surface is to stir the depths."

—Deane Juhan

STUDENT OBJECTIVES

After completing this chapter, the student should be able to:

- Recall the six functions of the integumentary system
- Discuss the structures in the epidermis and the dermis
- Define several factors that contribute to skin color
- Name the main parts of a nail
- Differentiate between sebaceous glands and sudoriferous glands
- Name types of skin pathologies, giving characteristics and massage considerations of each
- Explain first-, second-, and third-degree burns
- Define three types of skin cancer
- Identify four ways to assess moles for possible changes
- List all the known sensory receptors associated with the skin and name what type of sensation they detect
- Discuss the possible implications that touch research, as presented in this chapter, has on massage therapy

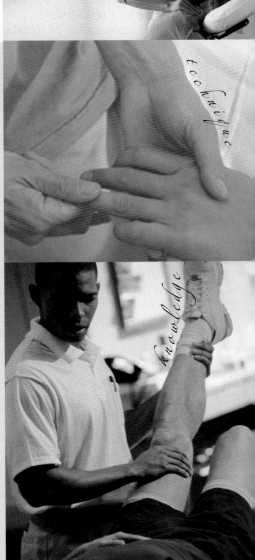

INTRODUCTION

The integumentary system consists of the skin and all of its derivatives, including hair, nails, and related glands. By weight, the skin is the largest organ of the body and houses the tactile system. Sensory receptors receive perceptual stimuli (e.g., heat, cold, movement, touch, pressure, pain). In fact, more than a half million sensory receptors from the skin are found entering the spinal cord.

The skin, like a cell membrane, defines our parameters. Housed within its layers are various tissues that carry out special functions such as waste elimination and temperature regulation. The skin forms natural openings such as the mouth, external ear canal, nose, urethra, vagina, and anus. These passageways to the digestive, respiratory, urinary, and reproductive systems can be seen as extensions of the external environment. No other body system is more easily exposed to infections, disease, pollution, or injury than the skin, yet no other body system is as strong and resilient.

The appearance of the skin reflects our physiology. At a glance, something about a person's nutrition, hygiene habits, circulation, age, immunity, parents (genetics), and environmental factors can be noted by the condition of the skin. Healthy skin is soft, flexible, moist, acidic, and blemish-free. People spend millions each year on products from companies that profess using their product will give them a more youthful appearance. Millions are also spent on surgical and nonsurgical procedures to darken the skin, remove wrinkles, lighten freckles, minimize scars, smooth out cellulite, remove unwanted hair, restore lost hair, and treat acne.

Not only does it reveal vital physiological data (e.g., circulation, fever), the skin also mirrors our emotional self. Through muscular expression and neurological impulses, the skin has the power to reflect an ever-changing stream of emotions. How people feel about themselves and others is reflected on the surface of the skin.

This chapter examines the skin, its structures and functions, and the concept of touch. By understanding the skin's embryonic origins and its connection with the nervous system, the relationship of touch to massage therapy can be appreciated.

For Your Information

The skin covers an area of about 22 square feet (ft²) and weighs approximately 9 pounds (lb), making up 7% percent of body weight. A piece of skin the size of a quarter contains more than 3 million cells, 100 sweat glands, 50 nerve endings, and 3 ft of blood vessels. The skin is thinnest over the eyelids and thickest on the soles of the feet. The fingertips have approximately 700 touch receptors on 2 square millimeters (mm²) of surface area. ⇨ ☐

FUNCTIONS

The skin has numerous functions, as is described in the following:

- **Protects.** One of the primary functions of the skin is protecting the organism by acting as a physical, biological, and chemical barrier. The skin's physical barrier is essential for protecting the underlying tissues from abrasion. The skin also provides waterproofing from a protein called *keratin* and limited protection from ultraviolet (UV) radiation through a substance called *melanin*. As a biological barrier, intact skin is an effective barrier against many foreign agents such as bacteria and viruses. The skin's acidic secretions inhibit the growth of these foreign agents by providing an acid mantle. This surface acidity provides the skin with a chemical barrier.
- **Absorbs.** The skin has limited properties of absorption. Substances that can be absorbed by the epidermis are lipid-soluble substances (oxygen, carbon dioxide), fat-soluble vitamins (A, D, E, and K), steroids, resins of certain plants (poison ivy and poison oak), organic solvents (paint thinner, which can cause brain and kidney damage), and salts of heavy metals (lead, mercury, and nickel). The use of medicated transdermal patches is based on the absorption properties of the skin.
- **Receives stimuli.** The skin is considered an extension of the nervous system. It receives stimuli such as pressure, pain, and temperature from the external environment and brings this information to the central nervous system. The most fundamental of all the senses is touch. The very concept of touch encompasses emotional and physical aspects of well-being; physical dimensions such as sensory receptors are covered later (see the section on Skin and Its Sensory Receptors). A separate section of this chapter has been set aside to examine touch in greater detail, especially as it relates to our emotional needs (see the section on Skin and the Importance of Touch).
- **Regulates body temperature.** An increase in blood circulation to the skin's surface creates a property of temperature regulation. As the blood moves to the skin's surface and blood vessels dilate, heat is discharged into the atmosphere. In this way, our bodies radiate to release internal heat. Heat can also be dissipated through the evaporation of perspiration produced by specialized glands called *sudoriferous glands*.
- **Eliminates waste.** The skin functions as a mini-excretory system, eliminating wastes through perspiration. Sweat, a waste product, is a mixture of

Terms and Their Meanings Related to the Skin

Term	Meaning
acne vulgaris	common acne
contusion	bruise
corium	leather, skin
cutaneous	skin
cuticle	little skin
decubitus	lying down
dermis	skin
eczema	to boil out
epidermis	upon or over skin
follicle	sac, small
furuncle	boil
granulosum	grain, small
integument	a covering, to cover over
Krause	German anatomist (1833-1910)
lacrimal	tear
lucidum	clear
Meissner	German histologist (1829-1905)
melano	black
Pacini	Italian anatomist (1812-1883)
palpate	stroke or touch
papule	pimple
pruritus	itching
psoriasis	an itching
pustule	blister
Ruffini	Italian anatomist (1864-1929)
scleroderma	hard, skin
seborrhea	tallow, to flow
sebum	grease, tallow
senile lentigo	old freckle
stratum	a layer, cover, or spread
sudoriferous	sweat, to carry or bear
verruca	wart

98% water and 2% solids (salt ions, lactic acid, and other metabolic wastes). By contrast, urine is 96% water and 4% solids.

- **Synthesizes vitamin D.** Located in the skin are precursor molecules that are converted by the UV rays in sunlight to vitamin D (with the help of liver and kidney enzymes). Vitamin D is important because it stimulates the absorption of calcium and phosphorus from food. Little UV light is required for this synthesis to occur, so prolonged sunbathing is actually unnecessary.

ANATOMICAL REGIONS AND STRUCTURES OF THE SKIN

The skin is divided into two distinct regions: epidermis and dermis. The epidermis consists of four or five layers and contains skin pigmentation cells, nails, and pores. The dermis and epidermis are firmly cemented together. However, a severe friction abrasion such as the rubbing of an improperly fitting shoe may cause the dermis and the epidermis to separate, resulting in a blister. The surrounding cells secrete a protective fluid to insulate themselves from the abrasive heat of the friction. The dermis is located under the epidermis and contains the blood vessels, many nerve receptors, hair follicles, and skin glands. Underneath the skin is a layer of tissue known as the *subcutaneous layer*. The following sections examine these layers more closely.

Epidermis

The **epidermis** is derived from ectoderm, the same embryonic cell layer that gives us the brain, spinal cord, and special senses. Contained in its layers are melanocytes, which contribute to the color of the skin, hair, and eye iris, and absorption of UV light. The epidermis also contains pores; these openings allow passage for hair and specialized glands.

Composed solely of epithelial tissue, the epidermis is relatively avascular. Therefore all oxygen and nutrients must reach the epidermal cells by diffusion of tissue fluids from the underlying dermis. The cells of the epidermis are formed in the deepest epidermal layer, where they multiply and eventually push themselves up toward the surface, like a seedling or a budding tooth. As they move farther away from their source of nutrition, they become starved and eventually die. The superficial epidermal cells are constantly being sloughed off in an endless renewal process. The entire life cycle of skin cells from birth to death is 21 to 27 days.

Epidermal Layers

Four epidermal layers are typically found. However, in areas where friction is greatest, namely the soles of the feet and palms of the hands, an extra layer of skin is evident. From deepest to most superficial, these layers are the stratum germinativum, stratum spinosum, stratum granulosum, stratum lucidum, and stratum corneum (Figure 12-1).

1. **Stratum germinativum.** This is the deepest layer of the epidermis. The stratum germinativum, or stratum basale, undergoes continuous cell division and generates all other layers. This layer also contains Merkel disks, which are nerve endings responding to superficial pressure.
2. **Stratum spinosum.** The stratum spinosum, or "prickly layer," is a bonding and transitional layer between the stratum granulosum and the stratum germinativum possessing cells of both these layers.
3. **Stratum granulosum.** A layer of cells containing an accumulation of keratin granules distinguishes the stratum granulosum under a microscope. This layer is three to five cells deep, depending on the thickness of the skin. This layer marks the beginning of change before the drying of the tissue.

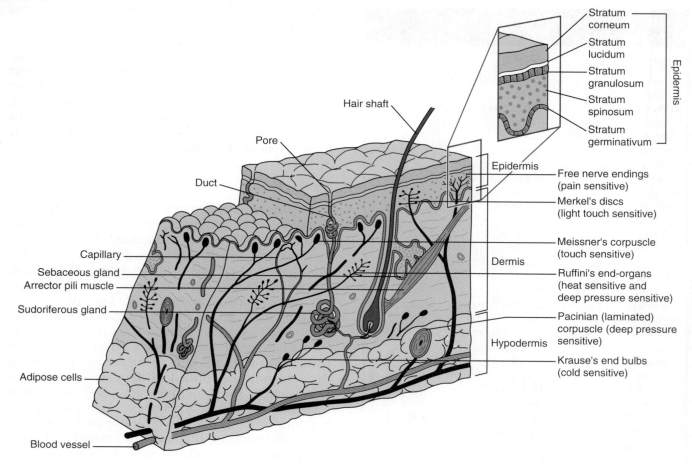

Figure 12-1 A cross-section of skin.

4. **Stratum lucidum.** In the thick skin of the hands and the feet, a translucent layer is found between the stratum corneum and the stratum granulosum. Like the stratum corneum, the stratum lucidum contains cells that are keratinized. In thin skin, the stratum lucidum is absent.

5. **Stratum corneum.** This is the outermost layer of the skin. By the time these epithelial cells reach the surface, they are no longer living cells. These cells have become completely keratinized; ready to be sloughed off.

Two special cells found in the epidermis are keratinocytes and melanocytes. Produced by keratinocytes, **keratin**, an extremely tough, fibrous protein, provides protection by waterproofing the skin's surface (it is insoluble in water) and contributing to the body's immune defenses. Its waterproofing properties serve a dual purpose; keeping water in and water out. These cells are dead and begin shedding at the skin's surface, only to be replaced by cells from the deeper epidermal layers.

Melanocytes are specialized cells in the epidermis where the yellow, brown, or black skin pigment, or melanin, is synthesized. **Melanin** contributes to the color of the skin but is also found in the hair and iris of the eye. Melanin granules serve to protect the underlying cells from the sun's UV radiation. Both the melanocyte-producing hormone from the pituitary and genetics determines the amount of melanin produced in an individual.

UV light stimulates the formation of this pigment and causes darkening of the melanin granules. Melanin serves as a protective shield for the skin from the damaging effects of sunlight and is activated by sunbathing (tanning). Freckles and moles are present when melanin is concentrated in one area.

Albinism is a genetic condition in which the individual cannot produce melanin. An albino's hair and skin appear white or pale and the iris of the eye appears pink or red because of the easy visibility of blood vessels. Vitiligo (Figure 12-2), or leukoderma, is the partial or total loss of skin pigmentation, which occurs in patches. This may be as the result of a deep burn or scar that damages the melanocytes in a given area of the body. The skin in this area remains white and will not tan. **Skin pallor** refers to an unnatural paleness or lack of color of the skin.

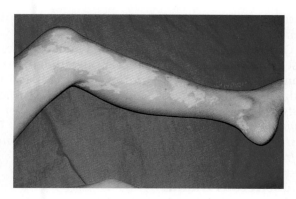

Figure 12-2 Vitiligo (leukoderma) is loss of skin pigmentation occurring in patches.

Certain hormones such as those secreted during pregnancy can stimulate the synthesis of melanin. This can produce a dark line between the navel and pubic area or give the childbearing woman a "mask of pregnancy" by darkening the skin of the face and throat.

Skin Color. Skin color variations are the result of the following several factors:
1. Melanin
2. Amount of oxygen present in the capillaries of the dermis, which can give the skin a rosy cast to a blue or purple cast of cyanosis (excessive amounts of deoxygenated blood)
3. Presence of the pigment bilirubin in the blood, which can produce the yellowish appearance of jaundice
4. Presence of the pigment carotene in the skin, which produces the yellowish appearance of Asians

Nails

Nails are heavily keratinized, nonliving tissue forming the thin hard plates that are found on the distal surfaces of the fingers and toes. The two main functions of the nails are (1) protection of the ends of the fingers and (2) use as a tool for tasks such as digging, scratching, and manipulation of objects. Nails are typically transparent but appear pinkish because of blood vessels present in the dermis below. If the blood contains an insufficient amount of oxygen, the nails appear cyanotic. Nail changes, like ridges and white spots, may occur as a result of poor nutrition or disease.

The **nail body** is the main visible part of the nail. Other nail structures are the nail bed, nail root, lateral nail folds, eponychium (cuticle), lunula, and the free edge of the nail. Nail production takes place in the **nail root**. Nail growth occurs at approximately 1 mm per week. The **nail bed** is the skin beneath the nail; it appears through the clear nail, often as a

series of longitudinal ridges. The **lateral nail folds** are the edges of the nail where they meet the skin at the sides of the nail. This is the area where hangnails occur. The **eponychium**, or cuticle, is the tough ridge of skin that grows out over the nail from its base. Also located here is the **lunula**, which is the whitish half-moon shape at the base of the nail. The most distal portion of the nail is the **free nail edge**, which is what is trimmed as a result of nail growth (Figure 12-3).

Dermis

Also known as the corium, or "hide," the **dermis** is the true skin. Leather products are the treated dermis of an animal. The dermis contains adipose tissue, many blood vessels, and nerve endings such as Meissner and Pacinian corpuscles, and it is generally thicker on the posterior aspect of the body. It is also thicker in men than in women; this may be the result of presence of certain hormones. More specifically, dermis is thickest on the palms of the hands and soles of the feet and quite thin over the eyelids.

Collagen, the main component of connective tissue, is an insoluble, fibrous protein that constitutes about 70% of the dermis and offers supports to the nerves, blood vessels, hair follicles, and glands. Within the collagen fibers are pliable fibers called *elastin,* which gives the skin its elasticity and resilience. As we age, fat is lost under the skin, which results in sags and wrinkles.

The loss of elasticity can be accelerated by excessive exposure of ultraviolet rays; perhaps one of the best ways to prevent premature wrinkling is to protect the skin from the sun. It is impossible to avoid aging, but good nutrition, plenty of fluids, and daily skin care can retard the process.

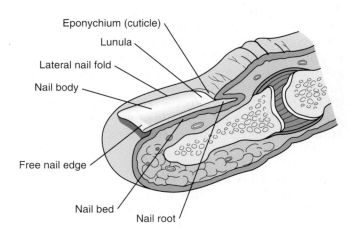

Figure 12-3 A cross-section of a nail.

Hair and Related Structures

Hair is made up of keratin filaments arising from a specialized follicle in the dermis. Its function is primarily protection. **Hair follicles** are pouchlike depressions in the skin that enclose the hair shaft. Hair and hair follicles cover almost the entire body but most are barely visible to the naked eye. Hair is typically absent on the palms of hands, sides of fingers, soles and sides of feet and toes, lips, eyelids, navel, and parts of the genitalia. Heavier concentrations of hair are found in the axillae, scalp, on external genitalia, and above eyes and eyelids. Because of male hormones, men typically have extra hair growth on their face and chest.

Hair comes in a variety of sizes and shapes. Hair is short and stiff in the eyebrow and flexible and long on the top, sides, and back of the head. A round shaft of hair produces straight hair. When the hair shaft is oval, the person usually has wavy hair. If the hair shaft is flat and ribbonlike, the hair is curly or kinky. In fine hair, no medulla (inner core) is present in the hair follicle. Genetics determine most of our hair characteristics, from hair color to texture.

All shades of hair come from one or a combination of the three colors of melanin: brown, yellow, and black. Red hair is a combination of brown and yellow pigment. White hair often is the result of air in the hair follicle itself. Gray hair occurs when the amount of melanin deposited in the hair decreases or is absent. Aging, emotional distress, certain chemical treatments (chemotherapy), radiation, excessive vitamin A, and certain fungal diseases can cause both graying and/or hair loss.

Hair follicles can sometimes become irritated during a massage. This may be caused by the following:
- *Having an allergic reaction to the massage lubricant*
- *Pulling of the hair*
- *Not using enough lubricant on the skin, causing undue friction*

Arrector Pili Muscle

Arrector pili are the muscles of the hair. These tiny muscles contract when you are cold or experiencing emotions such as fright or anxiety. The hair is pulled upright, dimpling the skin surface with goose bumps. If an animal is cold, this creates an insulating layer of air in the fur. Because most humans do not have fur, this effect is relatively useless. If an animal is frightened, this added volume allows the animal to appear larger and possibly deter an enemy.

Sebaceous Glands

Sebaceous glands, also known as *oil glands,* are attached to the hair follicle. Sebaceous glands secrete **sebum**, a mixture of fats, cholesterol, proteins, and inorganic salts, which are mildly antibacterial and antifungal, lubricating both the hair and the epidermis.

Overproduction of sebum, caused by hormones or disease, can make the skin appear oily; underproduction of sebum caused by nutritional factors and UV radiation makes the skin appear dry. *Massage therapists can use massage to stimulate the production of sebum, which adds additional natural oils to the skin. The best massage movement for sebaceous gland stimulation is friction.*

Sudoriferous Glands

Sudoriferous glands, located in the dermis, are exocrine glands that secrete sweat, or perspiration. They are regulated by the sympathetic nervous system and can be stimulated in response to excess heat or emotional arousal. The skin's surface possesses approximately 2 million sweat glands.

The primary functions of sudoriferous glands are to regulate body temperature and to eliminate waste products. As perspiration evaporates, it carries large amounts of body heat away from the skin surface. The most rapid process of heat dissipation is evaporation of perspiration.

Approximately 1 pint of fluid and impurities is lost in each 8-hour period when a person is visibly sweating. When sweat production is high, replacement of lost minerals is essential. When the sweating is low, most of the sodium chloride present in the perspiration is reabsorbed in the skin. In this case, mineral depletion is minimal.

MINI-LAB

Spray the back of your hand with tap water. Blow on the damp surface and describe the sensation as the water evaporates. Speculate how evaporation of water (sweat) from the skin surface can regulate the temperature of the body. Repeat the experiment with alcohol, which evaporates at a lower temperature than water, and compare the results.

Subcutaneous Layer

Also known as **superficial fascia** or **hypodermis**, the subcutaneous layer is not a true region of skin, but a connective tissue layer that connects the dermis to underlying structures. This layer contains nerve receptors called *Krause end bulbs* and *Ruffini end organs.* Also found in the subcutaneous layer is a band of adipose tissue called the *panniculus adiposus.* The thickness of the panniculus adiposus varies with age, gender, and health. Infants and children have a uniform fat layer under the skin. Females have an extra thickness of adipose over the breasts, hips, and inner thighs. Males have an accumulation of fat on the nape of the neck, deltoid and triceps muscles, and abdominal region of the body.

SKIN AND ITS SENSORY RECEPTORS

The skin functions as a large conductor of information such as heat, cold, pressure, pain, movement, and touch. The sense of touch is actually a complex composition of seven specialized receptors found in the skin (Table 12-1). Touch is an amalgamation of many sensations and is the least understood of all the senses. Touch provides sensory input and physical information about our surroundings. This sense also warns the body of impending damage such as a hot pot on the stove or knife about to slice a finger. The following is a list of all the currently known receptors and their functions:

Meissner corpuscles. These receptors detect light touch (pressure), responding to both the actual movement and the length of the movement across the skin. More specifically, Meissner corpuscles monitor vibration (onset and removal of pressure) and adapts to stimuli quickly. Meissner corpuscles are located in the dermis just below the epidermis.

Pacinian corpuscles. These deep pressure-sensitive receptors respond to skin displacement and vibration. These receptors also perceive proprioceptive information about joint positions. Unlike Meissner corpuscles, Pacinian corpuscles adapt quickly to stimuli. Notice how quickly we stop noticing the band around our waist. The corpuscles are located in the deeper layers of the dermis and their shape resembles an onion slice.

Free nerve endings. Free nerve endings are bare nerve endings that detect pain. Also known as *nociceptors,* free nerve endings are located in all parts of the body, especially in the skin. They can be stimulated by extremes in temperature, intense mechanical stimulation, and specific chemicals in extracellular fluid, including ones released by injured cells.

Merkel disks. Located in the epidermis, these receptors respond to superficial pressure and skin displacement. Merkel disks do not adapt quickly and possess the capacity for a longer, more continuous response.

Hair-follicle receptors. Each hair follicle is wrapped by a nerve that responds briefly to hair movement. These receptors, also called *hair root plexuses,* may alert us to goose bumps or inform us of a small breeze or intrusive insect.

Krause end bulbs. Although the operating mechanism of Krause end bulbs is not exactly known, they are believed to be stimulated by lowering temperatures (cold) and are found widely distributed in the subcutaneous layer.

Ruffini end organs. These receptors alert us when the skin comes into contact with deep or continuous pressure and the stretch of adjacent tissues. Some references indicate that these receptors detect the increase of temperature (e.g., warmth and heat). Ruffini end organs are located in the subcutaneous layer and are also known as *type II cutaneous mechanoreceptors.*

The Brain's Role in Touch

The brain detects the sensation of touch in the parietal lobe of the cerebral cortex. The postcentral gyrus, an elevated area of brain tissue located in the parietal lobe, is where the axons that detect touch terminate. Keep in mind that the right postcentral gyrus represents the left side of the body and vice versa. It is interesting just how much gray matter is dedicated to each surface area (Figure 12-4). The hands, face, lips,

TABLE 12-1

Skin Receptors

Type	Stimuli Received
Meissner corpuscles	Detect light touch (pressure) and vibration; responds to actual movement and length of movement across the skin
Pacinian corpuscles	Detects deep pressure and vibration; responds to skin displacement; perceives proprioceptive information; adapts quickly
Free nerve endings	Nerve endings that detect pain; also known as *nociceptors*
Merkel disks	Responds to superficial pressure and skin displacement; does not adapt quickly; has capacity for a longer response
Hair follicle receptors	Responds to hair movement
Krause's end bulbs	Not known; believed to respond to cold
Ruffini end organs	Responds to deep or continuous pressure, the stretch of adjacent tissues, and heat

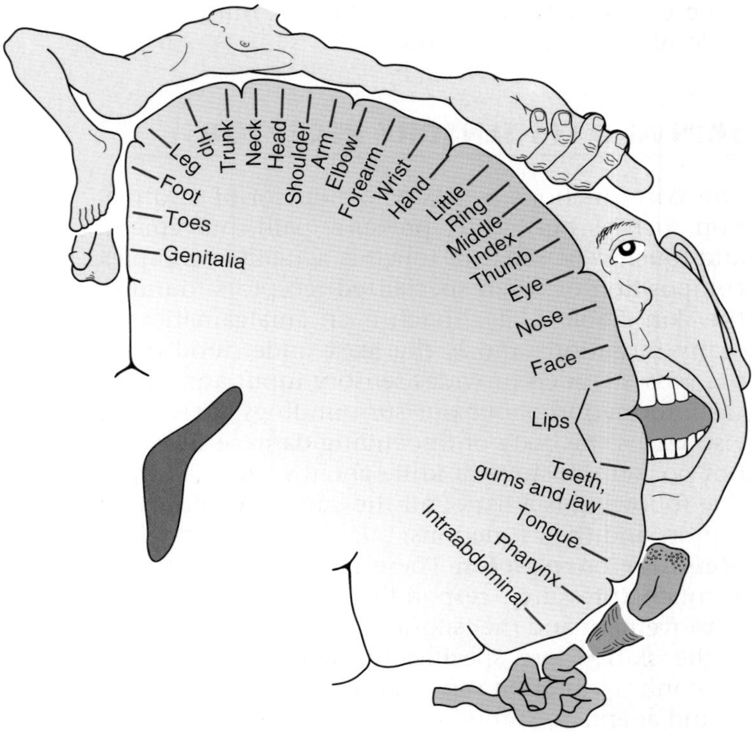

Figure 12-4 Illustration of the *homunculus,* meaning *little man,* in the postcentral gyrus.

jaw, and tongue take up about 80% of this neural space. The more space devoted to an area in the post-central gyrus, the more sensory touch receptors are found in the corresponding part of the body. The more sensory receptors that are located in that part of the body, the more sensitive is the body part.

INTEGUMENTAL PATHOLOGIES

Acne. A bacterial infection of the sebaceous glands, acne causes inflammation and pus formation. Acne usually begins at puberty and may continue through adolescence. Whiteheads are accumulations of dead bacteria, cell debris, and dead white blood cells. Blackheads are accumulations of dried sebum and bacteria in the gland and its duct. The black appearance results from oxidation of the sebum.

Massage over the infected area is contraindicated if there is extensive inflammation. The client may prefer facial massage without oil. It is important that massage therapists wash their hands thoroughly before massaging areas with acne.

Age spots. Also referred to as *senile lentigo* or liver spots, age spots are tan or brown patches found on the skin of older people, especially those who have excessive exposure to the sun.

Massage is fine for clients with age spots.

Athlete's foot. Athlete's foot is a contagious superficial fungal infection of the foot characterized by

discoloration of the skin and a ring or ridge of red tissue (Figure 12-5). The skin may also break, bleed, or ooze clear tissue fluids. The infected foot often has an unpleasant odor. The same fungus may also cause jock itch or ringworm in other areas of the body (Box 12-1).

Local massage is contraindicated because this fungal infection is contagious and spreads easily.

Blister. A blister is a collection of fluid below the epidermis sometimes caused by pressure or friction. Draining a blister constitutes medical treatment and therefore is not in the massage therapist's scope of practice.

Local massage is contraindicated.

Bruise. Also known as a *contusion,* a bruise is an injury that does not break the skin. It is caused by a blow and is characterized by swelling, discoloration, and pain. The color of a bruise is caused by blood from broken vessels that has leaked into the interstitial spaces.

BOX 12-1

Contagious Skin Pathologies

- Athlete's foot
- Herpes simplex
- Impetigo
- Lice
- Papule (if a wart)
- Ringworm
- Scabies
- Warts

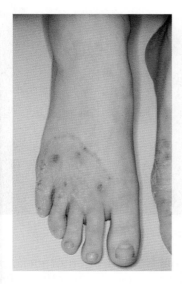

Figure 12-5   Athlete's foot.

Local massage is contraindicated until it begins to turn yellowish. Massage around the bruise while it is bluish or purple may help facilitate its healing by increasing nutrition to and removal of wastes from the area.

Burns. When the skin is damaged by heat, radiation, electricity, or chemical agents, skin cells perish. The damage that results is called a *burn*. Burns can be classified into three categories, depending on the severity of damage to the tissues and the area of involvement.

- A first-degree burn damages the epidermis. Symptoms are redness and mild pain. An example of a first-degree burn is a mild sunburn, which typically heals in 2 to 3 days.
- A second-degree burn damages the epidermis and the upper layers of the dermis. Some symptoms associated with second-degree burns are swelling, blistering, and pain. Hair follicles and sweat glands usually remain functional. Healing time can be from 7 days to 4 weeks. Once the burn heals, a mild scar may remain.
- A third-degree burn destroys the epidermis, dermis, hair follicles, and associated glands. Because of the damage to the glands and follicles, the functions of the skin are reduced or nonexistent. Because of injury of the lymph capillaries and nerve endings, little swelling and pain occurs. A client with third-degree burns may experience limited mobility because of the restrictive effect of scar tissue. Almost all third-degree burns require skin grafting.

Massage should be performed only when tissue is fully healed and can withstand pressure. Unhealed skin is pink, thin, and delicate and should not be massaged. Gentle massage is indicated, and no movements should be forced. Friction and cross-fiber friction over healed and scarred tissue may help break up adhesions. Gentle range of motion can help increase mobility. Massage for clients with healed skin grafts should be to soften and loosen the graft and improve circulation. Massage over the graft should occur only after complete healing. Use a good quality lubricant, preferably one with cocoa butter, aloe vera, and vitamin E.

Corns. Corns are thickened cone-shaped skin resulting from repeated friction or pressure. They occur primarily over toe joints and between the toes.

Massage is fine. Avoid sustained direct pressure. Lemon or peppermint essential oils may help reduce corns.

Decubitus ulcers. Decubitus ulcers, or bed sores, are caused by constant deficiency of blood to tissues that have been subjected to prolonged pressure. This restriction of the normal blood supply to the skin results in cell necrosis (death). The weight of the body puts pressure on the skin (especially over bony projections). As cells die, ulcers form. Decubitus ulcers occur in bedridden patients who are not turned regularly and in people who use wheelchairs, braces, or have casts.

Local massage is contraindicated. Light massage in a wide area encircling the ulcer may be beneficial to increase blood flow to an area that has been deprived. Gentle active and passive range-of-motion exercises in bedridden clients help with joint mobility. The client's caregiver should be advised of any redness, blistering, or ulcers the massage therapist notices.

Eczema. Eczema, a chronic dermatitis, is an acute or chronic superficial inflammation of the skin characterized by redness, watery discharge, crusting, scaling, itching, and burning (Figure 12-6). This disorder may be hereditary and is not contagious.

Massage is fine for clients with eczema. Massage over affected areas is contraindicated if there are open areas and watery discharge.

Furuncle. A furuncle is a boil or an abscess caused by the staphylococcal bacteria in a skin gland or hair follicle. It is characterized by pain, redness, and swelling. Necrosis forms a core of dead tissue that may extrude (Figure 12-7).

Local massage is contraindicated. Lymph nodes in the area may be painfully enlarged, so massage over them should be avoided.

Herpes simplex. Also known as *cold sores* or *fever blisters*, herpes simplex is a highly contagious viral infection that has the ability to lie dormant for extended periods without expressing any signs or symptoms of disease. Flare-ups are characterized by cold sores on the skin and mucous membranes. The appearance of cold sores can be triggered by stimuli such as UV radiation from the sun, hor-

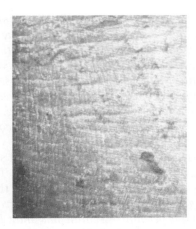

Figure 12-6   Eczema.

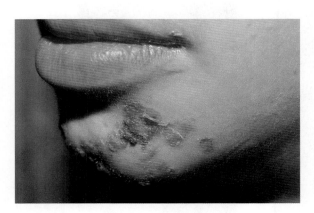

Figure 12-8   Impetigo.

monal changes that occur during menstruation and pregnancy, or emotional upset.

Local massage is definitely contraindicated.

Impetigo. This is an inflammatory skin infection caused by staphylococci or streptococci bacteria. It is characterized by raised, fluid-filled sores that itch or burn (Figure 12-8). This condition is most common in children, and it occurs mainly around the mouth, nose, and hands. Impetigo is highly contagious and can be spread by hand contact and handling contaminated objects such as linens, doorknobs, and toothbrushes.

Local massage is definitely contraindicated.

Lice. The body louse is a parasitic insect that is highly contagious (Figure 12-9). These are typically found in hair and are diagnosed with the presence of egg sacs on the hair shaft.

Massage is definitely contraindicated.

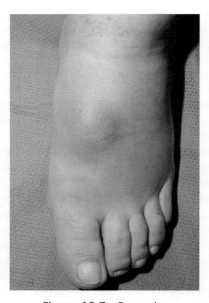

Figure 12-7   Furuncle.

Moles. A mole is a collection of melanocytes. Most moles are present at birth (often referred to as a *birth mark*), and some can become cancerous if visible changes occur. Please note the section on mole changes.

Massage is fine over noncancerous moles.

Papule. This is a small, round, firm, elevated area in the skin varying in size from a pinpoint to that of a small pea. An example of a papule is a wart.

Local massage may be contraindicated, depending on the cause. For instance, if it is a wart, it can be contagious.

Pruritus. Pruritus is severe itching of the skin caused by dryness, sweat retention on the skin, kidney failure, allergic reactions, fungi, or parasites such as scabies or body lice. Pruritus can also be caused by bile salts in the skin, cancer, or psychogenic disorders such as emotional stress.

Local massage may be contraindicated, depending on the cause. For instance, if it is a fungi or a parasite, it can be contagious.

Psoriasis. Psoriasis is characterized by red, flaky skin elevations covered by thick, dry, silvery scales (Figure 12-10). A chronic form of dermatitis, psoriasis is marked by periods of remission and exacerbation. In severe forms it is a disabling and disfiguring affliction and can involve the scalp, elbows, knees, back, and buttocks. Often psoriasis is genetic; it is not contagious. Stress can exacerbate the condition.

Massage is fine for clients with psoriasis. Some of the scales may dislodge during treatment.

Pustule. This skin condition is a small, raised elevation of the skin, often with a "head" containing lymph or pus such as a pimple.

Local massage may be contraindicated, depending on cause (e.g., chicken pox, acne, impetigo).

Ringworm. Ringworm is not a worm at all, but a group of fungal diseases characterized by itching, scaling, and sometimes painful lesions manifested as a raised red-ringed patch (Figure 12-11).

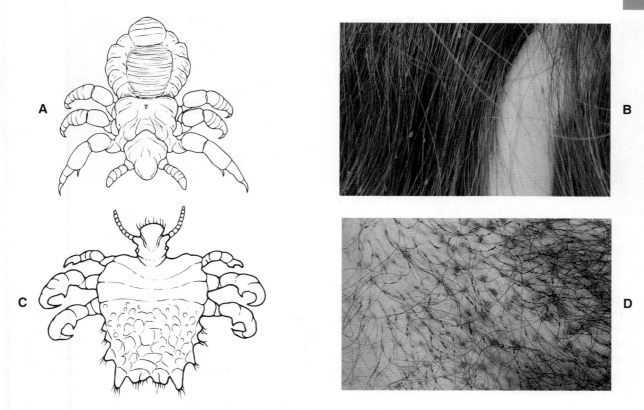

Figure 12-9 **A,** Head louse; **B,** lice nits; **C,** pubic louse; **D,** pubic lice rash.

Massage is contraindicated.

Rosacea. A chronic form of acne, usually involving the middle third of the face, rosacea is characterized by persistent redness and swelling (Figure 12-12).

Massage is fine for clients with rosacea.

Scabies. Scabies is a highly contagious infection caused by parasitic mites that crawl under the skin's surface (cannot be seen by the naked eye). The female mite (Figure 12-13, *A*) excretes a material that causes dreadfully intense itching (typically at night).

Massage is definitely contraindicated.

Scleroderma. Scleroderma is an autoimmune disorder affecting blood vessels and connective tissue. Fibrous degeneration of the connective tissue occurs in the skin, lungs, and internal organs. The skin tightens and becomes fixed to underlying tissues. Scleroderma is most common in middle-age women. Death may occur because of cardiac, renal, pulmonary, or intestinal involvement. Localized forms are present with just small patches of the skin involved. Scleroderma is not contagious.

Massage is contraindicated for the severe forms. In less severe forms, massage can be beneficial. Friction

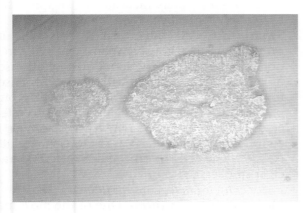

Figure 12-10 Psoriasis.

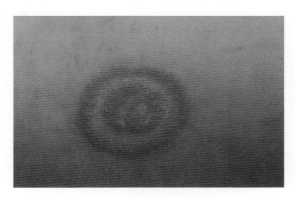

Figure 12-11 Ringworm.

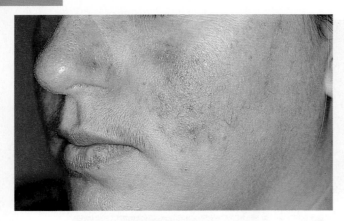

Figure 12-12 Rosacea. (From Callen JP et al: *Color atlas of dermatology,* ed 2, Philadelphia, 2000, WB Saunders.)

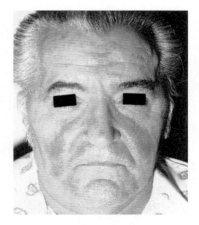

Figure 12-14 Seborrhea.

and cross-fiber friction may help reduce adhesions. Deep strokes can increase local circulation and improve nutrition and drainage for the tissues. Passive and active range of motion can help retain joint mobility.

Seborrhea. Seborrhea is a skin disease of the sebaceous glands, marked by an increase in the amount of oily secretions (Figure 12-14). Also known as *cra-*

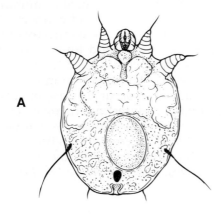

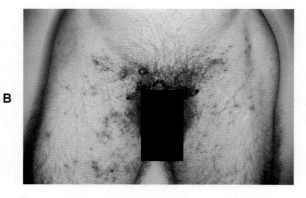

Figure 12-13 **A,** Scabies mite; **B,** scabies mite rash.

dle cap in infants, seborrhea begins as a pink raised patch that gradually turns yellow and scaly.

Local massage is contraindicated.

Skin cancer. Ninety percent of all reported skin cancers can be abated through early detection and treatment. The best preventive measure anyone can take to reduce skin cancer is to avoid overexposure to the sun. This is more important for light-skinned people. Darker-skinned people have fewer incidents of skin cancer because they have more pigment, or melanin, to protect their cells from UV radiation. Using a sunscreen lotion with a sun protection factor (SPF) of 15 or more is advisable. The three most common types of skin cancer are basal cell carcinoma, squamous cell carcinoma, and malignant melanoma.

1. **Basal cell carcinoma.** This accounts for about 75% of all cancers of the skin. This type of skin cancer is slow growing and is characterized by lesions that begin as small, raised nodules that ulcerate (Figure 12-15, *A*). The primary cause of basal cell carcinoma is excessive exposure to sunlight. Basal cell carcinoma is the least dangerous and rarely metastasizes, or spreads.
   See entry for malignant melanoma.

2. **Squamous cell carcinoma.** This type of cancer is more aggressive than basal cell carcinoma and accounts for about 20% of all cases of cancer. Squamous cell carcinoma also arises from the epidermis, beginning as a scaly pigmented area that may develop into a ulcerated crater (Figure 12-15, *B*). This type of cancer is common on sun-exposed areas or in the mouth (tobacco chewers) or on the lips (cigarette and cigar smokers).
   See entry for malignant melanoma.

3. **Malignant melanoma.** One of the most malignant and lethal skin cancer types, melanoma

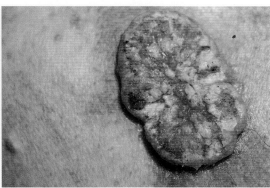

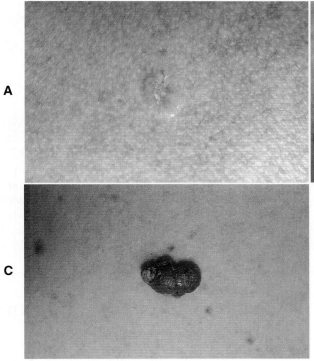

Figure 12-15 Any mole change must be brought to the client's attention. **A**, Basal cell carcinoma; **B**, squamous cell carcinoma; **C**, malignant melanoma.

is a group of melanocytes that has mutated into cancer. Accounting for about 5% of all skin cancers, it typically begins as a raised dark lesion with irregular borders and appears uneven in color (Figure 12-15, *C*). It typically occurs in light-skinned people who are exposed to UV radiation over many years. Melanoma is more likely to metastasize than any other form of cancer and can kill within months of diagnosis.

Bring to the client's attention any changes in color, size, shape, and texture of moles. Consult with the client's physician about the indication of massage as the spread and treatment of cancer varies according to they type and stage of cancer.

Skin tags. Skin tags are just tiny little flaps of skin. These are most common in middle-age women and are typically located around the neck, upper chest, armpit, and groin. Some are genetic; others are a result of friction such as clothes rubbing on skin.

Massage is okay. Take care not to pull skin tags during the massage.

Stretch marks. Also called *striae*, stretch marks begin as red to pink linear scars that eventually fade to silvery white. These streaks often result from extreme stretching of the skin. This can be the result of pregnancy, bodybuilding, sudden weight gain, or severe swelling resulting from accident or surgical complications.

Deep massage is contraindicated on stretch marks. Massage will not remove or reduce stretch marks because they are not a buildup of scar tissue. They are tearing, thinning, or overstretching of skin that actually reduces its thickness.

Warts. Also known as a *verruca,* a wart is a mass of cutaneous elevations caused by a contagious virus, the papillomavirus (Figure 12-16). Most warts are not cancerous, although some can be.

Local massage is contraindicated because warts are contagious.

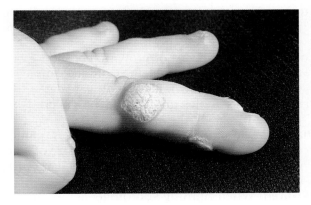

Figure 12-16   Warts.

Transdermal patches are used for conditions such as hormone replacement therapy and by clients who are trying to stop using tobacco products. Because the massage lubricant will weaken the adhesive, avoid up to 2 inches around the patch area.

If an area of complaint is under the transdermal patch, consult with the client's physician and obtain permission to remove the patch. Proceed with the massage as usual. After the massage, clean the area with alcohol and reapply the patch.

Mole Changes

Observing any changes and reporting those changes to the client is an added service in massage therapy. Because this profession uses the skin as the primary organ of contact, we have the unique opportunity to notice any changes in the skin's surface. These changes are noted both visually and tactilely.

Mole changes may occur more often with people who are exposed to natural and artificial UV light. Mole changes may also be associated with friction or irritation from clothing (particularly bra straps), elastic waistbands, eyeglasses, or hard hats. Changes in moles should be noted and discussed with the client. A referral may be made to a medical doctor for diagnosis and possible treatment.

Common moles and melanoma do not look alike. Using the ABCDEF method of mole assessment listed below, you will be able to detect changing moles as they occur. Point these moles out to your clients and ask them to continue checking their moles at home. A mirror can be used for hard-to-see places on the body. If moles have any of the abnormal characteristics listed below, see a physician immediately.

Asymmetry. Asymmetry means that if a line were drawn down the middle, it does not create two equal halves. Common moles are symmetrical and round. Malignant moles are asymmetrical.

Border. The edges or borders of early malignant melanoma are uneven, often containing scalloped or notched edges.

Color. Different shades of brown or black are often the first sign of a problem. Common moles are evenly shaded brown. Black moles are darker than surrounding moles and should be checked by a physician.

Diameter. Common moles are usually less than one quarter inch in diameter (6 mm), the size of a pencil eraser. Early melanomas tend to be larger than common moles.

Elevated. When running your finger across the skin, common moles are smooth and malignant moles are elevated.

Fast-growing. Common moles do not grow fast, if at all. Malignant moles change their size rapidly, indicating metastasis.

Also, look for a sore that does not heal properly. This may indicate skin cancer. Ask your client to check with his or her physician.

MINI-LAB

Take the bottom of a clear glass and press it into the heel of your hand. Describe the color changes and possible explanation for these changes. What would happen to the skin cells if the pressure were prolonged? How does this experiment reflect what happens to the skin when clients are bedridden? How can massage, with its circulatory effects, aid to prevent decubitus ulcers (bedsores)?

SKIN AND THE IMPORTANCE OF TOUCH

 There are so many other forms of communication that can be and should be used. Not just pictures and melodies, but touch, dance, and food.

—Pete Seeger

Although comprehension of anatomy and physiology is vital to the understanding of the skin, it is the sense of touch itself that enables us to actually experience this knowledge. *The sense of touch is the massage therapist's main avenue used to affect another human being and is the body's main method of gathering information about itself. In contrast, an artist uses the sense of vision, and a musician uses the sense of hearing to communicate with others. Touching can affect us physically, intellectually, psychologically, and emotionally.*

Aristotle was the first to enumerate the five senses. Of all the senses, only touch involves the entire body. The other four senses reside in the head. Indeed, touch is not one sense, but many. Touch can detect deep pressure or light stroking. It can differentiate between the weight of a feather and the skin's immersion in water.

The skin is temperature sensitive. It can distinguish between the warmth of wooden bleacher seats on a summer day and the cool shade found beneath the live oaks lining the still bayous of the South. It communicates intrusions, from the tickle of a kitten's fur to the intense pain of a nail piercing your shoe sole.

Touch is the most primitive of all sensations. Among the many studies that have been conducted, touch is the earliest sensory system to become functional in the human embryo. When the embryo

ASHLEY MONTAGU, PhD

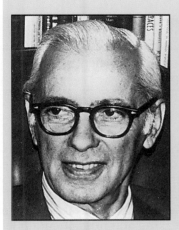

Born: June 28, 1905; died:
November 16, 1999.

*"To be kind, to be, to do,
and to depart gracefully."*

Born in London, Ashley Montagu studied at the University of London and the University of Florence before coming to the United States in 1927. He earned his doctorate from Columbia University in 1937. That same year, he published his first book, *Coming into Being Among the Aborigines.* Between 1937 and 1988, he authored more than 50 books, most of which are in their second or third editions.

Montagu's long and distinguished academic career included positions at some of the most respected schools in the country. He was a professor of anatomy at Hahnemann Medical College and Hospital, Philadelphia from 1938 to 1949, chairman of the Department of Anthropology at Rutgers University from 1940 to 1955, and a lecturer at Princeton University from 1978 to 1983. During this period, Montagu also held many other concurrent positions in education, professional associations, the United Nations, and the media.

Montagu realized that touch is an enormously important experience for every human being, not only from birth but also from the moment that life begins in the womb. As a professor of anatomy and anthropology, he was inspired to begin researching the effects of touch and nurturing after reading an article on the effects of thyroid surgery on two groups of rodents. The first group, with a 75% survival rate, was cared for by a woman doctor who caressed each rodent at feeding time. In the second group, the animals all died very rapidly. They were cared for by a male laboratory attendant who threw food into the cages and roughly clanged the door. The article noted this but attached no significance to it, but Montagu did. In sharing this study with a class he was teaching, a student from a farming area told Montagu that everyone knows that newborn animals must be licked by their mother or they soon die. These were the clues that led him to begin his research on effective nurturing. As a scientist, Montagu scientifically solved the mysteries concerning the attributes that make up what we understand to be love. In his own words, "It [love] is the communication to another, by demonstrative acts, of your profound involvement in their welfare."

His works have emphasized that a healthy mental state results from effective nurturing. Of his own findings, he says that "the most surprising of all things was that doctors had rarely understood this."

Most of Montagu's written work deals in some way with the human condition. His book, *Touching: the Human Significance of the Skin,* is a must-read for all massage therapists. He is also well known for *The Elephant Man* and *Man's Most Dangerous Myth: the Fallacy of Race,* now in its sixth edition.

Montagu's awards included the following:

- Distinguished Achievement Award from American Anthropological Association (1987)
- Darwin Award from the American Association of Physical Anthropologists (1994)
- American Humanist of the Year Award (1995)

He received more than a dozen major awards and two honorary doctorate degrees during his long and prolific career. When asked once what he would like future massage therapists to remember, he said, "To understand that what they are doing is very important indeed. That by caressing another human being's body, in which you are trained to do, I hope, by communicating this involvement in their welfare, what you are doing is what human beings should always be doing, all the days of their lives—caressing other people."

is less than 6 weeks old, measuring less than an inch long from crown to rump, light stroking of the upper lip or wings of the nose will cause bending of the neck and trunk away from the source of stimulation. At this stage of gestation, neither the eyes nor ears have developed.

The skin and the brain arise from ectoderm, the same cells that give rise to the entire nervous system, including the sense organs of smell, taste, hearing, and vision—all of which keeps the organism informed about what is going on in its environment. Because of the ectoderm connection, the skin is considered exposed neural tissue, and, in contrast, the brain is immersed skin. We can therefore regard the skin as a superficial nervous system.

Perhaps the fact that touch is such a primal sensation is precisely what makes it such a powerful therapeutic tool. Our first lessons about love and tenderness are learned through the medium of touch. Whether breast- or bottle-fed, our first meals were touch centered. Touch communicated some of our early experiences with pain. Quite often, this sense played a major role in the physical and emotional healing of those same wounds. Everyone, whether nurse or patient, massage therapist or client, parent or child, lover or friend, can look back on a time when touch played a personal role that was extremely important.

Touch is our first means of communication, and the skin is our main organ of sensation. We can see, hear, and think about something, but it is through touch that the event becomes part of our personal experience. Touch can alter how we perceive the world. Touch can also stimulate us to action.

Our intention during a massage can alter the result of the session. If you approach the massage with too many personal or therapeutic agendas, you may not be able to listen to what the body is telling you. This is very similar to having a one-sided conversation with someone; when you do all the talking, all you hear is yourself! Sometimes in massage therapy our desire to "help" interferes with our actual ability to observe what the client needs to happen. It helps to be willing to approach the massage table as a blank slate, willing to listen.

In massage, touch is not a monologue but rather dialogue. The client's body leads you in a certain direction, and you follow. Your hands, in turn, communicate with the client's tissue, and it responds accordingly. Spoken communication and the tissue response you feel in the client's skin give you the information you need to create therapeutic impact. Your hands become sensitive miniature microphones sensing restrictions in the tissue. With this information, you can verify or discard your original therapeutic assessment and offer the client the fullness of your therapeutic abilities.

Then if we combine the approaches of the two preceding paragraphs, we can create a session that is client focused and experience led. In this time of being both full and empty, the massage therapist can actually bring awareness to the clients and initiate the dialogue that can effect positive change.

MINI-LAB

Write about a time in your life when touch was meaningful to you in a personal way.

Touch Research

Many doctors, nurses, biochemists, and psychologists have developed studies on the effects of touch (see Box 12-2 for effects of massage on the skin). These studies address physical, intellectual, psychological, and emotional themes. Several studies discussed here are considered groundbreaking and fundamental. Below are brief summaries from research that focus on touch as a medium of communication. As you read them and draw your own conclusions, apply the concepts you develop to your attitude about massage and to your role as a caregiver.

BOX 12-2

Effects of Massage on the Skin and Related Structures

- **Increases skin temperature.** Warming of the skin indicates a reduction of stress and other benefits as described in the following.
- **Improves skin condition.** As superficial blood vessels dilate and circulation increases, the skin appears hyperemic. This brings added nutrients to the skin, improving the skin's condition, texture, and tone. Clinical observations have determined that massage also improves the appearance (i.e., color and texture) of the skin.
- **Stimulates sebaceous glands.** Stimulation of the sebaceous (oil) glands causes an increase in sebum production. This added sebum improves the skin's condition.
- **Stimulates sudoriferous glands.** Sudoriferous (sweat) gland stimulation increases insensible perspiration. Insensible perspiration is the constant evaporative cooling that occurs as microscopic beads of perspiration evaporate from the skin's surface.
- **Improves skin pathologies.** Unless a condition contraindicates massage, skin pathologies may improve by decreasing redness, reducing thickening or hardening of the skin, increasing healing of skin abrasions, and reducing itching.
- **Reduces superficial keloid formation.** Massage applied to scar tissue helps reduce the formation of superficial keloids in the skin and excessive scar formation in the soft tissues beneath the site of massage application.

Harry Harlow

In 1958, Dr. Harry Harlow, a pioneer in touch deprivation research, conducted experiments at the University of Wisconsin that involved the isolation of monkeys during their early developmental stages. After a period, these touch-deprived monkeys exhibited evidence of emotional and social impairment. The lack of touch during their early developmental years had left them neurotic and socially retarded. Most female monkeys refused mating, becoming hostile and aggressive when approached. The monkeys that did mate rejected or harmed their young. Harlow observed that during periods of isolation, the infant monkeys valued tactile stimulation more than they did nourishment. Harlow then created two artificial surrogate "mothers." One was a bare wire sculpture of a monkey that housed a bottle of formula. The other was a fur-covered wire monkey that felt and smelled like other monkeys, but offered no food. The infant monkeys preferred to cling to the "mother" who provided a semblance of physical contact without nourishment rather than to the wire models that provided food (Figure 12-17).

Bernard Grad

Dr. Bernard Grad, a Canadian biochemist, conducted his groundbreaking touch research on mice and barley seedlings in the early 1960s. In the first of his double-blind studies, 300 mice were selected and injured in the same manner. One third were allowed to heal without intervention, one third were held by medical students who did not profess to heal, and one third were held by a faith healer. After just 2 weeks, the mice held by the faith healer recovered remarkably faster than the mice in both of the other groups.

For the barley seed study, Grad soaked the seeds in a saline solution to get them off to a bad start. The seeds were then divided into three equal groups. The first group was watered with tap water. The second group was soaked using water held by disinterested students, and the last group was irrigated with water that was held by a renowned healer. The seeds that were watered by the healer held water sprouted faster, grew taller, and contained more green chlorophyll than either of the other two groups.

Delores Krieger

In the 1970s, Dr. Delores Krieger, a professor at New York University, became interested in touch healing through studies like Grad's. She was fascinated with the idea that intent was so important in healing touch. Using noninvasive techniques, Krieger wanted to apply the concepts of Grad's work in a way that could help her patients.

Through Krieger's research a tangible relationship emerged between touching and healing. She was able to measure an increase in the hemoglobin content of the blood, which directly corresponded to levels of touching. Hemoglobin is the oxygen-carrying molecule in red blood cells. In Krieger's study, when a healthy person placed his hands on or near an ill person for 10 to 15 minutes with the intent to heal, this was enough to cause the measurable increase.

MINI-LAB

Touching with Intent

1. Locate a partner.
2. Assign one person to be the giver and one person to be the receiver. Sit facing each other.
3. The receiver extends his or her hands, palms up. The giver places his or her hands on the receiver's hands, palm down. Both the giver and the receiver close their eyes.
4. The giver becomes unfocused, disinterested, and mentally distracted as the receiver stays open and passive for 2 minutes.
5. After that time, the giver becomes very aware, interested, and concerned about the receiver. This attitude is maintained for 2 minutes.
6. Reverse roles and repeat.
7. Share your experiences with each other. Did you notice any differences when the attitudes changed? Does intent really alter how touch is received? How can you use this information during a massage therapy session?

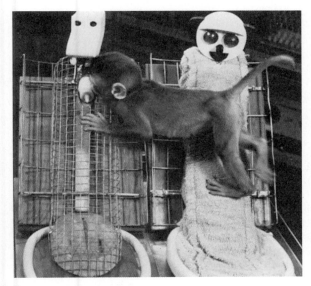

Figure 12-17 Harlow's monkeys. (Courtesy of Harlow Primate Laboratory; Madison, Wis.)

Tiffany Field

Dr. Tiffany Field, professor of pediatrics, psychology, and psychiatry of the University of Miami School of Medicine, began a research project to study the effects of massage on 40 premature babies. Half of the group was massaged three times a day for 15 minutes for 10 days. The massaged infants gained 47% more weight. They spent less time in the hospital than the babies who were not massaged, even though both groups of babies had the same number of feedings and averaged the same intake per feeding. The massaged babies were also more active, alert, and stayed about 6 days less in the hospital. The massaged babies were also more socially active, more responsive, and had better coordination and motor skills than the nonmassaged babies (1986).

Field found that individuals who received a 15-minute seated massage twice a week showed increased cognitive ability, performed better on math tests, and completed problems with increased accuracy and speed. These individuals also experienced a significant decrease in tension over individuals who practiced traditional relaxation techniques without massage (1997).

Many additional research studies are being conducted by the Touch Research Institute.

Wayne Dennis

In the 1950s, Dr. Wayne Dennis published his findings on what he called *infant* and *child retardation*. His research was based on his experience at an orphanage in Beirut, Lebanon. He found that the facility that contained the orphanage was more than adequate, but because of the orphanage's meager income, personnel was limited to one employee to 10 infants. The children were only taken out of the cribs for feedings, diaper changing, and a daily bath. The children remained in the crib until they began to pull up on the sides. From that point, they were placed in a playpen during the daylight hours with two other children. Opportunities for touch were very limited. A large number of these children died, even though they were receiving adequate nutrition and hygiene. The children who did survive were dwarfed or deformed.

The explanation Dennis gave for his findings of marasmus (wasting away) combined with the tragic death rates of the Lebanese orphanages were the result of touch deprivation and lack of physical stimulation and learning opportunities. The employees were so busy providing for their physical needs, they did not have time to hold and caress the infants. When aides were hired to rock and sing to these children, mortality rates dropped 70%.

Abraham Maslow

In the 1960s, Maslow, a renowned psychologist, placed the needs of human beings in a sequential order, from the most basic and concrete to the most ideal and abstract. He believed that these needs directed all human behavior and as these basic needs

are met, other needs of the hierarchy begin to emerge until the individual reaches what he terms *self-actualization*. Maslow called this progression the *Theory of Human Motivation*.

Maslow states that we have basic human needs, beginning from the concrete, biological needs of food and water to abstract needs of self-actualization. Maslow characterized the self-actualized person as self-accepting, striving to help others, and engaging in activities that will help the person achieve the highest potential. His model was later redesigned, with the help of other psychologists, to a more comprehensive list of human needs (Box 12-3). It is interesting to note that touching and skin contact are ranked very high on the list, just below the individual's needs for a safe shelter. *Many massage therapists attest to the fact that clients often receive massage to get their touch needs met.*

BOX 12-3

Hierarchy of Human Needs

1. Survival
2. Safety
3. Touching, skin contact
4. Attention
5. Mirroring and echoing
6. Guidance
7. Listening
8. Being real
9. Participating
10. Acceptance
    - Others are aware of, take seriously and admire the Real You
    - Freedom to be the Real You
    - Tolerance of your feelings
    - Validation
    - Respect
    - Belonging and love
11. Opportunity to grieve losses and to grow
12. Support
13. Loyalty and trust
14. Accomplishment
    - Mastery, "power," "control"
    - Creativity
    - Having a sense of completion
    - Making a contribution
15. Altering one's state of consciousness, transcending the ordinary
16. Sexuality
17. Enjoyment or fun
18. Freedom
19. Nurturing
20. Unconditional love (including connection with a Higher Power)

Data from Glasser, 1985; Maslow, 1962; Miller, 1981; Weil, 1973.

SUMMARY

The skin is so much more than an external covering. It is a highly sensitive boundary between our body and the environment. It offers protection, heat exchange, vitamin synthesis, waste removal and serves as a membrane of interfacing. We can survive without sight, taste, smell, or hearing, but to lose our sense of touch would leave us walled off from our environment and from contact with others.

Touch offers us a sense of nourishment and a feeling of belonging. The need for touch intensifies during periods of stress and cannot be addressed without the participation of another person. Without touch, we experience profound psychological pain. If massage does nothing more than nurture the human race through touch, our profession will be providing a great service. Scientific research shows it does that and more.

MATCHING I

List the letter of the answer next to the term or phrase that best describes it.

A. Epidermis
B. Sudoriferous glands
C. Melanocytes
D. Keratin

E. Cuticle
F. Arrector pili
G. Dermis
H. Sebaceous glands

I. Melanin
J. Nails
K. Hair follicles
L. Superficial fascia (subcutaneous layer)

_____ 1. The tough ridge of skin that grows out over the nail's base

_____ 2. True skin, containing adipose tissue, blood vessels, and nerve endings

_____ 3. A tough, fibrous protein that provides protection by waterproofing the skin

_____ 4. Tiny muscles that pull the hair upright

_____ 5. Skin layer that contains melanocytes, nails, and pore openings

_____ 6. Granules that gives color to the skin, hair, and the iris of the eye

_____ 7. Glands whose primary functions are to regulate temperature and eliminate wastes

_____ 8. Connective tissue layer that connects the dermis to underlying structures

_____ 9. Specialized cells in the epidermis where skin pigment is synthesized

_____ 10. Thin hard plates found on the distal ends of the fingers and toes

_____ 11. Can become irritated during a massage due to allergies, hair pulling, and inadequate amount of lubricant

_____ 12. Glands that secrete a fatty substance, lubricating both the hair and the epidermis

MATCHING II

List the letter of the answer next to the term or phrase that best describes it. One will be used twice.

A. Free nerve endings
B. Ruffini end organs

C. Pacinian corpuscle
D. Merkel disk

E. Meissner corpuscles
F. Krause end bulb

_____ 1. Detects light pressure, adapts slowly, and is located in the dermis

_____ 2. Deep pressure-sensitive receptor; shape resembles an onion slice; adapts quickly

_____ 3. Responds to heat and deep, continuous pressure

_____ 4. Detects light pressure, adapts slowly, and is located in the epidermis

_____ 5. Pain receptors

_____ 6. Receptor that is believed to respond to cold

_____ 7. Also known as *nociceptors*

MATCHING III

List the letter of the answer next to the term or phrase that best describes it.

A. Acne
B. Eczema
C. Impetigo
D. Ringworm

E. Malignant melanoma
F. Athlete's foot
G. Herpes simplex

H. Psoriasis
I. Seborrhea
J. Warts

_____ 1. An inflammatory skin infection caused by staphylococci or streptococci bacteria characterized by raised, fluid-filled sores that itch or burn; highly contagious

_____ 2. A mass of cutaneous elevations caused by the papillomavirus

_____ 3. Skin disease of the sebaceous glands marked by an increase in the amount of oily secretions

_____ 4. A fungal infection of the foot characterized by discoloration of the skin and a ridge of red tissue

_____ 5. A chronic skin disease characterized by red, flaky skin elevations which typically involve the scalp, elbows, knees, back, and buttocks; not contagious

_____ 6. One of the most malignant and lethal skin cancer types

_____ 7. A chronic type of dermatitis characterized by redness, watery discharge, crusting, scaling, itching, and burning; not contagious

_____ 8. A bacterial infection of the sebaceous glands

_____ 9. A group of fungal diseases characterized by itching, scaling, painful lesions characterized by a raised red-ringed patch

_____ 10. A viral infection also called *cold sores* or *fever blisters*

Bibliography

Applegate EJ: *The anatomy and physiology learning system,* ed 2, Philadelphia, 2000, WB Saunders.

Clarke AM, Clarke AD: *Early experience: myth and evidence,* London, 1976, Open Books.

Crawley J, Van De Graaff, KM: *A photographic atlas for anatomy and physiology,* Englewood, Colo, 2002, Morton.

Dennis W: Causes of retardation among institutionalized children, *J Genet Psychol* 96(7):1-12, 1960.

Field T, Bauer C, Nystrom J: Tactile/kinesthetic stimulation effects on preterm neonates, *Pediatrics* 77(5):654-658, 1986.

Frazier MS, Drzymkowski JW: *Essentials of human diseases and conditions,* ed 2, Philadelphia, 2000, WB Saunders.

Gerson J: *Standard textbook for professional estheticians,* Albany, 1992, Delmar.

Gould BE: *Pathophysiology for the health-related professionals,* Philadelphia, 1997, WB Saunders.

Grad B: The influence of an unorthodox method of treatment on wound healing in mice, *Int J Parapsychol* 3:5-24, Spring, 1961.

Grafelman T: *Graf's anatomy and physiology guide for the massage therapist,* Aurora, Colo, 1998, DG Publishing.

Guyton A: *Human physiology and mechanisms of disease,* ed 3, Philadelphia, 1982, WB Saunders.

Harlow H, Harlow M: Learning to love, *Am Sci* 54:244-272, 1966.

Haubrich WS: *Medical meanings: a glossary of word origins,* New York, 1984, Harcourt Brace Jovanovich.

Jacob S, Francone C: *Elements of anatomy and physiology,* Philadelphia, 1989, WB Saunders.

Juhan D: *Job's body: a handbook for bodyworkers,* Barrington, NY, 1987, Station Hill Press.

Kalat JW: *Biological psychology,* ed 2, Belmont, Calif, 1984, Wadsworth.

Kapit W, Elson LM: *The anatomy coloring book,* ed 3, New York, 2002, Benjamin Cummings.

Kendall F, McCreary E: *Muscles: testing and function,* Baltimore, 1983, Williams and Wilkins.

Kordish M, Dickson S: *Introduction to basic human anatomy,* Lake Charles, La, 1985, McNeese State University.

Krieger D: Therapeutic touch: the imprimatur of nursing, *Am J Nurs* 75(5):784-787, 1975.

Marieb EN: *Essentials of human anatomy and physiology,* ed 4, New York, 1994, Benjamin Cummings.

McAleer N: *The body almanac,* Garden City, NY, 1985, Doubleday.

Merck and Company: *Merck manual,* ed 17, Whitehouse Station, NJ, 1998, Research Laboratories, Merck.

Montagu A: *Touching: the human significance of the skin,* ed 2, New York, 1978, Harper and Row.

Mosby's medical, nursing, and allied health dictionary, ed 4, St Louis, 1994, Mosby.

Newton D: *Pathology for massage therapists,* ed 2, Portland, Ore, 1995, Simran.

Olsen A, McHose C: *BodyStories: a guide to experiential anatomy,* Barrytown, NY, 1991, Station Hill Press.

Premkumar K: *Pathology A to Z: a handbook for massage therapists,* Calgary, Canada, 1996, VanPub Books.

Skin Cancer Foundation, The: *The ABCD's of moles and melanomas,* New York, 1985, The Foundation.

Solomon EP, Phillips GA: *Understanding human anatomy and physiology,* Philadelphia, 1987, WB Saunders.

Spitz R: Hospitalism: an inquiry into the genesis of psychiatric conditions of early childhood, *Psychoanal Study Child* 2:53-74, 1945.

Taber's cyclopedic medical dictionary, ed 13, Philadelphia, FA Davis.

Thibodeau G, Patton K: *Structure and function of the body,* ed 11, St Louis, 2000, Mosby.

Tortora GJ: *Introduction to the human body: the essentials of anatomy and physiology,* ed 3, New York, 1994, HarperCollins.

Tortora GJ, Grabowksi SR: *Principles of anatomy and physiology,* ed 9, New York, 2000, John Wiley.

Werner R: *A massage therapist's guide to pathology,* ed 2, Baltimore, 2002, Lippincott Williams & Wilkins.

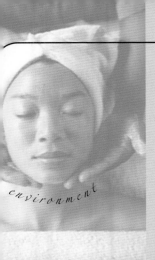

environment

Skeletal System

13

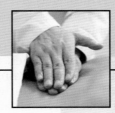

"What a piece of work is man."

—Shakespeare

pressure

STUDENT OBJECTIVES

After completing this chapter, the student should be able to:

- Recall the functions of the skeletal system
- Group the bones into classifications, according to their shape
- Determine if a bone is part of the axial skeleton or the appendicular skeleton
- List and describe the surface markings located on bones
- Compare synarthrotic, amphiarthrotic, and diarthrotic joints
- Identify the six types of synovial joints and give an example of each
- Demonstrate all the possible movements of the synovial joints
- Name types of skeletal pathologies, giving characteristics and massage considerations of each

technique

knowledge

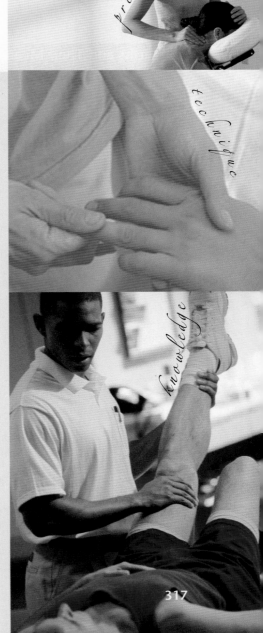

INTRODUCTION

The skeletal system is composed of bones, cartilage, ligaments, and joints. Not only do they provide protection and support movement, they also store minerals such as calcium and phosphorus.

Bone is living tissue. The skeletons in anatomy classes, laboratories, and museums are the mineral salts that remain after death. Bones are one of the hardest materials in the body, yet they are relatively light, somewhat flexible, and able to resist tension and other forces of stress.

The human body has 206 bones. Bones are the "steel girders" of the body, forming its internal framework. Mammals ranging from humans to bats to elephants have remarkably similar skeleton systems. For example, seven vertebrae are in the human cervical spine and also in the long-necked giraffe and the no-necked whale.

The skeletal system is of the utmost importance to the massage therapist because it constitutes the road map for locating muscles. Muscles attach to bones at various bony markings known as *origins* and *insertions*. Because bones are hard, most markings are easy to palpate. Learn your bony markings well in the next chapter because they will guide you into locating the muscles that are causing your clients the most difficulty. Muscles are located between their attachment points.

The study of the skeletal system is multifaceted. Besides the basic structure and function of bone, we will also study movement and leverage, types of joints and articulations, skeletal pathologies, and the general bony markings.

FUNCTIONS

The skeletal system serves a wide variety of functions. They are as follows:
- Supports the body through a bony framework.
- Protects the body's vital organs.
- Provides movement by giving leverage through muscle attachments.
- Blood cell production occurs in the red marrow of long bones and is called **hemopoiesis** (blood cell formation), producing both red and white blood cells.
- Fats storage occurs in yellow bone marrow and is released when needed.
- Mineral storage takes place in bone tissue. Minerals such as calcium phosphate, calcium carbonate, phosphorus, magnesium, and sodium are stored and released when the body needs them. This is accomplished through vascular interfacing with the bones.

CLASSIFICATION OF BONES

Bones are scientifically classified according to their shape. These categories are long bones, short bones, flat bones, irregular bones, and sesamoid bones (Figure 13-1). A brief description follows.

Long. These bones are longer than they are wide. Examples are the humerus, radius, ulna, femur, tibia, fibula, metacarpals, metatarsals, and phalanges.

Short. Short bones are generally cube-shaped, such as the carpals and tarsals.

Flat. Flat bones are thin and flattened like pancakes. The sternum, ribs, scapula, and certain skull bones are flat bones.

Irregular. Consider this a catch-all category for bones that do not fit in other categories. Irregular bones are certain cranial bones, facial bones, the vertebrae, and the hyoid bone.

Terms and Their Meanings Related to the Skeletal System

Term	Meaning
amphi	on both sides
arthric	joint
blast	germ cell or bud
bursa	a leather sac
clast	to break
condyle	knuckle
crepitus	a rattle
diarthrotic	two; joint
epiphysis	epi—upon, over; to grow
facet	small face
foramen	a passage
fossa	depression
Haversian	British physician and anatomist (1650-1702)
kyphosis	humpbacked condition
ligament	band
lordosis	bent backward
meatus	a passage
ossification	bone; to make
osteo; osseo	bone
periosteum	around, about; bone
process	going before
ramus	a branch
sesamoid	sesame seed–like; shaped
scoliosis	crooked condition
skeleton	dried up
symphysis	together with, joined; to grow
synarthrotic	together; joint
trochanter	a wheel or runner
tubercle	a hump, knob, or swelling; small
tuberosity	a swelling
Volkmann	German physician (1800-1877)

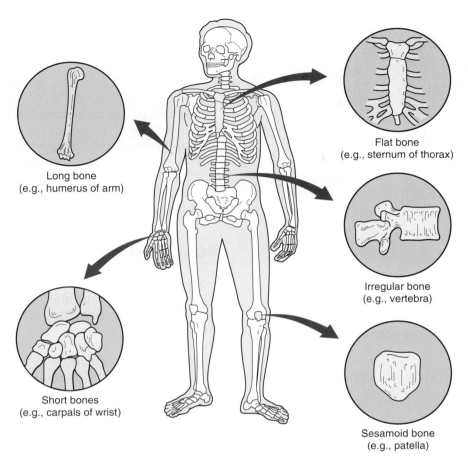

Figure 13-1   Examples of long, short, flat, irregular, and sesamoid bones.

Sesamoid. Sesamoid bones are small, round bones that are embedded in certain tendons. Often, they are found in the hands and feet. The largest sesamoid bone is the patella (kneecap), which is embedded in the quadriceps femoris tendon.

ANATOMY OF A LONG BONE

The following is a detailed discussion on the long bone (Figure 13-2):

Diaphysis: The shaft of a long bone

Epiphysis: The two ends of a long bone

Metaphysis: In mature bone, this is where the diaphysis and the epiphysis meet; in immature bone, it is where the *epiphyseal plate,* or "growth plate," exists

Epiphysial line: Replaces the epiphyseal plate when bone growth is complete

Periosteum: The fibrous, dense, vascular connective tissue sheath around the bone; the life support system of the bone, containing blood and lymphatic vessels, nerves, and bone-forming cells (osteoblasts) for growth and fracture healing; is absent on articular surfaces

Medullary cavity: The hollow space in the bone's center containing the marrow

Articular cartilage: The hyaline cartilage that is associated with joints and covers the epiphysis

Interosseous ligament: A tough membrane that interconnects select bones (e.g., ulna/radius, tibia/fibula) by attaching to their periosteum; it is also referred to as the *interosseus membrane*

The following two canal networks form the system of vascular channels in bone tissue. Blood reaches the medullary cavity by these systems of vessels. Blood cells that are formed in the red bone marrow can exit the bone and enter the general circulation through the two types of canal systems: (1) *Haversian canals* (minute vascular canals that run longitudinally through the bone) and (2) *Volkmann's canals* (connect the Haversian canals, running horizontally through the bone; see Figure 13-3).

HISTOLOGY

The skeletal system is composed of five types of connective tissue: osseous tissue, cartilage, ligaments, periosteum, and bone marrow. These tissue types have

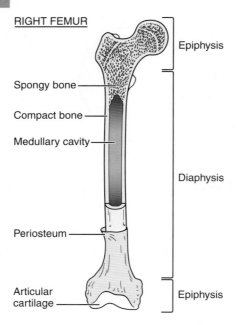

RIGHT FEMUR

Epiphysis

Spongy bone

Compact bone

Medullary cavity

Diaphysis

Periosteum

Epiphysis

Articular
cartilage

Figure 13-2   Long bone anatomy.

been introduced in Chapter 11. Osseous tissue can be classified according to its texture, differing only in bone density (see Figures 13-2 and 13-3). The categories include (1) *spongy bone*, which is the lighter of the two and is a latticelike network found in the center of long bones that are typically filled with red and yellow bone marrow, and (2) *compact bone*, which is more dense for added strength, forming the periphery of all bones and a portion of the shaft of long bones.

The rest of this section introduces the following microscopic cells within the skeletal system:

Osteoblasts are bone-forming cells found in the periosteum.

Osteoclasts are cells in bone that break down bone tissue to maintain homeostasis of calcium and phosphates and to repair bone.

Osteocytes are mature osteoblasts that soon become embedded in the bone matrix.

BONE DEVELOPMENT

Bones develop by a process known as **ossification**. The two types of ossification are *intramembranous ossification*, or the formation of bone from a membrane, and *intracartilaginous ossification*, or the formation of bone from cartilage. Intramembranous ossification is found on the roof and sides of the skull, and intracartilaginous ossification is found in the bones of the extremities. Ossification begins between the sixth and seventh week of embryonic life and continues throughout adulthood. Both mechanisms of ossification replace preexisting connective tissue with osseous connective tissue.

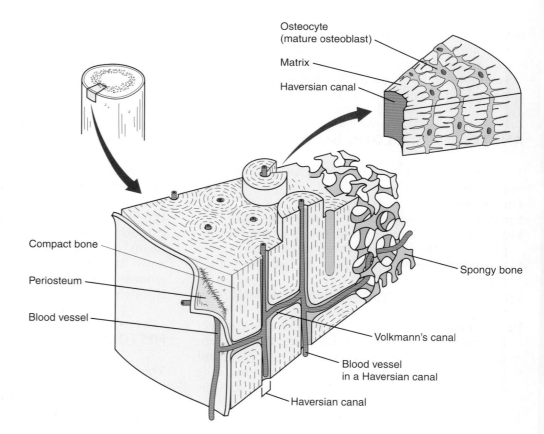

Figure 13-3   Haversian and Volkmann's canal, and periosteum.

Osteocyte
(mature osteoblast)

Matrix

Haversian canal

Compact bone

Periosteum

Blood vessel

Spongy bone

Volkmann's canal

Blood vessel
in a Haversian canal

Haversian canal

BONE HEALTH, EXERCISE, AND AGING

When you exercise, the skeletal system becomes stressed by pulling forces (e.g., gravity, tendons, and ligaments). The body responds to the demand of physical activity by secreting a hormone (calcitonin), which moves calcium into the bones. Osteoblasts are also stimulated to create more bone tissue and hence stronger bones. It cannot be emphasized enough that bones must be physically stressed to remain healthy. When we remain physically active and when muscles and gravity exert force on our skeleton, the bones respond by becoming stronger.

To maintain mineral homeostasis, the osteoclasts break down the bone's minerals and move it into the blood while osteoblasts replace the bone lost to metabolism. Both processes occur at about the same rate, so we constantly have the same amount of bone tissue. As we age, the osteoclasts in our bones breakdown bone faster than the osteoblasts can rebuild it. This lack of bone replacement makes the bones porous (osteoporosis). This condition is more common in postmenopausal women because of the body's drop in estrogen.

SKELETAL DISTRIBUTION

To make the study of the skeletal system easier, it can be divided into the following two distinct regions (Figure 13-4): (1) *axial skeleton,* consisting of the bones associated with the central axis of the body (skull, vertebrae, sternum, ribs) and (2) *appendicular skeleton,* comprising the extremities (arms, legs, and girdles).

☐ Axial skeleton
☐ Appendicular skeleton

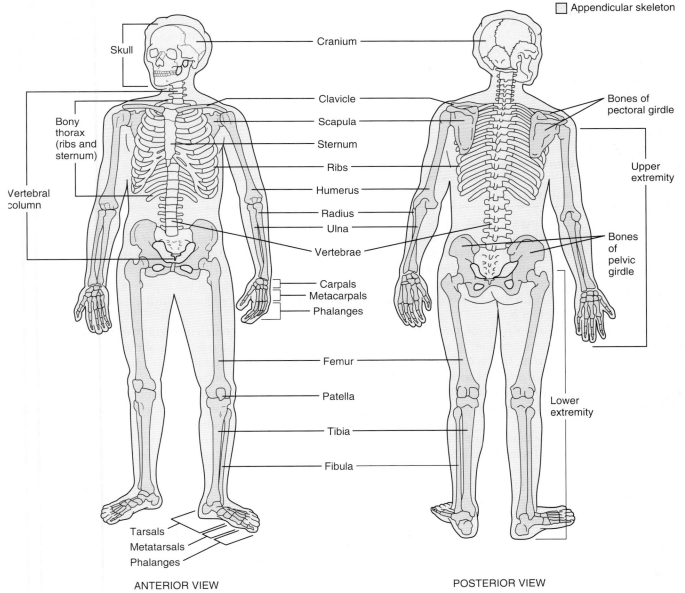

ANTERIOR VIEW

POSTERIOR VIEW

Figure 13-4　Skeletal bones with axial and appendicular divisions.

Axial Skeleton

The axial skeleton contains 80 bones, including the following:

- **Skull:** Total of 29 bones (eight bones in the cranium, 14 bones in the face, six ear ossicles, and one hyoid bone)
- **Vertebral column:** Total of 26 in an adult and 31 or 33 unfused bones in the embryo, depending on how many bones are present in the coccyx
- **Sternum:** One fused bone in the adult and three unfused bones in the embryo
- **Ribs:** Total of 24 bones or 12 pairs of bones, which are located in the thorax

Extremities or Appendicular Skeleton

The appendicular skeleton contains 126 bones, including the following:

- **Pectoral** or **shoulder girdle:** The clavicle and scapula on both sides totaling four bones
- **Upper limbs:** Total of 60 bones with 30 bones in each upper limb, including the humerus, ulna, radius, eight carpals, five metacarpals, and 14 phalanges
- **Pelvic girdle:** Often referred to as the *hip bone*, consisting of a left and right ilium, ischium, and pubis; the two bones in the adult pelvis were once six unfused bones in the embryo
- **Lower limbs:** Total of 60 bones with 30 bones in each lower limb, including the femur, patella, tibia, fibula, seven tarsals, five metatarsals, and 14 phalanges

BONY MARKINGS

Bones are not smooth but are marked with bumps, holes, and depressions. These markings are located where muscles, tendons, and ligaments attach and where nerve and blood vessels pass. These exterior marks are called **bony markings**, *bony landmarks,* or *surface markings.* Even though specific bones have not been introduced, examples for each surface marking are given to make the connection between the word and an example of a bony marking (Table 13-1). Use

TABLE 13-1

Bony Marking Terminology

Bony Marking	Description	Example
Angle	Projecting corner of a bone	Mandibular angle
Border	Linear bony ridge, often the edge of a bone	Medial border of the scapula
Condyle	Rounded projection that forms a joint; knuckle-shaped	Lateral condyle of the femur
Crest	Very prominent linear elevation	Iliac crest
Epicondyle	Projection over a condyle	Medial epicondyle of the humerus
Facet	Small, smooth, shallow depression articulating with another bone	Vertebral articular facet
Foramen	Hole or opening for blood vessels and nerves to pass	Foramen magnum of the occipital bone
Fossa	Shallow depression in a bone	Glenoid fossa of the scapula
Groove	Depression that accommodates a structure	Intertubercular groove
Head	Rounded end of a bone	Fibular head
Line	A narrow bony ridge that is less prominent than a crest	Superior nuchal line
Meatus	Tubelike opening in a bone that forms a tunnel or canal	External auditory meatus of the temporal bone
Notch	Deep indention or a narrow gap in a bone	Trochlear notch
Process	General term for any prominence or prolongation from a bone	Styloid process of the radius
Protuberance	Knoblike protrusion of a bone	External occipital protuberance
Ramus	Long branchlike bony prolongation of a bone	Superior pubic ramus
Ridge	Elongated projection from a bone	Supracondylar ridge
Spine	Sharp, slender projection of a bone	Spine of the scapula
Trochanter	Large rough process found only on the femur	Greater trochanter
Tubercle	Rounded projection usually blunt and irregular	Lesser tubercle of the humerus
Tuberosity	Large, rounded rough projection	Deltoid tuberosity

this information to remember specific markings on bones when they are presented in Chapter 14.

ARTICULATIONS

Articulations, or joints, are the meeting places for bones. Every bone in the human skeleton articulates with at least one other bone, except the hyoid bone. Where a joint exists, so do joint movements. This movement may be limited, such as sutures in the cranium; or it may be very mobile such as the ball-and-socket joint of the shoulder. Joints serve the following two purposes: (1) they hold the bones together through the ligaments, and (2) they allow a rigid skeletal system to become somewhat flexible by changing their relative positions to one another when acted on by muscles or outside forces.

Articulations can be classified according to how the joint functions.

Three Types of Articulations

These joints take into account the range or degree of movement that is allowed physiologically. The three types of joints are synarthrotic, amphiarthrotic, and diarthrotic. Use the mnemonic SAD to recall the terms *s*ynarthrotic, *a*mphiartic, and *d*iarthrotic (Figure 13-5).

Synarthrotic. Movement in these joints is absent or extremely limited. Examples of synarthrotic joints are the sutures found in the cranium.

Amphiarthrotic. These joints are slightly movable, such as intervertebral joints or the sternoclavicular joints, and move apart only a few millimeters. Many amphiarthrotic joints are classified as gliding diarthrotic joints.

Diarthrotic. Also known as *synovial joints,* these are freely movable joints. Diarthrotic joints allow movement in one, two, or three dimensions and feature articular cartilage and synovial membranes. Many synovial joints also contain bursa sacs (bursae) filled with synovial fluid. Examples of synovial joints include knees, elbows, hips, shoulders, wrists, and knuckle joints of the fingers and toes.

Diarthrotic/Synovial Joints

The following structures are associated with synovial joints (Figure 13-6):

Articular cartilage. The articulating surfaces of the bones that participate in the joint structure are covered with hyaline cartilage. This allows gliding movements to occur more easily.

Joint capsule. Diarthrotic joints are enclosed with a joint capsule in the shape of a sleeve. The joint

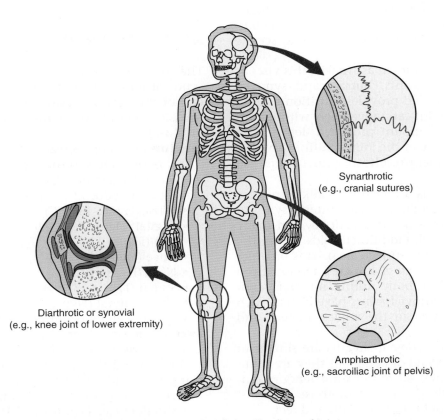

Diarthrotic or synovial
(e.g., knee joint of lower extremity)

Synarthrotic
(e.g., cranial sutures)

Amphiarthrotic
(e.g., sacroiliac joint of pelvis)

Figure 13-5 Functional classifications of joints.

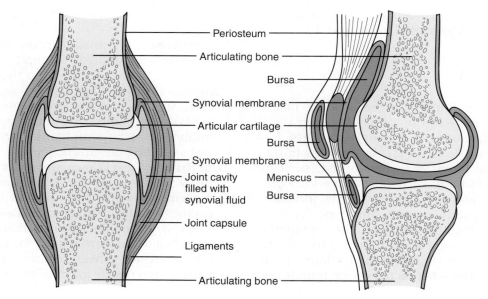

Figure 13-6   A joint.

capsule is a continuation of the periosteum of the bones involved in the joint. The sleeve is lined with a synovial membrane that produces synovial fluid, hence the name synovial joint.

Joint cavity. The joint cavity is the enclosed space between the bones of the joint filled with lubricating (synovial) fluid.

Synovial membrane. The synovial membrane lines the interior of the joint capsule and the bursae. The function of the membrane is to secrete synovial fluid.

Synovial fluid. Also known as *synovia,* this viscous fluid is found in joints, bursae, and synovial sheaths. Synovial fluid provides nutrition and lubrication so the joint can move freely without undue friction. The amount produced depends on the physical activity of the joints. Stiffness and reduction of movement results in synovial fluid deficiency.

Bursae. A bursa sac is a collapsed saclike structure with a synovial membrane that contains synovial fluid. It looks like a deflated balloon, and many bursae also have villi (additional folds within the bursae to increase the surface area). This provides a cushion that protects a muscle's tendon from rubbing against the bone during muscular contraction. Not all synovial joints have bursae, such as the joints located in the ankles, fingers, and toes.

Synovial sheaths. Synovial sheaths are similar to bursae except, instead of being flat they are tubular. These structures surround long tendons, increasing the gliding capacity of those tendons, and are mainly found in the hands and feet.

Ligaments. Ligaments reinforce and stabilize the joint. Bursae are often found between the ligaments and the joint capsule. Ligaments are connective tissues that connect bone to bone. Functionally, ligaments are an extension of the bone to allow lightness, flexibility, and added strength.

ACTION TERMINOLOGY

The following are the movements provided by the synovial joints of the body. Use the activity at the end of this section as an educational dramatization to assist you in learning these joint movements (Figure 13-7).

Flexion bends or decreases the angle of a joint. *Lateral flexion* refers to the direction of flexion.
- Shoulder (Figure 13-7, *A*)
- Elbow (Figure 13-7, *B*)
- Wrist (Figure 13-7, *C*)
- Digital (Figure 13-7, *D*)
- Hip (Figure 13-7, *E*)
- Knee (Figure 13-7, *F*)
- Neck (Figure 13-7, *G*)
- Spinal (Figure 13-7, *H*)
- Neck: Lateral (Figure 13-7, *I*)
- Spinal: Lateral (Figure 13-7, *J*)

Extension straightens or increases the angle of a joint. *Hyperextension* is a continuation of extension beyond the anatomical position, as in bending the head backward and may or may not be used by some textbook authors.
- Shoulder (see Figure 13-7, *A*)
- Elbow (see Figure 13-7, *B*)

IDA PAULINE ROLF, PhD

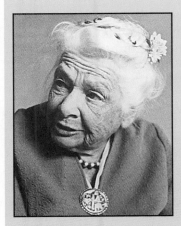

Courtesy of the Rolf Institute, Boulder, Colo. Photo by David Kirk Campbell.

Born: May 18, 1896; died: March 19, 1979.

"God didn't come down and tell me; I had to find it out through many years of experience. The work came first; the inspiration came later."

It was the middle of World War II, and most of America's men were far from home. Women began to fill roles they had never dreamed they would. One such young woman, Ida Pauline Rolf, accepted a position with the Rockefeller Institute, even though her father was dead set against it. War or peace, a proper lady stayed home where she belonged. After all, her family had money; she did not need to earn her way.

Rolf had a mind of her own, however, going on to earn a doctorate in biochemistry. She was just as passionate about philosophy and general semantics as she was about studying the science of the body, so she explored homeopathy, was heavily influenced by osteopathy, and practiced yoga under the direction of a tantric yogi. Perhaps even more integral to her success than any other factor was that she was not afraid to pursue new directions.

Her studies led her to Amy Cochran, an osteopath who claimed to have received her special abilities through a psychic encounter with Dr. Benjamin Rush, the physician who signed the Declaration of Independence. When Rolf returned to New York, she began work on a 45-year-old woman who had physical disabilities since the age of 8. Within a few years, the woman was up and walking.

Rolf believed that bodies are created balanced and comfortably supported by gravity, but injuries, overwork of one muscle group, or other postural dysfunctions result in fascia that are too tight or loose. Thus our bodies expend energy less efficiently and fight gravity rather than being supported by it. She also believed that anything that made individuals feel fear or guilt could manifest itself in bad physiology. For her, both mental and physical health make up two sides of the same coin.

Rolfing methodically restructures connective tissue through work on one body section at a time, gradually working deeper and deeper. The massage that we know today as rolfing was first called structural integration. When the container is aligned properly, the "stuff" inside functions as it should. Structural integration helps achieve homeostasis. Rolf's vision went beyond physical change because she believed that this tissue reorganization of the body was necessary to achieve spiritual growth.

Rosemary Feitis, Rolf's longtime assistant, writes, "[Ida] was not interested in curing symptoms; she was after a bigger game. She wanted nothing less than to create new, better human beings. The ills would cure themselves; the symptoms would melt as the organisms became balanced."*

To achieve this Nirvana, Rolf used her fingers, elbows, and forearms to loosen myofascial restrictions, moving tissue until it was "in the right place." Then she would proceed to the next problem area, asking for feedback as she went along. Eventually she developed a sequence of 10 progressive sessions now referred to as the *Basic Ten*.

One of the most lasting impressions of Rolfing seems to be that sessions must be painful to be effective. This was never Rolf's goal, and because of the body's reactive mechanism to pain, too much force may have a negative effect on results. In fact, Feitis quotes her as saying: "Don't just go in there as though you were a locomotive charging in at a 100 miles an hour. In general, if there is trouble going on inside the body, fascia on the outside will be so tight it will tend to protect the area that's in trouble. So don't barge through fascia. If you are doing the right thing, and there isn't some deep pathology, the fascia will let go—let you in."

Continued

IDA PAULINE ROLF, PhD—cont'd

Rolf tried to teach others what she had discovered and, at the same time, attempted to preserve the integrity of her work, but her commitment was singular. Not everyone shared her enthusiasm, work ethic, or understanding of the body. According to Feitis, Rolf did not want "mechanicalness." She taught whomever she could and cautioned them to wait until they were experienced before considering themselves *rolfers*.

Eventually, an invitation to present her work at Esalen, a California resort proving ground for new movements, landed Rolf in the midst of a new type of student. She began to teach her work to those with no preconceived notions and a variety of backgrounds. The world began to take notice of her work. Research established its effectiveness. Articles were published. The Rolf Institute, formerly the Guild for Structural Integration, was created in the early 1970s.

Today, rolfing has undergone some change. Not all practitioners accept Rolf's notion of the perfect or ideal body. Others plan sessions according to clients' needs instead of the Basic Ten. It is hard to say what Rolf would think about this evolution.

*From Feitis R: *Ida Rolf talks about rolfing and physical reality,* New York, 1978, Harper and Row.

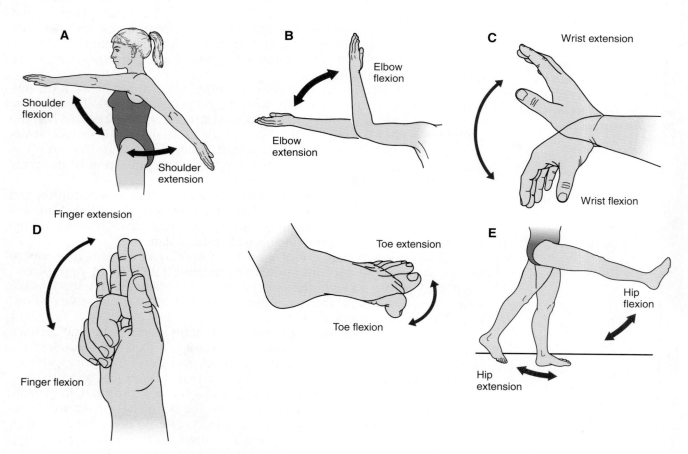

Figure 13-7   A, Shoulder flexion and extension; **B,** elbow flexion and extension; **C,** wrist flexion and extension; **D,** digital flexion and extension; **E,** hip flexion and extension.

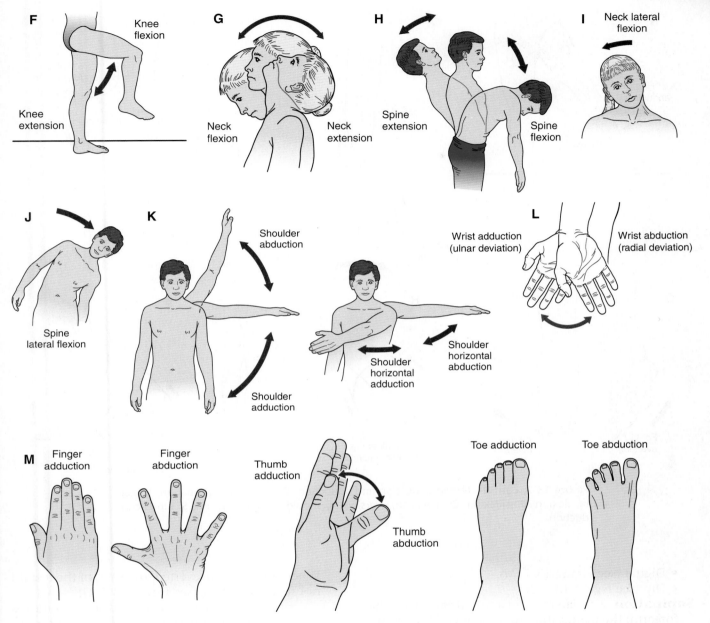

Figure 13-7, cont'd F, Knee flexion and extension; **G,** neck flexion and extension; **H,** spinal flexion and extension; **I,** neck: lateral flexion; **J,** spinal: lateral flexion; **K,** shoulder abduction and adduction; horizontal abduction and adduction; **L,** wrist abduction and adduction; **M,** digital abduction and adduction. *Continued*

- Wrist (see Figure 13-7, *C*)
- Digital (see Figure 13-7, *D*)
- Hip (see Figure 13-7, *E*)
- Knee (see Figure 13-7, *F*)
- Neck (see Figure 13-7, *G*)
- Spinal (see Figure 13-7, *H*)

Abduction is movement away from the median plane. *Horizontal abduction* refers to the direction of abduction.

- Shoulder (Figure 13-7, *K*)

- Wrist, also referred to as *radial deviation* (Figure 13-7, *L*)
- Digital (Figure 13-7, *M*)
- Hip (Figure 13-7, *N*)

Adduction is movement toward the median plane. *Horizontal adduction* refers to the direction of adduction.

- Shoulder (see Figure 13-7, *K*)
- Wrist: Also referred to as *ulnar deviation* (see Figure 13-7, *L*)

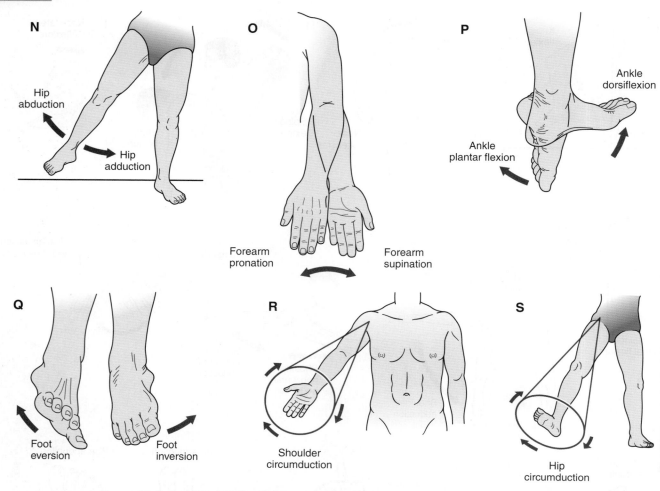

Figure 13-7, cont'd   N, Hip abduction and adduction; **O**, supination, pronation; **P**, plantar flexion, dorsiflexion; **Q**, inversion, eversion; **R**, shoulder circumduction; **S**, hip circumduction.

- Digital (see Figure 13-7, *M*)
- Hip (see Figure 13-7, *N*)

Supination is a lateral (outward) rotation of the forearm; the palm is turned up so it can hold a cup of "soup" (Figure 13-7, *O*).

Pronation is medial (inward) rotation of the forearm; the palm is turned down so it is prone to spill (see Figure 13-7, *O*).

Plantar flexion is extension of the ankle so that the toes are pointing downward, increasing the ankle angle anteriorly (Figure 13-7, *P*).

Dorsiflexion is flexing the foot dorsally so that the toes are moving toward the shin, as in walking on the heels (see Figure 13-7, *P*).

Inversion is elevation of the medial edge of the foot so that the sole is turned inward (or medially). When both feet are inverted, the soles of the feet face each other (Figure 13-7, *Q*).

Eversion is elevation of the lateral edge of the foot so that the sole is turned outward (or laterally).

When both feet are everted, the soles of the feet do not face each other (see Figure 13-7, *Q*).

Circumduction occurs when the distal end moves in a circle and the proximal end is relatively fixed; it can be described as cone-shaped range of motion, but is actually a combination of several movements such as flexion, extension, adduction, and abduction.

- Shoulder (Figure 13-7, *R*)
- Hip (Figure 13-7, *S*)
- Digital (Figure 13-7, *T*)

Rotation is circular movement when a bone moves around its own central axis. *Lateral* and *medial rotation* refer to direction of rotation. *Upward* and *downward* rotation are terms reserved for the scapula. The knee can be rotated slightly when flexed.

- Head/neck (Figure 13-7, *U*)
- Spinal (Figure 13-7, *V*)
- Shoulder (Figure 13-7, *W*)
- Hip (Figure 13-7, *X*)

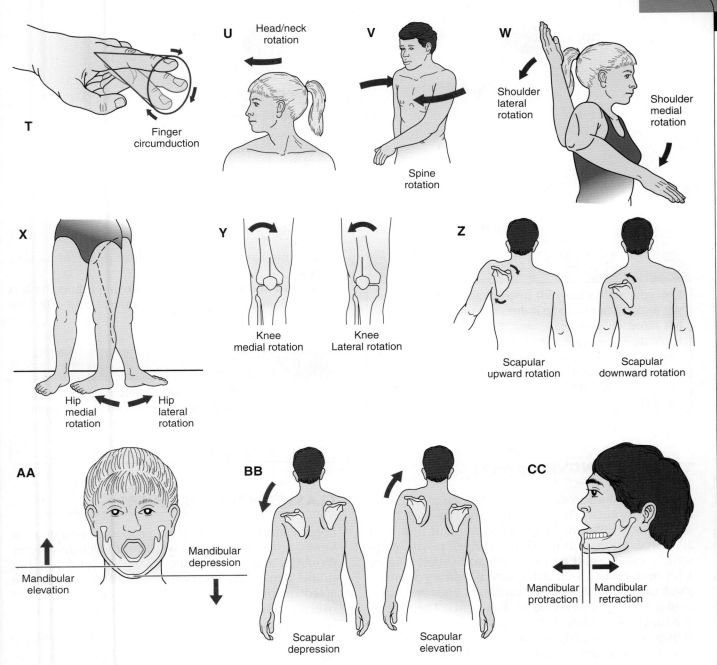

T, Digital circumduction; **U,** head/neck rotation; **V,** spinal rotation; **W,** shoulder rotation; **X,** hip rotation; **Y,** knee rotation; **Z,** scapular rotation; **AA,** mandibular elevation and depression; **BB,** scapular elevation and depression; **CC,** mandibular protraction and retraction.

Continued

Figure 13-7, cont'd

- Knee (Figure 13-7, *Y*)
- Scapular (Figure 13-7, *Z*)

Elevation is raising or lifting a body part.
- Mandibular (Figure 13-7, *AA*)
- Scapular (Figure 13-7, *BB*)

Depression is lowering or dropping a body part.
- Mandibular (see Figure 13-7, *AA*)

- Scapular (see Figure 13-7, *BB*)

Protraction is movement forward.
- Mandibular (Figure 13-7, *CC*)
- Scapular (Figure 13-7, *DD*)

Retraction is movement backward.
- Mandibular (see Figure 13-7, *CC*)
- Scapular (see Figure 13-7, *DD*)

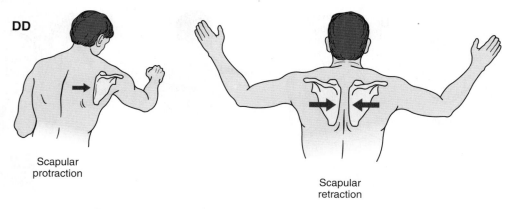

Scapular
protraction

Scapular
retraction

Figure 13-7, cont'd   **DD**, scapular protraction and retraction.

MINI-LAB

Flex your right elbow 90 degrees and affix your upper arm to your torso so it does not move. Place your left hand on your right ulna. Begin to pronate and supinate your right hand. Notice how your ulna never moves. Also notice how the thumb moves 180 degrees. Pronation and supination results from the radius rotating over the distal end of the ulna. The hand follows the movement of the radius.

TYPES OF SYNOVIAL JOINTS

Synovial or diarthrotic joints are the largest classification of joints. The following six types of these joints allow different ranges of movement in one or all three known dimensions: hinge, pivot, ellipsoidal, saddle, gliding, and ball-and-socket (Figure 13-8 and Table 13-2). All synovial joints contain a joint capsule and articular cartilage. They may also contain bursae and accessory ligaments. The following further describes these joints:

Hinge (monoaxial) joint movements are limited to flexion and extension, such as the knee, elbow, and interphalangeal joints.

Pivot (monoaxial) joints allows movement that is limited to rotation, such as the atlantoaxial or the proximal radioulnar joint.

Ellipsoidal (biaxial) joints are essentially a reduced ball-and-socket joints. Ellipsoidal joints allow flexion, extension, abduction, and adduction, but rotation is not permitted. Examples of ellipsoidal joints are radiocarpal joints located in the wrist.

Saddle (biaxial) joints allow movements of flexion, extension, abduction, adduction, opposition, reposition, circumduction, but rotation is not permitted. An example of a saddle joint is the carpometacarpal of the thumb.

Gliding (triaxial) joints permit all movements but are limited to gliding; gliding is present in acromioclavicular and intertarsal joints, to name a few.

Ball-and-socket (triaxial) joints, such as the hip and shoulder, permit all movements and offer the greatest range of motion.

MINI-LAB

Perform the different joint movements such as abduction of the arm and hip, rotation of the cervical region, flexion of the elbow and knee, and so on, until all joint movements have been experienced. Shout each movement as it is performed.

CLASSIFICATION OF LEVERS

For the muscular system to produce movement at joints, it uses the skeletal system for leverage. A lever (bone) is a rod that is moved by use of a fulcrum (joint). For a lever to be set in motion, it must be acted on by two forces. These forces are resistance (weight of body and/or an object) and effort (muscular contraction).

Levers are categorized into the following three classes according to how the fulcrum, effort, and resistance are arranged (Figure 13-9):

Class 1 lever. Class 1 levers resemble a seesaw. The fulcrum is positioned between the effort and the resistance. The cranium sitting on top of the vertebrae is an example of a class 1 lever. This is the least common type of lever in the body.

Class 2 lever. Class 2 levers function like a wheelbarrow. The fulcrum is at one end, the resistance is in the middle, and the effort is at the opposite end. One example of a class 2 lever is raising up on the toes.

Class 3 lever. Class 3 levers are the most common. The fulcrum is at one end, the effort is located in the central portion, and the resistance is at the opposite end. Two examples of a class 3 lever are flexing the arm and the elbow.

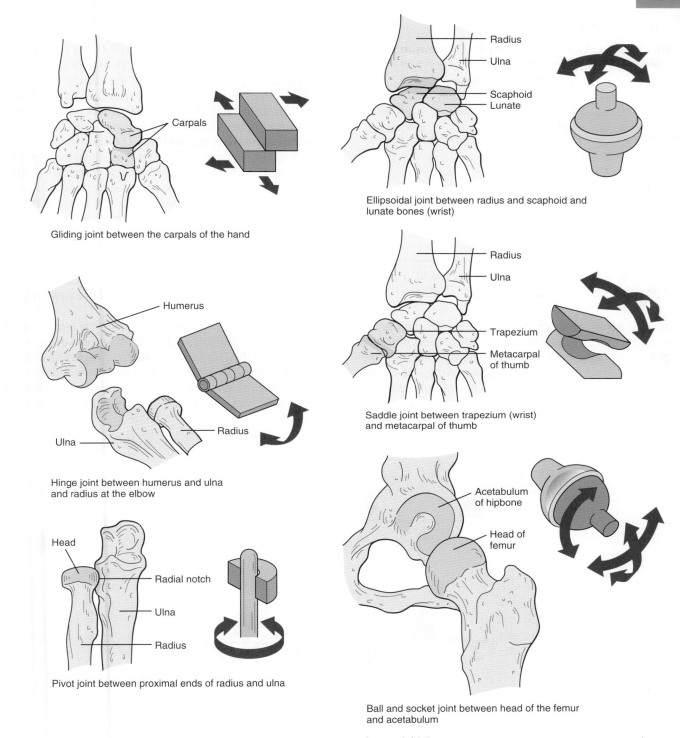

Gliding joint between the carpals of the hand

Carpals

Ellipsoidal joint between radius and scaphoid and lunate bones (wrist)

Radius
Ulna
Scaphoid
Lunate

Hinge joint between humerus and ulna and radius at the elbow

Humerus
Ulna
Radius

Saddle joint between trapezium (wrist) and metacarpal of thumb

Radius
Ulna
Trapezium
Metacarpal of thumb

Pivot joint between proximal ends of radius and ulna

Head
Radial notch
Ulna
Radius

Ball and socket joint between head of the femur and acetabulum

Acetabulum of hipbone
Head of femur

Figure 13-8   Types of synovial joints.

SKELETAL PATHOLOGIES

Ankylosing spondylitis. This is an inflammatory disease leading to calcification and fusion of the joints between vertebrae or in the sacroiliac joint. It is more common in males between the ages of 20 and 40. Pain and stiffness is present in the hips and lower back that can progress upward along the spine. Inflammation can lead to loss of movement of the joints (ankylosis) and kyphosis (hunchback). When the joints between the thoracic vertebrae and the ribs are involved, the person may have difficulty in expanding the rib cage for inhalation.

Clients need to be positioned for their comfort. Clients who have kyphosis may need extra cushioning

TABLE 13-2

Joint Classification According to Movement

	Abduction/ Adduction (Frontal Plane)	Flexion/ Extension (Sagittal Plane)	Rotation (Horizontal Plane)
Hinge (monoaxial)		×	
Pivot (monoaxial)			×
Ellipsoidal (biaxial)	×	×	
Saddle (biaxial)	×	×	
Gliding (triaxial)	×	×	×
Ball and socket (triaxial)	×	×	×

Modified from Grafelman S: *Graf's anatomy and physiology guide for the massage therapist,* Aurora, Colo, 1998, DG Publishing.

in the upper anterior thorax. Massage treatments should retain joint mobility, strengthen weak muscles, and stretch tight ones. Ankylosed joints should not be forced into movement. The back and limbs should be massaged gently. Heat packs help ease pain. Breathing exercises may help mobilize the thorax.

Arthritis. *Arthritis* refers to several chronic joint diseases characterized by inflammation, swelling, and pain in the joints. More than 100 types of arthritis are known, and it usually affects the smaller joints first, such as those found in the hands and feet. The three most common types of arthritis are rheumatoid arthritis, osteoarthritis, and gouty arthritis. Lyme disease can also cause arthritis.

- **Rheumatoid arthritis**. Rheumatoid arthritis (RA) is a systemic arthritis that destroys the synovial membranes of joints, especially the hands and feet. These membranes are replaced by fibrous tissues that add to the joint stiffness already present. This process greatly reduces the person's range of motion. Usually, bilateral involvement occurs with a high incident of crippling deformity. The cause of RA is unknown, but it is believed to be an autoimmune disease. People who have RA experience flare-ups and remissions.

  Massage is contraindicated when a client has a flare-up. When the client's RA is in remission, massage can be administered safely. Massage can help reduce stress, and gentle range of motion can help increase joint mobility. A shorter massage is indicated because the client may be on painkillers and/or

MECHANICAL ASPECT　　COMMON EXAMPLE　　MUSCULOSKELETAL COMPONENT

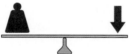

First-class lever

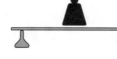

Second-class lever

Figure 13-9   Three classes of levers.

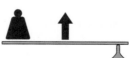

Third-class lever

Weight　Fulcrum　Force

antiinflammatory drugs that may result in inadequate feedback.

- **Osteoarthritis**. Osteoarthritis (OA) is a chronic, progressive erosion of the articular cartilage resulting from chronic inflammation. Often called the *wear and tear arthritis,* the most commonly affected areas are weight-bearing joints, which may eventually become immovable. OA, which is more common than RA, is most often seen in the elderly population.

  When applying massage techniques, do not use excessive pressure. Deep massage and range of motion are contraindicated because these movements may injure the client.

- **Gouty arthritis**. Gouty arthritis is characterized by an abnormal accumulation of uric acid in the body. Uric acid is produced when nucleic acids are metabolized; the uric acid is then converted to monosodium urate crystals. In most cases, uric acid is eliminated in urine. Some individuals, usually males, either produce excessive amounts or are unable to excrete the uric acid, resulting in abnormally high levels of uric acid in the bloodstream. The sodium urate crystals eventually settle in the soft tissue around joints, typically the feet and toes, causing irritation, pain, and swelling. Typically, the first joint affected is the metatarsophalangeal joint of the great toe. Initial bouts may just last a few days; later bouts may last several weeks.

  Local massage is contraindicated.

- **Lyme disease**. Also called *Lyme arthritis,* Lyme disease is a recurrent form of arthritis caused by a bacterium *Borrelia burgdorferi,* which is transmitted by a tick bite. The condition was originally described in the community of Lyme, Conn., but has been reported throughout North America and in other countries. Large joints such as the knee and hip are most commonly involved, with local inflammation and swelling. Headaches, fever, and a scaly red skin eruption (erythematous), often precede the joint manifestations.

  Because the disease is chronic (lasting months or years), the massage needs to be tailored to the client's individual symptoms. Massage is contraindicated if the client is experiencing widespread inflammation. Generally, a gentle, full-body massage is indicated. Passive range of motion retains joint mobility.

Bunions. Bunions are an abnormal medial tilting and enlargement of the joint between the first metatarsal of the great toe and the associated proximal phalanx. However, bunions can also be found on the lateral side of the foot. They are caused by chronic irritation and pressure from poorly fitted shoes or inflammation of the plantar fascia.

Local massage is contraindicated because of the pain, but general massage is all right.

Bursitis. Acute or chronic inflammation of the bursae is called *bursitis.* It is most often caused by direct trauma or chronic overuse of the tendon located over the bursae. The most common types of bursitis are subacromial bursitis, subcoracoid bursitis, subscapular bursitis, olecranon bursitis, trochanteric bursitis, ischial bursitis, prepatellar bursitis, and calcaneal bursitis.

Cold packs can be applied to reduce swelling. Local massage is contraindicated until swelling has subsided. Friction can then be done, with ice packs applied afterward.

Crepitus. A noisy discharge that may resemble a cracking sound and is produced by the body. Examples of crepitus are popping joints, rubbing of bone fragments, and flatulence. It can be the result of air present in subcutaneous tissue and can often be palpated.

If the crepitus is not resulting from a structural disorder, massage is fine. If associated anomalies are present, massage must be tailored accordingly.

Dislocation. A dislocation (luxation) occurs when bones are forced out of their normal position in the joint cavity. Associated ligaments, tendons, joint capsules, and blood vessels are torn in the process. An incomplete or partial dislocation is known as a subluxation.

Local massage, especially range of motion, is contraindicated. However, once the inflammation is gone and the healing is complete, range of motion, deep specific friction, and cross-fiber friction can help increase mobility of the joint.

Fractures. A fracture is a break, chip, crack, or rupture in a bone. Osseous tissue is highly vascularized, but healing sometimes takes months because sufficient calcium and phosphorus are deposited slowly in new bone. The three most common types of fractures are simple fractures, compound fractures, and stress fractures (Figure 13-10).

- **Simple**. Also known as *closed fractures,* in simple fractures, the bone is broken but does not protrude through the skin.
- **Compound**. Also known as *open fractures,* a broken end of the bone breaks through the skin and soft tissue.
- **Stress**. Stress fractures are accumulated microfractures (small cracks in a bone). These fractures are commonly a result of repeated activity, such as running on a hard surface or high-impact aerobic dance. A common place for stress fractures is the metatarsal bones.

  While the healing bone is immobilized, massage can help maintain circulation, joint mobility, and muscle tone and reduce edema. Elevate the affected limb to help with drainage. Massaging muscles close to the immobilized part can decrease spasms and reduce pain. A full-body, gentle massage can help reduce

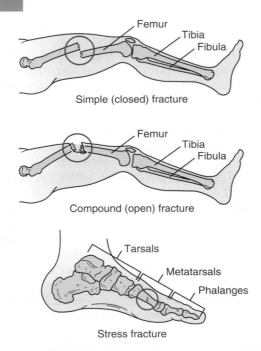

Simple (closed) fracture

Compound (open) fracture

Stress fracture

Figure 13-10   Three of the most common types of fractures.

client stress. Once healing is complete, massage and range of motion can help the client regain joint mobility and increase tone in muscles that have atrophied. Massage should begin slowly and gently, about a week after the cast has been removed. Gradually, range of motion can increase and massage can be deeper.

Herniated disk. Protrusion of the nucleus pulposus from the annulus fibrosus of an intervertebral disk is called a herniated disk. The protruding disk may impinge on nerve roots, causing numbness and pain. This may be a result of improper lifting or direct trauma. A herniated disk is also called a ruptured disk or a slipped disk.

Massage does little for a herniated disk. It can relieve pain from the muscles splinting around the area, which functions to limit movement. Muscles to treat are the iliopsoas, erector spinae, transversospinalis, quadratus lumborum. Heat can be used for its analgesic affect, as long as you follow its use with 20 minutes of ice.

Kyphosis. Often called hunchback or hyperkyphosis, kyphosis is an exaggeration of the normal posterior thoracic curve (Figure 13-11, A). Typically, the chest appears caved in, the arms tend to hang in the front of the body, and the head moves forward. Kyphosis may be caused by rickets (vitamin D deficiency), degeneration of the intervertebral disks in older adults, tuberculosis of the spine, chronic spasticity of the pectoralis major and minor and serratus anterior muscles, or weak rhomboid major and minor muscles. Mild to moderate back pain often accompanies this spinal condition. Rounded shoulders and a Dowager's hump

are occasionally classified as a mild form of kyphosis.

Some relief can be gained by massage of the involved muscles (pectoralis major/minor, serratus anterior, rhomboids major/minor). Take care not to overstretch the spine.

Lordosis. Often regarded as hyperlordosis, lordosis, or swayback, is an exaggeration of the anterior curvature of the lumbar concavity (see Figure 13-11, B). A tightening of the back muscles followed by a weakening of the abdominal muscles is typical. Increased weight gain or pregnancy may cause or exacerbate this spinal condition. Because of the anterior tilt of the pelvis, hamstring problems are common.

Treat the muscle of both anterior and posterior tilt. Remind the client to strengthen the abdominal muscles and not to gain excess weight.

Osteoporosis. Osteoporosis is characterized by decreased bone mass and increased susceptibility to fractures. As women and men age, they produce much smaller amounts of estrogen (estrogen helps keep calcium in bones). The decreased hormone levels result in osteoblasts becoming less active, so a decrease in bone mass occurs. Bone mass becomes so depleted the skeleton can no longer withstand mechanical stress. Osteoporosis is responsible for hip fractures, shrinkage of the backbone, height loss, hunched backs, other bone fractures, and considerable pain.

Gentle massage, avoiding undue pressure over bones, is indicated. Avoid or limit joint mobilizations.

Scoliosis. Scoliosis is the lateral deviation or curvature in the normally straight vertical line of the vertebral column, usually in the thoracic region (see Figure 13-11, C). Causes of scoliosis include congenital malformations of the spine; poliomyelitis; paralysis; chronic spasticity of the iliopsoas, quadratus lumborum, and the paraspinal

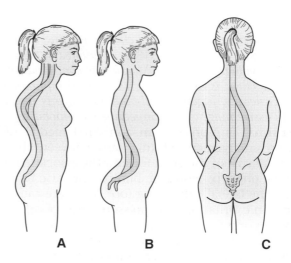

A   B   C

Figure 13-11   **A,** Kyphosis; **B,** lordosis; **C,** scoliosis.

muscles; and postural deviations such as poor posture, distorted rib cage, and leg length discrepancy. Unequal position of the hips or shoulders may be one indication of this condition. Early detection and intervention may prevent progression of the curvature. The vast majority of people who have scoliosis are female (80%).

Massage is indicated and should include the iliopsoas, quadratus lumborum, and the paraspinal muscles. Deep muscle stripping, fascial work, and gentle stretches are indicated. Take care not to overstretch the spine.

Separation. A separation is almost the same as a dislocation, but the joint structure is simply pulled and stretched; the bone is not displaced out of the joint capsule.

Gentle massage, avoiding undue pressure over the separated bones, is indicated.

Spondylolisthesis. Spondylolisthesis is an anteriorly displaced vertebra, usually the fifth lumbar vertebra over the first sacral vertebra. This condition can range from mild to severe. Severe cases deform the spine.

Gentle massage of the back is indicated. Tight muscles in the area can be stretched, but should not be forced.

Spondylosis. This is a general term for degenerative of the spinal column resulting from OA, often called *arthritis of the spine*.

Gentle massage, avoiding undue pressure over the spine, is indicated.

Sprain. Joint trauma that stretches or tears the ligamentous attachments without bone displacement is called a sprain. Sprains cause pain and possible temporary disability. Depending on the severity of the injury, it is not uncommon for a ligamentous sprain to take 6 months to a year to completely rehabilitate because ligaments have few blood vessels.

Acute ligament sprains can be classified into the following three grades or degrees of severity (Figure 13-12):

- **First degree** is the stretching of the ligament without tearing or up to a 20 percent tearing of fibers with no palpable defects. The joint structures can maintain efficient motion and hold against resistance.
- Between 20% and 75% tearing of a ligament with a defect felt in the structure is **second degree**. The joint structures cannot hold against moderate resistance. Edema is typically found and the muscles surrounding the sprain are splinted to restrict painful movement.
- In a **third-degree** tear, 75% to a complete rupture of the structure (100%) is noted and a "snap" is often heard at the time of injury. A piece of the bone also may be torn away (sprain fracture). A depression in the area of the torn muscle can be

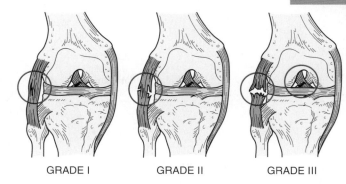

GRADE I   GRADE II   GRADE III

Figure 13-12   Three degrees of sprains.

felt and is usually painful to touch. Function is greatly altered in third-degree tears.

Once a joint is sprained, use RICE (rest, ice, compression, elevation) to bring down the swelling. Seventy-two hours after the initial injury, light effleurage and light friction are helpful massage techniques. Cross-fiber friction is an excellent rehabilitation technique. Do not begin the massage until the client receives medical clearance and DO NOT STRETCH the injured area.

Temporomandibular joint dysfunction. Temporomandibular joint (TMJ) dysfunction is a common ailment afflicting the jaw joint, its musculature, or both. Its chief symptoms are pain (e.g., jaw pain, toothache, headache, or earache), clicking of the joint, and limited range of motion. Causes of TMJ (Figure 13-13) dysfunction include trauma to the joint, chewing hard objects, especially if only on one side of the mouth, biting fingernails, teeth clenching or grinding (bruxism) whether awake or asleep, poor alignment of the upper and lower teeth, and emotional stress. It is estimated that 60% of the population either clench or grind their teeth, but only 25% of these are aware of it.

TMJ dysfunction can be treated with massage. Advanced techniques require the donning of rubber gloves to enter the oral cavity and use ischemic compression to treat the muscles of the jaw (masseter, temporalis, medial and lateral pterygoids), neck, and shoulders (trapezius, rhomboids, levator scapula, scalenes, splenius muscles, and suboccipitals). General massage techniques can benefit the individual because the majority of all TMJ dysfunction is associated with clenching or bruxism, which is often stress related.

Whiplash. Whiplash is a sprain/strain of cervical spine and spinal cord at the junction of the fourth and fifth cervical vertebrae that occurs as a result of rapid acceleration (causing extension) or deceleration (causing flexion) of the body. Because of their greater mobility, the four upper vertebrae act as the lash, and the lower three act as the handle of the whip. Symptoms may include headaches, dizziness, pain, dysphagia (difficulty swallowing), and inflammation.

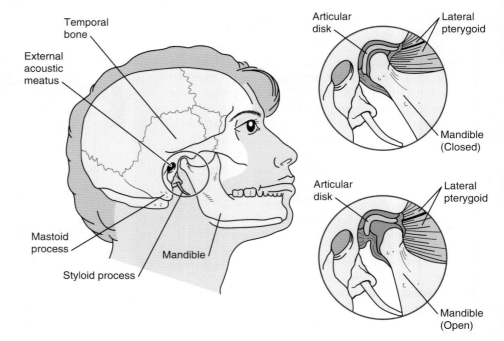

Figure 13-13   Temporomandibular joint.

Wait at least 72 hours after initial injury and treat the scalenes, splenius muscles, and sternocleidomastoid with broad strokes and gentle stretches. Muscles of the upper back should also be addressed. Follow up the session with ice for 20 minutes. Suggest use of ice at home to control inflammation.

See Box 13-1 for the effects of massage on bones.

BOX 13-1

Effects of Massage on Bones

- **Increases mineral retention in bone.** Massage increases the retention of nutrients such as nitrogen, sulfur, and phosphorus in bones.
- **Promotes fracture healing.** When a bone is fractured, the body forms a network of new blood vessels at the break site. Massage increases circulation around the fracture, promoting fracture healing. Increased circulation around a fracture leads to increased deposition of callus to the bone. A callus is formed between and around the broken ends of a fractured bone during healing and is ultimately replaced by compact bone.

SUMMARY

The intricate structures of bone, cartilage, ligament, and joints are what comprise our skeletal system. The skeleton acts as a supportive framework for the rest of our body systems. It protects our delicate internal organs and acts as a storehouse for fats, vital minerals, and blood cell production.

Bones are living tissue that is strong, flexible, and relatively light. The bones of the human body number 206. The study of the skeletal system is not limited to bone alone. It includes the tissue of the bone itself, types of joints, movement, leverage, skeletal pathologies, and the specific bony markings.

Finally, bones are the massage therapist's landmarks to muscle location. Although the various soft tissues are at times indistinguishable from each other, bone is easily palpated. Because muscle attachment is fairly consistent from one person to the next, the bones act as reference points for locating muscles.

MATCHING I

Write the letter of the best answer in the space provided.

A. Pivot
B. Axial skeleton
C. Periosteum
D. Bursae
E. Epiphysis
F. Articulation

G. Synovial fluid
H. Ball and socket
I. Diaphysis
J. Sesamoid
K. Synovial joints
L. Osteoclasts

M. Haversian canals
N. Hemopoiesis
O. Hinge
P. Bony markings
Q. Osteoblasts
R. Medullary cavity

_____ 1. Minute vascular canals running longitudinally down the bone

_____ 2. Lubricating fluid of freely movable joints

_____ 3. Meeting place for bones

_____ 4. Bone forming cells

_____ 5. Shaft of a long bone

_____ 6. Synovial joints with the greatest range of motion

_____ 7. Hollow space within the bone

_____ 8. Blood cell formation

_____ 9. Where muscles, tendons, and ligaments attach

_____ 10. Connective tissue covering around a bone

_____ 11. Freely movable joints

_____ 12. Bone destroying cells

_____ 13. Joint movements are limited to rotation

_____ 14. Small, round bones embedded in tendons

_____ 15. Bones associated with the body's central axis

_____ 16. Ends of a long bone

_____ 17. Joint movements are limited to flexion and extension

_____ 18. Saclike structure containing synovial fluid

MATCHING II

Write the letter of the best answer in the space provided.

A. Flexion	G. Elevation	L. Dorsiflexion
B. Abduction	H. Protraction	M. Eversion
C. Supination	I. Extension	N. Rotation
D. Plantar flexion	J. Adduction	O. Depression
E. Inversion	K. Pronation	P. Retraction
F. Circumduction		

_____ 1. Raising or lifting a body part

_____ 2. Elevation of the medial edge of the foot so that the sole is turned inward

_____ 3. Circular movement; when a bone moves around its own central axis

_____ 4. Movement toward the median plane

_____ 5. Lateral (outward) rotation of the forearm

_____ 6. Straightening or increasing the angle of a joint

_____ 7. Extension of the ankle so that the toes are pointing downward

_____ 8. Elevation of the lateral edge of the foot so that the sole is turned outward

_____ 9. Flexing the foot dorsally so that the toes are moving toward the shin

_____ 10. Medial (inward) rotation of the forearm

_____ 11. Cone-shaped range of motion

_____ 12. Lowering or dropping a body part

_____ 13. Bending or decreasing the angle of a joint

_____ 14. Movement forward

_____ 15. Movement away from the median plane

_____ 16. Movement backward

Bibliography

Applegate EJ: *The anatomy and physiology learning system,* ed 2, Philadelphia, 2000, WB Saunders.

Crawley J, Van De Graaff KM: *A photographic atlas for anatomy and physiology,* Englewood, Colo, 2000, Morton.

Dominguez R, Gajda R: *Total body training,* New York, 1982, Warnerbooks.

Goldberg S: *Clinical anatomy made ridiculously simple,* Miami, 1984, Medmaster.

Grafelman T: *Graf's anatomy and physiology guide for the massage therapist,* Aurora, Colo, 1998, DG Publishing.

Haubrich WS: *Medical meanings, a glossary of word origins,* New York, 1984, Harcourt Brace Jovanovich.

Jacob S, Francone C: *Elements of anatomy and physiology,* Philadelphia, 1989, WB Saunders.

Kapandji IA: *The physiology of the joints,* New York, 1982, Churchill Livingstone.

Kapit W, Elson LM: *The anatomy coloring book,* ed 3, New York, 2002, Benjamin Cummings.

Kordish M, Dickson S: *Introduction to basic human anatomy,* Lake Charles, La, 1985, McNeese State University.

Luttgens K, Wells K: *Kinesiology: scientific basis of human motion,* ed 7, Philadelphia, 1982, Saunders College Publishing.

Marieb EN: *Essentials of human anatomy and physiology,* ed 4, New York, 1994, Benjamin Cummings.

McAleer N: *The body almanac,* Garden City, NY, 1985, Doubleday.

McAtee R: *Facilitated stretching,* Colorado Springs, Colo, 1993, Human Kinetics.

Merck and Company: *Merck manual,* ed 17, Whitehouse Station, NJ, 1998, Research Laboratories, Merck.

Moore KL: *Clinically oriented anatomy,* ed 2, Baltimore, 1985, Williams and Wilkins.

Mosby's medical, nursing, and allied health dictionary, ed 4, St Louis, 1994, Mosby.

Newton D: *Pathology for massage therapists,* ed 2, Portland, Ore, 1995, Simran Publications.

Platzer W: *Color atlas and textbook of human anatomy: locomotor system,* vol 1, ed 3, New York, 1984, Thieme.

Premkumar K: *Pathology A to Z: Handbook for massage therapists,* Calgary, Canada, 1996, VanPub Books.

Solomon EP, Phillips GA: *Understanding human anatomy and physiology,* Philadelphia, 1987, WB Saunders.

Southmayd W, Hoffman M: SportsHealth: the complete book of athletic injuries, New York and London, 1981, Quick Fox.

Taber's cyclopedic medical dictionary, ed 13, Philadelphia, 1977, FA Davis.

Thibodeau G, Patton K: *Structure and function of the body,* ed 11, St Louis, 2000, Mosby.

Tortora GJ: *Introduction to the human body: the essentials of anatomy and physiology,* ed 3, New York, 1994, HarperCollins.

Tortora GJ, Grabowksi SR: *Principles of anatomy and physiology,* ed 9, New York, 2000, John Wiley.

Werner R: *A massage therapist's guide to pathology,* ed 2, Baltimore, 2002, Lippincott Williams & Wilkins.

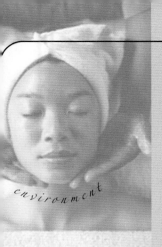

environment

Skeletal Nomenclature

14

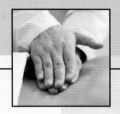

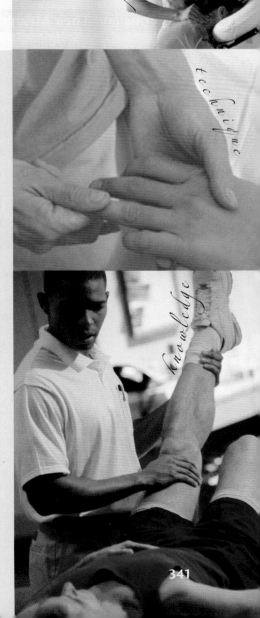

pressure

technique

knowledge

"Pain is inevitable. Suffering is optional."

—Kathleen Casey Theisen

STUDENT OBJECTIVES

After completing this chapter, the student should be able to:

- Describe the general locations of each bone listed in the chapter
- Locate each bony marking listed in the chapter
- Define each bony marking according to its significance in massage therapy
- Identify bony markings that are endangerment sites in massage therapy
- Under teacher supervision, examine the bony markings on yourself or a classmate
- Name and locate each joint listed in lesson five of this chapter

INTRODUCTION

Massage therapists come to know the skeleton well. Bones are landmarks for locating muscles and other soft tissues. Bony structures may also be areas to avoid in massage therapy (endangerment sites). Many of the terms in earlier chapters are repeated here. For example, the thighs are called the *femoral region* because the thigh bones are the femurs. This information is a prerequisite to learning muscular nomenclature, which is one of the main focuses for the study of massage therapy.

This chapter is divided into the anatomical regions of the body, and each region is subdivided into the bones of that region or a discussion on joints (Figure 14-1). Along with the bone names and locations are bony markings. Not all of the bones and their surface markings or joints are listed—only those that are the most important in the practice of massage therapy. Each bone is listed in chart form with the bony markings on the left and its significance on the right. When a structure such as the head, breastbone, or foot bones is discussed, the bones are listed to the left with important information to the right. Illustrations are included to locate the markings. Use anatomical models and a classmate to locate these bones and markings in class (Figure 14-2).

Your own body and all the bodies with which you will be working are the best teachers. Instead of thinking, "I am massaging the arm," repeat to yourself the terms *humerus, radius,* and *ulna.* This continually reinforces your new vocabulary. Try using scapula instead of shoulder blade or olecranon process instead of tip of the elbow. The sooner you begin to incorporate this new language into your massage work, the sooner you will have the confidence to progress into the world of muscles.

Terms and Their Meanings Related to the Skeleton

Term	Meaning	Term	Meaning
acetabulum	vinegar, saucer, or bowl; small	metacarpal	after or beyond; wrist
acromion	extremity; topmost; the shoulder	metatarsal	after or beyond; foot
aspera	rough	navicular	a ship; small
atlas	to bear; as the giant of Greek mythology holding up the world	obturator	to obstruct, close, block up, or plug
axis	an axis; an axle	odont	toothlike
bifid	cleaved or split in two; twice	olecranon	skull or head of the elbow
carpus	wrist	ossicle	small bone
calcaneus	heel	parietal	a wall or partition
clavicle	little key	patella	a little dish
coracoid	like a crow's beak	pectoral	the breast or chest
coronal	shaped like a corona or crown around the head	pedicle	small foot
costa	rib	pelvis	a basin
crural	leg	phalanx	a battle line or a closely knit row
cuneiform	wedge-shaped	pisiform	pea shaped
digit	resembling a finger or toe	poples	ham
dens, dent	toothlike	prominens	prominent or projecting
ethmoid	sievelike; shaped	pterygoid	winglike; shaped
femur	thigh	pubic	grownup
glenoid	like a socket; shaped	sacrum	sacred
hamate	to possess a small hook	sagittal	an arrow
humerus	upper arm	scaphoid	boatlike; shaped
hyoid	U shaped	sinus	a recess or cavity
ilium	flank	sphenoid	wedgelike; shaped
ischium	hip	spine	spiny or thorny plant
lambdoidal	shaped like the Greek letter Λ	stapes	a stirrup
lamina	a thin plate	suture	to sew; a seam
linea	line	styloid	a pillar; shaped
malleolus	hammer or mallet; small	talus	ankle
mandible	lower jawbone	tarsal	broad, flat surface; foot
manubrium	a handle	temporal	time
mastoid	breastlike; shaped	ulna	elbow
meniscus	moon; small	vertebrae	turning joint
		xiphoid	swordlike; shaped
		zygomatic	a yoke or bar

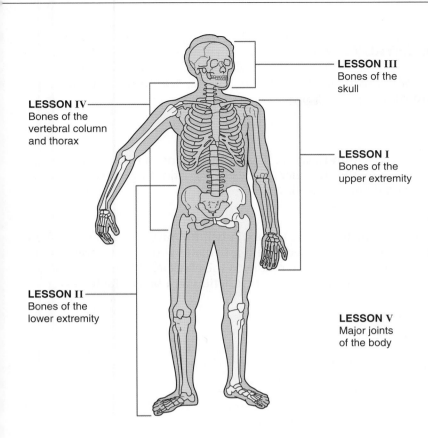

LESSON III
Bones of the
skull

LESSON IV
Bones of the
vertebral column
and thorax

LESSON I
Bones of the
upper extremity

LESSON II
Bones of the
lower extremity

LESSON V
Major joints
of the body

Figure 14-1   The relationship of the five lessons of this chapter to the human skeleton as a whole.

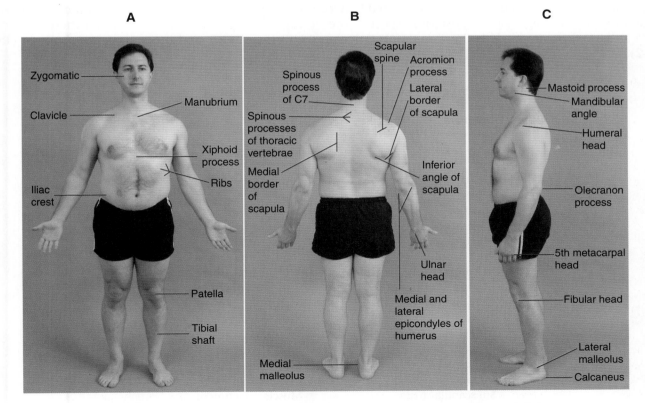

A

B

C

Zygomatic

Clavicle

Manubrium

Xiphoid process

Ribs

Iliac crest

Patella

Tibial shaft

Scapular spine   Acromion process

Spinous process of C7

Lateral border of scapula

Spinous processes of thoracic vertebrae

Medial border of scapula

Inferior angle of scapula

Ulnar head

Medial and lateral epicondyles of humerus

Medial malleolus

Mastoid process

Mandibular angle

Humeral head

Olecranon process

5th metacarpal head

Fibular head

Lateral malleolus

Calcaneus

Figure 14-2   Miscellaneous bony marking locations: **A**, anterior; **B**, posterior; and **C**, lateral views.

LESSON ONE—BONES OF THE UPPER EXTREMITY

Clavicle, scapula, humerus, ulna, radius, carpals (pisiform, triquetrum, lunate, scaphoid, hamate, capitate, trapezoid, trapezium), metacarpals, and phalanges

Shoulder Girdle

The bones of the shoulder (pectoral) girdle are the clavicle and scapula (Figure 14-3). One of the reasons the upper extremity has such a wide range of motion is because the shoulder girdle and the adjoining arm are attached to the axial skeleton at only one junction, the medial end of the clavicle.

Clavicle

The clavicle acts as a brace to hold the arm away from the top of the thorax. A helpful mnemonic to recall these two bones is "C and C" (collarbone is the *c*lavicle). The clavicle's medial end articulates with the sternum and its lateral end articulates with the scapula. The most commonly fractured bone is the clavicle. When the clavicle is broken, the entire shoulder region caves in medially. This demonstrates its function as a brace (Table 14-1).

TABLE 14-1

Clavicle

Bony Marking	Significance
Sternal (medial) end	Joint formation
Acromial (lateral) end	Joint formation

Scapula

The scapula is a triangular-shaped bone located between the second and seventh ribs. When the scapula is set in motion, it floats against the posterior aspect of the rib cage. A helpful mnemonic to recall these two bones is "S and S" (shoulder blade is the *s*capula). It articulates with the clavicle and humerus at the shoulder (Table 14-2).

TABLE 14-2

Scapula

Bony Marking	Significance
Medial (vertebral) border	Muscle attachment
Lateral (axillary) border	Muscle attachment
Superior angle	Muscle attachment
Inferior angle	Muscle attachment
Scapular spine	Muscle attachment
Root of spine	Muscle attachment
Acromion process	Muscle attachment and joint formation
Coracoid process	Muscle attachment
Supraglenoid tubercle	Muscle attachment
Infraglenoid tubercle	Muscle attachment
Glenoid fossa	Joint formation
Supraspinatus fossa	Muscle attachment
Infraspinatus fossa	Muscle attachment
Subscapular fossa	Muscle attachment

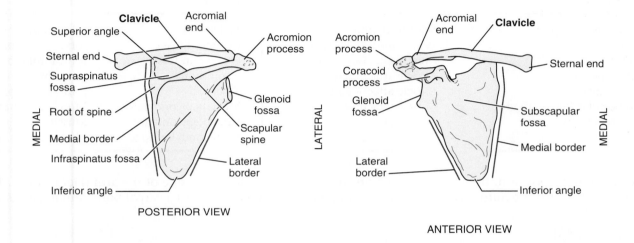

POSTERIOR VIEW

ANTERIOR VIEW

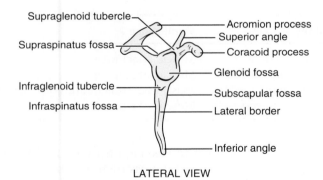

LATERAL VIEW

Figure 14-3 Right scapula and right clavicle with surface markings.

Arm

Humerus

The humerus is the upper arm bone (Figure 14-4), which is also known as the *funny bone* or *crazy bone* because hitting the elbow in a certain way makes it feel funny, or "humorous." The sensation felt when hitting the funny bone is the ulnar nerve as it passes superficially over the medial epicondyle of the humerus. The proximal end of the humerus articulates with the scapula at the shoulder, and the distal end of the humerus articulates with the radius and the ulna at the elbow (Table 14-3).

TABLE 14-3

Humerus

Bony Marking	Significance	Bony Marking	Significance
Humeral head	Joint formation	Radial fossa	Joint formation
Surgical neck	Where most fractures occur	Coronoid fossa	Joint formation
Humeral shaft	Muscle attachment	Olecranon fossa	Joint formation
Greater tubercle	Muscle attachment	Capitulum	Joint formation
Lesser tubercle	Muscle attachment	Trochlea	Joint formation
Intertubercular (bicipital) groove	Muscle attachment	Medial epicondyle	Muscle attachment
Deltoid tuberosity	Muscle attachment	Lateral epicondyle	Muscle attachment
		Supracondylar ridge	Muscle attachment

Ulna

In the anatomical position, the ulna is located on the medial, or little finger, side of the arm (Figure 14-5). The ulna articulates with the humerus at its proximal end, which is wider, and with a carpal bone (lunate) at its distal end (Table 14-4).

TABLE 14-4

Ulna

Bony Marking	Significance	Bony Marking	Significance
Olecranon process	Muscle attachment	Ulnar tuberosity	Muscle attachment
Trochlear (semilunar) notch	Joint formation	Coronoid process	Muscle attachment
Radial notch	Joint formation	Ulnar head	Muscle attachment and joint formation
Ulnar shaft	Muscle attachment	Styloid process	Muscle attachment

Radius

The radius is the lateral forearm bone, located on the thumb side of the arm (see Figure 14-5). To differentiate the radius from the ulna, locate the radial pulse. You palpate the radial pulse by pressing it into the radial bone. Another way to remember the name of this bone is to remember that the *r*adius always *r*otates on the ulna (during supination and pronation). The radius articulates with the humerus at its proximal end and with carpal bones (triquetrum, lunate, scaphoid) at its wide distal end.

An interosseous membrane weaves the ulna and the radius with bands of tough connective tissue. This anatomical arrangement gives the forearm lightness and mobility and provides attachment sites for the many muscles of the hand (Table 14-5). Imagine how heavy the arm would be if the ulna and radius were just one solid bone!

TABLE 14-5

Radius

Bony Marking	Significance	Bony Marking	Significance
Radial head	Joint formation	Radial (bicipital) tuberosity	Muscle attachment
Radial neck	Nonapplicable	Ulnar notch	Joint formation
Radial shaft	Muscle attachment	Styloid process	Muscle attachment

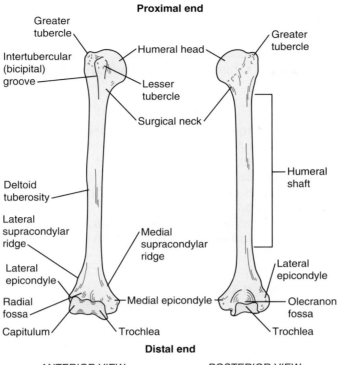

Proximal end

Greater tubercle

Intertubercular (bicipital) groove

Humeral head

Greater tubercle

Lesser tubercle

Surgical neck

Humeral shaft

Deltoid tuberosity

Lateral supracondylar ridge

Medial supracondylar ridge

Lateral epicondyle

Lateral epicondyle

Radial fossa

Medial epicondyle

Olecranon fossa

Capitulum

Trochlea

Trochlea

Distal end

ANTERIOR VIEW   POSTERIOR VIEW

Figure 14-4   Right humerus with surface markings.

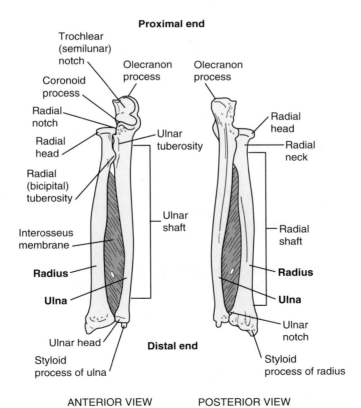

Proximal end

Trochlear (semilunar) notch

Olecranon process

Olecranon process

Coronoid process

Radial notch

Ulnar tuberosity

Radial head

Radial head

Radial neck

Radial (bicipital) tuberosity

Interosseus membrane

Ulnar shaft

Radial shaft

Radius

Radius

Ulna

Ulna

Ulnar notch

Ulnar head

Distal end

Styloid process of ulna

Styloid process of radius

ANTERIOR VIEW   POSTERIOR VIEW

Figure 14-5   Right ulna and radius with surface markings.

Hands

Each hand contains 27 bones: eight carpals, five metacarpals, and 14 phalanges (Figure 14-6). Opposing thumbs make human hands vastly different from those of other mammals; it can be rotated in front of the palm in the opposite direction of the other four digits for grasping. It is this flexibility that gives us the ability to create and use tools.

Carpals

The eight carpal bones of the wrist are arranged in two rows of four bones (proximal row and a distal row) that are linked together by ligaments and bound in a joint capsule. The carpal bones function like eight ball bearings. For centuries, they were simply numbered one through eight. In the early 1800s, each bone was named individually. The names of the carpal bones in the proximal row from medial to lateral are the pisiform, triquetrum, lunate, and scaphoid. The names of the carpal bones in the distal row from medial to lateral are the hamate, capitate, trapezoid, and trapezium.

A tunnel is produced by the carpal bones and bound by the *transverse carpal ligament*. This structure creates a flexor pulley system important for hand functions. Many muscles of the thumb and little finger originate on the transverse carpal ligament (Table 14-6).

TABLE 14-6

Carpals

Bony Marking	Significance
Scaphoid	Largest bone in the proximal row; most commonly fractured carpal bone
Lunate	Crescent moon-shaped bone
Triquetrum	Triangular or pyramid-shaped bone
Pisiform	Pea-shaped bone; smallest carpal bone
Trapezium	Triangular-shaped bone
Trapezoid	Four-sided bone with two parallel sides
Capitate	Largest carpal bone; has a round head
Hamate	Bone has an anterior hook

Metacarpals

The metacarpals are also referred to as the *hand bones,* with five in each hand, numbered I through V, starting from the thumb (I) to the little finger (V). When the hand is clenched to make a fist, the distal ends of the metacarpal heads become obvious as the knuckles.

Phalanges

Each hand has 14 phalanges. Each finger has three, and each thumb has two. Depending on their location, the phalanges are referred to as *proximal, middle,* and *distal;* the thumb is also referred to as *pollicis.*

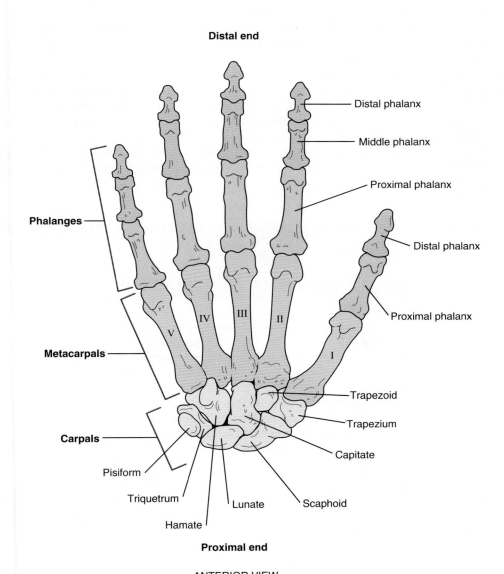

Distal end

Distal phalanx

Middle phalanx

Proximal phalanx

Phalanges

Distal phalanx

Proximal phalanx

V   IV   III   II   I

Metacarpals

Trapezoid

Trapezium

Carpals

Capitate

Pisiform

Triquetrum   Lunate   Scaphoid

Hamate

Proximal end

ANTERIOR VIEW

Figure 14-6   Carpals, metacarpals, and phalanges of right hand.

LESSON TWO—BONES OF THE LOWER EXTREMITY

Ilium, ischium, pubis, femur, patella, tibia, fibula, tarsals (talus, cuneiforms, navicular, cuboid, calcaneus), metatarsals, and phalanges

Pelvic Girdle

The pelvic girdle is also known as the *os coxa, coxal bones, hip bones,* or *innominate bones.* Each pelvic bone is made up of three fused embryonic bones: ilium, ischium, and pubis. In contrast, the pelvis is formed by the two matched pelvic bones, anteriorly connected by the pubic bones at the pubic symphysis, and the sacrum, posteriorly connected to the ilium, where the lower extremity joins the axial skeleton (Figure 14-7). The sacrum is not part of the pelvic girdle, but it must be included when discussing the pelvis.

The hip socket, or *acetabulum,* receives the femoral head. The ilium, ischium, and pubic bones all contribute equally to its makeup. This allows equal force from all three dimensions to pass into the acetabulum. The *obturator foramen* is located inferior to the acetabulum. The obturator membrane "obstructs" the foramen. This membrane provides attachment sites for the muscles of the hip and thigh. The superior opening of the pelvis is called the *pelvic inlet,* and the *pelvic outlet* is the inferior opening of the pelvis. The digestive, urinary, and reproductive systems use the latter opening to empty their products externally. *It is helpful, in massage, to have a notion where the external genitalia are in men and women.* See Figure 14-8 for these structures in relation to the bones of the pelvis.

Ilium

The ilium is the most superior pelvic bone in the pelvic girdle and looks like a broad, expanding blade (Table 14-7).

TABLE 14-7

Ilium

Bony Marking	Significance
Iliac crest	Muscle attachment
Iliac fossa	Muscle attachment
Anterior superior iliac spine (ASIS)	Muscle attachment
Anterior inferior iliac spine (AIIS)	Muscle attachment
Posterior superior iliac spine (PSIS)	Muscle attachment
Posterior inferior iliac spine (PIIS)	Muscle attachment
Superior gluteal line	Muscle attachment
Inferior gluteal line	Muscle attachment
Greater sciatic notch	Passage of sciatic nerve

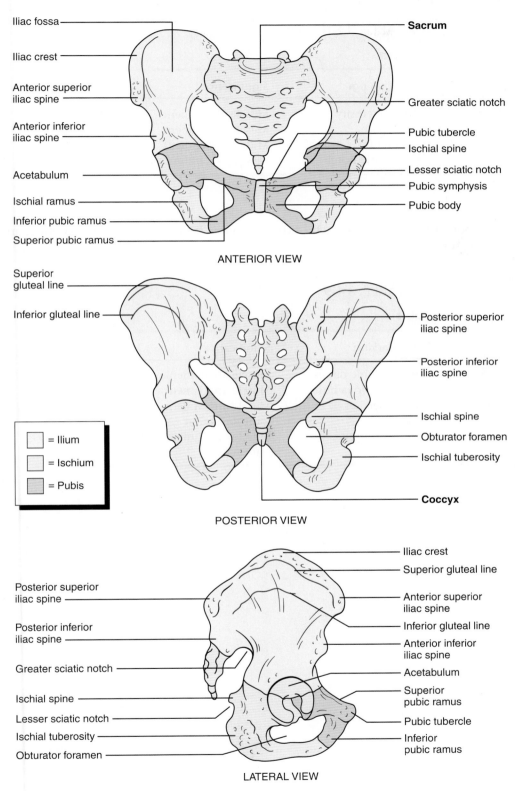

Iliac fossa

Iliac crest

Anterior superior
iliac spine

Anterior inferior
iliac spine

Acetabulum

Ischial ramus

Inferior pubic ramus

Superior pubic ramus

Sacrum

Greater sciatic notch

Pubic tubercle

Ischial spine

Lesser sciatic notch

Pubic symphysis

Pubic body

ANTERIOR VIEW

Superior
gluteal line

Inferior gluteal line

Posterior superior
iliac spine

Posterior inferior
iliac spine

Ischial spine

Obturator foramen

Ischial tuberosity

Coccyx

POSTERIOR VIEW

= Ilium

= Ischium

= Pubis

Posterior superior
iliac spine

Posterior inferior
iliac spine

Greater sciatic notch

Ischial spine

Lesser sciatic notch

Ischial tuberosity

Obturator foramen

Iliac crest

Superior gluteal line

Anterior superior
iliac spine

Inferior gluteal line

Anterior inferior
iliac spine

Acetabulum

Superior
pubic ramus

Pubic tubercle

Inferior
pubic ramus

LATERAL VIEW

Figure 14-7   Pelvis with surface markings.

Ischium

The ischium is the inferior and most posterior part of the pelvic girdle. Correcting sitting posture involves the ischial tuberosity (Figure 14-9; Table 14-8).

TABLE 14-8

Ischium

Bony Marking	Significance
Ischial tuberosity	Muscle attachment
Ischial spine	Muscle attachment
Ischial ramus	Muscle attachment
Lesser sciatic notch	Passage of obturator internus

Pubic Bone

In the most anterior portion of the pelvis, each of the two pubic bones resembles a wishbone, and they are collectively referred to as the *pubis* (Table 14-9).

TABLE 14-9

Pubis

Bony Marking	Significance
Superior pubic ramus	Muscle attachment
Inferior pubic ramus	Muscle attachment
Pubic tubercle	Muscle attachment
Pubic body	Joint formation
Pubic symphysis	Muscle attachment and joint formation

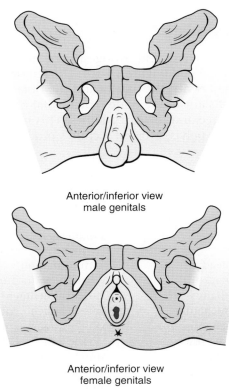

Anterior/inferior view
male genitals

Anterior/inferior view
female genitals

Figure 14-8   Pelvis and external genitalia.

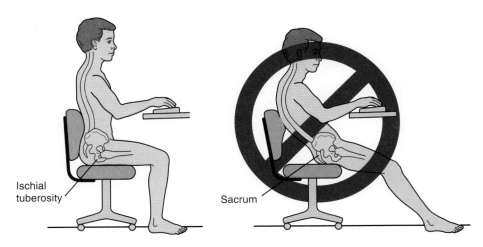

Ischial
tuberosity

Sacrum

Figure 14-9   Sitting on your ischial tuberosity versus sitting on your sacrum.

Leg

Femur

The femur (thigh bone) is the longest, heaviest, and strongest bone in the body. It has a curved ball at the proximal end and two curved balls at its distal end (Figure 14-10). The femur articulates proximally with the acetabulum, forming the hip joint, and distally with the patella and the tibia, forming the knee joint. When looking at the femur, you will notice a distinct slant to the bone. The medial course of the femoral shaft is necessary to bring the hips back in line with the knee and lower leg bones. This medial direction of the femur is more noticeable in females because of the wider pelvis. Most of a child's production of red blood cells occurs in the femur (Table 14-10).

TABLE 14-10

Femur

Bony Marking	Significance
Femoral head	Joint formation
Femoral neck	Where most fractures occur
Femoral shaft	Muscle attachment
Greater trochanter	Muscle attachment
Lesser trochanter	Muscle attachment
Gluteal tuberosity	Muscle attachment
Linea aspera	Muscle attachment
Adductor tubercle	Muscle attachment
Medial condyle	Joint formation
Lateral condyle	Joint formation
Medial epicondyle	Muscle attachment
Lateral epicondyle	Muscle attachment
Intercondylar fossa	Joint formation
Popliteal fossa	Joint formation
Patellar surface	Joint formation

Patella

The patella, or kneecap, is the largest sesamoid bone in the body and articulates with the distal end of the femur. It arises from the tendon of the quadriceps femoris muscle and can provide additional leverage for knee extension. However, the patella is not always considered part of the knee joint. Its main function is to provide stabilization and protect the knee by shielding it from impact.

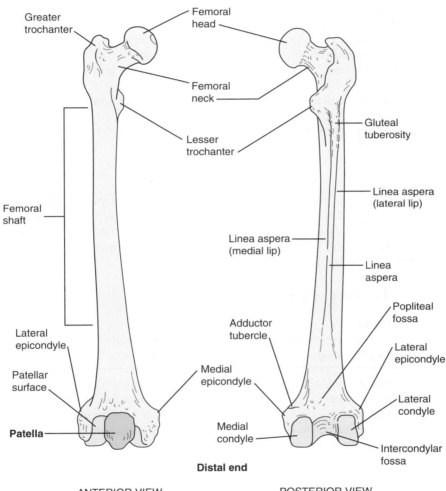

Figure 14-10   Right femur and patella with surface markings.

Tibia

The tibia, or shin bone, is the most stout and straight bone in the body and is located below the femur on the medial side of the lower leg (Figure 14-11). The proximal aspect of the tibia articulates with the femur, and its distal end articulates with the talus bone. The top of the tibia is relatively flat and the shaft has a triangular shape (Table 14-11).

TABLE 14-11

Tibia

Bony Marking	Significance
Tibial plateau	Joint formation
Tibial shaft	Muscle attachment
Anterior crest	Nonapplicable
Tibial (patellar) tuberosity	Muscle attachment
Soleal line	Muscle attachment
Medial malleolus	Joint formation
Medial condyle	Muscle attachment and joint formation
Lateral condyle	Muscle attachment and joint formation

Fibula

The fibula is located on the lateral side of the lower leg and is about the same length as the tibia. The fibula is smaller in diameter than the tibia and supports only about 10% of the body's weight. The proximal end of the fibula attaches to the tibia below the tibial plateau and is not involved with the knee joint. The distal end of the fibula articulates with the talus bone. Like the ulna and radius of the upper extremity, an interosseous membrane connects the tibia and the fibula (Table 14-12).

TABLE 14-12

Fibula

Bony Marking	Significance
Fibular head	Muscle attachment
Fibular neck	Nonapplicable
Fibular shaft	Muscle attachment
Lateral malleolus	Joint formation

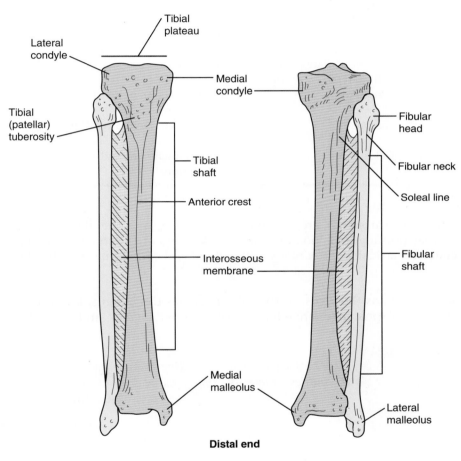

Proximal end

Tibial plateau

Lateral condyle

Medial condyle

Fibular head

Tibial (patellar) tuberosity

Fibular neck

Soleal line

Tibial shaft

Anterior crest

Interosseous membrane

Fibular shaft

Medial malleolus

Lateral malleolus

Distal end

ANTERIOR VIEW   POSTERIOR VIEW

Figure 14-11   Right tibia and fibula with surface markings.

Feet

Each foot contains 26 bones: seven tarsals, five metatarsals, and 14 phalanges (Figure 14-12).

Tarsals

Each tarsal is an irregular bone that slides minutely over the next bone to collectively provide motion. This is similar to the way the spine creates movement. *In massage therapy, range-of-motion exercises can help keep the tarsal bones mobile. If the tarsal bones become immobile or stuck, the foot cannot move properly or absorb shock* (Table 14-13).

TABLE 14-13

Tarsals

Bones	Significance
Talus (Astragalus)	Joint formation
Cuneiforms: I (medial), II (intermediate), III (lateral)	Muscle attachment and joint formation
Navicular	Muscle attachment and joint formation
Cuboid	Muscle attachment and joint formation
Calcaneus	Muscle attachment and joint formation

Metatarsals

Five metatarsals, numbered I through V are in each foot. The length of the metatarsals determines shoe size. When you flex your toes dorsally and look at your knuckles, you are actually looking at the heads of the metatarsals. The metatarsals articulate proximally with cuboid and cuneiforms and distally with the phalanges.

Phalanges

The phalanges are also known as the *digits,* or toes. Each toe has three digits, and the great toe has two. Depending on their location, the phalanges are referred to as *proximal, middle,* and *distal.* The great toe is also referred to as the *hallux.*

 Thinking is more interesting than knowing, but less interesting than looking.

—Goethe

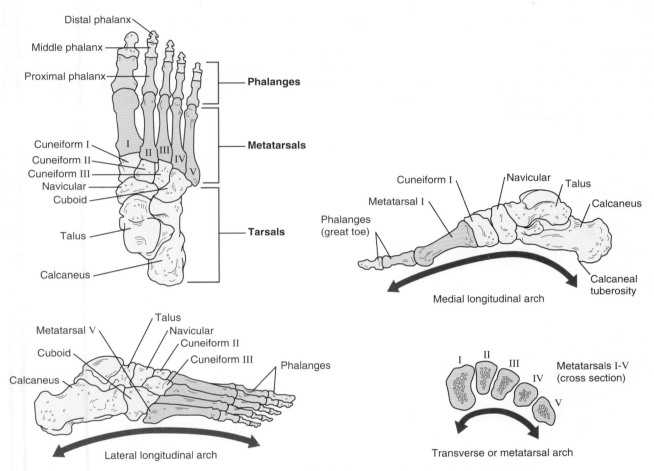

Figure 14-12 Tarsals, metatarsals, phalanges, and arches of the right foot.

Foot Arches

For walking, running, and jumping to be springy, our feet must absorb shock. To help accomplish this, the foot uses a system of arches to prevent the plantar surface of the foot from becoming flat (see Figure 14-12).

The posterior bones of the foot lie over each other, and the anterior and middle bones of the foot lie side to side. This arrangement produces the three arches of the foot. Together, these three arches resemble a geodesic dome.

The three bony points that are in contact with the ground are (1) the calcaneal tuberosity, (2) the head of the first metatarsal, and (3) the head of the fifth metatarsal. The three points of contact make the shape of a triangle (Figure 14-13).

Because the names of the arches are descriptive, they are easy to learn. Weak arches are referred to as *fallen arches* or *flat feet.* To strengthen these arches and the intrinsic muscles of the foot, pick up marbles or rocks with your toes. The three arches are the *medial longitudinal arch, lateral longitudinal arch,* and *transverse (metatarsal) arch.*

The imprint of a healthy foot arch looks like Figure 14-14, *A* and *B*. If the imprint is wide and flattened, the arches, namely the medial longitudinal arch, have "fallen," often as a result of overextension of foot ligaments and weakness of the deep (intrinsic) plantar musculature (Figure 14-14, *C*). If the imprint shows only two unconnected sections, the foot arches are "high," often as a result of the positions of foot bones rather than weak foot muscles and ligaments (Figure 14-14, *D*).

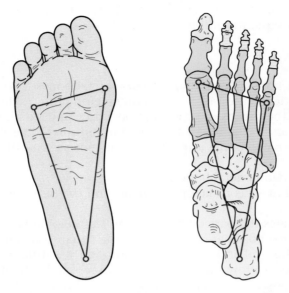

Figure 14-13   Foot with three points of contact with the ground.

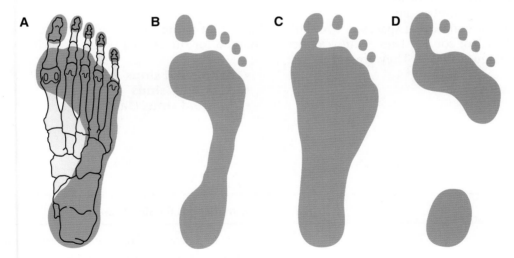

Figure 14-14   **A,** Footprint with skeletal overlay; **B,** imprint of a healthy foot arch; **C,** imprint of a person with a flat foot; **D,** imprint of a person with a high arch.

LESSON THREE—BONES OF THE STRUCTURES OF THE SKULL

Frontal, parietal, temporal, ethmoid, sphenoid, occipital, hyoid, nasal, vomer, zygomatic, lacrimal, inferior nasal concha, palatine, maxilla, mandible

Cranial Bones

The cranial vault contains eight bones: frontal bone, two parietal bones, two temporal bones, ethmoid bone, sphenoid bone, and occipital bone (Figure 14-15). This bony region protects the brain and related nerves; it also provides a bony passageway for the organs of sight, taste, hearing, and smell. Except for one synovial joint located at the jaw, all skull bones and facial bones are joined by sutures (Table 14-14).

Sutures are located anywhere cranial bones join and are classified as synarthrotic joints. Very little movement exists in these sutural regions.

- The **sagittal suture** joins the two parietal bones.
- This **coronal suture** is shaped like a corona, or crown, around the head and separates the frontal bone from the parietal bones.
- The **lambdoidal suture** separates the parietal bones from the occipital bone.
- The parietal bones and temporal bones are separated by the **squamosal suture.**

The fontanels are located in the fetal and neonatal cranium in the sutural regions. These membrane-covered spaces exist in the neonatal head to allow the head to be compressed during delivery and permit rapid growth of the brain. The anterior and posterior fontanels are also called *soft spots.* Obstetricians and midwives find these helpful in determining the position of babies during delivery. Although many fontanels exist in the newborn's head, the following two are the most prevalent:

- The **anterior fontanel** is diamond-shaped and is the largest of all the fontanels. It is located where the coronal suture and sagittal sutures meet. The anterior fontanel completely ossifies by 18 to 24 months. You can often see a pulse under the membrane in this region of the head.
- The **posterior fontanel** is located where the sagittal and lambdoidal sutures meet. It typically closes by the time the infant is 2 months old.

The sinuses are air-containing spaces in the skull and face that lighten the head, provide mucus, and act as resonance chambers for sound. These sinus cavities are named for the cranial bones or facial bones by which they are located (Figure 14-16). They are as follows:

- **Frontal sinus**
- **Sphenoidal sinus**

- **Ethmoidal sinus**
- **Maxillary sinus**
- **Mastoid sinus** (Table 14-14)

TABLE 14-14

Cranial Bones

Bones	Bony Markings and Significance
Frontal bone (1)	No relevant bony marking or endangerment site
Parietal bones (2)	No relevant bony marking or endangerment site
Temporal bones (2)	Styloid process (ligament attachment and endangerment site)
	External auditory meatus (ear ossicles)
	Mastoid process (muscle attachment)
Ethmoid bone (1)	No relevant bony marking or endangerment site
Sphenoid bone (1)	Sella turcica (pituitary gland location)
	Pterygoid plate (muscle attachment)
	Greater wings (muscle attachment)
Occipital bone (1)	Foramen magnum (passage for spinal cord)
	Superior nuchal lines (muscle attachment)
	Inferior nuchal lines (muscle attachment)
	External occipital protuberance (muscle attachment)
	Occipital condyles (joint formation)

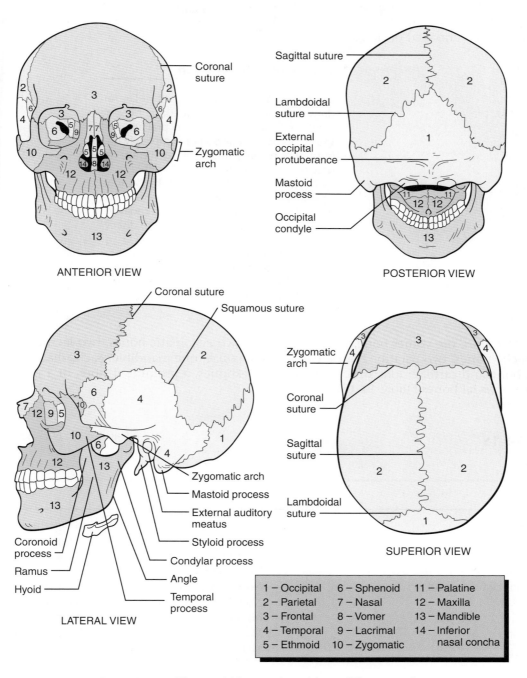

Figure 14-15 The cranial bones viewed from different angles.

Continued

Related Skull Bone

Hyoid

The hyoid bone is shaped like a miniature mandible with two incisor teeth and is usually found at the level of C3. This bone does not articulate directly with any other bone. It is suspended from the styloid process of the temporal bone by ligaments, serves as a support for the tongue, and provides muscle attachments for the tongue, neck, and pharynx. This bone is important in forensic medicine. When it is found broken, it usually means the victim was strangled or hanged.

For Your Information

Dr. William Sutherland, a student of Dr. Andrew Still (father of osteopathy), became convinced through study and practice that the bones of the skull do not completely fuse but rather retain a small, yet significant, degree of motion relative to one another.

This idea was expounded on by Dr. John Upledger and was proven when he took pictures of sutural contents from fresh cadavers. Connective and vascular tissues were discovered between the sutures.

From his finding, Upledger developed a system of nonintrusive diagnosis and treatment called craniosacral therapy. (See Chapter 17 for his biography.)

Facial Bones

The face has 14 bones: the vomer bone, two nasal bones, two zygomatic bones, two lacrimal bones, two inferior nasal concha bones, two palatine bones, two fused maxillae, one mandible. Facial features are largely a result of facial bone and cartilaginous structures. High cheekbones, a prominent nose, or a pointed chin are all representative of facial bones (Table 14-15).

TABLE 14-15

Facial Bones

Bony Marking	Significance
Nasal bones (2)	No relevant bony marking or endangerment site
Vomer bone (1)	No relevant bony marking or endangerment site
Zygomatic bones (2)	No relevant bony marking or endangerment site
Lacrimal bones (2)	No relevant bony marking or endangerment site
Inferior nasal concha bones (2)	No relevant bony marking or endangerment site
Palatine bones (2)	No relevant bony marking or endangerment site
Maxillae (2)	Muscle attachment
Mandible (1)	Mandibular ramus (muscle attachment)
	Mandibular angle (muscle attachment)
	Coronoid process (muscle attachment)
	Condylar process (muscle attachment and joint formation)

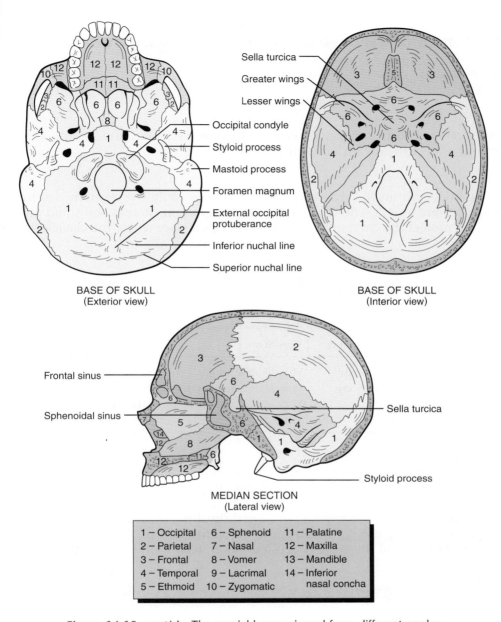

BASE OF SKULL
(Exterior view)

- Occipital condyle
- Styloid process
- Mastoid process
- Foramen magnum
- External occipital protuberance
- Inferior nuchal line
- Superior nuchal line

BASE OF SKULL
(Interior view)

- Sella turcica
- Greater wings
- Lesser wings

MEDIAN SECTION
(Lateral view)

- Frontal sinus
- Sphenoidal sinus
- Sella turcica
- Styloid process

1 – Occipital	6 – Sphenoid	11 – Palatine
2 – Parietal	7 – Nasal	12 – Maxilla
3 – Frontal	8 – Vomer	13 – Mandible
4 – Temporal	9 – Lacrimal	14 – Inferior
5 – Ethmoid	10 – Zygomatic	nasal concha

Figure 14-15, cont'd   The cranial bones viewed from different angles.

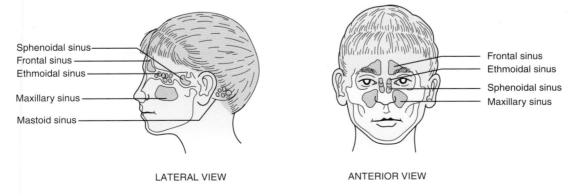

- Sphenoidal sinus
- Frontal sinus
- Ethmoidal sinus
- Maxillary sinus
- Mastoid sinus

- Frontal sinus
- Ethmoidal sinus
- Sphenoidal sinus
- Maxillary sinus

LATERAL VIEW   ANTERIOR VIEW

Figure 14-16   The sinuses.

LESSON FOUR—BONES OF THE VERTEBRAL COLUMN AND THORAX

Sternum, ribs, vertebrae

Thorax

The thorax, or chest cavity, consists of the sternum, 12 thoracic vertebrae, and 24 ribs. These bony structures support the body and protect the organs inside the thorax.

Sternum

The sternum, or breastbone, forms the anterior chest wall. In the adult, the sternum is a single bone made up of three fused bones (Figure 14-17). These bones are the manubrium, sternal body, and xiphoid process. Not only does the sternum protect the chest organs, it also provides a place where the clavicle and most ribs attach (Table 14-16).

TABLE 14-16

Sternum

Bony Marking	Significance
Manubrium	Muscle attachment and joint formation
Sternal body	Muscle attachment and joint formation
Xiphoid process	Muscle attachment and endangerment site

Ribs

The ribs are 24 individual (12 pairs) of long, slender, curved bones that articulate posteriorly with the thoracic vertebrae. Mobility of the rib cage is a precursor for proper respiration. Anteriorly, the first seven pairs of ribs have their costal cartilages articulate directly with the sternum and are known as the *true ribs*. The next three pairs of ribs attach to the sternum by borrowing the costal (hyaline) cartilage of the seventh rib and are called the *false ribs*. The last two pairs of ribs do not attach to the sternum at all. These are known as the *floating ribs*. The first rib is short and thick, and the great vessels and main nerves run over it (Table 14-17).

TABLE 14-17

Ribs

Bony Marking	Significance
True ribs (7 pairs)	Attach directly to sternum
False ribs (3 pairs)	Attach to sternum by costal cartilage
Floating ribs (2 pairs)	Do not attach to sternum and endangerment site

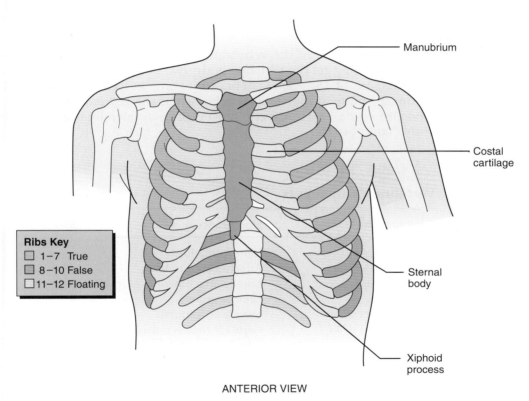

Manubrium

Costal
cartilage

Sternal
body

Xiphoid
process

Ribs Key
☐ 1−7 True
☐ 8−10 False
☐ 11−12 Floating

ANTERIOR VIEW

Figure 14-17   The sternum and ribs.

Vertebral Column

The vertebral (spinal) column consists of 26 individual bones in the adult and 33 to 35 in the embryo. The bones of the vertebral column are called the *vertebrae*. Each weight-bearing portion of the vertebra gradually increases in size so that the larger lumbar vertebrae and sacral vertebrae form a stable base. The *supraspinous ligament* connects the spinous process of C7 to L5 and offers strength and stability. The vertebral column encloses the spinal cord and provides support for the spinal cord and the head and an attachment site for the ribs and muscles of the back. Located in the posterior region of the neck, the *nuchal ligament,* attaches from the occipital bone (external occipital protuberance) to all the spinous processes of the cervical vertebrae and offers the neck both stability and muscle attachment sites. In reference, the supraspinous ligament lies on top of the nuchal ligament.

The vertebral column allows us to bend forward and backward, lean sideways, and twist or rotate through the three planes of movement. All these spinal movements are a result of collective action. The spinal column of an infant is U-shaped, arching posteriorly. It soon becomes S-shaped when learning to walk on two feet. This S-shaped curve is required for a functional upright posture, providing better balance and better shock absorption qualities.

Parts of a Typical Vertebra

All vertebrae (except C1) have two main regions: the vertebral body and the arch. Collectively, these regions possess eight basic vertebral elements. They are the vertebral body, two pedicles, two transverse processes, two laminae, and the spinous process (Figure 14-18). Each vertebra varies only in location, shape, and size. The circle of bone that extends out from the body of the vertebra is known as the *vertebral arch,* which is formed by the pedicles and the laminae on either side. The transverse process projects laterally from the arch and the spinous process projects posteriorly (Table 14-18).

TABLE 14-18

Vertebral Components

Bony Marking	Significance
Vertebral body	Joint formation
Pedicle	Attaches arch to body
Transverse processes	Muscle attachment
Lamina	Lamina groove
Spinous process	Muscle attachment
Intervertebral disks	Cartilage between vertebral bodies; contains annulus fibrosus and nucleus pulposus
Vertebral canal	Passage for spinal cord
Articular facet (superior and inferior)	Joint formation
Intervertebral foramen	Passage of spinal roots

Between each unfused vertebra is a fibrocartilage disk called the *intervertebral disk*. The functions of these disks are to maintain the joint spaces, assist with spinal movements, and absorb vertical shock. Weight and gravity compresses these disks and, once they are released, they regain their original shape. The disk has two parts: *annulus fibrosus* (outer ring for shock absorption) and *nucleus pulposus* (soft, gel-like center that adjusts to weight distribution throughout the column). The disk can lose some of its elasticity with age; it can also become compressed and herniate. Just posterior to the intervertebral disk is a large central hole, or canal, for the spinal cord to pass. This opening in the vertebrae is known as the *vertebral canal.* Each vertebra articulates to other vertebrae by *articular facets.* As vertebrae are stacked as a column, an opening is created at the pedicles for spinal roots to pass. This is called the *intervertebral foramen.* These stacked vertebrae also create a trench in the lamina region of the spine, or the *lamina groove.*

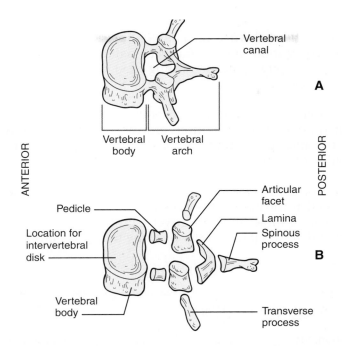

ANTERIOR

POSTERIOR

Vertebral canal

Vertebral body

Vertebral arch

A

Pedicle

Location for intervertebral disk

Vertebral body

Articular facet

Lamina

Spinous process

B

Transverse process

Figure 14-18   A, Parts of a typical vertebra. **B,** Exploded view.

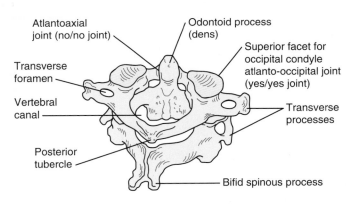

ANTERIOR

Atlantoaxial joint (no/no joint)

Transverse foramen

Vertebral canal

Posterior tubercle

Odontoid process (dens)

Superior facet for occipital condyle atlanto-occipital joint (yes/yes joint)

Transverse processes

Bifid spinous process

POSTERIOR

Figure 14-19   The atlas and axis—atlanto-occipital joint and atlantoaxial joint.

Atypical Vertebrae

C1.   The first cervical vertebra, also known as the *atlas,* or *C1,* is shaped like a bony ring. The atlas possesses no body, pedicles, or laminae. The spinous process has been reduced to a posterior tubercle. Facets on the superior surface articulate with the occipital bone, permitting head nodding. On the inferior surface, facets articulate with the second cervical vertebrae.

C2.   The second cervical vertebra is often referred to as the *axis,* or *C2.* The axis has a spinous process that is thick and strongly bifurcated (forked). The odontoid process, or dens, is a bony extension that projects superiorly through the ring of the atlas, permitting the rotation of the head (Figure 14-19). It is speculated that the dens evolved from the old body of the atlas.

C7.   The *vertebral prominens,* or *C7,* has a spinous process that is long and projects posteriorly. The vertebral prominens can be easily palpated at the base of the neck (Figure 14-20). This is the only cervical vertebra that does not possess a *transverse foramen* (holes in the transverse processes for the passage of blood vessels located in most cervical vertebrae); blood vessels pass directly over the transverse process.

Effects of Massage on Connective Tissues

- **Reduces keloid formation.** Massage applied to scar tissue helps reduce keloid formation in scar tissue.
- **Reduces excessive scar formation.** Deep massage reduces excessive scar formation, helping create an appropriate scar that is strong yet does not interfere with the muscle's ability to broaden as it contracts.
- **Decreases adhesion formation.** The displacement of scar tissue during massage helps to reduce formation of adhesions. This, in turn, facilitates normal, pain-free motion of the affected muscles and joints.
- **Releases fascial restrictions.** Pressure, and the heat it produces, converts fascia from a gel-state to a sol-state (thixotropy), reducing hyperplasia. Fascia loosens and melts, becoming more flexible and elastic. Softening of the fascia surrounding muscles allows them to be stretched to their fullest resting length, increasing joint range of motion, and freeing the body of restricted movements.
- **Improves connective tissue healing.** Occurring only with deep pressure massage, proliferation and activation of fibroblasts was noted, which leads to improved tensile strength of healed tissue.

LATERAL VIEW

SUPERIOR VIEW

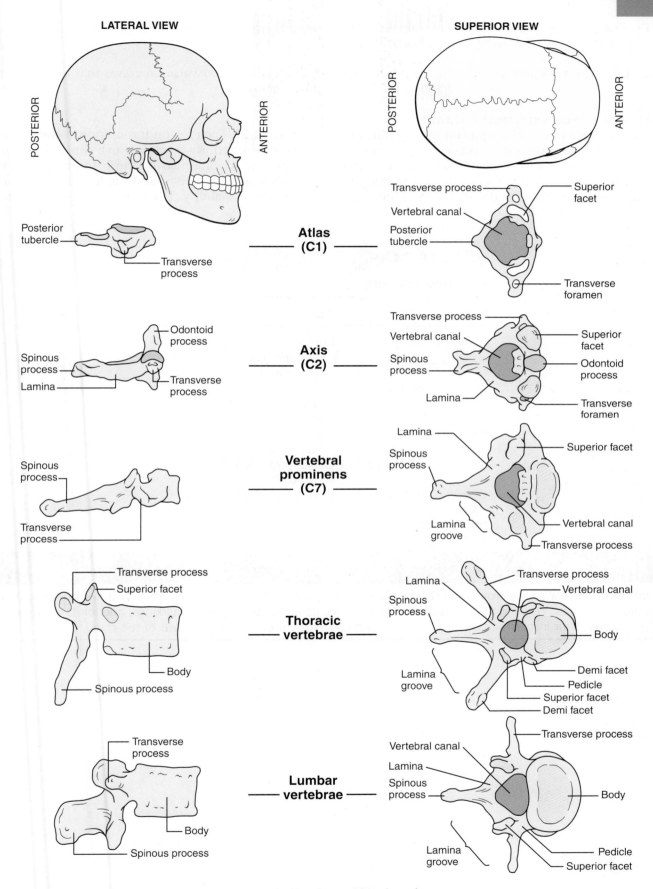

Figure 14-20   Vertebrae within the column.

T1-T12.   Located on the body and transverse processes of the thoracic vertebrae (except T11-T12) is an extra pair of facets called *demifacets* for articulating ribs.

L1-L5.   The large lumbar vertebrae contain a spinous process and transverse processes that are short and thick.

Divisions of the Vertebral Column

The five regions of the vertebral column are illustrated in Figure 14-21. Each region has unique characteristics. The vertebral column bends anteriorly to posteriorly and back to anteriorly a total of five times (in normal spines). Many ligaments join the vertebrae to other structures. The *sacrotuberous ligament*, running from the sacrum to the ischial tuberosity, provides stability to the vertebrae and the pelvis, and the *iliolumbar ligament*, running from the ilium to the transverse process of L5, also provides stability. The different vertebral regions are listed in Table 14-19.

TABLE 14-19

Vertebral Column

Regions	Traits
Cervical (C1-C7)	Curves anteriorly; possesses bifid spinous processes and transverse foramina
Thoracic (T1-T12)	Curves posteriorly; possess demifacets for articulating ribs
Lumbar (L1-L5)	Curves anteriorly; large vertebral bodies
Sacrum (S1-S5—fused)	Curves posteriorly; triangular-shaped
Coccyx (Co1-Co3 to Co5—fused)	Curves posteriorly; tail-shaped

MINI-LAB

Obtain an articulated skeleton and a disarticulated skeleton. Most high schools, colleges, or universities use them in biology classes. Working in groups of two or three, locate all the bones, bony markings, and joints discussed in this chapter. Your instructor may add or delete particular structures to suit the needs of the class.

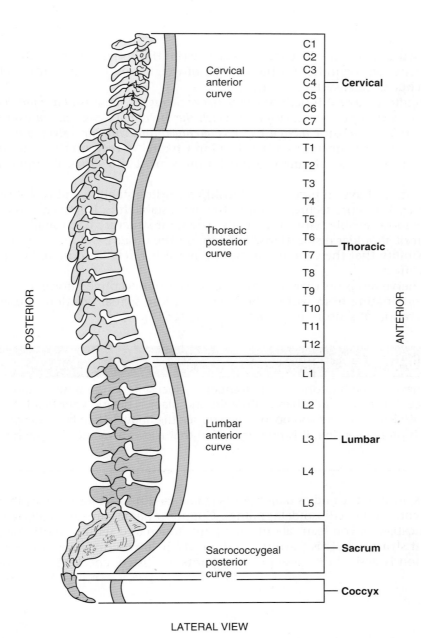

Cervical anterior curve

C1
C2
C3
C4 — **Cervical**
C5
C6
C7

Thoracic posterior curve

T1
T2
T3
T4
T5
T6 — **Thoracic**
T7
T8
T9
T10
T11
T12

Lumbar anterior curve

L1
L2
L3 — **Lumbar**
L4
L5

Sacrococcygeal posterior curve

— **Sacrum**

— **Coccyx**

POSTERIOR

ANTERIOR

LATERAL VIEW

Figure 14-21   The vertebral column with its curves and divisions.

LESSON FIVE—MAJOR JOINTS OF THE BODY

Glenohumeral, iliofemoral, temporomandibular, humeroulnar, humeroradial, tibiofemoral, talocrural, interphalangeal, atlantoaxial, radioulnar, carpometacarpal, radiocarpal, metacarpophalangeal, metatarsophalangeal, atlanto-occipital, intervertebral, acromioclavicular, sternoclavicular, intercarpal, pubic symphysis, sacroiliac, lumbosacral, patellofemoral, tarsometatarsal, intertarsal

Articulations

Articulations, also known as *joints,* are the connections between the bones (Figure 14-22). Joints provide a space where one bone articulates with another for the transfer of weight and energy. Joints not only help us move, they also help us keep our skeletal system together.

The shape of a joint affects how it functions. *As massage therapists, we often have problems in the joints of our hands because we expect them to function in ways for which they were not designed. For example, the wrist is not a weight-bearing structure. When a massage therapist spends too much time with the weight of his body on a flexed wrist, it gets injured.* This concept is explained in greater detail in Chapter 6. Feet, on the other hand, are designed to bear the body's weight. The feet contain many joints for movement and shock absorption, and they provide a stable base.

All the body's articulations have an inverse relationship regarding stability and mobility, where one function is sacrificed for the other. The more secure the joint, the more stable it is; however, it is less mobile. For example, the shoulder is the most flexible joint in the body. The joint structure has a shallow socket and hence sustains a greater incident of shoulder dislocations. The hip, on the other hand, has a deep socket. The hip joint does not have the flexibility that the shoulder possesses, but it is rarely dislocated. Often, the femur fractures before the hip joint is affected.

Each joint contains nerve receptors that constantly give us proprioceptive information. These proprioceptive nerves detect stimuli originating from within the body regarding spatial position, muscular activity (motion and resistance), or activation of sensory receptors (see Chapter 17).

MINI-LAB

Proprioceptive awareness can be brought to our attention by focusing on the position of our joints and their relative positions in space. Close your right hand into a fist and place it behind your head. Now open any one finger of this closed fist. Which finger did you open? Can you see the finger? Then how do you know which one you opened? The answer is proprioception. It is proprioception that allows awareness of the position of each joint of the body.

This section features most of the body's major joints (Table 14-20). Each joint is classified by its synovial type (ball/socket, hinge, pivot, saddle, ellipsoidal, gliding). Common names are given along with the joints scientific name, when applicable. As you learn about each joint, touch and set into motion each joint while imagining the internal joint structures. This learning method will help you understand the mechanisms involved. If additional information is desired on these joints or joints not listed, check the references at the end of the chapter.

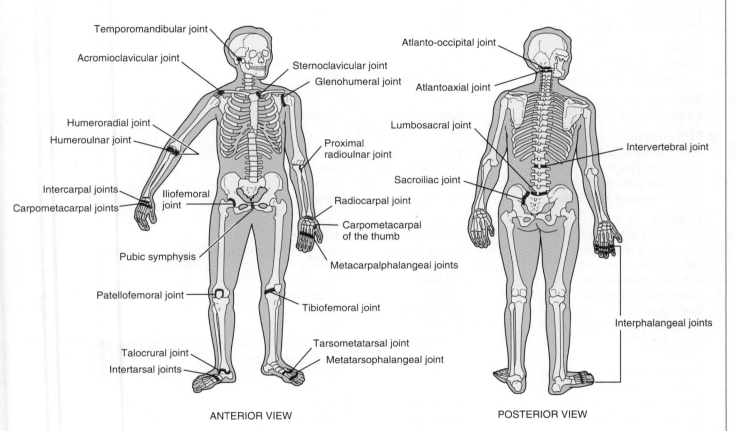

Figure 14-22 Synovial joints of the body.

TABLE 14-20

Articulations

Scientific Name	Common Name	Location
Ball and Socket		
Glenohumeral (scapohumeral) joint	Shoulder joint	Shoulder
Iliofemoral (coxal) joint	Hip joint	Hip
Hinge		
Temporomandibular joint	TMJ	Face/jaw
Humeroulnar/humeroradial joint	Elbow joint	Elbow
Tibiofemoral joint	Knee joint	Knee
Talocrural joint	Ankle joint	Ankle
Interphalangeal joint	IP joint	Fingers and toes
Pivot		
Atlantoaxial joint	"No-no" joint	Upper neck
Radioulnar joint (proximal)	Elbow joint	Elbow
Saddle		
Carpometacarpal of the thumb	Nonapplicable	Thumb
Ellipsoidal		
Temporomandibular joint	TMJ	Face/jaw
Radiocarpal joint	Wrist joint	Wrist
Metacarpophalangeal joint	MP joint	Hand
Metatarsophalangeal joint	MP joint	Foot
Gliding		
Atlanto-occipital joint	"Yes-yes" joint	Upper neck
Intervertebral joint	Nonapplicable	Spine/between vertebral bodies and arches
Temporomandibular joint	TMJ	Face/jaw
Acromioclavicular joint	AC joint	Shoulder
Sternoclavicular joint	SC joint	Upper chest
Intercarpal joint	Wrist joint	Wrist
Carpometacarpal joint	CM joint	Hand
Pubic symphysis	Nonapplicable	Pubis (synarthrotic, gliding during pregnancy as a result of hormones)
Sacroiliac joint	SI joint	Low back
Lumbosacral joint	Nonapplicable	Low back
Patellofemoral joint	Nonapplicable	Knee
Tarsometatarsal joint	Nonapplicable	Foot
Intertarsal joint	Nonapplicable	Foot

MINI-LAB

Nod your head slowly as if to say yes, then shake your head slowly as if to say no. Now repeat these movements while concentrating on the cervical-occipital area at the back of the neck. Which movement feels higher? Which one feels lower? Is the atlanto-occipital joint, also known as the yes/yes joint, more superior? Or is the atlantoaxial joint, also known as the no-no joint, more superior?

Knee Joint

The knee has an internal and external ligament system (Figure 14-23). The internal ligament system is composed of the anterior and posterior cruciate ligaments. The external ligament system is the medial (tibial) collateral ligament and the lateral (fibular) collateral ligament. The internal and external ligament systems are for

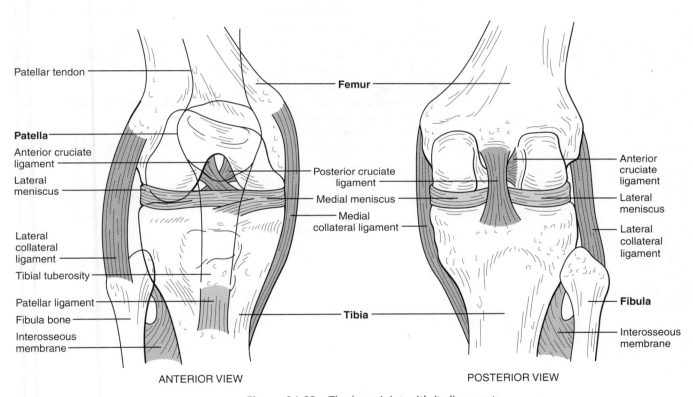

Figure 14-23   The knee joint with its ligaments.

static stabilization. Muscles and related tendons are dynamic stabilizers, supporting the knee joint in motion. Although many ligaments are in the joint capsule of the knee, the focus here is on the most important ones (Table 14-21).

TABLE 14-21

Connective Tissue Structures of the Knee

Structure	Commentary
Patellar (quadriceps) tendon	Attaches the quadriceps femoris muscle to the patella; the entire patella is embedded in this tendon, which continues to the tibia as the patellar ligament
Patellar ligament	Ligament between the patella and the tibia
Meniscus (medial and lateral)	Each concave meniscus is composed of half-ringed fibrocartilage attaching to the tibia; the two femoral condyles are convex and articulate with the medial and lateral menisci during knee movements
Collateral ligaments (medial, or MCL, and lateral, or LCL)	Provide external support and help prevent side-to-side movements
	MCL connects the femur to the tibia and may tear during lateral blows to the knee; MCL and the medial meniscus are commonly torn together
	LCL connects the femur to the fibula
Cruciate ligaments (anterior, or ACL, and posterior, or PCL)	Provide internal support and help prevent front to back movements; anchor the tibia to the femur; cross in the middle of the knee joint
	ACL often torn in knee injuries

Arthrometric Model

The arthrometric model was developed by John Wilson of the University of Arizona in Tucson. It describes the body's joint placement in radial symmetry. Radiating from the center of the circle are zones or perimeters that describe movement. The joints toward the center of this circle, or the central zone, are suited for directional movement. Going from the center toward the periphery, range, not direction, is involved. For example, the hand may grasp the apple from the tree branch, but the shoulder must position the arm in space so that this task may be achieved. This model stimulates the imagination and wisdom behind the articulate design of the human skeleton (Figure 14-24).

1. **Central zone.** The function of the central zone is to position the body. Motion in all three dimensions from gliding joints is available, but motion from a single joint is limited.
2. **First perimeter.** The first perimeter includes the ball-and-socket joints of the shoulder and hip, which are involved with directional movements.
3. **Second perimeter.** The synovial joints of the elbow and knee are located in the second perimeter and allow movement in only one dimension. Note that the joints cannot change the direction of motion, but they allow for some fulfillment of the motion intended by the organism.
4. **Third perimeter.** The third perimeter includes both ellipsoid and gliding joints. These are biaxial joints and allow movement in two or three dimensions. The joints in the third perimeter cannot change the direction of movement established by the central zone and the first perimeter, but can assist in the refinement of movement.
5. **Peripheral zone.** The peripheral zone includes the most diverse arrangements of synovial joints. Hinge joints, ellipsoid joints, gliding joints, and saddle joints help the organism to express, manipulate, maneuver, and complete the motion that originated toward the center of the arthrometric model.

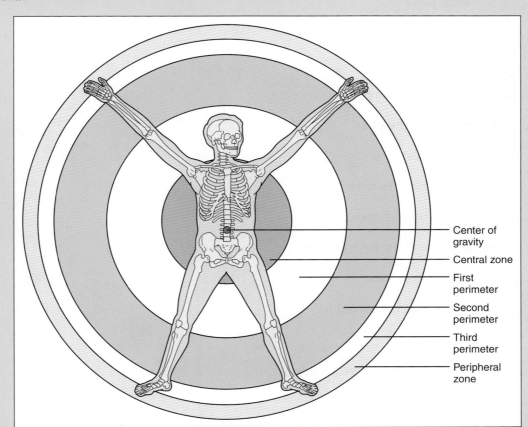

Figure 14-24 The arthrometric model.

- Center of gravity
- Central zone
- First perimeter
- Second perimeter
- Third perimeter
- Peripheral zone

SUMMARY

Skeletal nomenclature is the prerequisite to the muscular system and therefore fundamental to the study of massage. The bony skeleton provides a road map to the muscles, with its signs being the bony markings that are the sites of tendon attachment. The 206 bones of the skeleton have been divided regionally: bones of the upper extremity, bones of the lower extremity, bones of the skull, bones of the vertebral column and thorax, and major joints of the body. In each region, the specifics of each bone are detailed in regard to name, location, joint involvement, and important bony markings.

MATCHING—LESSON ONE

Write the letter of the best answer in the space provided. Some may be used more than once.

A. Clavicle   D. Metacarpals   G. Carpals
B. Humerus   E. Scapula   H. Phalanges
C. Radius   F. Ulna

_____ 1. Greater tubercle

_____ 2. Lateral forearm bone

_____ 3. Capitulum

_____ 4. Trochlea

_____ 5. Bicipital tuberosity

_____ 6. Collar bone

_____ 7. Acromion process

_____ 8. Ulnar tuberosity

_____ 9. Deltoid tuberosity

_____ 10. Rotates on the ulna

_____ 11. Glenoid fossa

_____ 12. Supraglenoid tubercle

_____ 13. Medial forearm bone

_____ 14. Collective term for wrist bones

_____ 15. Olecranon process

_____ 16. Hand bones numbered I-V

_____ 17. Shoulder blade

_____ 18. Located in the fingers/thumb

_____ 19. Coracoid process

_____ 20. Infraspinatus fossa

MATCHING—LESSON TWO

Write the letter of the best answer in the space provided. Some may be used more than once.

A. Ilium
B. Pubis
C. Patella
D. Fibula

E. Metatarsals
F. Ischium
G. Femur

H. Tibia
I. Tarsals
J. Phalanges

_____ 1. Greater trochanter

_____ 2. Bones located in the toes

_____ 3. Talus, cuneiforms, calcaneus

_____ 4. Lateral malleolus

_____ 5. Most superior pelvic bone

_____ 6. Longest bone in the body

_____ 7. Most inferior pelvic bone

_____ 8. Soleal line

_____ 9. Superior gluteal line

_____ 10. Sesamoid bone

_____ 11. Lateral lower leg bone

_____ 12. Tibial tuberosity

_____ 13. Iliac fossa

_____ 14. Anterior superior iliac spine

_____ 15. Linea aspera

_____ 16. Foot bones numbered I-V

_____ 17. Ischial tuberosity

_____ 18. Medial malleolus

_____ 19. Gluteal tuberosity

_____ 20. Most anterior pelvic bones

MATCHING—LESSON THREE

Write the letter of the best answer in the space provided. Some may be used more than once.

A. Frontal   E. Mandible   H. Hyoid
B. Temporal   F. Parietal   I. Maxilla
C. Occipital   G. Sphenoid   J. Sinuses
D. Zygomatic

_____ 1. Foramen magnum

_____ 2. Condylar process

_____ 3. External auditory meatus

_____ 4. Styloid process

_____ 5. Sagittal suture joins these bones

_____ 6. Superior nuchal lines

_____ 7. Forehead bone

_____ 8. Sella turcica

_____ 9. Mandibular angle

_____ 10. Air-containing spaces in head

_____ 11. Mastoid process

_____ 12. Cheek bones

_____ 13. Coronoid process

_____ 14. Does not join directly with a bone

_____ 15. Upper jaw bone

_____ 16. Mandibular ramus

_____ 17. External occipital protuberance

_____ 18. Bone where the sphenoidal sinuses are located

_____ 19. Pterygoid plate

_____ 20. Occipital condyles

MATCHING—LESSON FOUR

Write the letter of the best answer in the space provided. Some may be used more than once.

A. Sternum
B. Vertebrae
C. Pedicles
D. Laminae
E. Atlas
F. Cervical

G. Lumbar
H. Coccyx
I. True ribs
J. Ribs
K. Vertebral body
L. Transverse processes

M. Spinous process
N. Axis
O. Thoracic
P. Sacrum
Q. Floating ribs
R. False ribs

_____ 1. Xiphoid process

_____ 2. Spinal region that contains demifacets

_____ 3. Posterior projections of vertebrae

_____ 4. C2

_____ 5. Superior region of spinal column

_____ 6. Joins the vertebral body to the lamina

_____ 7. Ribs that attach by costal cartilage

_____ 8. Long, slender, curved bones

_____ 9. Part of pelvis

_____ 10. Lamina groove

_____ 11. Bones of the spinal column

_____ 12. Ribs that do not attach to sternum at all

_____ 13. Contains the intervertebral disk

_____ 14. Possesses the odontoid process

_____ 15. Inferior bone of spinal column

_____ 16. Ribs that attach directly to sternum

_____ 17. Breastbone

_____ 18. Low back region of spinal column

_____ 19. C1

_____ 20. Lateral projections of vertebrae

MATCHING—LESSON FIVE

Write the letter of the best answer in the space provided. Some may be used more than once.

A. Ball and socket   C. Ellipsoidal   E. Saddle
B. Pivot   D. Hinge   F. Gliding

_____ 1. Atlanto-occipital joint

_____ 2. Humeroulnar joint

_____ 3. Talocrural joint

_____ 4. Iliofemoral joint

_____ 5. Metatarsophalangeal joint

_____ 6. Radiocarpal joint

_____ 7. Patellofemoral joint

_____ 8. Intercarpal joint

_____ 9. Sternoclavicular joint

_____ 10. Atlantoaxial joint

_____ 11. Carpometacarpal of the thumb

_____ 12. Tibiofemoral joint

_____ 13. Interphalangeal joint

_____ 14. Intervertebral joint

_____ 15. Proximal radioulnar joint

_____ 16. Lumbosacral joint

_____ 17. Metacarpophalangeal joint

_____ 18. Glenohumeral joint

_____ 19. Humeroradial joint

_____ 20. Acromioclavicular joint

Bibliography

Ardoin W: From a lecture on temporomandibular joint dysfunction given at the Louisiana Institute of Massage Therapy, Lafayette, La, 1994, personal contact.

Biel A: *Trail guide to the body: how to locate muscles, bones, and more,* Boulder, Colo, 1997, Author.

Bowden B, Bowden J: *An illustrated atlas of the skeletal muscles,* Englewood, Colo, 2002, Morton.

Brossman AB: *Some of the finer points about temporomandibular joint anatomy and physiology,* Wheeling, WV, 1997. Available at: *http://www.ovnet.com/userpages/rebross/tmjoints.html.*

Crawley J, Van De Graaff KM: *A photographic atlas for anatomy and physiology,* Englewood, Colo, 2002, Morton.

Goldberg S: *Clinical anatomy made ridiculously simple,* Miami, 1984, Medmaster.

Grafelman T: *Graf's anatomy and physiology guide for the massage therapist,* Aurora, Colo, 1998, DG Publishing.

Gray H, Pick TP, Howden R: *Gray's anatomy,* ed 29, Philadelphia, 1974, Running Press.

Guyton A: *Human physiology and mechanisms of disease,* ed 3, Philadelphia, 1982, WB Saunders.

Haubrich WS: *Medical meanings: a glossary of word origins,* New York, 1984, Harcourt Brace Jovanovich.

Hoppenfeld S: *Physical examination of the spine and extremities,* Norwalk, Conn, 1976, Appleton-Century-Crofts.

Jacob S, Francone C: *Elements of anatomy and physiology,* Philadelphia, 1989, WB Saunders.

Juhan D: *Job's body: a handbook for bodyworkers,* Barrington, NY, 1987, Station Hill Press.

Kapandji IA: *The physiology of the joints,* New York, 1982, Churchill Livingstone.

Kapit W, Elson LM: *The anatomy coloring book,* ed 3, New York, 2002, Benjamin Cummings.

Kordish M, Dickson S: *Introduction to basic human anatomy,* Lake Charles, La, 1985, McNeese State University.

Marieb EN: *Essentials of human anatomy and physiology,* ed 4, New York, 1994, Benjamin Cummings.

McAleer N: *The body almanac,* Garden City, NY, 1985, Doubleday.

Moore KL: *Clinically oriented anatomy,* ed 2, Baltimore, 1985, Williams and Wilkins.

Olsen A, McHose C: *Bodystories: a guide to experiential anatomy,* Barrytown, NY, 1991, Station Hill Press.

Platzer W: *Color atlas and textbook of human anatomy: locomotor system,* vol I, New York, 1984, Thieme.

Taber's cyclopedic medical dictionary, ed 13, Philadelphia, 1977, FA Davis.

Thibodeau G, Patton K: *Structure and function of the body,* ed 11, St Louis, 2000, Mosby.

Tortora GJ: *Introduction to the human body: the essentials of anatomy and physiology,* ed 3, New York, 1994, HarperCollins.

Wilson JM: *Doctoral dissertation: a natural philosophy of movement styles for theatre performers,* Madison, Wis, 1973, University of Wisconsin-Madison.

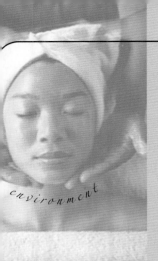

environment

Muscular System

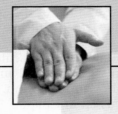

15

"One cannot step twice into the same river."

—Herakleitos

pressure

STUDENT OBJECTIVES

After completing this chapter, the student should be able to:

- Recall the functions of the muscular system
- Identify three classifications of muscle tissue and basic characteristics of each
- Categorize the connective tissue components of the muscular system
- List the parts of a skeletal muscle
- Explain the sliding filament theory including how muscles contract and relax
- Compare and contrast fast and slow twitch muscle fibers
- Identify how skeletal muscles interact to coordinate movement
- Demonstrate all types of skeletal muscle contraction
- Distinguish the difference between eccentric and concentric contractions
- Discuss the receptors involved in stretch reflexes
- Name types of muscular pathologies, giving characteristics and massage considerations of each

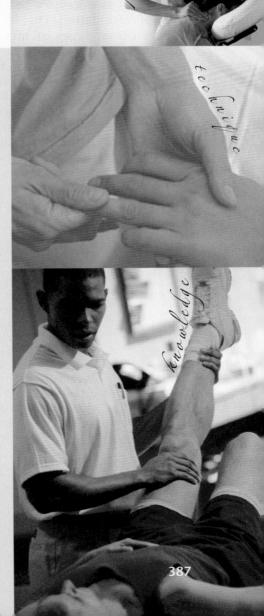

technique

knowledge

INTRODUCTION

Everything you have learned until now was in preparation for learning and understanding the muscular system. This knowledge is essential to massage therapists because the muscles and the related connective tissue (fascia) are the primary focus of massage.

The thought of being alive brings to the forefront the idea of movement—the heartbeat, muscle twitches, and the rise and fall of the chest with each breath. These visible signs of life are all created by muscle contraction.

This chapter examines the muscular system, exploring the mechanism of skeletal muscle contraction. The individual origin, insertion, and action of the muscles are discussed in Chapter 16.

In massage schools, the depth of knowledge regarding the muscular system exceeds that of many other health care fields. Beyond a basic understanding of the anatomy and physiology of the muscles, it is necessary to consider a broad spectrum of information. This includes the histology of muscle tissue; types of muscle tissue; connective tissue components; structures of skeletal muscles; anatomy, neurology, and chemistry of muscular contraction; muscular relaxation; types of skeletal muscle; muscle stretching; types of skeletal muscle contractions; muscle fiber arrangement; parts of a skeletal muscle; how the body coordinates movement; and muscular pathologies. This comprehensive study of muscles provides the massage therapist with a complex array of information that can be used to address muscular dysfunction resulting from stress, illness, or injury.

For Your Information

Muscle comes from the Latin word musculus, which means "a little mouse." How "little mouse" came to mean "muscle" seems to be explained by the appearance of movement of muscles under the skin to the scurrying of little mice. Dissected muscle may have looked like small rodents, and the tissue was named for this appearance. Anatomists of the pre-Galenic time had little knowledge of muscles. Plato and Aristotle, among other ancient authorities, regarded muscle tissue as part of the covering of the body, like skin.

FUNCTIONS

External mobility. Skeletal muscles create visible movement. This includes both motion and locomotion. *Motion* is defined as a change in position resulting from movement (e.g., manipulation); *locomotion* is defined as movement from one place to another.

Internal mobility. Internal mobility refers to the movement resulting from the contraction of smooth muscles. An example is peristalsis of the intestines. The special name given to the movement resulting from smooth muscle contractions is *motility*.

Produce heat. All muscle contractions produce and release heat. Muscles are the most metabolic structures in the body, producing a significant amount of heat. This physiological mechanism of thermogenesis is also important to maintain internal body temperature. Additionally, when the body becomes chilled, muscles contract rapidly (shivering) to produce additional heat.

Maintain posture. To maintain static positions such as sitting and standing, the skeletal muscles periodically contract to hold us in these postures. Muscles also contribute to joint stability.

HISTOLOGY

A muscle is composed of muscle bundles, or *fasciculi*, which is a group of muscle fibers. A muscle fiber is called a *myofibril* and is made up of *myofilaments* (e.g., actin, myosin). Groups of these muscle cells are

Terms and Their Meanings Related to the Muscular System	
Term	**Meaning**
antagonist	to struggle against
alba	white
aponeurosis	away from; nerve; condition
atrophy	lacking, without, not; to grow
concentric	toward the middle
eccentric	away from the middle
fatigue	to tire
fascia	strong central structural unit or band
fasciculi	little bundle
flaccid	flabby
Golgi tendon organs	Italian histologist (1844-1926)
hypertrophy	over, above, excessive; to grow
isometric	same or equal measure
isotonic	same or equal tension
myo	muscle
pennate	feather
retinaculum	a halter
sarco	flesh
spasm	a convulsion
synergist	together, work
tendon	to stretch

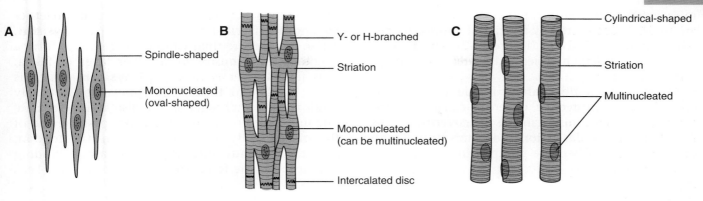

Figure 15-1 **A**, Smooth; **B**, cardiac; and **C**, skeletal muscle illustrations.

organized into muscular tissues. The progression from microscopic to macroscopic looks like this:

Myofilaments (actin/myosin) → Myofibrils (muscle fibers) → Fasciculi (muscle bundles) → Muscle

The three types of muscle tissue in the body are smooth muscle, cardiac muscle, and skeletal muscle (Figure 15-1) and are commonly referred to by their features or characteristics. Table 15-1 summarizes each type of muscle tissue according to its distinctive traits. Smooth muscle is found in the viscera of the body and includes blood vessels and the organs of digestion, excretion (urinary), and reproduction. Cardiac muscle is found in the heart, and skeletal

muscles generally attach to the bones of the skeleton either directly or indirectly. Each muscle tissue type is discussed, but the skeletal muscles are studied in detail. More information on cardiac muscle can be found in Chapter 19; smooth muscle receives additional coverage in Chapters 21 and 22.

CONNECTIVE TISSUE COMPONENTS AND OTHER RELATED STRUCTURES OF SKELETAL MUSCLES

Muscle fibers are generally arranged in parallel rows. Some individual muscle fibers may be more than 12 inches long. Muscles are considered to be tough, but

TABLE 15-1

Muscle Histological Table

Histological Characteristics	Smooth	Cardiac	Skeletal
Synonyms	Visceral	Heart	Voluntary
Striations	No	Yes	Yes
Number of nuclei	Mononucleate	Mononucleate (can be multinucleate)	Multinucleate
Location of nuclei	Centrally located	Centrally located	Peripherally located
Shape of nuclei	Oval shaped	Oval shaped	Small, elongated
Shape of fibers	Spindle shaped	Y or H shaped	Cylindrical shaped
Voluntary or involuntary	Involuntary	Involuntary	Voluntary
Fatigue rate: rapid, slow, or none	Slow	None	Rapid
Discussion	Forms the walls of hollow organs and tubes (e.g., stomach, bladder, blood vessel; controls the transport of materials, moving them along or restricting their flow	Located in the myocardium; possesses intercalated disks, which operate like an electrical synapse	Attaches to bones or related structures; is the "flesh" of the body; must be stimulated by a nerve impulse to contract

muscle fibers are quite fragile. Therefore they are arranged and protected by a series of connective tissue wrappings, or **fascia** (Figure 15-2). **Myofascial** refers to the skeletal muscles and related fascia in the muscular system.

Because muscle fibers are so fragile, each fiber is enclosed in a protective covering called the **endomysium**. This important fascial covering allows for muscular vascularization and innervation. Many of these muscle fibers are grouped into bundles of

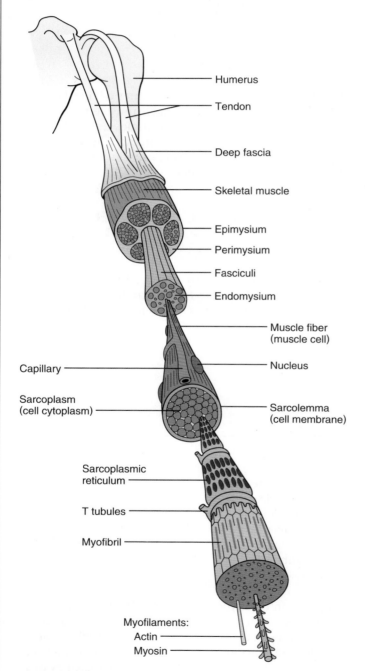

Capillary ──────────

Sarcoplasm
(cell cytoplasm) ──────

Sarcoplasmic
reticulum ──────

T tubules ──────

Myofibril ──────

Myofilaments:
    Actin ──────
    Myosin ──────

Humerus
Tendon
Deep fascia
Skeletal muscle
Epimysium
Perimysium
Fasciculi
Endomysium
Muscle fiber
(muscle cell)
Nucleus
Sarcolemma
(cell membrane)

Figure 15-2 Connective tissue components and anatomy of skeletal muscle.

tissue known as **fasciculi**, and are bound together by another fascia layer known as **perimysium**. These bundles are then wrapped together to form a single specific muscle by another layer of fascia. This fascial layer is called **epimysium**, which is quite tough and thick. The epimysium not only binds the fasciculi together but also acts to separate one muscle from another. It reaches past the end of the muscle belly, also encompassing the tendon, and then blends into the deep fascia, binding muscles into the following functional groups. Let's review:

Endomysium (wraps around muscle fibers) → Perimysium (wraps around muscle fiber bundles/fasciculi) → Epimysium (wraps around entire muscle) → Deep fascia (wraps muscle groups)

When organization of deep fascia forms a cord, anchoring the ends of muscle to bone, it is called a **tendon**. A broad, flat tendon is called an **aponeurosis** and attaches skeletal muscle to bone, another muscle, or skin. A muscle's more movable attachment is known as its *insertion,* whereas its more fixed (or immovable) attachment is known as its *origin* (both discussed later in this chapter). Tendons and aponeuroses are tough, collagenous structures and differ only in shape; tendons are cords, whereas aponeuroses are sheetlike. When tendons cross multiple joints, as in the hands and feet, they are wrapped in **tendon sheaths**. These tubular-shaped structures look like little sleeves and are lined with a synovial membrane. Synovial fluid reduces friction as the tendons glide back and forth within the sheath.

To keep tendons and tendon sheaths in place, **retinacula**, bandagelike retaining bands of connective tissue, are found primarily around the knees, ankles, and wrists. The retinaculum may also act as a pulley for the tendon at the joints of the wrist, ankle, and digits.

HOW DO MUSCLES CONTRACT?

Muscles possess the following characteristics that give them the ability to shorten and lengthen:
Contractility: Shortening of muscle fibers
Extensibility: Lengthening of muscle fibers
Elasticity: Ability of muscle fibers to return to its original shape after movement
Excitability: For muscles to contract, a nerve stimulus must be present
Years ago, physiologists believed that skeletal muscles contracted by folding like an accordion or by changes in the diameter of each cell. Some hypothe-

sized that muscles just grew or perhaps moved like springs. To understand this *shortening,* or contractile mechanism of the muscle, the muscle fibers must be examined themselves.

Sliding Filament Theory

In 1969, Hugh Huxley discovered that contraction does not occur by folding or "springing." Shortening or lengthening of a muscle results from a change in the relative positions of one muscle fiber to another. Myofilaments slide past each other in order to create a change in the length of muscle fibers, resulting in a change in the muscle length. This was appropriately named the **sliding filament theory**.

Think of these filaments as parts of a sliding glass door. The sliding door has two sections that sit side by side in adjacent tracks. Usually one door is permanently secured, and the other is movable. The entire glass door, when fully closed, represents a muscle at rest. The individual sections of the door represent muscle filaments. As the movable part of the door glides past the fixed door section, the length of the whole structure is shortened. As the door is pulled closed, the whole structure lengthens. Muscle contractions are similar. The lengths of the individual sections of filaments never change. Instead, they just slide over each other, changing the length of the muscle's contractile unit, or **sarcomere**. Other examples of this concept are a tele-

scoping car antenna or collapsible shower curtain rod. All these objects change their overall length by this sliding mechanism, as in muscle contraction.

THE ANATOMY OF MUSCULAR CONTRACTION

The three parts of a cell (membrane, cytoplasm, organelles) are all present in muscle cells, but they have specialized names and functions. The cell membrane is called the **sarcolemma** (Figure 15-3), and it encases the cytoplasm and organelles. The cytoplasm is called the **sarcoplasm** and surrounds the organelles. In addition to the regular organelles of other cells, a muscle cell contains two specialized organelles, the **sarcoplasmic reticulum** and **transverse** or **T tubules**. The sarcoplasmic reticulum is a fluid-filled system of cavities that contain the sarcomeres. The sarcoplasmic reticulum plays a crucial role in muscular contraction by storing and releasing calcium ions. The T tubules are channels that run transversely across the sarcoplasmic reticulum at the level of the Z-lines (mentioned in the following section). These T tubules invaginate the cell, and spread the action potential of the nerve impulse by transporting stored ions into and out of the cell.

Sarcomeres are composed of bundles of protein threads called **myofilaments**, or contractile proteins. The two types of myofilaments are **actin** and

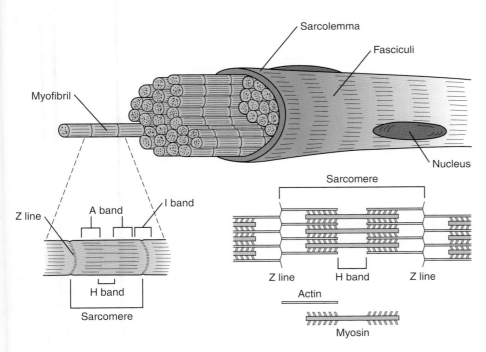

Figure 15-3   A myofibril with sarcomere, Z lines, H, I, and A bands. Sarcomere with actin and myosin.

myosin. The thin actin filaments are pulled over the thick myosin filaments to produce muscular contraction.

For Your Information

An easy way to remember that actin is the thinner myofilament and myosin is the thicker myofilament is that actin is a shorter/thinner word. Myosin is a longer/thicker word and is the thicker myofilament.

The sarcomeres are bundled together and lie in parallel rows in a honeycomb arrangement. These are stacked end to end in a continuous chain of repeating compartments. Defining the ends of the sarcomere are Z-lines, named because of their jagged appearance. Actin bundles are connected to the Z-lines at the end of the sarcomere. Myosin filaments do not run the entire length of the sarcomere. Because the filament arrangement is slightly staggered, the myofilaments overlap in some areas (dark stripe) and not in others (light stripe), giving it a striated appearance. The central region of a resting sarcomere is devoid of actin filaments, giving it a lighter color, and is known as the *H-band*. The dark red area on either side of the H-band, containing both actin and myosin, is known as the *A-band*. The absence of the myosin filament at either end of the sarcomere is known as the *I-band,* which has a light appearance. As the muscle contracts and the filaments slide, the white H- and I-bands become narrow.

The actin filaments resemble a twisted double strand of beads, and are dotted with protein molecules called **troponin** and **tropomyosin**. Together, tropomyosin and troponin regulate interactions of actin and myosin during muscle contractions. The binding sites on actin filaments are covered by troponin and tropomyosin. Here, they wait for calcium ions to move them off, which exposes the binding sites. When the binding sites are exposed, the myosin filaments can attach and contraction can occur (Figure 15-4). The myosin threads are the thicker protein filaments and are easily recognizable under a microscope because of the presence of cross-bridges or **myosin heads**. To understand neuroanatomy, a review of the following terms is necessary:

Sarcomere: Contractile unit
A-band: Actin and myosin overlapping
H-band: Myosin only; center of sarcomere
I-band: Actin only
Z-line: Ends of the sarcomere

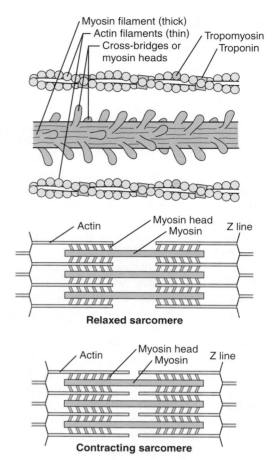

Figure 15-4   The drawing cross-bridge attachment process.

MINI-LAB

Hold your hands 18 inches from your face, palms facing you. Extend your thumbs up and interlace your fingers. Let your thumbs represent the Z-lines, and your fingers represent thick and thin myofilaments. Slide your fingers toward the middle. Notice how the space between your thumbs, or Z-lines, moves closer together. As the spaces between the thumbs shorten, do your fingers shorten? This illustrates how the sarcomere within a muscle creates movement by shortening.

THE NEUROLOGY OF MUSCLE CONTRACTION

The contraction of skeletal muscle begins with a nerve impulse that stimulates the conversion of chemical energy into mechanical energy. This nerve impulse may be initiated by either a reflex or a conscious desire to change the body's position. This stimulus travels down the **motor neurons** to the muscle. Motor neurons are responsible for carrying messages of contraction (or in some cases, inhibition of contraction) to a muscle. One motor neuron may branch off and connect to 10 or 1000 individual muscle fibers. A single motor neuron and all its associated skeletal muscle fibers are known as a **motor unit**. A single muscle is composed of many motor units. The axons of the motor neurons terminate at the sarcolemma of muscle fibers to form the **neuromuscular junction**. This gap, filled with interstitial fluid, is called the **synaptic cleft** and is between the neuron and muscle fiber; the neuron does not make physical contact with the muscle.

When a motor neuron delivers a stimulus, all the muscle fibers of the motor unit receive the signal to contract at the same time. If the stimulus lacks sufficient intensity (subthreshold stimulus), the motor neuron is not activated, and contraction does not occur. In the absence of sufficient stimuli, each muscle fiber relaxes to its full resting length. Likewise, each individual muscle fiber, when sufficiently stimulated, contracts to its fullest extent. Within the muscle fibers of motor units, no partial contraction takes place. This is known as the **all-or-none response**.

This all-or-none response is true only for motor units, not the entire muscle. Thousands of motor units are in a single muscle. The nervous system regulates the amount of muscular contraction by activating only the motor units needed to perform a given action. If more strength is required, additional motor units are stimulated, and the muscle contrac-

tion is stronger. More motor units are required to pick up a hammer than to pick up a nail. This process of motor unit activation based on need is known as **recruitment**.

THE CHEMISTRY OF MUSCLE CONTRACTION

When the nerve impulse travels through a motor neuron and enters the neuromuscular junction through the axon terminal, a chemical messenger stored in vesicles, is released (Figure 15-5). This chemical is called **acetylcholine** (ACh) and is stored in synaptic vesicles at the **axon terminal** (where the axon of the motor neuron terminates). When ACh crosses the synaptic cleft to the sarcolemma, it binds with receptor sites on the **motor end plate** like a key in a lock. When this connection is made with the sarcolemma, it temporarily becomes permeable to sodium ions, which enter the cell. The excess of positive sodium ions disrupts the electrical environment inside the cell and actually generates an electrical impulse or **action potential**.

The impulse travels across the surface of the sarcolemma and is carried into the cell through the T tubules, causing sodium ions (Na) to enter and potassium ions (K) to leave the muscle cell. The introduction of sodium triggers calcium ions (Ca) to be released from storage in the sarcoplasmic reticulum.

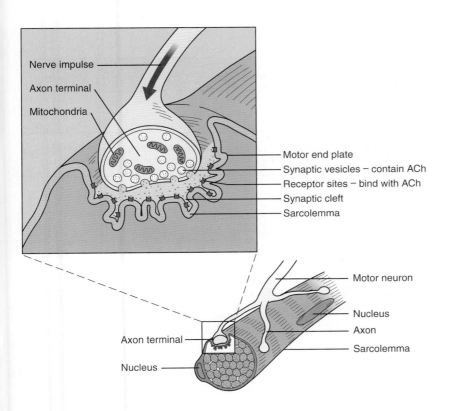

Nerve impulse
Axon terminal
Mitochondria

Motor end plate
Synaptic vesicles – contain ACh
Receptor sites – bind with ACh
Synaptic cleft
Sarcolemma

Motor neuron
Nucleus
Axon
Sarcolemma

Axon terminal
Nucleus

Figure 15-5 Neuromuscular junction.

Calcium ions are the chemical driving force behind contraction because it assists actin and myosin to connect so contraction can occur.

To review, positioned on the actin filaments are two regulatory proteins called *troponin* and *tropomyosin.* They cover the myosin binding site, preventing attachment of myosin so that muscles are not in a constant state of contraction. However, when calcium ions enter the sarcomere, these ions bond with the troponin-tropomyosin complex, altering them in a way that leaves an exposed site for the heads of the myosin filaments to attach.

The connection between the myosin heads and the actin filaments creates a cross-bridge effect. The myosin heads are hinged at their base, and during contraction, toggle like a light switch. If energy from adenosine triphosphate (ATP) is present, the myosin heads toggle several times, pulling the attached actin filaments toward the H-band (center of the sarcomere). This process repeats itself; actin and myosin filaments draw Z-lines closer together, causing the entire sarcomere to shorten (Figure 15-6). Hence muscle contraction has occurred, and this process takes just a few thousandths of second.

Figure 15-6   Muscular contraction simplified.

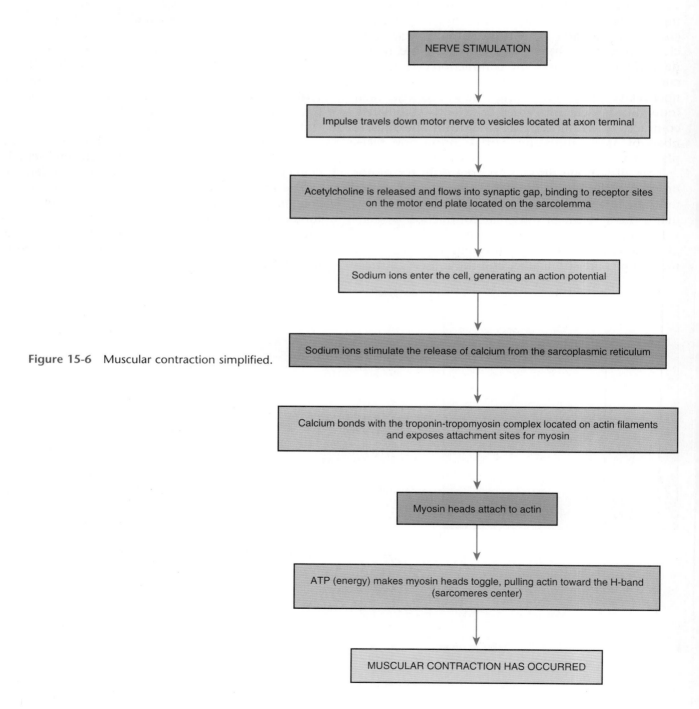

NERVE STIMULATION

Impulse travels down motor nerve to vesicles located at axon terminal

Acetylcholine is released and flows into synaptic gap, binding to receptor sites on the motor end plate located on the sarcolemma

Sodium ions enter the cell, generating an action potential

Sodium ions stimulate the release of calcium from the sarcoplasmic reticulum

Calcium bonds with the troponin-tropomyosin complex located on actin filaments and exposes attachment sites for myosin

Myosin heads attach to actin

ATP (energy) makes myosin heads toggle, pulling actin toward the H-band (sarcomeres center)

MUSCULAR CONTRACTION HAS OCCURRED

Muscular Relaxation

When the nerve stimulus stops, ACh is no longer released from the axon terminal vesicles of the motor neuron. To clean up any residual ACh in the synaptic cleft, the enzyme **acetylcholinesterase** (AChE) is secreted. This stops the flow of sodium ions into the muscle cell. Without the sodium ions, flow of calcium ions is shut down. Existing calcium ions are returned to the sarcoplasmic reticulum by an ATP transport pump. Sodium and potassium ions are actively transported back to their initial positions through a sodium/potassium pump. Freed from its chemical bond with the calcium ions, the troponin-tropomyosin complex recovers the attachment sites on the actin filaments. This action releases the myosin filaments, which return to their relaxed state (Figure 15-7). The muscle is now at rest.

A goal in massage is to release muscular spasm. One of the components of a spasm is a leak of calcium from the sarcoplasmic reticulum without nerve stimulation. This can occur as a result of a tear from an injury or exercise. The calcium triggers contraction and this sets up a condition of spasm, unless something flushes the calcium out of the cells. Massage creates a flushing affect, and not only removes

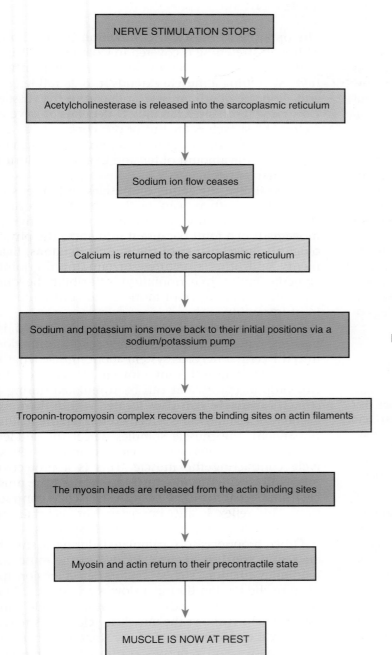

Figure 15-7   Muscular relaxation simplified.

calcium but also metabolic wastes. As an added bonus, massage also brings oxygen and other essential nutrients to the tissues.

THREE TYPES OF SKELETAL MUSCLE FIBERS

Smooth and cardiac muscle tissue is the same throughout the body; no variations are evident. However, skeletal muscle is classified into three types of fibers: **slow twitch**, **fast twitch A**, and **fast twitch B**. This terminology is used to describe how fast the muscle fibers use the energy stored in muscle, or ATP, and how fast they convert adenosine diphosphate (ADP) to ATP. ADP is produced by the use of ATP and is converted back to ATP once energy is produced. Slow twitch fibers accomplish this aerobically (with O_2) while fast twitch fibers conduct this process anaerobically (without O_2). The ratio of slow twitch to fast twitch is unique to each individual, but some commonalities exist, as is described in the following:

1. **Slow twitch.** Also known as *red muscle,* slow twitch fibers are fatigue-resistant fibers, are small in diameter, are very vascular, and have copious amounts of mitochondria and a red respiratory pigment called *myoglobin*. **Myoglobin** is chemically similar to the hemoglobin molecule present in red blood cells. Slow twitch fibers generate large amounts of ATP aerobically, but break down the ATP slowly to reduce the rate of muscle contraction so muscles are not easily fatigued. Most postural muscles are slow twitch muscles. A high ratio of slow twitch muscles is present in the legs of world-class long-distance runners.

For Your Information

The presence of myoglobin in skeletal muscles makes them appear darker. Notice that the dark meat of chickens are the legs and the thighs. Ducks, on the other hand, have dark breast meat. This is because, in general, chickens run around a chicken yard and ducks fly powered by their breast muscles.

2. **Fast twitch A.** Fast twitch muscles are also fatigue-resistant fibers and are intermediate in diameter; they are referred to a *pink muscle*. They contain large amounts of myoglobin, many mitochondria, and numerous capillaries. These fibers also generate copious amounts of ATP aerobically. However, they break down ATP quickly. Fast twitch A fibers are resistant to fatigue but not as much as slow twitch fibers. Many world-class sprinters have a high ratio of fast twitch A in their leg muscles and world-class

boxers have a high ratio of fast twitch A in their arms. Although legs are involved in maintaining posture, they also have some slow twitch fibers.

3. **Fast twitch B.** Also known as *white muscle,* fast twitch B are rapidly fatigable fibers. They possess the largest diameters, have the lowest amount of myoglobin, few mitochondria, and few capillaries, so they appear white. Fast twitch B fibers generate ATP anaerobically in short bursts, and these fibers fatigue quickly. However, their contractions are powerful and rapid. Muscles of the arm contain many fast twitch B fibers.

STRETCHING

The opposite of muscular contraction is stretching. Although stretching is covered in Chapter 7, it is important enough to warrant another brief mention here. Stretching a muscle extends it to its full length and elongates both muscle and connective tissue. How far you can stretch a muscle depends on several factors. Most factors are out of our control (e.g., genetics, movement capability of a joint). What can be changed is the amount of tension in a muscle during a voluntary stretch.

Extensibility, the ability of muscles and other soft tissues to lengthen, can be improved by regular stretching. Stretching can also improve the range of movement of a joint because it influences the physiological characteristics of the muscle, tendons, ligaments, and other structures surrounding the joint. Hyperflexibility (hypermobility) is flexibility beyond a joint's normal range of motion and contributes to joint instability.

Proprioceptors are sensory receptors located in muscles, tendons, and joints. They send information into the central nervous system about muscle length, muscle tension, and joint movements. One of the two proprioceptors that can be stimulated during a stretch is **muscle spindles** located within the muscle belly. If the muscle is stretched too rapidly (ballistic stretch), the muscle spindles detect the sudden motion, and the nervous system responds by reflexively contracting the muscle. This is a protective mechanism which is intended to safeguard the muscle from overstretching by causing muscular contraction. This reflex is also important for maintaining posture, which is mediated by muscle spindles.

Other proprioceptors stimulated during a stretch are **Golgi tendon organs**, located in the musculotendinous junction. These receptors detect tension applied to the tendon during a slow, static stretch. The nervous system responds by inhibiting muscle contraction, which allows the muscle to relax and stretch. It works the exact opposite of the stretch reflex mentioned above and represses contraction to prevent tearing of a muscle or avulsion of the tendon from its attachment.

Massage therapists can use this information when applying or instructing clients in stretching. To enhance flexibility, apply only slow, static stretches. Movements that are perceived by the nervous system as "dangerous" will be met with resistance.

MINI-LAB

Hold a shoestring by the two coated ends with both of your hands. Slowly begin to pull the ends apart. Watch what happens to the individual strands in the string. Do the fibers spread apart or draw closer together? Imagine that this string is a muscle and the two ends are tendinous attachments. Within this muscle is a spasm. Pull the ends again. As the muscle is being stretched, is the spasm released? Note that separation in the muscle fibers does not occur when the muscle is stretched. This explains why stretching does not release local muscle spasms.

TYPES OF SKELETAL MUSCLE CONTRACTIONS

Isotonic contractions. During isotonic, or dynamic, contractions, the muscle changes length against resistance, and movement occurs. This is the most common type of muscle contraction. Isotonic contractions result from increased nerve activity and increased blood supply to the muscles being contracted (Figure 15-8, *A*). When a muscle is involved in isotonic contractions, it can shorten or lengthen. In fact, lengthening contractions are as much a part of coordinated motion as shortening contractions. Without the ability of a muscle to shorten and lengthen during contractions, we could not lower objects after we lifted them. Shortening contractions are called concentric and lengthening contractions are called eccentric.

- **Concentric contractions**. This type of isotonic contraction occurs as the muscle shortens and pulls on a bone to produce movement. When movement occurs as the muscle is shortening, it is called a concentric or shortening contraction. An example of a concentric contraction is the lifting phase of a biceps curl (flexing the elbow). Muscles involved in concentric contractions are also known as accelerators or spurt muscles. They may provide a forward acceleration in locomotion.

- **Eccentric contractions**. Eccentric contractions, or lengthening contractions, occur when the muscle lengthens during contraction. For example, during the lowering phase of a biceps curl, the biceps brachii muscle will be eccentrically contracted as you extend the elbow. The biceps brachii is contracting, but it is getting longer. Repeated eccentric contraction causes more muscle damage and muscle soreness than concentric contraction, such as running downhill. These muscles are also known as decelerators or shunt muscles because they slow down the powerful concentric contractors. Unless the body compensates with some corrective braking action, injuries are likely to occur.

Isometric contractions. Muscles do not always shorten or lengthen when they contract (Figure 15-9). If you attempt to pick up a weight that is too heavy, do the muscles still shorten? No. In isometric muscle contractions, the muscle increases in tension by contraction but does not change its length or angle of the joint. Isometric contractions are important because they stabilize some joints as others are moved (Figure 15-8, *B*).

Isometrics are the therapy of choice when a client fears pain during movement or refuses to move an in-

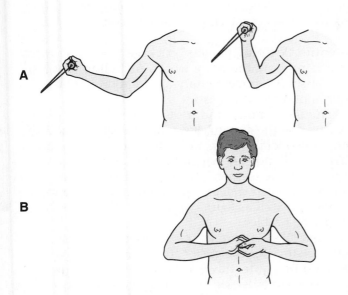

Figure 15-8 Isotonic **(A)** vs. isometric **(B)** contractions.

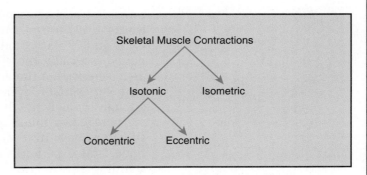

Figure 15-9 Skeletal muscle contractions.

JON ZAHOUREK

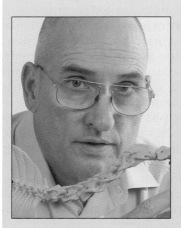

Born: January 5, 1940.

"The mind cannot forget what the hands have learned."

Artists dream of creating a work designed to last. Jon Zahourek is no exception. What makes him unique, however, is that his masterpiece could influence the way future generations learn how the body—especially the muscles—works.

It was a painful process for Zahourek, but not your typical artistic angst. For years Zahourek, a sculptor, artist, and Parson's School of Design instructor, was plagued with debilitating back pain. As a drawing teacher he taught a detailed anatomy class. "The names of some of the muscles scared me to death," he laughs. So, like a lot of teachers, he would gloss over these and go on. But a new way to teach anatomy led to a revelation for Zahourek, who began building clay muscles—layer by layer—on a model skeleton.

"It was like 'whoosh,' a wind rushed through me and suddenly everything that I had been trying to teach about how the muscles work became integrated within me. I spent all weekend trying to understand what happened," he says. "What most of us grasp about how our bodies work is either very childlike or dead wrong."

But he wasn't able to see this—or feel it in his own body—until he actually modeled each muscle in space. By building each muscle, one by one, and learning how it connected to bone and worked with or against other muscles, Zahourek moved from the ability to point to a muscle, name it, and tell his students which action it performed to a deeper level of knowing. Suddenly his body understood and felt how each muscle worked. "It set me free physically! My back problems of 20 years were gone. It wasn't the pain that was disabling me. It was the fear and lack of knowledge. I didn't understand what was causing the pain until I began to see the conflicts between the muscles."

If this could have such a liberating effect on him, it could also help others. So, what started as the perfect way to instruct art students became a creative work in itself. At first he intended to build clay muscles on a life-sized wooden skeletal model, then realizing the weight would be not only unwieldy but downright deadly if it toppled over on someone, he began to create scaled-down models. When these were perfected, Zahourek Systems, Inc., was born. A complete system package contains detailed videos, workbooks, clay, sculpting tools, and mannequins (skeletons of varying degrees of complexity and price ranges).

He began marketing his entire "learning process" package to anyone who could benefit from understanding how the body works, including physical therapists, college anatomy classes, even elementary-aged children, massage therapy schools, and of course, massage therapists.

For massage therapists, Zahourek's model and ideas have several implications. For massage schools who use the system, it's a guaranteed method to learn—really learn—the musculoskeletal system, not just about where a muscle is and its name and shape. It's hands-on, which benefits all massage students, especially those who are tactile learners, as many massage therapists are. Otherwise, a therapist may complete a degree program and merely work on a very surface level—literally, as well as figuratively—and often that's not enough for a client with a specific problem.

There's also the chance, that like Zahourek, the massage therapist will somehow have his or her own chance for the great "aha" to rush through his body, and experience the opportunity to travel from a conceptual understanding of how the muscles work to a deeper, cognitive level—to know the

JON ZAHOUREK—cont'd

body from the inside out. Massage therapists lucky enough to have had this experience can often tell from the moment the client walks into the office, what's happening with her body. The therapist doesn't just see it, he senses it or even feels it.

Massage therapists absolutely and unequivocally must understand their own bodies. Massage therapy can be such physically demanding work, many therapists don't last for more than 5 years. Not understanding their own bodies—and their hands in particular—is occupational suicide. As Zahourek says, "It's like working hard for a diploma and someone telling you, 'Congratulations, in 4 years you'd better find something else to do.'" Massage therapists need to understand how it all works. Zahourek offers the analogy: If you were a runner and you woke up one morning and your legs were sore, you wouldn't stop running, would you?

One way to stay strong? "Socrates was right," says Zahourek. "Know thyself." As massage therapists we must return again and again to the learning laboratory—our own minds and bodies, peeling layer from layer, then rebuilding layer upon layer until we get it right. Jon Zahourek, in his attempt to teach art students how to draw more lifelike figures, stumbled upon a new lease on life for himself and a model that allows massage therapists to learn how the body works in a way that will never be forgotten.

jured part. However they only strengthen muscles in the position of the actual contraction. Isometric contractions are the key component of Muscle Energy Techniques and are used when a muscle does not respond to massage. Isometrics are great for building muscle bulk or increasing strength in certain positions, but these exercises do not increase the efficiency or endurance of skeletal muscles.

Isometric contraction can also be used clinically to reset tone on muscles weak from nonuse. It is often the first method of rehabilitation after surgery or injury, because isometric contractions are relatively painless and increase local blood circulation without stretching tissues.

PARTS OF A SKELETAL MUSCLE

The gross structures of a skeletal muscle come in a range of shapes and sizes, but all possess a central portion of the muscle and at least two points of attachment. At the simplest level, a muscle shortens, one attachment moves toward the other, and movement occurs. These attachment sites can also be referred to as the "origin" and "insertion," which are terms that indicate movement caused by muscle contraction. Generally, insertion moves toward origin; however, the roles can be reversed. Some muscles

possess a property of *functional reversibility*. An example of this is the psoas major muscle that can flex the trunk by bringing the trunk down or by lifting the lower leg up. Following are the parts of a muscle:

Belly. The belly of the muscle is also referred to as the gaster (Figure 15-10). This wide central portion comprises the bulk of the muscle. The belly of the muscle produces movement of the joint by the shortening of its fleshy mass during contraction. This action pulls the tendons attaching the muscle to the bone closer together. The tissue of the muscle belly contains sarcomeres, the functional contractile unit of the muscle discussed earlier.

The arrangement of the muscle belly is dependant on the available space; typically in the central portion of a limb. Long tendons attached to muscle bellies are advantageous if there is a shortage of space, such as the hands and feet. Hence, the muscles that have the most influence on movement in the hands and feet are located in the forelimbs.

Origin. The tendinous attachment of the muscle on the less movable bone or attachment during contraction is its origin. It is usually located on the medial or proximal end of the skeleton.

Insertion. The insertion, usually located lateral or distal, is the muscle attachment on the more movable bone or attachment during contraction.

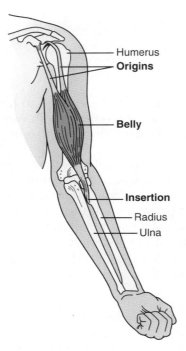

Figure 15-10   Parts of a skeletal muscle.

When a muscular contraction occurs, the insertion commonly moves toward the origin.

As you learn individual skeletal muscles, the origins and insertions will help you to think about muscles causing a desired action. When a muscle crosses a joint, it acts on that joint. Muscles may cross one or more joints and are referred to as uniarticular, biarticular, and multiarticular.

Uniarticular: Muscles that cross one joint.
Biarticular: Muscles that cross two joints, acting on both joints.
Multiarticular: Muscles that cross more than two joints.

MUSCLE FIBER ARRANGEMENT

Muscle fibers are arranged in several ways, typically due to the relationship between the muscle fibers and its tendons. The differences between muscle fiber arrangements affect its shape and the resulting strength (Figure 15-11). Parallel muscle fiber arrangements have greater range of motion but are less powerful. The multipennate shape allows more force in contraction but offers less range of motion. Muscle fiber arrangements are as follows:

Parallel: The fibers in this arrangement run in a parallel arrangement down a long axis. These can be quadrilateral (four-sided) or triangular (fan-shaped).
Fusiform: These muscles are spindle-shaped with the fibers tapering at both ends.
Circular: Muscles that form a circular arrangement describe this arrangement.
Pennate: These muscles are short and are arranged with a central tendon and muscle fibers extending from the tendon diagonally, giving the muscle a feather-like appearance. Types of penniform muscles are a unipennate (fibers come off one side of the tendon), bipennate (fibers arranged on both sides of a central tendon) and multipennate (have several tendons within the belly with fibers run diagonally between them).

Furthermore, a muscle may have more than one origin, or head. For example, a muscle may be two-, three-, or four-headed. Each "head" represents a muscle belly. These individual insertions merge into a single muscle belly and terminate into a common insertion. Examples of this type of arrangement are the biceps (brachii and femoris), triceps (brachii and surae), and the quadriceps femoris.

For Your Information

The two worst things for your muscular system are overuse and no use.
    Somewhere in between is the right use.

HOW DOES THE BODY COORDINATE MOVEMENT?

Muscles work most of the time to maintain posture and to help keep joints stabilized. This continuous, partial contraction is called muscle tone or **tonus**. Posture can be static (not moving) or dynamic (in

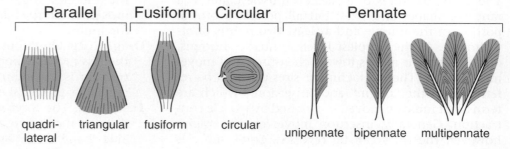

Figure 15-11   Muscle fiber arrangements.

motion). Muscles do not simply contract simultaneously to achieve motion. Even the simplest movements would be impossible with all the muscles fully contracted. Instead, muscles assume different responsibilities to carry out a variety of movements. A muscle may function as agonist, antagonist, synergist, or fixator depending on its role in performing a particular task. Agonists are also called prime movers, and fixators are also referred to as stabilizers.

Most skeletal muscles are arranged in pairs. The muscle that is most responsible for causing desired joint action is the **agonist**. The opposing muscle, or **antagonist**, must stretch, resist, or yield to the joint motion initiated by the agonist. The antagonist usually lies on the opposite side of the joint and causes the opposite joint action. Imagine what movement would be like without the antagonist opposing the pull of the prime mover. The upper fibers of the trapezius muscle would contract, creating extension of the head. When the movement task is fulfilled, your head would fall, uncontrolled, in response to the pull of gravity. The antagonist allows movements to be more controlled and refined. Examples of an agonist/antagonist relationship are the biceps brachii/triceps brachii.

To help things run smoothly, other muscles, called **synergists**, aid by causing the same movement. For example, the peroneus longus and peroneus brevis are synergistic as well as the gastrocnemius and soleus.

Fixators are specialized synergists. They stabilize the joint over which the prime mover exerts its action. This allows the prime mover to perform a motion more efficiently. For example, the postural muscles stabilize the vertebral column so the iliopsoas and the rectus femoris can flex the thigh. Let's review:

Agonist/prime mover: Muscle causing desired action

Antagonist: Muscle opposing agonist

Synergist: Muscle aiding by causing same movement

Fixators/stabilizers: Muscles stabilizing joints so agonist can exert its action

When the central nervous system sends a message for the agonist (muscle causing movement) to contract, the tension in the antagonist (muscle opposing movement) is inhibited by impulses from motor nerves, and thus must simultaneously relax. *This neural phenomenon is called reciprocal inhibition (Sherrington's Law).*

This information can be used to ease the pain of an acute muscle spasm or cramp. Contract the muscle opposite (antagonist) of the muscle spasm and the muscle spasm will let go. This conscious contraction may have to be repeated several times, and the contraction must be isometrically resisted. It is as if the brain is turning off the message of contraction, and relaxation is the result. A further discussion can be found in Chapter 17.

Strain between body segments alters patterns of movement. Tight muscles can affect movement partly because antagonists cannot fully elongate. Any given movement evokes response not only from the prime movers but also from the antagonists, synergists, and fixators. Imagine watching a baseball player throw a baseball. His foot goes forward, one hip swings back, then forward as his entire upper torso and arm are propelling the baseball. Full, powerful motion is a synchronized wave of smaller motions rather than a single movement.

Let's apply one of these concepts to a clinical setting. One rehabilitative approach for musculoskeletal problems is to strengthen the antagonist. This corrects positional and postural distortions by creating balanced motion on both sides of the joint. For example, if poor posture is due to hypercontracted back muscles, strengthening the abdominals can create a change in the resting length of these tight muscles. Don't be surprised if a client with a low back condition comes home from a doctor's appointment with a recommended daily routine of proper abdominal exercises.

MUSCULAR PATHOLOGIES

Atrophy. A decrease in the size of muscle fibers or a wasting away of muscles from poor nutrition, lack of use, motor unit dysfunction, or lack of motor nerve impulses is called muscular atrophy.

Massage strokes should be slow, superficial, and soothing with intermittent use of vibration and cross fiber tapotement.

Contracture. Also known as ischemic contracture, contracture is an abnormal, usually permanent condition of a joint in which the muscle is fixed in a flexed position. It may be the result of spasm, paralysis, or fibrotic tissue surrounding a joint. A contracture can be brought on by heat or medication.

Use broad strokes to increase blood flow in the affected area. Friction, followed by the application of ice, can be used to reduce adhesions. The muscles should be kneaded thoroughly to stretch the fascia. Myofascial release would also be helpful. Slow and gentle stretches may help elongate the muscles.

Fibromyalgia. Also known as fibrositis, or muscular rheumatism, fibromyalgia is a chronic inflammatory disease that affects muscle and related connective tissues. Pain, joint stiffness, and the presence of "tender points" and "trigger points" are involved in this condition. During diagnosis, the physician evaluates 18 tender points on the body; if 11 of these 18 points are painful, the diagnosis of fibromyalgia is often made. This condition frequently develops after emotional trauma (client may not have dealt with an emotional situation and it manifests as physical pain), local or general infections, or even changes in climate. The symptoms vary from individual to individual and may range from pain, insomnia, headaches, depression, GI and urinary disturbances, to lethargy. Fibromyalgia may go into remission, only to flare up at a later date.

Massage should be tailored to how the client is feeling at the time of the treatment because symptoms vary from day to day. Some clients want deep pressure and others can withstand only light pressure. Massage is currently the best treatment for this condition.

Flaccid. Muscles lacking normal tone are loose and appear flattened rather than rounded are flaccid muscles. Flaccidity is often considered the first stage of muscular atrophy. Muscles will become flaccid if they are not used and exercised regularly.

Friction, effleurage, and pétrissage may help increase muscle tone with intermittent use of vibrating and cross fiber tapotement.

Hernia. A hernia is a protrusion of an organ or part of an organ through its surrounding connective tissue membranes or cavity wall. This condition may be congenital, resulting from failure of structures to completely close after birth, or a hernia may be developmental due to obesity, chronic illness, or surgery. There are many types of hernias and they are named for their location (e.g., hiatal, inguinal).

Local massage is contraindicated. General massage is okay to do. If the client is experiencing pain in the area of the hernia, refer him immediately to his healthcare professional.

Hypertrophy. An increase in the size and diameter of muscle fibers without cell division is known as hypertrophy. Exercise and weight lifting may cause muscular hypertrophy, which increases the number of actin and myosin filaments in the sarcomere.

Massage is fine for hypertrophy.

Muscle fatigue. Muscle activity cannot be sustained indefinitely. The inability of a muscle to contract even though it is still being stimulated is called muscle fatigue. Insufficient oxygen, exhaustion of energy supply, or the accumulation of lactic acid can cause muscles to lose their ability to contract efficiently. A muscle may become fatigued if it generates wastes faster than the circulatory system can carry them away. When muscle fatigue occurs, muscle strength and coordination decrease.

Massage can increase local circulation to a muscle, helping to reduce muscle fatigue by bringing nutrition to the cells and transporting wastes away.

Muscle spasm/cramp. An increase in muscle tension with or without shortening due to excessive motor nerve activity may result in a rigid zone (knot) in the muscle called a spasm. Muscle spasms cannot be alleviated by voluntary relaxation. Cramping is often associated with mineral deficiency or muscle fatigue and is usually short-lived.

Massage can increase local circulation to a muscle spasm/cramp and mechanically lengthen and spread muscle fibers apart.

Muscular dystrophy. A collection of genetic diseases, muscular dystrophy is characterized by the progressive atrophy of skeletal muscles without any indication of neural degeneration or damage. All forms of muscular dystrophy involve a loss of muscular strength, disability, and deformity.

Massage may slow muscular atrophy. Also, active and passive range of motion of the joints may be helpful. Abdominal massage may help with constipation because this disorder also affects involuntary muscles, including those of the large intestine.

Myasthenia gravis. Myasthenia gravis is a weakness in the muscles characterized by chronic fatigability. This is an autoimmune disorder, resulting in a deficiency of acetylcholine, causing a malfunction at the neuromuscular junction. The onset of myasthenia gravis is gradual, with an initial drooping of the upper eyelids, throat, and facial muscles. The weakness may extend to the respiratory muscles. Muscular exertion may exacerbate this condition and is not advised.

Clearance for massage from the client's physician is necessary. Massage may slow the muscle atrophy. Also, active and passive range of motion of the joints may be helpful.

Plantar fasciitis. This is inflammation of the plantar fascia at the calcaneus, medial aspect of the foot, and insertions of tibialis posterior. Symptoms are "pain in the heel," and/or pain on dorsiflexion. Clients will often state that they cannot walk comfortably on their heels for several hours after waking. The pain frequently goes away, only to return the next morning.

Massage is okay. If the condition is prolonged, the client may not be able to withstand pressure applied to the heel. Suggest ice to combat the inflammation and an activity that does not involve putting pressure on the heel, such as biking or swimming. Cross fiber friction on the calcaneus may reduce adhesions, and muscles of the leg should be massaged thoroughly.

Shin splints. Shin splints are strain of the either anterior or posterior tibial muscles marked by pain along the shin bone. It is often the result of running or jumping on hard surfaces. During these activities, the tibia and fibula are jarred on top of the talus bone, causing the tibia and fibula to migrate laterally. This action tears the interosseous membrane between the two lower leg bones as well as the muscles attaching to all three structures (tibia, fibula, and interosseous membrane). Pain is referred to the anterior tibial shaft (shin).

Massage of the tibialis anterior is helpful. Tibialis posterior is too deep of a muscle to easily access; deep massage of the calf may bring some pain relief. Suggest ICE (ice, compression, elevation), rest, proper athletic shoes, and performing their athletic activity on a yielding surface.

Spasticity. Spasticity is characterized by increased muscle tone and stiffness and is associated with an increase in tendon reflexes. A spastic muscle will resist stretching and typically involves the arm flexors and leg extenders and effects can range from mild to severe. In severe cases, movement patterns become uncoordinated or impossible and usually involve a neurological dysfunction.

Clearance from the client's physician is necessary. Use caution during the massage since sensations are impaired and client may not be able to give accurate feedback. Move the joints through as wide a ROM as possible without using force. Cross fiber friction can be used around joints to prevent adhesions and contractures. Concentrate on the spastic muscles as well, using a gentle pressure. Ongoing massage treatments can be very helpful.

Strain. A strain, commonly called a pull, is an injury of a muscle or tendon due to a violent contraction, forced stretching, or synergistic failure. Most muscle strains occur on the antagonist, or the muscle that must resist the muscle creating the action. When the antagonist is tight or spasmed, it cannot stretch easily and may become injured. Acute muscle strains can be classified into the following three grades or degrees of severity (Figure 15-12):

1. **First-degree** strains involve up to 20% of stretching or a partial tear of fibers with no pal-

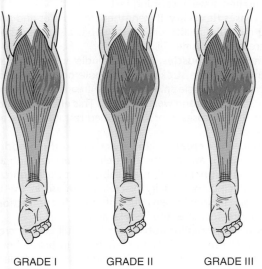

GRADE I   GRADE II   GRADE III

Figure 15-12 Three degrees of strain.

pable defects. There is typically mild pain at the time of injury and there may be mild swelling and localized tenderness. The joint structures can maintain efficient motion and hold against resistance.

2. When the muscle or tendon is torn between 20 and 75%, it is classified as a **second-degree** strain. A palpable defect is noted and the joint structures cannot hold against moderate resistance. Edema is typically found, and the muscles surrounding the strain splint to restrict painful movement.

3. In **third-degree** tears, 75% to 100% of the fibers are torn. Third-degree tears may represent a complete rupture of the involved structures. An avulsion fracture is when a tendon is pulled away from a bone, taking a bone fragment with it. A depression in the area of the torn muscle can be palpated and is usually painful to touch. Function is greatly altered in third-degree tears.

Use ice therapy in the first 72 hours to reduce pain and swelling. Massage around the affected area can reduce muscle spasms. Don't massage distal to injury site. Move joints passively to maintain ROM. Be careful not to stretch the injured area. After the acute stage, cross fiber friction can prevent adhesion formation. Gentle stretches to realign fibers can be done. Initially, treatments of shorter duration are indicated, and can become longer as injury heals.

Tendinitis. Inflammation of the tendon, accompanied by pain and swelling, is called tendinitis. This may be a result of chronic overuse, direct trauma, or even a sudden pull of the muscle. When inflammation also involves the tendon sheath, it is referred to as tenosynovitis.

If tendinitis is the result of injury, wait 72 hours. Afterward, massage should include stripping the muscle, cross fiber friction on the involved tendons, and a follow-up with 20 minutes of ice.

Torticollis. Torticollis, or wryneck, involves spasms of the sternocleidomastoid muscles. The scalenes, trapezius, and the splenius muscles may also be involved. This condition may cause vertigo because of the many sensory and positional receptors located in the SCM. Because this muscular condition is often unilateral, a tilt or rotation of the head is often noted.

Local massage is indicated and treatment should include not only SCM but also the trapezius, the scalenes, and the splenis muscles. Moist heat can reduce spasms and loosen connective tissues. Firm, but light strokes along the muscles may help loosen them as well.

See Box 15-1 for the effects of massage on muscles.

SUMMARY

The understanding of structures and functions of muscle tissue and its related fascia is vital to the practice of massage therapy. Physiologically, muscles serve four basic functions; they provide external mobility and internal motility, produce heat, and maintain posture. It takes three different types of muscle tissue to perform these various functions: smooth, cardiac, and skeletal.

Each skeletal muscle is composed of bundles of muscle fibers known as fasciculi. These are bound together individually and collectively with layers of fascia, which is a tough, white, protective membrane. The main part of the muscle is the belly, which is attached to the bone by two or more tendons, which are known as its origin and insertion. The shortening of the muscle belly draws the tendons closer together to produce movement. This shortening is produced by a change in the relative size of the basic contractile unit known as the sarcomere. An explanation of the cellular processes of muscular contraction is known as the sliding filament theory.

In the coordination of movement, muscles work in pairs or groups. Muscles involved in these groups are classified by function as agonists (prime movers), antagonists, synergists, and fixators (stabilizers). The muscle tissue can also be classified by its chemistry as slow twitch or fast twitch (A and B).

Biomechanically, muscles do one of two things: stretch or contract. Muscular contractions can be isometric or isotonic. Isotonic contractions may be further classified as either concentric or eccentric. The opposite of contracting is stretching, which extends the muscle.

With an understanding of the theory and actual mechanics of the muscular system, as well as the structure and location of the individual muscles, the application and effectiveness of the massage strokes can be greatly enhanced.

BOX 15-1

Effects of Massage on Muscles

- **Relieves muscular tension.** Massage relieves muscular restrictions, tightness, stiffness, and spasms. These effects are achieved by direct pressure and by increasing circulation, resulting in more flexible, supple, and resilient muscle tissues.
- **Relaxes muscles.** Muscles relax as massage reduces excitability in the sympathetic nervous system.
- **Reduces muscle soreness and fatigue.** Massage enhances blood circulation thus increasing the amount of oxygen and nutrients available to the muscles. Increased oxygen and nutrients reduce muscle fatigue and post-exercise soreness. Massage promotes rapid disposal of waste products, further reducing muscle fatigue and soreness. A fatigued muscle recuperates 20 percent after 5 minutes of rest and 100 percent after 5 minutes of massage. A reduction in post-exercise recovery time was indicated by a decline in pulse rate and an increase in muscle "work" capacity.
- **Reduces trigger point formation.** Trigger point formation is greatly reduced by the pressure applied to tissues during a massage, affecting trigger points in both muscle and fascia.
- **Manually separates muscle fibers.** Compressive strokes and cross fiber friction strokes separate muscle fibers, reducing muscle spasms.
- **Increases range of motion.** When muscular tension is reduced, range of motion is improved. The freedom of the joints is dictated by the freedom of the muscles.
- **Improves performance (balance and posture).** Many postural distortions are removed when trigger points are released and when muscle tension is reduced. Range of motion increases, gait becomes more efficient, the posture is more aligned and balanced, and improved performance is the net result.

- **Improves motor skills.** Not surprisingly, if a massage was found to improve performance, balance, and posture, motor skills are enhanced as well.
- **Lengthens muscles.** Massage mechanically stretches and broadens tissue, especially when combined with Swedish Gymnastics (joint mobilization and stretches). These changes are detected by Golgi tendon organs, which inhibit a contraction signal, further lengthening muscles. Massage retrains the tissue from a contracted state to an elongated state, increasing resting length.
- **Increases flexibility.** By lengthening muscles and promoting muscular relaxation, massage has also been shown to increase muscle flexibility.
- **Tones weak muscles.** Muscle spindle activity is increased during massage strokes (e.g., tapotement, vibration). An increase in muscle spindle activity creates muscle contractions, helping tone weak muscles. This effect is particularly beneficial in cases of prolonged bed rest, flaccidity, and atrophy.
- **Reduces the creatine kinase activity in the blood.** Creatine kinase is an enzyme that helps ensure enough adenosine triphosphate (ATP) is available for muscle contraction. By reducing the activity of creatine kinase in the blood, massage indirectly helps decrease muscle contraction and, therefore, increase muscle relaxation.
- **Improves muscular nutrition.** As a result of an increase in blood-transported nutrients, massage improves muscular nutrition. This hastens muscle recovery and enables muscles to function at maximum capacity.
- **Decreases electromyography (EMG) readings.** This signifies a decrease in neuromuscular activity and a reduction of neuromuscular complaints.

MATCHING I

Write the letter of the best answer in the space provided.

A. Cardiac muscle   F. Extensibility   K. Aponeurosis
B. Myofascial   G. Retinacula   L. Sarcomere
C. Actin   H. Skeletal muscle   M. Contractility
D. Myosin   I. Tendon   N. Epimysium
E. Fasciculi   J. Smooth muscle   O. Myofibril

_____ 1. Muscle found in blood vessels and some organs

_____ 2. Thin myofilament

_____ 3. Fascial covering of entire muscle

_____ 4. Flat, broad tendon

_____ 5. Cordlike structure attaching muscle to bone

_____ 6. Bundles of muscle fibers

_____ 7. Ability of a muscle to shorten

_____ 8. Voluntary, striated muscle

_____ 9. Muscle of the heart

_____ 10. Retaining bands of connective tissue around knees, ankles, and wrists

_____ 11. Thick myofilament

_____ 12. Muscles contractile unit

_____ 13. A muscle fiber, made up of actin and myosin filaments

_____ 14. Term referring to skeletal muscles and related fascia

_____ 15. Ability of a muscle to lengthen

MATCHING II

Write the letter of the best answer in the space provided.

A. Z-lines
B. Troponin/tropomyosin
C. Sarcolemma
D. Agonist
E. H-Band

F. Recruitment
G. Motor unit
H. Slow twitch fibers
I. Neuromuscular junction
J. Acetylcholinesterase

K. All-or-none response
L. Insertion
M. Eccentric contractions
N. Muscle spindles
O. Origin

_____ 1. Central region of resting sarcomere

_____ 2. Enzyme that cleans up acetylcholine left in the synaptic cleft after muscle contraction

_____ 3. Fatigue resistant fibers

_____ 4. Cell membrane of muscle fiber

_____ 5. Muscle attachment undergoing the greatest movement during contraction

_____ 6. Muscle causing desired action

_____ 7. Ends of a resting sarcomere

_____ 8. Attachment of the muscle that is relatively fixed and immovable during contraction

_____ 9. Lengthening contractions

_____ 10. A single motor neuron and all its associated skeletal muscle fibers

_____ 11. Stimulated during ballistic stretching and muscle contracts

_____ 12. Point where the axon terminates at the sarcolemma

_____ 13. Muscles contract to their fullest extent or not at all

_____ 14. Process of motor unit activation based on need

_____ 15. Regulatory proteins that prevent myosin attachment and, therefore, muscle contraction

Bibliography

Applegate EJ: *The anatomy and physiology learning system,* ed 2, Philadelphia, 2000, WB Saunders.

Ardion C: Certified manual lymphatic drainage practitioner, 1996, personal contact.

Crawley J, Van De Graaff KM: *A photographic atlas for anatomy and physiology,* Englewood, Colo, 2002, Morton.

Goldberg S: *Clinical anatomy made ridiculously simple,* Miami, 1984, Medmaster.

Grafelman T: *Graf's anatomy and physiology guide for the massage therapist,* Aurora, Colo, 1988, DG Publishing.

Guyton A: *Human physiology and mechanisms of disease,* ed 3, Philadelphia, 1982, WB Saunders.

Haubrich WS: *Medical meanings: a glossary of word origins,* New York, 1984, Harcourt Brace Jovanovich.

Jacob S, Francone C: *Elements of anatomy and physiology,* Philadelphia, 1989, WB Saunders.

Kapit W, Elson LM: *The anatomy coloring book,* ed 3, New York, 2002, Benjamin Cummings.

Kordish M, Dickson S: *Introduction to basic human anatomy,* Lake Charles, La, 1985, McNeese State University.

Marieb EN: *Essentials of human anatomy and physiology,* ed 4, New York, 1994, Benjamin Cummings.

Mattes A: *Active isolated stretching,* Sarasota, Fla, 1995, Author.

McAleer N: *The body almanac,* Garden City, NY, 1985, Doubleday.

Merck: *Merck manual,* ed 17, Whitehouse Station, NJ, 1998, Merck and Co.

Moore KL: *Clinically oriented anatomy,* ed 2, Baltimore, 1985, Williams and Wilkins.

Mosby's medical, nursing, and allied health dictionary, ed 4, St Louis, 1994, Mosby.

Newton D: *Pathology for massage therapists,* ed 2, Portland, Ore, 1995, Simran.

Platzer W: *Color atlas and textbook of human anatomy: locomotor system,* vol 1, ed 3, New York, 1984, Thieme.

Premkumar K: *Pathology A to Z: a handbook for massage therapists,* Calgary, Canada, 1996, VanPub Books.

Solomon EP, Phillips GA: *Understanding human anatomy and physiology,* Philadelphia, 1987, WB Saunders.

Southmayd W, Hoffman M: *Sportshealth: the complete book of athletic injuries,* New York and London, 1981, Quickfox.

Taber's cyclopedic medical dictionary, ed 13, Philadelphia, 1977, FA Davis.

Thibodeau G, Patton K: *Structure and function of the body,* ed 11, St Louis, 2000, Mosby.

Tortora GJ: *Introduction to the human body: the essentials of anatomy and physiology,* ed 3, New York, 1994, HarperCollins.

Tortora GJ, Grabowksi SR: *Principles of anatomy and physiology,* ed 9, New York, 2000, John Wiley.

Travell JG, Simons DG: *Myofascial pain and dysfunction: the trigger point manual,* Baltimore, 1983, Williams and Wilkins.

Werner R: *A massage therapist's guide to pathology,* ed 2, Baltimore, 2002, Lippincott Williams & Wilkins.

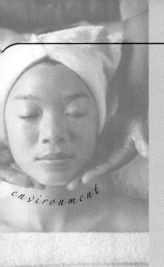

Muscular Nomenclature and Kinesiology

16

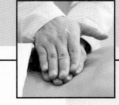

"How can you think and hit at the same time?"

—Yogi Berra

STUDENT OBJECTIVES

After completing this chapter, the student should be able to:

- Describe the general locations of each muscle listed in the chapter
- Explain the location of each muscle listed in the chapter according to its muscle attachment sites
- Demonstrate the actions of each muscle listed in the chapter
- Apply the knowledge gained in your practice as a massage therapist

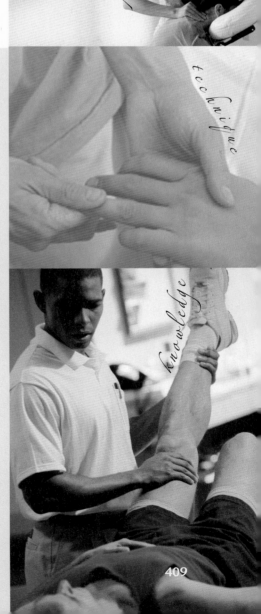

INTRODUCTION

This chapter examines 122 of the major muscles of the body (Figure 16-1). To get the most out of this chapter, you must look at how the material is organized. This chapter is divided into two separate sections and nine individual lessons. The first section, Muscles of the Appendicular Skeleton, consists of six lessons: Muscles of Scapular Movement (6 muscles featured); Muscles of Shoulder Movement (9 muscles featured); Muscles of Elbow Movement (5 muscles featured); Muscles of the Forearm, Wrist, and Hand (24 muscles featured); Muscles of Hip and Knee Movement (25 muscles featured); and Muscles of Foot Movement (13 muscles featured).

The second section, Muscles of the Axial Skeleton, consists of three lessons: Muscles of the Head and Neck (24 muscles featured); Muscles of the Trunk and Vertebral Column (11 muscles featured); and Muscles of Respiration (5 muscles featured).

The muscles should be learned in the sequence presented because these are generally the order in which muscles are addressed during a massage. This system supports students of massage to gain a strong foundation of musculoskeletal anatomy, muscle

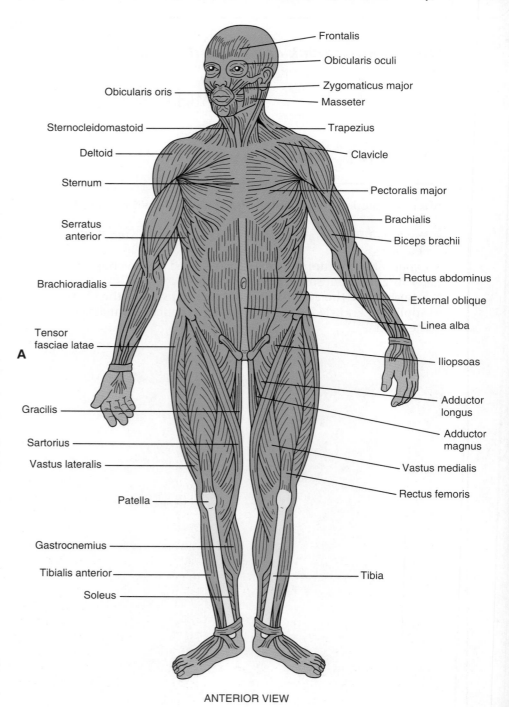

Figure 16-1 Anterior **(A)** and posterior **(B)** view of muscles of the body.

A

Frontalis
Obicularis oculi
Zygomaticus major
Masseter
Obicularis oris
Sternocleidomastoid
Trapezius
Deltoid
Clavicle
Sternum
Pectoralis major
Brachialis
Serratus anterior
Biceps brachii
Brachioradialis
Rectus abdominus
External oblique
Linea alba
Tensor fasciae latae
Iliopsoas
Gracilis
Adductor longus
Sartorius
Adductor magnus
Vastus lateralis
Vastus medialis
Rectus femoris
Patella
Gastrocnemius
Tibialis anterior
Tibia
Soleus

ANTERIOR VIEW

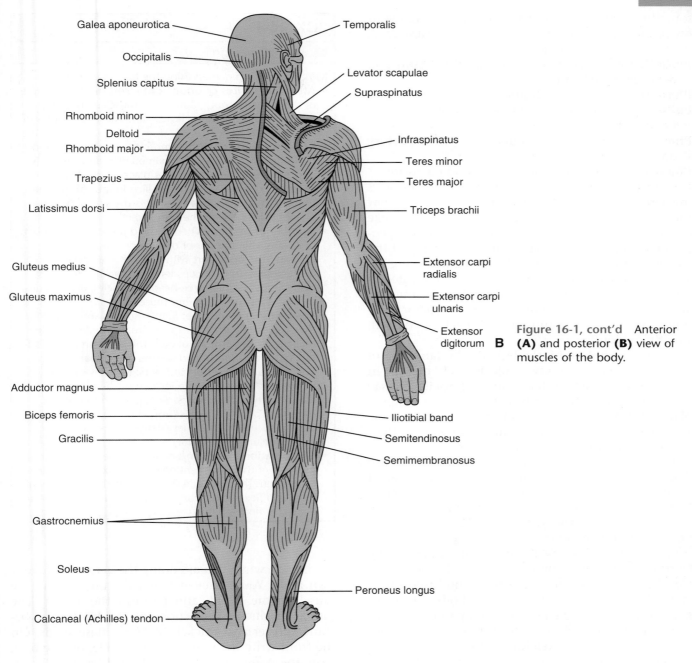

Galea aponeurotica
Occipitalis
Splenius capitus
Rhomboid minor
Deltoid
Rhomboid major
Trapezius
Latissimus dorsi
Gluteus medius
Gluteus maximus
Adductor magnus
Biceps femoris
Gracilis
Gastrocnemius
Soleus
Calcaneal (Achilles) tendon

Temporalis
Levator scapulae
Supraspinatus
Infraspinatus
Teres minor
Teres major
Triceps brachii
Extensor carpi radialis
Extensor carpi ulnaris
Extensor digitorum **B**
Iliotibial band
Semitendinosus
Semimembranosus
Peroneus longus

POSTERIOR VIEW

Figure 16-1, cont'd Anterior **(A)** and posterior **(B)** view of muscles of the body.

nomenclature, and kinesiology. **Kinesiology** is the study of human motion.

Muscles commonly attach to the bony markings covered in Chapter 14. However, muscles can also attach to ligaments (i.e., nuchal, inguinal, transverse carpal), fascia (i.e., palmar, superficial, abdominal, thoracolumbar, iliotibial band), membranes (i.e., obturator, interosseous), and tendinous structures (i.e., galea aponeurotica, linea alba).

Muscles can be arranged and classified into many groups. They can be grouped regionally (e.g., arm, leg, abdomen), according to their attachment sites (i.e., clavicle, ribs, femur), or by how they move the joints (actions). Muscles in these units are grouped in

regions, and the muscles of each lesson are grouped according to actions. Muscles can be examined individually or in the bigger context of motion. At the end of each lesson, a chart is provided to further your study of kinesiology.

One of the best approaches to learning the muscles is to reduce the task into bite-size pieces. Five learning phases are presented to assist you in this endeavor. Understanding is a process, like learning a new dance. First, you must hear the music, then you observe others, and then you follow them with your body, until you are moving through space. This muscle-learning system uses the building-block approach to learning, on which a foundation is laid before something is built. However, feel free to design your own learning system and use this system as a starting point for further exploration.

Phase I: Decode muscle names in each lesson and learn pronunciations.

Phase II: Learn general locations of muscles.

Phase III: Learn specific muscle locations using attachment sites.

Phase IV: Study muscle actions using a multisensory approach.

Phase V: Application of knowledge and repetition.

In Phase I, spend time looking over all the muscles in each lesson of the chapter and learn exactly how they were named. Do not be surprised if it feels like a history lesson. Try to imagine a small group of people dissecting a cadaver and having to name all the structures they find. All muscles are named using descriptive words. Read over the information located in Box 16-1 to familiarize yourself with ways muscles are named. Listen to how your instructor pronounces each muscle and repeat it back to yourself, silently or aloud.

Once you feel comfortable with the language of musculoskeletal anatomy, look at each muscle in each lesson, place your hand on the muscle, and say its name. As your teacher is instructing this chapter, place your hand on the muscle and repeat its name silently or aloud. Phase II familiarizes you with their general locations on the body.

Phase III adds a very important dimension to understanding muscle location for a massage therapist by focusing on attachment sites. Using an articulated skeleton, find each bony attachment site. Using a piece of colorful yarn or cording, touch both bony markings at once. This gives you a graphic idea of the muscles. Make up flash cards; on the front of each card, write the name of the each muscle; the back then states the origin and insertion. It is helpful to draw muscles on a real body; this body may be one of your classmates, or you can recruit someone. Use nontoxic, water-soluble markers. Use a plastic model of a skeleton and clay to build the muscles on the model, focusing on attachment sites. A large picture of a skeleton may be used if a skeletal model is not available; use a color marker and draw in the muscle, going from origin to insertion. You can also practice this activity in pairs or groups. As a learning tip, *origins are generally located medial or proximal to their insertions.*

Phase IV is to learn the action of muscles. Typically, the insertion, or *I,* moves toward the origin, or *O.* You can learn them by rote memory or by a multisensory approach. If you have chosen the latter, go back to the Phase III learning strategy, the yarn on the articulated skeleton, and shorten the string. This will produce the action of the muscle because muscles produce movement by contracting their fibers. Another useful technique is to say aloud the name of

BOX 16-1

Muscle Naming

Most muscles are named using the following methods:

- **Attachment sites or origin and insertion:** An example of this is the sternocleidomastoid muscle, which is attached to the sternum, clavicle, and mastoid process of the temporal bone.
- **Action or function:** When muscles are named by function, the function is usually named first, and the body part on which the action takes place is usually named second. Examples are flexor pollicis longus (flexes the thumb), levator scapulae (elevates the scapula), and erector spinae (keeps the spine erect).
- **Number of origins:** When naming muscles by number of origins, the number of origins, or heads, is given first, and the body part with which it is associated is given second (e.g., biceps femoris [two-headed muscle], triceps brachii [three-headed muscle], and quadriceps femoris [group of four muscles]).
- **Relative shape and size:** Some muscles are named for their geometric shape or gross size. Examples are gluteus maximus (largest), gluteus minimus (smallest), adductor longus (long), and deltoid (triangular).
- **Location and direction of fibers:** Muscles can be named for where they are located or the direction of the majority of their fibers. Examples are temporalis (temporal bone), frontalis (frontal bone), rectus femoris (straight), internal obliques (slanted), and latissimus dorsi (dorsum or posterior).
- **Combinations:** Many muscles are named using a combination of the aforementioned (e.g., extensor digitorum longus [long muscle that extends the digits or fingers] and flexor digitorum profundus [deep muscle that flexes the fingers]).

the muscle while you are doing the action with your own body. You can even touch the muscle, say the muscle name aloud, and perform the action. The muscle producing the action will feel harder and become shorter and thicker. Make up flash cards. On the front write the name of the muscle; on the back write the name of the action. To assist you in learning the muscle actions, please review the following information; ask your instructor for additional suggestions:

- Muscles located on the anterior side of the body generally flex (except the thigh).
- Muscles located on the posterior side of the body generally extend (except the thigh).
- Muscles located on the medial side of the body generally adduct.
- Muscles located on the lateral side of the body generally abduct.
- Muscles with fibers running superior to inferior generally flex and extend.
- Muscles with oblique running fibers generally rotate.

- If a muscle crosses two joints, it has an action on both joints.
- Most muscles have two actions: a primary and a secondary.
- The antagonist and agonist are generally situated opposite of each other, typically with the same insertion.
- Synergist generally has parallel fiber directions.

Phase V is to APPLY, APPLY, APPLY! With your instructor's help, learn how to palpate these muscles using the information in Box 16-2, wherever possible. Use all of this anatomical information in massage class and use the names of these muscles with your clients. Use the anatomical terminology as much as you can so it becomes part of *you*. As the names, locations, and actions of the muscles become more fixed in your brain, your confidence will grow. Remember, repetition is the key to learning; repetition is the key to learning; repetition is the key to learning.

For Your Information

In researching muscle origin, insertion, action, and nerve supply information, the authors discovered numerous variations, inconsistencies, and disagreements on the subject of muscle nomenclature. It should be noted as you read and work with the information found in this chapter. Collect the books mentioned in the reference section and many other books concerning this fascinating subject to aid in the process of learning.

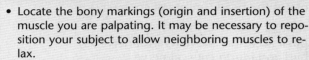

BOX 16-2

How to Palpate Muscles

- Locate the bony markings (origin and insertion) of the muscle you are palpating. It may be necessary to reposition your subject to allow neighboring muscles to relax.
- Do not push too hard. In palpation, make contact with the skin and allow your hand to sink into the tissues. Now you can go for depth slowly and with purpose.
- Once you are in the neighborhood of the structure you wish to palpate, allow your fingers to move back and forth. This strumming motion allows for better identification as the structure moves under your fingertips.
- Ask your subject to perform the action of the muscle. The muscle contraction will probably be the muscle you are trying to locate. Apply resistance to the movement. Palpate the muscle in its contracted state. Ask your subject to relax and repeat the contraction.

Some muscle names are in a shaded box. These are words that are commonly used when discussing a group of muscles. An example of muscle groups are the hamstrings and the adductors.

All muscles do is contract and relax and contract and relax, so relax your brain and enjoy this part of the book by learning through application. The retention of this knowledge comes with reinforcement.

Unit ONE—Muscles of the Appendicular Skeleton

Lesson ONE—Muscles of Scapular Movement (Trapezius, Levator Scapulae, Rhomboids Major and Minor, Serratus Anterior, Pectoralis Minor)

Trapezius

Greek:
trapezoeides—tablelike

ORIGINS
external occipital protuberance
superior nuchal lines
nuchal ligament
spinous processes of C7-T12

INSERTIONS
lateral one third of the clavicle
acromion process
scapular spine

ACTIONS
extends the neck and head (upper fibers)
elevates the scapula (upper fibers)
upwardly rotates the scapula (upper fibers)
retracts the scapula (middle fibers)

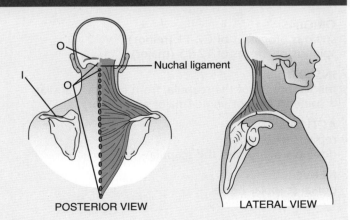

POSTERIOR VIEW   LATERAL VIEW

Figure 16-2

Trapezius—cont'd

depresses the scapula (lower fibers)
laterally flexes the neck (unilateral contraction)
rotates the head (unilateral contraction)

NERVES
spinal accessory nerve (cranial nerve XI)
third and fourth cervical nerve

Notes: Also known as the *coat hanger muscle* because clothes hang from the trapezius, like a coat hanger, the trapezius muscle behaves like three muscles in one. Covering more than half the back, the upper, middle, and lower fibers contract to perform three separate actions. The trapezius, or *traps,* is to the neck and head what the erectors are to the back. Note that this muscle can be an antagonist to itself. This muscle was once called *musculus cucullaris* (Latin for *muscle hood*) because the entire trapezius resembled a monk's hood.

Levator Scapulae

Latin:
levator—a lifter
scapulae—shoulder blade

ORIGINS
transverse processes of C1-C4

INSERTION
medial border of the scapula (superior angle to root of spine)

ACTIONS
elevates the scapula
downwardly rotates the scapula
laterally flexes the neck

NERVES
dorsal scapular nerve
cervical nerves

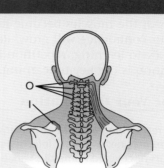

POSTERIOR VIEW

Figure 16-3

Notes: This muscles lies between two muscles discussed later, the splenius capitis and the scalenus posterior. Often, the body shifts its fascial structure from sol- to gel- to reinforce this muscle's actions. In its gel-state, it will feel like crunches as it is flipped over the insertion. The levator scapulae is the only neck muscle that moves the scapula.

Rhomboids Major and Minor

Latin:
rhombos—all sides even
major—larger
minor—smaller

ORIGINS
spinous processes of C7-T1 (minor)
spinous processes of T2-T5 (major)

INSERTION
medial border of the scapula, from root of scapular spine to inferior angle (major and minor)

ACTIONS
retracts the scapula
downwardly rotates the scapula

NERVE
dorsal scapular nerve

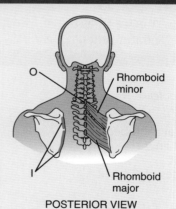

Rhomboid minor

Rhomboid major

POSTERIOR VIEW

Figure 16-4

Rhomboids Major and Minor—cont'd

Notes: Rhomboids is the name given for the rhomboid major and rhomboid minor, but they occasionally fuse to form one muscle. Both lie deep to the trapezius; the rhomboid minor is superior to the rhomboid major. They are also known as the *Christmas tree muscles* because the fiber direction is obliquely arranged, like Christmas tree branches.

Serratus Anterior

Latin:
serratus—notched or jagged like a saw
ante—before

ORIGINS
ribs 1-8 (lateral to costal cartilage)

INSERTION
anterior medial border of the scapula

ACTIONS
protracts the scapula
upwardly rotates the scapula

NERVE
long thoracic nerve

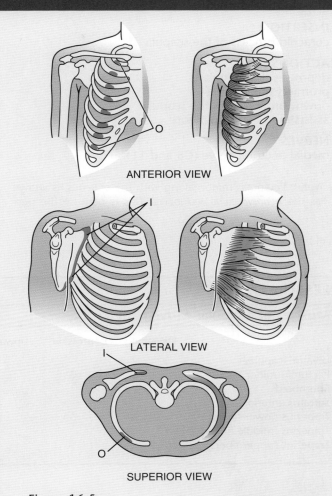

ANTERIOR VIEW

LATERAL VIEW

SUPERIOR VIEW

Figure 16-5

Notes: This, along with the triceps brachii, is called the *boxer's muscle* because the forward movement of the scapula enables a boxer to deliver a punch. Note that this muscle is antagonist to the rhomboids. The serratus anterior interlaces with the external obliques on the lateral aspect of the trunk. Full or partial paralysis of the serratus anterior produces a *winged scapula,* making it impossible for the person who has this condition to lift the affected arm laterally beyond 90 degrees.

Pectoralis Minor

Latin:
pectoralis—pertaining to the chest
minor—smaller

ORIGINS
ribs 3-5 (lateral to costal cartilage)

INSERTION
coracoid process of the scapula

ACTIONS
depresses the scapula
protracts the scapula
downwardly rotates the scapula
assists in forced inspiration

NERVES
medial pectoral nerve (C8 and T1)

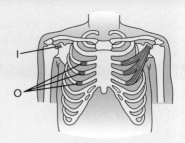

ANTERIOR VIEW

Figure 16-6

Notes: Pectoralis minor, along with the scalenes, is known as the *neurovascular entrappers.* This is because the pec- toralis minor forms a bridge over the axillary artery and the distal portion of the brachial plexus.

LESSON ONE

Muscles of Scapular Movement

	Elevation	Depression	Upward Rotation	Downward Rotation	Protraction	Retraction
Levator scapulae	×			×		
Pectoralis minor		×		×	×	
Rhomboids				×		×
Serratus anterior			×		×	
Trapezius (lower fibers)		×				
Trapezius (middle fibers)						×
Trapezius (upper fibers)	×		×			

Unit ONE—Muscles of the Appendicular Skeleton

Lesson TWO—Muscles of Shoulder Movement (Latissimus Dorsi, Teres Major, Supraspinatus, Infraspinatus, Teres Minor, Subscapularis, Deltoid, Pectoralis Major, Coracobrachialis, Biceps Brachii [Lesson Three], Triceps Brachii [Lesson Three])

Latissimus Dorsi

Latin:
latus—broad
dorsum—back

ORIGINS
spinous processes of T6-L5
ribs 9-12 (posterior surface)
posterior iliac crest
posterior sacrum

INSERTION
intertubercular groove of the humerus (medial region)

ACTIONS
extends the shoulder
medially rotates the shoulder
adducts the shoulder

NERVE
thoracodorsal nerve

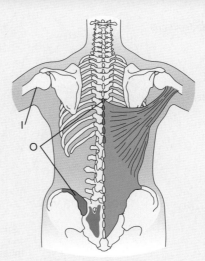

POSTERIOR VIEW

Figure 16-7

Notes: Also known as the *swimmer's muscle* because this muscle allows us to extend our arm and propel us in water. The latissimus dorsi is the widest muscle of the body and one of the major muscles involved with back pain. Because of its iliac attachments, improper lifting can cause trauma and tearing in the iliosacral region, resulting in low back pain.

The latissimus dorsi interlaces with the external obliques on the lateral aspect of the trunk.

Teres Major

Latin:
teres—round
major—larger

ORIGIN
inferior half of the lateral border of the scapula

INSERTION
intertubercular groove of the humerus (medial region)

ACTIONS
extends the shoulder
medially rotates the shoulder
adducts the shoulder

NERVE
lower subscapular nerve

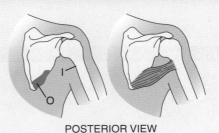

POSTERIOR VIEW

Figure 16-8

Notes: The teres major muscle is a synergist to the latissimus dorsi muscle and may merge with it. In some cases, it may be completely absent.

Musculotendinous Cuff Also known as the *rotator cuff,* musculotendinous cuff is a group of muscles deep to the deltoids. Three of the four muscles arise from scapular fossas (supraspinatus, infraspinatus, subscapularis). Three of the four muscles attach to the greater tubercle (supraspinatus, infraspinatus, teres minor). They do a great deal for the stability of the glenohumeral joint and may function as ligaments. They are also called the *SITS muscles:* *s*upraspinatus, *i*nfraspinatus, *t*eres minor, and *s*ubscapularis.

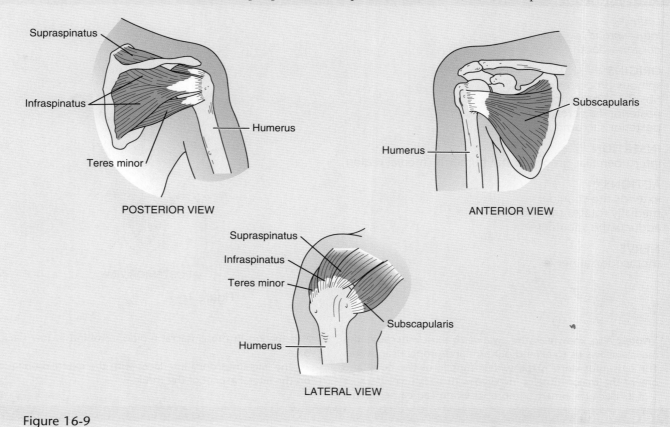

POSTERIOR VIEW

ANTERIOR VIEW

LATERAL VIEW

Figure 16-9

Supraspinatus

Latin:
supra—above
spinatus—spine

ORIGIN
supraspinatus fossa of the scapula

INSERTION
greater tubercle of the humerus

ACTION
abducts the shoulder

NERVE
subscapular nerve

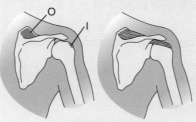

POSTERIOR VIEW

Figure 16-10

Notes: The supraspinatus muscle is the only muscle of the musculotendinous cuff that does not rotate the humerus.

The supraspinatus prevents downward dislocation of the humerus when carrying a heavy portable massage table.

Infraspinatus

Latin
infra—beneath
spinatus—spine

ORIGIN
infraspinatus fossa of the scapula

INSERTION
greater tubercle of the humerus

ACTION
laterally rotates the shoulder

NERVE
subscapular nerve

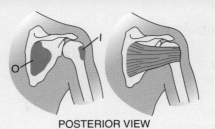

POSTERIOR VIEW

Figure 16-11

Teres Minor

Latin:
teres—round
minor—smaller

ORIGIN
superior half of the lateral border of the scapula

INSERTION
greater tubercle of the humerus

ACTIONS
adducts the shoulder
laterally rotates the shoulder

NERVE
axillary nerve

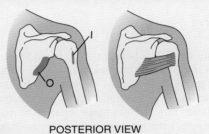

POSTERIOR VIEW

Figure 16-12

Notes: The teres minor muscle is the synergist to the infraspinatus muscle and may fuse with it.

Subscapularis

Latin:
sub—below
scapulae—shoulder blade

ORIGIN
subscapular fossa of the scapula

INSERTION
lesser tubercle of the humerus

ACTIONS
medially rotates the shoulder

NERVE
subscapular nerve

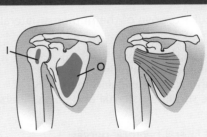

ANTERIOR VIEW

Figure 16-13

Notes: Dr. Janet Travell, author of *Myofascial Pain and Dysfunction,* refers to the subscapularis muscle as the *frozen shoulder* muscle.

Deltoid

Greek:
delta—triangular-shaped

ORIGINS
lateral one third of the clavicle
acromion process
scapular spine

INSERTION
deltoid tuberosity

ACTIONS
flexes the shoulder (anterior fibers)
medially rotates the shoulder (anterior fibers)
abduct the shoulder (middle fibers)
extends the shoulder (posterior fibers)
laterally rotates the shoulder (posterior fibers)

NERVE
axillary nerve

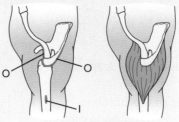

SUPERIOR VIEW

Figure 16-14

Notes: Mary Kordish, a biology professor at McNeese State University, Lake Charles, La., said that if the deltoids were discovered today, they would be considered three independent muscles. The anterior, middle, and posterior fibers of the deltoids function like three separate muscles. Structurally, they resemble the gluteals. To get a better understanding of this concept, get on your hands and knees and imagine yourself as a four-legged animal. The deltoid is the most important abductor of the shoulder and can be antagonist to itself.

Pectoralis Major

Latin:
pectoralis—pertaining to the chest
major—larger

ORIGINS
medial half of the clavicle
edge of the sternal body
ribs 1-8 (costal cartilages)

INSERTION
intertubercular groove of the humerus (lateral region)

ACTIONS
adducts the shoulder
medially rotates the shoulder
flexes the shoulder (clavicular fibers only)
extends the shoulder (sternal and costal fibers)

NERVES
medial and lateral pectoral nerves

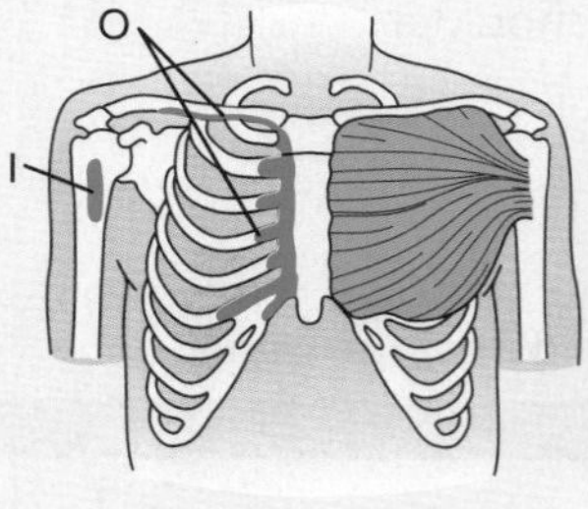

ANTERIOR VIEW

Figure 16-15

Notes: The pectoralis major muscle, or *pecs*, forms the upper anterior chest wall and anterior axillary fold. This muscle possesses a clavicular portion, sternal portion, and costal portion. Tightness in this muscle may cause constriction of chest and angina pectoralis-like pain or postural distortions such as rounded shoulders.

Coracobrachialis

Greek:
korax—crow's beak
Latin:
bracchium—arm

ORIGIN
coracoid process of the scapula

INSERTION
medial humeral shaft (middle region)

ACTIONS
flexes the shoulder
adducts the shoulder

NERVE
musculocutaneous nerve

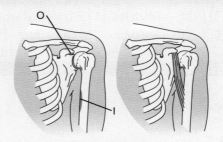

ANTERIOR VIEW

Figure 16-16

LESSON TWO

Muscles of Shoulder Movement

	Flexion	Extension	Medial Rotation	Lateral Rotation	Abduction	Adduction
Biceps brachii	×					
Coracobrachialis	×					×
Deltoids (anterior fibers)	×		×			
Deltoids (middle fibers)					×	
Deltoids (posterior fibers)		×		×		
Infraspinatus				×		
Latissimus dorsi		×	×			×
Pectoralis major	×		×			
Pectoralis major (sternal/costal portion)		×				×
Subscapularis			×			
Supraspinatus					×	
Teres major		×	×			×
Teres minor				×		×
Triceps brachii		×				

Unit ONE—Muscles of the Appendicular Skeleton

Lesson THREE—Muscles of Elbow Movement (Biceps Brachii, Brachialis, Brachioradialis, Triceps Brachii, Anconeus, Pronator Teres [Lesson Four]) NOTE: All of these muscles, except for the anconeus and pronator teres, have the Latin word root *brachi* in them.

Biceps Brachii

Latin:
bis—twice + caput—head
bracchium—arm

ORIGINS
supraglenoid tubercle of the scapula (long head)
coracoid process of scapula (short head)

INSERTION
radial tuberosity

ACTIONS
flexes the elbow
supinates the forearm
flexes the shoulder

NERVE
musculocutaneous nerve

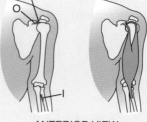

ANTERIOR VIEW

Figure 16-17

Notes: The biceps brachii muscle is called the *corkscrew muscle* because two of its actions resemble how you uncork a wine bottle. This muscle may have an additional head attaching to the midshaft of the humerus (about 10% of cadavers).

Brachialis

Latin:
bracchium—arm

ORIGIN
distal anterior humeral shaft

INSERTION
ulnar tuberosity

ACTION
flexes the elbow

NERVE
musculocutaneous nerve

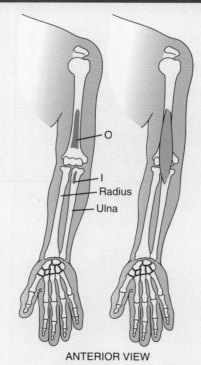

ANTERIOR VIEW

Figure 16-18

Notes: The brachialis is the most effective arm flexor because of its mechanical advantage, lying deep to the biceps brachii.

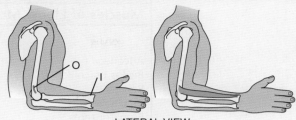

Brachioradialis

Latin:
bracchium—arm
radialis—spoke of a wheel

ORIGIN
lateral supracondylar ridge of the humerus

INSERTION
styloid process of the radius

ACTION
flexes the elbow

NERVES
radial nerve

LATERAL VIEW

Figure 16-19

Notes: The bulge you can palpate on the radial side of your forearm is the brachioradialis. The radial pulse is located between the tendons of the brachioradialis and the flexor carpi radialis.

Triceps Brachii

Greek:
treis—three
Latin:
bracchium—arm

ORIGINS
infraglenoid tubercle of the scapula (long head)
posterior proximal humeral shaft (lateral head)
posterior distal humeral shaft (medial head)

INSERTION
olecranon process

ACTIONS
extends the elbow
extends the shoulder

NERVE
radial nerve

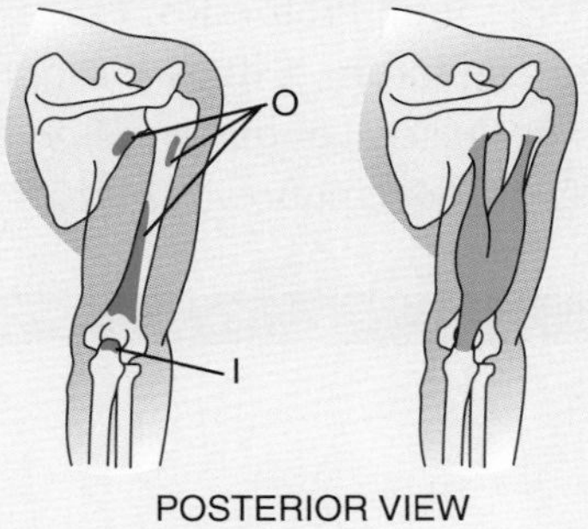

POSTERIOR VIEW

Figure 16-20

Notes: This, along with the serratus anterior, is called the *boxer's muscle,* because it delivers a straight-arm knockout punch.

Anconeus

Greek:
eln + boga—forearm, bend

ORIGIN
lateral epicondyle of the humerus

INSERTION
olecranon process
superior one eighth of ulnar shaft

ACTIONS
extends the elbow

NERVE
radial nerve

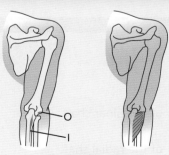

POSTERIOR VIEW

Figure 16-21

LESSON THREE		
Muscles of Elbow Movement		
	Flexion	Extension
Anconeus		×
Biceps brachii	×	
Brachialis	×	
Brachioradialis	×	
Pronator teres	×	
Triceps brachii		×

Unit ONE—Muscles of the Appendicular Skeleton

Lesson FOUR—Muscles of the Forearm, Wrist, and Hand (Pronator Teres, Pronator Quadratus, Supinator, Flexor Carpi Radialis, Flexor Carpi Ulnaris, Palmaris Longus, Flexor Digitorum Superficialis, Flexor Digitorum Profundus, Extensor Carpi Radialis Longus and Brevis, Extensor Carpi Ulnaris, Extensor Digitorum, Extensor Digiti Minimi, Extensor Indicis, Extensor Pollicis Longus and Brevis, Flexor Pollicis Longus and Brevis, Opponens Pollicis, Abductor Pollicis Longus and Brevis, Flexor Digiti Minimi Brevis, Abductor Digiti Minimi, Opponens Digiti Minimi, Biceps Brachii [Lesson Three])

Pronator Teres

Latin:
pronus—downward
teres—round

ORIGINS
medial epicondyle of the humerus
coronoid process of the ulna

INSERTION
lateral proximal radial shaft

ACTIONS
pronates the forearm
flexes the elbow

NERVE
median nerve

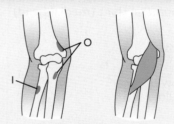

ANTERIOR VIEW

Figure 16-22

Pronator Quadratus

Latin:
pronus—downward
quadratus—four sided

ORIGIN
anterior distal one eighth of the ulnar shaft

INSERTION
anterior distal one eighth of the radial shaft

ACTION
pronates the forearm

NERVE
median nerve

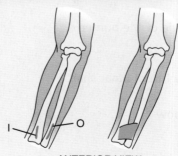

ANTERIOR VIEW

Figure 16-23

Supinator

Latin:
supinatus—bent backward

ORIGINS
lateral epicondyle of the humerus
proximal one eighth of ulnar shaft
radial collateral ligament
annular ligament

INSERTION
proximal lateral radial shaft

ACTION
supinates the forearm

NERVE
radial nerve

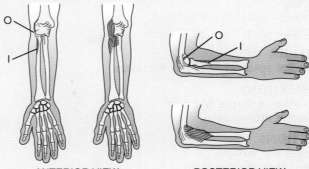

ANTERIOR VIEW   POSTERIOR VIEW

Figure 16-24

Flexor Carpi Radialis

Latin:
flexus—bent
karpos—wrist
radialis—spoke of a wheel

ORIGIN
medial epicondyle of the humerus

INSERTION
bases of metacarpals II-III

ACTIONS
flexes the wrist
abducts the wrist

NERVE
median nerve

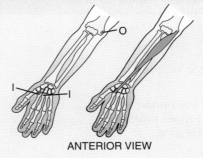

ANTERIOR VIEW

Figure 16-25

Notes: Notice how this muscle and the next three (flexor carpi ulnaris, palmaris longus, flexor digitorum superficialis) all flex the wrist and all originate on the medial epicondyle of the humerus. The flexors lie on the fleshy side of the forearm. In fact, wrist flexion is a more powerful movement than wrist extension, abduction, or adduction. The radial pulse is located between the tendons of the flexor carpi radialis and the brachioradialis.

Flexor Carpi Ulnaris

Latin:
flexus—bent
karpos—wrist
ulna—elbow

ORIGIN
medial epicondyle of the humerus

INSERTIONS
base of metacarpal V
pisiform
hamate

ACTIONS
flexes the wrist
adducts the wrist

NERVE
ulnar nerve

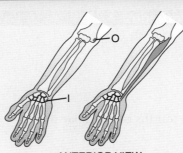

ANTERIOR VIEW

Figure 16-26

Palmaris Longus

Latin:
palma—hand
longus—long

ORIGIN
medial epicondyle of the humerus

INSERTIONS
transverse carpal ligament
palmar aponeurosis

ACTIONS
flexes the wrist
cups (tenses) the palm

NERVE
median nerve

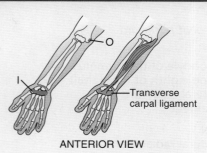

ANTERIOR VIEW

Figure 16-27

Notes: This muscle is absent in about 10% of cadavers.

Flexor Digitorum Superficialis

Latin:
flexus—bent
digitus—finger
superficialis—toward the surface

ORIGINS
medial epicondyle of the humerus
proximal radial shaft (upper region)
coronoid process of the ulna

INSERTIONS
middle phalanges of fingers 2-5

ACTIONS
flexes the wrist
flexes the fingers at the PIP and MP joints

NERVE
median nerve
ulnar nerve

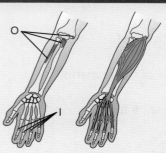

ANTERIOR VIEW

Figure 16-28

Notes: Of all the movements allowed at the forearm, wrist, and hand, finger flexion is the most powerful.

Flexor Digitorum Profundus

Latin:
flexus—bent
digitus—finger
profundus—deep

ORIGIN
anterior proximal three fourths of the ulnar shaft

INSERTIONS
distal phalanges of fingers 2-5

ACTION
flexes the fingers at the DIP, PIP, MP joints

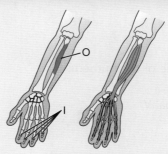

ANTERIOR VIEW

Figure 16-29

Flexor Digitorum Profundus—cont'd

NERVES
ulnar nerve
median nerve

Notes: Of all the movements allowed at the forearm, wrist, and hand, finger flexion is the most powerful. Flexor digitorum may also flex the wrist.

Extensor Carpi Radialis Longus and Brevis

Latin:
extensio—to extend
karpos—wrist
radialis—spoke of a wheel
longus—long
brevis—brief

ORIGINS
supracondylar ridge of the humerus (longus)
lateral epicondyle of the humerus (brevis)

INSERTIONS
base of metacarpal II (longus)
base of metacarpal III (brevis)

ACTIONS
extends the wrist
abducts the wrist

NERVE
radial nerve

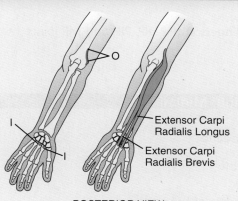

POSTERIOR VIEW

Figure 16-30

Notes: Extensor carpi radialis brevis often becomes inflamed at its origin (epicondylitis) in tennis elbow. Notice how these muscles and the next two (extensor carpi ulnaris, extensor digitorum) all extend the wrist and all originate on the lateral epicondyle of the humerus. The extensors lie on the hairy side of the forearm. These two muscles are also referred to as the *fist clenchers;* for the finger flexors to fully make a fist, the wrist must be slightly extended.

Extensor Carpi Ulnaris

Latin:
extensio—to extend
karpos—wrist
ulna—elbow

ORIGIN
lateral epicondyle of the humerus

INSERTION
base of metacarpal V

ACTIONS
extends the wrist
adducts the wrist

NERVE
radial nerve

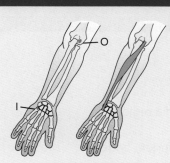

POSTERIOR VIEW

Figure 16-31

Extensor Digitorum

Latin:
extensio—to extend
digitus—finger

ORIGIN
lateral epicondyle of the humerus

INSERTIONS
middle phalanges of four fingers

ACTIONS
extends the wrist
extends the fingers at the DIP, PIP, and MP joints

NERVE
radial nerve

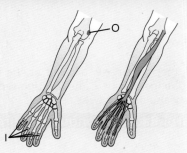

POSTERIOR VIEW

Figure 16-32

Extensor Digiti Minimi

Latin:
extensio—to extend
digitus—finger
minimum—least

ORIGIN
lateral epicondyle of the humerus

INSERTION
proximal phalanx of fifth finger

ACTION
extends the little finger

NERVE
radial nerve

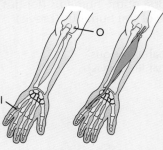

POSTERIOR VIEW

Figure 16-33

Notes: Also known as the *tea drinker's muscle,* because it extends the little finger while you raise the tea cup to your lips.

Extensor Indicis

Latin:
extensio—to extend
indices—forefinger

ORIGIN
posterior ulnar shaft (middle region)

INSERTION
distal phalanx of second (index) finger

ACTION
extends the index finger

NERVE
radial nerve

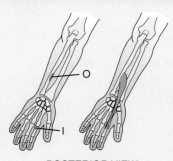

POSTERIOR VIEW

Figure 16-34

Extensor Pollicis Longus and Brevis

Latin:
extensio—to extend
pollex—thumb
longus—long
brevis—brief

ORIGINS
posterior ulnar shaft middle region (longus)
posterior radial shaft middle region (longus)
posterior radial shaft distal region (brevis)
interosseous membrane (brevis and longus)

INSERTIONS
distal phalanx of the thumb (longus)
proximal phalanx of the thumb (brevis)

ACTION
extends the thumb

NERVE
radial nerve

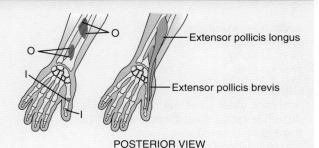

POSTERIOR VIEW

Figure 16-35

Flexor Pollicis Longus and Brevis

Latin:
flexus—bent
pollex—thumb
longus—long
brevis—brief

ORIGINS
anterior radial shaft middle region (longus)
interosseous membrane (longus)
anterior ulnar shaft middle region (longus)
trapezium (brevis)
transverse carpal ligament (brevis)

INSERTIONS
distal phalanx of the thumb (longus)
proximal phalanx of the thumb (brevis)

ACTION
flexes the thumb

NERVE
median nerve
ulnar nerve

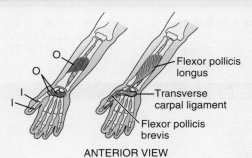

ANTERIOR VIEW

Figure 16-36

Opponens Pollicis

Latin:
opponens—opposing
pollex—thumb

ORIGINS
trapezium
transverse carpal ligament

INSERTION
proximal phalanx of the thumb

ACTIONS
flexes the thumb
adducts the thumb (moves the thumb into opposition)

NERVE
median nerve

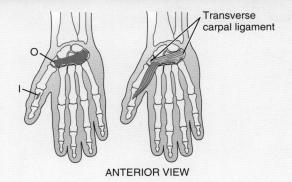

ANTERIOR VIEW

Figure 16-37

Abductor Pollicis Longus and Brevis

Latin:
abductus—led away
pollex—thumb
longus—long
brevis—brief

ORIGINS
posterior ulnar shaft middle region (longus)
posterior radial shaft middle region (longus)
trapezium (brevis)
scaphoid (brevis)
transverse carpal ligament (brevis)

INSERTIONS
base of metacarpal I (longus)
proximal phalanx of the thumb (brevis)

ACTION
abducts the thumb

NERVE
median nerve

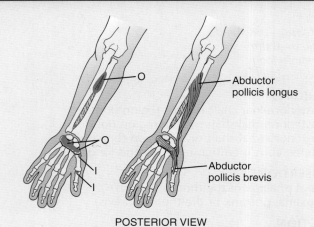

POSTERIOR VIEW

Figure 16-38

Thenar Eminence
Greek:
thenar—palm of hand
minere—to hang on

The thenar eminence is the thumb pad on the anterior surface of the hand. It is made up of three individual muscles called the *opponens pollicis, abductor pollicis brevis,* and the *flexor pollicis brevis.*

Flexor Digiti Minimi Brevis

Latin:
flexus—bent
digitus—finger
minimum—least
brevis—brief

ORIGIN
transverse carpal ligament

INSERTION
proximal phalanx of the fifth finger

ACTION
flexion of the fifth (little) finger

NERVE
ulnar nerve

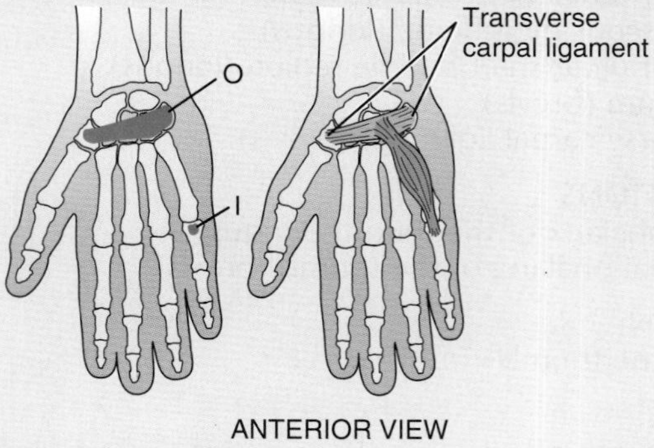

ANTERIOR VIEW

Figure 16-39

Notes: This muscle is often absent.

Abductor Digiti Minimi

Latin:
abductus—led away
digitus—finger
minimum—least

ORIGIN
transverse carpal ligament

INSERTION
proximal phalanx of the fifth finger

ACTION
abduction of the fifth (little) finger

NERVE
ulnar nerve

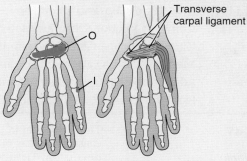

ANTERIOR VIEW

Figure 16-40

Opponens Digiti Minimi

Latin:
opponens—opposing
digitus—finger
minimum—least

ORIGIN
transverse carpal ligament

INSERTION
metacarpal V

ACTION
adducts the little finger (moves the little finger into opposition)

NERVE
ulnar nerve

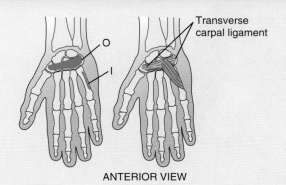

ANTERIOR VIEW

Figure 16-41

Hypothenar Eminence
Greek:
hypo—under
thenar—palm of hand
minere—to hang on

The hypothenar eminence is the little finger pad on the anterior surface of the hand. It consists of three individual muscles called the opponens digiti minimi, flexor digit minimi brevis, and abductor digiti minimi.

LESSON FOUR

Muscles of the Forearm, Wrist, and Hand Movement

	Flexion	Extension	Medial Rotation	Lateral Rotation	Abduction	Adduction
Biceps brachii						X
Extensor carpi radialis			X			
Extensor carpi radialis brevis		X	X			
Extensor carpi radialis longus		X	X			
Extensor carpi ulnaris		X		X		
Extensor digitorum		X				
Flexor carpi radialis	X					
Flexor carpi ulnaris	X			X		
Flexor digitorum superficialis	X					
Palmaris longus	X					
Pronator quadratus					X	
Pronator teres					X	
Supinator						X

Unit ONE—Muscles of the Appendicular Skeleton

Lesson FIVE—Muscles of Hip and Knee Movement (Psoas Major, Iliacus, Piriformis, Gemellus Superior, Gemellus Inferior, Obturator Internus, Obturator Externus, Quadratus Femoris, Gluteus Maximus, Gluteus Medius, Gluteus Minimus, Tensor Fascia Lata, Rectus Femoris, Vastus Intermedius, Vastus Medialis, Vastus Lateralis, Sartorius, Semimembranosus, Semitendinosus, Biceps Femoris, Gracilis, Adductor Magnus, Adductor Longus, Adductor Brevis, Pectineus, Gastrocnemius [Lesson Six], Plantaris [Lesson Six], Popliteus [Lesson Six])

Iliopsoas

Latin:
ilium—flank
Greek:
psoa—muscle of the loin

The psoas major, psoas minor, and iliacus are usually referred to as the *iliopsoas*. Because the psoas minor is absent in about 60% of cadavers, it will not be included for discussion. Tightness in the iliopsoas muscle can play a significant role in functional lordosis and scoliosis. A filet mignon is the iliopsoas muscle of a cow, which is the main flexor of the hip, the muscle that initiates walking (it lifts the leg), and the major cause of muscular low back pain.

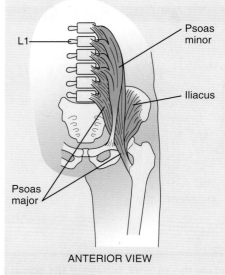

ANTERIOR VIEW

Figure 16-42

Psoas Major

Greek:
psoa—muscle of the loin
major—larger

ORIGINS
transverse processes of T12-L5
vertebral bodies of T12-L5

INSERTION
lesser trochanter

ACTIONS
laterally rotates the hip (unilateral contraction)
flexes the hip (bilateral contraction)
flexes the vertebral column (bilateral contraction)

NERVE
lumbar nerve

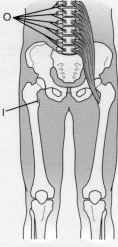

ANTERIOR VIEW

Figure 16-43

Psoas Major—cont'd

Notes: The psoas major is the strongest hip flexor. Because of its dual origins, the psoas major can be subdivided into two sections, with the lumbar plexus running through them.

Iliacus

Latin:
iliacus—ilium

ORIGINS
iliac fossa
anterior inferior iliac spine

INSERTION
lesser trochanter

ACTIONS
flexes the hip
laterally rotates the hip

NERVE
femoral nerve

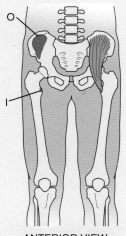

ANTERIOR VIEW

Figure 16-44

Deep Hip Outward Rotators

The six deep lateral rotators are located beneath the gluteals and correspond to some degree to the rotator cuff muscles of the shoulder joint. Each rotator is synergistic to the other. To help you learn the names of these muscles, from superior to inferior, use the mnemonic phrase, *"Pieced goods often go on quilts"*: *p*iriformis, *g*emellus superior, *o*bturator internus, *g*emellus inferior, *o*bturator externus, and *q*uadratus femoris. These are the six deep lateral rotators, and all of them have an insertion on the greater trochanter. The hip lateral rotators are stronger than the hip medial rotators. Note how the foot is turned slightly outward when lying down or in normal gait.

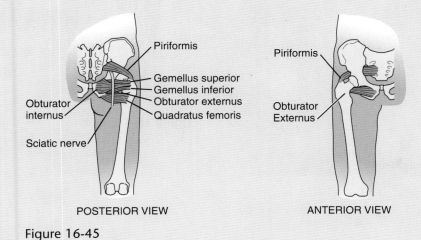

POSTERIOR VIEW   ANTERIOR VIEW

Figure 16-45

Piriformis

Latin:
pirum—pear
forma—shape

ORIGIN
anterior sacrum

INSERTION
greater trochanter

ACTIONS
laterally rotates the hip
abducts the hip

NERVE
sciatic nerve

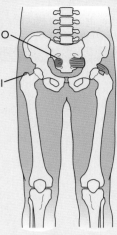

ANTERIOR VIEW

Figure 16-46

Notes: The piriformis is the largest of all the lateral rotators and the most likely to become chronically shortened. Of the population, 15% has all or part of the sciatic nerve running *through* this muscle. The piriformis may be in spasm if one or both feet are laterally rotated, in a ducklike position.

Gemellus Superior

Latin:
gemellus—twin
superus—upper

ORIGIN
ischial spine

INSERTION
greater trochanter

ACTION
laterally rotates the hip

NERVE
sciatic nerve

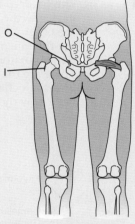

POSTERIOR VIEW

Figure 16-47

Notes: This muscle is occasionally absent.

Gemellus Inferior

Latin:
gemellus—twin
inferus—beneath

ORIGIN
superior ischial tuberosity

INSERTION
greater trochanter

ACTION
laterally rotates the hip

NERVE
sciatic nerve

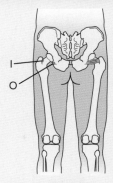

POSTERIOR VIEW

Figure 16-48

Notes: This muscle is occasionally absent.

Obturator Internus

Latin:
obturare—obstruct
internus—within

ORIGIN
obturator membrane

INSERTION
greater trochanter

ACTION
laterally rotates the hip

NERVE
sciatic nerve

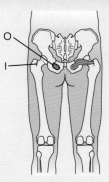

POSTERIOR VIEW

Figure 16-49

Notes: The obturator internus passes through, and almost fills, the lesser sciatic notch.

Obturator Externus

Latin:
obturare—obstruct
externus—outside

ORIGINS
obturator membrane
superior pubic ramus
inferior pubic ramus

INSERTION
greater trochanter

ACTION
laterally rotates the hip

NERVE
obturator nerve

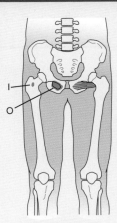

ANTERIOR VIEW

Figure 16-50

Quadratus Femoris

Latin:
quadratus—four-sided
femoralis—pertaining to the femur

ORIGIN
lateral ischial tuberosity

INSERTION
greater trochanter

ACTION
laterally rotates the hip

NERVE
sciatic nerve

Notes: This muscle is occasionally absent or fused with the adductor magnus.

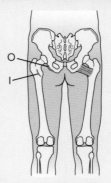

POSTERIOR VIEW

Figure 16-51

Gluteals

The gluteals, or *glutes*, refer to the gluteus maximus, gluteus medius, and gluteus minimus. Note that these muscles can be antagonists to themselves. The iliotibial band is an insertion for both the gluteus maximus and the tensor fascia lata, helping stabilize the knee. Also known as the *iliotibial tract*, the iliotibial band (ITB) is a thickened strap of a fascial tube that surrounds the thigh. The ITB stretches from the iliac crest to the tibia.

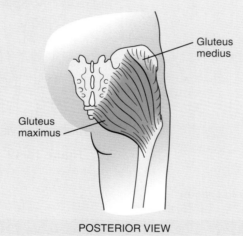

Gluteus medius

Gluteus maximus

POSTERIOR VIEW

Figure 16-52

Gluteus Maximus

Greek:
gloutos—buttock
Latin:
maximus—greatest

ORIGINS
posterior sacrum
posterior coccyx
posterior iliac crest

INSERTIONS
gluteal tuberosity (25%)
iliotibial band (75%)

ACTIONS
extends the hip
laterally rotates the hip
adducts the hip

NERVE
gluteal nerve

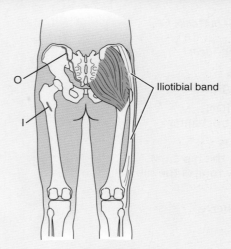

POSTERIOR VIEW

Figure 16-53

Notes: The gluteus maximus is the strongest hip extensor and one of the strongest muscles of the body; it is often more than 1 inch thick. This muscle is mainly used for power, as in climbing stairs, rising from a seated position, or running instead of walking. This muscle also helps tense the fascia lata, the fascial tube around the thigh.

Gluteus Medius

Greek:
gloutos—buttock
Latin:
medius—middle

ORIGIN
superior gluteal line

INSERTIONS
greater trochanter

ACTIONS
abducts the hip
medially rotates the hip

NERVE
gluteal nerve

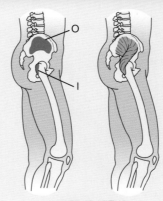

LATERAL VIEW

Figure 16-54

Notes: This muscle stabilizes the hip to give us the ability to stand on one leg.

Gluteus Minimus

Greek:
gloutos—buttock
Latin:
minimum—least

ORIGIN
inferior gluteal line

INSERTION
greater trochanter

ACTIONS
abducts the hip
medially rotates the hip

NERVE
gluteal nerve

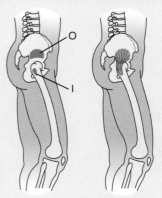

LATERAL VIEW

Figure 16-55

Notes: The gluteus minimus is the synergist to the gluteus medius and is a weak hip abductor, compared with the gluteus medius.

Tensor Fascia Lata

Latin:
tensor—stretching
fascia—band
lata—broad

ORIGINS
anterior iliac crest
anterior superior iliac spine

INSERTION
iliotibial band

ACTIONS
abducts the hip
flexes the hip
medially rotates the hip

NERVE
gluteal nerve

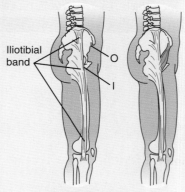

LATERAL VIEW

Figure 16-56

Notes: As the name implies, this muscle also helps tense the fascia lata, which is the fascial tube around the thigh.

Quadriceps Femoris

Latin:
quattuor—four
caput—head
femoralis—pertaining to the femur

The quadriceps femoris is a group of four muscles sharing a common attachment site on the tibia. The four muscle heads, which are often listed as four individual muscles, are the rectus femoris, vastus intermedius, vastus medialis, and vastus lateralis. Lengthening and softening of the quadriceps femoris may provide quick relief from knee problems because the quadriceps tendon crosses the knee joint. Conversely, overuse of quads may create knee problems.

Quadriceps Femoris—cont'd

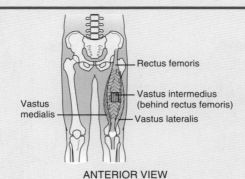

ANTERIOR VIEW

Figure 16-57

Rectus Femoris

Latin:
rectus—straight
femoralis—pertaining to the femur

ORIGIN
anterior inferior iliac spine

INSERTION
tibial tuberosity

ACTIONS
flexes the hip
extends the knee

NERVE
femoral nerve

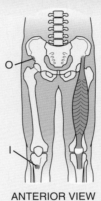

ANTERIOR VIEW

Figure 16-58

Notes: The rectus femoris runs in a channel formed by the vastus muscles, and it overlies the vastus intermedius. It is the only muscle in the quadriceps femoris group that crosses two joints (hip and knee) and has two actions.

Vastus Intermedius

Latin:
vastus—immense
inter—internal
medius—middle

ORIGINS
anterior lateral femoral shaft

INSERTION
tibial tuberosity

ACTION
extends the knee

NERVE
femoral nerve

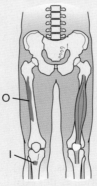

ANTERIOR VIEW

Figure 16-59

Vastus Medialis

Latin:
vastus—immense
medius—middle

ORIGIN
linea aspera (medial lip)

INSERTION
tibial tuberosity

ACTION
extends the knee

NERVE
femoral nerve

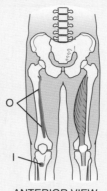

ANTERIOR VIEW

Figure 16-60

Vastus Lateralis

Latin:
vastus—immense
lateralis—toward the side

ORIGINS
linea aspera (lateral lip)
gluteal tuberosity

INSERTION
tibial tuberosity

ACTION
extends the knee

NERVE
femoral nerve

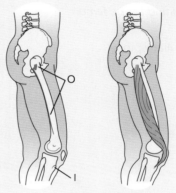

LATERAL VIEW

Figure 16-61

Sartorius

Latin:
sartor—tailor

ORIGIN
anterior superior iliac spine

INSERTION
medial proximal tibial shaft (at pes anserinus)

ACTIONS
flexes the hip
laterally rotates the hip
abducts the hip
medially rotates the knee (when knee is flexed)
laterally rotates the knee (when knee is flexed)

NERVE
femoral nerve

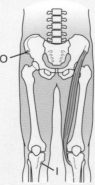

ANTERIOR VIEW

Figure 16-62

Notes: Also known as the *tailor's muscle* because in older times, tailors sat cross-legged while they sewed. The sartorius is the longest muscle in the body, crossing both the hip and knee joints, running superficially and obliquely across the quadriceps femoris muscle.

Hamstrings
Anglo-Saxon:
haun—haunch

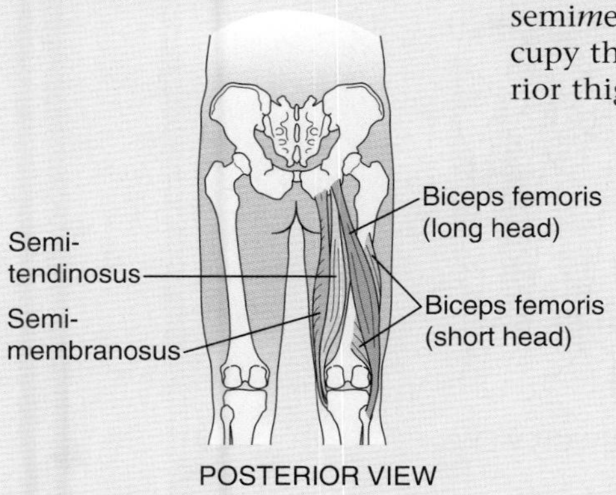

The term *hamstrings* comes from the fact that butchers in the eighteenth century used the tendons of the thighs and hips of pig carcasses to hang ham. Use the mnemonic BMT to indicate their location on the posterior thigh: *b*iceps femoris, semi*m*embranosus, semi*t*endinosus. Both semimembranosus and semitendinosus occupy the medial posterior thigh with the biceps femoris occupying the lateral posterior thigh.

Semi-
tendinosus

Semi-
membranosus

Biceps femoris
(long head)

Biceps femoris
(short head)

POSTERIOR VIEW

Figure 16-63

Semimembranosus

Latin:
semis—half
membrana—membrane

ORIGIN
ischial tuberosity

INSERTION
medial condyle of the tibia (posterior surface)

ACTIONS
flexes the knee
medially rotates the knee (when knee is flexed)
extends the hip
medially rotates the hip
posteriorly tilts the pelvis

NERVE
tibial nerve

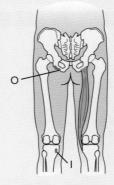

O

I

POSTERIOR VIEW

Figure 16-64

Notes: Use the mnemonic M&M to remember that the semi*m*embranosus is the most *m*edial hamstring muscle.

Occasionally, this muscle is absent or may fuse with the semitendinosus.

Semitendinosus

Latin:
semis—half
tendinosus—tendinous

ORIGIN
ischial tuberosity

INSERTION
medial proximal tibial shaft (at the pes anserinus)

ACTIONS
flexes the knee
medially rotates the knee (when knee is flexed)
extends the hip
medially rotates the hip
posteriorly tilts the pelvis

NERVE
tibial nerve

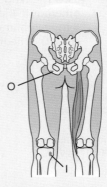

POSTERIOR VIEW

Figure 16-65

> *Notes:* The semitendinosus is superficial to, or on *top* of, the semimembranosus. This muscle may contain obliquely arranged tendinous intersections within its belly.

Biceps Femoris

Latin:
bi—twice
caput—head
femoralis—pertaining to the femur

ORIGINS
ischial tuberosity (long head)
linea aspera-lateral lip (short head)

INSERTION
fibular head

ACTIONS
flexes the knee
laterally rotates the knee (when knee is flexed)
extends the hip
laterally rotates the hip
posteriorly tilts the pelvis

NERVE
sciatic nerve (long head) and tibial nerve (short head)

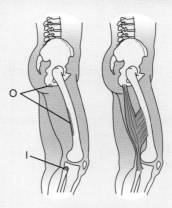

LATERAL VIEW

Figure 16-66

> *Notes:* The biceps femoris occupies the lateral side of the posterior thigh. The short head of the biceps femoris does not cross the hip joint and occasionally may be absent.

Adductors

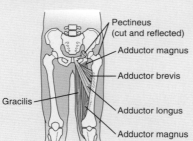

Pectineus
(cut and reflected)

Adductor magnus

Adductor brevis

Gracilis

Adductor longus

Adductor magnus

ANTERIOR VIEW

Figure 16-67

The adductors are a group of muscles forming the inner thigh; all have their origins on the pubis and insertions on the linea aspera except for the gracilis. They are the gracilis, adductor magnus, adductor longus, adductor brevis, and pectineus.

Gracilis

Latin:
gracilis—slender

ORIGIN
inferior pubic ramus

INSERTION
medial proximal tibial shaft (at the pes anserinus)

ACTIONS
adducts the hip
flexes the hip
flexes the knee
medially rotates the knee (when knee is flexed)

NERVE
obturator nerve

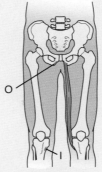

ANTERIOR VIEW

Figure 16-68

Notes: The femoral shaft and gracilis form the letter V. The gracilis is the most medial adductor and the only adductor that crosses both the hip and knee.

Adductor Magnus

Latin:
adductus—brought toward
magnum—large

ORIGINS
ischial tuberosity
inferior pubic ramus
ischial ramus

INSERTIONS
linea aspera
adductor tubercle of the femur

ACTIONS
adducts the hip
flexes the hip
extends the hip

NERVE
sciatic and obturator nerves

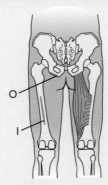

POSTERIOR VIEW

Figure 16-69

Notes: The adductor magnus lies deep to the hamstrings and is divided into two sections: one on the linea aspera and one on the adductor tubercle. Between these two sections is an opening called the *adductor hiatus* for passage of the femoral artery and vein.

Adductor Longus

Latin:
adductus—brought toward
longus—long

ORIGIN
pubic tubercle

INSERTION
linea aspera (medial lip)

ACTIONS
adducts the hip

NERVE
obturator nerve

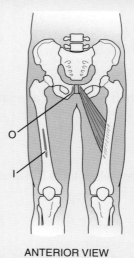

ANTERIOR VIEW

Figure 16-70

Adductor Brevis

Latin:
adductus—brought toward
brevis—brief

ORIGIN
inferior pubic ramus

INSERTION
linea aspera (medial lip)

ACTIONS
adducts the hip

NERVE
obturator nerve

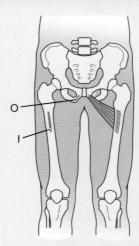

ANTERIOR VIEW

Figure 16-71

Pectineus

Latin:
pecten—comb

ORIGIN
superior pubic ramus

INSERTION
linea aspera (inferior to the lesser trochanter)

ACTIONS
flexes the hip
adducts the hip

NERVE
femoral nerve

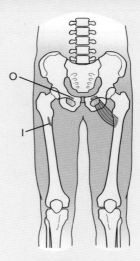

ANTERIOR VIEW

Figure 16-72

Notes: In relationship to the pectineus, the femoral artery may lie medial to the muscle; or, in some cases it may cross the pectineus superficially. Additionally, this muscle is often regarded as an extension of the iliopsoas muscle because of its insertion and action.

Pes Anserinus
Latin:
pedes—footlike
anserinus—goose

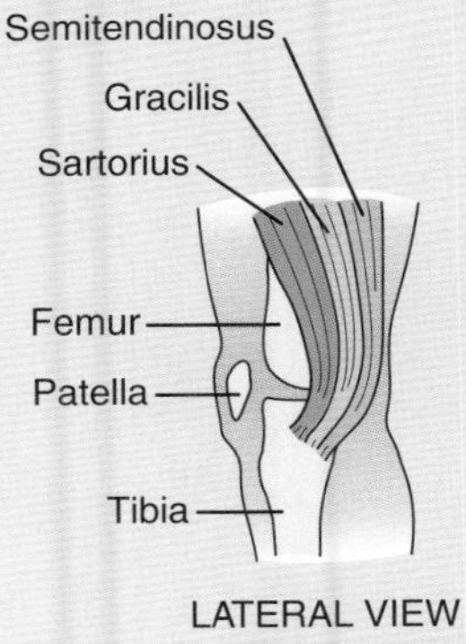

Semitendinosus
Gracilis
Sartorius

Femur
Patella

Tibia

LATERAL VIEW

Figure 16-73

The pes anserinus is the tendinous expansions of the sartorius, gracilis, and semitendinosus inserting at the medial proximal tibial shaft. Use the mnemonic phrase, "*Say grace* before *tea*," to assist you in remembering the three muscles that contribute to this structure.

LESSON FIVE

Muscles of Hip Movement

	Flexion	Extension	Medial Rotation	Lateral Rotation	Abduction	Adduction
Adductor brevis						×
Adductor longus						×
Adductor magnus	×	×				×
Biceps femoris		×		×		
Gemellus inferior				×		
Gemellus superior				×		
Gluteus maximus		×		×		×
Gluteus medius			×		×	
Gluteus minimus			×		×	
Gracilis	×					×
Iliacus	×			×		
Obturator externus				×		
Obturator internus				×		
Pectineus	×					×
Piriformis				×	×	
Psoas major	×			×		
Quadratus femoris				×		
Rectus femoris	×					
Sartorius	×			×	×	
Semimembranosus		×	×			
Semitendinosus		×	×			
Tensor fascia lata	×		×		×	

Muscles of Knee Movement

	Flexion	Extension	Medial Rotation	Lateral Rotation	Abduction	Adduction
Biceps femoris	×			×		
Gastrocnemius	×					
Gracilis	×		×			
Plantaris	×					
Popliteus	×		×			
Rectus femoris		×				
Sartorius			×	×		
Semimembranosus	×		×			
Semitendinosus	×		×			
Vastus intermedius		×				
Vastus lateralis		×				
Vastus medialis		×				

Unit ONE—Muscles of the Appendicular Skeleton

Lesson SIX—Muscles of Foot Movement (Tibialis Anterior, Extensor Digitorum Longus and Brevis, Extensor Hallucis Longus, Peroneus Longus, Peroneus Brevis, Gastrocnemius, Plantaris, Soleus, Popliteus, Tibialis Posterior, Flexor Digitorum Longus, Flexor Hallucis Longus)

Tibialis Anterior

Latin:
tibialis—shinbone
ante—before

ORIGINS
lateral tibial shaft
interosseous membrane

INSERTIONS
base of metatarsal I
cuneiform I (plantar surface)

ACTIONS
dorsiflexes the ankle
inverts the foot

NERVE
common peroneal nerve

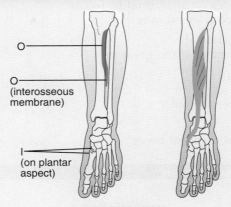

ANTERIOR VIEW

Figure 16-74

Notes: The tibialis muscle is strengthened after an inversion sprain is healed to aid in rehabilitation. It is referred to as the *stirrup muscle,* along with peroneus longus.

Extensor Digitorum Longus and Brevis

Latin:
extensio—to extend
digitus—finger or toe
longus—long
brevis—brief

ORIGINS
fibular head (longus)
proximal two thirds of the fibular shaft (longus)
lateral condyle of the tibia (longus)
calcaneus (brevis)

INSERTIONS
middle phalanges two through five (longus)
distal phalanges two through five (longus)
tendons of extensor digitorum longus (brevis)

ACTIONS
extends digits two through five
dorsiflexes the ankle (longus)

NERVE
common peroneal nerve

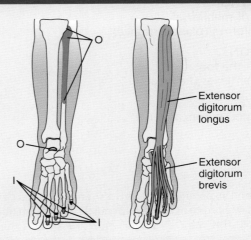

ANTERIOR VIEW

Figure 16-75

Notes: Individual tendons may be absent. The tendon for the fifth phalanx is only occasionally present.

Extensor Hallucis Longus

Latin:
extensio—to extend
hallex—large toe
longus—long

ORIGINS
anterior fibular shaft (middle region)
interosseous membrane

INSERTION
distal phalanx of the great toe

ACTIONS
extends the great toe
dorsiflexes the ankle

NERVE
common peroneal nerve

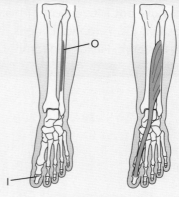

ANTERIOR VIEW

Figure 16-76

Peroneus Longus

Greek:
perone—pin
Latin:
longus—long

ORIGINS
fibular head
lateral proximal two thirds of the fibular shaft

INSERTIONS
base of metatarsal I
cuneiform I (plantar surface)

ACTIONS
everts the foot
plantar flexes the ankle

NERVE
common peroneal nerve

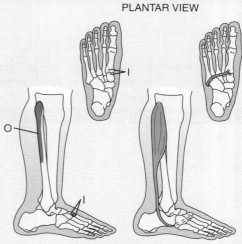

PLANTAR VIEW

LATERAL VIEW

Figure 16-77

Notes: The peroneus longus is also known as *fibularis longus* and is referred to as the stirrup muscle along with tibialis anterior. This muscle's tendon now lies behind the lateral malleolus but originally lay in front. The latter tendon arrangement is present in predators.

Peroneus Brevis

Greek:
perone—pin
Latin:
brevis—brief

ORIGIN
lateral distal two thirds of the fibular shaft

INSERTION
base of metatarsal

ACTIONS
everts the foot
plantar flexes the ankle

NERVE
common peroneal nerve

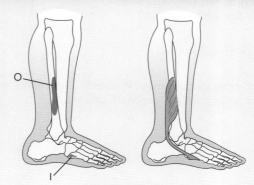

LATERAL VIEW

Figure 16-78

Peroneus Brevis—cont'd

Notes: The peroneus brevis is also known as *fibularis brevis.* This muscle's tendon now lies behind the lateral malleolus but originally lay in front. The latter tendon arrangement is present in predators.

Triceps Surae

Greek:
treis—three
Latin:
sura—pertaining to the calf of the leg

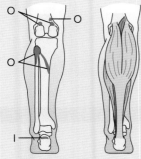

POSTERIOR VIEW

Figure 16-79

The triceps surae is another name for the gastrocnemius, plantaris, and soleus (some references include only the two heads of the gastrocnemius and the soleus as the triceps surae). These three muscles share a common tendon and are viewed as the triceps brachii of the lower extremity. The triceps surae lifts the weight of the body when moving forward, as in walking or running, and make up the superficial layer of the posterior lower leg.

Gastrocnemius

Greek:
gaster—belly
kneme—leg

ORIGINS
medial epicondyle of the femur
lateral epicondyle of the femur

INSERTION
calcaneus via the Achilles tendon

ACTIONS
plantar flexes the ankle
flexes the knee

NERVE
tibial nerve

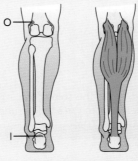

POSTERIOR VIEW

Figure 16-80

Notes: The gastrocnemius is also known as the *toe dancer's muscle* because it helps a ballerina stand on toe. The two actions of this muscle, ankle plantar flexion and knee flexion, are an either/or situation—the gastrocnemius cannot perform both actions simultaneously. Occasionally, origins of this muscle are found on the joint capsule of the knee.

Plantaris

Latin:
planta—sole

ORIGIN
lateral epicondyle of the femur

INSERTION
calcaneus via the Achilles tendon

ACTIONS
plantar flexes the ankle
flexes the knee

NERVE
tibial nerve

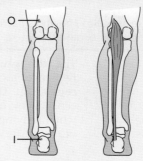

POSTERIOR VIEW

Figure 16-81

Notes: The plantaris is regarded as a mini-gastrocnemius because of a common insertion and is occasionally missing in cadavers (about 10%).

Soleus

Latin:
solea—sole of the foot

ORIGINS
superior posterior one third the fibular shaft
soleal line of the tibia

INSERTION
calcaneus via the Achilles tendon

ACTION
plantar flexes the ankle

NERVE
tibial nerve

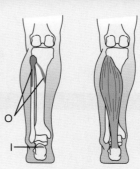

POSTERIOR VIEW

Figure 16-82

Notes: According to one source, the soleus was so named because it looks like a sole fish from the Mediterranean sea.

Popliteus

Latin:
poples—hollow behind the knee

ORIGIN
lateral condyle of the femur

INSERTION
posterior proximal tibial shaft

ACTIONS
flexes the knee
medially rotates the knee (when knee is flexed)

NERVE
tibial nerve

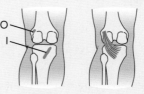

POSTERIOR VIEW

Figure 16-83

Notes: The popliteus is a weak knee flexor, but its function of unlocking the extended knee to begin flexion is vital to the other stronger knee flexors. For this, it gets the nickname the *key that unlocks the knee.*

Tibialis Posterior

Latin:
tibialis—shinbone
posterus—behind

ORIGINS
posterior tibial shaft
posterior fibular shaft
interosseous membrane

INSERTIONS
navicular bone (plantar surface)
cuneiform III
cuboid
bases of metatarsals II, III, and IV

ACTIONS
inverts the foot
plantar flexes the ankle

NERVE
tibial nerve

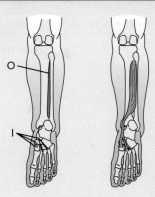

POSTERIOR VIEW

Figure 16-84

Notes: This muscle may be completely absent.

Flexor Digitorum Longus

Latin:
flexus—bent
digitus—finger or toe
longus—long

ORIGIN
posterior tibial shaft-middle region

INSERTIONS
distal phalanges II-V (plantar surface)

ACTIONS
flexes digits 2-5 at the DIP, PIP, and the MP joints
plantar flexes the ankle

NERVE
tibial nerve

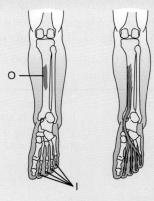

POSTERIOR VIEW

Figure 16-85

Flexor Hallucis Longus

Latin:
flexus—bent
hallex—large toe
longus—long

ORIGIN
posterior fibular shaft-middle region

INSERTION
distal phalanx of the great toe (plantar surface)

ACTIONS
flexes great toe
plantar flexes the ankle (longus)
inverts the foot (longus)
supports the longitudinal arch (longus)

NERVE
tibial nerve

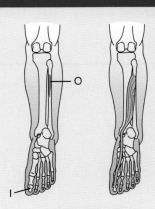

POSTERIOR VIEW

Figure 16-86

LESSON SIX

Muscles of Ankle and Foot Movement

	Plantar Flexion	Dorsiflexion	Inversion	Eversion
Extensor digitorum longus		X		
Extensor hallucis longus		X		
Flexor digitorum longus	X			
Flexor hallucis longus	X			
Gastrocnemius	X			
Peroneus brevis	X			X
Peroneus longus	X			X
Plantaris	X			
Soleus	X			
Tibialis anterior		X	X	
Tibialis posterior	X		X	

Unit TWO—Muscles of the Axial Skeleton

Lesson SEVEN—**Muscles of the Head and Neck** (Frontalis, Occipitalis, Orbicularis Oculi, Orbicularis Oris, Zygomaticus Major and Minor, Buccinator, Platysma, Temporalis, Masseter, Lateral Pterygoid, Medial Pterygoid, Longus Capitis, Longus Colli, Sternocleidomastoid, Scalenus Anterior, Scalenus Medius, Scalenus Posterior, Splenius Capitis, Splenius Cervicis, Rectus Capitis Posterior Major, Rectus Capitis Posterior Minor, Oblique Capitis Superior, Oblique Capitis Inferior, Levator Scapulae [Lesson One], Trapezius [Lesson One], Spinalis [Lesson Eight], Longissimus [Lesson Eight])

Occipitofrontalis

The occipitofrontalis, a two-bellied muscle containing the occipitalis and the frontalis, is connected by an extensive network of cranial fascia called the *galea aponeurotica* or the *epicranius*. The galea aponeurotica is firmly connected to the hypodermis and slides over the periosteum of the cranium.

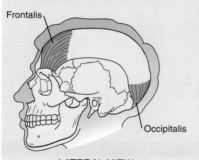

Frontalis

Occipitalis

LATERAL VIEW

Figure 16-87

Frontalis

Latin:
frons—brow or referring to the frontal bone

ORIGIN
galea aponeurotica

INSERTION
superficial fascia beneath the eyebrows

ACTIONS
elevates the eyebrows
horizontally wrinkles skin on your forehead

NERVE
facial nerve (cranial nerve VII)

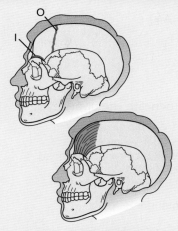

LATERAL VIEW

Figure 16-88

Notes: The frontalis muscle contributes to tension headaches. Contraction of many muscles of the head and neck simply displace skin, which is the basis of facial ex-pression. The frontalis muscle produces the expression of worry or concern.

Occipitalis

Latin:
occipitalis—pertaining to the back of the head

ORIGIN
lateral two thirds of the superior nuchal line

INSERTION
galea aponeurotica

ACTION
moves scalp over the cranium

NERVE
facial nerve (cranial nerve VII)

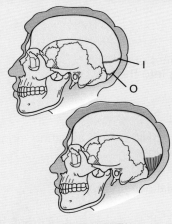

LATERAL VIEW

Figure 16-89

Orbicularis Oculi

Latin:
orbiculus—little circle
oculus—eye

ORIGIN
orbital margin

INSERTION
superficial fascia beneath the upper eyelids

ACTIONS
closes the eyelids
vertically wrinkles skin on your forehead
squints the eyelids

NERVE
facial nerve (cranial nerve VII)

Notes: Also known as the *winking or blinking muscle,* it closes the eyelid.

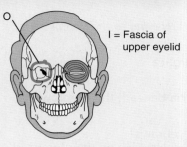

I = Fascia of upper eyelid

ANTERIOR VIEW

Figure 16-90

Orbicularis Oris

Latin:
orbiculus—little circle
oris—mouth

ORIGINS
maxilla
mandible
buccinator

INSERTIONS
mucous membranes of the lips
muscles inserting into the lips

ACTIONS
closes the lips
protrudes the lips
allows dozens of activities such as eating, drinking, talking, and sucking

NERVE
facial nerve (cranial nerve VII)

Notes: Also known as the *kissing muscle,* it protrudes the lips for a kiss.

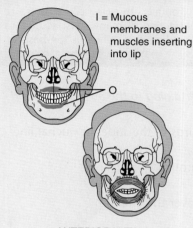

I = Mucous membranes and muscles inserting into lip

ANTERIOR VIEW

Figure 16-91

Zygomaticus Major and Minor

Latin:
zygotos—yoked or to connect
major—larger

ORIGINS
zygomatic arch (major)
zygomatic arch (minor)

INSERTIONS
lateral angle of the mouth (major)
lateral angle of the mouth (minor)

ACTION
lifts corners of the mouth upward and outward

NERVE
facial nerve (cranial nerve VII)

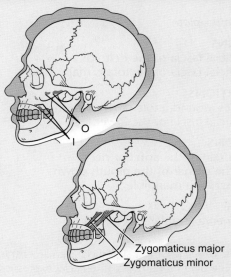

Zygomaticus major
Zygomaticus minor

LATERAL VIEW

Figure 16-92

Notes: Contraction of these muscles produce the facial expression of a smile and are called the *smiling* or *laughing muscles.* The zygomaticus minor inserts just medial to the zygomaticus major.

Buccinator

Latin:
buccinator—trumpeter

ORIGINS
maxilla
mandible

INSERTION
orbicularis oris

ACTIONS
compresses the cheeks
retracts angles of the mouth

NERVE
facial nerve (cranial nerve VII)

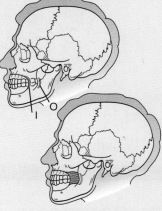

LATERAL VIEW

Figure 16-93

Notes: This muscle creates the shape of the mouth for the action of blowing. It also aids in mastication as it pulls food toward the teeth.

Platysma

Greek:
platysma—plate

ORIGINS
superficial fascia of the deltoids
superficial fascia of pectoralis major

INSERTIONS
muscles around angle of the mouth
superficial fascia of the lower face

ACTIONS
tenses skin of the anterior neck
pulls the corner of the mouth down
depresses the mandible

NERVE
facial nerve (cranial nerve VII)

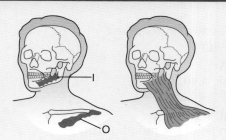

ANTEROLATERAL VIEW

Figure 16-94

Notes: This is the most superficial muscle of the anterior neck. The platysma produces the facial expression of pouting and is often called the *pouting muscle.*

Muscles of Mastication (Temporalis, Masseter, Medial and Lateral Pterygoids)

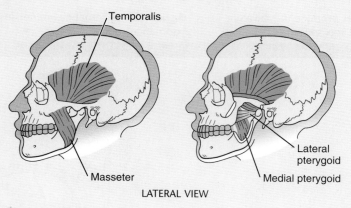

Temporalis

Masseter

Lateral pterygoid

Medial pterygoid

LATERAL VIEW

Figure 16-95

Temporalis

Latin:
temporalis—pertaining to the temporal bone

ORIGIN
temporal fossa

INSERTION
coronoid process of the mandible

ACTIONS
elevates the mandible
retracts the mandible

NERVE
trigeminal nerve (cranial nerve V)

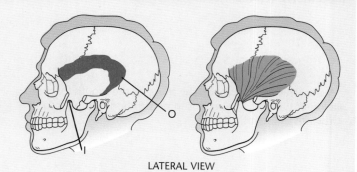

LATERAL VIEW

Figure 16-96

Notes: The temporalis is the strongest elevator of the mandible.

Masseter

Greek:
masseter—chewer

ORIGIN
zygomatic arch

INSERTIONS
mandibular angle (exterior surface)
mandibular ramus (exterior surface)

ACTIONS
elevates the mandible
protracts mandible

NERVE
trigeminal nerve (cranial nerve V)

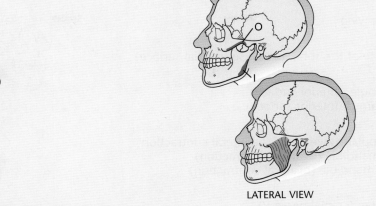

LATERAL VIEW

Figure 16-97

Notes: Masseter is the mirror image of medial pterygoid.

Lateral Pterygoid

Latin:
lateralis—toward the side
Greek:
pterygodes—a wing

ORIGINS
pterygoid plate of the sphenoid bone (lateral surface)
greater wing of the sphenoid bone

INSERTIONS
condylar process of the mandible
temporomandibular joint capsule

ACTIONS
lateral mandibular movements (unilateral contraction)
depresses the mandible (bilateral contraction)
protracts the mandible (bilateral contraction)

NERVE
trigeminal nerve (cranial nerve V)

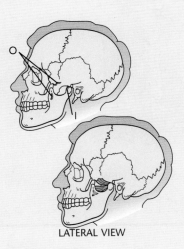

LATERAL VIEW

Figure 16-98

Medial Pterygoid

Latin:
medialis—toward the midline
Greek:
pterygodes—a wing

ORIGIN
pterygoid plate of the sphenoid bone (medial surface)

INSERTIONS
mandibular angle (interior surface)
mandibular ramus (interior surface)

ACTIONS
lateral mandibular movements (unilateral contraction)
elevates the mandible (bilateral contraction)
protracts the mandible (bilateral contraction)

NERVE
trigeminal nerve (cranial nerve V)

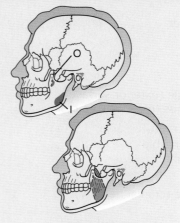

LATERAL VIEW

Figure 16-99

Notes: The medial pterygoid is the mirror image of the masseter.

Longus Capitis and Longus Colli

Two important muscles of the anterior neck are the longus capitis and longus colli, helping maintain an anterior curve of the cervical spine.

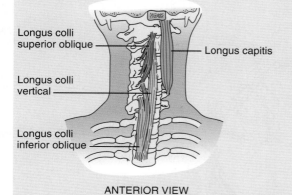

Longus colli superior oblique

Longus colli vertical

Longus colli inferior oblique

Longus capitis

ANTERIOR VIEW

Figure 16-100

Longus Capitis

Latin:
longus—long
caput—head

ORIGINS
transverse processes of C3-C6

INSERTION
inferior base of the occipital bone

ACTIONS
rotates the head
flexes the neck

NERVE
anterior rami

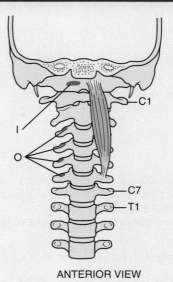

ANTERIOR VIEW

Figure 16-101

Longus Colli

Latin:
longus—long
colli—collar

ORIGINS
anterior transverse processes of C3-C5 (superior
   oblique portion)
bodies of T1-T3 (inferior oblique portion)
vertebral bodies of C5-T3 (vertical portion)

INSERTIONS
anterior tubercle of C-1 (superior oblique portion)
anterior transverse processes C5-C6 (inferior oblique
   portion)
vertebral bodies C2-C4 (vertical portion)

ACTIONS
rotates the head
flexes the neck
laterally flexes the neck

NERVE
anterior rami

ANTERIOR VIEW

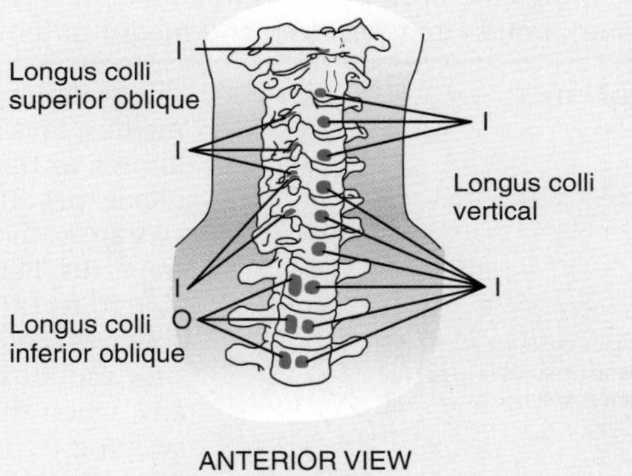

Figure 16-102

Notes: The longus colli, like the iliopsoas of the lower extremity, contains three different muscles: longus colli superior oblique, longus colli inferior oblique, and longus colli
vertical.

Sternocleidomastoid

Greek:
sternon—sternum
cleido—clavicle
mastos—breastlike

ORIGINS
manubrium of the sternum
medial one third of the clavicle

INSERTION
mastoid process

ACTIONS
laterally flexes neck (unilateral contraction)
rotates head to opposite side (unilateral contraction)
flexes the neck (bilateral contraction)
assists in forced inspiration (bilateral contraction)

NERVE
spinal accessory nerve (cranial nerve XI)

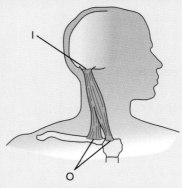

ANTEROLATERAL VIEW

Figure 16-103

Notes: The sternocleidomastoid (SCM) feels like a cable on both sides of the neck. A condition called *torticollis,* or *wry-neck,* involves spasms of the SCM. Spasm in this muscle may also cause vertigo because of the many sensory and positional receptors located here. The SCM is the only muscle that moves the head but does not attach to any vertebrae.

The carotid artery lies deep and medial to the SCM, and the external jugular vein lies on top of it. SCM is the mirror image of splenius capitis.

Note the close relationship between the SCM and the trapezius; both attach to the base of the skull and the clavicle. Both muscles laterally flex the neck and rotate the head. One muscle flexes the neck, and the other extends it.

Scalenes

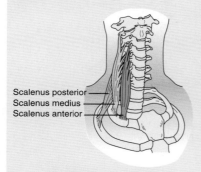

Scalenus posterior
Scalenus medius
Scalenus anterior

ANTEROLATERAL VIEW

Figure 16-104

The scalenes are a group of muscles consisting of the scalenus anterior, scalenus medius, and scalenus posterior. These muscles, along with the pectoralis minor, are known as the *neurovascular entrappers* because the subclavian artery and brachial plexus pass between the scalenus anterior and the scalenus medius. All scalene muscles are palpable in the posterior triangular of the neck between the SCM and the trapezius. Place your hands in this triangle and take a deep breath. You should be able to feel these muscles shortening. Because of the effect on respiration, the scalenes represent the cranial continuation of the intercostals. Acting unilaterally, they mobilize the neck; acting bilaterally, they actively aid in respiration.* Additionally, when the body is in motion, the scalenes stabilize the neck by preventing side swaying.

In about 30% of all cadavers, another scalene muscle, the scalenus minimus, is found.

*From Platzer, 1977.

Scalenus Anterior

Greek:
skalenos—uneven
Latin:
ante—before

ORIGINS
transverse processes of C3-C6

INSERTION
rib 1 (superior surface)

ACTIONS
laterally flexes the neck (unilateral contraction)
rotates the head (unilateral contraction)
elevates the first rib during inhalation (bilateral contraction)

NERVE
posterior rami of C3-C8

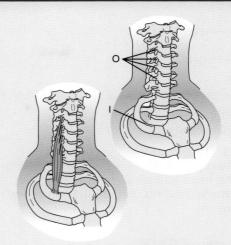

ANTEROLATERAL VIEW

Figure 16-105

Scalenus Medius

Greek:
skalenos—uneven
Latin:
medialis—toward the midline

ORIGINS
transverse processes of C2-C7

INSERTION
rib 1 (superior surface)

ACTIONS
laterally flexes the neck (unilateral contraction)
rotates the head (unilateral contraction)
elevates first rib during inhalation (bilateral contraction)

NERVE
posterior rami of C3-C8

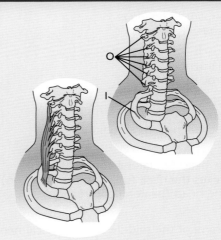

ANTEROLATERAL VIEW

Figure 16-106

Scalenus Posterior

Greek:
skalenos—uneven
Latin:
posterus—behind

ORIGINS
transverse processes of C4-C6

INSERTION
rib 2 (superior lateral surface)

ACTIONS
laterally flexes the neck (unilateral contraction)
rotates the head (unilateral contraction)
elevates the second rib during inhalation (bilateral contraction)

NERVE
posterior rami of C3-C8

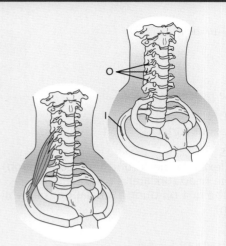

ANTEROLATERAL VIEW

Figure 16-107

Splenius Capitis

Greek:
splenion—splint or bandage
caput—head

ORIGINS
nuchal ligament
spinous processes of C7-T3

INSERTIONS
mastoid process
inferior nuchal line-lateral region

ACTIONS
rotates the head (unilateral contraction)
laterally flexes the neck (unilateral contraction)
extends the head (bilateral contraction)

NERVE
posterior rami of the middle lower cervical nerves

Notes: Splenius capitis is the mirror image of SCM.

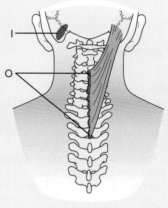

POSTERIOR VIEW

Figure 16-108

Splenius Cervicis

Greek:
splenion—splint or bandage
cervicalis—neck

ORIGINS
spinous processes of T3-T6

INSERTIONS
transverse processes of C1-C3

ACTIONS
rotates the head (unilateral contraction)
laterally flexes the neck (unilateral contraction)
extends the head (bilateral contraction)

NERVE
posterior rami of middle lower cervical nerves

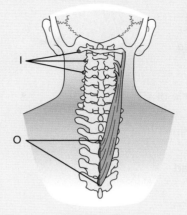

POSTERIOR VIEW

Figure 16-109

Suboccipitals

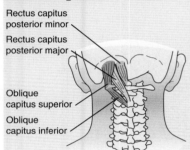

Rectus capitus posterior minor
Rectus capitus posterior major
Oblique capitus superior
Oblique capitus inferior

POSTERIOR VIEW

Figure 16-110

The suboccipital muscles include the rectus capitis posterior major, rectus capitis posterior minor, oblique capitis inferior, and oblique capitis superior. Dr. Janet Travell (see her biography in Chapter 18) refers to the suboccipitals as the *ghost headache muscles* because the pain referred from these muscles seems to penetrate the skull and is difficult to locate. All suboccipitals attach on C1-C2 and are responsible for initiating most of the head movements.

Rectus Capitis Posterior Major

Latin:
rectus—straight
caput—head
posterus—behind
major—larger

ORIGIN
spinous process of C2

INSERTION
inferior nuchal line

ACTIONS
extends the head
rotates the head

NERVE
suboccipital nerve

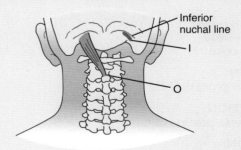

Inferior nuchal line

POSTERIOR VIEW

Figure 16-111

Rectus Capitis Posterior Minor

Latin:
rectus—straight
caput—head
posterus—behind
minor—smaller

ORIGIN
posterior tubercle of C1

INSERTION
inferior nuchal line

ACTION
extends the head

NERVE
suboccipital nerve

> *Notes:* This muscle also attaches to the dura mater. Tension in this muscle may cause headaches of a vascular and neurological nature.

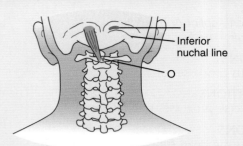

POSTERIOR VIEW

Figure 16-112

Oblique Capitis Superior

Latin:
obliquus—slant
caput—head
superus—upper

ORIGIN
transverse process of C1

INSERTION
inferior nuchal line

ACTIONS
extends the head
rotates the head

NERVE
suboccipital nerve

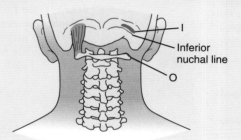

POSTERIOR VIEW

Figure 16-113

Oblique Capitis Inferior

Latin:
obliquus—slant
caput—head
infra—beneath

ORIGIN
spinous process of C2

INSERTION
transverse process of C1

ACTION
rotates the head

NERVE
suboccipital nerve

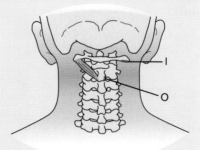

POSTERIOR VIEW

Figure 16-114

LESSON SEVEN

Muscles of Mandibular Movement

	Elevation	Depression	Protraction	Retraction	Lateral Movement
Masseter	✕		✕		
Platysma		✕			
Pterygoid lateralis		✕	✕		✕
Pterygoid medialis	✕		✕		✕
Temporalis	✕			✕	

Muscles of Head and Neck Movement

	Flexion	Extension	Lateral Flexion	Rotation
Levator scapulae			✕	
Longissimus		✕		
Longus capitis	✕			✕
Longus colli	✕		✕	✕
Oblique capitis superior		✕		✕
Rectus capitis posterior major		✕		✕
Rectus capitis posterior minor		✕		
Scalenus anterior			✕	✕
Scalenus medius			✕	✕
Scalenus posterior			✕	✕
Spinalis		✕		
Splenius capitis		✕	✕	✕
Splenius cervicis		✕	✕	✕
Sternocleidomastoid	✕		✕	✕
Trapezius		✕	✕	

Unit TWO—Muscles of the Axial Skeleton

Lesson EIGHT—Muscles of the Trunk and Vertebral Column (Rectus Abdominis, External Obliques, Internal Obliques, Transverse Abdominis, Quadratus Lumborum, Semispinalis, Rotatores, Multifidus, Spinalis, Longissimus, Iliocostalis)

Abdominals

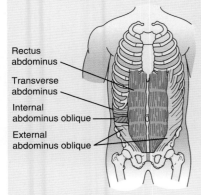

Rectus abdominus

Transverse abdominus

Internal abdominus oblique

External abdominus oblique

ANTERIOR VIEW

Figure 16-115

The abdominal muscles are the rectus abdominis, external and internal obliques, and transverse abdominis. The fiber arrangement of the abdominal muscles runs in four different directions. Think of this organization as the "plywood" principle of anatomy, used for added strength to hold in internal abdominal organs. You can feel how these muscles compress the abdominal contents by placing your hands on your belly while you laugh, cough, defecate, or vomit. The abdominals are also involved in forced exhalation.

Rectus Abdominis

Latin:
rectus—straight
abdomen—belly

ORIGINS
pubic symphysis
pubic tubercle

INSERTIONS
ribs 5-7 (costal cartilage-anterior surface)
xiphoid process

ACTIONS
flexes the vertebral column
compresses abdominal contents
posteriorly tilts the pelvis

NERVE
anterior rami of intercostal nerves (T7-T12)

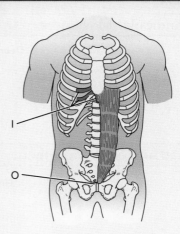

ANTERIOR VIEW

Figure 16-116

Notes: The rectus abdominis goes a long distance without any skeletal attachment, so physiology has provided a way of keeping its length constant by including a horizontal layer of connective tissue every few inches. This band of con- nective tissue is called a *tendinous intersection.* Separation of this muscle, which may occur during advanced pregnancy, is called *rectus diastasis.*

External Obliques

Latin:
externus—outside
abdomen—belly
obliquus—slant

ORIGINS
ribs 5-12 (anterior lateral surface)

INSERTIONS
iliac crest
abdominal fascia
linea alba

ACTIONS
laterally flexes the vertebral column (unilateral contraction)
rotates the vertebral column (unilateral contraction)
flexes the vertebral column (bilateral contraction)
compresses abdomen contents (bilateral contraction)

NERVE
anterior rami of intercostal nerves (T7-T12)

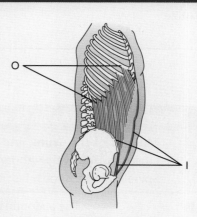

LATERAL VIEW

Figure 16-117

Notes: The fiber direction of this muscle is similar to the direction of your fingers when your hands are in the pockets of a jacket. The pockets of most jackets do not reach the midline. Likewise, the external obliques do not reach the midline. They insert into the sheath of the rectus abdo- minis instead. Tendinous intersections such as those present in the rectus abdominis may be present.

The external obliques interlace with the serratus anterior and latissimus dorsi on the lateral aspect of the trunk.

Internal Obliques

Latin:
internus—within
abdomen—belly
obliquus—slant

ORIGINS
iliac crest
thoracolumbar fascia
inguinal ligament

INSERTIONS
ribs 7-12 (anterior lateral surface)
linea alba

ACTIONS
laterally flexes the vertebral column (unilateral contraction)
rotates the vertebral column (unilateral contraction)
flexes the vertebral column (bilateral contraction)
compresses abdominal contents (bilateral contraction)

NERVE
anterior rami of intercostal nerves

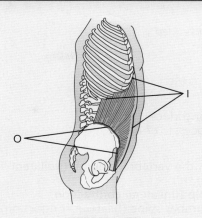

LATERAL VIEW

Figure 16-118

Notes: The fiber direction of the internal obliques ascends like a fan, with the majority of the fibers laying in the direction of your fingers when your thumbs are hooked behind suspenders and your fingers are resting on your chest.

Transverse Abdominis

Latin:
transversus—lying across
abdomen—belly

ORIGINS
ribs 7-12 (costal cartilage-inner surface)
iliac crest
thoracolumbar aponeurosis
inguinal ligament

INSERTIONS
abdominal aponeurosis
linea alba

ACTION
compresses abdominal contents

NERVE
anterior rami of intercostal nerves

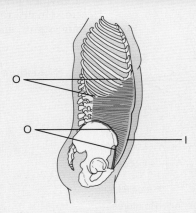

LATERAL VIEW

Figure 16-119

Notes: The transverse abdominis is the deepest abdominal muscle and wraps around the internal organs like a cummerbund, helping stabilize the lumbar spine. The lower fibers of the rectus abdominis are enclosed by the transverse abdominis, probably for added strength. The inferior portion of this muscle may fuse completely with the internal obliques. Because of its frequent variance, the transverse abdominis is often called the *complex muscle.*

Quadratus Lumborum

Latin:
quadratus—four-sided
lumbus—loins

ORIGIN
posterior iliac crest

INSERTIONS
rib 12 (inferior surface)
transverse processes of L1-L4

ACTIONS
laterally flexes the vertebral column (unilateral
  contraction)
elevates the hip (unilateral contraction)
extends the lumbar spine (bilateral contraction)
anteriorly tilts pelvis (bilateral contraction)

NERVES
thoracic nerve
lumbar nerve

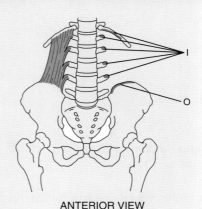

ANTERIOR VIEW

Figure 16-120

Notes: Also known as the *hip hiker muscle,* it hikes up the hip.

Paraspinals
Greek:
para—beside
Latin:
spinatus—spine

The paraspinals are the collective term given to a group of back muscles composed of two groups: the transversospinalis (deep paraspinals) and erector spinae (superficial paraspinals). Important in maintaining the posture, each muscle group can be subdivided into smaller branches (Table 16-1). Transversospinalis' subgroups are semispinalis, rotatores, and multifidus. Erector spinae's subgroups are spinalis, longissimus, and iliocostalis.

Figure 16-121

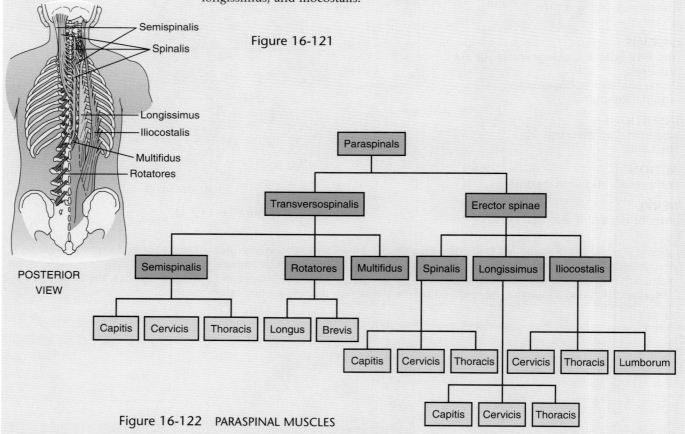

Figure 16-122   PARASPINAL MUSCLES

Transversospinalis

Latin:
transversus—lying across
spinatus—spine

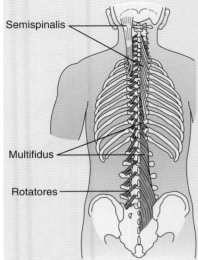

Semispinalis

Multifidus

Rotatores

POSTERIOR VIEW

Figure 16-123

The term *transversospinalis* refers to the vertebral processes to which most of the muscles in this group attach; all originate on the transverse processes and insert on the spinous processes. Two of the three muscle groups, the semispinalis and rotatores, can be further subdivided. These subgroupings are the semispinalis capitis, semispinalis cervicis, semispinalis thoracis, rotatores longus, and rotatores brevis. The multifidi has no subgroup. All of these muscles are stacked on top of each other and are comprised of many short diagonal fibers.

Two other muscles, called *segmental muscles,* lie deep in the back. These muscles are the interspinales and intertransversarii. They are called *segmental muscles* because the traverse a single vertebral segment. The interspinales attach to the spinous processes and the intertransversarii attach to the transverse processes.

Semispinalis

Latin:
semis—half
spinatus—spine

ORIGIN
transverse process of one vertebral segment (cervical and thoracic regions)

INSERTIONS
spinous processes of the fifth, sixth, and seventh vertebral segments above (cervical and thoracic regions except C1)

ACTIONS
rotates the vertebral column (unilateral contraction)
extends the vertebral column (bilateral contraction)

NERVE
posterior rami of spinal nerves

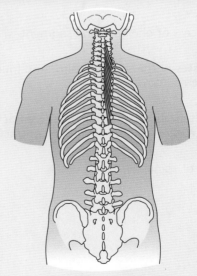

POSTERIOR VIEW

Figure 16-124

Notes: This group of muscles runs in only the thoracic and cervical regions of the vertebral column. This is the most superficial of the transversospinalis and is one of the strongest muscles of the neck.

Rotatores

Latin:
rotare—to turn

ORIGIN
transverse process of one vertebral segment

INSERTION
spinous process of the second vertebral segment
   above

ACTIONS
rotates the vertebral column (unilateral contraction)
extends the vertebral column (bilateral contraction)

NERVE
posterior rami of spinal nerves

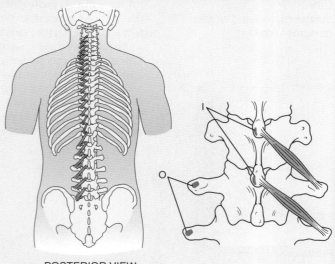

POSTERIOR VIEW

Figure 16-125

Notes: The rotatores span one to two vertebrae. This muscle is the deepest of the transversospinalis group.

Multifidus

Latin:
multus—many
fidus—to split

ORIGIN
transverse process of one vertebral segment

INSERTIONS
spinous processes of the second, third, and fourth vertebral segments above

ACTIONS
rotates the vertebral column (unilateral contraction)
extends the vertebral column (bilateral contraction)

NERVE
posterior rami of spinal nerves

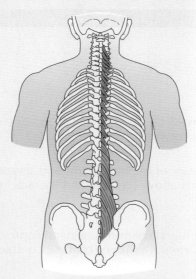

POSTERIOR VIEW

Figure 16-126

Notes: The multifidus spans two to four vertebrae and lies over the rotatores.

Erector Spinae

Latin:
erigere—to erect
spinatus—spine

The term *erector spinae* refers to the action of this muscle group—erection of the spine. These muscles fill the osseous canal formed by the vertebral arches (lamina groove). Each subgroup (spinalis, longissimus, iliocostalis) can be further subdivided. These groups are the spinalis capitis, spinalis cervicis, spinalis thoracis, longissimus capitis, longissimus cervicis, longissimus thoracis, iliocostalis cervicis, iliocostalis thoracis, iliocostalis lumborum.

Also known as the *sacrospinalis muscle,* the erector spinae runs parallel to the spine and erects it like a silo. The word *SILO* can be used as a mnemonic phrase to recall the names of the erector spinae muscles: spinalis, iliocostalis, and longissimus. These muscles lie next to each other, compared with the transversospinalis, which lies on top of each other.

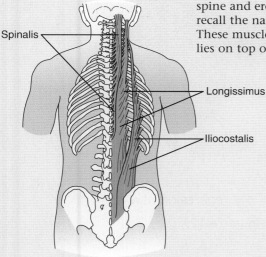

Spinalis

Longissimus

Iliocostalis

POSTERIOR VIEW

Figure 16-127

Spinalis

Latin:
spinatus—spine

ORIGINS
spinous processes of C4-T12
nuchal ligament

INSERTIONS
spinous processes of C2-T8
occipital bone (between the superior and inferior
  nuchal lines)

ACTIONS
laterally flexes the vertebral column (unilateral
  contraction)
extends the vertebral column (bilateral contraction)
extends the head (bilateral contraction)

NERVE
posterior rami of spinal nerves

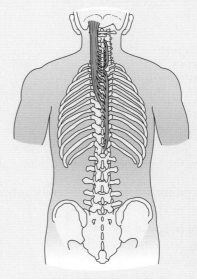

POSTERIOR VIEW

Figure 16-128

Notes: The spinalis is the medial tract of the erector spinae and interconnects the upper 80% of the vertebral column with the skull. The *spin*alis hugs the *spin*e and lies in the lamina groove.

Longissimus

Latin:
longus—long

ORIGINS
posterior sacrum
spinous processes of T1-L5
transverse processes of C4-T12

INSERTIONS
mastoid process
transverse processes of C2-T12
ribs 4-12 (posterior surface)

ACTIONS
laterally flexes the vertebral column (unilateral contraction)
extends the vertebral column (bilateral contraction)
extends the head (bilateral contraction)

NERVE
posterior rami of spinal nerves

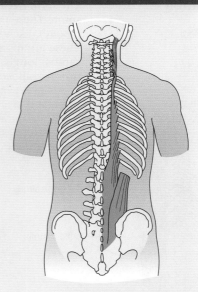

POSTERIOR VIEW

Figure 16-129

Notes: The *longissimus* is the intermediate tract of the erector spinae and covers a *long* territory stretching from sacrum to skull.

Iliocostalis

Latin:
ilium—flank
costae—rib

ORIGINS
posterior iliac crest
posterior sacrum
ribs 1-12 (posterior surface)

INSERTIONS
ribs 1-12 (posterior surface)
transverse processes of C4-C6

ACTIONS
laterally flexes the vertebral column (unilateral contraction)
extends the vertebral column (bilateral contraction)

NERVE
posterior rami of spinal nerves

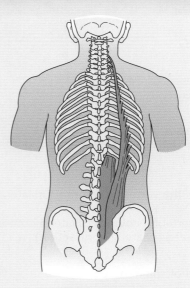

POSTERIOR VIEW

Figure 16-130

Notes: The iliocostalis is the lateral tract of the erector spinae. The ilio*costalis* hugs the *costals* (ribs).

LESSON EIGHT

Muscles of Vertebral Column Movement

	Flexion	Extension	Lateral Flexion	Rotation
External obliques	X		X	X
Iliocostalis		X	X	
Internal obliques	X		X	X
Longissimus		X	X	
Multifidus		X		X
Psoas major	X			
Quadratus lumborum		X	X	
Rectus abdominis	X			
Rotatores		X		X
Semispinalis		X		X
Spinalis		X	X	

Unit TWO—Muscles of the Axial Skeleton

Lesson NINE—Muscles of Respiration (Diaphragm, Internal Intercostals, External Intercostals, Serratus Posterior Superior, Serratus Posterior Inferior, Pectoralis Minor [Lesson One], Scalenus Anterior [Lesson Seven], Scalenus Medius [Lesson Seven], Scalenus Posterior [Lesson Seven], Sternocleidomastoid [Lesson Seven])

Diaphragm

Greek:
diaphragma—a partition

ORIGINS
L1-L3
lower six costal cartilages
xiphoid process

INSERTION
central tendon (cloverleaf-shaped aponeurosis)

ACTION
expands the thoracic cavity during inspiration

NERVE
phrenic nerve

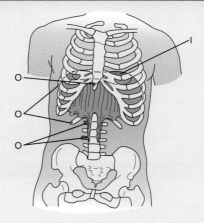

ANTERIOR VIEW

Figure 16-131

Notes: The diaphragm divides the thoracic from the abdominal cavity and is the prime mover of inspiration. Because of its origins, the diaphragm possesses lumbar, costal, and sternal portions.

Internal Intercostals

Latin:
internus—within
costae—rib

ORIGIN
superior border of rib (below)

INSERTION
inferior border of rib (above)

ACTIONS
depresses the rib cage during exhaling
maintains intercostal spaces

NERVE
intercostal nerves

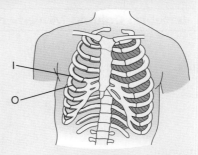

ANTERIOR VIEW

Figure 16-132

Notes: The fiber direction of the internal intercostals is the same as the internal obliques.

External Intercostals

Latin:
externus—outside
internus—within
costae—rib

ORIGIN
inferior border of rib (above)

INSERTION
superior border of rib (below)

ACTIONS
elevates the rib cage during inhalation
maintains intercostal spaces

NERVE
intercostal nerves

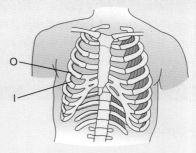

ANTERIOR VIEW

Figure 16-133

Notes: As the name implies, the external intercostals are external, or superficial, to the internal intercostals and in between the ribs. The fiber direction of this muscle is the same as the external obliques.

Serratus Posterior Superior

Latin:
serratus—notched or jagged like a saw
posterus—behind
superus—upper

ORIGINS
nuchal ligament
spinous processes of C7-T2

INSERTIONS
ribs 2-5 (posterior surface)

ACTIONS
elevates ribs during inspiration

NERVE
intercostal nerves

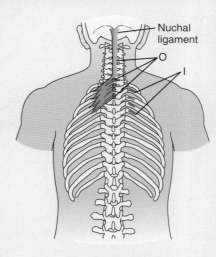

Nuchal ligament

POSTERIOR VIEW

Figure 16-134

Serratus Posterior Superior—cont'd

Notes: Deep to the rhomboids, these two muscles aid in the process of labored breathing; however, many notable anatomy texts such as *Myofascial Pain and Dysfunction: the* *Trigger Point Manual,* by Janet Travell and David Simons, do not consider these muscles as respiratory muscles, because they appear to remain passive during normal respiration.

Serratus Posterior Inferior

Latin:
serratus—notched or jagged like a saw
posterus—behind
infra—beneath

ORIGINS
spinous processes of T11-L2

INSERTIONS
ribs 9-12 (posterior surface)

ACTIONS
depresses ribs during exhalation

NERVE
intercostal nerves (T9-T12)

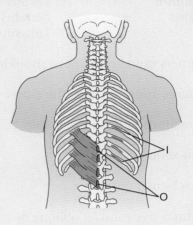

POSTERIOR VIEW

Figure 16-135

For Your Information

Smallest muscle: stapedius muscle of the middle ear
Largest muscle: latissimus dorsi
Longest muscle: sartorius
Thickest muscle: gluteus maximus
Strongest muscle: masseter, tunge (tongue), or gluteus maximus

SUMMARY

Muscular nomenclature deals with the names, locations, attachment points, actions, and nerve supply of individual skeletal muscles. The muscles of the appendicular skeleton are divided into the following groups: Muscles of Scapula Movement; Muscles of Shoulder Movement; Muscles of Elbow Movement; Muscles of the Forearm, Wrist, and Hand; Muscles of the Hip and Knee Movement; and Muscles of Foot Movement.

The muscles of the axial skeleton are broken down into the following groups: Muscles of the Head and Neck, Muscles of the Trunk and Vertebral Column, and Muscles of Respiration.

For each muscle in these groups, the origin of its name is broken down, synonyms are listed, and specific actions, origins, and insertions are detailed.

NOTE: Many of the figures in the charts in this chapter have been modified with permission from Bates A, Hanson N: *Aquatic exercise therapy,* Philadelphia, 1996, WB Saunders.

MATCHING—LESSONS ONE, TWO, AND THREE

Write the letter of the best answer in the space provided. Some may be used more than once.

A. Trapezius
B. Rhomboids major/minor
C. Pectoralis minor
D. Supraspinatus
E. Deltoid

F. Coracobrachialis
G. Brachialis
H. Levator scapulae
I. Serratus anterior
J. Latissimus dorsi

K. Subscapularis
L. Pectoralis major
M. Biceps brachii
N. Triceps brachii

____ 1. Swimmers muscle; action of shoulder extension

____ 2. Corkscrew muscle; flexes the elbow and supinates the forearm

____ 3. Contractions of this muscle may cause angina-like pain

____ 4. Frozen shoulder muscle

____ 5. Neurovascular entrapper

____ 6. Christmas tree muscle; oblique fiber arrangement

____ 7. The two boxer's muscles

____ 8. Muscles that attach to the coracoid process of the scapula and ribs 3 to 5

____ 9. Coat hanger's muscle

____ 10. Most effective arm flexor because of its mechanical advantage

____ 11. Muscle that attaches to the deltoid tuberosity

____ 12. Muscle named for elevating the scapula

____ 13. Musculotendinous cuff muscle that does not actually rotate

____ 14. Musculotendinous cuff muscle that attaches on the lesser tubercle of the humerus

____ 15. Most superficial muscle of the posterior upper back

____ 16. Muscle that attaches to the coracoid process and the humerus.

MATCHING—LESSON FOUR

Write the letter of the best answer in the space provided. Some may be used more than once.

A. Pronator quadratus
B. Flexor carpi ulnaris
C. Extensor digiti minimi

D. Opponens pollicis
E. Flexor digiti minimi brevis
F. Supinator

G. Extensor carpi ulnaris
H. Extensor indicis
I. Flexor carpi radialis

____ 1. Only muscle listed in this group that supinates the forearm

____ 2. Muscle that extends the index finger

_____ 3. Muscles that flex the wrist

_____

_____ 4. Muscle that pronates the hand

_____ 5. Tea drinker's muscle; extends the little finger

_____ 6. Muscle that performs abduction of the wrist

_____ 7. Muscles that moves the thumb into opposition

_____ 8. Muscle that extends the wrist

_____ 9. Muscles that adduct the wrist

_____

_____ 10. Muscle that flexes the little finger

MATCHING—LESSONS FIVE AND SIX

Write the letter of the best answer in the space provided.

A. Iliopsoas
B. Rectus femoris
C. Biceps femoris
D. Tibialis anterior
E. Popliteus

F. Piriformis
G. Sartorius
H. Gracilis
I. Gastrocnemius
J. Peroneus longus

K. Gluteus maximus
L. Semitendinosus
M. Adductor magnus
N. Soleus
O. Plantaris

_____ 1. Tailor's muscle

_____ 2. Hamstring that attaches to the fibular head

_____ 3. Quadriceps femoris muscle that crosses two joints

_____ 4. Muscle that initiates walking

_____ 5. Largest outward rotator of the hip

_____ 6. Strongest extender of the hip

_____ 7. Hamstring that is also part of the pes anserinus

_____ 8. Adductor that forms the letter V with the femoral shaft

_____ 9. Mini-gastrocnemius; missing in about 10% of cadavers

_____ 10. Muscle that dorsiflexes the ankle and inverts the foot

_____ 11. Muscle that plantar flexes the ankle and everts the foot

_____ 12. Muscle called *the key that unlocks the knee*

_____ 13. Muscle of plantar flexion that attaches below the knee joint

_____ 14. Toe dancer's muscle

_____ 15. Adductor muscle that attaches to the linea aspera and the adductor tubercle

MATCHING—LESSON SEVEN

Write the letter of the best answer in the space provided.

A. Frontalis
B. Orbicularis oris
C. Buccinator
D. Temporalis

E. Lateral pterygoid
F. Sternocleidomastoid
G. Orbicularis oculi
H. Zygomaticus major and minor

I. Platysma
J. Masseter
K. Rectus capitis posterior minor
L. Scalenus medius

_____ 1. Muscle for blowing

_____ 2. Winking muscle

_____ 3. Muscle of mastication attaching to the coronoid process of the mandible

_____ 4. Spasms of this muscle are involved in torticollis

_____ 5. Muscle of mastication that attaches to the temporomandibular joint capsule

_____ 6. Muscle that lifts the corners of the mouth into a smile

_____ 7. Muscle of mastication that is the mirror image of the medial pterygoid

_____ 8. Scalene muscle that runs behind the brachial plexus

_____ 9. Muscle that is called the *pouting muscle*

_____ 10. Muscle that lies across the frontal bone and contributes to tension headaches

_____ 11. Muscle that attaches to the dura mater

_____ 12. Kissing muscle

MATCHING—LESSONS EIGHT AND NINE

Write the letter of the best answer in the space provided.

A. Rectus abdominis
B. Rotatores
C. Spinalis
D. Iliocostalis

E. Diaphragm
F. Quadratus lumborum
G. Multifidus

H. Longissimus
I. Internal intercostals
J. External obliques

_____ 1. Hip hiker's muscle; elevates the hip

_____ 2. Deepest transversospinalis muscle

_____ 3. Medial erector spinae muscle

_____ 4. Abdominal muscle with oblique fiber arrangement

_____ 5. Main muscle of respiration

_____ 6. Most lateral erector spinae muscle

_____ 7. Abdominal muscle that attaches to the xiphoid process and the ribs

_____ 8. Part of the transversospinalis named for the muscles many attachments

_____ 9. Muscle that depresses the rib cage during exhalation

_____ 10. Intermediate tract of the erector spinae group that attaches to the occipital bone

Bibliography

Applegate EJ: *The anatomy and physiology learning system,* ed 2, Philadelphia, 2000, WB Saunders.

Biel A: *Trail guide to the body: how to locate muscles, bones, and more,* Boulder, Colo, 1997, Author.

Bowden B, Bowden J: *An illustrated atlas of the skeletal muscles,* Englewood, Colo, 2002, Morton.

Crawley J, Van De Graaff KM: *A photographic atlas for anatomy and physiology,* Englewood, Colo, 2002, Morton.

Grafelman T: *Graf's anatomy and physiology guide for the massage therapist,* Aurora, Colo, 1998, DG Publishing.

Goldberg S: *Clinical anatomy made ridiculously simple,* Miami, 1984, Medmaster.

Guyton A: *Human physiology and mechanisms of disease,* ed 3, Philadelphia, 1982, WB Saunders.

Haubrich WS: *Medical meanings: a glossary of word origins,* New York, 1984, Harcourt Brace Jovanovich.

Hoppenfeld S: *Physical examination of the spine and extremities,* Norwalk, Conn, 1976, Appleton-Century-Crofts.

Jacob S, Francone C: *Elements anatomy and physiology,* Philadelphia, 1989, WB Saunders.

Juhan D: *Job's body: a handbook for bodyworkers,* Barrington, NY, 1987, Station Hill Press.

Kapit W, Elson LM: *The anatomy coloring book,* ed 3, New York, 2002, Benjamin Cummings. Kapit W, Macey R, Meisami E: *The physiology coloring book* New York, 1987, HarperCollins.

Kendall FP, McCreary EK: *Muscles: testing and function,* ed 3, Baltimore, 1983, Williams and Wilkins.

Kordish M, Dickson S: *Introduction to basic human anatomy,* Lake Charles, La, 1985, McNeese State University.

Lauderstein D: *Putting the soul back in the body: a manual of imaginative anatomy for massage therapists,* Chicago, 1985, the Author.

Lowe WW: *Functional assessment in massage therapy,* Corvallis, Ore, 1995, Pacific Orthopedic Massage.

Marieb EN: *Essentials of human anatomy and physiology,* ed 4, New York, 1994, Benjamin Cummings.

Mattes A: *Active isolated stretching,* Sarasota, Fla, 1995, Author.

McAleer N: *The body almanac,* Garden City, NY, 1985, Doubleday.

McLaughlin C: *The bodyworker's muscle reference guide,* Bellevue, Colo, 1996, Bodyguide.

Moore KL: *Clinically oriented anatomy,* ed 2, Baltimore, 1985, Williams and Wilkins.

Mosby's medical, nursing, and allied health dictionary, ed 4, St Louis, 1994, Mosby.

Myers TW: *Anatomy trains: myofascial meridians for manual and movement therapists,* New York, 2001, Churchill Livingstone.

Olsen A, McHose C: *Bodystories: a guide to experiential anatomy,* Barrytown, NY, 1991, Station Hill Press.

Platzer W: *Color atlas and textbook of human anatomy: locomotor system,* vol 1, ed 3, New York, 1984, Thieme.

Rolf IP: *Rolfing: the integration of human structures,* New York, 1977, Harper and Row.

Sieg K, Adams S: *Illustrated essentials of musculoskeletal anatomy,* ed 3, Gainesville, Fla, 1996, Megabooks.

Solomon EP, Phillips GA: *Understanding human anatomy and physiology,* Philadelphia, 1987, WB Saunders.

St. John P: *St. John neuromuscular therapy seminars: manual I,* Largo, Fla, 1995, Author.

Taber's cyclopedic medical dictionary, ed 13, Philadelphia, 1977, FA Davis.

Thibodeau G, Patton K: *Structure and function of the body,* ed 11, St Louis, 2000, Mosby.

Tortora GJ: *Introduction to the human body: the essentials of anatomy and physiology,* ed 3, New York, 1994, HarperCollins.

Travell J, Simons D: *Myofascial pain and dysfunction: the trigger point manual,* vol I, Baltimore, 1983, Williams and Wilkins.

Travell J, Simons D: *Myofascial pain and dysfunction: the trigger point manual,* vol II, Baltimore, 1992, Williams and Wilkins.

Warfel JH: *The extremities: muscles and motor points,* ed 5, Philadelphia, 1985, Lea and Febiger.

Warfel JH: *The head, neck, and trunk,* ed 5, Philadelphia, 1985, Lea and Febiger.

Nervous System

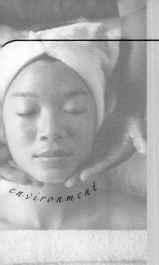

environment

17

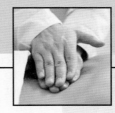

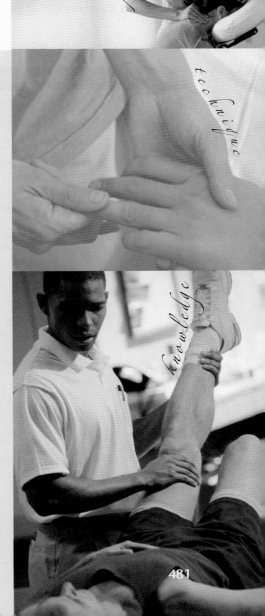

pressure

technique

knowledge

"The greatest undeveloped territory in the world lies under your hat."

—Anonymous

STUDENT OBJECTIVES

After completing this chapter, the student should be able to:

- List functions of the nervous system
- Discuss basic organization of the nervous system
- Identify types of nerve tissue
- Label parts of a neuron
- Classify neurons according to their function
- Describe how nerves initiate, receive, and transmit impulses
- Name important neurotransmitters of the nervous system
- List structures of the central nervous system, identifying regions of the brain and spinal cord
- List structures of the peripheral nervous system
- Explain the mechanisms involved in a reflex arc
- Name the cranial nerves
- Name the cranial and spinal nerves that are relevant for massage therapists
- Name and discuss sensory receptors
- List physiological effects of the sympathetic and parasympathetic nervous systems
- Briefly discuss the special senses (taste, smell, hearing, and vision)
- Name types of nervous pathologies, giving characteristics and massage considerations of each

INTRODUCTION

The human body has two specialized centers of control that make important adjustments to maintain homeostasis. The endocrine system, which is discussed later, is the slower of these two centers. The faster control system is the nervous system, a complex and fascinating system of the body. It is the body's master controlling and communicating system; it even monitors and regulates aspects of the endocrine system. Every thought, action, and sensation reflect its activity. We are what our brain has experienced. If all past sensory input could be completely erased, we would be unable to walk, talk, or communicate; we would remember no pain or pleasure.

The study of the functions and disorders of the nervous system is referred to as **neurology**. This chapter explores neurology, examining the structural and functional classifications of the nervous tissue. It begins with an overview of nerves and the chemistry behind nerve impulses and synaptic transmissions and then examines the two divisions of the nervous system itself—the central and peripheral nervous systems. Nerves may also be areas to avoid in massage therapy (endangerment sites) and are also discussed here. Finally, the chapter reviews specialized nerve receptors that provide the five senses and nervous system pathologies, some of which may affect the application of massage.

FUNCTIONS

Sensory input. The sensory receptors of the body detect **stimuli** (any change in the internal or external environment) such as pressure, temperature, and motion, both inside and outside the body.

Interpretive and integrative functions. After registering these changes, the nervous system interprets the perceived information to provide a response. Integration occurs between the sensory input of information and the motor output.

Terms and Their Meanings Related to the Nervous System

Term	Meaning	Term	Meaning
arachnoid	spider; shaped	neurotransmitters	nerve; a sending across
autonomic	self; law	nociceptor	hurt; to receive
axon	axis	nodes of Ranvier	French pathologist (1835-1922)
baroreceptor	weight; to receive	oligodendrocytes	little; tree; cell
Broca's area	French surgeon (1824-1880)	otolith	ear; stone
cauda equina	tail-like; horse	palsy	paralysis
cerebellum	little brain	papilla	nipple
cerebrum	brain	parasympathetic	by the side of, sympathetic
chemoreceptors	chemical; to receive	photoreceptors	light; to receive
cochlea	land snail	pia mater	tender, soft; mother
corpus callosum	body; hard or callused	plexus	braid
cortex	bark or rind	proprioceptor	one's own; a receiver
cyton	cell	pons	bridge
dendrites	treelike	reciprocal inhibition	alternate; to restrain
Diencephalon	two or second; brain	reflex	bent back
dura mater	hard or tough; mother	retina	a net
encephal	brain	Schwann cell	German anatomist (1810-1882)
filum terminale	threadlike; at the end	soma	body
ganglion	knot	stapes	stirrup
gyri	circle	stimuli	a goad (a pointed rod or spear); to urge on
incus	anvil		
internuncial	between; together, midst; messenger	sulci	groove
		summation	adding
macula	spot	sympathetic	sympathy
mechanoreceptors	machine; to receive	synapse	point of contact
medulla oblongata	marrow or middle; long	thalamus	chamber
meninges	membrane	thermoreceptors	heat; to receive
myelin	marrow	tympanic	drum
neurilemma	nerve; husk	vagus	wandering
neuro	sinew; nerve	vermis	wormlike
neuroglia	nerve; glue	Wernicke's area	German neurologist (1848-1905)

Motor output. Once the nervous system has received and interpreted the stimuli, a motor response may be activated in the form of muscular contractions or glandular secretions.

Higher mental functioning and emotional responsiveness. The nervous system is also responsible for mental processes (cognition and memory) and emotional responses (joy, excitement, anger, anxiety, and so on).

BASIC ORGANIZATION OF THE NERVOUS SYSTEM

The nervous system is complex. Divisions exist that possess unique structural and functional characteristics (Figure 17-1).

The **central nervous system** (CNS) occupies a central or medial position in the body. It is primarily concerned with interpreting incoming sensory information and issuing instructions in the form of motor responses. It is also the major control center for thoughts and emotional experiences. The major components of the CNS include the brain (cerebrum, cerebellum, diencephalon, and brain stem), meninges, cerebrospinal fluid, and spinal cord. These structures are surrounded by the bones of the skull or spinal column.

The **peripheral nervous system** (PNS) is composed of the cranial and spinal nerves emerging from the CNS. **Cranial nerves** originate from the brain, and **spinal nerves** exit the spinal cord at the intervertebral foramen of the spinal column. These are openings at the pedicles for spinal roots to pass. The PNS has 43 pairs of nerves: 12 pairs of cranial nerves and 31 pairs of spinal nerves.

Within the PNS are special divisions, the somatic and the autonomic nervous systems. The **somatic nervous system** is a voluntary system governing impulses from the CNS to the skeletal muscles. The **autonomic nervous system** is an involuntary system, supplying impulses to smooth muscle, cardiac (heart) muscle, and glands. The autonomic nervous system consists of a sympathetic and parasympathetic division, each of which possesses complementary responses. For example, if the sympathetic nervous system speeds up heart rate, the parasympathetic nervous system slows it down to a normal heart rate.

NERVE TISSUE

The two types of nerve tissue are neuroglia and neurons. **Neuroglia**, or glial cells, are connective tissue that supports, nourishes, protects, insulates, and organizes the neurons. Neuroglia are smaller and more numerous than neurons. More than 50% of the CNS is made up of these cells. Neuroglia are unable to transmit impulses and never lose their ability to divide. For this reason, most brain tumors are made up of glial cells. The six types of neuroglia are as follows (four are located in the CNS [astrocytes, ependymocytes, microglia, oligodendrocytes], and two are located in the PNS [satellite cells and Schwann cells]):

1. **Astrocytes** are located between the neurons in CNS for structural support of delicate neurons; part of the blood-brain barrier.
2. **Ependymocytes** line the cranial ventricles and central canal of the spinal cord and assist in the circulation of cerebrospinal fluid.
3. **Microglia** protect CNS by destroying pathogens.
4. **Oligodendrocytes** produce the myelin around axons in CNS.
5. **Satellite cells** are located between the neurons in PNS for structural support of delicate neurons.
6. **Schwann cells** produce the myelin around axons in PNS. Neurilemma (sheath of Schwann) is a layer of Schwann cells enclosing the myelin

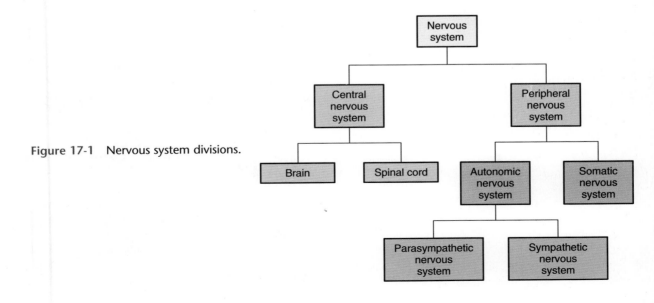

Figure 17-1   Nervous system divisions.

sheath. This sheath plays an important role in the regeneration of PNS nerve fibers.

Neurons (Figure 17-2) are nerve cells. They are the basic impulse-conducting cells and have the following two major properties:

1. **Excitability** is the ability to respond to a stimulus and convert it to a nerve impulse.
2. **Conductibility** is the ability to transmit the impulses to other neurons, muscle, and glands.

Neurons act like tiny sense organs. Many of these neurons organize themselves into bundles of tissue called *nerve fascicles*. A collection of these impulse-carrying fascicles, or nerve fibers, is called a **nerve**. Let's review:

Neuron (nerve cell) → Nerve fascicles → Nerve

CONNECTIVE TISSUE COMPONENTS OF NERVES

Each nerve has a series of connective tissue wrappings as muscles do. **Endoneurium** surrounds each nerve fiber. Groups of nerve fibers are bound together by

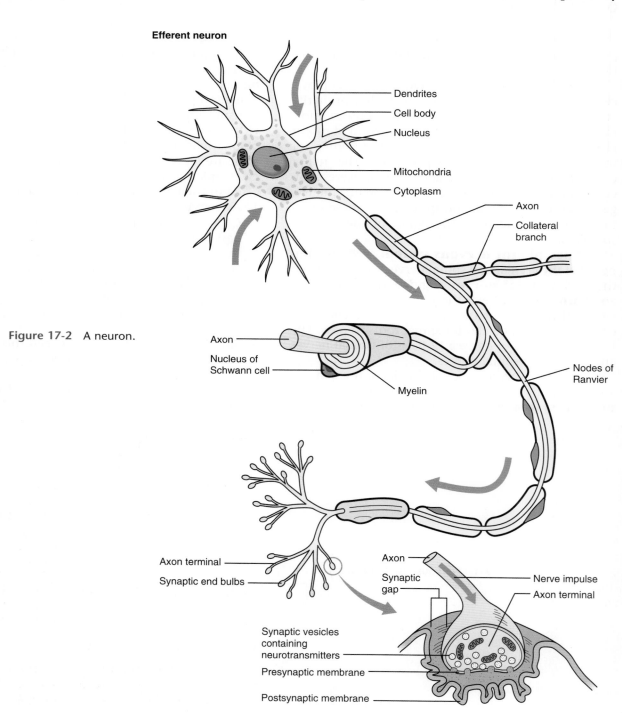

Efferent neuron

Dendrites
Cell body
Nucleus
Mitochondria
Cytoplasm
Axon
Collateral branch
Axon
Nucleus of Schwann cell
Myelin
Nodes of Ranvier
Axon terminal
Synaptic end bulbs
Axon
Synaptic gap
Nerve impulse
Axon terminal
Synaptic vesicles containing neurotransmitters
Presynaptic membrane
Postsynaptic membrane

Figure 17-2 A neuron.

perineurium, forming nerve fascicles (Figure 17-3). The perineurium binds the fasciculi together, but it also acts to separate one compartment from another. Nerves are bound together by another connective tissue layer known as the **epineurium**. Let's review:

Endoneurium (wraps nerve fiber) → Perineurium (wraps nerve fascicle) → Epineurium (wraps entire nerve)

Parts of a Neuron

Even though neurons vary widely in shape and size to accommodate a number of neural connections, they all have three basic parts: a cell body and two or more cytoplasmic extensions (dendrite and axon). These extensions are often referred to as the *nerve fibers.*

Cell body (cyton). The cyton contains the nucleus and other standard equipment (organelles) of the cell. In addition to the usual organelles, neurons posses a unique organelle called *Nissl bodies,* which make protein for the cell. Neural cell bodies are also the gray matter of the nervous system. In the brain, gray matter is found on the outer layer (cortex) and in the very deep part of the brain; in the spinal cord, it is centrally located and forms regions called *horns.*

Dendrites. Dendrites are typically short, narrow, and highly branched extensions of the nerve cell. These neural extensions receive and transmit stimuli toward the cell body.

Axons. Axons are typically single cylindrical extensions of the cell. Their job is to transmit impulses away from the cell body. Axons can possess collateral extensions. As axons terminate, they branch into many fine filaments called **axon terminals**. The ends of axon terminals have **synaptic end bulbs**; these bulblike structures contain sacs called **synaptic vesicles**. These vesicles store neurotransmitters, chemicals that facilitate, arouse, or inhibit the transmission of nerve impulses between neurons and across synapses (junction between two

neurons). Most axons are wrapped by a fatty insulating sheath called a **myelin sheath**. The myelinated axons are known as white matter. Myelin not only electrically insulates the neuron (preventing signal leakage to adjacent neurons) but also increases the speed of nerve impulse conduction. At certain intervals along an axon, the myelin sheath has gaps called **nodes of Ranvier**. During neural activity, impulses jump from one node to another, resulting in an increased rate of conduction.

For Your Information

A mnemonic device for remembering that axons carry neural impulses away from the cell body is that both *a*xon and *a*way begin with the letter *A.*

CLASSIFICATION OF NEURONS AND GROUPINGS OF NERVE TISSUE

Classification of Neurons

Neurons can be classified functionally (based on the direction that the impulse is traveling in relation to the CNS) as either sensory, association, or motor.

Sensory (afferent) neurons. Sensory nerves are said to be afferent—that is, they carry impulses from nerve receptors to the brain or spinal cord. Some receptors are close to the surface of the skin, such as Meissner corpuscles. Some sensory receptors lie deep within the body, such as proprioceptors. A map of the distribution of these nerves is called a *dermatome map.* A **dermatome** is an area of skin that a specific sensory nerve root serves (C2-S5) or one of three branches of the fifth cranial (trigeminal) nerve. Dermatomes (Figure 17-4) are roughly the same from person to person, although sometimes a significant overlap in innervation is found between adjacent dermatomes.

Interneurons (association) neurons. Interneurons nerves connect sensory to motor neurons and vice versa. They integrate (process) sensory information, analyze and store some of it, and then make decisions about appropriate responses. Interneurons make up most of the neurons in the body and are found in both the brain and spinal cord.

Motor (efferent) neurons. Motor nerves are classified as efferent, which means that they carry messages from the brain or spinal cord. These neurons transmit impulses that activate (or inhibit) a muscle or gland.

Grouping of Nerve Tissue

A group of neurons is called a *nerve.* These fibers connect the brain and spinal cord with other parts of the body. A collection of nerves running up and down

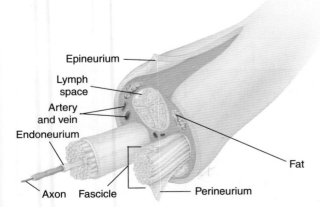

Epineurium
Lymph space
Artery and vein
Endoneurium
Axon   Fascicle   Perineurium
Fat

Figure 17-3   Structure of a nerve with connective tissue coverings.

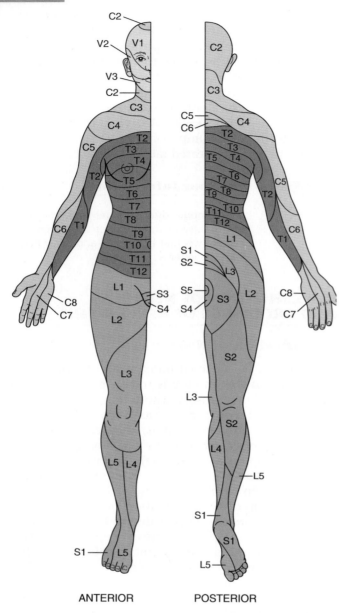

Figure 17-4 Dermatome map.

the spinal column in the CNS is called a **tract**. Afferent signals travel up the cord in ascending tracts, and efferent signals travel down the cord in descending tracts.

A cluster of nerve cell bodies located in the PNS is called a **ganglion**. Most ganglia are located next to the spinal cord. A network of intersecting nerves in the PNS is called a **plexus**. The body contains many plexuses; the four most important ones are as follows:

- **Cervical plexus** (C1-C5) supplies the head and neck
- **Brachial plexus** (C5-T1) supplies the arm and hand
- **Lumbar plexus** (L1-L4) supplies the abdomen, low back, and genitalia

- **Sacral plexus** (L4-S4) supplies the posterior hip, legs, and feet

NERVE IMPULSES

Nerve impulses are the messages or signals of the nervous system that travel along the neuron(s) from dendrite to axon, and these impulses are electrochemical in nature. The nerve impulse is the body's quickest way of controlling and maintaining homeostasis. Ions are electrically charged particles that pass through the ion channels of the neural cell membrane during a nerve impulse.

Nerves may become excitable because of a stimulus (Figure 17-5). Any alteration in the environment (e.g., pain, pressure, movement, heat, light, aroma of foods, release of hormones) can initiate a nerve impulse. The strength and frequency of stimuli determine whether a nerve impulse is generated. When the stimulus is of sufficient intensity to generate a nerve impulse, threshold stimulus is the result. Any single stimulus below the threshold level does not result in the creation of a nerve impulse. However, if a subthreshold stimulus (one lower than the threshold) should be repeated in succession, the summation of these small stimuli may act cumulatively to create a nerve impulse. **Summation** is the amount of stimuli needed (both in frequency and number of fibers stimulated) to reach threshold stimulus and create a nerve impulse.

When a stimulus generates a nerve impulse, the impulse is conducted along the entire neuron at maximum capacity. This principle is referred to as

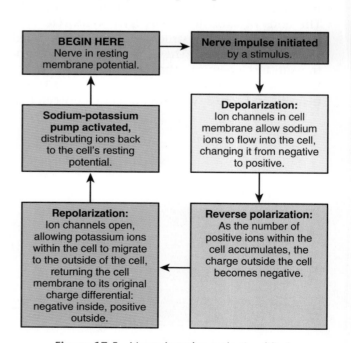

Figure 17-5 Nerve impulse cycle simplified.

the **all-or-none response**. For example, a fire-cracker with an 8-foot fuse can be lit by a match or torch. These are two vastly different stimuli in intensity, yet both methods result in the same rate of fuse burning (impulse) and in the same result or response—explosion of the firecracker.

When such a stimulus is constant, over time, **adaptation**, a decrease in sensitivity to a prolonged stimulus, may occur. Adaptation tends to be rapid regarding pressure, touch, and smell. We become accustomed to the weight of our clothes during the day, and an odor that offended us when we first entered the room is no longer detected at the end of the day.

Adaptation occurs more slowly with pain and body position. This is a protective mechanism that prevents us from "becoming used to severe pain," or from keeping our bodies in awkward, potentially harmful, body positions.

Now that the relationship between stimulus and impulse is understood, it is time to examine the dynamics of the nerve impulse itself. **Action potential** is a measurement of electrical difference between the charge inside the cell (negatively charged) and the charge outside the neural cell membrane (positively charged). The difference in voltage is created by the presence of ions. The resting neuron is one that is not conducting a nerve impulse at a given time; this state is referred to as a *resting membrane potential*. This potential means that the neuron is cocked, ready to fire.

As mentioned earlier, a system of gateways controls the flow of ions both into and out of the neuron through the cellular membrane. When a stimulus is applied, the cell responds by changing the membrane's level of ion permeability. The main ions related to nerve cells are sodium and potassium ions, which are both positively charged and existing inside and outside the membrane. The concentration of sodium ions is greater outside the membrane, and the concentration of potassium ions is greater inside the resting cellular membrane. The membrane is *polarized* when the inside of the membrane bears a negative charge and the outside of the membrane bears a positive charge (an action potential).

When a threshold stimulus is added to a neuron, the sodium ion channels open, permitting sodium ions to flow into the cell. This reduces the polarization of the cell membrane, changing it from negative to positive, in a process known as *depolarization*. This occurs in segments along the axon (Figure 17-6). This flow of ions is the electricity of a nerve impulse.

As the large migration of sodium ions across the neural membrane continues, the polarity of the cell membrane reverses as a result of the increased presence of positive ions inside the cell. This is referred to as *reverse polarization*. The cell's interior is now positive from the higher concentration of positive ions. This creates a differential in charge, which translates to a negative charge on the outside of the membrane, causing the sodium ion channels to close.

Once this change has occurred, the cellular membrane once again becomes impermeable to sodium ions. The potassium ion channels open and allow potassium to leave the cell. As the positive potassium ions leave the cell, the outside once again becomes positively charged, and the inside of the membrane resumes its negative charge. This is known as *repolarization*.

It is the reverse polarization in the initial section of the cell membrane that acts as the stimulus for the adjacent sections of the neuron. The initial stimulus has created a ripple or wave effect that travels down the cell as the depolarization–reverse polarization–repolarization process is repeated. Much like a line of dominoes, the ripple of current travels the length of the neuron until it reaches its destination. This is true for sensory neurons that may be bringing temperature information to the brain, for motor neurons that may be sending a message to the eyelids to blink, and for chains of neurons that stimulate adjacent neurons. Therefore the nerve impulse is simply a matter of ions changing places, creating different electrical charges along the cell membrane.

After the cell has returned to its normal polarized state during the repolarization process, the resting membrane potential is reinstated, but the distribution of sodium and potassium ions is reversed. This distribution is set back to normal by means of the sodium-potassium pump.

The Sodium-Potassium Pump

The **sodium-potassium pump** redistributes the sodium-potassium ions to their original positions. The pump actively transports sodium and potassium, maintaining cell membrane polarity. The sodium-potassium pump is easier to understand if it is pictured as a sprocket. The sodium and potassium ions attach between the spokes or teeth of the sprocket that will move them from one side of the cell membrane to the other, just as a revolving door moves people between the inside and outside of a building.

The sodium ions inside the cell membrane attach themselves to the spaces between the "teeth" of the pump, triggering the breakdown of adenosine triphosphate into adenosine diphosphate and a free phosphate. The free phosphate attaches itself to the pump, and this action changes the shape of the pump in a way that moves the sodium ions to the outside of the cellular membrane. At this point, the potassium ions outside the cellular membrane attach to the pump, releasing the phosphate. The pump reverts to its original shape, drawing the potassium ions into the cell where they are released, and the cycle perpetuates itself.

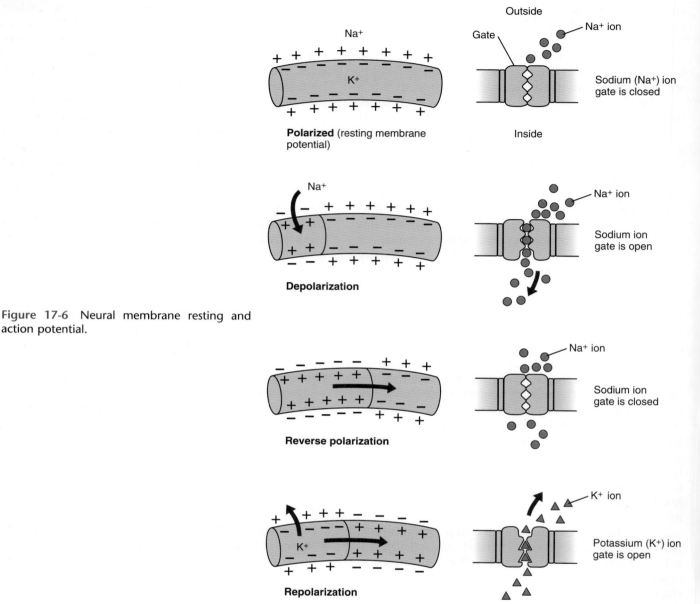

Figure 17-6 Neural membrane resting and action potential.

Nerve Impulse Conduction

Nerve fibers with larger diameters conduct impulses faster than those with smaller diameters. However, if the axons were all large, they would be cumbersome and create a packaging problem. The problem is solved by keeping axon diameters small and by using another means, myelin sheaths, to achieve rapid conduction velocities. A myelin sheath is a fat and protein insulator surrounding sections of the axon. The myelin aids in conduction and insulation and prevents the leaking of microcurrent from one neuron to influence another. Signals conducted down unmyelinated axons are slower; this is called *continuous conduction*. Signals conducted down myelinated axons are faster; this is called *saltatory conduction*.

Located along the axon are unmyelinated gaps called nodes of Ranvier. Because the myelinated segments of the axon are insulated, the action potential or depolarization process occurs only where myelin is absent (at the nodes of Ranvier). The impulse then jumps across the myelinated section of the axon to the next node and so on. This is further enhanced by the presence of an increased number of ion channels. This jumping effect enables the impulse to traverse a much longer distance in a much shorter time. In a game of checkers, you can move your checker across the board one square at a time, or you can jump the opposing pieces and make it across the board much quicker. In this way, myelinated fibers conduct impulses faster than unmyelinated.

SYNAPSE AND SYNAPTIC TRANSMISSION

The **synapse** is the junction between two neurons or between a neuron and a muscle or gland, where they connect to transmit information. This junction is actually more of a fluid-filled space than an actual connection. **Synaptic transmission** is the electrochemical method by which the nerve impulse from one neuron bridges the synaptic cleft to convey the nerve impulse to the next neuron (Figure 17-7). This is a one-way nerve impulse conduction from the axon of one cell to the dendrite of another. Another term for synapse, **synaptic cleft**, is the gap between neurons.

The axon carries the nerve impulse away from the nerve cell body. At the distal end of each axon are clusters of short branches called *axon terminals*. Each axon terminal ends with a small bud known as a *synaptic end bulb,* which contains synaptic vesicles that produce and store neurotransmitters. These neurotransmitters are released into the synapse and bond with postsynaptic receptor sites on the adjacent dendrite.

Neurotransmitters

Neurotransmitters is a collective term for a vast range of chemicals that facilitate, arouse, or inhibit the transmission of nerve impulses across synapses. These chemical messengers are stored in vesicles at the synaptic end bulbs, and each vesicle may store as many as 10,000 different molecules. Neurotransmitters depart the synaptic end bulbs and cross the synaptic cleft, thereby bridging the space between the neurons. The neurotransmitter then attaches itself to a receptor site on the postsynaptic neuron. The receptor sites are located adjacent to the ion channels. The action of chemical bonding at the receptor site acts as a stimulus on the adjacent neuron by affecting sodium and potassium movement across the neural membrane.

Neurotransmitters can be either excitatory or inhibitory. Excitatory neurotransmitters decrease the negativity of postsynaptic membrane potentials, thereby increasing the impulse rate. Inhibitory neurotransmitters increase membrane potentials, which increases the threshold needed to create the nerve impulse.

The action of the neurotransmitter does not persist for a long time because it is continuously removed from the synaptic cleft by either enzymes or reuptake (the drawing up of a substance) into axon terminals.

Types of Neurotransmitters

About 30 known neurotransmitters are in the body. The following is a list of some of the more important ones:

Acetylcholine, which is vital for stimulating muscle contraction. This neurotransmitter stimulates vagus nerve and parasympathetic nervous system activity and is rapidly destroyed by the enzyme acetylcholinesterase.

Catecholamines are a chemical family containing norepinephrine, epinephrine, and dopamine. The major functions of catecholamines include the excitation and inhibition of certain muscles, cardiac excitation, metabolic action, and endocrine action. Catecholamines act directly on sympathetic cells to cause the desired action.

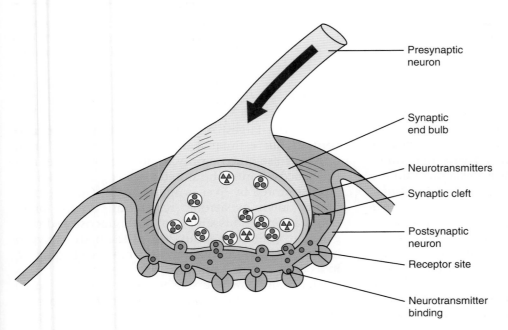

Presynaptic neuron

Synaptic end bulb

Neurotransmitters

Synaptic cleft

Postsynaptic neuron

Receptor site

Neurotransmitter binding

Figure 17-7 Synaptic cleft and neurotransmitter action.

- **Epinephrine** is a hormone and a neurotransmitter secreted by the adrenal medulla, and this chemical simulates the functions of the sympathetic nervous system.
- **Norepinephrine**, like epinephrine, is both a hormone and a neurotransmitter secreted by the adrenal medulla; this chemical mediates several physiologic and metabolic responses that follow the stimulation of the sympathetic nerves. For example, norepinephrine acts to increase blood pressure by vasoconstriction but does not affect cardiac output. This neurotransmitter may be related to arousal, dreaming, and mood regulation.
- **Dopamine** is a neurotransmitter that is the precursor of norepinephrine and may have an inhibitory effect on movement. Dopamine is also implicated in attention and learning. A depletion of dopamine produces the symptoms of rigidity, tremors, and uncoordinated and slower than normal movement.

Serotonin, a naturally occurring derivative of tryptophan (an amino acid), acts as a potent vasoconstrictor. It is theorized to be important for sensory perception, mood regulation, and normal sleep.

Gamma-aminobutyric acid (GABA) is an amino acid with neurotransmitter activity; found in the brain, it has an inhibitory effect of nerve transmission.

Histamine, a compound found in all cells, causes dilation of capillaries, decreased blood pressure, and constriction of smooth muscles of the bronchi. The release of histamine is stimulated by allergic, inflammatory reactions.

CENTRAL NERVOUS SYSTEM

The CNS, surrounded and protected by the cranium and vertebral column, is located in the dorsal cavity. The CNS is further protected by a liquid called *cerebrospinal fluid* and a connective tissue membranous covering called the *meninges*.

Cerebrospinal Fluid

Circulating around the brain and spinal cord is a clear fluid called **cerebrospinal fluid** that functions as a shock absorber and provides a medium for nutrient exchange and waste removal. Cerebrospinal fluid is produced in chambers called the *choroid plexus* within the ventricles of the brain and is similar in composition to blood, minus the blood cells. Cerebrospinal fluid is sensitive to glucose and electrolyte balance and to changes in the carbon dioxide content.

Massage therapists can enhance the flow of cerebrospinal fluid and reduce fascial restrictions with craniosacral therapy (CST). This is achieved by applying light

pressure along with specific directions on the cranial bones. CST has been effective in treating a variety of conditions, from chronic headaches, and earaches, to lower back pain. For more information, see the biography in this chapter on John Upledger.

Meninges

The entire CNS (brain and spinal cord) is enveloped by special connective tissue membranes: the **meninges**. The innermost layer is called the **pia mater**, which is thin and vascular and hugs the CNS; this covering is so tight that it is difficult to remove the pia mater without damaging the CNS's surface (Figure 17-8).

The middle layer is called the **arachnoid**, which possesses many threadlike strands, giving it a webbed appearance. The outermost layer, the thick and tough **dura mater**, lies against the bone and contains a double layer of connective tissue with the outer layer resembling periosteum. Within the two layers are thick venous channels called *sinuses*. The dura mater dips down between the cerebral hemispheres (falx cerebri), separates the cerebrum and cerebellum (tentorium cerebelli) and divides the paired cerebellar hemispheres (falx cerebelli).

The subdural space, filled with circulating serous fluid, lies between the dura mater and the arachnoid. Between the pia mater and the arachnoid is the subarachnoid space, filled with cerebrospinal fluid. The epidural space lies between the dura and the vertebral canal; this space, which is the safest place for injections such as saddle blocks, contains adipose tissue, connective tissue, and blood vessels.

For Your Information

A mnemonic device to recall the three layers of the meninges, from deep to superficial is *PAD: p*ia mater, *a*rachnoid, and *d*ura mater.

BRAIN

One of the largest organs in the body, the **brain** contains an estimated 100 billion neurons. Brain cells can use glucose only as an energy source, and this glucose cannot be stored as glycogen, unlike the glucose stored by liver or muscle cells. Glucose only breaks down by aerobic respiration, so the brain needs a continuous supply of both glucose and oxygen. The brain uses about 20% of the body's oxygen intake. Oxygen deprivation kills brain cells quickly, in as little as 1 to 2 minutes.

The brain is where sensory information is fused into character and behavior. The brain's unimpressive appearance gives no hints of its remarkable abilities. In the embryo, the skull forms before the brain

JOHN UPLEDGER, DO, OMM

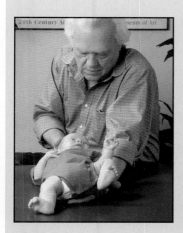

Born: February 10, 1932.

"Trust the universe . . . accept its messages . . . and keep your motives clean. The client's body will tell you which way to go."

From what might be called humble beginnings, John Upledger burst forth unto the world like a firecracker wanting to touch everything, a task on which he fared well. Aside from being an accomplished osteopathic physician, surgeon, and researcher, he was a musician, soldier, and scholar, primarily known for observing a whole new physiological system and developing the form of massage called *craniosacral therapy.* Growing up poor in an Italian neighborhood in Detroit, Upledger endured threats on his life from the junior Mafia, hanging out with gangs, and playing the piano in bars.

He once dreamed of becoming a criminal lawyer, but he graduated with a psychology degree instead and joined the U.S. Coast Guard. Rowing a boat in the dead of winter off the coast of Long Island, N.Y., was less than rewarding. As the only enlisted man with a college education, he took a lot of ribbing. Unsatisfied with the rigorous lifestyle of a soldier, he enrolled in the Hospital Corpsman School. While assisting a neurosurgeon during a very risky neurological membrane operation, Upledger's job was to hold the dura mater membrane perfectly still so that the surgeon could remove a spot of calcium plaque from its surface. A slip of the knife might injure the dura and open an avenue for infection. Here, Upledger details the experience:

It wouldn't hold still no matter what I did. It kept moving toward and away from us rather slowly but rhythmically and irresistibly. My pride was hurt. I was embarrassed at my own ineptitude. But I also became very curious. Wonder of wonders, I was experiencing the privilege of seeing firsthand the physiological performance of an as-yet-undiscovered bodily system. It would turn out to be another system just like the cardiovascular system, the digestive system, and the like.

—From *Your inner physician and you* by John Upledger, 1991.

As early as the 1900s, Dr. William Sutherland had been studying the possibility of skull bone movement and developed cranial osteopathy. Using his experience in the operating room and Sutherland's work as a beginning point, Upledger forged on to document support of this physiological phenomenon. At Michigan State University he supervised a team of anatomists, physiologists, biophysicists, and bioengineers in the study of the craniosacral system for almost a decade.

The result of these endeavors is craniosacral therapy. The craniosacral system consists of the membranes and cerebrospinal fluid that surround and protect the brain and spinal cord. It extends from the bones of the skull, face, and mouth, which make up the cranium, down to the sacrum.

Upledger, who sounds more like a metaphysic guru than a scientist, has spent much of his life trying to demystify what happens during a craniosacral therapy session. However, he abhors the term *healer,* preferring to say that we are all facilitators of our own healing. "Everyone is born with healing abilities," says Upledger. "It's trained out of us by society as we grow to rely on external health care methods." It is actually much more complex than this, but in Upledger's book, *Craniosacral Therapy,* co-written with Jon D. Vredevoogd, the craniosacral system is described as a *semi-closed hydraulic system.* It is the therapist's job to "feel" for restrictions in the motion of this system and facilitate their release. Craniosacral therapy practitioners assess the entire body to discover restrictions that may be caused by inflammation, adhesion, somatic dysfunction, and neuroreflexes. These restrictions keep the body from obtaining complete homeostasis or optimal health. The touch is extremely light, and the pressure applied usually no heavier than the weight of a nickel.

Continued

JOHN UPLEDGER, DO, OMM—cont'd

Results have been phenomenal at times. Mentally retarded children have been mainstreamed. One child, spastic and paralyzed, walked into his fourth session. Craniosacral therapy has helped women through difficult labor, eased chronic pain, and helped an Olympic athlete recover from vertigo.

If, as a massage therapist, you feel as though your own results have been less than miraculous, Upledger urges you to remember simple things, like how massage stimulates serotonin, the body's own tranquilizer. Asked how he likes to feel after a Swedish massage, Upledger replied, "Good . . . tingly . . . vibrant . . . mobile . . . warm . . . energized . . . as though everything is circulating."

Upledger's techniques have be used in a wide variety of occupations, including osteopaths, medical doctors, psychiatrists, psychologists, dentists, physical therapists, and occupational therapists. Additionally, the Upledger Institute, Inc., in Palm Beach Gardens, Fla., promises that craniosacral study will continue to expand its reach because the possibilities of this therapy seem limitless.

is finished; this results in the forebrain turning in on itself and mushrooming. **Sulci** are grooves in the outer layer of the brain (cortex), and **gyri** are elevated ridges of tissue. Fissures are specialized deep sulci that divide the brain into hemispheres and lobes. Twelve pairs of cranial nerves originate in the brain and travel to the periphery.

The brain is divided into four major areas: cerebrum, diencephalon, cerebellum, and brain stem (stalk) (Figure 17-9).

Cerebrum

Shaped like a boxing glove, the **cerebrum** is divided by the longitudinal fissure into two large (right and left) cerebral hemispheres. The cerebrum governs all higher functions (i.e., language, memory, reasoning, and some aspects of personality) and is the largest region of the brain. Connecting the two cerebral hemispheres are large fibrous bundles of transverse fibers, the **corpus callosum**, which provides a

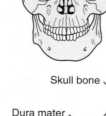

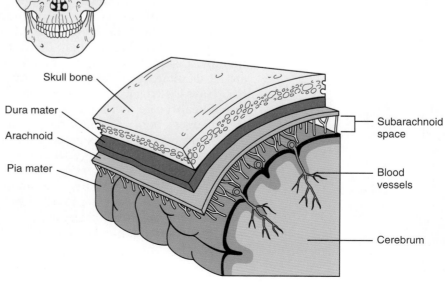

Figure 17-8 The meninges around the brain.

Skull bone

Dura mater

Arachnoid

Pia mater

Subarachnoid space

Blood vessels

Cerebrum

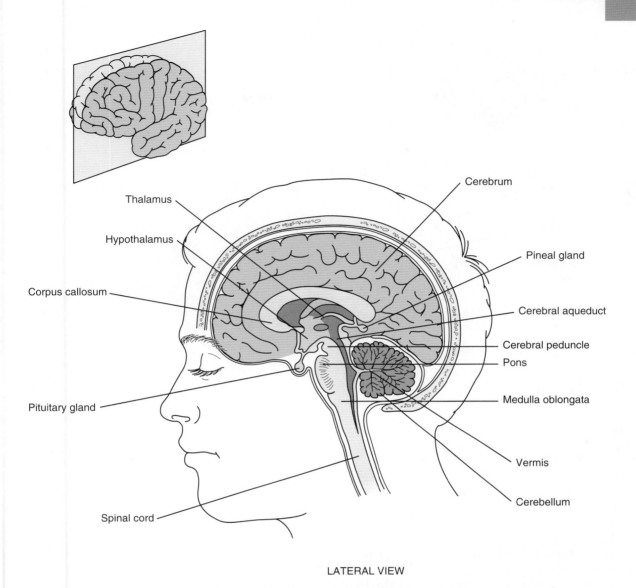

Thalamus

Hypothalamus

Corpus callosum

Pituitary gland

Spinal cord

Cerebrum

Pineal gland

Cerebral aqueduct

Cerebral peduncle

Pons

Medulla oblongata

Vermis

Cerebellum

LATERAL VIEW

Figure 17-9   Sagittal slice of the brain.

communicative pathway for impulses to move from one hemisphere to another.

The **cerebral cortex** is a thin gray layer covering the outer portion of the cerebrum. White matter, which constitutes most of the cerebrum, lies beneath the cerebral cortex.

Within each hemisphere of the cerebrum are **lobes**, which are named for the bone each hemisphere lies beneath (Figure 17-10). The *frontal lobe* regulates motor output, cognition, and speech production (Broca's area; typically the left hemisphere only). The *parietal lobes* govern somatosensory input (namely the skin and muscles). The *temporal lobes* house an auditory and an olfactory area and Wernicke's area (an area critical to language comprehension that is typically the left hemisphere only), and the *occipital lobe* contains a center for visual input.

Hidden by parts of the frontal, parietal, and temporal lobes is a structure called the *insula (island of Reil)*, which is sometimes considered a fifth lobe of the cerebrum.

Diencephalon

Located in the center of the brain, the **diencephalon** houses two primary structures: thalamus and hypothalamus. The **thalamus**, which is nearly 80% of the diencephalon, is a relay station and interpretation center for all sensory impulses except olfaction.

The **hypothalamus** is a small structure that governs many important homeostatic functions. It regulates the autonomic nervous system and endocrine system by governing the pituitary gland, and it controls hunger, thirst, temperature regulation, anger,

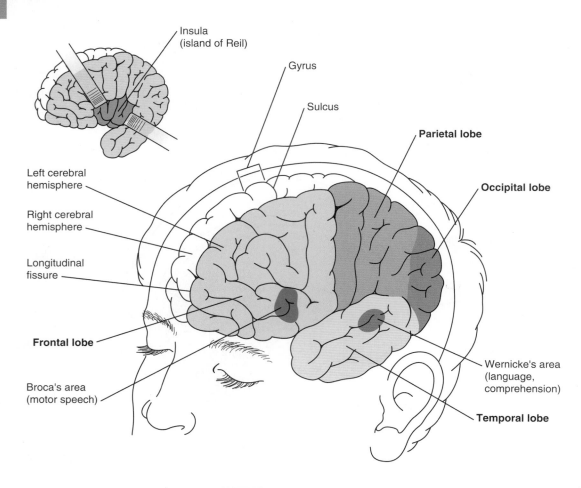

ANTEROLATERAL VIEW

Figure 17-10   Cerebrum outlining lobes and insula.

aggression, hormones, sexual behavior, sleep patterns, and consciousness.

The **pituitary gland** is connected to the hypothalamus by a slender stalk (infundibulum). It sits in the sella turcica of the sphenoid bone and was once considered the master gland of the endocrine system because its hormones control and stimulate all other glands to produce their individual products. However, the hypothalamus is the true master gland because it controls secretions of the pituitary gland. The **pineal gland** is located below the corpus callosum. Although its function is not clear, the pineal gland produces and secretes the hormone melatonin. Both of these glands are discussed in the endocrine chapter.

Cerebellum

The **cerebellum** is a cauliflower-shaped structure located posterior and inferior to the cerebrum. The cerebellum is the second largest part of the brain and consists of two cerebellar hemispheres connected by a middle section, the *vermis*. Like the cerebrum, the cerebellum consists of a **cerebellar cortex** (thin

outer layer of gray matter). White matter lies beneath the cerebellar cortex and is structured as the *arbor vitae* (tree of life).

The cerebellum is concerned with muscle tone, coordinates skeletal muscles and balance (posture integration and equilibrium), and controls fine and gross motor movements.

Brain Stem

The **brain stem** contains three main structures: midbrain, pons, and medulla oblongata.

The most superior structure of the brain stem, the **midbrain** (mesencephalon), contains two *cerebral peduncles* that house the voluntary motor tracts descending from the cerebral cortex to the spinal cord. The *cerebral aqueduct*, a narrow canal conveying cerebrospinal fluid, is located in the midbrain.

The large rounded area below the midbrain is the **pons**, which relays messages from the cerebral cortex to the spinal cord. The pons can be compared with the thalamus in the sense that both are relay stations. Four pairs of cranial nerves branch off the pons.

The most inferior portion of the brain stem is the **medulla oblongata**, which continues downward to connect to the spinal cord. The medulla oblongata contains much of the crossing-over fibers that cause the left cerebral hemisphere's association with the body's right side. Conversely, the right hemisphere is associated with the left side of the body.

The medulla, often considered the most vital part of the brain, contains the respiratory, cardiovascular, and vasomotor centers. The medulla also controls gastric secretions and reflexes such as sweating, sneezing, swallowing, and vomiting. Five pairs of cranial nerves branch from the medulla.

Blood-Brain Barrier

The **blood-brain barrier** is a selective semipermeable wall of blood capillaries with a thick basement membrane and neuroglial cells (astrocytes). The function of the blood-brain barrier is to prevent or slow down the passage of some chemical compounds and disease-causing organisms such as viruses from traveling from the blood into the CNS. Blood itself contains chemicals that can damage neurons; if blood comes into contact with neurons, they die.

Spinal Cord

The **spinal cord**, located in the vertebral canal of the vertebral column, is an extension of the brain stem. It exits the skull through the foramen magnum and extends to about the L2 region. The spinal cord stops growing before the spinal column, hence a difference in length. The functions of the spinal cord are to carry sensory impulses to the brain and motor impulses from the brain and to mediate reflex responses.

Two enlargements are located in the length of the spinal cord: one in the cervical region and one in the lumbar region. The lower end of the spinal cord is marked by the threadlike **filum terminale**, which is anchored to the coccyx. The ends of the cord fan out like a horse's tail, and form a structure appropriately called the **cauda equina** (Figure 17-11).

The spinal cord consists of 31 segments, each of which gives rise to a pair of spinal nerves. Beginning at the top of the cord are 8 cervical nerves, 12 thoracic nerves, 5 lumbar nerves, 5 sacral nerves, and 1 coccygeal nerve.

The cross-section of the spinal cord reveals white matter on the periphery surrounding gray matter (H-shaped) at the center of the cord. In the center gray is a structure properly named the *central canal,* which runs the entire length of the spinal cord and contains cerebrospinal fluid. The sides of the H are called *horns,* which are divided into the anterior, lateral, and posterior horns. White matter is organized into regions called *columns* (anterior, lateral, and poste-

Electrical Brain Waves and States of Consciousness

Brain waves are rhythmic electric impulses produced in the cerebral cortex. Scientists have noted four different types of brain wave patterns and have associated them with various states of consciousness. Most patterns are similar for all people with normal brain functions. Identified by Greek letters, these wave patterns are called *beta, alpha, theta,* and *delta.*

Beta
Beta (13 to 30 Hz) is associated with wakeful consciousness and being mentally active. Attention is focused on external surroundings, and activity is typified by rational thinking, some scattered thought patterns, and occasional distractions. High-intensity beta waves are associated with extreme stress. Dreaming while sleeping (rapid eye movement [REM]) appears as beta waves.

Alpha
The alpha state (8 to 12 Hz) is regarded as awake but relaxed; focused awareness with synchronization is between the right and left cerebral hemispheres. Alpha activity is related to inner consciousness and is associated with relaxation, self-healing, creativity, and meditation.

Theta
Theta (4 to 8 Hz) is associated with deep relaxation, unfocused attention, dreamlike awareness, sleep, the collective subconscious, and out-of-body experiences. This state of consciousness is used to access deep-rooted memories.

Delta
Delta (0.5 to 4 Hz) patterns are associated with deep sleep or comalike states.

rior), within which are groups of myelinated axons called *nerve tracts.* Sensory impulses travel up the cord to the brain on ascending tracts, and motor impulses travel down and out the cord on descending tracts.

The spinal dura mater is the outermost layer of the meninges. The space between the dura mater and the bone of the spinal column, known as the *epidural space,* is filled with adipose and connective tissue.

Reflex Arc and Reflexes

A **reflex** is an instantaneous, automatic response to a stimulus originating from either inside or outside the body. Instead of the sensory impulse going all the way to the brain where it would be analyzed and a correct motor response being selected, a reflex allows a shorter and quicker response because it is processed in the spinal cord (Figure 17-12).

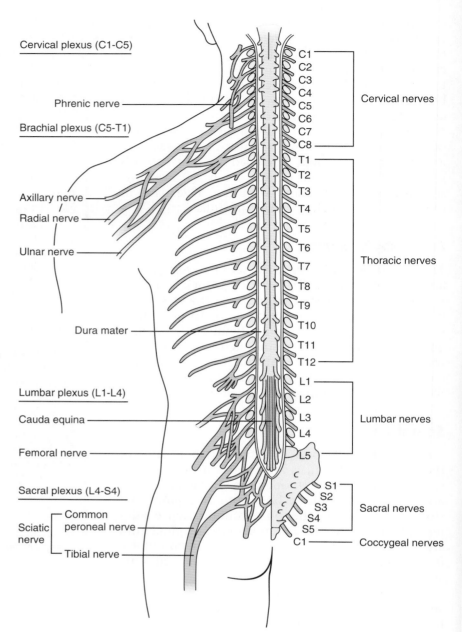

Cervical plexus (C1-C5)

Phrenic nerve

Brachial plexus (C5-T1)

Axillary nerve

Radial nerve

Ulnar nerve

Dura mater

Lumbar plexus (L1-L4)

Cauda equina

Femoral nerve

Sacral plexus (L4-S4)

Sciatic nerve { Common peroneal nerve

Tibial nerve

C1
C2
C3
C4
C5
C6
C7
C8

T1
T2
T3
T4
T5
T6
T7
T8
T9
T10
T11
T12

L1
L2
L3
L4
L5

S1
S2
S3
S4
S5

C1

Cervical nerves

Thoracic nerves

Lumbar nerves

Sacral nerves

Coccygeal nerves

POSTERIOR VIEW

Figure 17-11   The spinal cord.

Fortunately, we do not have to wait to process the information consciously. When intense stimuli (e.g., contact with direct heat) comes in on the sensory nerve, some of this electrical energy is diverted directly back out the motor nerve from the spinal cord, causing the skillet to be dropped without any conscious thought. The sensory information does reach the brain but only after the motor responses have responded to the stimulus, thereby protecting us.

Reflexes are essentially a protective neural shortcut and can be a reaction to stimuli such as pain, pressure, or even loud noises. **Somatic reflexes** are those that are responsible for the contraction of skeletal muscle such as the patellar tendon is tapped with a rubber hammer (knee-jerk or patellar reflex). Examples of somatic reflexes are muscle spindles producing the stretch reflex and Golgi tendon organs producing the tendon reflex, both of these are discussed later in this chapter. **Visceral (autonomic) reflexes** maintain homeostasis through coughing, sneezing, blinking, and correcting the heart rate, respiratory rate, and blood pressure.

Although the neuron is a structural unit of the nervous system, a functional component of the nervous system is the reflex arc. The **reflex arc**, which consists of two or more neurons (afferent/sensory

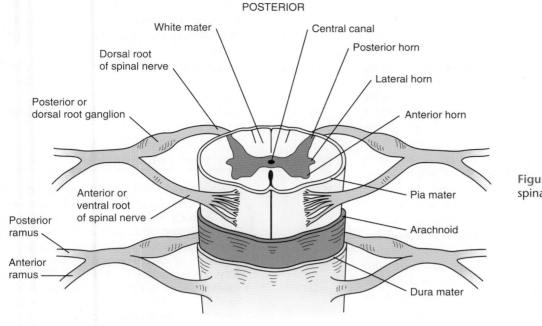

POSTERIOR

White mater

Central canal

Posterior horn

Dorsal root
of spinal nerve

Lateral horn

Anterior horn

Posterior or
dorsal root ganglion

Anterior or
ventral root
of spinal nerve

Pia mater

Posterior
ramus

Arachnoid

Anterior
ramus

Dura mater

ANTERIOR

Figure 17-11, cont'd   The spinal cord.

and efferent/motor neurons), is the smallest, simplest portion of the nervous system capable of receiving stimuli and yielding a response. Sensory receptors respond to stimuli and produce action potentials in afferent neurons. The nerve impulses stimulated by action potentials travel into the posterior horn of the spinal cord, exciting interneurons (internuncial pool). The interneurons interface with efferent neurons to elicit motor response that can range from increases in muscle tone to changes of organ or gland function to movement. All this occurs in a normal reflex arc.

An abnormal, or **physiopathological reflex arc**, is caused by increased stimuli or an increase in the amount of afferent impulses entering the cord. This creates a disturbance in the interneurons, resulting in vasoconstriction, increased muscle tone, increased intrajoint pressure, and decreased visceral functions. The increased stimuli could be the result of pain from an accident, emotional stress,

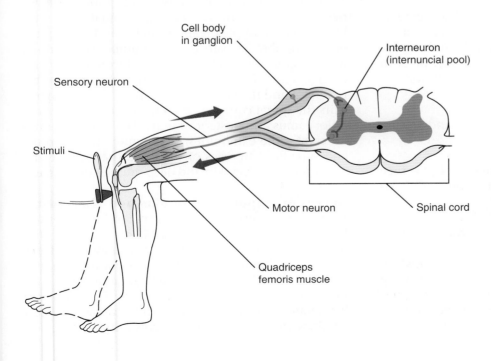

Cell body
in ganglion

Interneuron
(internuncial pool)

Sensory neuron

Stimuli

Motor neuron

Spinal cord

Quadriceps
femoris muscle

Figure 17-12   A reflex arc (somatic reflex).

biomechanical dysfunction, or poor posture. The increased muscle tonus, which causes vasoconstriction, begins to starve the muscles for oxygen and nutrition by limiting their blood supply. This ischemic condition generates cellular waste products, many of which are irritants to the tissues, and increases the perception of pain. Trigger points form in the tissues. Pain from the trigger points is referred to adjacent tissues and the pain-spasm-pain cycle continues.

Massage therapy aids in breaking the physiopathological reflex arc and helps reestablish equilibrium and a normal reflex arc. As the tissues are warmed, the fascia, which encases the muscle, is softened, allowing the muscles to more easily lengthen. As the muscles lengthen, the intrajoint pressure is decreased. The massage stimulates increased local circulation by forcing blood through dormant capillary beds. This brings oxygen and nutrition and removes accumulated waste products and toxins. Massage can also stimulate the release of natural pain killers in the body, such as endorphins. It can also inhibit the sensation of pain by activation of the gate theory, in which the experience of one type of stimulation (pressure, cold, heat) can act to exclude the experience of other sensations (pain) that are all vying for the same gate to the brain.

PERIPHERAL NERVOUS SYSTEM

The PNS contains all the nerves outside the CNS. The PNS can be subdivided into the somatic nervous system and the autonomic nervous system.

Cranial Nerves

The cranial nerves number 12 pairs. They emerge from the inferior surface of the brain and are named by Roman numerals or the areas that the nerves supply. Cranial nerves can be sensory, motor, or both (Figure 17-13). The cranial nerves are as follows:

I   **Olfactory:** senses smell
II **Optic:** employs vision
III **Oculomotor:** moves the eyeball and eyelid; constricts the pupil
IV **Trochlear:** moves the eyeball
V   **Trigeminal (great sensory nerve of the face and head):** contains three branches for chewing, pain, and temperature
VI **Abducens:** moves the eyeball
VII **Facial:** makes facial expression; produces saliva and tears
VIII **Vestibulocochlear (auditory or acoustic):** conveys messages of equilibrium and hearing (two branches to the inner ear)
IX **Glossopharyngeal:** produces saliva; employs taste and swallowing

X   **Vagus:** receives sensations from the external ear and external auditory canal and thoracic and abdominal organs; aids digestion; helps regulate heart activity
XI **Accessory (spinal accessory):** controls the tongue for speech and swallowing; innervates the trapezius and sternocleidomastoid
XII **Hypoglossal:** moves the tongue for speech and swallowing

For Your Information

The mnemonic device for remembering the names of the 12 cranial nerves is, *"Oh, oh, oh! To touch and feel very green vegetables, ah!"* (olfactory, optic, oculomotor, trochlear, trigeminal, abducens, facial, vestibulocochlear, glossopharyngeal, vagus, accessory, and hypoglossal), or *"On old Olympus's towering tops, a Finn and German viewed some hops"* (olfactory, optic, oculomotor, trochlear, trigeminal, abducens, facial, auditory, glossopharyngeal, vagus, spinal accessory, and hypoglossal).

Spinal Nerves

Each pair of spinal nerves joins the spinal column at two points: one on the left and another on the right. Each spinal nerve of each pair has anterior and posterior roots. The anterior, or ventral, root contains motor neurons, and the posterior, or dorsal, root contains sensory neurons. The posterior root of the spinal nerve contains a swelling called the *posterior or dorsal (sensory) root ganglion,* which is a collection of cell bodies of sensory neurons.

All spinal nerves have sensory and motor components. When the nerves leave the spinal cord, they branch out to supply organs, muscles, and skin. Spinal nerves number 31 pairs and are numbered according to the region and level of spinal cord from which they emerge (e.g., C7, T5, L4, S2). The first pair emerges between C1 and the occipital bone. When a spinal nerve exits the spinal cord, it divides into two branches: anterior ramus and posterior ramus. The anterior ramus innervates the extremities, lateral and anterior trunk, and superficial muscles of the back; the posterior ramus innervates the skin and deep muscles of the back.

Nerves of Importance to Massage Therapists

Some cranial nerves, spinal nerves, and plexuses can be compressed during massage (Figure 17-14). During manual compression, the client may experience numbness, tingling, burning, or a shooting pain. It is doubtful that this will damage the nerve, but it may make your client feel uncomfortable. The following list details innervated muscles and organs:

Axillary nerve: Deltoids and teres minor

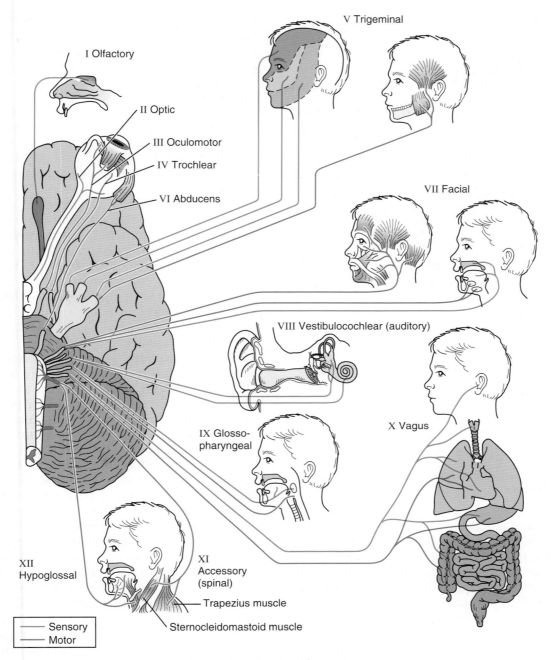

Figure 17-13 Cranial nerves.

Brachial plexus: C5 to T1 (supplies the arm and hand)

Common peroneal nerve: Tibialis anterior, peroneus longus/brevis, extensor digitorum longus/brevis, extensor hallucis longus

Facial nerve: Frontalis, occipitalis, orbicularis oris and oculi, buccinator, platysma, zygomaticus major and minor

Femoral nerve: Iliacus, pectineus, sartorius, quadriceps femoris

Median nerve (great flexor): Flexor digitorum superficialis/profundus, flexor carpi radialis, pronator teres/quadratus, palmaris longus, flexor pollicis longus/brevis, opponens pollicis, abductor pollicis longus/brevis,

Lumbar plexus: L1 to L4 (supplies the abdomen, low back, and genitalia)

Musculocutaneous nerve: Biceps brachii, brachialis, coracobrachialis

Obturator nerve: Obturator externus, gracilis, adductor magnus, adductor longus, adductor brevis

Radial nerve (great extensor): Triceps brachii, anconeus, brachioradialis, extensor carpi ulnaris,

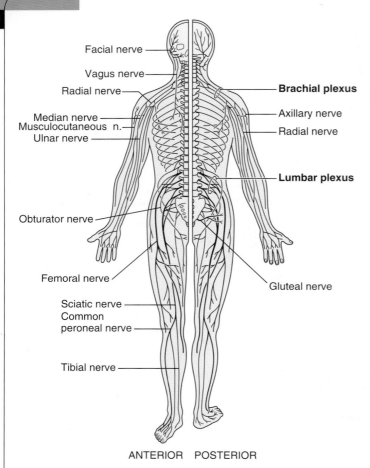

Facial nerve
Vagus nerve
Radial nerve
Brachial plexus
Median nerve
Musculocutaneous n.
Ulnar nerve
Axillary nerve
Radial nerve
Lumbar plexus
Obturator nerve
Femoral nerve
Gluteal nerve
Sciatic nerve
Common
peroneal nerve
Tibial nerve

ANTERIOR   POSTERIOR

Figure 17-14 Cranial and spinal nerves identification for massage therapists.

extensor carpi radialis longus/brevis, extensor digitorum, extensor indicis, extensor pollicis longus/brevis, extensor digiti minimi, supinator

Sciatic nerve: Adductor magnus, bicep femoris (long head), piriformis, quadratus femoris, gemellus superior/inferior, obturator internus

Tibial nerve: Gastrocnemius, soleus, plantaris, popliteus, tibialis posterior, flexor digitorum longus, flexor hallicis longus, bicep femoris (short head), semimembranous, semitendinosus

Ulnar nerve (accessory flexor): Flexor digitorum superficialis/profundus, flexor carpi ulnaris, flexor digiti minimi brevis, flexor pollicis longus/brevis, opponens digiti minimi, abductor digiti minimi

Vagus nerve: Heart, lungs, kidneys, gastrointestinal tract (accessory organs of digestion)

Types of Sensory Receptors

Special sensory receptors in the body detect certain types of sensory information. These are chemoreceptors, mechanoreceptors (proprioceptors, baroreceptors), thermoreceptors, photoreceptors, and nociceptors (Figure 17-15). All initiate nerve impulses in sensory neuron membranes but differ in the nature of the stimuli that initiates an impulse (e.g., chemical, pressure, light, heat, and pain).

Chemoreceptors

Located in the nose, tongue, within the walls of certain arteries and the brain, **chemoreceptors** are activated by chemical stimuli and detect smells, tastes, and chemistry changes in the blood. To create an action potential, certain molecules fit into certain receptor sites.

Chemoreceptors that are sensitive to changes in pH and carbon dioxide concentration are located in the aorta, carotid arteries, and medulla oblongata. These receptors are occasionally sensitive to low oxygen levels in the blood. If oxygen is low or carbon dioxide is high, the chemoreceptors stimulate the respiratory center in the medulla oblongata to increase respiration rate.

Mechanoreceptors

Mechanoreceptors are sensory receptors that respond to mechanical stimuli and are located in the skin, ears, muscles, tendons, joints, and fascia. They detect tactile sensations such as touch, pressure, blood pressure, vibration, stretching, muscular contraction, proprioception, sound, and equilibrium. Examples of mechanoreceptors are Meissner's and Pacinian corpuscles and proprioceptors (Table 17-1). Mechanoreceptors detect mechanical forces on the cellular membrane and initiate action potentials. A discussion of many of these receptors can be found in Chapter 12.

A special type of mechanoreceptor detecting stimuli within the body is called a **proprioceptor**. Proprioceptors respond to changes in muscle length and tension, body position, and blood pressure; these receptors are located in muscles, joints, walls of certain arteries, and inner ear. **Proprioception** is a kinesthetic sense that aids in consciously orienting the body in space without the use of vision. Examples of proprioceptors are muscle spindles and Golgi tendon organs.

Muscle spindles are stretch-sensitive receptors wrapped around intrafusal muscle fibers (striated muscle fiber), which monitor changes in the length of a muscle and the rate of this change. When the muscle is stretched quickly or overstretches (ballistic stretch), the muscle spindle elongates and conducts action potentials to the spinal cord. This causes motor neurons to produce muscle contraction. Referred to as a *stretch reflex,* this protective mechanism guards against muscle damage (tearing) by counteracting the sudden or overstretch with muscle contraction. This mechanism provides the basis for reflexes such as the knee-jerk reflex.

A massage therapist may use the stretch reflex when strengthening a weak antagonist. For example, if a client

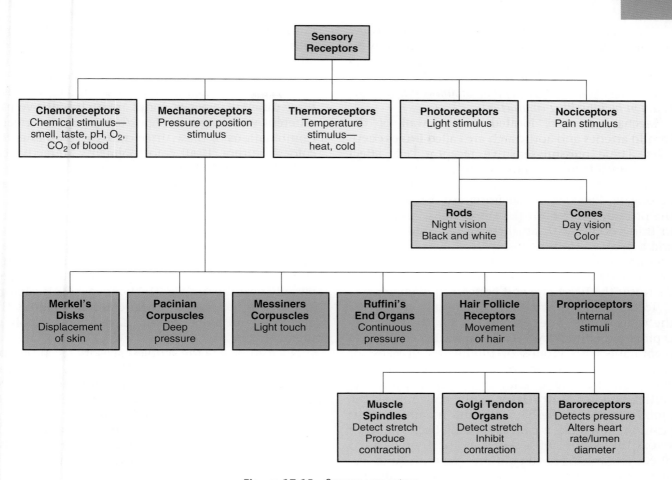

Figure 17-15   Sensory receptors.

has rounded shoulders, the pectoralis major may be tight while the rhomboids are weak. During treatment, use hacking tapotement across the fibers of the rhomboids to create minute muscle contractions. Over time, strengthening of the rhomboids may pull the shoulders back for a more balanced posture.

Receptors that are stimulated by both tension and excessive stretch are called **Golgi tendon organs** (GTOs). They are located at the musculotendinous junction of skeletal muscles and activate a reflex response to inhibit the motor neuron if tension is too high. Referred to as a *tendon reflex*, this protective mechanism helps ensure that muscles do not contract too strongly and damage their tendons. The stimulated GTOs cause inhibition of contraction throughout the entire muscle.

TABLE 17-1

Types of Mechanoreceptors

Types	Stimuli Received
Hair follicle receptors	Detect hair movement
Meissner corpuscles	Detect light touch (pressure); respond to actual movement and length of movement across skin
Pacinian corpuscles	Detect deep pressure; respond to skin displacement and high-frequency vibration
Merkel disks	Respond to pressure and skin displacement
Ruffini end organs	Respond to deep or continuous pressure
Proprioceptors	Respond to changes in muscle length and tension, limb position, and pain
Baroreceptors	Detect pressure in vessels; respond by altering heart rate and vessel wall diameter
Muscle spindles	Detect stretch; respond by producing contraction
Golgi tendon organs	Detect tension and excessive stretch; respond by inhibiting contraction

The tendon reflex may also be used during massage treatment. Plucking the tendons perpendicularly tricks the GTOs into thinking a load is present and reduces muscular tension. This technique is also called the transverse tendon technique (triple T) *and enhances muscular relaxation by inhibiting contraction.*

Mechanoreceptors located in the wall of the carotid arteries and aortic arch are called **baroreceptors**. These pressure-sensitive receptor cells affect blood pressure by sending impulses to the cardiac center and to the vasomotor center in the medulla oblongata. Rates of neural firing are determined by the pressure exerted on the vessel walls. An increase in firing occurs with an increase in blood pressure, and a decrease in firing results from decreased blood pressure. The CNS responds by stimulating the autonomic nervous system; this action either increases or decreases the heart rate and vessel wall diameter.

To determine orientation with respect to gravity, the walls of the inner ear are lined with special receptors called *maculae.* Each **macula** contains a membrane with groups of modified hair cells, or cilia, that are attached to sensory nerves. Floating above the membrane is layer of calcium carbonate particles known as **otoliths**. As the body moves, the otoliths and the underlying otolithic membrane shift position, much like a pancake sliding back and forth across the bottom of a skillet as the frying pan is tilted. The weight of the otoliths responds to movement and changes in inertia. As they move, the cilia are disturbed, initiating a nerve impulse.

The three fluid-filled semicircular canals located within the inner ear help orient the position of the body in different planes. Tips of cilia protrude in the gelatin-filled canals and rotation of the head causes movement of fluid, which bends the cilia and creates action potential. This process helps maintain the position of the body in space and aids in equilibrium.

Photoreceptors

Photoreceptors are receptors that are sensitive to light stimuli. The two types of photoreceptors are rods and cones, which are located in the retina. The **retina** is a delicate nervous tissue membrane of the eye, which is continuous with the optic nerve. The cellular structures of both types of photoreceptors are similar. Each retina possesses more than 100 million rods and 3 million cones.

Rods are thin cellular structures with slender rod-like projections that are very sensitive to dim light (night vision) and shades of black, white, and gray. Notice how difficult it is to determine color and detail in dim light. When light hits a rod photoreceptor, a nerve impulse is triggered.

Cones are needed for color vision; they are short and thick with blunt projections. Most cones are found in the center of the retina where very few rod cells are located. This area is designated for acute, detailed vision partly because blood vessels do not exist there and so color vision is not hindered.

Cones and rods function in a similar way. The three different types of cones are each sensitive to a different wavelength of light (blue, red, and green). Combinations of these three colors give us an entire color spectrum. If all color pigments are activated, white is perceived; if no color pigments are activated, black is seen. To see color, more light is required; color vision is also known as *daytime vision.*

Nociceptors

Receptors for detecting pain are **nociceptors**. These free nerve endings are actually bare dendrite endings and are located in almost every tissue of the body, especially near the surface. The brain lacks nociceptors; however, other tissues of the cranium, such as the meninges and blood vessels, have a large supply of them.

Nociceptors are the simplest sensory receptors and serve a protective function. They rarely adapt and may continue to fire once the painful stimulus is removed. Otherwise, pain would stop being sensed, and irreparable damage could result.

Nociceptors respond to stimuli that cause tissue damage, irritants (e.g., ones released by injured cells), and extreme stimuli (e.g., excessive heat, bright light, loud sound, and intense mechanical stimulation such as excessive pressure). The painful sensation may cause reflexive withdrawal of the involved body segments if from an external source and stimulation of the sympathetic nervous system, such as changes in heartbeat and blood pressure.

In most instances, pain is felt at the point of nociceptive stimulation. However, a client may have referred pain, which can be experienced as sensations such as tingling, numbness, itching, aching, heat, or cold. Visceral pain may be sensed in the area over the organ or projected to another area of the body. Often, these areas are innervated by the same spinal segment (Hilton's Law). For example, the pain of angina may cause pain down the left arm resulting from a common spinal nerve connection. A massage therapist may apply pressure to a trigger point, and the client may feel a referred pain in another area. All trigger points found in the area of the referred pain should be treated (Box 17-1).

Thermoreceptors

Located immediately under the skin, **thermoreceptors** include two types of free nerve endings: one that detects cold and one for heat. Cold receptors are 10 times more numerous than heat receptors and are stimulated by lowering temperatures. Heat receptors are stimulated by rising temperatures. Once

BOX 17-1

Neurological Laws: Presentation and Discussion

Arndt's Law (Rudolf Arndt, German Psychiatrist, 1835-1900)

Weak stimuli excite physiological activity, moderately strong ones favor it, strong ones retard it, and very strong ones arrest it.

Arndt's law applies directly to the physiological effects of stress and relaxation (massage). Strong stimuli such as pain and trigger points disrupt normal functioning of body systems. Muscle tonus may become increased, digestive functions may be inhibited, and blood pressure may rise. Massage, being a weak but pleasurable stimulus, returns the body to homeostasis.

Davis's Law

If muscle ends are brought closer together, then the pull of tonus is increased, thereby shortening the muscle, which may even cause hypertrophy. If muscle ends are separated beyond normal, then tonus is lessened or lost, thereby weakening the muscle.

Davis's law is an example of the body preferring balance to extremes and can be observed in various situations. The increase in muscle tonus gained by weight lifting is the result of repetitive contractions. However, chronic shortening can produce spasms, such as a muscle that has stayed in a shortened position for long periods (e.g., sleeping on the stomach with ankles in full extension or wearing shoes with high heels). The opposite extreme can occur when muscles have been overstretched in an accident, exceeding their normal limit (e.g., whiplash). The microtrauma of tearing many muscle fibers often causes a loss of strength and increase in flaccidity of the muscle. Each of these scenarios can effectively be addressed with massage and joint mobilizations.

Hilton's Law (John Hilton, English Surgeon, 1804-1878)

A nerve trunk that supplies a joint also supplies the muscles of the joint and the skin over the insertions of such muscles.

Hilton's law is significant for the massage therapist, especially when combined with Arndt's law. Each nerve trunk supplies both sensory information and motor control for joints, muscles, vessels, skin, and organs in a given area. Pain in this area results in a physiopathological reflex arc, which generates a spontaneous increase in motor impulses, sending signals of the pain to the cord. The increased motor stimuli cause vasoconstriction, a decrease in visceral function, an increase in muscular tonus, and an increase in intrajoint pressure. Arndt's law states that strong stimuli retard or arrest physiological activity.

The advantage of Hilton's law for the massage therapist is that not only does massage have the direct effects of increasing local circulation, relaxing muscle fiber, and calming stimulated nerves, but it has the indirect effect of interrupting the physiopathological reflex arc. As the pain subsides because of disruption of strong stimuli, normal function returns.

Pfluger's Laws (Edward Friederich Wilhem Pfluger, German Physiologist, 1829-1910)

Although not specifically stated, Pfluger's laws are (1) progressive in nature and (2) dependent on the degree of irritation to the nerve. *Progressive* refers to the fact that the laws are experienced *in order*—that is, a client begins experiencing the Law of Unilaterality and, if left untreated, can proceed through each of the succeeding laws until the Law of Generalization is reached. This does not mean that every client experiences the effects of all five laws; progression is dependent on the degree of neural irritation to the nerve. Clients with minor injuries may only experience the Law of Unilaterality, whereas others may progress to the Law of Symmetry, Law of Intensity, and so on.

Law of Unilaterality

If a mild irritation is applied to one or more sensory nerves, the movement takes place usually on one side only—the side that is irritated.

The word *movement* in Pfluger's laws refers primarily to motor reflexes responding to a nerve stimulus. Increased tonus occurs first on the side of the body reporting pain or injury. Motor reflexes tighten the muscles on the affected side, limiting range of motion as a protective mechanism, preventing further injury (muscular splint). Constriction of vessels prevents internal bleeding in muscular tears.

Law of Symmetry

If the stimulation is sufficiently increased, motor reaction is manifested not only by the irritated side but also in similar muscles on the opposite side of the body.

When an injury is left untreated on one side of the body, the symptoms begin to migrate to the opposite side of the body. Spasms in the right levator scapulae, if not addressed, increase in intensity. Eventually, the body seeks to reduce some of this sensory input (pain) by directing it down motor nerves on the opposite side of the body. The result is a general increase of tonus in the left levator scapula and other muscles that the nerve innervates.

Law of Intensity

Reflex movements are usually more intense on the side of irritation. At times, the movements of the opposite side equal them in intensity, but they are usually less pronounced.

Pfluger's Law of Intensity states that irritation (pain) increases in intensity on both ides of the body, but the pain is greater on the initial side of irritation and discomfort.

Law of Radiation

If the excitation continues to increase, it is propagated upward, and reactions take place through centrifugal nerves coming from the cord segments higher up.

Again, if left untreated, the discomfort grows, and the client proceeds from one law to the next. The body seeks to dissipate more sensory input (pain), directing it to motor nerves higher up the cord, such as a tight shoulder radiating to the neck musculature.

Law of Generalization

When the irritation becomes very intense, it is propagated in the medulla oblongata, which becomes a focus from which stimuli

Continued

BOX 17-1

Neurological Laws: Presentation and Discussion—cont'd

radiate to all parts of the cord, causing a general increase of tonus in all muscles of the body.

This law represents a client in chronic pain, having a long-standing history of pain and limited range of motion. The Law of Generalization seldom applies for something like a tight levator and is usually reserved for clients with problems such as chronic low back pain. Once the medulla is involved, the internuncial pool of the entire spinal cord is excited, causing pain and increased tonus to all muscles. Chronic pain clients may experience severe headaches, neck and shoulder stiffness, arm pain, and the expected back and sciatic pain. The goal of the massage therapist is to reduce the sensory stimulation and muscle tonus to a point where the client begins to back down the scale of Pfluger's Laws and symptoms abate. Thermotherapy, in conjunction with massage therapy, is an excellent modality for clients who have advanced to this stage of pain.

Sherrington's Law (Sir Charles Scott Sherrington, English Physician, 1857-1952)

When a muscle receives a nerve impulse to contract, its antagonist simultaneously receives an impulse to relax.

Sherrington's law is also known as *reciprocal inhibition*. It would be difficult to move if all muscles contracted at the same time. In fact, if opposing muscles could both contract simultaneously, the weaker of the two would be torn. Reciprocal inhibition ensures that when the prime mover (agonist) is creating movement, its antagonist cooperates by elongating. In a client with normal neurological function, these two impulses automatically occur simultaneously.

Massage therapists can apply this principle to turn off messages of contraction in acute muscle cramps. For example, when the hamstrings are experiencing a muscle cramp,

the cramp could be relieved by forcibly contracting their antagonists, the quadriceps femoris. This is best accomplished through isometric contraction (contraction against resistance). Instruct the prone client to extend his flexed knee while the massage therapist applies resistance. Maintain the contraction for 10 to 20 seconds, then release. Repeat 3 times (Figure 17-16).

Law of Facilitation

When an impulse has passed once through a certain set of neurons to the exclusion of others, it tends to take the same course on future occasions, and each time it traverses this path, the resistance is less.

The repetition of a particular action ingrains a habit between the brain and muscles. Pain from postural distortions and improper movement patterns are often habitual. The best way to break a bad habit is to replace it with a good one. Massage reprograms the body with new information. The client can move differently because he or she has felt something different. It really does not matter what form of massage is used, as long as it is not perceived as painful to the client because pain triggers a protective response.

A client with a first-degree tear of his or her right supraspinatus may not be able to actively raise an arm above shoulder level. Even after the tear has healed, the previous experience of pain sometimes limits the range of motion. However, if the therapist treats the injury with massage and passively ranges the arm without going into the pain barrier, the brain is reprogrammed to accept the movement pattern once again. By repeating passive movements several times, neural messages are forced to cross certain synapses repeatedly. The message can then easily begin taking that particular route.

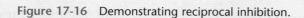
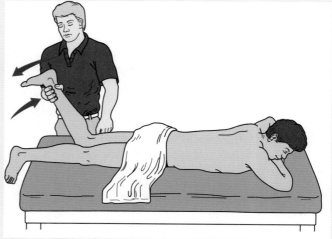

Figure 17-16 Demonstrating reciprocal inhibition.

temperature falls below 10° C (50° F) or rises above 45° C (113° F), nociceptors rather than thermoreceptors are activated.

Another way in which physiologists classify sensory receptors is by where the receptor is located and not what type of sensory information it receives. These alternate classifications are exteroceptors, proprioceptors, and interoceptors.

Exteroceptors

These sensory nerve endings are located in the skin, mucous membranes, and sense organs, responding to stimuli originating from outside of the body, such as touch, pressure, or sound.

Proprioceptors

In this grouping, proprioceptors represent the same description is mechanoreceptor, mentioned earlier; sensory receptors respond to movement and position and are located in the skin, ears, muscles, tendons, joints, and fascia.

Interoceptors

These receptors respond to stimuli originating from within the body regarding the function of the internal organs, such as digestion, excretion, and blood pressure, and are located in the viscera.

The word crisis is written with two characters in Chinese. One symbol represents danger and the other stands for opportunity.
—Robert Cantor

AUTONOMIC NERVOUS SYSTEM

The autonomic nervous system, together with the endocrine system, regulates the body's internal organs. The autonomic nervous system innervates smooth muscle, cardiac muscle, and glands, and it controls the circulation of blood, activity of the gastrointestinal tract, body temperature, respiration rate, and many other functions. The autonomic nervous system is regarded as a visceral efferent system because motor signals are sent to the visceral organs. Most of these motor activities are not under conscious control and thus are involuntary (Figure 17-17). The hypothalamus regulates the activity of the autonomic nervous system.

Within the autonomic nervous system are two divisions: sympathetic nervous system and the *parasympathetic nervous system*. Their effects on the visceral organs are complementary (one system excites, and the other system inhibits) because nerves from both divisions supply many the same organs. This complementary relationship controls the body's internal organs in a way to maintain homeostasis (Table 17-2).

Some structures have only sympathetic innervation (adrenal glands and blood vessels); some structures have only parasympathetic innervation (lacrimal apparatus). In extreme fear, both systems may act simultaneously, producing involuntary emptying of the bladder and rectum and a generalized sympathetic response.

Sympathetic Nervous System

The **sympathetic nervous system** as a whole is a catabolic system and is involved with spending body resources and with preparing the body for emergency situations. However, the sympathetic nervous system is activated anytime an alarm reaction is experienced (anger, fright, anxiety, or any other type of emotional upset, real or imagined). The sympathetic division is also stimulated in situations of physical stress. Stress may be viewed as homeostasis interrupted and disease as homeostasis malfunctioning.

All reactions of the sympathetic division occur quickly. The nerves of this system cause the adrenal gland to secrete epinephrine, which sustains the actions of the sympathetic nervous system through the endocrine system. Body responses while being in sympathetic mode include pupil dilation, increase in heart rate and the force of contraction, airway dilation, mobilization of glucose and fats for energy. Processes that are not needed for meeting the stressful situation, like movements and secretions of the digestive tract, are suppressed.

Most of the cell bodies of the sympathetic system lie just outside the spinal cord at the level of T1 to L2. For this reason, the sympathetic nervous system is often called **thoracolumbar outflow**.

Parasympathetic Nervous System

The **parasympathetic nervous system** in general is an anabolic system, conserving the body's resources. Representing the body's calmness and the relaxation response, the parasympathetic nervous system's actions are complementary to the sympathetic system. Because the parasympathetic nervous system is most active under calm conditions and stimulates visceral organs for normal functions as it maintains homeostasis, it is referred to as the *housekeeping system*. Body processes in parasympathetic mode include salivation, urination, digestive processes, defecation, and storing nutrients to be used later.

The fibers of the parasympathetic nervous system occupy spaces at the spinal cord level S2 to S4 and

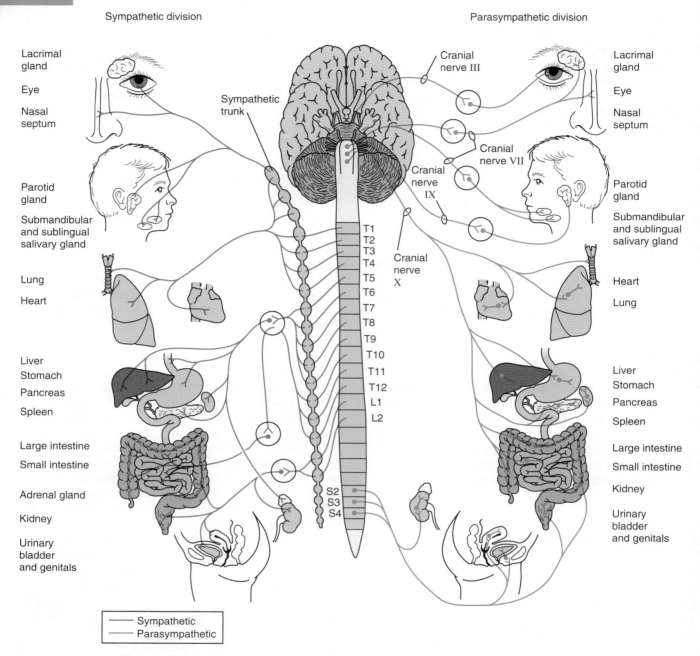

Sympathetic division

Parasympathetic division

Lacrimal gland

Eye

Nasal septum

Parotid gland

Submandibular and sublingual salivary gland

Lung

Heart

Liver
Stomach
Pancreas
Spleen

Large intestine

Small intestine

Adrenal gland

Kidney

Urinary bladder and genitals

Sympathetic trunk

Cranial nerve III

Cranial nerve VII

Cranial nerve IX

Cranial nerve X

T1
T2
T3
T4
T5
T6
T7
T8
T9
T10
T11
T12
L1
L2

S2
S3
S4

Lacrimal gland

Eye

Nasal septum

Parotid gland

Submandibular and sublingual salivary gland

Heart

Lung

Liver
Stomach
Pancreas
Spleen

Large intestine

Small intestine

Kidney

Urinary bladder and genitals

Sympathetic
Parasympathetic

Figure 17-17 The autonomic nervous system: sympathetic and parasympathetic branches.

cranial nerves 3, 7, 9, and 10. For this reason, the parasympathetic nervous system is often called **craniosacral outflow**.

During stressful situations, the sympathetic nervous system narrows the perceptual field to facilitate the fight-or-flight response. In contrast, during times of rest and relaxation, the parasympathetic nervous system broadens the perceptual field. One gift of parasympathetic response that occurs during a massage is that often, in the client's relaxed state, he can contemplate more options or solutions to life's challenges.

SPECIAL SENSES

All sense receptors arise from ectoderm (the cellular layer from which the brain and spinal cord arise). Receptors for general senses (e.g., pain, pressure, temperature, proprioception) are distributed throughout the body. They are part of the nervous system and are made up of special sensory neurons that receive stimuli from the outside environment, such as vibration, light, and chemicals.

TABLE 17-2

Effects of the Autonomic Nervous System

Sympathetic Activity	Parasympathetic Activity
Increased heart rate	Maintains resting heart rate
Increased respiratory rate	Maintains resting respiratory rate
Bronchiolar dilation	Maintains homeostasis
Glucose released from liver	Maintains homeostasis of glucose levels
Increased blood pressure	Maintains resting blood pressure
Pupillary dilation	Maintains homeostasis
Increased perspiration and oil gland activity	Stimulates tearing
Inhibited salivation	Stimulates salivation
Vasoconstriction	Maintains homeostasis of vasomotor activity
Decreased gastrointestinal motility (inhibits digestion)	Increases gastrointestinal motility and pancreatic secretions of digestive enzymes (stimulates digestion)
Inhibited elimination	Stimulates elimination
Stimulation of adrenal glands to release epinephrine and norepinephrine	Nonapplicable

In this section, the special senses (taste, olfaction, vision, hearing, and equilibrium) are briefly discussed. Information on the touch sense is located in Chapter 12 because it is considered a general sense rather than a special sense.

Taste

Mediated by taste buds (gustatory organs), taste is a collection of chemosensitive receptors concentrated on projections on the tongue called **papillae**. Within each papilla are taste hairs extending from taste pores. These hairs are attached to a gustatory receptor that supports a chemoreceptor, which becomes aroused when a molecule of a particular size and shape enters a receptor site, like a lock-and-key mechanism. Controversy exists whether these receptors detect four primary tastes (salty, sweet, bitter, and sour) or whether a continuum of many tastes exists. Most textbooks assert that these four primary tastes are localized in specific regions on the tongue, but new research indicates that more taste receptors exist than the four primaries. The perception of taste is a combination of impulses from many taste receptors. The input from one receptor means little without the combined information from other receptors, just as the letter K is relatively meaningless without surrounding letters to form a word.

Taste is strongly influenced by sense of smell. It is difficult to taste food without scent molecules rising up to the nostrils (cold food does not have as much taste as hot food). A condition such as a cold often interferes with the sense of smell, and taste is inhibited (Figure 17-18).

Olfaction

Olfaction (sense of smell) uses chemoreceptors to detect odors. The cell bodies of olfactory receptors are found in the olfactory mucosa, and dendritic extensions or cilia (hair cells) are located in the nasal mucosa. The act of inhalation forces airborne molecules up to the mucous layer where they dissolve and come into contact with the chemosensitive receptors. Once certain gaseous chemical molecules fit into the correct receptor site, action potentials are created, and impulses of odor are sent to the olfactory bulb and temporal lobe of the cerebrum. Scientists that have suggested that humans can detect between seven and 32 primary odors (e.g., ether, camphor, musk, floral, mint, pungent, putrid). Regarded as the most primitive of all senses, smell plays an important role in sexual behavior for most mammals (Figure 17-19) and is the strongest sense linked to memories.

Vision

Vision uses photoreceptors (rods and cones) that are located in the eye. Light enters the eye through the pupil (opening in the center of the iris) and strikes the retina, which is essentially a membranous screen composed of delicate nervous tissue at the rear of the eye (Figure 17-20).

The photoreceptors on the retina convert light energy into action potentials, which are transmitted to the brain through the optic nerve for visual interpretation. A blind spot exists where the optic nerve exits the retina, but this does not affect vision because there are two eyes, and the blind spots do not coincide with each other.

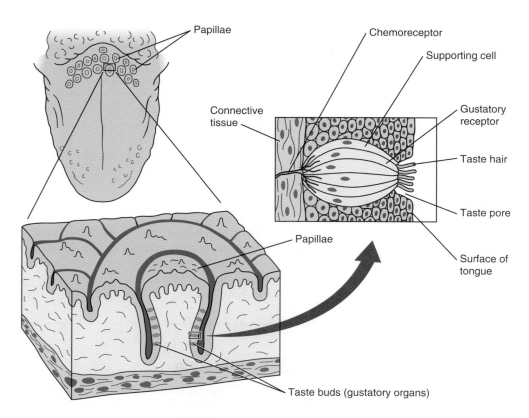

Figure 17-18   Taste buds on the tongue.

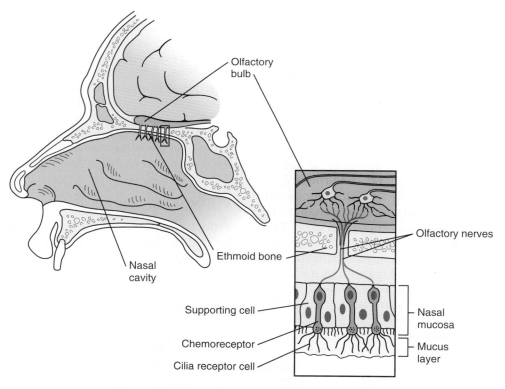

Figure 17-19   Nasal cavity and the olfactory bulb.

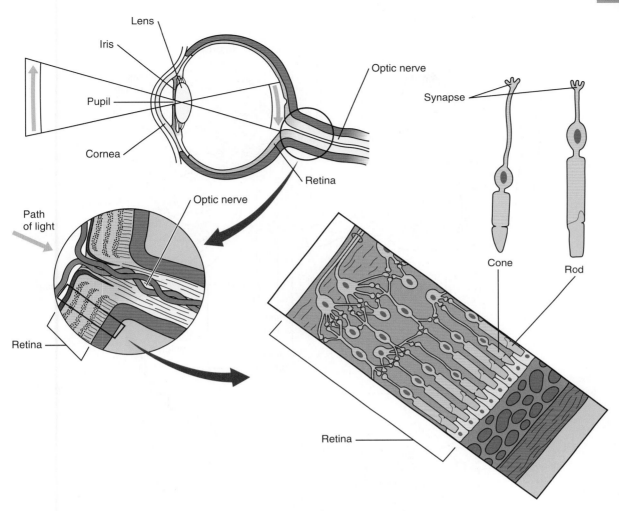

Figure 17-20   Rods and cones in the retina.

Hearing

Hearing responds to air vibrations that are detected by mechanoreceptors. Air vibrations, or sound waves, are transmitted into neural messages in an indirect, roundabout process.

Sound waves hit the **tympanic membrane** (eardrum) at the back of the auditory canal. The membrane, which separates the outer ear from the middle ear, vibrates like a drum at the same frequency as the sound waves that strike the membrane. These waves are transmitted through three small bones (ossicles) in the middle ear: malleus (hammer), incus (anvil), and stapes (stirrup). The vibration of these three small bones causes a domino effect, relaying this auditory information to the oval window.

The **oval window** is a membrane that covers the opening to a coiled, fluid-filled cavity (cochlea) of the inner ear. It then transfers the sound vibrations to the fluid of the cochlear duct (endolymph). Within the cochlea are three fluid-filled canals. The **cochlea** con-

tains a **basilar membrane** (sensory cells are located on top of this basilar membrane where hair cells attach to the auditory nerve). Bending of the hair cells sends action potential through the auditory nerve to the brain, and it is interpreted as sound. The moving fluid essentially "plucks" the hair cells in the lining, producing the impulses for sound (Figure 17-21).

Two aspects of sound are pitch and volume. **Pitch** is the quality of a tone or sound, which is dependent on the relative rapidity of the vibrations (slow vibrations produce deep sounds, and fast vibrations produce high sounds). The ability to hear high-pitched sounds declines with age. **Volume** is the loudness of sound; volume can change without altering pitch.

NERVOUS PATHOLOGIES

Carpal tunnel syndrome. Carpal tunnel syndrome is a painful repetitive strain injury (RSI) of the hand and wrist caused by compression of the

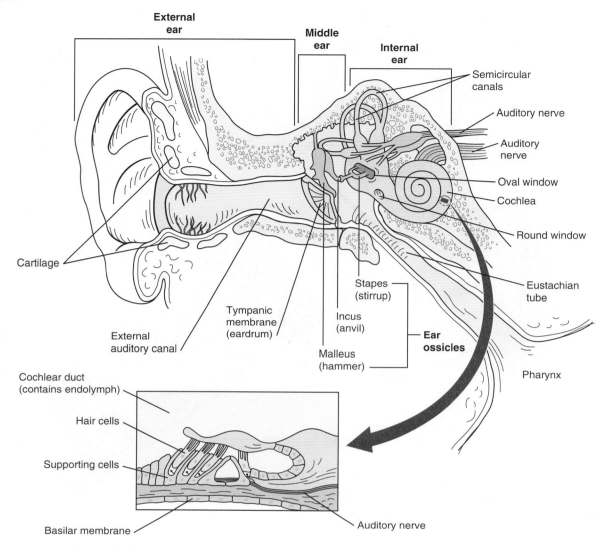

Figure 17-21   Tympanic membrane, oval window, ear ossicles, cochlea, and mechanoreceptors.

median nerve by the transverse carpal ligament. Tendinous sheaths may become swollen and irritated through an improper arm-to-wrist angle and overuse. As these tendons become irritated, extra synovial fluid is secreted. The accumulated fluid compresses the median nerve. Chronic inflammation causes the tendon sheath to thicken, compounding the problem.

Because this is an occupational hazard for massage therapists, take preventive measures like keeping your wrists neutral while you work, massaging your forearms and hands regularly, and stretching and doing range-of-motion exercises for your hands, shoulders, and neck. To prevent RSIs, strengthen your forearm and hand muscles using isometric and isotonic contractions; also, use a variety of strokes, rest your hands by spacing out your clients, stretch between sessions, and adjust the height of the massage table.

For clients with this syndrome, local massage over the wrist is contraindicated if acute inflammation is present. In chronic conditions, edema can be reduced by elevating the limb and using centripetal effleurage or lymphatic drainage techniques. Penetrating moist heat can help soften and allow stretching of fibrous adhesions. Cross-fiber friction loosens scar tissue. Passive movement of the elbow, wrist, and finger joints maintains range of motion. It is also essential to massage the neck, shoulders, upper chest, and arms. Massage therapists should help the client identify and avoid risk factors such as improper arm-to-wrist angle and excessive wrist flexion.

Encephalitis. Inflammation of the brain, or encephalitis, is an infectious disease typically transmitted by the bite of an infected mosquito. Encephalitis may be the result of hemorrhage, lead or other type of poisoning, or as a secondary complication of another condition. This condition is characterized by headaches, fever, vertigo, nausea, and vomiting. In severe cases, encephalitis causes seizures, paralysis, and coma.

Massage is contraindicated.

Epilepsy. Epilepsy, or seizure disorder, is the presence of abnormal and irregular discharges of cerebral electrical activity; billions of neurons in the brain fire at once. During these episodes, the individual may experience sensory disturbances, seizures, abnormal behavior, and loss of consciousness. The causes of most epileptic cases are unknown, but it has been linked to cerebral trauma, brain tumors, cerebrovascular disturbances, or chemical imbalances. It is viewed as a "lightning storm in the brain."

Massage is fine for clients who have a history of epilepsy. However, it is important to have the address and phone number of a contact person in case a seizure occurs during a massage treatment. If this occurs, move all objects away so the client cannot injure herself. You may choose to begin the massage on the floor if your client has a history of seizures. Certain types of epilepsy can be triggered by specific smells, so aromatherapy can serve as a trigger and is therefore contraindicated.

Hyperesthesia. Hyperesthesia is hypersensitivity to touch. Often touch is perceived as a painful sensation. The irritation to touch may be caused by emotional stress, chronic pain, shingles, or nerve compression.

Clients with hyperesthesia most likely do not schedule a massage. Massage in warm water, such as Watsu, may be indicated because the pressure of the water on the skin is usually tolerated well. Daily light, but brisk, frictioning of the skin with a plush towel can help reduce hypersensitivity.

Meningitis. Meningitis is an infection or inflammation of the meninges, often characterized by a sudden severe headache, vertigo, stiffness of the neck, and severe irritability. As the condition progresses, individuals experience nausea, vomiting, and mental disorientation. An elevated body temperature, pulse rate, and respiration rate are often noted. Meningitis can be life threatening.

Massage is contraindicated.

Multiple sclerosis (MS). MS is an autoimmune disorder in which a progressive destruction of myelin sheaths occurs in the CNS (similar to an electrical wire stripped of its insulation). The myelin sheaths deteriorate to sclerosis (plaques). The symptoms depend on what areas of the CNS are most laden with plaque. It usually begins slowly in young adulthood, worsening throughout life with periods of flare-ups and remission. Remission occurs because the damaged axons heal and normal function resumes. Intervals be-

tween flare-ups grow shorter as the disease advances.

Massage is contraindicated during flare-ups. Clients should be assessed thoroughly at every visit because symptoms may change from day to day. The goal of massage is to lessen exacerbations, relax the client, decrease tone in rigid muscles, and prevent stiffness and contractures. Heat and cold therapies are contraindicated because temperature extremes can make symptoms worse. Treatments should be slow and gentle and of shorter duration because clients may tire easily.

Nerve compression. Nerve compression is also known as *nerve impingement* and is caused by pressure against the nerve resulting from contact with hard tissues such as bone or cartilage. Common nerve compressions are found when vertebral disks slip from between the bodies of adjacent vertebrae and migrate into the nerve root branching from the spinal cord. The symptoms of nerve compressions are sharp, radiating pain; burning; numbness; tingling; and weakness and may occasionally result in loss of all strength or dexterity.

Deep pressure should not be applied to vertebral disks and bony surfaces, but massage may be indicated for the muscles in the area of the compression or muscles that are innervated by the nerve being compressed. However, a physician's clearance is needed.

Nerve entrapment. Nerve entrapments are a dysfunction of a nerve as a result of pressure against it by adjacent soft tissues such as muscle, tendon, fascia, and ligaments. The entrapment can be caused by muscle tightness and shortening resulting from injury or overuse. These tight soft tissues can affect the nerve two ways. They may press an underlying nerve against hard tissues such as bone, disrupting normal nerve function (e.g., thoracic outlet syndrome caused by either the scalene or pectoralis minor muscles pressing the brachial plexus against the ribcage). The other type of entrapment occurs when a nerve actually passes through the belly of a muscle and is constricted by the tightening muscle, much like a rubber band stretched between two fingers (e.g., triceps brachii entrapment of the radial nerve or piriformis entrapment of the sciatic nerve). Both types of entrapment may have symptoms of sharp, radiating pain, especially in the extremities; burning; numbness; pins and needles; or weakness in the affected muscles.

The main goal of the massage treatment is the release of the muscles involved. It is helpful to have a library that includes trigger point manuals and charts. Many clients will already have a medical diagnosis that may name the nerve or muscles implicated. Work deeply, but briefly, to release the tissues responsible for the entrapment; overworking the affected area further traumatizes it.

Palsy is an abnormal condition characterized by paralysis. The three most common forms are Bell's, cerebral, and Erb's.

- **Bell's palsy**. Bell's palsy manifests as unilateral facial paralysis of sudden onset resulting from inflammation of the facial nerve. Paralysis causes distortion of the face and may be so severe that the person may not be able to close an eye or control salivation on the affected side. The symptoms may be transient (lasting only a few months) or permanent.

  Light strokes on the face directed upward are indicated. Light kneading, tapotement, and vibration may help stimulate paralyzed muscles. The client could also massage her own face 2 to 3 times a day to maintain muscle tone.

- **Cerebral palsy**. This is a group of motor disorders resulting in muscular incoordination and loss of muscle control. It is caused by damage to the brain's motor areas during fetal life, birth, or infancy. Causes include rubella infection, toxemia, or malnutrition during pregnancy or damage during birth in which oxygen to the fetus is reduced. Cerebral palsy is not progressive, meaning it does not worsen as time goes on; however, the damage is irreversible. Intelligence is usually not affected, but speech is impaired. The muscles may be spastic and hyperexcitable. Even small movements, touch, muscle stretch, pain, or emotional stress can increase spasticity.

  Relaxing massage treatments with light pressure help reduce spasms and involuntary movements. Passive movements and range-of-motion exercises prevent muscle contractures. Force should not be used to stretch muscles in spasm. Pressure sores may form in clients who use wheelchairs. Avoid massaging ulcer areas and bring them to the attention of the client's caregiver.

- **Erb's palsy**. Often caused by birth injury, Erb's palsy is caused by injury to the upper brachial plexus, causing paralysis in the arm. One or more cervical nerve roots may also be involved.

  Massage is indicated for clients with Erb's palsy, assisting with muscle function, reduction of swelling, and reducing contracture. Because these clients cannot give feedback about their affected limbs, a lighter pressure is indicated.

Paralysis. Paralysis is the loss of muscle function and/or the loss of sensation. This condition can be caused by trauma during a vehicular accident, sporting incidents, gunshot wounds, disease, and poisoning. Paralysis of the lower extremities and trunk is called *paraplegia,* whereas paralysis of the arms and legs is called *quadriplegia.* When the paralysis is restricted to one side of the body, it is called *hemiplegia.*

Massage is fine for clients with paralysis. Because these clients cannot give feedback about their affected limbs, a lighter pressure is indicated. They may also be prone to pressure sores. Avoid massaging the ulcer area and bring it to the notice of the client's caregiver. See also flaccidity and spasticity in muscular pathologies.

Parkinson's disease. Parkinson's disease is a progressive, degenerative, neurological disorder marked by the destruction of the dopamine-producing neurons of the brain and depletion of the neurotransmitter dopamine. Symptoms are stooped posture, shuffling gait, and an expressionless face. Muscles may alternately contract and relax, causing tremors, while other muscles contract continuously, causing rigidity in the involved part. Injections of dopamine are useless because the blood-brain barrier does not permit passage of this neurotransmitter. Levodopa, a dopamine precursor that does cross the blood-brain barrier, is often used to treat this disease.

The goal of massage treatments is to reduce rigidity. Gentle, slow massages of shorter duration are indicated. Passive movements of joints after the massage are also indicated, but force should not be used. Symptoms are reduced, although only temporarily.

Poliomyelitis. Poliomyelitis, or polio, is an infectious disease transmitted through fecal contamination or nasal secretions. It is caused by one of the three polioviruses and can range in severity from relatively asymptomatic to severe paralysis. Factors that influence the susceptibility to the viruses are gender, stress, and age. In spinal poliomyelitis, the virus replicates in the anterior horn of the spinal cord, causing inflammation and eventual destruction of the spinal neurons.

Massage therapists are most likely to encounter adults in the chronic noninfective stage. A lighter massage is indicated because the skin may be dry and fragile. Massage treatments should increase joint mobility and prevent contractures. The paralysis of one group of muscles causes antagonist muscles to increase in tone. The increased tone results in excessive stretch and adhesions of the affected muscle group. Passive range-of-motion exercise helps with joint mobility. Cross-fiber friction over joints and atrophied muscle helps loosen adhesions. It is important to remember that the loss of motor function is irreversible. Pressure sores may be evident in clients who wear braces or use crutches. Avoid massaging the ulcer area and bring it to the attention of the client's caregiver.

Reflex sympathetic dystrophy. Reflex sympathetic dystrophy (RSD) is a complex disorder or group of disorders affecting the limbs. It may develop as a result of trauma (accident, repetitive motion, or surgery). It is characterized by pain, sensory and motor dysfunction, and localized abnormal blood flow.

Massage treatments need to be tailored to the client's specific needs, depending on the extent of the disorder. If the client is experiencing acute symptoms, massage is contraindicated. With less severe symptoms, a gentle massage is indicated, with passive range-of-motion exercise to increase joint mobility.

Sciatica. Inflammation of the sciatic nerve, or sciatica, is a type of neuritis often experienced as a dull pain and tenderness in the buttock region with sharper radiating pain or numbness down the leg. The pain is felt along the path of the sciatic nerve. As inflammation increases, motor function may be affected, with the knee becoming "rubbery" or unstable. Branches of the sciatic nerve may also be affected. Sciatica may be a result of nerve compression from bone or cartilage or nerve entrapment from muscle/soft tissues (most likely the piriformis and other hip outward rotators). It may be unilateral or bilateral and can be brought on by injury, overuse, or excessive emotional stress.

It is a good idea to assess the motor and sensory function and keep a record of it. Treatment needs to be modified according to the cause. For example, if the sciatica is the result of a herniated disk, massage in the area of the disk is contraindicated. However, treatment of quadratus lumborum and psoas major may be helpful. If the sciatica is the result of a tight piriformis muscle, deep specific work in the area is indicated. Deep work right over the sciatic nerve is contraindicated. The aim is to relax muscles, reduce atrophy, prevent spasms, and reduce edema.

Shingles. Shingles is an acute infection of the PNS caused by the reactivation of a latent herpes zoster (chickenpox) virus. Affecting mainly adults, shingles presents itself as painful, blisterlike eruptions in a striplike pattern along the affected nerves of a dermatome (Figure 17-22). Scarring may result. The distribution of the blisters is usually unilateral, typically affecting the thoracic area and sometimes the face, although both sides of the body may be involved. The skin in the area of the blisters is hypersensitive.

Local massage is contraindicated. General massage, if the client feels up to it, is fine. The blisters resulting from shingles contain the chickenpox virus, which is contagious. If you, the therapist, have not had chicken pox, do not massage this area because it is a local contraindication for you.

Spina bifida. Spina bifida is a congenital defect characterized by a lack of osseous development in the lamina (posterior vertebral arch). This condition may be mild (only a small, deformed lamina), or it may be associated with the complete absence of laminae surrounding a large area (usually the lumbar spine). In the more severe cases, the meninges and spinal cord protrude, producing a

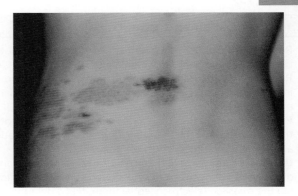

Figure 17-22   Shingles.

saclike appearance in the region. The severe forms cause weakness or paralysis of the legs.

In the less severe forms, general massage is fine, but local massage in the lumbosacral area is contraindicated. The more severe forms cause neurological problems. The aim is to prevent contractures, prevent pressure ulcers, and reduce spasticity. Passive range-of-motion exercise helps prevents contractures; force should not be used to stretch muscles that are in spasm. These clients may be prone to pressure ulcers and edema in the legs or sacral region. Avoid massaging the ulcer area and bring it to the notice of the client's caregiver.

Stroke/cerebrovascular accident. See this section in Chapter 19.

Thoracic outlet syndrome. Thoracic outlet syndrome (TOS) is caused by compression of the brachial nerve, often between the clavicle and the first rib. Nerve compression may be muscular in origin. Pain and weakness down the arm are common symptoms. Some clients also experience pain in the chest and neck.

Massage is indicated to reduce muscle compression, especially the scalenes (pulling the rib upward) and pectoralis minor (compressing the brachial plexus into the rib cage). Massage treatment should also include the entire shoulder girdle, the arm, and the neck.

Transient ischemic attack. Transient ischemic attack (TIA) is an event of temporary cerebral dysfunction caused by ischemia or reduced blood circulation. TIAs are characterized by abnormal vision in one or both eyes, vertigo, shortness of breath, general loss of sensation, or unconsciousness. Common causes are occlusion by embolus, thrombus, or atherosclerotic plaque. The attack is typically sudden and brief (lasting only a few minutes), leaving no long-term neurological damage.

If the client is on anticoagulant therapy, he may be prone to bruising and internal bleeding so a lighter massage is indicated.

See Box 17-2 for the effects of massage on the nervous system.

BOX 17-2

Effects of Massage on the Nervous System

- **Reduces stress.** Stress is reduced by activation of the parasympathetic nervous system.
- **Reduces anxiety.** Ironically, a reduction in anxiety is noted in both the people who received the massage and the massage therapist.
- **Promotes relaxation.** General relaxation is promoted through activation of the relaxation response. Relaxation also has a diminishing effect on pain.
- **Decreases beta wave activity.** Associated with relaxation, a decrease in beta wave activity occurred during and following the massage (electroencephalogram [EEG] determined).
- **Increases delta wave activity.** Increases in delta wave activity are linked to sleep and relaxation; both are promoted with massage (EEG determined).
- **Increases alpha wave activity.** Confirmed by an EEG, an increase in alpha wave activity during massage indicates relaxation.
- **Decreases pain.** Massage relieves local and referred pain caused by hypersensitive trigger points, presumably by increasing circulation, thereby reducing ischemia. Massage also stimulates the release of endorphins (endogenous morphine), enkephalins, and other pain-reducing neurochemicals. General relaxation brought on by massage therapy also has a diminishing effect on pain. The pressure of a massage interferes with pain information entering the spinal cord by stimulating pressure receptors, further reducing pain (Gate Theory). Massage interrupts the pain cycle by relieving muscular spasms, increasing circulation, and promoting rapid disposal of waste products. Massage also improves sleep patterns. During deep sleep, a substance called *somatostatin* is normally released. Without this substance, pain is experienced.

- **Reduces analgesic use.** Because pain is reduced with massage so is the need for pain medication.
- **Activates sensory receptors.** Depending on factors such as stroke choice, direction, speed, and pressure, massage can stimulate different sensory receptors, impacting the massage outcome. For example, cross-fiber tapotement stimulates muscle spindles, which activates muscular contraction, whereas slow, passive stretches activate Golgi tendon organs, which inhibit muscular contraction. Stimulation of sensory pressure receptors reduces pain.
- **More quickly and elaborately develops the hippocampal region of the brain.** Development of the hippocampal region, which is part of the limbic system, is related to superior memory performance.
- **Increases vagal activity.** Increased vagal activity lowers physiological arousal and stress hormones. A decrease in stress hormones leads to enhanced immune functions. One of the branches of the vagus nerve found to be stimulated during massage is the nucleus ambiguus branch, or "smart" branch. Stimulation of this nerve branch increases facial expression and vocalization, which reduces feelings of depression.
- **Shifts EEG activation from right frontal to left frontal.** Right frontal EEG activation is associated with a sad affect and left frontal EEG activation is associated with a happy affect. This implies that the client experienced an improvement of mood during the massage.
- **Decreases H-amplitude levels during massage.** A decrease of 60% to 80% was noted. This reduction is crucial for the comfort of spinal cord injuries patients as it signifies a decrease of muscle cramps and spasm activity.

SUMMARY

A study of the nervous system includes the details of the anatomy and physiology of individual nerve fibers and nerve transmission and a look at the system as a whole.

The neurons are the functional unit of the nervous system and can be classified according to functional (sensory, association, or motor). The interneurons neurons are found in the brain and spinal cord where they connect the sensory and motor neurons. The sensory nerve runs from a remote nerve receptor and enters the posterior horn of the spine. The motor neuron originates at the anterior horn of the same spinal segment and runs until it reaches its target muscle or gland.

The nerve impulse generated when the receptor senses input is an electrochemical reaction to stimuli. This occurs when the stimulus reaches the threshold limit of the neuron, and a nerve impulse is created. This all-or-none response is fueled by a process in which the polarized membrane of the nerve cell becomes depolarized, reverse polarized, and then repolarized. This is accomplished by a complex exchange of sodium and potassium ions across the cellular membrane, which is driven by a mechanism known as the sodium-potassium pump. Nerve impulses are affected by neurotransmitters. The neurotransmitters may facilitate, arouse, or inhibit nerve impulse transmission.

The nervous system as a whole is divided into the CNS and the PNS. The CNS is composed of the brain, spinal cord, cerebrospinal fluid, and meninges.

The PNS consists of the intricate network of many millions of branching nerve fibers that leave and return to the brain and spinal cord, some of which are sensory and some of which are motor. Nerves leaving directly from the brain are referred to as cranial nerves; spinal nerves are those originating from and terminating at the spine. Types of sensory receptors include chemoreceptors, mechanoreceptors, photoreceptors, nociceptors, and thermoreceptors; these provide the specialized senses of taste, olfaction, vision, hearing, and touch.

A subdivision of the PNS is the autonomic nervous system, which in turn is divided into the sympathetic nervous system and the parasympathetic nervous system.

MATCHING I

Write the letter of the best answer in the space provided.

A. Neuron
B. Peripheral nervous system
C. Dendrite
D. Nerve
E. Parasympathetic nervous system

F. Myelin
G. Autonomic nervous system
H. Neuroglia
I. Reflex
J. Sympathetic nervous system

K. Nodes of Ranvier
L. Synapse
M. Central nervous system
N. Neurotransmitter
O. Axon

_____ 1. Division of the autonomic nervous system that creates the alarm reaction; also known as thoracolumbar outflow

_____ 2. Contains the brain, spinal cord, cerebrospinal fluid, and meninges

_____ 3. Nerve cell classified as connective tissue that supports, nourishes, protects, insulates, and organizes the neurons

_____ 4. A group of impulse carrying fibers

_____ 5. Extensions of a nerve cell that receives and transmits stimuli toward the cell body

_____ 6. Contains the cranial and spinal nerves

_____ 7. An impulse-conducting cell possessing the properties of excitability and conductibility

_____ 8. Cell extension transmitting impulses away from the cell body

_____ 9. Junction between two neurons

_____ 10. Chemicals that facilitate, arouse, or inhibit the transmission of nerve impulses

_____ 11. Division of the autonomic nervous system that is involved with the relaxation response; also known as craniosacral outflow

_____ 12. Division of the PNS that is involuntary, supplying the smooth muscles, heart muscle, skin, special senses, some proprioceptors, organs, and glands

_____ 13. Fat- and protein-insulating substance around some axons to assist conduction

_____ 14. An instantaneous, involuntary response to a stimulus

_____ 15. Interruptions in the myelin along an axon that increase neural conduction rate

MATCHING II

Write the letter of the best answer in the space provided.

A. Alpha
B. Nociceptors
C. Golgi tendon organs
D. Cerebrospinal fluid
E. Medulla oblongata

F. Muscle spindles
G. Plexus
H. Proprioceptors
I. All-or-none response
J. Adaptation

K. Dermatome
L. Cerebellum
M. Action potential
N. Ganglion
O. Meninges

_____ 1. Special connective tissue membranes covering the brain and spinal cord

_____ 2. Part of the brain that governs muscle tone, coordination, balance, fine and gross motor movements

_____ 3. When a stimulus generates a nerve impulse, the impulse is conducted along the entire neuron at maximum capacity

_____ 4. A cluster of nerve cell bodies located in the PNS, typically next to the spinal cord

_____ 5. Tendon reflex receptors that respond by inhibiting muscle contraction

_____ 6. Part of the brain stem containing the respiratory, cardiac, and vasomotor centers

_____ 7. The measurement of electrical difference between the inside and outside of the neural cell membrane

_____ 8. A network of intersecting nerves in the PNS

_____ 9. An area of skin that a specific sensory nerve root serves

_____ 10. Clear fluid circulating around the brain and spinal cord

_____ 11. Receptors for detecting pain

_____ 12. The brain wave state that represents a person who is awake but relaxed

_____ 13. Stretch reflex receptors that respond by contracting the muscle

_____ 14. A decrease in sensitivity to a prolonged stimulus

_____ 15. General term for receptors responding to changes in muscle length and tension, and body position

Bibliography

Applegate EJ: *The anatomy and physiology learning system,* ed 2, Philadelphia, 2000, WB Saunders.

Crawley J, Van De Graaff KM: *A photographic atlas for anatomy and physiology,* Englewood, Colo, 2002, Morton.

Crooks R, Stein J: *Psychology: science, behavior, and life,* New York, 1988, Holt, Rinehart, and Winston.

Damjanov I: *Pathology for the health-related professions,* Philadelphia, 1996, WB Saunders.

Gould BE: *Pathophysiology for the health-related professions,* Philadelphia, 1997, WB Saunders.

Grafelman T: *Graf's anatomy and physiology guide for the massage therapist,* Aurora, Colo, 1998, DG Publishing.

Gray H: *Gray's anatomy,* ed 29, Philadelphia, 1974, Running Press.

Haubrich WS: *Medical meanings: a glossary of word origins,* New York, 1984, Harcourt Brace Jovanovich.

Jacob S, Francone C: *Elements of anatomy and physiology,* Philadelphia, 1989, WB Saunders.

Juhan D: *Job's body: a handbook for bodyworkers,* Barrington, NY, 1987, Station Hill Press.

Kalat JW: *Biological psychology,* ed 2, Belmont, Calif, 1984, Wadsworth.

Kapit W, Elson LM: *The anatomy coloring book,* ed 3, New York, 2002, Benjamin Cummings.

Kordish M, Dickson S: *Introduction to basic human anatomy,* Lake Charles, La, 1995, McNeese State University.

Marieb EN: *Essentials of human anatomy and physiology,* ed 4, New York, 1994, Benjamin/Cummings.

McAleer N: *The body almanac,* Garden City, NY, 1985, Doubleday.

McAtee R: *Facilitated stretching,* Champaign, Ill, 1993, Human Kinetics.

Melzack R, Wall PD: *The challenge of pain,* New York, 1982, Basic Books.

Merck Research Laboratories: *Merck manual,* ed 17, Whitehouse Station, NJ, 1998, Author.

Mosby's medical, nursing, and allied health dictionary, ed 4, St Louis, 1994, Mosby.

Newton D: *Pathology for massage therapists,* ed 2, Portland, 1995, Simran.

Premkumar K: *Pathology A to Z: a handbook for massage therapists,* Calgary, 1996, VanPub Books.

Solomon EP, Phillips GA: *Understanding human anatomy and physiology,* Philadelphia, 1987, WB Saunders.

St. John P: *St. John neuromuscular therapy seminars,* manual I, Largo, Fla, 1995, Author.

Taber's cyclopedic medical dictionary, ed 13, Philadelphia, 1977, FA Davis.

Thibodeau G, Patton K: *Structure and function of the body,* ed 11, St Louis, 2000, Mosby.

Tortora GJ: *Introduction to the human body: the essentials of anatomy and physiology,* ed 3, New York, 1994, Harper-Collins.

Tortora GJ, Grabowksi SR: *Principles of anatomy and physiology,* ed 9, New York, 2000, John Wiley.

Travell JG, Simons D: *Myofascial pain and dysfunction: the trigger point manual,* Baltimore, 1983, Williams and Wilkins.

Voss DE, Ionta MK, Myers BJ: *Proprioceptive neuromuscular facilitation,* Philadelphia, 1985, Harper and Row.

Werner R: *A massage therapist's guide to pathology,* ed 2, Baltimore, 2002, Lippincott Williams & Wilkins.

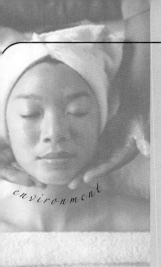

environment

Endocrine Glands and Hormones

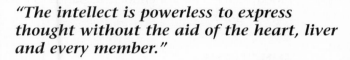

18

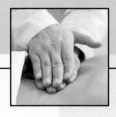

pressure

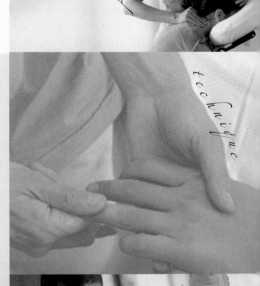

technique

"The intellect is powerless to express thought without the aid of the heart, liver and every member."

—Wordsworth

STUDENT OBJECTIVES

After completing this chapter, the student should be able to:

- Identify the four functions of the endocrine system
- Describe the types of hormones
- Explain the hormonal control systems
- Identify specific endocrine glands
- Name the hormones produced and secreted by each endocrine gland
- Discuss the function of each glandular hormone
- Name types of endocrine pathologies, giving characteristics and massage considerations of each

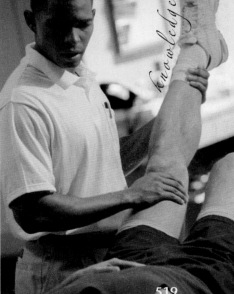

knowledge

INTRODUCTION

The two types of glands of the body are exocrine and endocrine. **Exocrine glands** contain cells that produce secretions and use ducts to transport these products to their site of action. Examples of exocrine glands are sudoriferous, sebaceous, and salivary glands. **Endocrine glands** have cells that produce glandular secretions called *hormones*. Also known as *ductless glands,* endocrine glands empty their products directly in the bloodstream, which carries the hormones to the sites of action. Some glands such as the pancreas and ovaries are both endocrine and exocrine glands. The gastric mucosa possesses both endocrine and exocrine cells (G cells, parietal, and chief cells). The placenta, an organ of pregnancy, also produces and secretes hormones (human chorionic gonadotropin [HCG], estrogen, and progesterone).

The endocrine system is the second major controlling and communicating system of the body. The first the nervous system, and its activity is relatively fast. The nervous and endocrine systems work together to integrate body activities. The endocrine system regulates processes that continue for relatively long periods, and its effects are more widespread, in comparison to the nervous system.

In contrast, the nervous system detects a stimulus and reports it to the brain, which produces a response (the exception is a reflex). The endocrine system is stimulated through feedback systems and gives a report to the hypothalamus and/or the pituitary, which produces a response. Instead of an electrical response (like the nervous system), however, it is a hormonal response.

Terms and Their Meanings Related to the Endocrine System

Term	Meaning
adenohypophysis	gland; below; to grow
adrenal	kidney
antidiuretic	against; urine; production
diabetes	overflow; passing through
endocrine	within; to separate
exocrine	away from; to separate
hormone	to excite, arouse, or urge on
insipidus	not; tasty
mellitus	sugar; honey
oxytocin	swift; childbirth
pancreas	all flesh
pineal	pine cone
polydipsia	much or many; thirst
suprarenal	above; kidney
thyroid	shield; shaped

Compared with other body systems, which are made up of fairly large organs, the glands of the endocrine system may seem small and unimportant. Although the total weight of all the endocrine glands is less than one half pound, normal functioning of the endocrine system is vital to the body's physiology, which becomes apparent when hormone levels are too low or high; drastic changes in the body's metabolism occur when hormonal levels are out of balance.

The endocrine system consists of the endocrine glands and glandular secretions called *hormones*. Endocrine glands are surrounded by rich capillary networks. The purpose of the vascularity of the endocrine glands is to assist the delivery of hormones to their sites of action. Hormones are carried by the blood, so it is vital for endocrine glands to have good blood supply.

FUNCTIONS

The functions of the endocrine system are as follows:
1. To produce and secrete hormones
2. To regulate body activities such as growth, development, metabolism, and fluid, mineral, and electrolyte balance
3. To help the body to adapt during times of stress, such as infection, trauma, dehydration, emotional stress, and starvation
4. To contribute to the reproductive process

Each hormone has its own specific role to play in regulating body activities. Each of the endocrine glands and the functions of their hormones are discussed in Individual Endocrine Glands.

HORMONES

The word *hormone* means to set in motion or to arouse. **Hormones** are internal secretions that are chemical messengers of the endocrine system. They act as catalysts in biochemical reactions and regulate the physiological activity of other cells in the body. Because hormones circulate freely in the blood, they have the potential of coming into contact with every type of cell in the body. However, hormones *do not affect* every cell they may encounter. Each type of hormone is specifically programmed to seek out a corresponding type of cell, called **target cells**. The target cells contain *receptor sites,* which are chemically compatible with their corresponding hormone. When the hormone comes into contact with the receptor site of the target cell, they lock together like puzzle pieces, and the resulting chemical change produces the desired effect on the cell. This arousal of the target cell usually increases or decreases the rate of its primary metabolic function.

Types of Hormones

Hormones may be grouped according to their chemical makeup. The four most common types of hormones are steroids, peptides, biogenic amines, and eicosanoids.

Steroid hormones alter cell activity by turning genes on or off. Hormones of the adrenal cortex and gonads are steroid hormones.

Peptide hormones introduce a series of chemical reactions to alter the cell's metabolism. Hormones of the pituitary gland, parathyroid glands, and some of the hormones of the thyroid glands are peptide hormones.

Biogenic amines function as neurotransmitters. Hormones of the adrenal medulla and thyroid gland are both biogenic amines and the catecholamines histamine, serotonin, and dopamine. These substances regulate blood pressure, waste elimination, body temperature, and many other functions.

Eicosanoids alter smooth muscle contractions, blood flow, nerve impulse transmission, and immune responses. Also called *tissue hormones,* eicosanoids are produced by almost every cell in the body.

Hormonal Control Systems

The body uses three mechanisms to control the amount of hormones secreted by the endocrine glands. These are the negative feedback system, hormonal control system, and neural control system.

Negative feedback system. Most hormone levels in the body are regulated by a negative feedback system. Information about blood hormone levels is relayed back to the endocrine gland, and the gland responds by secreting more or less hormone. This process is known as the *negative feedback system* because the stimulus triggers the negative, or opposite, response (Figure 18-1). For example, when a low level of calcium is in the bloodstream, it triggers an increase of parathyroid hormone from the parathyroid gland, releasing stored calcium from the bones into the bloodstream. This increase continues until the level of calcium exceeds the target value or becomes high; the parathyroid then responds negatively by decreasing production. This principle may be confusing unless we apply it to something that we use every day.

A more familiar example would be a home's central-air unit that controls the climate by using a negative feedback system. When the temperature rises above a set point (target value), the air-conditioning unit is activated and cold air blows through vents to cool the dwelling. When the room temperature drops below the set point, the cooling system is shut down. Conversely, the central heat unit will work in the opposite direction; it will warm the house when the temperature drops too low. In comparing the two, remember that the direction of change is not important; the effect is always opposite the stimulus. The temperature is thus controlled in a narrow range by responding negatively to the input.

Hormonal control system. Hormones themselves can stimulate or inhibit the release of other

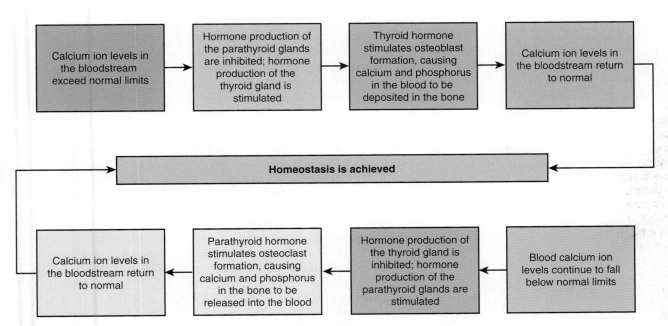

Figure 18-1 Negative feedback regulation of the endocrine system.

JANET TRAVELL, MD

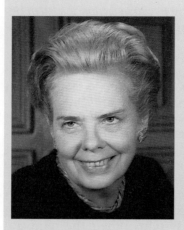

Born: December 17, 1901;
died: August 1, 1997.

"It is obvious that our potential for optimal health depends not alone on the pathology of disease, but on the fiber of our personalities."

At the 1949 American Medical Association (AMA) convention, a renowned British rheumatologist and author was introduced to Dr. Janet Travell. His response was, "Oooh! Dr. Travell! Soooo, you're the Trigger Queen."

Most massage therapists today are familiar with Travell's groundbreaking work, but mapping previously uncharted patterns of pain is only part of this extraordinary woman's legacy. In addition to her unceasing study of the human body, she was a poet, mother, and the first female physician in the White House.

As a youngster, Travell loved the process of learning but especially enjoyed the sciences. During her school days, one of her roles was to supply the class with earthworms for dissection. Summer months were spent at the farm engrossed in education of a different sort: tree climbing, storm watching and of course, earthworm collecting. Her mother taught her basket making, tooling leather, sewing, tatting lace, and knitting.

Her father was responsible for teaching her how to shoot—and how to think. He also showed her how to make the best use of her time. "Over and over, he pointed out the value of time and the importance of concentration," she has been quoted as saying. "If I could do a piece of homework well in fifteen minutes, I should not dawdle over it for thirty. I learned to shut out extraneous matters and to accelerate the pace of my thinking. Another technique of learning that my father taught me to focus on was to focus my attention on things I did not know—new ideas, strange words, and my own mistakes."

Travell wanted to follow in her father's footsteps and become a physician "because he was a magician and everything he did was wonderful." It did not surprise Travell when learned through her mother that he regularly set off giant firecrackers in the fireplace at 3 AM. "I think that he must have been born with a firecracker in one hand and a lighted match in the other," she wrote in her autobiography.

Travell's daughter, Virginia P. Wislon, says this about her grandfather: "I think my mother's energy was inherited from her father, Dr. Willard Travell, an early pioneer in the field of physical medicine. My sister has the same energy. We call it 'the Travell energy' in the family. Those who possess it walk fast so it is difficult to keep up with them, and they get an enormous amount done in a day. They never waste time. They are trim, never overweight, organized people who plan their work, recreation, and activities well."

Travell completed tasks too quickly to suit one of her medical school professors. Again and again, he accused her of hurrying through her dissection. Travell came up with the idea of doing the dissection with her left hand, to slow her down enough to match the speed of the rest of the students. Not only did this appease her professor, she delighted at her newfound ambidexterity.

To better balance career and family, Travell scaled her practice of medicine back to part time. However, it did not really slow her down much; she simply earned less money. Jack Powell, her husband, said that before they married, he had thought carefully about the consequences of starting a life with someone whose career made her quite different from most of the women of her time. He knew he could not make her into something other than who she was, so he accepted her wholly and completely, including her rigorous daily

JANET TRAVELL, MD—cont'd

schedule, offering her support when and where she needed it the most. In a reunion address 45 years after her medical school graduation, Travell commended him and the importance of the man behind every successful woman.

Travell's part-time schedule did give her the freedom to practice at home. Her initial investigation into muscular pain rose out of this additional time to do research, her father's physical medicine experience, and her own shoulder injury at age 38.

When working in a cardiac clinic, she had also treated patients with life-threatening pulmonary disease. Common among both the heart and lung patients were complaints of persistent, acute pain in the shoulder area. Travell came up with enough published findings, mostly from outside the United States, to begin her own study.

She researched, ignored skeptics, looked at muscle tissue under a microscope, injected, poked, prodded, and sprayed but did not even stop there. She recognized the role of body mechanics and quizzed patients about how they stood, worked, or turned. She discovered that muscles have memory and can stay contracted for long periods. She found evidence of existing myofascial pain from old injuries that responded to trigger point therapy. Although the prevailing protocol in her time was heat for sore muscles, she successfully experimented with the use of cold. She developed a method for painless needle injections and even meandered into chair design for a time. She was a "whole body practitioner" who listened carefully to her patients, preached preventative medicine, and made pain go away, even for those whose pain had been diagnosed for years by stumped doctors as psychosomatic.

She bemoaned the fact that so many of us are willing to accept average health. With this intense dedication and track record for success, it is no wonder that word of her reputation reached the young Senator John F. Kennedy for whom Travell is credited with getting in good enough shape to launch a presidential race. In return, he appointed her White House Physician. After his assassination, Travell remained on staff at President Lyndon Johnson's request. During her tenure in the position, she missed only 1 day due to illness. "Although my health was not a problem, I took the precautions of having thorough medical checkups and of taking a sensible dose of regular exercise," she stated in her autobiography. On her departure the Johnsons presented her with a token of their appreciation—a framed, "Prescription for Happiness" that stated at the top, "OFFICE HOURS Day & Night." That indeed had been my life," she said in the book she later named after the plaque, "and my happiness was founded on hard work."

Travell left the White House in 1965, and although she was 64, she was in no way considering retirement. She published her autobiography in 1968, and in 1992, she and David G. Simons published *The Trigger Point Manuals*.

Wilson describes her mother as "a true humanitarian who wanted to solve the pain problems of as many people as she could and didn't stop answering letters and reading her journals until a few weeks before her death at [age] 95, on August 1, 1997." Richard and Kathryn Weiner of the American Academy of Pain Management wrote a tribute to Travell that included the following line: "She loved those whom she encountered and in return received that special gift of knowing that her life mattered."

hormones in the endocrine system. For example, thyroid-stimulating hormone, released by the anterior lobe of the pituitary, activates the thyroid gland to secrete thyroxine and triiodothyronine.

Neural control system. Some hormones are secreted as a result of direct nerve stimulation, the most classic example being the release of epinephrine and norepinephrine from the adrenal medulla. Sympathetic arousal, also known as the *stress response,* releases epinephrine and norepinephrine into the bloodstream to maintain the fight-or-flight response. The neural control system has a much faster response time than the negative feedback or the hormonal control systems.

INDIVIDUAL ENDOCRINE GLANDS

The nine individual endocrine glands are the pituitary, pineal, thyroid, parathyroid, thymus, and adrenal glands; pancreas, female ovaries, and male testes (Figure 18-2). The pituitary's posterior lobe and the adrenal medulla are not technically endocrine glands because they contain neurosecretory cells (specialized nervous tissue that secretes hormones).

Pituitary gland. The bilobed pituitary gland sits in the sella turcica of the sphenoid bone and extends from the hypothalamus by a stalklike structure known as the *infundibulum.* Approximately the size of a small grape, the pituitary gland is protected on all sides by osseous tissue and is considered to be the most protected gland in the body. The pituitary gland was once known as the *master*

gland because its hormones control and stimulate other glands to produce and secrete their hormones (Figure 18-3). The pituitary itself also has a master—the hypothalamus, which sends hormones and nerve impulses to control secretions of the pituitary gland; the hypothalamus is the true master gland. The pituitary gland consists of anterior and posterior lobes.

- **Anterior lobe.** Also known as the *adenohypophysis,* the anterior lobe of the pituitary constitutes about 75% of the total weight of the entire gland. Of the nine hormones secreted by the pituitary gland, seven are produced by the anterior lobe. The anterior lobe and the hypothalamus are interconnected by a rich vascular network. Hormones from the hypothalamus travel this network to stimulate or inhibit the release of hormones from the pituitary's anterior lobe (Table 18-1).

For Your Information

To memorize the hormones of the anterior pituitary, use the mnemonic phrase, *Flat miles per gallon:* follicle-stimulating hormone, luteinizing hormone, adrenocorticotropic hormone, thyroid stimulating hormone, melanocyte-stimulating hormone, prolactin, and human growth hormone.

- **Posterior lobe.** Also known as *neurohypophysis,* the posterior lobe of the pituitary is not technically an endocrine gland because it does not

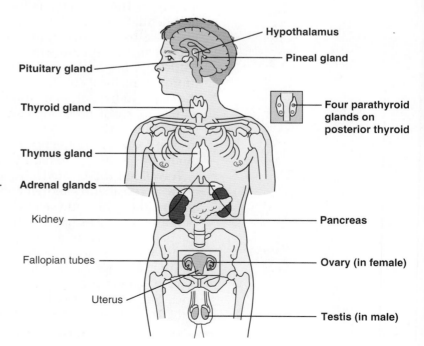

Figure 18-2 Location of all endocrine glands.

Hypothalamus

Pineal gland

Pituitary gland

Thyroid gland

Four parathyroid glands on posterior thyroid

Thymus gland

Adrenal glands

Kidney

Pancreas

Fallopian tubes

Ovary (in female)

Uterus

Testis (in male)

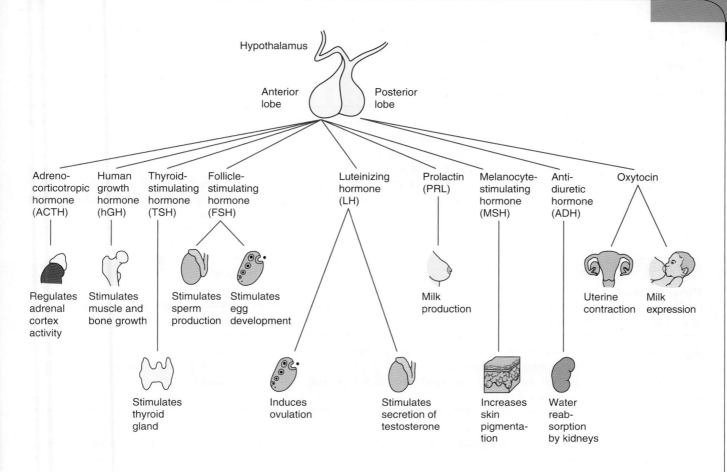

Figure 18-3   The pituitary gland with all hormones.

TABLE 18-1

Anterior Pituitary

Hormone	Abbreviation	Action(s)
Adrenocorticotropic hormone	ACTH	Regulates endocrine activity of the adrenal cortex, especially cortisol secretions.
Human growth hormone (somatotropin)	hGH	Stimulates protein synthesis for muscle/bone growth and maintenance; plays a role in metabolism.
Thyroid-stimulating hormone	TSH	Stimulates the thyroid gland to produce and secrete triiodothyronine (T_3) and thyroxine (T_4).
Follicle-stimulating hormone	FSH	Stimulates estrogen production and egg development in the ovaries; stimulates sperm production in the testes.
Luteinizing hormone	LH	Stimulates ovulation and the production of estrogen and progesterone by the ovaries; stimulates testosterone secretion by the testes.
Prolactin	PRL	Stimulates milk production in the mammary glands.
Melanocyte-stimulating hormone	MSH	Increases skin pigmentation by stimulating the distribution of melanin granules.

TABLE 18-2

Posterior Pituitary

Hormone	Abbreviation	Action(s)	Commentary
Antidiuretic hormone (vasopressin)	ADH	Decreases urine output by stimulating the kidneys to reabsorb water to prevent dehydration; raises blood pressure by constricting arteries.	Alcohol consumption inhibits secretion of ADH, increasing urine production.
Oxytocin	Not applicable	Involved in milk expression from the mammary glands and in uterine contractions.	A synthetic version of oxytocin, Pitocin, is used to stimulate labor in pregnant women.

TABLE 18-3

Pineal Gland

Hormone	Action(s)	Commentary
Melatonin	Involved in the control of circadian rhythms (occurring daily, such as sleeping and eating) and in the growth and development of sexual organs.	When injected into the body, melatonin produces drowsiness; inhibits the secretion of luteinizing hormone.

produce the hormones it releases. It stores and releases hormones produced by the hypothalamus. The cellular makeup of the posterior lobe is similar to the neuroglia cells of the nervous system and are called *neurosecretory cells* (Table 18-2).

Pineal gland. The pineal gland is a pine cone-shaped structure in the brain, attached to the roof of the third ventricle and inferior to the corpus callosum. Although its function is not clear, the pineal gland produces and secretes the hormone melatonin (Table 18-3).

Thyroid gland. Located at the base of the throat, posterior and inferior to the larynx, is the butterfly-shaped thyroid gland (Figure 18-4). The thyroid gland is a bilobed gland connected in the center by a mass of tissue known as the *isthmus* (Table 18-4).

Parathyroid glands. Usually four in number, the tiny parathyroid glands are located on the posterolateral surface of the thyroid lobes (Table 18-5; see Figure 18-4).

Thymus gland. The thymus gland is a bilobed gland posterior to the sternum (see Figure 18-4).

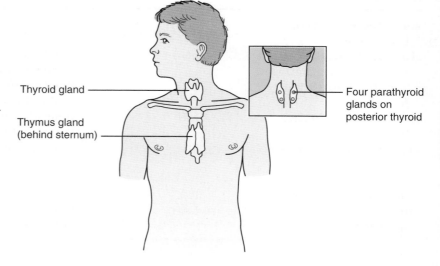

Figure 18-4   The thyroid, parathyroid, and thymus glands.

Thyroid gland

Thymus gland (behind sternum)

Four parathyroid glands on posterior thyroid

TABLE 18-4

Thyroid Gland

Hormone	Abbreviation	Action(s)	Commentary
Triiodothyronine	T_3	Regulates growth and development and influences mental, physical, and metabolic activities.	This hormone consists of a small peptide molecule bound to iodine; therefore it cannot be made without iodine. Some good sources of iodine are iodized salt and seafood.
Thyroxine	T_4	See T_3.	See T_3.
Calcitonin	CT	Decreases blood calcium and phosphorus levels by stimulating osteoblasts to make bone matrix, causing calcium and phosphorus to be deposited in the bones.	Low calcitonin production contributes to insufficient calcium in the body. Calcitonin production decreases in older adults, which may explain why many older people experience an increase in the decalcification of bones.

TABLE 18-5

Parathyroid Gland

Hormone	Abbreviation	Action(s)
Parathyroid hormone	PTH	Blood calcium levels are increased by stimulating osteoclast activity, breaking down bone tissue; the liberated calcium is released in the bloodstream, raising blood calcium levels; PTH also increases calcium reabsorption from urine and the intestines back into the blood.

TABLE 18-6

Thymus

Hormone	Action(s)	Commentary
Thymosin	Plays a role in the body's growth and development; sexual maturation; growth and maturation of antibodies, namely T cells.	T cells are a type of white blood cell that destroys bacteria and viruses; thymosin appears to be present in copious amounts in young children and decreases throughout life.
Thymopoietin	Same as thymosin.	

Large in infancy, the thymus reaches its maximum size at puberty; it then atrophies and is replaced by adipose tissue in adulthood (Table 18-6).

Adrenal glands. The adrenal glands (suprarenals) are located superior to each kidney and are among the most vascular organs in the body. These important glands are divided into two regions and, like the pituitary gland, possess two types of tissue, each producing different hormones (Figure 18-5).

1. The **adrenal cortex** is the outer region and makes up most of the gland. It arises from the embryonic tissue endoderm, which is similar

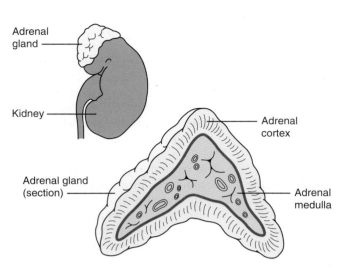

Figure 18-5   The adrenal cortex and medulla.

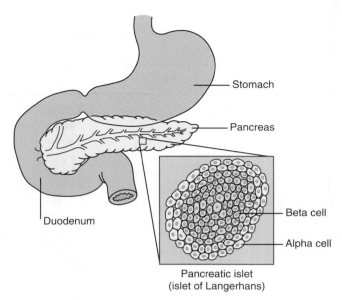

Figure 18-6   Beta cells of alpha cells of the islets of Langerhans.

to that of the kidneys. The hormones of the adrenal cortex are steroid hormones (Table 18-7).

2. The **adrenal medulla** is the inner region of the adrenals, which arises from ectoderm. The hormones of the adrenal medulla, also called *neurohormones*, mimic the effects of the sympathetic nervous system and account for the sudden emergency energy required for the stress response (Table 18-8).

TABLE 18-7

Adrenal Cortex

Hormone	Action(s)
Aldosterone	Stimulates the retention of sodium and water in kidney filtration; helps maintain proper mineral balance; monitors blood volume.
Cortisol	Affects carbohydrate, protein, and fat metabolism; produces an antiinflammatory response.
Androgen	Promotes male secondary sex characteristics.

TABLE 18-8

Adrenal Medulla

Hormone	Action(s)	Commentary
Epinephrine (adrenaline)	Increases blood pressure by stimulating vasoconstriction, rather than affecting cardiac output; occurs in response to stress.	Epinephrine is broken down slowly, so the effects on the sympathetic nervous system are long lasting.
Norepinephrine (noradrenaline)	Helps the body maintain the stress response by increased heart rate, blood pressure, and blood glucose levels and by dilation of the bronchi; results in more oxygen and glucose in the blood and a faster circulation of blood to the body organs and most importantly, to the brain, muscles, and heart.	Norepinephrine is also broken down slowly, so the effects on the sympathetic nervous system are long lasting.

TABLE 18-9

Pancreas

Hormone	Action	Commentary
Insulin	Decreases blood glucose levels (hypoglycemic).	Insulin, secreted by beta cells, is the only hormone that decreases blood glucose levels and is necessary for metabolism. Because this hormone is deactivated by digestive enzymes, it cannot be administered orally. If an individual requires insulin, it must be given by injection.
Glucagon	Increases blood glucose levels (hyperglycemic).	Glucagon, secreted by the alpha cells, is stimulated by low blood levels of glucose, causing the liver and the skeletal muscles to break down stored glycogen into glucose.

For Your Information

Although it is a commonly used term, *Adrenalin* is a registered trademark for epinephrine held by the Parke-Davis Company.

Pancreas. The pancreas, or pancreatic gland, is located inferior to the stomach and is both endocrine and exocrine. Within the pancreas are islands of specialized cells called the **islets of Langerhans** or **pancreatic islets**. The pancreas contains more than 1 million islets, each consisting of *alpha* and *beta cells* (Figure 18-6) that function like an organ within an organ. Both hormones of the pancreas help regulate carbohydrate metabolism (Table 18-9).

Gonads. The ovaries and testes, or gonads, are the reproductive glands. They function both as endocrine and exocrine glands. The testes are located in the male scrotum, and the ovaries are located in the pelvic cavity of the female body. The hormones of both glands stimulate the growth and development of primary sex organs and secondary sex characteristics and play a very important role in reproduction (Figure 18-7).

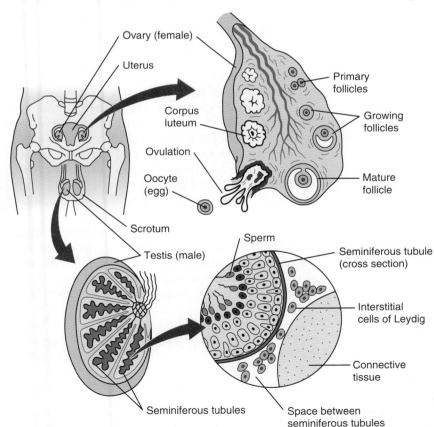

Figure 18-7   The gonads and hormonal function of each.

TABLE 18-10

Ovaries

Hormone	Action(s)	Commentary
Estrogen	Responsible for female secondary sex characteristics; during menstrual cycles, estrogen triggers the preparation of the female organs for fertilization and implantation of the early embryo. Helps keep calcium in bones.	Estrogen is also produced in the placenta.
Progesterone	Prepares the endometrium for pregnancy and helps maintain the corpus luteum once conception and implantation occurs.	One cause of spontaneous abortion (miscarriage) is a drop in progesterone levels.
Relaxin	Softens the connective tissue in the body of a pregnant woman, especially the pelvic ligaments, for fetal delivery; helps dilate the cervix during labor and delivery.	*Because relaxin loosens connective tissue during pregnancy, all range of motion and stretching modalities must be kept to a minimum and performed with caution.*

- **Ovaries**. Within the ovaries, a structure called the *corpus luteum* produces the hormones estrogen, progesterone, and relaxin (Table 18-10).

For Your Information

The first oral contraceptive, Enovid, was approved by the Food and Drug Administration in 1960. It was manufactured and distributed that same year. More than 9 million women in the United States and Europe use oral contraceptives (birth control pills) every year.

- **Testes**. Within the testes are groups of specialized cells called the *interstitial cells of Leydig*. These cells produce and secrete androgens, namely testosterone (Table 18-11).

ENDOCRINE PATHOLOGIES

Acromegaly. Acromegaly, or acromegalia, is caused by the overproduction of growth hormone during the adult years. It is characterized by elongation and enlargement of the bones of the extremities, face, and jaw. The condition mainly affects middle-age and older persons.

A gentle massage is permissible, after obtaining clearance from the client's physician.

Addison's disease. Addison's disease is caused by failure of adrenal functions, often resulting from an autoimmune disease, local or general infection, or adrenal hemorrhage. The disease is characterized by general weakness, reduced endurance, and an increase in pigmentation of the skin and mucous membranes (called *bronzing*). Loss of appetite, anxiety, lethargy, depression, and other emotional disturbances often accompany this disease.

A gentle, relaxing full body massage of shorter duration is indicated.

Cretinism. A congenital deficiency in the secretion of the thyroid hormones, cretinism is characterized by a lack of physical and mental development. This condition is typical in countries where the diet is deficient in iodine and where goiters are common. The addition of iodized salt reduces the occurrence of cretinism.

A gentle, relaxing massage is indicated, avoiding the neck region.

Cushing's disease. Classified as a metabolic disorder, Cushing's disease is caused by an overproduction of adrenocortical steroids. An overabundance of these hormones causes an accumulation of fluids and fat on the face, neck, and upper back.

TABLE 18-11

Testes

Hormone	Action(s)
Testosterone	Promotes secondary male sex characteristics, libido (sex drive), and sperm production.

Other conditions that may develop are muscle weakness, purplish streaks on the skin, acne, osteoporosis, and diabetes mellitus. The person bruises easily, and wound healing is poor.

A very gentle massage is indicated.

Diabetes. Diabetes refers to a family of metabolic disorders that alter the fluid balance of the body. The four main types of diabetes are as follows:

1. **Diabetes mellitus**. This is a group of disorders that lead to elevated blood glucose levels (hyperglycemia). Glucose appears in the urine and is accompanied by polyuria (excessive excretion of urine), excessive eating (polyphagia), and polydipsia (excessive thirst), and peripheral neuropathy. Type I diabetes entails a deficiency of insulin, and regular injections of insulin are needed. It is thought to be an autoimmune disease because the beta cells of the pancreas, which produce insulin, are destroyed. Type II diabetes represents more than 90% of all cases. Long-term complications such as **peripheral vascular disease** (decreased circulation in the hands and feet) and **neuropathy** (decrease/change in sensation in hands and feet) may develop as the disease progresses. Other complications are atherosclerosis, high blood pressure, blindness, and thrombosis. It usually occurs later and can be controlled by diet, exercise, and weight loss.

   Relaxing and gentle massage is indicated for clients with diabetes mellitus. Sometimes clients cannot give accurate feedback about pressure because of accompanying neuropathy, so lighter pressure is indicated. Inform the clients of any bruises or breaks in the skin. If your client is taking insulin, massage should not be done on or around the injection site. The increased circulation speeds up insulin absorption and may cause a low blood sugar reaction. Vigorous massage, especially tapotement and vibration, must be carefully administered because it can damage already compromised blood vessels. It is important that clients have their necessary medications (e.g., insulin, antidiuretic hormone [ADH]) with them when they come for treatment in the event of a diabetes-related emergency.

2. **Diabetes insipidus**. This is caused by a posterior pituitary gland dysfunction that results in deficient production of ADH. Diabetes insipidus has absolutely nothing to do with insulin production or pancreatic dysfunction, but like diabetes mellitus, it results in polyuria, thus reducing fluid volume in the body and increasing thirst.

   The same considerations apply as in diabetes mellitus.

3. **Nephrogenic diabetes insipidus**. This is much the same as diabetes insipidus, except that the cause results from kidney dysfunction, often as a result of disease or damage, rather than pituitary gland dysfunction. Blood levels of ADH are normal, but the kidneys do not respond to it. Instead of concentrating impurities into a small amount of urine, the kidneys filter large amounts of water with impurities, resulting in dilute urine and excessive fluid loss.

   The same considerations apply as in diabetes mellitus.

4. **Gestational diabetes mellitus**. This usually occurs in women in the second and third trimesters of pregnancy. Hormones secreted by the placenta disturb the function of insulin, causing expectant mothers to become glucose intolerant. This condition is temporary, usually diminishing after the baby is born.

   A gentle, relaxing massage is indicated.

Goiter. An enlarged thyroid gland, or goiter, is associated with hyperthyroidism, hypothyroidism, inflammation, infection, or lack of iodine in the diet. Goiters are more prevalent in countries where dietary iodine intake is inadequate. Iodized salt reduces the occurrence of goiters.

Massage is fine for clients who have goiters. However, the throat region should be avoided.

Graves' disease. Graves' disease is characterized by hyperthyroidism, related anxiety, fatigue, tremors of the hands, loss of appetite, and increased metabolic rate. An enlarged thyroid and lymph nodes and an unusual protrusion of the eyeballs often accompany this condition. This disease is thought to be an autoimmune disorder.

A gentle full-body massage is indicated. Massage over the throat region and any enlarged lymph nodes is contraindicated.

Hyperthyroidism. Hyperactivity of the thyroid gland, hyperthyroidism is characterized by an enlarged thyroid, nervousness and tremor, heat intolerance, increased appetite with weight loss, rapid forceful pulse, and increased respiration rate.

Massage is fine for clients with hyperthyroidism. However, the throat region should be avoided.

Hypoglycemia. Hypoglycemia is almost the opposite of diabetes, although it too can be related to pancreatic dysfunction. *Hypoglycemia* refers to an excessive loss in blood glucose levels that can result in a variety of symptoms including weakness, light-headedness, headaches, excessive hunger, visual disturbances, anxiety, and sudden changes in personality. If left untreated, the result may be delirium, coma, and death. Causes of hypoglycemia can be an overdose of prescribed insulin, an excessive level of insulin production by the pancreas, or extreme dietary deficiencies.

Massage is fine for clients with hypoglycemia. However, they may experience light-headedness when getting up from the massage table, so they may need assistance.

TABLE 18-12

Hormonal Functions

Hormone	Gland	Primary Action(s)
Adrenocorticotropic hormone (ACTH)	Pituitary (anterior lobe)	Regulates endocrine activity of the adrenal cortex.
Aldosterone	Adrenals (cortex)	Stimulates the reabsorption of sodium and water in kidney filtration.
Androgen	Adrenals (cortex)	Maintains male sex characteristics.
Antidiuretic hormone (ADH)	Pituitary (posterior lobe)	Decreases urine output and raises blood pressure.
Calcitonin (CT)	Thyroid	Decreases blood calcium and phosphorus levels.
Cortisol	Adrenals (cortex)	Produces an antiinflammatory response and affects carbohydrate, protein, and fat metabolism.
Epinephrine	Adrenals (medulla)	Increases blood pressure by stimulating vasoconstriction.
Estrogen	Ovaries	Prepares female genital tract for fertilization and implantation embryo and helps keep calcium in bones.
Follicle stimulating hormone (FSH)	Pituitary (anterior lobe)	Stimulates ovarian egg development and production; stimulates sperm production in testes.
Glucagon	Pancreas	Increases blood glucose levels.
Human growth hormone (hGH)	Pituitary (anterior lobe)	Stimulates protein synthesis for muscle and bone growth.
Insulin	Pancreas	Decreases blood glucose levels.
Luteinizing hormone (LH)	Pituitary (anterior lobe)	Stimulates ovulation and production of estrogen and progesterone in ovaries; stimulates testosterone secretion in testes.
Melanocyte stimulating hormone (MSH)	Pituitary (anterior lobe)	Stimulates distribution of melanin, increasing skin pigmentation.
Melatonin	Pineal	Controls circadian rhythms and growth and development of sexual organs.
Norepinephrine	Adrenals (medulla)	Helps body maintain the stress response.
Oxytocin	Pituitary (posterior lobe)	Involved in milk expression and uterine contractions.
Parathyroid hormone (PTH)	Parathyroid	Increases blood calcium levels.
Progesterone	Ovaries	Prepares endometrium for pregnancy.
Prolactin (PRL)	Pituitary (anterior lobe)	Stimulates milk production.
Relaxin	Ovaries	Softens connective tissue of a pregnant woman for fetal delivery.
Testosterone	Testes	Promotes secondary male sex characteristics, libido, and sperm production.
Thymopoietin	Thymus	Play a role in the body's growth and maturation of antibodies.
Thymosin	Thymus	Play a role in the body's growth and maturation of antibodies.
Thyroid stimulating hormone (TSH)	Pituitary (anterior lobe)	Stimulates thyroid to produce and secrete triiodothyronine and thyroxine.
Triiodothyronine (T_3)	Thyroid	Regulates growth and development and influences mental, physical, and metabolic activites.
Thyroxine (T_4)	Thyroid	Regulates growth and development and influences mental, physical, and metabolic activities.

Hypothyroidism. A deficiency of thyroid activity, hypothyroidism is marked by fatigue and lethargy; weight gain; slowed mental processes; skin dryness; and slow digestive, heart, and respiration rates. More common in women, this condition may lead to cretinism.

Massage is fine for clients with hypothyroidism. However, the throat region should be avoided.

See Box 18-1 for the effects of massage on the endocrine system.

BOX 18-1

Effects of Massage on the Endocrine System

- **Increases dopamine level.** Linked to decreased stress levels and reduced depression.
- **Increases serotonin level.** Suggests a reduction of both stress and depression. It is believed that serotonin inhibits transmission of noxious signals to the brain, indicating that increased levels of serotonin may also reduce pain.
- **Reduces cortisol level.** Reduces cortisol level by activating the relaxation response. Elevated levels of cortisol not only represent heightened stress but also inhibited immune functions.
- **Reduces norepinephrine level.** Reduces norepinephrine, which is linked to the relaxation response.
- **Reduces epinephrine level.** Reduced with massage.
- **Reduces feelings of depression.** Both chemical and electrophysiological changes from a negative to a positive mood were noted and may underline the decrease in depression after massage therapy.

SUMMARY

The endocrine glands and the hormones they secrete make up the endocrine system (Table 18-12). The endocrine glands are ductless and discharge directly into the bloodstream through their surrounding network of capillaries. The functions of the endocrine system are to regulate growth, development, metabolism, and fluid balance; maintain homeostasis; and contribute to the reproductive process.

Hormones are the chemical messengers and act as catalytic agents that affect the physiological activity of other cells in the body. Types of hormones are steroids, peptides, biogenic amines, and eicosanoids. The amount of hormone secreted into the bloodstream is governed by negative feedback systems, other hormones, and the nervous system.

Hormones are produced by the following glands: pituitary, pineal, thyroid, parathyroids, thymus, adrenals, pancreas, ovaries, and testes. Abnormal hormone production may result in diseases such as diabetes, hypoglycemia, and obesity.

MATCHING I

Write the letter of the best answer in the space provided. Some will be used more than once.

A. Adrenal cortex
B. Adrenal medulla
C. Pituitary (anterior lobe)

D. Pituitary (posterior lobe)
E. Ovaries
F. Thyroid gland

G. Pancreas
H. Parathyroid glands

_____ 1. Prolactin

_____ 2. Aldosterone

_____ 3. Insulin

_____ 4. Thyroxin and triiodothyronine

_____ 5. Estrogen and progesterone

_____ 6. Cortisol

_____ 7. Calcitonin

_____ 8. Parathyroid hormone

_____ 9. Adrenocorticotropic hormone

_____ 10. Glucagon

_____ 11. Oxytocin

_____ 12. Epinephrine and norepinephrine

_____ 13. Human growth hormone

_____ 14. Antidiuretic hormone

_____ 15. Contains neurosecretory cells in pituitary

_____ 16. Follicle stimulating hormone

MATCHING II

Write the letter of the best answer in the space provided. Some will be used more than once.

A. Adrenocorticotropic hormone
B. Oxytocin
C. Antidiuretic hormone
D. Insulin

E. Prolactin
F. Luteinizing hormone
G. Human growth hormone
H. Thyroid stimulating hormone

I. Melanocyte stimulating hormone
J. Glucagon
K. Thyroxine

_____ 1. Stimulates secretion and production of thyroid hormones

_____ 2. Regulates endocrine functions of the adrenal cortex

_____ 3. Stimulates ovulation

_____ 4. Is involved in uterine contractions

_____ 5. Decreases urine output

_____ 6. Decreases blood glucose levels

_____ 7. Stimulates protein synthesis for muscle/bone growth

_____ 8. Stimulates the mammary glands to produce milk

_____ 9. Stimulates milk expression

_____ 10. Increases blood glucose levels

_____ 11. Influences mental, physical, and metabolic activities

_____ 12. Stimulates the distribution of melanin granules in the skin

Bibliography

Applegate EJ: *The anatomy and physiology learning system,* ed 2, Philadelphia, 2000, WB Saunders.

Crawley J, Van De Graaff KM: *A photographic atlas for anatomy and physiology,* Englewood, Colo, 2002, Morton.

Guyton A: *Human physiology and mechanisms of disease,* ed 3, Philadelphia, 1982, WB Saunders.

Haubrich WS: *Medical meanings: a glossary of word origins,* New York, 1984, Harcourt Brace Jovanovich.

Jacob S, Francone C: *Elements of anatomy and physiology,* Philadelphia, 1989, WB Saunders.

Kalat JW: *Biological psychology,* ed 2, Belmont, Calif, 1984, Wadsworth.

Kapit W, Elson, LM: *The anatomy coloring book,* ed 3, New York, 2002, Benjamin Cummings.

Kordish M, Dickson S: *Introduction to basic human anatomy,* Lake Charles, La, 1985, McNeese State University.

Marieb EN: *Essentials of human anatomy and physiology,* ed 4, New York, 1994, Benjamin Cummings.

McAleer N: *The body almanac,* Garden City, NY, 1985, Doubleday.

Merck Research Laboratories: *Merck manual,* ed 17, Whitehouse Station, NJ, 1998, Author.

Mosby's medical, nursing, and allied health dictionary, ed 4, St Louis, 1994, Mosby.

Newton D: *Pathology for massage therapists,* ed 2, Portland, Ore, 1995, Simran.

Premkumar K: *Pathology A to Z: a handbook for massage therapists,* Calgary, Canada, 1996, VanPub.

Solomon EP, Phillips GA: *Understanding human anatomy and physiology,* Philadelphia, 1987, WB Saunders.

Taber's cyclopedic medical dictionary, ed 13, Philadelphia, 1977, FA Davis.

Thibodeau G, Patton K: *Structure and function of the body,* ed 11, St Louis, 2000, Mosby.

Tortora GJ: *Introduction to the human body: the essentials of anatomy and physiology,* ed 3, New York, 1994, HarperCollins.

Tortora GJ, Grabowksi SR: *Principles of anatomy and physiology,* ed 9, New York, 2000, John Wiley.

Werner R: *A massage therapist's guide to pathology,* ed 2, Baltimore, 2002, Lippincott Williams & Wilkins.

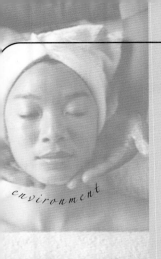

Circulatory System

19

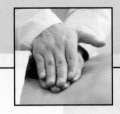

"A man is only as old as his arteries."

—Pierre Cabanis

STUDENT OBJECTIVES

After completing this chapter, the student should be able to:

- List the functions of the circulatory system (cardiovascular and lymphatic)
- Describe blood's characteristics and physical composition (plasma and blood cells)
- Identify how oxygen is transported in the blood
- Explain three blood-clotting mechanisms
- Identify and discuss blood types
- Trace blood through the heart, identifying each chamber
- Discuss the heart's conduction system
- List three main types of blood vessels, identifying characteristics of each
- Discuss blood pressure and factors that influence both blood pressure and heart rate
- Name and locate all major arteries, pulse points, and veins of the body
- Identify the lymphatic organs and vessels of the body
- Trace lymph flow from the lymphatic capillaries to the major lymphatic ducts
- Name types of cardiovascular and lymphatic/immune pathologies, giving characteristics and massage considerations of each
- Discuss natural and acquired immunity

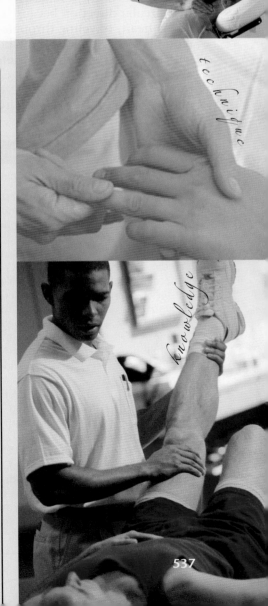

INTRODUCTION

The body is 60% to 80% fluid (by volume). This fluid requires circulation to maintain the body's health. The circulatory system consists of the cardiovascular and lymphvascular, or lymphatic, systems. The cardiovascular system circulates blood, and the lymphvascular system circulates lymph. Both subsystems are regarded as "pick-up and delivery" systems because their primary function is transportation.

CARDIOVASCULAR SYSTEM

The cardiovascular system consists of the blood, heart, and blood vessels. This section examines the characteristics of blood, such as plasma and blood cells, its clotting function, blood typing, and its main function of transport. Blood is the primary transport medium for a variety of substances that travel through the body. It makes its way through the body in a circular direction because of the pumping action of the heart, traveling through thousands of miles of blood vessels. Some of the blood vessels are areas in which caution needs to be exercised in massage therapy (endangerment sites). Circulation is accomplished by a vast network of vessels, and each vessel plays a different role in the circulatory process.

FUNCTIONS OF THE CARDIOVASCULAR SYSTEM

The functions of the cardiovascular system are the following:

1. Transportation and distribution of the respiratory gases, nutrients from the digestive tract, antibodies, waste materials, and hormones from endocrine glands; blood also transports heat from active muscles to the skin where the heat can be dissipated through vasodilation and perspiration.
2. Protection of the body through disease-fighting white blood cells and the removal of impurities and pathogens
3. Prevention of hemorrhage through clotting mechanisms; prevention of loss of body fluids from damaged vessels

BLOOD

Blood is classified as a liquid connective tissue and is essential for human life because the body's tissues can get oxygen and nutrients only from its blood supply. Representing about 8% of total body weight, blood is composed of a liquid (plasma) in which cells and cell fragments possessing different functions are

Terms and Their Meanings Related to the Circulatory System

Term	Meaning	Term	Meaning
aorta	a strap; to suspend	lumen	light
atrium	corridor	lupus wolf	wolf
bicuspid	two; pointed	mediastinum	standing in the middle
brady	slow	mitral	headdress
capillary	hairlike	phagocytosis	to eat; cell; condition
cardio, cardia	heart	phleb	vein
chordae tendineae	cordlike; tendon	pinocytosis	to drink; cell; condition
cisterna chyli	a reservoir or cavity; juice	plasma	a thing formed
coagulation	to curdle	platelet	flat
coronary	shaped like a crown or circle	Purkinje fibers	Bohemian anatomist (1787-1869)
cyanosis	dark blue; condition		
diastole	to expand	saphenous	the hidden
edema	swelling	semilunar	half; moon
erythrocyte	red; cell	sphygmomanometer	pulse; thin; measure
fibrinogen	fiber; to produce	systole	contraction
hemo	blood	tachy	rapid, fast, or swift
hemocytopoiesis/ hemocytogenesis	blood; cell; formation or birth	thrombocytes	clot; cell
		tricuspid	three; pointed
hemoglobin	blood; globe	tunica	a sheath
hemorrhage	blood; to burst forth	vascular	a vessel or duct
hemostasis	blood; stopping	vasoconstriction	vessel; a binder
intercalate	between; to put in place	vasodilation	vessel; to widen
intima	innermost	vena cava	vein; cavity
ischemia	to hold; blood	ventricle	little belly
leukocytes	white; cell		

suspended. Blood volume in the average-size male is approximately 5 to 6 liters (L) (6 quarts or 12 pints); blood volume in average-size females is approximately 4 to 5 L. Under normal circumstances, a blood cell makes a round trip through the circulatory system every 60 seconds.

Characteristics of Blood

The following is a list of the characteristics of blood:
- Blood is a viscous fluid that is thicker and more adhesive than water.
- Its pH is slightly alkaline.
- The color varies from bright scarlet red to dull maroon, depending on oxygen content.
- Blood is warmer (100° F) than the rest of the body.

Components of Blood

Plasma
Plasma is a straw-colored liquid that helps transport the blood cells. Approximately 55% of blood is plasma, but plasma itself is 90% water and 10% solutes (substances dissolved in a solution). One of

the solutes is **fibrinogen**, which functions in blood clotting. When necessary, fibrinogen is converted to fibrin, forming the foundations of a blood clot. Other solutes include plasma proteins, hormones, enzymes, and wastes.

Blood Cells
Blood cells are formed primarily in the red bone marrow of long, flat, and irregular bones. All types of blood cells are produced from a single, undifferentiated cell called a *pluripotent stem cell* (Figure 19-1). The three blood cells (erythrocytes, leukocytes, and thrombocytes) comprise approximately 45% of blood, each cell performing a different function.

Erythrocytes. The primary function of **erythrocytes**, or red blood cells (RBCs), is to transport oxygen in the blood. They also carry carbon dioxide. RBCs are the most numerous of all cells in the blood, and they are the major factor contributing to blood viscosity. These cells do not have a nucleus, which keeps them from reproducing or carrying out extensive metabolic activities. Each functional erythrocyte is biconcave to allow greater surface area for more

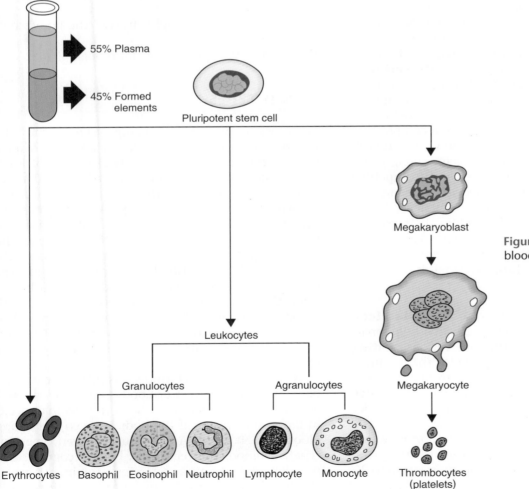

Figure 19-1 Different kinds of blood cells.

efficient diffusion of oxygen molecules and ease of movement through tiny capillaries (minute blood vessels). Erythrocytes are occupied by a red respiratory pigment called **hemoglobin**, giving blood its characteristically red color. Hemoglobin, an iron-based protein, combines with oxygen and carbon dioxide so that these gases can be transported to body tissues. Hemoglobin carries oxygen or carbon dioxide, but not both, at any given time. The different blood types (A, B, AB, or O) are determined by special proteins on the surfaces of RBCs. The life span of an erythrocyte is between 100 to 120 days, after which it begins to fragment, and the remains are eliminated by the spleen and liver.

For Your Information

Cigarette smoking damages about 20% of the smoker's hemoglobin because of the presence (and crowding) of carbon monoxide. Carbon monoxide binds to hemoglobin 200 times stronger than does oxygen, thus leaving no room for oxygen to bind.

Leukocytes. **Leukocytes**, white blood cells (WBCs), serve as part of the body's immune system by protecting the body from invading bacteria, viruses, and other pathogens. Think of these cells as the blood's defensive "mobile army." WBCs begin to mobilize and destroy the invader in processes known as *phagocytosis* and *pinocytosis* (see Chapter 11). Some WBCs combat irritants by producing **histamine**, a compound released in allergic, inflammatory reactions that in extreme cases causes dilation of capillaries, decreased blood pressure, and constriction of smooth muscles of the bronchi. Other WBCs produce antimicrobial substances such as antibodies. Antibodies are produced in response to specific foreign substances such as bacteria, viruses, or an incompatible blood type. Leukocytes are formed in bone marrow, and some mature in the thymus. Whenever WBCs mobilize for action, the body doubles their production within a short time. Their life span lasts from a few hours to a few days. Specialized leukocytes include basophils, eosinophils, neutrophils, lymphocytes, and monocytes.

Thrombocytes. Also known as **platelets**, **thrombocytes** are fragmented cells that help repair leaks in the blood vessels through various clotting mechanisms. Their jagged shape helps them adhere to torn surfaces more easily, such as from a vessel. A thrombocyte life span is from 5 to 9 days. The three main mechanisms for blood clotting are a platelet plug, vascular spasm, and coagulation.

1. **Vascular spasm**. When the smooth muscle in a vessel is torn, it begins to spasm, reducing the blood flow. This process can continue for up to 30 minutes.

2. **Platelet plug**. When platelets come into contact with the damaged blood vessel, their physical characteristics change by becoming larger and sticky, causing them to clump together and form a plug. This plug helps seal damaged vessels.

3. **Coagulation**. Coagulation, or clot formation, is the process of transforming fibrinogen into fibrin threads that tighten the platelet plug into a clot. Many plasma proteins are needed to transform fibrinogen into fibrin threads; vitamin K is needed to make many of these proteins. Once a clot is formed, it goes through a process of retraction (tightening) that draws the injured vessel walls closer together for repair and reduces, and later stops, blood loss. At the time a clot is formed, an enzyme is formed, which has the ability to slowly dissolve the clot over time.

If your client has clotting difficulties, is on anticoagulant therapy, or is taking prescription or nonprescription blood thinners (e.g., aspirin, ibuprofen, or Coumadin [warfarin]), a deep massage is contraindicated. These clients are more prone to bruising, which can result from pressure. Discuss this with your client during the intake before the massage.

Let's review blood cells:

- Erythrocytes (RBCs): transport oxygen and carbon dioxide
- Leukocytes (WBCs): fight disease (the body's mobile army)
- Thrombocytes (platelets): clot blood

BLOOD TYPES

The most common blood typing system is the ABO system, which uses the absence or presence of proteins to classify blood groups. The surfaces of RBCs contain genetically determined proteins called *agglutinogens*. Two blood agglutinogens are A and B. People with agglutinogen A are type A, and those with agglutinogen B are type B. Those with both agglutinogens are type AB, and those with neither of the agglutinogens are type O. Additionally, people with type A blood have antibodies against type B in their plasma. People with type B blood have antibodies against type A in their plasma. People with type AB blood do not have antibodies against either type A or type B in their plasma. People with type O blood have antibodies against both type A and type B in their plasma.

When a foreign agglutinogen is introduced to the body, its corresponding antibody recognizes the foreigner as an intruder and attacks it. This may occur in blood transfusion if the body is given the wrong blood type. If a type A individual is given type B or type AB blood, the recipient's body recognizes the type B agglutinogens as a foreign protein, attacks it, clumps the foreign cells together, and slices them open. Widespread inflammatory response occurs, and the iron released from the sliced open hemoglobin can cause organ failure and death.

Because type AB has no antibodies for agglutinogen A or B, it can receive all other blood types and is referred to as a **universal recipient**. Type O has neither of the agglutinogens and does not react to any other blood types and hence is referred to as a **universal donor**. Blood transfusions must be made with compatible blood types because mismatching can cause severe medical problems or death.

The Rh blood group system depends on the presence or absence of the Rh protein on erythrocytes. **Rh factor** is so named because the theory was refined in the blood of rhesus monkeys. Rh positive (about 85% of the population) describes the presence of the Rh protein and is not a health problem. Rh negative (about 15% of the population) indicates the absence of the Rh protein and can become a problem

during pregnancy. If the pregnant mother is Rh negative and the fetus is Rh positive, blood incompatibility may occur if the blood interacts, such as through a ruptured vessel. The mother's Rh-negative blood develops antibodies against the fetus's Rh-positive blood. These antibodies then attack the fetus's RBCs. Because of medical advances, this situation is now rarely life threatening for the fetus.

THE HEART

The heart is located in the mediastinum region of the thoracic cavity and rests on the diaphragm. About the size of a clenched fist, the **heart** possesses four hollow chambers: two **atria** (superior chambers) and two **ventricles** (inferior chambers). A septum separates the ventricles and extends up between the atria (Figure 19-2, *A*). These hollow chambers function as a

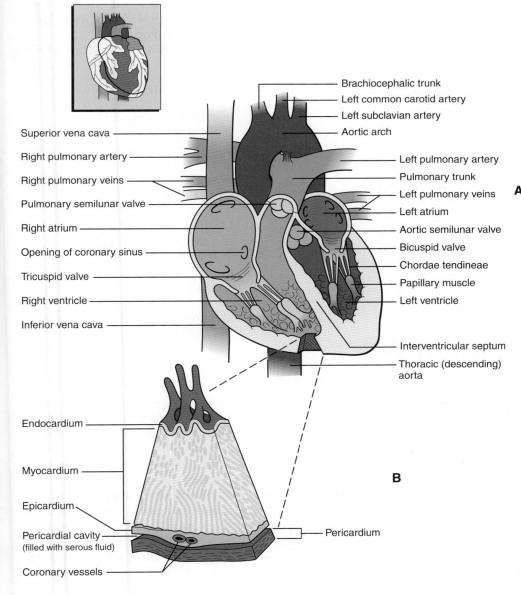

Superior vena cava
Right pulmonary artery
Right pulmonary veins
Pulmonary semilunar valve
Right atrium
Opening of coronary sinus
Tricuspid valve
Right ventricle
Inferior vena cava

Brachiocephalic trunk
Left common carotid artery
Left subclavian artery
Aortic arch
Left pulmonary artery
Pulmonary trunk
Left pulmonary veins
Left atrium
Aortic semilunar valve
Bicuspid valve
Chordae tendineae
Papillary muscle
Left ventricle

A

Interventricular septum
Thoracic (descending) aorta

Figure 19-2   A, The heart, chambers, and valves. **B,** Heart wall.

Endocardium
Myocardium
Epicardium
Pericardial cavity (filled with serous fluid)
Coronary vessels

Pericardium

B

double pump; the right-hand pump forces oxygen-depleted blood to the lungs, whereas the left-hand pump squeezes oxygen-rich blood out to the rest of the body. Pumping blood is the heart's primary function. When the heart contracts, the heart muscle (myocardium) forces blood out of the ventricles while valves open and shut to keep it on its course. The heart pumps blood intermittently, on the average of 70 beats per minute (BPM) in a resting person.

For Your Information

The heart beats an average of more than 100,000 times a day. The blood is pumped through 60,000 miles of blood vessels, or roughly 2.5 times around the world at the equator.

Heart Coverings and Heart Wall

Surrounding and protecting the heart is a structure called the **pericardium** (see Figure 19-2, *B*). Within the pericardium is the pericardial cavity filled with serous fluid; this fluid reduces friction between the pericardium and the heart as it contracts and expands.

The heart wall possesses the following three layers: epicardium, myocardium, and endocardium (see Figure 19-2, *B*). The **epicardium** is a thin outer layer of serous membrane. This protective layer possesses adipose tissue and the blood vessels that nourish the heart (coronary vessels). The **myocardium** is the thick cardiac muscle layer that makes up the bulk of the heart wall. Contraction of the myocardium forces blood out of the ventricles (see Chapter 15 for a discussion of cardiac muscle). The **endocardium** is the thin, inner lining of the heart and is continuous with the endothelial lining of the heart chambers and blood vessels, as well as the valves of the heart.

Heart Chambers

The hollow heart is subdivided into four chambers that receive and pump blood. The superior chambers are called the *atria* and take in blood from the body through large veins and then pump it to the inferior chambers. The lower chambers, or ventricles, pump blood to the body's organs and tissues. The septum separating the right and left atria is called the *interatrial septum,* and the septum separating the right and left ventricles is called the *interventricular septum.* The heart chambers are described as follows:

- **Right atrium:** Atria, in general, are thin-walled because they only need enough cardiac muscle to deliver the blood into the ventricles. The right atrium receives blood from all parts of the body except the lungs. Blood is received from the superior and inferior vena cava and the coronary sinus.

The superior vena cava returns blood from the chest area, arms, and head. The inferior vena cava returns blood from the abdominal area and the legs. The coronary sinus returns blood from the heart itself. Blood from the right atrium is delivered into the right ventricle beneath it.

- **Right ventricle:** The right ventricle receives blood from the right atrium and pumps blood through the pulmonary trunk and into the right and left pulmonary arteries. Blood is routed to the lungs to release carbon dioxide and pick up oxygen. The oxygenated blood is returned to the heart via the pulmonary veins.
- **Left atrium:** The oxygen-rich blood from the pulmonary veins enters the left atrium. During an atrial contraction, blood passes from the left atrium to the left ventricle.
- **Left ventricle:** This ventricular structure has the thickest heart wall because it pumps blood into the aorta and then through miles of blood vessels throughout the body. The amount of blood ejected from the left ventricle during each contraction is called **stroke volume**.

In review, blood travels through the heart as follows (Figure 19-3):

Blood enters the right atrium,

↓

is delivered to the right ventricle,

↓

moves into the right and left pulmonary arteries,

↓

enters the lungs (releases CO_2 [exhale] and obtains O_2 [inhale]),

↓

travels into the right and left pulmonary veins,

↓

moves into the left atrium,

↓

is delivered to the left ventricle,

↓

and flows into the aorta to all parts of the body via the arteries.

Heart Valves

The heart valves are little flaps of endothelium located between the chambers of the heart (atria and ventricles) and also between the ventricles and some of the great vessels. These valves work to keep blood flowing in one direction as the pressure exerted on the blood changes during heart contraction. These valves include the **atrioventricular valves** (AV valves) and the **semilunar valves** (SL valves). The characteristic *lubb-dupp* sound of the heart is from the movement of these valves.

The AV valves separate the atria from the ventricles; these valves are held in place by tendonlike

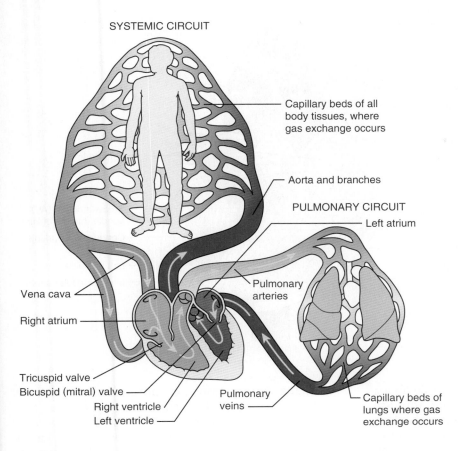

SYSTEMIC CIRCUIT

Capillary beds of all
body tissues, where
gas exchange occurs

Aorta and branches

PULMONARY CIRCUIT

Left atrium

Figure 19-3   Blood circulation.

Vena cava

Right atrium

Pulmonary
arteries

Tricuspid valve
Bicuspid (mitral) valve

Right ventricle
Left ventricle

Pulmonary
veins

Capillary beds of
lungs where gas
exchange occurs

cords called *chordae tendineae,* which attach to the ventricular walls through cardiac muscle projections called *papillary muscles.* The *lubb* sound of the heart is from blood turbulence when the AV valves close. The **tricuspid valve** is the right AV valve and possesses three flaps or cusps. The **bicuspid valve,** or mitral valve, is the left AV valve and possesses two flaps or cusps.

The SL valves are located between both ventricles and their adjacent arteries; each valve consists of three half moon-shaped cusps; named for the vessels to which they lead. The *dupp* sound is from blood turbulence when the SL valves close. The **pulmonary semilunar valve** lies between the right ventricle and the pulmonary trunk, and the **aortic semilunar valve** lies between the left ventricle and the aorta.

Heart Rate and the Heart's Conduction System

The heart's rate of contraction is controlled by a system of modified cardiac cells that conduct impulses through the muscle tissue of the heart. The purpose of this conduction system is to coordinate and synchronize the heart's activity. Cardiac muscle is autorhythmic (capable of self-excitation). Thus the heart has the ability to generate its own independent

muscle contraction without outside innervation. The main parts of this system are the **sinoatrial node** (SA node) and the **atrioventricular node,** (AV node) the **atrioventricular bundle,** (AV bundle) and the **Purkinje fibers,** which are conducting fibers (Figure 19-4).

The SA node lies within the right atrium and initiates the cardiac impulse, stimulating both the right and left atria to contract. Blood in these chambers is then pushed into the ventricles and the impulses from the SA node immediately arrive at the AV node. The purpose of the SA node is to initiate the heartbeat cycle because it initiates the cardiac impulse faster than anywhere else in the heart. This is accomplished without the input of the nervous system, but the rate at which the contractions are generated is influenced by the nervous system. The SA node would generate impulses at 90 BPM; the parasympathetic division of the autonomic nervous system keeps the resting rate down to about 70 BPM.

The AV node is designed to work at a slower rate than the SA node to give the atria plenty of time to empty themselves of blood. It is this brief delay that causes the slight pause between two sounds of the heart (*lubb-dupp*). The AV node relays the impulses to the AV bundle (bundle of His). The AV bundle divides into right and left bundles, which run in the interventricular septum to the right and left ventricles.

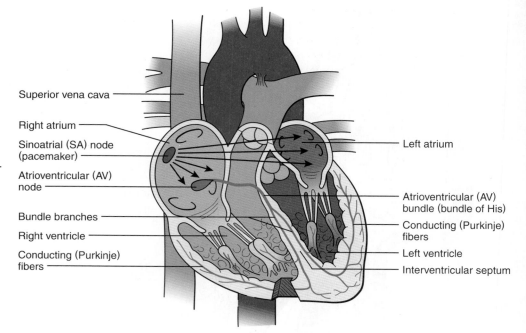

Figure 19-4 The heart's conduction system.

Superior vena cava

Right atrium

Sinoatrial (SA) node (pacemaker)

Atrioventricular (AV) node

Bundle branches

Right ventricle

Conducting (Purkinje) fibers

Left atrium

Atrioventricular (AV) bundle (bundle of His)

Conducting (Purkinje) fibers

Left ventricle

Interventricular septum

These bundles branch out to form the Purkinje fibers; the function of which is to spread the impulse throughout the myocardium of the ventricles. This second stimulation through the myocardium causes the ventricles to simultaneously contract, expelling the blood from the ventricles to the arteries.

The cycle of events occurring with each alternating contraction and relaxation of the heart muscle, coordinated by the conducting system, is called the **cardiac cycle**. The firing action of the cardiac cycle remains constant when the SA node acts alone; however, other factors can regulate the cardiac cycle to increase or decrease the output of the heart to meet the demands of the body. The majority of heart rate changes are controlled by a specialized portion of the medulla oblongata known as the *cardiovascular center*. Other influencing factors are as follows:

Sympathetic division of the autonomic nervous system: Stress increases heart rate

Parasympathetic division of the autonomic nervous system: Relaxation decreases heart rate

Chemoreceptor input: High carbon dioxide levels increases heart rate while high oxygen decreases heart rate; exercise, emotional stress, and altitude changes alter oxygen/carbon dioxide levels

Temperature: Elevated temperatures increase heart rates whereas colder temperatures decrease heart rates

Age: Younger people have a higher heart rate

General health: Healthier individuals tend to have a lower heart rate

Any deviation from a normal heart rate pattern is termed **arrhythmia**. Pulse rate is the number of ventricular contractions per minute. Slow heart rate (under 50 to 60 BPM) is called **bradycardia**. The condition may be the result of disease; however, it is often normal for people who are physically fit. Rapid heart rate (more than 100 BPM) is called **tachycardia**. This condition may be the result of fever, strenuous exercise, or emotions such as anxiety. Tachycardia is the body's response to an increased demand for oxygen by the tissues.

Dr. Janet Travell (see Chapter 18) documents a myofascial trigger point in the right pectoralis major muscle whose pain referral zone refers noxious impulses into the SA node. This trigger point is related to cardiac arrhythmia. Releasing the trigger point with massage techniques can often end symptoms of tachycardia or "runaway" heartbeat. It is important to note that this procedure is only performed while the client is asymptomatic. A client experiencing tachycardia while in your office should be referred immediately to a physician.

For Your Information

An **electrocardiogram** (ECG or EKG) is a graphic tracing of the variations in electrical potential caused by the excitation of the heart muscle and detected at the body's surface.

BLOOD VESSELS

Blood vessels are a closed network of tubular structures connected to the heart that transport blood to all the cells of the body. These blood vessels are divided into three main groups based on their structure and function: arteries, veins, and capillaries. The walls of both arteries and veins possess three layers (tunics). The innermost layer is called the **tunica interna**, which is endothelial tissue fused with a small quantity of connective tissue. The middle layer is the **tunica media**, which contains quantities of both connective tissue and smooth muscle. The outer layer, possessing mostly dense connective tissue, is the **tunica externa** (Figure 19-5). Large blood vessels have their own blood supply called the *vasa-vasorum,* which are often referred to as the *vessels of the vessels,* and are located in the tunica externa layer of these vessels.

The walls of arteries and veins, being part muscle, possess two properties: elasticity and contractility. The levels of these properties differ greatly between the arteries and the veins; arterial walls are more elastic and have a thicker muscular layer than veins.

The muscular layer of the arteries and veins can dilate and contract to change the diameter of the vessel. The open space within the blood vessel is known as the **lumen**. When the diameter of the vascular lumen enlarges, the process is called **vasodilation**; when the diameter becomes narrower, it is called **vasoconstriction**. Vasodilation and vasoconstriction may be initiated by the following two sources: (1) *direct nerve stimulation* from the vasomotor center located in the medulla oblongata and (2) *local reflex response* resulting from a stimulus such as pressure (i.e., massage) or temperature (i.e., heat or cold application).

Arteries

By definition, **arteries** are vessels that move blood away from the heart. In general, blood within the arteries is oxygenated (has already been to the lungs to receive oxygen). The only artery that contains de-oxygenated blood is the pulmonary artery, moving blood from the right ventricle of the heart to the lungs; conversely, the pulmonary veins carry oxygenated blood. Because arteries are closer to the pumping action of the heart, their vascular walls are considerably thicker and stronger than veins to withstand higher blood pressure. Arteries continue to branch off into smaller and thinner vessels, becoming **arterioles**, as they lose their two outer layers. When the vessels are one layer thick, they are called *capillaries.*

Because arteries deliver oxygenated blood to the body's tissues, sustained pressure applied on these vessels could interfere with blood delivery and could damage tissues. Thus several important arteries must be avoided by the massage therapist (i.e., endangerment sites).

For Your Information

A mnemonic device to help you remember that arteries carry blood away from the heart is that both *a*rteries and *a*way begin with the letter *A.*

Arterial Pulse

The word **pulse** refers to the expansion effect that occurs when the left ventricle contracts, producing a wave of blood that surges through and expands the arterial walls. The **arterial pulse** can be felt in the arteries that are located close to the surface of the body or where they lie over bone or other firm tissue. Avoid using your thumb or index finger when taking someone's pulse because you may register your own pulse instead. Each pulse point is named for the region of the body in which it is located. The common

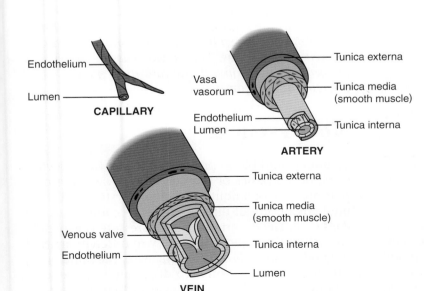

Endothelium

Lumen

CAPILLARY

Vasa vasorum

Endothelium
Lumen

ARTERY

Tunica externa

Tunica media (smooth muscle)

Tunica interna

Tunica externa

Tunica media (smooth muscle)

Tunica interna

Lumen

Venous valve

Endothelium

VEIN

Figure 19-5 Comparing arteries and veins: tunics of blood vessels.

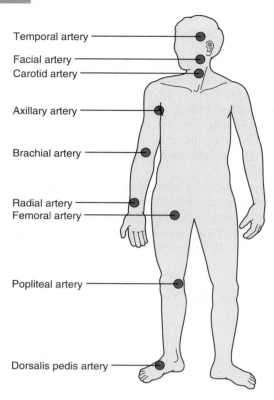

Figure 19-6   Map of pulse points.

pulse points are detailed in the following list (Figure 19-6):

Temporal artery: Anterior to the ear; temple region
Facial artery: Inferior to the corner of the mouth
Carotid artery: Sides of the throat
Axillary artery: Armpit region
Brachial artery: Antecubital region
Radial artery: Lateral aspect of the wrist
Femoral artery: Crease between lower abdomen and upper thigh
Popliteal artery: Posterior knee
Dorsalis pedis artery: Anterior medial foot

MINI-LAB

Using the map of pulse points, locate these areas on a partner or on yourself. Note that pressure must be used to feel the pulse, but too much pressure prevents blood from flowing in the vessel.

Capillaries

When the arterioles lose their two outer layers, leaving only endothelium, they become the **capillaries**, which possess a thin, permeable membrane for efficient gas exchange. RBCs carry oxygen in the blood on the hemoglobin molecule; these blood cells must move in a single file to squeeze through each capillary. The movement of blood in capillaries is the slowest of all the vessels, and its flow is intermittent, providing ample opportunity for an exchange to occur. Nutrients and oxygen are provided to the tissues and waste from cells is removed from interstitial fluid through a process called **capillary exchange**. The exchange of gases is referred to as *internal* or *tissue respiration*. Capillary exchange is the main function of the capillaries and is achieved by diffusion and filtration. Tissues and organs that have extensive capillary networks are the muscles, liver, spleen, kidneys, and connective tissue, although cartilage is avascular. Other areas of the body that are devoid of capillaries (and other blood vessels) are the epidermis, hair, nails, and lens and cornea of the eye.

Veins

Veins begin at the capillary level and gradually become larger; small veins are called **venules**. **Veins** drain the tissues and organs and return blood, which is now low in oxygen, back to the heart and lungs. Unlike arteries, no pulse is felt in veins, and they are considerably less elastic, possess thinner walls, and are easily collapsed. By the time blood leaves the capillaries and moves into the veins, it has lost a great deal of pressure. The blood pressure in veins is usually too low to force the blood back to the heart, and venous return is often flowing against gravity.

To assist venous flow, the lumina in veins are larger, and in small and medium-size veins, folds in the endothelium form the numerous valves that open in the direction of the heart. This one-way valve system functions to prevent backflow. The valve system, combined with the pumping action of muscular contraction in the limbs, is called the **venous pump**. Veins also depend on pressure changes in the thorax and abdomen during breathing (respiratory pump) to push blood back to the heart.

The veins are generally located superficially and near the skeletal muscles so that muscular contraction can assist venous blood flow. This is why massage movements are performed centripetally (toward the center) to assist the veins in their function.

BLOOD PRESSURE

To understand blood pressure, it is helpful to review some of the basics of physics. One law of physics is that pressure of a liquid in a closed system is distributed equally in all directions to the confines of the container. Hence, arterial blood pressure is generally consistent throughout the artery in different areas of the body at any given time. Likewise, the same holds true for venous pressure. To distribute itself equally, a liquid always flows from areas of high pressure to areas of low pressure. When a liquid such as blood flows into the heart, it does so because the empty chamber expands, creating a lower pressure or suction effect. Once the blood has filled the chamber, the contraction places force on the blood, and pressure builds. When the pressure inside the chamber of the heart overcomes the combination of the pressure outside the heart and the resistance of the valve, blood begins flowing out of the heart. Blood continues to move forward by the one-way action of the valves of the heart.

Blood pressure is the pressure exerted by blood on an arterial wall during the contraction of the left ventricle. Blood pressure is most often measured in the brachial artery using a **sphygmomanometer**, or blood pressure cuff. The reading gathered during the blood pressure measurement looks like a fraction or ratio. The top number represents the pressure exerted on the arterial wall during active ventricular contraction (**systole**). The bottom number represents the static pressure against the arterial wall during the rest or pause between contractions (**diastole**). Blood pressure is measured in millimeters of mercury (mm Hg). This is the pressure required to lift a column of mercury into the gauge to a given height (millimeters). A reading of 120/80 mm Hg is considered to be normal blood pressure for adults. Borderline high blood pressure is above 140/90 mm Hg. Readings over 160/95 mm Hg are considered high, requiring medical attention. The diastolic reading is considered to be the most critical in health considerations. The heart is designed for periodic exertion; it will work harder to supply the body with blood during times of high demands but cannot keep up a high rate for an extended period without resting. A high diastolic reading may indicate that the heart is working too hard, even during its resting phase.

Blood flow, the amount of blood passing through a vessel in a given amount of time, depends on two factors: blood pressure and the resistance of friction between the blood and vessel wall. When blood pressure rises, the friction resistance rises slightly because of the greater amount of blood being forced through the vessels. The main factor influencing blood flow is the blood pressure. The greater the difference between systolic and diastolic pressures, the higher is the flow rate. For example, a blood pressure of 120/80 mm Hg has a pressure difference of 40 mm Hg during the cardiac cycle. If the blood pressure is increased to 140/90 mm Hg because of physical exertion, the pressure difference has increased to 50 mm Hg. A greater quantity of blood is pushed through the vessel with the higher pressure drop or greater difference in pressures.

Increased local blood flow is called **hyperemia**, *causing the skin to become reddened and warm. This often occurs during massage or heat application. Local de-crease in blood flow is called* **ischemia** *and is often marked by pain and tissue dysfunction. Ischemia occurs when blood flow is disturbed, such as a sustained muscular contraction or spasm. Massage therapy, increasing blood flow to an area, reduces ischemia.*

Blood flow is directly influenced by blood pressure. Factors that influence blood pressure itself include resistance, cardiac output, blood volume, homeostatic regulation, and diseases.

Resistance. Resistance is the effect of friction between the blood and the vessel walls. Resistance is directly influenced by blood viscosity and the diameter of the blood vessel.

- **Viscosity.** The thicker the blood, then the more friction is created, causing blood pressure to rise. Blood thickness may be influenced by dehydration, which reduces blood plasma, causing blood volume to decrease and the blood to thicken. An increase in RBC count causes an increase in blood viscosity.

- **Diameter of the blood vessel.** The smaller the diameter of the blood vessel, the more resistance it offers the blood, raising blood pressure.

Cardiac output. Cardiac output represents the blood volume expelled by the ventricles of the heart (stroke volume), multiplied by the heart rate (number of BPM). The ventricles of the heart in a resting adult pump a volume of blood varying from about 4 to 8 L of blood per minute. Cardiac output is influenced by the cardiovascular center of the brain and certain blood chemicals, health, and genetics of the person.

Blood volume. The greater the volume of blood in the body, the higher the blood pressure, which might be the result of a condition such as pregnancy. As blood volume decreases (perhaps because of blood loss by hemorrhage), blood pressure decreases.

Homeostatic regulation. Homeostasis measures and attempts to maintain normal blood pressure through the nervous, endocrine, and urinary systems. These include the medulla oblongata (cardiac and vasomotor centers), chemoreceptor input, baroreceptor input, the presence of hormones (epinephrine, norepinephrine, antidiuretic hormone [ADH], aldosterone), and an enzyme (renin).

Diseases. Vascular diseases such as arteriosclerosis may raise systolic blood pressure resulting from the loss of elasticity in the arterial wall. Deposits of plaque on the vessel walls may result in an increase of resistance from friction or a diameter restriction, causing an increase in blood pressure. Conditions such as edema may cause extravascular pressure against the vessels, particularly the veins, causing the heart to work harder to achieve circulation.

JACK MEAGHER, PT, MsT

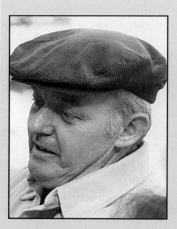

Born: July 6, 1923.

"Massage is the study of anatomy in Braille."

Jack Meagher is the father of sports massage. At age 74, with cancer at the time of this interview, he radiates the energy and demonstrates the quick wit rarely encountered in men half his age.

Before enlisting as U.S. Army medic for 4 years, Meagher took a course in Swedish massage, hoping eventually to get into physical therapy. When he was in Epernay, France, he experienced a different type of massage than he had learned back home. This massage, performed by a German prisoner of war, made Meagher move markedly better on the baseball field.

After his discharge, he was signed by the Boston Braves as a pitcher, but a wartime shoulder injury threw him a curve that landed him in physical therapy unable to continue a baseball career. That sent him looking for the same kind of massage he had received in France. He found another German therapist, an instructor at the Viennese Massage School in Connecticut, who relieved his pain to the extent that Meagher was able to play semiprofessional baseball in his hometown of Gloucester, Mass.

The success of his therapy did more than put Meagher's body into motion again, it got him thinking. The result was sports massage, the massage that can enhance athletic performance. Just as Swedish massage uses specific strokes, Meagher classified sports massage strokes as direct pressure, friction, compression, and percussion. He also recommends effleurage and kneading when necessary.

"It took me 15 years of putting it together," says Meagher. "I was at a YMCA working on professional athletes and people for whom exercise was a way of life. The sports massage helped them do more before they faded. A loose body uses less energy."

Soon Meagher discovered that what made man go farther and faster could also help horses. That is when sports massage really took off. "In the 1976 Olympics, the horses I'd worked on took two golds and a silver," remembers Meagher. "I was written up and asked to do a book. Then the American Massage Therapy Association became interested, and I was invited to speak at one of their conferences."

The classic sports massage text is *Sports Massage: A Complete Program for Increasing Performance and Endurance in Fifteen Popular Sports* (Doubleday, 1998). It more than introduces a specific massage to the reader. It provides a glimpse into the life of a warm, dedicated, and extremely results-oriented man with a sharp mind, who understands the intricate biomechanics of the body and is able to break it down into simple steps to make his life's work accessible to weekend warriors and professional athletes alike.

Meagher also has a wonderful sense of humor, exemplified in the title of his book, *Never Goose an Appaloosa*. Ticklish himself, he does not even receive Swedish massage, but regarding the horses he massages, Meagher says, "I would not get on a horse, but I do get along with horses. I've never been kicked. Horses understand when you're trying to help them." He is still massaging 40 to 50 horses per week but not the workload he did in his prime. "I used to do 55 people and 30 horses a week," he says.

When asked what characteristics should be present in a successful massage therapist, he cites that the desire to help people and the ability to know how to use ones hands are of utmost importance. Additionally, a massage therapist should possess the education for putting it all together.

JACK MEAGHER PT, MsT—cont'd

> When asked if he would do it all over again, he says, "I wouldn't do anything differently. It's taken years of hard work. One time a chief of orthopedics told me I had a real gift, and I had to disagree. Gifts come easily. What I do is not a gift. I work hard. I developed my instincts through my failures and my successes."

PATHS OF BLOOD CIRCULATION

As you may recall, the primary function of the circulatory system is transportation. Within the cardiovascular system are two paths or circuits based on the areas of the body that are served: pulmonary and systemic.

Pulmonary Circuit

The purpose of the pulmonary circuit is to replenish the oxygen supply of the blood and to eliminate gaseous waste products. The **pulmonary circuit** brings deoxygenated blood from the right ventricle to the alveoli of the lungs to release carbon dioxide and regain oxygen. Oxygenated blood returns to the left atrium of the heart and moves into the systemic circuit with the contraction of the left ventricle. When the pulmonary arteries carry blood away from the heart and the pulmonary veins carry blood back to the heart, the oxygen content of the blood is reversed—that is, the pulmonary arteries carry deoxygenated blood away from the heart to the lungs, and the pulmonary veins carry oxygenated blood back from the lungs to the heart.

Systemic Circuit

The **systemic circuit** brings the oxygenated blood from the left ventricle through numerous arteries into the capillaries. From here, blood moves back through the veins and returns the now deoxygenated blood to the right atrium to enter the pulmonary circuit. The function of this circuit is to bring nutrients and oxygen to all systems of the body and to carry waste materials from the tissues for elimination. The systemic circuit is the body's highway system consisting of hollow streets (arteries, capillaries, and veins).

Not all circulation routes begin with arteries and end with veins. Another circulatory network for transporting blood is located within the systemic circuit. *Venous portal systems* start and end with veins.

The main venous portal system is the **hepatic portal system**, which collects blood from the digestive organs (stomach, intestines, gallbladder, spleen, and pancreas) and delivers this blood to the liver for processing and storage. Because the liver is a key organ involved in maintaining the proper glucose, fat, and protein concentrations in the blood, the hepatic portal system allows the blood from the digestive organs to detour through the liver to process these substances before they enter the systemic circulation (Figure 19-7). The other venous portal system is located between the hypothalamus and the anterior pituitary of the brain.

Major Systemic Arteries

Arteries are named for their locations. Notice how the name of the artery changes as it progresses into a new region of the body, like a road crossing through a country. It is the same artery but, as it moves down the arm, the name changes from axillary to brachial to radial and ulnar and so on. Arteries generally lie deep and are well shielded within tissues and muscles; however, some are superficial enough that they can be palpated (see Figure 19-6). The following list contains the major systemic arteries with endangerment sites noted (Figure 19-8):

- Aorta (aortic arch, ascending, descending [thoracic and abdominal]): the descending and abdominal aorta are endangerment sites
- Axillary: this is an endangerment site
- Brachial: this is an endangerment site
- Brachiocephalic
- Carotid (internal, external, and common): external and common are endangerment sites
- Coronary
- Dorsalis pedis
- Facial: this is an endangerment site
- Femoral: this is an endangerment site
- Iliac (internal, external, and common)
- Peroneal
- Mesenteric (superior and inferior)
- Popliteal: this is an endangerment site
- Radial: this is an endangerment site
- Subclavian: this is an endangerment site

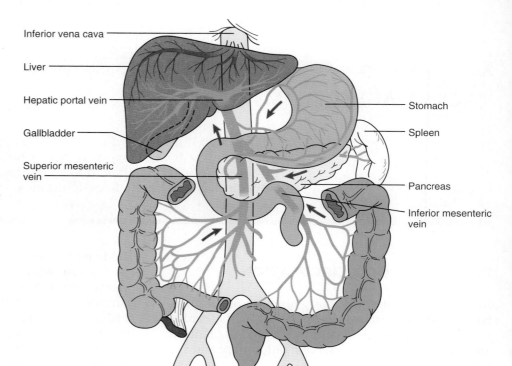

Inferior vena cava

Liver

Hepatic portal vein

Gallbladder

Superior mesenteric vein

Stomach

Spleen

Pancreas

Inferior mesenteric vein

Figure 19-7 Venous portal system.

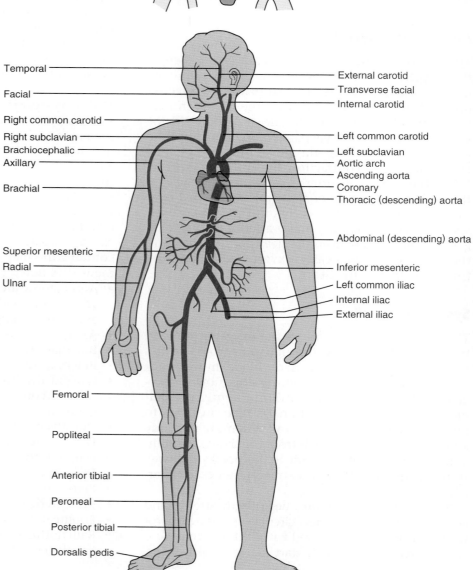

Temporal

Facial

Right common carotid

Right subclavian

Brachiocephalic

Axillary

Brachial

Superior mesenteric

Radial

Ulnar

External carotid

Transverse facial

Internal carotid

Left common carotid

Left subclavian

Aortic arch

Ascending aorta

Coronary

Thoracic (descending) aorta

Abdominal (descending) aorta

Inferior mesenteric

Left common iliac

Internal iliac

External iliac

Femoral

Popliteal

Anterior tibial

Peroneal

Posterior tibial

Dorsalis pedis

Figure 19-8 Major arteries.

- Temporal
- Tibial (anterior and posterior)
- Transverse facial: this is an endangerment site
- Ulnar: this is an endangerment site

When massaging an area where an arterial endangerment site is located, apply light pressure and feel for a pulse. If a pulse is felt, avoid prolonged pressure on the specific pulse location.

Major Systemic Veins

Veins, like arteries, are also named for their locations. The following list contains the major systemic veins found in the body with endangerment sites noted (notice how the names of the veins, like the arteries, change as they progress through body) (Figure 19-9):

- Axillary: this is an endangerment site
- Brachial: this is an endangerment site
- Brachiocephalic
- Femoral: this is an endangerment site
- Hepatic portal
- Iliac (internal, external, and common)
- Jugular (internal and external): this is an endangerment site
- Median cubital
- Mesenteric (superior and inferior)
- Peroneal
- Popliteal: this is an endangerment site
- Radial: this is an endangerment site
- Saphenous (great and small): this is an endangerment site
- Subclavian
- Tibial (anterior and posterior)
- Ulnar: this is an endangerment site
- Vena cava (superior and inferior)

When applying a deep stripping pressure over a superficial vein, always move from distal to proximal, or you

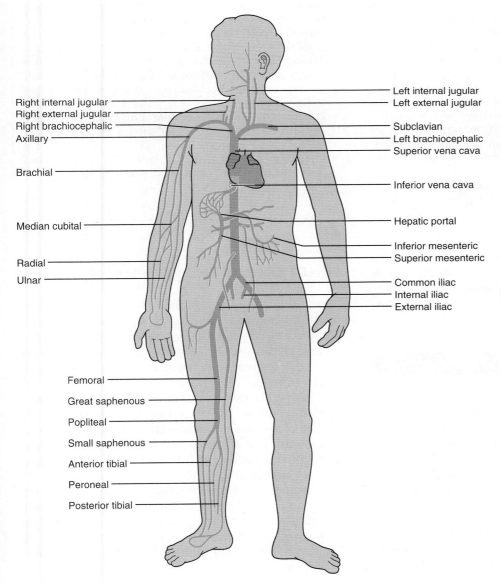

Right internal jugular
Right external jugular
Right brachiocephalic
Axillary

Brachial

Median cubital

Radial
Ulnar

Left internal jugular
Left external jugular

Subclavian
Left brachiocephalic
Superior vena cava

Inferior vena cava

Hepatic portal

Inferior mesenteric
Superior mesenteric

Common iliac
Internal iliac
External iliac

Femoral

Great saphenous

Popliteal

Small saphenous

Anterior tibial

Peroneal

Posterior tibial

Figure 19-9   Major veins.

BOX 19-1

Effects of Massage on the Cardiovascular System

- **Dilates blood vessels.** The body responds to massage by reflexively dilating the blood vessels. This in turn aids in improving blood circulation and lowering blood pressure.
- **Improves blood circulation.** Deep stroking improves blood circulation by mechanically assisting venous blood flow back to the heart. The increase of blood flow is comparable with that of exercise. It has been documented that local circulation increases during massage up to 3 times more than circulation at rest.
- **Creates hyperemia.** Increased blood flow creates a hyperemic effect, which is often visible on the surface of the skin.
- **Stimulates release of acetylcholine and histamine for sustained vasodilation.** These two substances are released as a result of vasomotor activity, helping prolong vasodilation.
- **Replenishes nutritive materials.** Another benefit of increased circulation, products such as nutrients and oxygen are transported to the cells and tissues more efficiently.
- **Promotes rapid removal of waste products.** Not only are nutrients brought to cells and tissues, but metabolic waste products are removed more rapidly through massage. It is often said that massage "dilutes the poisons."
- **Reduces ischemia.** Massage reduces ischemia and ischemic-related pain. Ischemia is also related to trigger point formation and their associated pain referral patterns.
- **Decreases blood pressure.** Blood pressure is decreased by dilation of blood vessels. Both diastolic and systolic readings decline and last approximately 40 minutes after the massage session.
- **Reduces heart rate.** Massage decreases heart rate through activation of the relaxation response.

- **Lowers pulse rate.** As one would expect, a reduced heart rate lowers pulse rate.
- **Increases stroke volume.** Stroke volume is the amount of blood ejected from the left ventricle during each contraction. As the heart rate decreases, more time is made for the cardiac ventricles to fill with blood. The result is a larger volume of blood pushed through the heart with each ventricular contraction, thereby increasing stroke volume.
- **Increases red blood cell count.** The number of functioning red blood cells and their oxygen carrying capacity are increased. It is speculated that this effect is achieved by (1) promoting the spleen's discharge of red blood cells (RBCs), (2) recruiting excess blood from engorged internal organs into general circulation, and (3) stimulating stagnant capillary beds and returning this blood into general circulation. All three events increase RBC count.
- **Increases oxygen saturation in blood.** When RBC count rises, a greater oxygen saturation occurs in the blood.
- **Increases WBC count.** The presence of white blood cells (WBCs) increases after massage. The body may perceive massage as a stressor (an event to which the body must adapt) and recruits additional WBCs. The increase in WBC count enables the body to more effectively protect itself against disease.
- **Enhances the adhesion of migrating WBC.** The surfaces of WBCs become more "sticky" after a massage, increasing their effectiveness.
- **Increased platelet count.** Gentle but firm massage strokes increase the number of platelets in the blood.

---

may promote varicosities. Varicose veins, or damaged veins, lack a sufficient interior valve system. Pressure in the wrong direction also promotes improper blood flow.

See Box 19-1 for the effects of massage on the cardiovascular system.

LYMPHATIC SYSTEM

The lymphatic system, or lymph/immune system, is a one-way system for drainage of excess fluid from the body's tissues, and is a complement to the circulatory system. Like the circulatory system, the lymphatic system has disease-fighting functions. The lymphatic system is composed of lymph fluid, lymph vessels, and specialized tissues and organs. **Lymph**, the fluid of the lymphatic system, is transported through progressively larger vessels that drain into two large veins near the neck. This portion of the chapter explores the structures, functions, and pathways of the lymphatic system and the body's immunological responses.

FUNCTIONS OF THE LYMPHATIC SYSTEM

The functions of the lymphatic system are as follows:
1. After draining the tissues of excess interstitial fluid, the lymphatic system returns this fluid to the cardiovascular system. This helps maintain blood volume and pressure and prevent edema (swelling).
2. The lymphatic system transports fats and some vitamins from the digestive tract to the blood. These specialized lymphatic vessels are called *lacteals*. The lymphatic system also returns proteins and cellular debris that have escaped from the blood back to the general circulation.
3. Through the filtering action of lymph nodes and organs, the lymphatic system provides immunity against disease. Many pathogens and other impurities are removed from the lymph and destroyed by disease-fighting lymphocytes and antibodies.

LYMPH

The body is primarily composed of a base fluid consisting of water with a few proteins and complex sugars. When this fluid is situated between cells it is referred to as *extracellular fluid*. When it is situated between tissues, it is referred to as *interstitial fluid*. When located in the blood, it is referred to as *blood plasma*. When found in the lymphatic system, it is referred to as *lymph*. Hence, the main difference between lymph, blood plasma, extracellular fluid, and interstitial fluid is location.

Unlike the cardiovascular system, which flows in a continuous circle, the lymphatic system moves in only one direction, toward the subclavian veins. Without a pump to assist flow, lymph moves only through pressure gradients from external sources. Transportation of lymph depends entirely on pressure exerted on its vessel walls. This pressure can come from the milking action of skeletal muscle contractions or on the pressure changes in the thorax and abdomen during breathing. Lymph moves slowly when compared with blood circulation. When lymph pools in an area, the condition is referred to as **lymphedema** or *edema*.

LYMPH VESSELS

Lymphatic vessels (lymphatics) include lymph capillaries, lymph vessels, lymphatic trunks, and two main collecting ducts (Figure 19-10, *A*).

Lymph capillaries have the same structures as blood capillaries, but they are larger, more irregular,

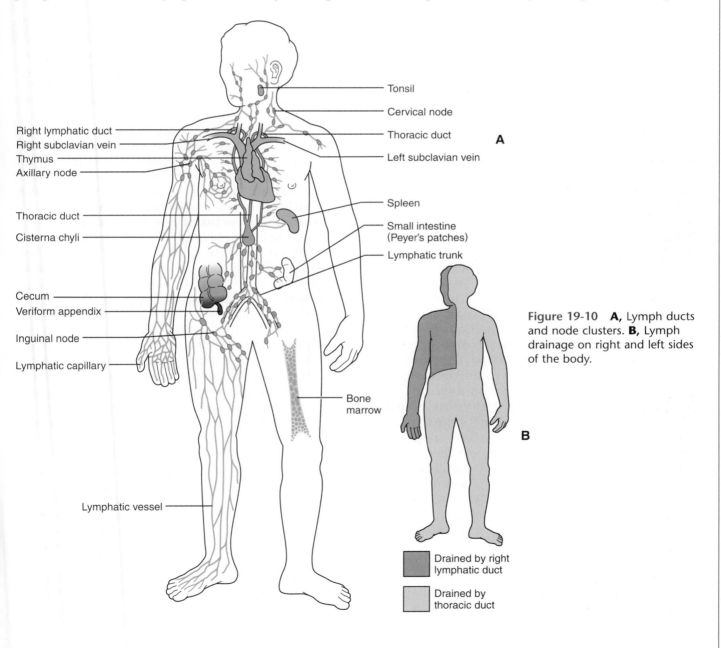

Tonsil

Cervical node

Thoracic duct

Left subclavian vein   **A**

Right lymphatic duct
Right subclavian vein
Thymus
Axillary node

Spleen

Thoracic duct

Small intestine
(Peyer's patches)

Cisterna chyli

Lymphatic trunk

Cecum
Veriform appendix

Inguinal node

Lymphatic capillary

Bone
marrow

Lymphatic vessel

B

Drained by right
lymphatic duct

Drained by
thoracic duct

Figure 19-10   A, Lymph ducts and node clusters. **B,** Lymph drainage on right and left sides of the body.

and more permeable. They start in the tissues and exist in all parts of the body except bone marrow, epidermis, central nervous system (brain and spinal cord), and the eyes. Lymph nodes are located throughout lymphatic tributaries to filter the lymph moving through the system.

Lymph capillaries become larger vessels called *lymph vessels.* Compared with veins, lymphatic vessels have thin walls and more valves that open up in only one direction. These merge along similar pathways to form region draining **lymphatic trunks**, which join to form one of two lymphatic ducts: right and thoracic. The **right lymphatic duct** drains lymph from the right arm and the right side of the head and the right half of the thorax into the right subclavian vein. The thoracic duct drains lymph from all remaining parts of the body into the left subclavian vein. The **thoracic duct** begins at the *cisterna chyli* (i.e., lymphatic sac located between the abdominal aorta and L2) and lies along the thoracic vertebrae.

LYMPH ORGANS

The primary lymphatic structures are the bone marrow and thymus (these are known as the *generative lymphatic organs* because they produce and mature lymphocytes). Secondary lymphatic structures include the spleen, lymph nodes, tonsils, Peyer's patches, and inside the vermiform appendix. These secondary lymphatic structures are populated by lymphocytes from the bone marrow and the thymus, which are described as follows:

1. **Bone marrow**, located in the hollow cavity of bones, produces the precursors to all lymphocytes. **Lymphocytes** are a type of WBC comprising about 25% of the total WBC count, increasing in number in response to infection. Some lymphocytes mature and become B lymphocytes, or B cells, within the red bone marrow. Other lymphocytes differentiate and travel to the thymus where they mature and become T lymphocytes or T cells.

2. Also an endocrine gland, the **thymus gland** is located in the mediastinal region of the thorax. As stated above, the thymus receives immature T cells. These lymphocytes complete their maturation and become T lymphocytes or T cells. Both T cells and B cells then travel to secondary lymphatic structures. Large in infants, the thymus reaches its maximum size at puberty, then atrophies and is replaced by adipose tissue in adults.

3. The largest lymphatic organ, the dark purple **spleen** lies within the left lateral rib cage (between the ninth and eleventh ribs) just posterior to the stomach. Functions of the spleen have baffled physiologist for hundreds of years, but recent

research indicates that it stores blood cells and destroys old, worn-out RBCs and platelets. Another major activity of the spleen is antibody production. As blood flows into the spleen, antigens are greeted and destroyed by T cells, B cells, phagocytes, and macrophages.

4. **Lymph nodes** are bean-shaped structures located along lymph vessels that collect and filter lymph. Lymph nodes are the only place where lymph is filtered in the lymphatic system. These are powerful defense stations that help protect the body from unwanted invaders. These nodes house phagocytes and lymphocytes (both B and T cells) that destroy bacteria, viruses, and other foreign substances in the lymph before it is returned to the blood. When the body is experiencing a local infection, the regional lymph nodes enlarge (Figure 19-11, *A*).

   Afferent vessels bring lymph into the lymph node to be filtered and cleaned. Efferent vessels take lymph out of the node. More afferent lymphatic vessels enter the node than efferent vessels leave the node, an imbalance that creates a pressure differential, slowing down the flow of lymph for filtering to occur.

   Although lymph nodes are located along all lymphatic vessels, nodes are clustered superficially in three areas on each side of the body and are palpated on routine physical examinations. They are named for their location: **cervical nodes**, **axillary nodes**, and **inguinal nodes**.

5. **Mucosal associated lymphoid tissue** (MALT) is a collection of lymphoid cells in the mucosa or submucosa of the digestive tract. These are tonsils, Peyer's patches, and inside the vermiform appendix.

   • **Tonsils** are a group of large specialized lymph tissues embedded in the mucus membranes around the throat. They include the adenoids or pharyngeal tonsils, palatine tonsils, and lingual tonsils. The function of the tonsils is to protect the body from airborne pathogens or other harmful substances that might enter through the nose or mouth. The lymphatic tissues use lymphocytes and macrophages to combat hostile intruders (see Chapter 21).

   • **Peyer's patches**, or intestinal tonsils, are groups of lymphatic nodules found in the mucus membrane of the small intestine, usually in the ileum and jejunum. These lymphatic cells constitute another member of the body's defense mechanisms by combating ingested pathogens.

   • Located inferior to the cecum, the **vermiform appendix** varies from 3 to 6 inches in length. Like other members of the lymphatic system, the appendix helps to fight pathogens and other bodily intruders.

Lymph node (enlargement)

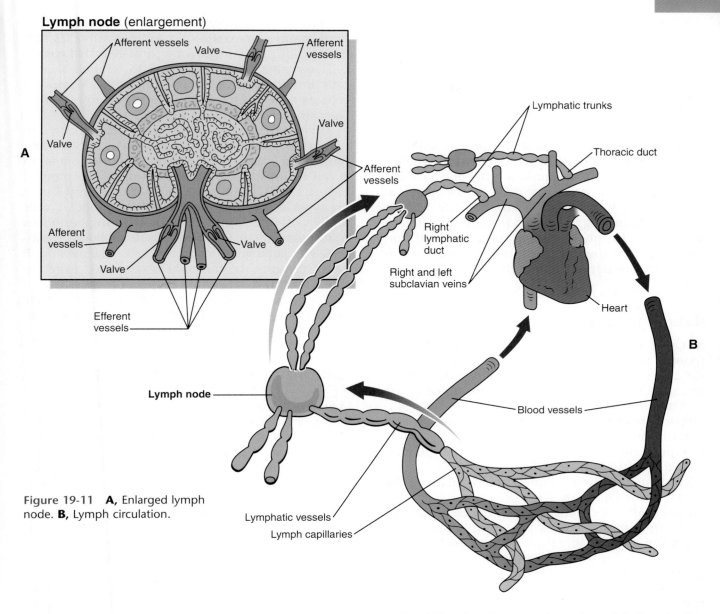

Figure 19-11   **A,** Enlarged lymph node. **B,** Lymph circulation.

PATHS OF LYMPH CIRCULATION

All lymph moves back toward the cardiovascular system. Lymph, which starts out as interstitial fluid, is collected by lymph capillaries and moves into lymph vessels, which become successively larger. Periodically along its one-way path, lymph flows into lymph nodes through afferent vessels and leaves through efferent vessels. Ultimately, lymph converges into either the right lymphatic duct or the thoracic duct and then enters the bloodstream through the right and left subclavian veins. The thoracic duct enters only the left venous circulation. In fact, most of the body's lymph empties on the left side (see Figure 19-11, *A*). Only the right side of the head and neck, the right upper extremity, and right half of the upper trunk empty into the right lymphatic duct (see Figure 19-11, *B*).

The following diagram shows lymph's flow in this pathway:

It starts out as tissue fluid,

↓

is collected by the lymphatic capillaries,

↓

moves into lymphatic vessels,

↓

moves through lymph nodes,

↓

moves through larger lymph vessels,

↓

collects in lymph trunks (either thoracic duct or right lymphatic duct),

↓

and is dumped in the right or left subclavian veins.

The deeper structures of the thorax, abdomen, pelvis, and perineum drain directly into the larger lymph vessels rather than passing through lymph capillaries.

IMMUNITY

Immunity is an anatomical and physiological defense reaction to invading microorganisms. The key components of this response are lymphocytes and WBCs, although structures such as the skin and chemicals such as digestive enzymes are also involved. Immunology is studied in the lymphatic system because lymphoid tissue is the anatomical component of the immune system. The two types of immunity are natural immunity and acquired immunity.

Natural Immunity

Natural immunity refers to the nonspecific responses to invading pathogens. Natural immunity can be affected by diet, mental health, environment, and metabolism. The following are examples of natural immune responses:

Physical barrier: Skin, mucosa, and cilia physically resist invaders.

Chemical barrier: Digestive enzymes, perspiration, vaginal secretions, acid mantel (on skin).

Complement proteins: Proteins found in blood that attack foreign agents.

Phagocytes: Cells that kill pathogens by phagocytosis. They approach their prey from the blood, engulfing and digesting them with lysomal enzymes. Primary phagocytic cells are neutrophils and macrophages. Phagocytes are involved with both natural and acquired immunity.

Inflammation: A protective mechanism that stabilizes and prepares the damaged tissue for repair and is involved in both natural and acquired immunity. Inflammatory symptoms are local heat, swelling, redness, pain, and decreased function (see Chapter 11).

Acquired Immunity

Acquired immunity involves diverse but specific responses to invaders involving lymphocytes. The cells involved in acquired immunity are specialized and possess memory (once they encounter and destroy the invader, they remember it and can destroy it quicker in the future). The two types of acquired immunity based on the type of lymphocyte involved are humoral immunity and cellular immunity. Humoral immunity involves B cells and cellular immunity involves T cells.

B Cells, T Cells, and Natural Killer Cells

Bone marrow–derived B cells secrete antibodies that destroy antigens. Antigens are pathogens that elicit B cell activation. They are slower to respond than T cells and are involved in immunization. Memory B cells stay after an infection is contained to recognize the pathogen if it invades again.

Thymus-derived T cells respond quickly to pathogens by attacking them directly. These cells puncture a hole in the pathogens cell membrane, so it can fill with tissue fluid, bursting in the process. Helper T cells, cytotoxic T cells, and memory T cells are types of T-cells. Helper T cells help both T cells and B cells fight an infection by secreting hormones to stimulate them. Cytotoxic T cells kill body cells infected by pathogens. Memory T cells, like memory B cells, stay after the infection is contained to recognize the pathogen if it invades again.

Natural killer cells are large lymphocytes and are neither B nor T cells. They bind to pathogens and tumor cells to kill them.

CARDIOVASCULAR PATHOLOGIES

Anemia. Anemia is a reduction of the oxygen-carrying capacity of the blood, a decrease in RBCs, or a reduced number of functional hemoglobin in the blood. It is usually a sign of other disorders. Characteristics of anemia include fatigue, vertigo, headaches, insomnia, paleness, and intolerance to cold.

Many types of anemia have been determined. The most common is iron-deficiency anemia resulting from lack of iron, and pernicious anemia in which not enough vitamin B_{12} is absorbed from the digestive tract into the blood.

Massage can help give rest and oxygenate an anemic client. However, if the anemia is the result of a bleeding disorder, lighter pressure should be used because the client may bruise easily as bleeding occurs under the skin.

Aneurysm. An aneurysm is a weakened section of a blood vessel wall that bulges outward. The most common causes are atherosclerosis, hypertension, and trauma, but it can also be the result of a congenital vascular weakness. The most common areas for aneurysms are the aorta and blood vessels in the brain, but they can occur in the extremities. Aneurysms may burst, causing hemorrhage, and possibly death.

If a client has a history of hypertension or atherosclerosis, the massage therapist should consult the client's physician before performing deep massage. If a client has been diagnosed with an abdominal aortic aneurysm, abdominal massage is contraindicated.

Angina pectoris. Often felt as chest pain, angina pectoris is commonly caused by constriction of coronary arteries and myocardial anoxia (lack of oxygen in the heart muscle). The pain originates from the chest and then radiates down the inner side of the left arm. The pain disappears with rest, and no lasting tissue damage occurs. Angina pectoris is often associated with physical overexertion, when the heart needs more oxygen. Emotional stress and exposure to intense cold can also trigger angina pectoris.

Massage can help clients by reducing stress. Massage also decreases the effects of the sympathetic nervous system, which is partially responsible for coronary artery vasoconstriction. Because sudden exposure to extreme cold or heat can bring on an attack, keep the client warm and avoid using heat or cold packs. If a client has an attack during a massage treatment, bring him to a sitting or standing position—gravity will help decrease the load of blood on the heart—then call for help. It is important that clients have with them their necessary medications (e.g., beta-blockers, nitroglycerin) when they come for treatment, in the event of a medical emergency.

Atherosclerosis. Arteriosclerosis is the thickening of arterial walls and the loss of arterial wall elasticity. Atherosclerosis is the narrowing of arteries resulting from the accumulation of hard lipid plaques in their walls. Atherosclerosis is often associated with obesity, hypertension, and diabetes. The narrowed arteries reduce blood flow, especially to the heart and brain. Because the plaque has a rough surface, platelets can snag on it, forming clots; this can further impede blood flow. Treatments include angioplasty, which is the insertion of a small balloon that, when inflated, squashes the plaque against the arterial walls to enlarge the hollow center of the artery. Lasers are also used to evaporate plaque. Catheter arthrectomy is a procedure that shaves the plaque off arterial walls. Clot-dissolving agents can be injected to remove thrombi.

If a client has atherosclerosis, she may be prone to thrombosis (blood clot) formation. Deep massage may dislodge the thrombus that could float as an embolus and lodge in smaller blood vessels in the lungs, heart, or brain, leading to difficulty breathing, heart attack, or stroke. Massage should be given only after consulting the client's physician. A lighter massage is indicated.

Cardiac arrest. A cardiac arrest is the sudden and complete cessation of the heartbeat, stopping all cardiac output, including pulmonary and systemic circulation. Once a cardiac arrest occurs, vascular delivery of oxygen and nutrients and removal of carbon dioxide and waste products is interrupted. Anaerobic metabolism begins and, if measures are not taken to stimulate the pumping action of the heart, damage to the brain, kidneys, heart, and lungs or even death can occur.

Massage is definitely contraindicated. The client needs immediate medical attention.

Congestive heart failure. In congestive heart failure (CHF), the heart is a failing pump. Causes include coronary artery disease, long-term hypertension, and myocardial infarcts (areas of dead heart tissue from previous heart attacks). If the left ventricle fails first, blood backs up in the lungs and can result in pulmonary edema. If the right ventricle fails first, blood backs up in peripheral blood vessels and can result in edema in the extremities, most noticeably the feet and ankles.

Massage should only be performed after obtaining clearance from the client's physician. A light massage of shorter duration is indicated because vigorous massage may tax an already debilitated heart.

Coronary artery disease. In coronary artery disease (CAD), the coronary arteries are narrowed and there is reduced blood flow to the heart. CAD is the leading cause of death in the United States, with symptoms ranging from mild angina to a full-scale heart attack. Usually symptoms start when about 75% of a coronary artery is blocked. The three main causes are atherosclerosis, coronary artery spasm, and blood clots.

Massage is same as for atherosclerosis.

Embolus. A blood clot, bubble of air, or any piece of debris transported by the bloodstream is an embolus. When an embolus becomes lodged in a vessel and cuts off circulation, it is then called an *embolism*.

Massage is definitely contraindicated.

Hemophilia. The three types of hemophilia are each genetically determined. In each case, only one clotting factor is missing, making it difficult or impossible for the blood to clot. Large hematomas can develop in the muscle or under the skin with mild trauma. Bleeding into the joints may occur, causing pain, swelling, and permanent joint stiffness. Often referred to as *free bleeders*, people with hemophilia receive transfusions of their missing clotting factor.

Massage is contraindicated for people with severe hemophilia. In milder forms, light massage is indicated, depending on the vitality of the client. Permission from the client's physician is needed.

Hemorrhage. Hemorrhaging is excessive bleeding, either internally (from blood vessels into tissues) or externally (from blood vessels directly to the surface of the body). The blood spillage may come from arteries, veins, or capillaries.

Massage is definitely contraindicated.

Hypertension. Hypertension is a common, often asymptomatic disorder of elevated blood pressure: 140/90 mm Hg is regarded as the threshold of hypertension, and 160/95 mm Hg is classified as serious hypertension. With sustained hypertension, arterial walls become inelastic and resistant to blood flow and, as a result, the left ventricle may become enlarged to maintain normal circulation. Risk factors for hypertension are cigarette smoking, obesity, lack of exercise, diabetes, and genetic predisposition.

People with hypertension that is not under control by diet, exercise, and/or medication should not have a massage. For clients who do have their hypertension under control, massage helps keep blood pressure lowered by reducing both stress and the activity of the sympathetic nervous system. Clients on antihypertensives may be prone to postural hypotension (a low blood pressure from the massage treatment). These clients will feel lightheaded and need to get up slowly from the massage table, perhaps needing assistance.

Leukemia. Also called *cancer of the blood,* leukemia is a cancer characterized by elevated WBC count. Generally, the two main categories of leukemia are acute and chronic. Acute leukemia is a malignant disease of blood-forming tissues resulting in uncontrolled production and accumulation of immature leukocytes. Chronic leukemia results in an accumulation of mature leukocytes that do not die at the end of their life span. Complications include anemia and bleeding problems because the immature WBCs crowd out functioning RBCs and platelets. Uncontrolled infection can also occur as a result of lack of mature or normal leukocytes.

Clearance from the client's physician is essential before performing massage. A gentle, relaxing massage is indicated because the client may bruise easily and have a tendency to bleed. Because enlargement of the spleen or liver may have occurred, abdominal massage is contraindicated.

Migraine headache. Also called *vascular headaches,* migraines are caused by dilation of extracranial blood vessels. Migraines may be triggered by foods (carbohydrates, iodine-rich foods, cheese, chocolate), alcohol (red wine), bright lights, loud noises, hormones (pregnancy hormones), or during a period of relaxation after physical or emotional stress. The acute phase may be accompanied by nausea, vomiting, chills, sweating, irritability, and extreme fatigue. After an attack the individual often has dull head and neck pains and a great need for sleep.

Massage is contraindicated during the migraine headache but can lessen the frequency and intensity of migraines between attacks. A full body, relaxation massage is indicated. Craniosacral therapy, biofeedback, and mediation have also been proven to be helpful.

Myocardial infarction. This is a heart attack. Death (necrosis) of myocardial tissue is the result of an interrupted coronary blood supply. Blood clots, atherosclerosis, and vascular spasms could lead to a myocardial infarction. Preceding symptoms are a viselike pain in the chest, which may radiate down the left arm, neck, or sternal region.

Massage considerations are the same as for angina pectoris.

Pericarditis. Pericarditis is an inflammation of the parietal pericardium and may be the result of trauma or infectious disease.

Massage is definitely contraindicated.

Phlebitis. Phlebitis, or thrombophlebitis, is an inflammation of the veins, often accompanied by a thrombus (blood clot). Phlebitis usually occurs after acute or chronic infection; surgery; pregnancy and childbirth; or prolonged sitting, standing, or immobilization. The affected area is hypersensitive to pressure and swollen and can be either hot or cold to the touch. It generally affects the arms or the calf area.

Local massage is contraindicated. A lighter, general massage is all right.

Raynaud's syndrome. Raynaud's syndrome is periodic attacks of vasospasm of blood vessels in the body's extremities, especially the most distal parts such as the fingers, toes, ears, and nose. It is most commonly caused by exposure to cold, emotional stress, or smoking (nicotine is a powerful vasoconstrictor). This condition can lead to ischemia, tissue necrosis, and nerve damage.

Massage helps increase local circulation. By reducing stress, massage helps reduce sympathetic stimulation and so relaxes the smooth muscle of blood vessels. Heat and ice packs are contraindicated.

Sickle cell disease. A genetic disorder, sickle cell disease is characterized by abnormal hemoglobin, which causes red blood cells to take on the shape of a sickle. This shape greatly reduces the amount of oxygen that can be supplied to the tissues, eventually causing extensive tissue damage. Sickle cell anemia is characterized by lethargy, fatigue, pain in the joints, thrombosis, and headaches. Treatments include analgesics to relieve pain, antibiotics to counter infections, and blood transfusions.

Clients with this disorder have periods of remission and flare-ups. Massage is contraindicated during flare-ups because the client is in pain and debilitated. During periods of remission, a lighter massage, paying close attention to the client's vitality, is indicated. Permission from the client's physician is needed.

Stroke. Also known as a *cerebrovascular accident (CVA),* a stroke is an occlusion (blockage) of cerebral blood vessels by an embolus or thrombus, or cerebrovascular hemorrhage. Muscular weakness or paralysis, an increase or decrease in sensation, speech abnormalities, or death may occur. Subsequent damage resulting from CVA depends on the location and extent of neurological damage.

Massage is indicated during the rehabilitation process, once the client's physician is consulted.

Thrombosis. This is thrombus (blood clot) formation in an unbroken blood vessel. Tissue damage can result from an interrupted blood supply. When the thrombus becomes dislodged and floats in the blood, it is referred to as an *embolus*.

Local massage is contraindicated. A lighter, general massage would be all right. Avoid deep massage in the inner thigh, especially in older clients. This area is referred to as the "valley of the clots."

Varicose veins. Varicose veins are dilated veins resulting from incompetent valves. In veins with weak valves, gravity prevents large amounts of blood from flowing upward. The back pressure overloads the vein and pushes its walls outward. The veins lose elasticity and become stretched and flabby. Thromboses may form in the varicose veins. They are typically caused by a congenital defect or repeated stress from overloading, such as pregnancy or obesity. This condition may worsen if the client is on her feet for long periods.

Because clients with varicose veins may be prone to thromboses, clearance from their physician may be necessary. Massage should be geared to reduce edema and prevent venous and lymphatic stasis. These clients' legs should be raised above the heart during treatment. The area involved may be sore to the touch.

LYMPHATIC/IMMUNE SYSTEM PATHOLOGIES

Acquired immunodeficiency syndrome. Acquired immunodeficiency syndrome (AIDS) is a disease caused by the human immunodeficiency virus (HIV). Transmission of the virus occurs through the exchange of bodily fluids such as blood, semen, vaginal secretions, and mother's milk. The average time between exposure to the virus and diagnosis is 8 to 10 years, but the incubation time is much shorter. Generally, there may be enlarged lymph nodes, weight loss, fatigue, night sweats, and fever. An AIDS diagnosis is made when a person has three or more opportunistic infections (e.g., tuberculosis, pneumonia, fungi) and/or a T-cell count below 200. A normal T-cell count is 1200.

It is unlikely that massage therapists will come in contact with client blood or body fluids. However, if a massage therapist has an open wound on her hands, she should not treat any client. Massage treatment for a client with AIDS needs to be tailored to that client's vitality, but a gentle massage is indicated. Care needs to be taken so that any infectious disorders of the client are not spread to the therapist, and vice versa.

Allergies. Allergies are a hypersensitivity and overreaction of the immune system to otherwise harmless agents (most are environmental or dietary). The person may experience inflammation or a runny nose from excess mucus secretion or,

more seriously, anaphylactic shock, in which air passageways constrict. A local allergic reaction could result in a rash or hives.

The massage therapist should make sure that the massage products and treatment room do not contain items to which the client is allergic (e.g., pet dander, lubricants that contain nut oils, and other possible allergens). Ask the client to review the ingredient list before applying massage lubricant on the skin.

Autoimmune diseases. Autoimmune diseases occur when the body's immune system fails to recognize its own tissues and attacks them as though they are foreign. Examples of autoimmune diseases are rheumatoid arthritis, lupus, and multiple sclerosis.

Massage is contraindicated during flare-ups. Massage for autoimmune diseases in remission depends on the individual disorder. Communication with the client and her health care provider on the client's vitality is essential for planning the massage treatment.

Chronic fatigue syndrome. Chronic fatigue syndrome (CFS) is characterized by the onset of disabling fatigue, sometimes after a viral infection. CFS is often accompanied by influenza-like symptoms such as low-grade fevers, sore throat, headaches. Memory deficits and sleep disturbances are also associated with this condition. Often resembling fibromyalgia, treatment is geared toward relieving symptoms. Counseling is often indicated because depression is common. CFS occasionally resolves spontaneously.

Massage can be very helpful for a client with CFS. It can soothe the nervous system, relieve muscle and joint pain, and give the client a chance to rest.

Hodgkin's disease. Hodgkin's disease is a cancer of the lymph nodes with painless, progressive enlargement of lymph nodes that may spread to other areas. Other symptoms include fever, night sweats, weight loss, fatigue, itching, and anemia. It is more common in young women between the ages of 15 and 35.

Clearance from the client's physician is necessary before performing massage. Massage is contraindicated if the client is debilitated. Otherwise, a gentle, relaxing massage is indicated.

Lupus. Lupus is an autoimmune, inflammatory disease of the connective tissues. It is not contagious. The cause of lupus is unknown. Its onset may be abrupt or gradual, but it primarily affects women age 20 to 40 years. A rash develops around the nose and check, resembling a wolf (often called a butterfly rash). Symptoms include painful joints, fever, fatigue, weight loss, enlarged lymph nodes and spleen, and sensitivity to light. There are periods of remission and exacerbation. Triggers for exacerbation include certain drugs, exposure to excessive sunlight, injury, and stress. Serious complications of the disease involve inflammation of the kidneys, liver, spleen, lungs, heart, and central nervous system. The three main types of lupus are as follows:

- **Discoid (DLE).** Skin disease; characterized by the presence of skin rash showing varying degrees of edema, redness, and scaliness
- **Systemic (SLE).** Most serious; body attacks connective tissue in joints, skin, and organs; this is a chronic, remitting, relapsing, inflammatory process and is often a multisystemic disorder
- **Drug-induced.** Medications used to treat hypertension and irregular heartbeat; can cause the onset of lupus; usually resolves after withdrawal of the medication

Massage is contraindicated when clients have a flare-up. During periods of remission, a gentle full body massage is indicated with special care taken of joints during stretches and ROM. Clients may be on corticosteroids and antiinflammatory drugs, so they may be more susceptible to bruising. Clients could also be on immunosuppressants, so care should be taken not to expose the clients to any form of infection.

Lymphedema. An abnormal accumulation of interstitial fluid tissues is referred to as lymphedema or *edema.* It is most often the result of lack of muscular activity (e.g., sitting in a car all day) but may be the result of local or general inflammation, obstruction, or removal of lymph vessels.

Massage can help lymphatic drainage by moving excess fluid into lymphatic vessels. The client's edematous limb should be supported and elevated. Elevation promotes dependent drainage (lymph drainage assisted by gravity). Proximal areas should be worked first to clear the path for lymph from distal areas.

Mononucleosis. Infectious mononucleosis is an acute viral infection that results from the Epstein-Barr virus (EBV). Symptoms are a slight to high fever, sore throat, red throat and soft palate, stiff neck, enlarged lymph nodes, coughing, and fatigue. It is highly contagious, transmitted by droplets that contain the virus. No cure has been found, and treatment is usually to allow it to run its course, treating any complications.

Massage is contraindicated until the client has recovered. Lighter abdominal massage is indicated after the client has recovered because the spleen may be enlarged. Gentle massage with heat packs may help relieve persistent body ache.

See Box 19-2 for the effects of massage on the lymphatic/immune system.

BOX 19-2

Effects of Massage on the Lymphatic/Immune System

- **Promotes lymph circulation.** Lymphatic circulation depends entirely on pressure; from muscle contraction, pressure changes in the thorax and abdomen during breathing, or pressure from a massage.
- **Reduces lymphedema.** Massage reduces lymphedema (swelling) by promoting lymph circulation, which helps remove waste from the system more effectively than either passive range of motion or electrical muscle stimulation.
- **Decreases the circumference of an area affected with lymphedema.** When an area swells, an increase in diameter occurs. When the swelling subsides, circumference decreases.
- **Decreases weight in patients with lymphedema.** Fluid retention adds weight to a patient. When lymphedema is addressed with massage, weight is consequently reduced.
- **Increases lymphocyte count.** Lymphocytes are types of WBCs. This indicates that massage supports immune functions.
- **Increases the number and function (or cytotoxicity) of natural killer cells.** Natural killer cells are also types of WBCs. This further suggests that massage strengthens immune functions and might help individuals with immune disorders.

SUMMARY

The cardiovascular and lymphvascular systems are the main transport mechanisms of the body for various fluids, gases, nutrients, wastes, antibodies, hormones, and heat. These two systems also play an important role in the body's defense system by fighting a variety of invaders. The clotting mechanism of the blood enables the body to make repairs to breaches of its tissues. The circulatory system also plays a part in water and chemical balance of the body. The main components of the cardiovascular system are the blood, heart, and vast network of arteries, capillaries, and veins that make up the circulatory vessels. The two main circuits of the cardiovascular system are pulmonary and systemic.

Although the cardiovascular system provides the liquid nourishment to the body's tissues, it is the lymphvascular system that collects and recycles that fluid back into circulation. Along with fluid conservation, the lymph system also transports fats, vitamins, lost proteins, and cellular debris, in addition to filtering the lymph and combating diseases with its own immune functions. The lymphatic system's major structures include lymph, bone marrow, thymus, spleen, lymph nodes, and MALT (e.g., tonsils, Peyer's patches, and inside the vermiform appendix). Lymphatic vessels route the collected fluids from all areas of the body and direct it to two main vessels, which return it into the cardiovascular system.

The two types of immunity are natural and acquired. Natural immunity is the nonspecific response to invaders. Acquired immunity involves specific responses to invaders involving lymphocytes, namely B cells and T cells.

MATCHING I

Write the letter of the best answer in the space provided.

A. Type AB
B. Leukocytes
C. Plasma
D. Hyperemia
E. Vasodilation
F. Blood pressure

G. Type O
H. Agglutinogens
I. Veins
J. Ischemia
K. Arteries
L. Erythrocytes

M. Atrium
N. Stroke volume
O. Platelets
P. Hemoglobin
Q. Ventricle
R. Carotid

____ 1. Local decrease in blood flow

____ 2. Straw-colored liquid that helps transport blood cells

____ 3. The amount of blood ejected from the left ventricle during each ventricular contraction

____ 4. Blood cells involved in blood clotting

____ 5. Superior heart chamber

____ 6. Enlargement of the vascular lumen

____ 7. Universal blood recipient

____ 8. Genetically determined proteins on the surfaces of RBCs

____ 9. Superficial artery in the throat region

____ 10. These blood cells serve as part of the body's immune system

____ 11. Most numerous blood cells and possesses hemoglobin

____ 12. An iron-based protein that is the red respiratory pigment in RBCs

____ 13. Thick-walled inferior heart chamber

____ 14. Vessels that drain the tissues, returning the deoxygenated blood back to the heart

____ 15. Increased local blood flow

____ 16. Vessels that move blood away from the heart

____ 17. Universal blood donor

____ 18. Pressure exerted by blood on arterial walls during contraction of the left ventricle

MATCHING II

Write the letter of the best answer in the space provided.

A. Mucosal associated lymphoid tissue
B. Spleen
C. Thymus
D. B cells
E. Right lymphatic duct

F. Acquired immunity
G. T cells
H. Natural immunity
I. Inflammation
J. Cisterna chyli
K. Vermiform appendix

L. Lymph
M. Lymph nodes
N. Bone marrow
O. Thoracic duct
P. Tonsils

_____ 1. Generative lymphatic structure that produces precursors of all lymphocytes

_____ 2. Lymphatic duct that drains the right arm, right side of head, and right half of thorax, dumping lymph into the right subclavian vein

_____ 3. Groups of specialized lymph tissues embedded in mucus membranes around the throat

_____ 4. Thymus derived cells that respond quickly to pathogens; types include helper cells, cytotoxic cells, and memory cells

_____ 5. Largest lymphatic organ

_____ 6. A protective mechanism that stabilizes and prepares the damaged tissue for repair; symptoms are local heat, swelling, redness, pain, and decreased function

_____ 7. Type of immunity that is a nonspecific response to invading pathogens

_____ 8. Lymphoid cells in the mucosa or submucosa of the alimentary canal

_____ 9. Filtering stations for lymph

_____ 10. Immunological response that is diverse but specific and involves lymphocytes

_____ 11. Lymphatic structure located inferior to the cecum

_____ 12. Fluid of the lymphatic system

_____ 13. Bone marrow–derived cells secreting antibodies that destroy antigens

_____ 14. Lymphatic duct that drains the majority of the body and dumps lymph into the left subclavian vein

_____ 15. Lymphatic sac located between the abdominal aorta and L2; inferior portion of the thoracic duct

_____ 16. Generative lymphatic organ receiving immature B-cells, maturing them into T cells

Bibliography

Applegate EJ: *The anatomy and physiology learning system,* ed 2, Philadelphia, 2000, WB Saunders.

Crawley J, Van De Graaff KM: *A photographic atlas for anatomy and physiology,* Englewood, Colo, 2002, Morton.

Damjanov I: *Pathophysiology for the health-related professions,* Philadelphia, 1996, WB Saunders.

Gould BE: *Pathophysiology for the health-related professionals,* Philadelphia, 1997, WB Saunders.

Gray H, Pickering P, Howden R: *Gray's anatomy,* ed 29, Philadelphia, 1974, Running Press.

Haubrich WS: *Medical meanings: a glossary of word origins,* New York, 1984, Harcourt Brace Jovanovich.

Jacob S, Francone C: *Elements of anatomy and physiology,* Philadelphia, 1989, WB Saunders.

Kalat JW: *Biological psychology,* ed 2, Belmont, Calif, 1984, Wadsworth.

Kapit W, Elson, LM: *The anatomy coloring book,* ed 3, New York, 2002, Benjamin Cummings.

Marieb EN: *Essentials of human anatomy and physiology,* ed 4, New York, 1994, Benjamin Cummings.

McAleer N: *The body almanac,* Garden City, NY, 1985, Doubleday.

Merck Research Laboratories: *Merck manual,* ed 17, Whitehouse Station, NJ, 1998, Author.

Mosby's medical, nursing, and allied health dictionary, ed 4, St Louis, 1994, Mosby.

Newton D: *Pathology for massage therapists,* ed 2, Portland, Ore, 1995, Simran.

Premkumar K: *Pathology A to Z: a handbook for massage therapists,* Calgary, Canada, 1996, VanPub.

Solomon EP, Phillips GA: *Understanding human anatomy and physiology,* Philadelphia, 1987, WB Saunders.

Taber's cyclopedic medical dictionary, ed 13, Philadelphia, 1977, FA Davis.

Thibodeau G, Patton K: *Structure and function of the body,* ed 11, St Louis, 2000, Mosby.

Tortora GJ: *Introduction to the human body: the essentials of anatomy and physiology,* ed 3, New York, 1994, HarperCollins.

Tortora GJ, Grabowksi SR: *Principles of anatomy and physiology,* ed 9, New York, 2000, John Wiley.

Travell JG, Simons DG: *Myofascial pain and dysfunction: the trigger point manual,* Baltimore, 1983, Williams and Wilkins.

Werner R: *A massage therapist's guide to pathology,* ed 2, Baltimore, 2002, Lippincott Williams & Wilkins.

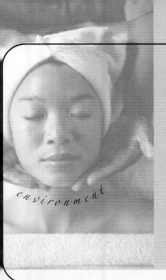

environment

Respiratory System

20

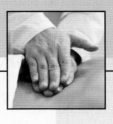

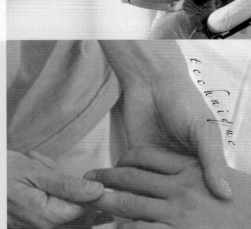

pressure

technique

"When you breathe, you inspire. When you don't, you expire."

—Popular Science

After completing this chapter, the student should be able to:

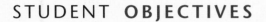

- List functions of the respiratory system
- Identify and discuss each respiratory structure
- Describe mechanisms of breathing
- Name the modified respiratory air movements
- Name types of respiratory pathologies, giving characteristics and massage considerations of each
- Discuss olfaction as it relates to the use of aromatherapy

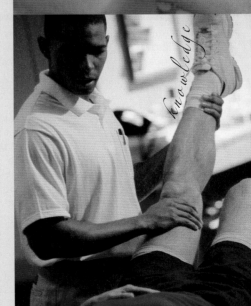

knowledge

INTRODUCTION

Breathing has long been the inspiration of poets and philosophers. Books have been filled with references to "his dying breath," "her breast rose and fell," "his breath quickened," and "he breathed life into them." Breath and the breathing process are synonymous with life itself. Breathing is the most easily observable of the body's vital signs. It is through respiration that we take in new air, extract oxygen from it, and expel carbon dioxide and other waste gases back into the atmosphere. Every cell of the body needs oxygen, and delivery is accomplished by way of the bloodstream. The respiratory and the circulatory systems both participate in this respiratory process. Failure of either system has the same effect on the body, including disruption of homeostasis and rapid cell death from oxygen deprivation.

The various life-sustaining mechanisms of the respiratory system are discussed in this chapter, along with some of the modified respiratory functions. The following topics are included in discussion: basic anatomy of the respiratory system, the respiratory system's role in the senses of smell and speech, mechanisms of breathing, internal and external respiration, and how breathing can aid massage.

FUNCTIONS

Exchange of gases. Oxygen and carbon dioxide exchange is the primary function of the respiratory system. A constant intake of oxygen is essential for maintaining life. Without oxygen intake and the elimination of carbon dioxide, the body's cells would start to perish within 5 minutes. This gas exchange occurs in the lungs and capillaries.

Olfaction. Olfaction refers to the sense of smell. Through the act of inhalation, scent molecules enter the nose and are forced against the mucosal lining in the nasal cavity. Receptors from the olfactory nerve are embedded in the nasal mucosa and, if stimulated, send impulses for the sense of smell to the brain.

Speech. The production of speech is a complex coordination of muscles and nerves. Sound is produced by air moving over the vocal cords. Movements of the facial muscles and tongue form words.

Homeostasis. The respiratory system helps maintain oxygen levels in the blood. It also helps maintain homeostasis through the elimination of wastes (e.g., carbon dioxide and heat). Excess carbon dioxide in the blood can lead to an acidic condition. When carbon dioxide is expelled through exhalation, the respiratory system helps regulate blood pH.

All things share the same breath.
—Chief Sealth, Duwamish tribe, 1885

ANATOMY AND PHYSIOLOGY

Air is conducted by a pathway of structures in the respiratory system. The following is a description of each structure (Figure 20-1).

Nose. The nose is port of entry for air and the beginning of the air conduction pathway. What we see and feel as the nose is primarily hyaline and elastic cartilage. The paired nasal bones and process of the maxillae bone form the central region of the nose. The bridge of the nose consists of the nasal bones and the frontal bone.

Nasal cavity. Just behind the nose is the nasal cavity. The nasal septum, formed by the vomer and the ethmoid bones and hyaline cartilage, divides the nasal cavity into right and left sides. The nasal cavity leads to the **nasal conchae**. The superior, middle, and inferior nasal conchae are the ridges that extend out of each lateral wall of the nasal cavity (Figure 20-2). The three conchae subdivide further into the creaselike passageways called **meatuses**. The nasal conchae terminate at the throat. The mucosal lining of the nasal cavity contains blood capillaries, cells with cilia, and goblet cells. As air flows over the nasal cavity mucosa, it becomes warm and moist. The nasal cavity tries to clean the air before it enters the lungs, so cilia trap air particles and move them up and out or down the throat.

Term	Meaning
allergy	other; work
apnea	not; breathing
auditory	to hear
bronchus	windpipe
cilia	hairlike
eustachian	Italian anatomist (1524-1574)
exudate	to sweat out
glottis	back of the tongue
meatus	passage
olfaction	to smell
phrenic	diaphragm
pleura	rib; side
pneumo, pneum	air; lungs
pulmo	lung
trachea	rough
ventilation	to air
volitional	will

Terms and Their Meanings Related to the Respiratory System

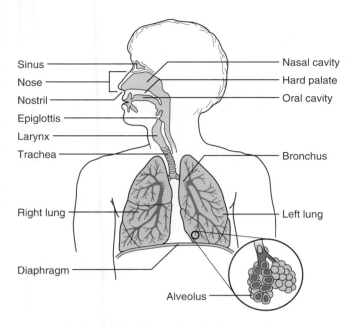

Figure 20-1   General respiratory structures.

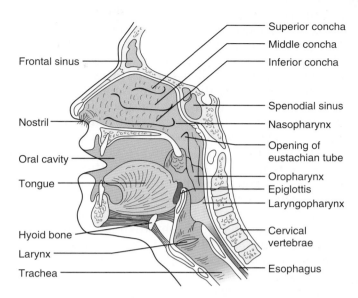

Figure 20-2   Upper respiratory anatomy.

Cilia are hairlike projections on the outer surfaces of certain cells. **Goblet cells** produce mucus that moistens the air and traps incoming foreign particles. Because of all of these functions, the nasal cavities are called the *air-conditioning chambers*.

Four of the paranasal sinuses (frontal, sphenoidal, ethmoidal, and maxillary) have openings into the nasal cavity. The mastoid sinus drains into the middle ear. The sinuses are featured in Chapter 14.

Pharynx. The pharynx, or throat, is a muscular tube approximately 5 inches long that is shared by the respiratory and the digestive systems. Located anterior to the cervical vertebrae, the pharynx extends from behind the nasal cavity (nasopharynx) to the back of the oral cavity (oropharynx) and down to the larynx (laryngopharynx). It contains the tonsils (pharyngeal, palatine, and lingual), which help our immune system by protecting against inhaled or ingested pathogens.

The eustachian tube opens into the superior pharynx. Because of this close proximity, respiratory infections can easily create middle ear infections and vice versa.

Larynx. The larynx, or voice box, is formed by three single and three paired cartilages. The single cartilages are the epiglottis, cricoid, and thyroid (Adam's apple), which is the largest. Enlargement of the thyroid cartilage occurs primarily in men because of the presence of testosterone. The three paired cartilages (arytenoid, corniculate, and cuneiform) attach to and support the vocal cords or folds.

The two sets of **vocal cords** are a superior pair called the *false vocal cords* and an inferior pair called the *true vocal cords,* or simply vocal cords. The true vocal cords are used for normal voice production; however, a person can train to use the false cords, as is shown in ventriloquism or singers who have two ranges.

The vocal cords are bands of elastic ligaments that are attached to the rigid cartilage of the larynx by skeletal muscle. At the space between the cords, air passes over them, causing vibration and producing sound. The tighter the skeletal muscles pull the vocal cords, the higher is the pitch of the voice.

One of the single laryngeal cartilages, the **epiglottis**, closes the trachea during swallowing (deglutition), preventing food from entering the inferior respiratory passageways. Because of this function, the epiglottis is referred to as the *guardian of the airways.*

Trachea. The trachea, or windpipe, is a tube from the larynx to the upper chest. Located anterior to the esophagus, it measures about 5 inches long and consists of 16 to 20 half-ring hyaline cartilages. These half-ring cartilages serve a dual purpose. The incomplete sections of the ring allow the esophagus to expand into the trachea when a food bolus is swallowed. The rings also keep the tracheal wall from collapsing during pressure changes that occur during breathing. The trachea bifurcates at its base into the right and left primary bronchi.

Bronchi. The right and left bronchi are the large air-conduction passageways leading from the trachea to each lung. Each tubelike structure is reinforced with hyaline cartilage, helping keep the airway open. The right primary bronchus is slightly wider and has a slightly steeper downward angle than the left; because of this, foreign bodies more often lodge on the right side. The right and left primary bronchi branch out like roots of a tree into even smaller divisions called **bronchioles**. As the airways branch out, they become smaller, with less cartilage and more smooth muscle.

Alveoli. Alveoli are tiny sacs attached to the distal ends of the bronchioles. They are made of a single layer of epithelial tissue blended with elastic connective tissue. The walls are so thin that it is hard to imagine their thinness, but a sheet of notepaper is much thicker. **Alveolar sacs** are two or more alveoli that share a common opening. The lungs contain approximately 300 million alveoli, providing an immense surface area of about 1000 square feet (ft^2), roughly the area of a handball court. Superficial to the alveoli are numerous capillaries, so many that 900 ml of blood are able to participate in gas exchange at any given time.

- **Surfactants**. Surfactants are phospholipids that assist in the exchange of gas in the alveoli, reduce surface tension, and contribute to the elasticity of pulmonary tissue. Lungs are the last organ to develop in utero. Infants born prematurely (before 28 gestational weeks) may not have produced enough surfactants to allow their lungs to expand with air.

Lungs. Lungs are spongy, highly elastic, paired organs of respiration. Although the lungs fill most of the thoracic cavity, they weigh less than 1 lb each. The inferior surface of the lungs is broad and concave to match the shape of the superior surface of the respiratory diaphragm. The right lung has three lobes; the left lung has two lobes because the heart is more localized on the left side. This depression in the left lung to accommodate the heart is called the *cardiac notch* (Figure 20-3). The external surfaces of the lungs are lined by a serous membrane, and both lungs are encased by a pleural membrane, which secretes a thin serous fluid. This fluid prevents friction, allowing the lungs to move easily in the doubled-walled pleural cavity during respiration.

Respiratory diaphragm. The respiratory diaphragm is a dome-shaped muscular partition that separates the thoracic cavity from the abdominal cavity. It is the main muscle of respiration. The diaphragm consists of both contractile muscular fibers and resistant, tendinous connective tissues, which serve to increase extensibility and help keep its firm shape. Passing through the transverse plane with an airtight seal and inserting into its central tendon, the diaphragm attaches around the circumference of the lower six ribs, connecting

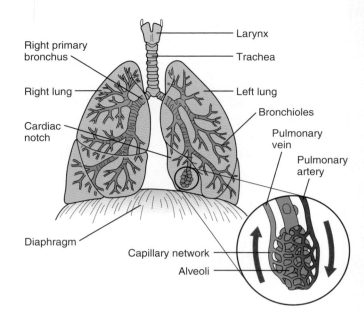

Figure 20-3   Lower respiratory anatomy.

the spine, ribs, and xiphoid process (three portions can be differentiated). The opening for the passage of the descending aorta, inferior vena cava, and the esophagus pierces the diaphragm. During contraction, the diaphragm is pulled down, creating a vacuum in the chest cavity, which sucks air down into the lungs. Relaxation of the diaphragm causes it to rise, allowing the lungs to deflate, and pushes out air as a result.

Because the respiratory diaphragm never stops contracting, the potential for trigger point development is tremendous. Tightening of the diaphragm's fibers can cause torquing of the rib cage around the spine and central tendon, thus limiting the efficiency of inhalation. Some rib cage mobilizations and deep-tissue diaphragmatic releases can actually increase the lungs vital capacity.

In review, air is conducted by the following pathway of structures:

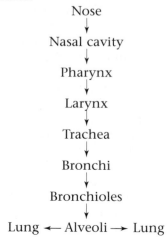

THE MECHANISMS OF BREATHING

Three processes are required to get oxygen from the atmosphere to the body's cells. They are breathing (the mechanics of inhaling and exhaling), external respiration (extraction of oxygen and disposal of carbon dioxide), and internal respiration (getting oxygen to the cells and removing carbon dioxide from the cells).

For Your Information

If an individual lives to be age 72, he or she will have taken more than 530 million breaths of air.

- **Breathing**, or pulmonary ventilation, is a mechanical process because muscular contraction and relaxation are required to move air in and out of the lungs. The two phases of breathing are inspiration and expiration.
- **Inspiration**, or **inhalation**, is the process that is responsible for drawing air into the lungs and can be divided into normal and forced inspiration. Normal inspiration occurs when the diaphragm contracts and descends into the abdominal cavity and when the external intercostal muscles simultaneously contract to raise the ribs. Forced or labored inspiration requires additional muscular contraction by the sternocleidomastoid, scalenes, and pectoralis minor. These muscles are considered accessory muscles of respiration.
- **Expiration**, or **exhalation**, is the process that is responsible for expelling air from the lungs back to the atmosphere. Expiration can also be classified as normal or forced. During normal expiration, the diaphragm relaxes and ascends back up toward the thoracic cavity. Air is forced out of the lungs because of elastic recoil of the alveoli (Figure 20-4). Forced or labored expiration is an active process, using voluntary muscular contractions of the internal intercostals and the abdominal muscles.

At rest, adults respire about 15 to 20 times a minute; children breathe twice as fast. Exercise can increase oxygen need up to 30 times. Respiration rates increase to match the oxygen needs of cells.

The respiratory center in the brain stem that controls the basic rhythm of breathing is influenced by the amount of carbon dioxide in the blood. It operates without conscious control and works by sending nerve impulses down the phrenic nerve to the diaphragm. These impulses are also sent to the other muscles of respiration.

Several other factors help regulate the respiratory center; for example, the cerebral cortex can modify our breathing patterns when laughing or crying and

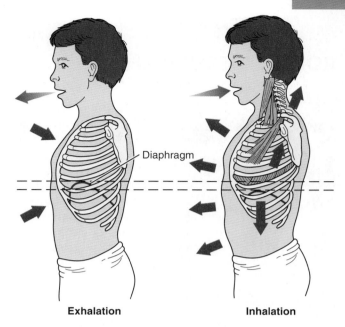

Figure 20-4   Air moving in and out of the lungs.

can initiate voluntary breathing. Voluntary breathing allows you to hold your breath during swimming under water and to take deep breath to project your voice during public speaking. However, if you control your breath by rapid breathing (hyperventilation) or holding your breath too long, you will

Aromatherapy and Olfaction

A person does not smell with the nose; she smells with the brain. Aromatherapy can be used to enhance relaxation or stimulate the nervous system. The olfactory bulb is part of the limbic system, which is regarded as the neurological seat of the emotions. Other parts of the limbic system are the hypothalamus, hippocampus, amygdala, thalamus, and a marginal section of the cerebral hemispheres close to the thalamus. Scientists believe that these structures work as a system to regulate emotional behaviors.

In 1937, J.W. Papez identified these structures and stated that the structures of the limbic system responded to smell, taste, sound, sight, and painful stimuli, all of which elicit emotional responses. When these structures are damaged, emotional experience decreases significantly. When these neurological structures are stimulated electrically, individuals experience emotions such as anger, aggression, fear, sadness, pleasure, happiness, and sexual arousal.

The easiest way to stimulate the limbic system is through the sense of smell. Massage therapists can use aromatherapy in conjunction with massage therapy to enhance therapeutic benefits. A list of essential oils and their effects is found in Chapter 3.

ROBERT TISSERAND

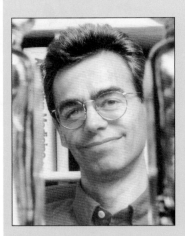

Born: November 11, 1948.

"Love what you do. Enjoy listening to people. It can be hard work, but the potential for helping people is tremendous."

Robert Tisserand, author and aromatherapist, was born in London to a father who made baskets and a mother who "did a little of this and that, but mostly raised three kids." Luckily for his "mum," the two girls were not quite as inquisitive as Tisserand, who shares his first "taste" of the aromatherapy experience.

"Curiously, I did actually drink a bottle of perfume when I was about 2 years old. My father bought it for my mother in a flea market in Paris in 1945, so the perfume would have been about 5 years old at the time. It was called *Creme de Zofali.* I survived, but the bottle has not."

Considering that it is often the smell and not the taste of foods that makes them appealing, it's easy to understand why a little boy would not think twice before turning up a bottle of slightly aged perfume. However, aromas affect more than our appetites. Odors of certain plants have been used to dedicate newborns, banish evil spirits, guide dearly departed souls to the other side, and heal all manner of ills in between. Long before frankincense and myrrh were offered to the Christ child, Egyptian physicians were using it in their practices. Greek mythology includes stories regarding the healing properties of aromatic plants, and Romans enjoyed massage with wonderfully scented, unbelievably expensive oils.

What has become a popular trend in the past few years was an academic area of study as far back as the Middle Ages. During this time, essential oils were classified according to the four elements or humors, the degree of "hotness" or "coldness" and also by the shape or color of the plant from which it was derived. For example, lungwort looks like lungs, so it was used for the respiratory system. Blue is a calming color, so plants with blue flowers were considered to have sedative properties. This way of cataloging plant essences was called the *doctrine of signatures.* Astronomy also helped play a role in organizing certain scents. Late in the sixteenth century, Nicholas Culpepper, an astrological physician, associated oils with planetary characteristics. For instance, ylang-ylang is identified as having Venus properties because it has a strong, sweet odor and a slightly yellow tint and is considered an aphrodisiac.

The first people to dispense aromatics were the priests. They were the first perfumers, or what we would call an *aromatherapist* today. Physicians picked up the practice soon thereafter.

Although aromatherapy (the use of essential oils distilled from plants for certain conditions) has been widely used in England for some time, only recently did its climb in popularity start in the United States. Lately, massage therapists are learning more about how aromatherapy can benefit their practices. At the very least, aromatherapy adds another sensory-pleasing dimension to the pleasure of receiving a massage. However, because of the strong connection between our sense of smell and mood, it can also add other benefits. For instance, lavender is thought to be calming. On the other end of the spectrum, mints and citrus oils have an energizing effect. Mixed with oil or lotion, essential essences are considered by many to work magic on a myriad of maladies, from clogged sinuses to diarrhea. Aromatherapy can also be ingested (only by trained aromatherapists) for treatment of some ailments.

When asked which five essential oils are most important for massage therapists to always have on hand, Tisserand hesitates, pointing out that ideally, no limit should be made. However, if it is necessary to choose only five, he recommends eucalyptus, lavender, rosemary, geranium, and ylang-ylang. He also advises therapists to practice the craft in as professional a manner as

ROBERT TISSERAND—cont'd

possible, experiment, and attend some type of training in aromatherapy. The Tisserand School of Aromatherapy requires 6 months' full-time attendance or 2 years' part-time attendance. Massage therapists should also be aware that some oils do have contraindications. For example, a popular essential oil for muscular aches and pains, bergamot, can cause photosensitivity.

Tisserand's "taste" for aromatherapy piqued around 1967 at age 19, when he attended a lecture on the subject along with his mother. She bought a book and had it signed by the speaker, Dr. Valnet. A couple of years later, Tisserand became interested in bodywork and did some training in that area. He soon made a conscious decision to pursue a career in aromatherapy. "Not for the money," he laughs, "or I would have given up a long time ago. Basically, I starved for 20 years."

Today, he teaches others the art of aromatherapy. He has also developed and distributes Tisserand essential oil products all over the world. His works include the quintessential *The Art of Aromatherapy* (Beekman, 1977); *Aromatherapy to Heal and Tend the Body, published* (Lotus Light, 1996); and *Essential Oil Safety* (Churchill Livingstone, 1995).

Tisserand still has his mother's signed copy of Valnet's French aromatherapy book, and after 30 years of hard work, audiences flock to his seminars, buy his books, seek his advice, and ask for his signature. The little boy who could not resist his mother's bottle of flea market perfume is finally able to sit back and enjoy the sweet smell of success.

become unconscious. How long the breath is held is limited by carbon dioxide buildup in the blood.

An increase in body temperature (e.g., fever, exercise) increases respiration whereas a decrease in body temperature (e.g., hypothermia, jumping into cool water) decreases respiration. Emotions such as anger or fear can also change respiration rates. A sudden, severe pain can temporarily stop breathing (apnea), and stretching the anal sphincter muscle increases the respiration rate (this technique is sometimes employed to stimulate respiration during medical emergencies).

The total amount of air that can be forcibly inspired and expired from the lungs in one breath is called **vital capacity**. This represents the greatest respiratory volume of an individual. Age, gender, physical fitness, and disease affect vital capacity. Average values range from 4000 to 5000 ml.

During massage, apply the downward pressure for an effleurage during an exhalation. When applying static pressure over a trigger point, wait for the client to exhale. Follow the wave of the client's breath; release pressure on the inhalation and apply pressure on the exhalation. This not only gives a sense of rhythm to your massage but also uses the client's natural ability to relax during an exhalation to enhance the effectiveness of your work.

Encourage your client to breathe properly during the massage. Invite him to focus on his breathing by placing your hand just below his navel while he is lying supine. Ask him to take a deep breath and to allow his belly to elevate your hand. Occasionally, a simple goal like using the breath to move the therapist's hand helps the client understand the abdominal changes that occur while breathing.

While your client is prone, place your hand on the small of her back and ask her to take a deep breath, elevating your hand during inhalation. After instructing your client how to breathe for relaxation, teach her to use this simple technique when she feels stress or fatigue. These types of client/therapist interactions help teach clients how to relax and be aware of their bodies.

External and Internal Respiration

Respiration takes place by *diffusion,* or the tendency of molecules to move from a region of higher concentration to an area of lower concentration. The main functions of the respiratory process are to supply the body with oxygen and dispose of carbon dioxide. Every cell needs oxygen to sustain life. Respiration occurs through two distinct processes: external and internal respiration.

MINI-LAB

Using a tape measure, note the change in the circumference as you measure the rib cage during inspiration and expiration. Measure parts of the body such as the upper and lower ribs and abdomen.

External (pulmonary) respiration is gas exchange in the lungs, between blood and air in the alveoli that came from the external environment. Oxygen diffuses from the air inside the alveoli across the alveolar walls into the blood capillaries. The oxygen binds to the hemoglobin inside red blood cells and is then transported to cells throughout the body. Carbon dioxide is transported by the blood from the cells of the body to the capillaries covering the alveoli. The carbon dioxide then diffuses from the blood across the alveolar walls into the air inside the alveoli, which will then be exhaled.

Internal (tissue) respiration is the gas exchange between blood and body's tissues. Oxygen diffuses from the blood into the cells, and carbon dioxide diffuses from the cells into the bloodstream. Each cell participates in absorption of oxygen and removal of waste materials in connection with this process.

MODIFIED RESPIRATORY AIR MOVEMENTS

Coughing is a sudden expulsion of air to clear the lungs and lower respiratory passageways of irritants or foreign materials. Coughing is a protective reflex but can be voluntarily induced or inhibited. The act of coughing occurs after a brief inspiration. The abdominal muscles contract, forcing air out of the lungs. Productive coughing helps clear the respiratory tract.

Crying is a response to emotions, such as grief, pain, fear, or joy. A common breath pattern while crying involves a sudden inspiration followed by the release of air in short breaths.

Hiccups, or hiccoughs, are intermittent contractions of the diaphragm followed by a spasmodic closure of the vocal cords. The sound occurs when inspired air hits the closed vocal cords. Hiccups have a variety of causes that appear to be linked to irritation of gastrointestinal sensory nerve endings.

Laughing involves the same modified respiratory patterns as crying and is usually a response to happiness, being tickled, or that something strikes us as funny. During laughter, the mouth is typically

Breathing and Massage Therapy

Breathing not only reflects our physiological and psychological states, it also creates them. Actors have known this for many years. Whenever a particular scene requires them to appear anxious, they take shallow, rapid breaths before the scene. Conversely, when a scene requires that they look calm and relaxed, they use slow, deep breaths to bring them to a state of relaxation. Massage therapists use breathing techniques themselves while they are giving a massage and often teach these techniques to their clients.

The most effective type of breathing to produce relaxation is deep, slow abdominal or diaphragmatic breathing. During deep breathing, the muscles of the abdominal wall expand when the diaphragm moves down during inhalation; the abdominal contents get a massage as they are compressed and released.

When we breathe deeply, it is a total body experience. Deep breathing can ease pain, relax tension, or introduce much-needed energy into the body. Shallow breathing does not encourage relaxation and can create tension in the neck and shoulders.

Breathing creates and reflects our emotional sphere, so deep, full breaths positively affect the free expression of our feelings. Restrictive breathing tends to constrict our expressions and wall off our feelings; we feel disconnected from the world around us.

The rhythm of breathing can give us an indication of how we feel about our surroundings. If we observe a slight pause before inhalation, this may announce a fear of new experiences. People inevitably stop breathing in an attempt to prevent something from happening. Clients hold their breath during a massage when the pressure is uncomfortable. A slight pause before exhalation may indicate a fear of the client's own personal expression.

Imagine that the air around you has a fluid quality. As you inhale, the bottom portion of your lungs fills up first (like a glass of water). This filling causes a depression of the diaphragm and an expansion of the abdomen and thorax. As air fills the upper lungs, the rib cage expands and elevates on all sides. The spine also moves to accommodate the thoracoabdominal expansion. To complete your inhalation, puff out your cheeks and tightly close your lips. Allow your breath to burst out of your lips and exhale through your mouth, nose, or both. Although exhalation is typically a passive event, you may force air out of your lungs by contracting your abdominal muscles and "kissing your belly button to your spine." As you breathe, you should feel your body, especially your spine, ribs, and abdomen, move. Subtle movements may be felt in the extremities.

Children and most animals breathe with their bellies. Observe a sleeping cat or a toddler running around in a diaper. Her belly moves in a wave as she breathes. On mornings when you can wake up naturally (without an alarm), notice how you are breathing; you will probably be doing abdominal breathing. Encourage your body to breathe this way throughout the day.

open in a grin. Laughing and crying can be so similar in sound that we typically have to look at a person's face to tell which emotion is being expressed.

Sneezing is a forceful involuntary expulsion of air through the nose and mouth to clear the upper respiratory passageways. Most sneezes occur as a result of irritation of the respiratory lining by foreign particles such as dust or pollen.

Snoring is audible breathing during sleep resulting from vibration of the uvula and soft palate. Snoring can be accompanied by harsh sounds and is common among individuals who sleep with their mouths open. When a person who snores sleeps on her back, the mouth opens because of gravity, and the tongue may rest in the back of the throat, partly blocking the air passage. In most cases, closing the mouth or simply rolling the snoring individual over stops the snoring.

A **yawn** is a very deep breath, initiated by opening the mouth wide and through movements of the upper torso to expand the chest. Some believe that yawning is triggered by the need to increase the oxygen content and decrease carbon dioxide in the blood or as a result of drowsiness, boredom, or depression, but the precise cause is unknown.

For Your Information

Cigarette smoking eventually destroys alveoli and reduces gas exchange in the lungs. Smoking also destroys respiratory cilia that remove particles in the nasal cavity and respiratory tract. As cilia die and the respiratory lining becomes irritated, the body produces excess mucus to trap the foreign particles in the cigarette smoke and to protect these delicate membranes and related tissues. This is why smokers often cough (trying to expel the extra mucus).

Smoking can also inhibit macrophage cells, which increases the likelihood of respiratory infections. The excess mucus is also a breeding ground for bacteria. Hence, smokers tend to be sick more often than nonsmokers. A recent medical discovery found that when smoking begins during early teen years, complete maturation of the lungs never occurs and those additional alveoli are lost forever.

As a result, individuals who smoke one pack of cigarettes a day will statistically take 7 years off their life expectancy.

RESPIRATORY PATHOLOGIES

Apnea is a temporary cessation (usually lasting 15 seconds) or absence of spontaneous breathing. Sleep apnea occurs during sleep.

Massage is fine for clients with apnea.

Asthma is a chronic, inflammatory disorder in which the smooth muscles of the smaller bronchi and bronchioles spasm to close, completely or partially, causing labored breathing. Asthma usually is preceded by emotional stress, respiratory infections, strenuous exercise, or inhalation of allergens (substances that promote allergic reactions).

Make sure from the client's intake form and pre-massage interview that no allergens are in the massage office that would trigger an attack. Side-lying position may be the most comfortable for the client. A full-body, relaxing massage is helpful. Focus on the accessory muscles of respiration and also the postural muscles because many clients with chronic asthma develop kyphosis. Vibration over the ribcage may help loosen mucus.

Bronchitis is inflammation of the bronchial mucosa that causes the bronchial tubes to swell and extra mucus to be produced. The two types of bronchitis are acute and chronic. Acute bronchitis, caused by an upper respiratory tract infection, results in a productive cough and high fever. Chronic bronchitis involves copious secretions of mucus with a productive cough that typically lasts 3 full months of the year for 2 successive years. Cigarette smoking is the most common cause of chronic bronchitis.

Postural drainage is helpful in clearing the respiratory tract of mucus. Position the client so her head is lower than the rest of her body. This can be done by putting pillows under the client's abdomen or making the head of the massage table lower than the foot of the table. A full-body relaxing massage is helpful, with tapotement and vibration on the ribcage for 10 to 20 minutes. Be sure to massage the accessory muscles of respiration.

Bronchogenic carcinoma, or lung cancer, is caused by a long-term irritant such as air pollution, cigarette smoke, asbestos, or coal dust. Initially, no symptoms are usually evident, and it is not detected until the late stages when symptoms include chronic cough, difficulty breathing, chest pain, coughing up blood, weight loss, and weakness.

Massage can be beneficial in reducing stress for the client. However, it is essential to consult with the client's physician before performing any massage. It is also very important to consider the client's vitality because a long and vigorous massage may in fact make the client feel weakened.

Carbon monoxide poisoning is a toxic, often lethal condition that is caused by the absorption of carbon monoxide through inhalation. Carbon monoxide binds at the same receptor sites as oxygen on the hemoglobin molecule, preventing oxygen from being carried by the hemoglobin. Carbon monoxide poisoning leads to oxygen starvation of cells. Its most common causes are automobile exhaust fumes and improperly functioning furnaces.

Massage is contraindicated. Medical attention is needed.

Cystic fibrosis is a genetic disorder involving over-secretion of all exocrine glands, especially the pancreas, and the respiratory mucosa. The bronchi secrete thick mucus, which obstructs and narrows the airway. The prognosis is poor, and no cure is known.

Postural drainage is helpful. Position the client so that his head is lower than his chest. Tapotement and vibration can help loosen phlegm. Massage of the accessory muscles of respiration is also very helpful.

Decompression sickness. When people work in a high-pressure region, such as below sea level, the blood and body tissues can absorb unusual amounts of nitrogen. Decompression sickness is harmless as long as the pressures inside and outside the body are equal. If divers or aviators move too quickly between areas of high and low pressure, a painful, often fatal syndrome called the *bends* may occur. When pressure is reduced too quickly, nitrogen cannot move from the tissues to the lungs fast enough for it to be dispelled through expiration. Nitrogen accumulates in the body as bubbles in tissues and impairs normal tissue oxygenation. Symptoms include joint pain, dizziness, shortness of breath, extreme fatigue, paralysis, and unconsciousness. The term *bends* comes from the fact that victims of decompression sickness double over from the extreme pain caused by the expansion of gases in the bloodstream. Gradual decompression is the safest way to normalize the gaseous condition.

Massage is contraindicated. Immediate medical attention is necessary.

Emphysema involves overinflation and destruction of the alveoli; this produces abnormally large air spaces that remain filled with air during expiration. With the loss of the elasticity of the alveoli, a person may inhale easily but has to labor to exhale. The added exertion increases the size of the rib cage, resulting in a barrel chest. Emphysema is caused by a long-term irritation such as cigarette smoking, air pollution, and exposure to industrial dust.

The client may need to be propped in a semireclining position for ease of breathing (Figure 20-5). The accessory muscles of respiration are especially tight, so focus massage on them. In particular, the sternocleidomastoid, intercostals, scalenes, and pectoralis minor need to be addressed.

Hypoxia is a decrease in the amount of oxygen in the blood, often characterized by rapid heart rate, excessive carbon dioxide levels in the blood, cyanosis, vertigo, and mental confusion. Mild hypoxia increases respiration; severe hypoxia can lead to heart failure and death. The organs most affected by hypoxia are the brain, heart, and liver.

Massage is contraindicated. Immediate medical attention is necessary.

Laryngitis is inflammation of the larynx that often results in loss of voice. Laryngitis is caused by respiratory infections or irritants such as cigarette smoke. Most long-term smokers acquire a permanent hoarseness from the damage created by chronic irritation and inflammation. Edema of the vocal cords often accompanies this disorder with coughing and a scratchy throat.

Massage is fine, unless the laryngitis is caused by an infectious disease.

Pleurisy is inflammation of the pleural membranes characterized by stabbing pain during breathing. The painful breathing is caused by friction created as the swollen pleural membranes rub against each other. Chronic pleurisy may result in permanent pleural adhesions.

Massage is contraindicated if the pleurisy is the result of bacterial infection. If it is from other causes, a full-body massage can be done to the client's tolerance. Attention should be paid to the accessory muscles of respiration.

Pneumonia is an infection or inflammation of the alveoli caused by the bacterium *Streptococcus pneumoniae,* but other infectious agents such as protozoans, viruses, and fungi may be responsible. During pneumonia, the alveoli fill with fluid and exudates such as dead white blood cells and pus. Exudates are substances that have been slowly discharged from cells or blood vessels as waste products. Pneumonia is the most common infectious cause of death in the United States, affecting, in particular, the elderly, infants, immunocompromised individuals, and cigarette smokers.

Massage is contraindicated during the acute phase because it is infectious. Once a client has recovered, massage can be beneficial. Tapotement and vibration on the ribcage can help drain secretions. Range of motion and massage on the extremities can help prevent muscle atrophy from prolonged bed rest.

Pulmonary edema is a condition involving an excessive amount of blood and interstitial fluid in the lungs. Common causes of pulmonary edema are near drowning, congestive heart failure, infection (i.e., pneumonia, tuberculosis), renal failure, and cerebrovascular accidents.

If the symptoms are severe, massage is contraindicated because the increased circulation can make the edema in the lungs worse. If the symptoms are less severe, a light, relaxing massage may be helpful as long as the client's physician approved it.

Respiratory distress syndrome (RDS), or hyaline membrane disease, is an acute lung disease characterized by inelastic lungs, respiration rate of more than 60 per minute, and nasal flaring. The

BOX 20-1

Effects of Massage on the Respiratory System

- **Reduces respiration rate.** Massage slows down the rate of respiration as a result of activation of the relaxation response.
- **Strengthens respiratory muscles.** The muscles of respiration have a greater capacity to contract, helping improve pulmonary functions.
- **Decreases the sensation of dyspnea.** Dyspnea is shortness of breath or difficult breathing, and is lessened because of massage.
- **Decreases asthma attacks.** Through increased relaxation and improved pulmonary functions, the client experiences fewer asthma attacks.
- **Reduces laryngeal tension.** Laryngeal tension may occur from excessive public speaking or singing. Massage reduces the stress on the larynx and tension on the muscles of the throat.
- **Increases fluid discharge from the lungs.** The mechanical loosening and discharge of phlegm in the respiratory tract increases with rhythmic alternating pressures. Tapotement (cupping) and vibration on the rib cage are often used to enhance this effect. Phlegm loosening and discharge is further enhanced when combined with pos-

tural drainage (promoting fluid drainage of the respiratory tract through certain body positions) and when the client is encouraged to cough.
- **Improves pulmonary functions.** Relaxation plays a big role in how massage improves pulmonary function, but massage also loosens tight respiratory muscles and fascia. The affected pulmonary functions are as follows:
  - *Increased vital capacity.* This is the amount of air that can be expelled at the normal rate of exhalation after a maximum inhalation, representing the greatest possible breathing capacity.
  - *Increased forced vital capacity.* This is the amount of air that can be forcibly expelled after a forced inhalation.
  - *Increased forced expiratory volume.* This is the volume of air that can be forcibly expelled after a full exhalation.
  - *Increased forced expiratory flow.* This is the volume of air that can be forcibly expelled after a full inhalation.
  - *Improved peak expiratory flow.* This is the greatest rate of airflow that can be achieved during forced expiration beginning with the lungs fully inflated.

condition occurs most often in premature babies because of inadequate pulmonary surfactants. Adult respiratory distress syndrome (ARDS) is characterized by hypoxia and is often the result of foreign objects (e.g., asbestos) aspirated into the lungs, cardiopulmonary bypass surgery, or pneumonia.

Massage is contraindicated. Immediate medical attention is necessary.

Sinusitis is an inflammation of the paranasal sinuses. Swelling of nasal mucosa may obstruct the openings from sinuses to the nose, resulting in an accumulation of sinus secretions, causing local tenderness, pain, headache, and fever.

Massage is fine. Local heat applications help relieve pain, and steam inhalation helps relieve congestion.

Tuberculosis is a chronic lung infection caused by the bacterium *Mycobacterium tuberculosis*. It is typically transmitted by the inhalation and exhalation (or consumption) of infected droplets. Even though the lungs are the primary target of the disease, the liver, bone marrow, and spleen also may be involved. During tuberculosis, lung tissue is destroyed by bacteria and replaced by fibrous connective tissue, limiting gas exchange.

Generally, tuberculosis is not infectious from 2 to 4 weeks after the start of treatment with antitubercular medications. Massage is contraindicated unless the client is no longer infective. Check with the client's physician to be sure.

See Box 20-1 for the effects of massage on the respiratory system.

For Your Information

A client receiving a massage in a recumbent position, when she is experiencing respiratory congestion, compounds the problem. This is because of gravity. The following pointers can make the client more comfortable:

1. When the client is in the supine position, elevate the upper body to assist drainage. Dr. Keith De Sonnier, an ear, nose, and throat physician, recommends a 30-degree incline to assist sinus drainage (see Figure 20-5).

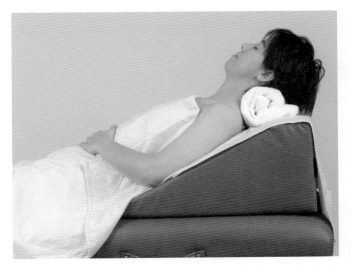

Figure 20-5 Client in the supine position supported by pillows to create a 30-degree incline.

2. After massaging in the prone position, lower the upper body by placing pillows or other supportive cushions under the hips and abdomen. Use cupping percussion delivered to the ribcage to loosen phlegm. Expect the client to cough as a natural reflex (Figure 20-6). Have tissues handy for client use.

3. Adjust the table legs so that you raise the head of the massage table higher than the foot of the table during the massage; then, turning the client 180 degrees while prone, percuss and vibrate the ribcage for the final few minutes.

4. You may elect not to massage the client in the prone position and instead may choose a side-lying position.

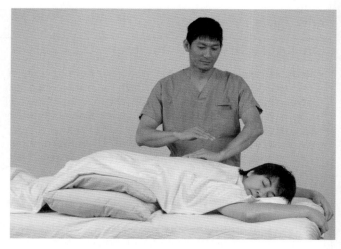

Figure 20-6   Client receiving percussion to loosen phlegm.

SUMMARY

The respiratory system is physiologically and poetically associated with the very concept of life itself. The main functions of this system include the exchange of gases, homeostasis, olfaction, and production of speech. This method of air movement and chemical exchange is accomplished by the anatomical structures of the respiratory system, including the nasal cavities, pharynx, larynx, trachea, bronchi, alveoli, lungs, and respiratory diaphragm. Breathing, external respiration, and internal respiration are the processes necessary to get oxygen to cells and eliminate gaseous wastes. The main mechanisms of air movement involved in the breathing process are inspiration and expiration. Several modified respiratory air movements are also evident, including yawning, sneezing, coughing, crying, laughing, snoring, and hiccupping. The main purpose of air movement is to take in oxygen, which is vital to sustain life and expel carbon dioxide, a waste product. Aromatherapy and massage therapy complement each other and benefit the client greatly.

MATCHING I

Write the letter of the best answer in the space provided.

A. Breathing
B. Internal respiration
C. Inspiration
D. Alveoli
E. Trachea
F. Epiglottis

G. Surfactants
H. Pharynx
I. Lungs
J. Cilia
K. Respiratory diaphragm

L. External respiration
M. Vital capacity
N. Bronchii
O. Larynx
P. Expiration

_____ 1. Tiny sacs attached to the distal ends of the bronchioles

_____ 2. Referred to as the *guardian of the airways* because it closes the trachea during swallowing

_____ 3. Process of drawing air into the lungs

_____ 4. Paired organs of respiration

_____ 5. Throat or muscular tube shared by the respiratory and digestive systems

_____ 6. Process responsible for expelling air from the lungs back to the atmosphere

_____ 7. Dome-shaped muscle of respiration

_____ 8. Process consisting of the two phases inspiration and expiration

_____ 9. Projections on the outer surfaces of certain cells

_____ 10. Right and left air-conduction passageways leading to each lung

_____ 11. Gas exchange in the lungs between blood and the external environment

_____ 12. Phospholipids that assist in the exchange of gas in the alveoli by reducing surface tension and contributing to lung elasticity

_____ 13. Voice box that houses the two sets of vocal cords

_____ 14. Windpipe; a tube from the larynx to the upper chest

_____ 15. Gas exchange between blood and body tissues

_____ 16. Total air amount that can be forcibly inspired and expired from the lungs in one breath

MATCHING II

Write the letter of the best answer in the space provided.

A. Cough   C. Hiccup   E. Sneeze
B. Cry   D. Snore   F. Yawn

_____ 1. A response to emotions such as grief, pain, fear, or joy that involves a sudden inspiration followed by the release of air in short breaths

_____ 2. A very deep breath, initiated by opening the mouth wide

_____ 3. A sudden expulsion of air to clear the lungs and lower respiratory passageways of irritants or foreign materials

_____ 4. Intermittent contractions of the diaphragm followed by a spasmodic closure of the vocal cords

_____ 5. A forceful expulsion of air through the nose and mouth to clear the upper respiratory passageways

_____ 6. Audible breathing during sleep because of vibration of the uvula and soft palate

Bibliography

Applegate EJ: *The anatomy and physiology learning system,* ed 2, Philadelphia, 2000, WB Saunders.

Crawley J, Van De Graaff KM: *A photographic atlas for anatomy and physiology,* Englewood, Colo, 2002, Morton.

Damjanov I: *Pathology for the health-related professions,* Philadelphia, 1996, WB Saunders.

Ford CW: *Where healing waters meet: touching mind and emotions through the body,* Barrytown, NY, 1992, Station Hill Press.

Gray H, Pick TP, Howden R: *Gray's anatomy,* ed 29, Philadelphia, 1974, Running Press.

Haubrich WS: *Medical meanings: a glossary of word origins,* New York, 1984, Harcourt Brace Jovanovich.

Jacob S, Francone C: *Elements of anatomy and physiology,* Philadelphia, 1989, WB Saunders.

Kalat JW: *Biological psychology,* ed 2, Belmont, Calif, 1984, Wadsworth.

Kapit W, Elson LM: *The anatomy coloring book,* ed 3, New York, 2002, Benjamin Cummings.

Kordish M, Dickson S: *Introduction to basic human anatomy,* Lake Charles, La, 1995, McNeese State University.

Marieb EN: *Essentials of human anatomy and physiology,* ed 4, New York, 1994, Benjamin/Cummings.

McAleer N: *The body almanac,* Garden City, NY, 1985, Doubleday.

Merck Research Laboratories: *Merck manual,* ed 17, Whitehouse Station, NJ, 1998, Author.

Mosby's medical, nursing, and allied health dictionary, ed 4, St Louis, 1994, Mosby.

Newton D: *Pathology for massage therapists,* ed 2, Portland, Ore, 1995, Simran.

Premkumar K: *Pathology A to Z: a handbook for massage therapists,* Calgary, Canada, 1996, VanPub Books.

Solomon EP, Phillips GA: *Understanding human anatomy and physiology,* Philadelphia, 1987, WB Saunders.

Taber's cyclopedic medical dictionary, ed 13, Philadelphia, 1977, FA Davis.

Thibodeau G, Patton K: *Structure and function of the body,* ed 11, St Louis, 2000, Mosby.

Tortora GJ: *Introduction to the human body: the essentials of anatomy and physiology,* ed 3, New York, 1994, HarperCollins.

Tortora GJ, Grabowksi SR: *Principles of anatomy and physiology,* ed 9, New York, 2000, John Wiley.

Werner R: *A massage therapist's guide to pathology,* ed 2, Baltimore, 2002, Lippincott Williams & Wilkins.

Digestive System

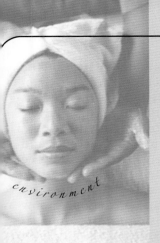

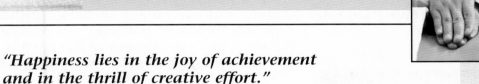

"Happiness lies in the joy of achievement and in the thrill of creative effort."

—Franklin D. Roosevelt

STUDENT OBJECTIVES

After completing this chapter, the student should be able to:

- Explain the functions of the digestive system
- Discuss basic anatomical structures of the digestive system
- Identify specific divisions of the alimentary canal
- Describe what happens to food when it enters the alimentary canal
- Trace the path food takes from the time it enters the mouth to the time wastes are eliminated
- Identify where products of the salivary glands, liver, gallbladder, and pancreas enter the alimentary canal
- Describe the disassembly of foods in the body
- Name types of digestive pathologies, giving characteristics and massage considerations of each

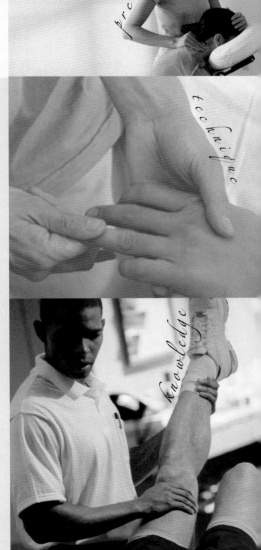

INTRODUCTION

People consume more than 40 tons of food in an average lifetime. The digestive system provides processes by which molecules such as proteins, carbohydrates, and fats are broken down into a state more easily assimilated into the body. Essentially, the digestive process is a "disassembly line." These digestive processes themselves consume a tremendous amount of bodily resources, but fortunately they produce more energy than they use.

Chapter 10 explained the two divisions of the autonomic nervous system: sympathetic and para-

Terms and Their Meanings Related to the Digestive System	
Term	**Meaning**
amylase	starch; enzyme
bolus	a lump
Brunner's glands	Swiss anatomist (1653-1727)
bucca	cheek
cecum	blindness
chol	bile
chyme	juice
deglutition	to swallow
dent	toothlike
duodenum	12
enzyme	leaven
fundus	base
gingiva	gums
gustatory	to taste
haustra	to draw, drink
hepato	liver
ileum	twisted
jejunum	empty
Kupffer's cells	German anatomist (1829-1902)
lacteal	of milk
mastication	to chew
mesentery	middle; intestine
omentum	a covering or apron
peristaltic	around; contraction
plicae circulares	a fold; a little ring
pylorus	gatekeeper
rectum	straight
rugae	a crease or fold
sacchar	sugar
sigmoid	the Greek letter *sigma*, meaning S-shaped
sphincter	a binder
sphincter of Oddi	Italian physician (1864-1913)
taenia coli	tape; colon
tonsils	almond
vermiform appendix	wormlike; hanger-on
villi	tuft of hair

sympathetic. Digestive functions are initiated by the parasympathetic nervous system during periods of low stress. Because digestion requires a tremendous expenditure of energy, it occurs during times of low activity. The body can then reallocate energy that would normally be spent on muscular activity and route it to the digestive system. Activation of the parasympathetic nervous system is also known as the *relaxation response,* or "rest and digest." Stress and emotions such as anger, fear, and anxiety may slow down digestion because they stimulate the sympathetic nervous system, or stress response. People in high-stress or high-responsibility positions are more likely to have problems with ulcers, heartburn, colitis, irritable bowel syndrome, and constipation because of frequent disruption of the digestive process.

The digestive system may be viewed as a refinery. An industrial refinery takes a product such as raw crude oil from the ground and fractionates or disassembles it into useful components such as gasoline, butane, and diesel. Likewise, the digestive system takes in the raw materials of food and drink and converts them both physically and chemically into highly refined fuel. Just as fuel oil or natural gas is transported to people's homes by pipes, digested materials are delivered to the body's cells through the vessels of the circulatory system. Many unneeded resources can be stored for future metabolism.

Study of the anatomy of the digestive system shows that it is primarily composed of a tube, which is linked to the outside world. This chapter identifies each tube section and organ and describes each by structure and function. Included are the various digestive secretions and the food types on which they act.

FUNCTIONS

The four functions of the digestive system are as follows:

1. **Ingestion** is the process of orally taking materials into the body. This term applies to taking in food, liquids, and oral medications.
2. **Digestion** is the mechanical and chemical processes that occur as food is mixed with digestive enzymes and converted into an absorbable state. Mechanical digestion includes chewing in the oral cavity, churning in the stomach, and the mixing movements of the intestinal tube (peristalsis). After digestion, food is capable of being taken into the bloodstream. An **enzyme** is a catalyst that accelerates chemical reactions.
3. **Absorption** is the process by which the products of digestion move into the bloodstream or lymph vessels and then into the body's cells.
4. **Defecation** is the process of eliminating indigestible or unabsorbed material from the body.

GENERAL DIGESTIVE ANATOMY AND RELATED PHYSIOLOGY

Alimentary Canal

The **alimentary canal**, also referred to as the *gastrointestinal (GI) tract,* is the mostly coiled, muscular passageway leading from the mouth to the anus. The alimentary canal is approximately 30 feet long and includes the oral cavity, pharynx, esophagus, stomach, small intestine, and large intestine (Figure 21-1). The tube itself has four layers, or **tunics**. From innermost to outermost, the layers are the mucosa, submucosa, muscularis, and serosa, all of which are host to blood vessels, lymphatic vessels, and glands that produce and secrete digestive enzymes. The alimentary canal is primarily smooth muscle, and this muscle tissue is responsible for most of the movement and mixing actions. Skeletal muscle is present only in parts of the pharynx, esophagus, and anus.

Within the muscular layer of the alimentary canal are two types of contractions: tonic and rhythmic. Tonic contractions are sustained contractions that occur in sphincter muscles. A **sphincter** is a ring of muscle fibers that regulate movement of materials from one compartment of the GI tract to another. Rhythmic or peristaltic contractions are the most common muscular contraction of the digestive system. These wavelike contractions mix and propel materials farther into the GI tract. **Peristalsis** occurs as a contraction just behind a **bolus** (a ball-like, masticated lump of food once swallowed). As the bolus approaches, the sphincter relaxes and then opens to allow passage. During mixing movements, peristaltic contractions occur as a rhythmic, sequential contraction of smooth muscle, moving the intestinal materials back and forth until they are thoroughly mixed.

Peritoneum

The **peritoneum**, which envelops the entire abdominal wall, is the largest serous membrane in the body. The free surface of the peritoneum is lubricated with a serous fluid, permitting the digestive structures and other visceral organs to glide easily against the abdominal wall without friction. Within the peritoneum are blood vessels, lymph vessels, and nerves. Sections of the peritoneum include the mesenteries, parietal and visceral peritoneum, and greater and lesser omentum. These structures are discussed later in this chapter in the section on the Small Intestine (Figure 21-2).

DIVISIONS OF THE ALIMENTARY CANAL

Oral Cavity

Also known as the *mouth,* the **oral cavity** is the port of entry for food and drink. The oral cavity contains the tongue, teeth, gums, and openings from the salivary ducts. Digestion begins in the oral cavity. **Mastication** (chewing) is aided by the tongue; digestive enzymes present in saliva break down food. **Saliva**, containing water, mucus, organic salts, and digestive enzymes, is a clear, nondigestible, viscous

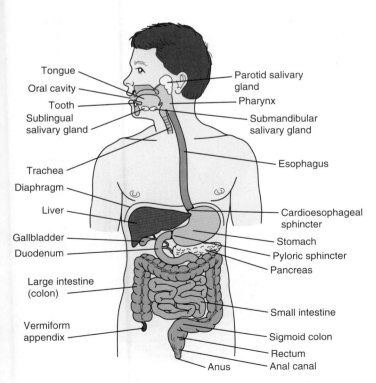

Figure 21-1   The digestive system and accessory organs.

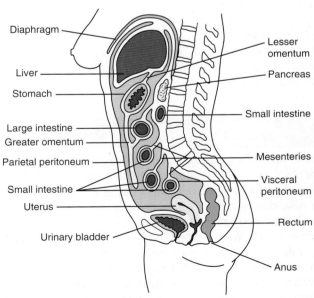

Figure 21-2   Lateral view of the peritoneum.

fluid secreted by the salivary and mucous glands in the mouth. The functions of saliva are to act as a lubricant and an adhesive by causing food to stick together, forming a bolus for **deglutition** (swallowing). Saliva stimulates the taste buds and protects the mucosa by acting as a buffer. With the exception of several medications, such as nitroglycerin, no absorption takes place in the oral cavity.

Saliva also serves to initiate the digestion of starches and fats through salivary amylase and lingual lipase. Salivary amylase, or ptyalin, begins the digestion of carbohydrates. Lingual lipase, secreted by glands located near the tongue, breaks lipids down into glycerol and fatty acids. Saliva is produced in one of the three pairs of salivary glands. They are the *submandibular glands,* the *sublingual glands,* and the *large parotid glands.*

The tongue aids in deglutition, by directing the bolus toward the back of the throat. Nestled in spherical pockets on the superior and lateral surfaces of the tongue are the **gustatory organs** (taste buds), chemoreceptors that detect the primary tastes of sweet, sour, bitter, and salty. However, taste is a response of many neurons and not just a signal from a single gustatory nerve. Even though the tongue is considered the primary organ of taste, the nose and the temperature of food play a significant role in how food tastes. Hot food tastes better than cold food because heat causes the aroma of the food to rise and enter our nose. Food does not taste as good when any type of condition affects sense of smell.

Within the adult oral cavity are 32 secondary or permanent teeth. Children possess only 20 primary or deciduous teeth that are usually shed between the ages of 6 and 12 years. Enamel, which is the hardest substance in the body, covers each tooth. Teeth are classified according to shape and function: incisors, cuspids (canines), bicuspids (premolars), and multicuspids (molars). The third molars are also called *wisdom teeth* because they evidently erupt when a person is "old enough to be wise" (usually between the ages of 17 and 25).

MINI-LAB

Most people can recall a biology experiment in elementary school in which different substances were placed on the tongue to grasp a better understanding of how different parts of the tongue detected tastes.

Gather a small container of sugar, a small container of salt, and a sliced lemon. Apply these foods on different areas of your tongue and notice the areas that clearly detect the tastes. Can you taste the lemon or the salt on the tip of your tongue? After wetting your finger, apply the sugar on the backside of the tongue. Can you taste the sweetness?

Pharynx

The **pharynx**, or throat, is the tube structure that transports food, liquid, and air to their respective destinations. In the digestive system, the pharynx takes food from the oral cavity to the esophagus during swallowing.

Esophagus

The **esophagus** (gullet) is the muscular tube that connects the pharynx to the stomach. The esophageal lining secretes mucus to aid in the transport of food. Bypassing the thoracic organs, the esophagus transports food to the stomach.

Stomach

The **stomach** is a J-shaped organ that is essentially an enlargement of the GI tract bound at both ends by sphincters. The superior sphincter, found at the junction between the esophagus and stomach, is the **cardioesophageal sphincter** or cardiac sphincter. The **pyloric sphincter** is located between the stomach and small intestine. The stomach is situated directly under the diaphragm in the left upper quadrant of the abdomen. Exteriorly, the shape of the stomach reveals a *greater curvature* and a *lesser curvature* (Figure 21-3).

The stomach receives partially digested food and drink from the esophagus. When empty, the stomach is about the size of a large sausage. Depending on body size, the stomach, when full, can hold up to 1 gallon of food. This expansion is permitted by the longitudinal folds in the lining of the stomach called **rugae**.

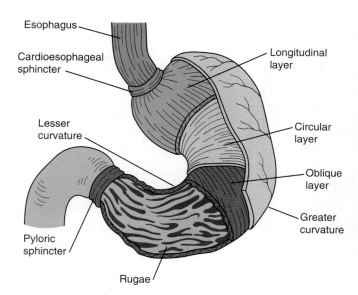

Figure 21-3   The stomach and its structures.

The muscular tunic of the stomach has three layers of muscle: *oblique, circular,* and *longitudinal.* The oblique layer adds a new dimension to the churning action of the stomach, giving it an extraordinary ability to mix food. Entering the stomach, food mixes with gastric enzymes to initiate protein digestion. As food is further blended and digested, a bolus of food is reduced to a thin viscous fluid called **chyme.**

The pyloric sphincter opens periodically to allow chyme to enter into the small intestine. The process of moving chyme into the small intestine may take up to 4 hours, so the stomach also serves as both a storage tank and digestive chamber. Because of this slow release of chyme into the small intestines, it is possible for the body to maintain energy needs with only two or three meals a day, instead of requiring a steady supply of food like grazing animals.

The gastric mucosa possesses both endocrine and exocrine cells. The endocrine cells are called **G cells** and secrete the hormone gastrin, which initiates the production and secretion of gastric juice and stimulates bile and pancreatic enzyme emissions into the small intestines (Table 21-1). The stomach produces about 2 to 3 quarts of gastric juice per day. The only substances that are absorbed by the lining of the stomach are water, some minerals, alcohol, and some medications such as aspirin.

Two types of exocrine cells in the stomach are the parietal and chief cells. The **parietal cells** produce intrinsic factor, a substance required for the absorption of vitamin B_{12} from the small intestine to the bloodstream. The parietal cells also produce hydrochloric acid, a compound of hydrogen and chlorine, which breaks down protein and activates many gastric enzymes. Hydrochloric acid, which kills bacteria and other pathogens, is so powerful that it can eat through wood. The gastric lining is protected from this strong acid by a thick layer of alkaline mucus produced by mucous cells within the gastric lining. **Chief cells** produce the gastric enzyme pepsinogen, which is a precursor to pepsin. Pepsin is

TABLE 21-1

Substances Affecting Digestion

Name and Substance	Location Produced	Action(s)
Bile (emulsifier)	Liver	Physically breaks apart large fat globules into smaller ones
Carboxypeptidase (enzyme)	Pancreas	Breaks down proteins
Cholecystokinin (hormone)	Small intestines	Stimulates the release of bile from the gallbladder and pancreatic enzyme secretion
Chymosin/rennin (enzyme)	Stomach (infants only)	Aids in milk curdling
Chymotrypsin (enzyme)	Pancreas	Breaks down proteins
Enterocrinin (hormone)	Small intestines	Stimulates the flow of intestinal juice
Enterokinase (enzyme)	Small intestines	Activates protein enzyme secretion from pancreas
Gastrin (hormone)	Stomach (G cells)	Initiates production and secretion of gastric juice; stimulates release of bile and pancreatic enzymes into the small intestines
Hydrochloric acid (compound)	Stomach (parietal cells)	Breaks down protein and activates gastric enzymes
Intrinsic factor (substance)	Stomach (parietal cells)	Required for the absorption of vitamin B_{12} from the small intestine into the bloodstream
Lactase (enzyme)	Small intestines	Promotes carbohydrate digestion
Lingual lipase (enzyme)	Oral cavity	Breaks lipids down into glycerol and fatty acids
Maltase (enzyme)	Small intestines	Promotes carbohydrate digestion
Pancreatic amylase (enzyme)	Pancreas	Converts polysaccharides into disaccharides
Pancreatic lipase (enzyme)	Pancreas	Converts triglycerides into monoglycerides and fatty acids
Pepsinogen/pepsin (precursor/enzyme)	Stomach (chief cells)	Begins chemical digestion of proteins by converting them into peptides
Peptidase (enzyme)	Small intestines	Promotes the digestion of proteins
Salivary amylase/ptyalin (enzyme)	Salivary glands	Begins carbohydrate digestion
Secretin (hormone)	Small intestines	Stimulates the production and secretion of pancreatic enzymes
Sucrase (enzyme)	Small intestines	Promotes carbohydrate digestion
Trypsinogen/trypsin (precursor/enzyme)	Pancreas	Breaks protein into smaller chains of amino acids

secreted in an inactive form to prevent the gastric lining from eroding from pepsin's protein digestion. Pepsinogen converts to pepsin when it comes into contact with hydrochloric acid and begins the chemical digestion of proteins by converting them into peptides.

Chymosin, or rennin, an enzyme found in the gastric juices of infants, is used to aid in milk curdling and is used commercially to produce cheese.

For Your Information

What causes hunger? Is it the need for food and energy? Heredity? Several theories are considered for why we get hungry. One theory is stomach contractions or stomach "growling," which may increase when the stomach is empty. Another idea is that the body detects a low level of blood sugar or a combined reduction of all available digestible foods. Additionally, the hypothalamus appears to regulate the sensation of hunger and the feeling of satiety (fullness). Other reasons besides hunger are often indicated when people are asked why they eat. Many individuals eat when they are lonely, depressed, or bored. Hunger is most likely a combination of several physiological and psychological events.

Small Intestine

The **small intestine** is actually the longest section of the alimentary canal and is situated in the central abdomen, framed by the large intestine. This muscular tube is bound at both ends by the pyloric sphincter (at the stomach) and the **ileocecal sphincter** (at the large intestine). The lumen of the small intestine possesses circular folds called **plicae circulares** (Figure 21-4). The lining of the small intestines contains numerous **villi**, fingerlike projections that house blood and lymph capillaries. The lymph capillaries in the villi are called **lacteals**, which assist in the absorption of fat. The plicae circulares and the villi increase the surface area of the small intestine for more efficient absorption.

The three divisions of the small intestines, from beginning to end, are the duodenum, jejunum, and ileum. The first section of the small intestine, the **duodenum**, is between 10 and 12 inches long and contains the sphincter of Oddi and the major duodenal papilla. The **sphincter of Oddi** regulates the flow of secretions from the pancreas, liver, and gallbladder; the **major duodenal papilla** is the site of entry for these secretions. The major duodenal papilla is a dilation that is formed by the juncture of the pancreatic and common bile ducts as they open into the small intestines.

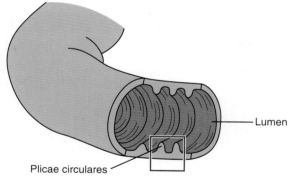

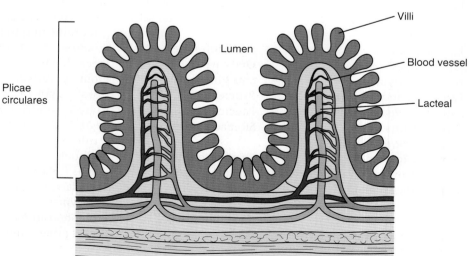

Figure 21-4 Cutaway of the small intestine exposing the plicae circulares and the villi and a close-up of a lacteal.

The intermediate portion of the small intestine, the **jejunum**, runs from the duodenum to the ileum and is approximately 6 feet long. The walls of the jejunum are slightly thicker than those of the ileum, and the jejunum possesses a smaller lumen. The villi are larger in this section, presumably to increase absorption.

For Your Information

The word *jejunum* is derived from the Latin adjective *jejunus* (fasting or hungry), meaning being empty or devoid of food. The ancient Greeks, during the practice of necropsy (examination of a dead body), found that the lumen of the middle small intestine was always empty.

The final division of the small intestine, the **ileum**, is approximately 9 feet long and terminates at the ileocecal sphincter, which connects the ileum of the small intestine to the cecum of the large intestine. This section of the small intestine contains numerous clusters of lacteals to enhance fat absorption.

All divisions of the small intestines are connected to each other and to the posterior abdominal wall by a section of the peritoneum called the **mesenteries**. The mesentery is a large, fan-shaped structure consisting of two omentums. Also referred to as the *fatty apron*, the **greater omentum** is a double-layered structure that connects to the greater curvature of the stomach and duodenum, drapes down over the coils of the small intestine, and then attaches to the transverse colon. The **lesser omentum** is a fatty, membranous extension of the peritoneum and attaches from the right side of stomach and first section of the duodenum to the liver (see Figure 21-2).

The length of the small intestine is responsible for 90% of all absorption (the other 10% occurs in the stomach and large intestine). Digested foodstuffs, absorbed through the intestinal walls, are transported by the blood, which takes care of sugars and proteins, and lymph, which is responsible for fats. If more food nutrients (e.g., fat, fat-soluble vitamins) are absorbed than the body requires, the extra is stored until needed.

Brunner's glands (duodenal glands) secrete alkaline mucus. Other intestinal glands secrete intestinal juice containing digestive enzymes such as enterokinase, peptidase, maltase, sucrase, and lactase. These enzymes promote the digestion of proteins and carbohydrates. Hormones secreted by the intestinal mucosa are enterocrinin, cholecystokinin, and secretin. Enterocrinin stimulates the flow of intestinal juice, and cholecystokinin stimulates contraction of the gallbladder and pancreatic enzyme secretion. Secretin stimulates the pancreas to secrete an alkaline liquid that neutralizes the acid chyme facilitating the action of the intestinal enzymes.

Large Intestine

The **large intestine**, or colon, is the final stretch that undigested and unabsorbed food takes before it is eliminated by the body. The lining of the large intestine does not produce digestive enzymes; instead it produces mucus that allows the developing fecal matter to move down more easily. With the exception of water, vitamins, and minerals, few substances are absorbed by the colon lining.

The large intestine is characterized by two structures: haustrum and taenia coli. Located in the muscularis tunic of the large intestine are thick, longitudinal bands called the **taenia coli**, which resemble a thread-gathering fabric. The gathers, or tucks, along the length of the colon make a series of pouches, called **haustra**. Once filled, these pouches contract to push the contents to the next haustrum.

The divisions of the large intestine are the cecum, colon proper, rectum, anal canal, and anus. The colon proper is further divided into the ascending, transverse, descending, and sigmoid colons. Flexures exist where the colon turns into an upside-down U shape (Figure 21-5).

The first section of the colon, the **cecum**, is a small saclike structure located in the right lower quadrant of the abdomen. The cecum is attached to the ileocecal sphincter. Suspended from and opening into the inferior portion of the cecum is a lymph gland called the **vermiform appendix**. The wormlike appendix varies from 3 to 6 inches in length and is discussed in Chapter 19.

The next segment of the colon is the ascending colon, continuing from the cecum up the lower right abdomen, turning from the hepatic or right colic flexure. After the hepatic flexure the colon moves horizontally from right to left, draping to form the transverse colon. The colon proper takes a downward turn at the splenic or left colic flexure, providing the path for the descending colon. At the level of the iliac crest, the descending colon turns back toward the right at the sigmoid flexure to become the sigmoid colon. Then, with a final S-shaped downward curve, the colon reaches the **rectum** and terminates at the **anal canal**, opening to the outside at the **anus**.

The rectum usually contains three circular folds that overlap when empty and grow in size as the rectum fills with waste to be excreted. The main function of the rectum and anal canal is storage.

The anal canal possesses two sphincters: an internal sphincter, containing visceral muscle, and an external sphincter, containing skeletal muscle. As the rectal contents move into the anal canal, the internal anal sphincter muscle distends, stimulating pressure-sensitive receptors and initiating the defecation reflex. If this urge is suppressed, it may dissipate, and it may be hours before the desire to defecate returns. If the urge to defecate is chronically suppressed,

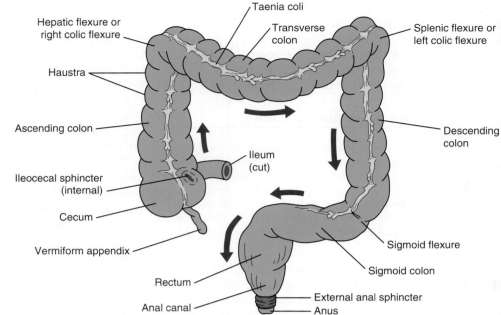

Figure 21-5   The large intestine.

copious amounts of water are absorbed from the colon, and constipation may result.

During defecation, the levator ani muscle raises the anus to eliminate fecal matter. Feces, or stool, is excrement from the GI tract formed in the intestine and released through the anus. Feces consist of indigestible foodstuffs, water, bacteria, and cells sloughed off the walls of the rectum and anal canal.

For Your Information

When the psoas major muscle is accessed through the abdominal wall, the therapist must work through both the large and small intestines. Small circular movements are done on the abdominal skin, using mild pressure, to allow the intestines to slide out of the way before deep pressure is applied.

ACCESSORY DIGESTIVE ORGANS

The accessory digestive organs produce substances that aid digestion in the small intestines. They are the liver, gallbladder, and pancreas (Figure 21-6). The digestive substances produced and secreted by these organs continue the chemical digestion of food.

Liver

The largest internal organ in the body, the **liver**, weighs about 3 pounds (lb). It is located in the upper right quadrant of the abdominal cavity. This reddish-brown organ consists of hepatocytes (liver cells) that are arranged around thousands of specialized venous

channels called **sinusoids**, which are larger than ordinary capillaries. Lining the sinusoids of the liver are phagocytic cells called **Kupffer's cells**. These specialized macrophages destroy pathogens and move other foreign material out of the blood before sending it through the hepatic vein. Blood flowing through the sinusoids originates from the stomach and the intestines through the hepatic portal system (see Chapter 19). Because of the vascularity of this organ, the liver holds approximately 1 pint of blood at any given moment.

One of the most complex organs of the body, the liver has more than 500 functions. One of its

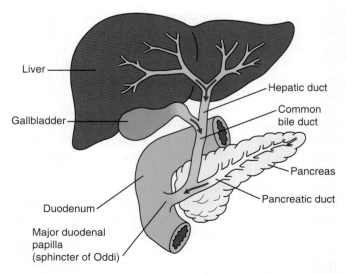

Figure 21-6   Liver, pancreas, and gallbladder in relationship to the duodenum.

DWIGHT BYERS

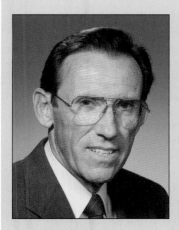

Born: February 10, 1929.

"You may be walking on the solution to many of your health problems."

Dwight Byers claims he was one of the guinea pigs for his aunt's early work in reflexology. His aunt, Eunice Ingham, a physical therapist and member of the New York Medical Massage Therapist Association, worked during the early 1930s for a doctor who had a passing interest in the art of zone therapy. Zone therapy was a predecessor of reflexology and was introduced in the early 1900s by Dr. William H. Fitzgerald, who successfully used different devices to place pressure on certain points on the hands to relieve pain.

Eunice Ingham took this work a step further and put her own mark on this ancient healing art, which was practiced as far back as 2330 BC. According to Byers, his aunt was strong-willed, extremely intuitive, and totally dedicated to easing suffering in her fellow man.

Along with a compassionate heart, Ingham had a keen mind. Her time-honored techniques are the result of experiment, research, and copious notes. She threw out what did not work and perfected what did. Her books, *Stories the Feet Can Tell Through Reflexology* (Ingham, 1984) and *Stories the Feet Have Told Through Reflexology* (Ingham, 1984) provide more details on this subject.

It was Ingham's dedication to helping relieve suffering that proved inspirational to her young nephew, who was at first skeptical. His skepticism, along with his hay fever and asthma, vanished after experiencing his aunt's healing touch firsthand.

"At first we kind of laughed at her," remembers Byers, as he shares the stories of traveling with his aunt as she conducted seminars on reflexology across the United States. "I helped her carry her bags and set up. But soon I became fascinated, and eventually my sister and I began helping her teach."

Byers's background as a medic in the U.S. Army and his later experience in mortuary science helped hone some of his anatomy skills as he began practicing reflexology part-time. When his aunt died in 1974, Byers formed the International Institute of Reflexology to help preserve the original Ingham method. In 1983 he published his book, *Better Health With Foot Reflexology* (Ingham, 2001), for the same reason.

This book defines reflexology as "the science that deals with the principle that there are reflex areas in the feet and hands which correspond to all the glands, organs, and parts of the body. Reflexology is a unique method of using the thumb and fingers on the reflex areas to help relieve stress and tension, improve blood supply, promote the unblocking of nerve impulses, and help nature achieve homeostasis" (p. 11).

Basically, every aspect of your body can be "found" on the bottom of your feet, and these locations correspond roughly with anatomy, thus the term *zone therapy.* For instance, the gallbladder is located in your upper torso to your right. On the bottom of the right foot, its corresponding point is to the upper portion of the right foot. However, it is not enough to know where particular organs are located. Reflexologists are also trained in physiology to understand how different body systems interface. For instance, while working with someone who might have gallstones, added emphasis is placed on the entire digestive system. Studying the correct pressure and type of motion to employ on the feet or hands is also vital.

"Reflexology sends a message to the organs to normalize, to decrease or increase hormonal levels," explains Byers. His results have been phenomenal, but even he admits that he does not have all the answers to why this method works.

DWIGHT BYERS—cont'd

In the foreword of Byers's text, Dr. Ray C. Wunderlich Jr. offers some compelling theories to account for reflexology's success:

Quite probably, it will eventually be shown that foot reflexology alters energy flow in the body.... There are 7,200 nerve endings in each foot. Perhaps this fact, more than any other, explains why we feel so much better when our feet are treated. Nerve endings in the feet have extensive interconnections through the spinal cord and brain with all areas of the body.

—From *Better Health With Foot Reflexology* by Dwight Byers, 1983.

Byers, whose favorite adage is "experience is the father of all knowledge," claims that the best results are obtained by those who practice, practice, practice. "You've got to work on thousands of feet," he says. "My advice for beginning massage therapists is to master your art. Don't be a jack-of-all-trades and master of none."

Byers feels that it is essential that the therapist is the type of person who wants to help people and not someone who thinks of money first. "You've got to give a lot," he says. This is not idle lip service from Byers. He has done his share of throwing in an extra free visit for clients and has helped senior citizen clients by providing them with discounted sessions.

Byers is a man who understands people. He is down to earth and pragmatic, and so are his seminars. The final is hands-on, and it is his feet that are up for grabs after a 200-hour program. His criterion for grading: "Would I pay to have this treatment done?"

Massage therapists who become certified in reflexology use it to enhance their business. Beginning the session with reflexology can induce relaxation and increase circulation, which benefits muscles, glands, and internal organs from the inside out.

digestive functions is the production of bile—approximately 1 quart of bile per day. **Bile** enters the left and right hepatic ducts, which join to form the common bile duct that leads to the duodenum of the small intestine. Produced from the hemoglobin in worn-out red blood cells, bile is not an enzyme but an emulsifier. It physically breaks apart large fat globules into smaller ones and provides a larger surface area for the fat-digesting enzymes to work. Bile gives urine and the stool their characteristic color.

Some other liver functions are the production, storage, and breakdown of glucose and hemoglobin. The liver produces amino acids, blood plasma proteins, fibrinogens (blood-clotting substances), and antibodies. It also processes absorbed nutrients and stores vitamins A, D, E, and K; minerals; iron; copper; and other compounds used by the body.

The liver detoxifies numerous toxic substances such as alcohol, nicotine, and other poisons, into nontoxic materials. Toxic substances that cannot be broken down and excreted are stored. One such substance is dichlorodiphenyltrichloroethane (DDT), which was banned in the United States in 1971.

Gallbladder

The **gallbladder**, which stores bile manufactured by the liver, is a pear-shaped sac located in a depression on the inferior surface of the liver. The sphincter of Oddi controls the release of bile into the duodenum. When the sphincter is closed, bile backs up into the gallbladder, where it is stored until needed. Recall that the intestinal mucosa secretes a hormone, cholecystokinin, which stimulates the release of bile from the gallbladder.

Pancreas

Both an endocrine and exocrine gland, the **pancreas** is a carrot-shaped organ located inferior and posterior to the greater curvature of the stomach. The pancreas is the most important digestive gland because it secretes enzymes that break down all categories of digestible foods, including proteins, carbohydrates, and fats. The main duct of the pancreas runs the length of the organ, draining the smaller ducts and emptying the pancreatic enzymes into the duodenum. Pancreatic enzymes are secreted in an alkaline fluid to neutralize the acid chyme from the stomach. Recall that secretin, a hormone produced by the intestinal mucosa, stimulates the production and secretion of pancreatic enzymes.

The pancreas produces about 1 to 1.5 quarts of digestive enzymes per day, including trypsinogen, chymotrypsin, carboxypeptidase, pancreatic amylase, and pancreatic lipase. Trypsinogen, a protein-splitting enzyme, is converted to trypsin when it enters the duodenum. Trypsin, activated by the intestinal enzyme enterokinase, breaks protein into smaller chains of amino acids called *peptides*. Chymotrypsin and carboxypeptidase also assist in the breakdown of proteins. Pancreatic amylase converts polysaccharides into disaccharides (maltose, sucrose, and lactose). Pancreatic lipase converts triglycerides into monoglycerides and fatty acids.

DISASSEMBLY OF FOODS

The major purpose of eating is to feed the body. This sounds simple enough, but the process is not quite so simple. Ultimately, nutrient delivery takes place at the cellular level. The previous discussion examined the how-to part of getting food broken down, but this next section explores what food becomes and how these products are used by our cells.

To be beneficial on the cellular level, food must be disassembled into its component parts: proteins, carbohydrates, fats, vitamins, minerals, and water (Table 21-2). Two functions of the digestive system are to disassemble these nutrients and eliminate the unused matter. Nutrients such as vitamins, minerals, and water do not have to be digested before they are used in the body, but proteins, carbohydrates, and fats need to be mechanically and chemically broken down.

Proteins

Proteins are naturally occurring organic compounds that contain large combinations of amino acids. Twenty identified amino acids are vital for proper growth, development, and health maintenance. Ten of the 20 amino acids are classified as nonessential, meaning that the body can synthesize them. The remaining 10 amino acids are essential amino acids, and these must be obtained from dietary sources (Table 21-3). Sources rich in protein are meat, poultry, seafood, eggs, soy products, and diary products (including yogurt and cheese).

Amino acids are the building blocks of protein. Amino acids are the major components for building muscles, blood, skin, hair, nails, and visceral organs. Protein is also essential for the formation of hormones, enzymes, and antibodies and is used by the

TABLE 21-2

Nutrients and Their Functions

Nutrient	Function
Proteins	Building and repairing muscles, blood, skin, hair, nails, and visceral organs
	Formation of hormones, enzymes, and antibodies
Carbohydrates	Preferred source of energy
	Metabolism of proteins and fats
Fats	Maintenance of cell membranes
	Storage and absorption of fat-soluble hormones and vitamins
	Cushioning and insulation of visceral organs
Vitamins	Normal physiologic and metabolic function, including the following:
	Antioxidants: E, C, and beta carotene
	Hormones: D
	Enhances the immune system: A
Minerals	Building of bone (calcium, magnesium, boron, etc.)
	Muscular activity (calcium and magnesium)
	Support for various organs such as the pancreas (manganese, chromium, and vanadium)
	Transportation of oxygen and carbon dioxide (iron)
Water	Maintenance of proper body pH, nutrient transport, lymphatic transport, and elimination

TABLE 21-3

Selected Nutrient Classifications

Nutrient	Classification
Amino acids: building blocks of proteins	Nonessential amino acids (can be synthesized by the body)
	Essential amino acids (must be obtained from dietary sources such as meat, poultry, seafood, eggs, soy products, and dairy products [including yogurt and cheese])
Carbohydrates	Monosaccharides (simple sugars)
	Glucose (blood sugar)
	Fructose (fruit sugar)
	Galactose (milk sugar)
	Disaccharides (union of two monosaccharides)
	Sucrose (table sugar)
	Lactose (milk sugar)
	Maltose (malt sugar)
	Polysaccharides (trisaccharides)
	Dextrins
	Glycogen (stored glucose)
	Cellulose and gums
Fats	Saturated (solid at room temperature)
	Lard (animal fats)
	Processed oils (hydrogenated or partially hydrogenated oils)
	Coconut oil
	Palm kernel oil
	Used restaurant oils
	Unsaturated (liquid at room temperature)
	Olive oil
	Peanut oil
	Flax seed oil
	Sesame oil
Vitamins	Fat-soluble vitamins can be stored by the body, including A, D, E, and K
	Water-soluble vitamins must be ingested regularly, including B and C

body to repair and rebuild tissues because the body is in a constant state of tearing down and rebuilding.

Carbohydrates

Also known as *starches* and *sugars,* **carbohydrates** are classified according to molecular structure as mono-, di-, and polysaccharides (see Table 21-3). Monosaccharides, or simple sugars, are glucose (blood sugar), fructose (fruit sugar), and galactose (milk sugar). Disaccharides, which are the union of two monosaccharides, are sucrose (table sugar), lactose (milk sugar), and maltose (malt sugar). Polysaccharides, or trisaccharides, which are carbohydrates containing three or more simple sugar molecules, are dextrins, glycogen (stored glucose), cellulose, and gums.

Carbohydrates are the body's preferred source of energy and are required for the metabolism of other nutrients such as proteins and fats. Ingested carbohydrates, mediated by the hormone insulin, are absorbed immediately by the cells of the body or stored as glycogen (stored glucose). Some dietary sources of carbohydrates are grains, cereals, vegetables, fruits, potatoes, and legumes.

Fats

Fats are composed of lipids or fatty acids and can range in consistency from a solid to a liquid. Stored fat (adipose tissue) helps cushion and insulate visceral organs. Fats are classified as saturated or unsaturated, depending on whether they are solid (saturated) or liquid (unsaturated) at room temperature (see Table 21-3). Examples of saturated fats are lard (animal fats), processed oils (hydrogenated or partially hydrogenated), coconut and palm kernel oil, and used restaurant oils. Examples of unsaturated fats are olive, peanut, flax seed, and sesame oils. The body requires fats to maintain cell membranes and steroid hormones.

Of all the nutrients, fats are probably the least understood of all. Good and bad fats are known, but discussion about each abounds as if no distinction can be made. Bad fats are saturated and include lard (animal fats), processed oils (hydrogenated or partially hydrogenated oils), and even unsaturated oils that have been used numerous times (many restaurant oils) because repeated heating breaks down their molecular structure. Good fats are unsaturated and include olive oil, peanut oil, flax seed oil, and sesame oil.

Vitamins

Vitamins are organic compounds essential for normal physiologic and metabolic functioning of the body. Many vitamins act as coenzymes. Most vitamins cannot be synthesized by the body and must be obtained from a healthy diet or vitamin supplements. Vitamins are either fat soluble or water soluble (see Table 21-3). The body can store fat-soluble vitamins, whereas water-soluble vitamins must be ingested regularly. Fat-soluble vitamins are A, D, E, and K; water-soluble vitamins are the B vitamins and vitamin C.

Vitamins have various functions. Vitamin E is an *antioxidant* (a substance that inhibits or retards oxidation), as are vitamin C and beta carotene (a precursor to vitamin A); vitamin D functions as a hormone; and vitamin A enhances the immune system. Vitamins are necessary micronutrients for the body, and the U.S. government has recognized their importance by establishing minimum daily requirements.

Minerals

Minerals are essential nonorganic compounds found in nature that the body uses. Minerals are needed in trace amounts and are used to build bone (calcium, magnesium, boron, etc.), during muscle activity (calcium and magnesium), to support various organs such as the pancreas (manganese, chromium, and vanadium), and to transport oxygen and carbon dioxide (iron). Minerals also play a vital role in regulating many body functions; many also function as coenzymes.

A mineral is usually referred to by the name of a metal, nonmetal, radical, or phosphate, rather than by the name of the compound (e.g., sodium chloride or table salt).

Water

Although water is not often thought of as food, it is an essential nutrient that every part of the body needs. Water-based fluids surround every cell in the body, except the outer layer in the skin, and all nutrients and wastes travel through fluids (blood, lymph, and interstitial fluid). These fluids require a continuous supply of fresh water for proper body pH, nutrient transport, lymphatic transport, and elimination. Each day, a person should drink at least 0.5 ounces (oz) of water per 1 lb of body weight (e.g., 128 lb = 64 oz [$\frac{1}{2}$ gallon] of water per day).

DIGESTIVE PATHOLOGIES

Anorexia nervosa. Classified as both an eating and emotional disorder, anorexia nervosa is the prolonged avoidance of eating. Lack of nutrients results in emaciation, amenorrhea (cessation of menstruation), decreased sleep, and psychological disturbance. When people with anorexia nervosa do eat, they often prefer foods low in calories. Although cases among young males are on the rise, most anorexia nervosa cases are young Caucasian females. Treatment consists of increasing dietary intake and psychological counseling.

Massage therapy can be a helpful adjunct to psychological counseling. Massage may help improve the client's self-image and may decrease anxiety.

Appendicitis. An inflammation of the vermiform appendix, appendicitis is often detected by acute pain in the lower right quadrant of the abdomen, vomiting, fever, and elevated white blood cell count. Intestinal disease, intestinal obstruction or adhesions, or parasites typically cause appendicitis. The most common treatment is an appendectomy.

Massage is contraindicated for appendicitis. Immediate medical attention is needed.

Bulimia. Bulimia is characterized by overeating (bingeing) and self-induced vomiting (purging). Like anorexia nervosa, bulimia is classified as an eating and emotional disorder treated by psychological counseling.

Massage considerations for a client with bulimia are the same as for a client with anorexia nervosa.

Cirrhosis of the liver. Cirrhosis of the liver is a chronic degenerative disease in which the hepatic cells are destroyed and replaced with fibrous connective tissue, giving the liver a yellow-orange color. Liver functions deteriorate as hepatic cells are destroyed. As the disease progresses, GI hemorrhage and kidney failure may also occur. Cirrhosis is usually the result of chronic alcohol abuse or severe hepatitis. The symptoms of cirrhosis are nausea, fatigue, and loss of appetite.

If the cirrhosis is caused by viral hepatitis, massage is contraindicated because of the risk of infection. Otherwise, a gentle, full-body massage is indicated. Reducing the edema in the legs is not recommended because the return of the lymph to the blood may stress the liver and its filtering capacity.

Colitis. Colitis is an inflammation of the mucosa of the large intestine and rectum and is characterized by weight loss, intestinal ulcerations, diarrhea, and bleeding of the colon wall. The origins of colitis are not known, although it is thought to be an autoimmune disease. Some treatment recommendations are increased fluid intake, dietary alterations, and antibiotics.

General massage is beneficial to the client, although the abdomen should be avoided.

Constipation. Constipation is infrequent or difficult passing of stools. Common causes of constipation are insufficient intake of fluid or dietary fiber, lack of physical activity, emotional disturbance, diverticulitis, pregnancy, enema abuse, and painful defecation.

Abdominal massage can help relieve constipation by stimulating the forward movement of intestinal contents.

Crohn's disease. A disease of unknown origin, Crohn's is a progressive inflammatory disease of the colon and/or ileum. Early symptoms are severe abdominal pain, diarrhea, fever, nausea, and loss of appetite. Typically, diseased colon segments are separated by normal colon segments. Crohn's disease is often confused with colitis.

General massage is beneficial to the client, although the abdomen should be avoided.

Diarrhea. The frequent passing of unformed, loose, watery stools is called diarrhea. Factors that cause diarrhea are stress, diet, infection, medication side effects, or inflammation. The stool may also contain blood, pus, or mucus. Other symptoms are abdominal pain, cramping, and intestinal crepitus. Diarrhea may also lead to dehydration.

Clients who have an acute onset of diarrhea should not be massaged until all symptoms are gone because this is often the result of infection. If a client has chronic diarrhea (lasting more than 3 weeks), it is usually the result of conditions such as inflammatory bowel disease. In these cases, abdominal massage is contraindicated, but general massage is all right, depending on the cause.

Diverticulosis. Diverticula are pouchlike herniations of the colon wall where the muscle has become weak. This condition is most likely to be found in individuals over age 50 who have a low-fiber diet. Even though people who have diverticulosis have no symptoms, 15% develop diverticulitis (inflammation of the diverticula).

General massage is beneficial to the client, although the abdomen should be avoided.

Gallstones. Gallstones result from the fusion of cholesterol crystals in bile. They gradually grow in size and number and may cause minimal to total obstruction of bile flow into the duodenum.

Massage is contraindicated during a gallbladder attack. Otherwise, general massage is all right, with abdominal massage contraindicated.

Gastroesophageal reflux disease. If the lower cardioesophageal sphincter fails to close normally after food has entered the stomach, hydrochloric acid from the stomach can enter the inferior portion of the esophagus. The hydrochloric acid irritates the esophageal wall and causes a burning sensation. Gastroesophageal reflux disease (GERD) is also known as *heartburn* because the sensation is near the heart, not because of cardiac problems. Antacids neutralize the hydrochloric acid and decrease the burning sensation. If food is eaten in smaller amounts and the person does not lie down right after a meal, symptoms are less likely to occur.

If a client is prone to GERD, urge him to not eat a large meal during the 2 hours before his appointment.

Hemorrhoids. Hemorrhoids, or *piles*, are varicosities of the rectal veins. The veins in the rectal area lack internal valves, which makes them particularly susceptible to vascular congestion. Prolonged sitting, pregnancy, obesity, constipation, and straining to defecate can contribute to hemorrhoid development.

Massage is fine.

Hepatitis. Hepatitis is an inflammation of the liver that can be caused by alcohol, drugs, toxins, and infection by the hepatitis virus, of which several types are known. Symptoms include muscle and joint pain, fatigue, loss of appetite, nausea, vomiting, diarrhea or constipation, abdominal discomfort, tea-colored urine, white stools, and jaundice. Severity ranges from mild and brief to chronic and life threatening and is detailed as follows:

- **Type A:** Viral transfer by fecal-contaminated food or water
- **Type B:** Viral transfer by blood or sexual contact
- **Type C:** Viral transfer by blood
- **Type D:** Viral transfer by blood or sexual contact; occurs only in patients infected with hepatitis B
- **Type E:** Viral transfer by fecal-contaminated food or water

Massage is contraindicated during the acute phases because it is infectious. If a client has chronic hepatitis (lasting more than 6 months) massage should be performed only after receiving a physician's clearance to make sure the client is not infectious and that the debilitated liver will not be stressed by massage. If clearance is given, abdominal massage is contraindicated.

Irritable bowel syndrome. Also known as *spastic colon*, irritable bowel syndrome is a condition of the large intestine characterized by abnormal muscular contraction (i.e., peristalsis is not working properly) and excessive mucus in stools. It is generally associated with young adults under extreme emotional stress. Early symptoms are diarrhea, nausea, and cramping in the lower abdomen. Because no disease is present, no cure is known either; however, many individuals benefit from adding roughage to their diets. Other positive steps to take in reducing irritable bowel syndrome are counseling, stress reduction, change in dietary habits, and antispasmodic medications.

General massage is beneficial to the client, although the abdomen should be avoided.

Mumps. Mumps is an acute infectious viral disease caused by a *paramyxovirus*, an airborne member of the herpes family. Symptoms are enlargement of the parotid salivary glands, fever, and extreme pain during swallowing. Transmitted by contact with infectious droplets, mumps is most likely to be contracted by children between ages 5 and 15, but the disease may occur in adults.

Massage is contraindicated.

Obesity. Obesity is characterized by an abnormal increase in subcutaneous fat tissue, primarily in visceral regions of the body. Generally, an individual is regarded as obese if his body fat content is ≥30%. Normal (nonathlete) body fat is 18% in men and 25% in women.

Approach the obese client compassionately and nonjudgmentally, making necessary accommodations for client comfort. Avoid deep pressure on areas containing high quantities of adipose tissue to reduce tissue damage and bruising. Provide a sheet or an extra-large towel as a top drape to provide adequate coverage. Have a footstool available and be willing to offer assistance if your client feels awkward or unsafe getting on and off the massage table. If the client does not feel comfortable on your massage table, provide a comfortable floor mat so he may receive his massage on the floor.

Pancreatitis. An inflammation of the pancreas, pancreatitis is usually the result of trauma, alcohol abuse, infection, or certain medications that damage the pancreas. Symptoms may be severe abdominal pain that refers to the back, fever, lack of appetite, nausea, vomiting, and a decreased production of pancreatic enzymes.

Acute pancreatitis needs medical attention. Abdominal massage is contraindicated in clients with chronic pancreatitis, but general massage is fine. Permission from the client's health care provider is a must.

Peritonitis. An acute inflammation of the peritoneum, peritonitis is produced by bacteria or irritating substances that gain access into the abdominal cavity. These substances are introduced into the cavity by a ruptured organ, a penetrating wound, perforation of the GI or urogenital tract (e.g., ectopic pregnancy), or a ruptured appendix.

Usually the client is too sick to be massaged. However, massage may be administered in the hospital to reduce stress and pain, but only after obtaining the physician's clearance. The massage should be gentle and soothing, avoiding the abdomen.

Ulcer. An ulcer is a lesion in a membrane. A peptic ulcer can develop in parts of the digestive tract exposed to acidic gastric juice. Those that occur in the first part of the duodenum are called *duodenal ulcers*. Some occur in the stomach and are called *gastric ulcers*. Symptoms of ulcers are a nonradiating pain in the upper abdominal region, dark fecal stools, and bleeding that could lead to anemia.

The three main causes of ulcers are (1) use of nonsteroidal antiinflammatory drugs (NSAIDs) such as aspirin, (2) hypersecretion of hydrochloric acid caused by a tumor of the pancreas, and (3) the bacterium *Helicobacter pylori* (the most common cause). Cigarette smoking, alcohol, caffeine, aspirin, and stress can exacerbate ulcers.

Massage is beneficial for clients with ulcers because massage is an effective stress management tool. Abdominal massage is contraindicated.

See Box 21-1 for the effects of massage on the digestive system.

BOX 21-1

Effects of Massage on the Digestive System

- **Promotes evacuation of the colon.** By increasing peristaltic activity in the colon through massage, bowel contents move toward the anus for elimination.
- **Relieves constipation.** Because evacuation of the colon is promoted, constipation is relieved.
- **Relieves colic and intestinal gas.** Increased peristaltic activity also helps to relieve colic and intestinal gas.
- **Stimulates digestion.** Massage also promotes activation of the parasympathetic nervous system, which stimulates digestion.

For Your Information

It is generally accepted that ulcers are attributed to stress, but the cause of ulcers is an overproduction of gastric enzymes, which is actually a parasympathetic response. Stress does the opposite; it stimulates a sympathetic nervous system response and reduces gastric secretions, making the condition of ulcers seem like an oxymoron.

Using monkeys as subjects, several experiments were conducted to study ulcers in 1971 and again in 1979. Situations were set up in which shocks were administered to monkeys at a predictive rate. One monkey, the executive monkey, could control whether or not the shock was administered by using a lever. Another monkey, the passive monkey, did not have the same control over the shock. If the executive monkey received a shock, both monkeys were shocked. Likewise, both were spared the shock if the executive monkey pressed the lever at the appropriate time.

So which monkey got the ulcers? The executive monkey was full of ulcers, but the passive monkey had none. Although this was not a perfect experiment, it appears that ulcers may develop after periods of emotional strain, excessive responsibility, and worrying. Because gastric enzymes do not freely flow during periods of stress, ulcers seem to form during periods of rest or parasympathetic activity. The body is attempting to "catch up" after frequent and prolonged stress.

66

In dwelling, live close to the ground
In thinking, keep it simple
In conflict, be fair and generous
In governing, don't to control
In work, do what you enjoy
In family life, be completely present
—Tao Te Ching

SUMMARY

The digestive system consists of a series of structures designed to break down food and liquids into usable body fuel by the processes of ingestion, digestion, absorption and defecation. To carry out these processes, the digestive system makes use of a series of specialized, interrelated structures collectively known as the *alimentary canal.* These structures include the oral cavity, pharynx, esophagus, stomach, small intestines, and large intestines. The alimentary canal makes use of a set of accessory organs that aid in the digestive processes. These accessory organs include the liver, gallbladder, and pancreas. The six types of nutrients are proteins, carbohydrates, fats, vitamins, minerals, and water.

MINI-LAB

Calculate your total caloric intake over a 24-hour period by using a simple caloric guide from any drugstore. Look at the distribution of the basic food groups and write a list of what improvements could (and should) be made in your eating habits.

MATCHING

Write the letter of the best answer in the space provided.

A. Stomach
B. Mastication
C. Pancreas
D. Absorption
E. Esophagus
F. Sphincter

G. Alimentary canal
H. Digestion
I. Villi
J. Large intestine
K. Liver
L. Gallbladder

M. Rugae
N. Vitamins
O. Deglutition
P. Duodenum
Q. Bolus
R. Peristalsis

_____ 1. Synonymous with the word chewing

_____ 2. The muscular tube connecting the pharynx to the stomach

_____ 3. A muscular ring regulating movement of materials from one compartment of the GI tract to another

_____ 4. The process of moving digested products into the bloodstream and then into the body's cells

_____ 5. The final stretch of intestine undigested and unabsorbed food takes before it is eliminated by the body

_____ 6. Synonymous with the word swallowing

_____ 7. Ball-like, masticated lump of food once swallowed

_____ 8. Organic compounds essential for normal physiological and metabolic functions

_____ 9. The process that occurs as food is mixed with digestive enzymes and converted into an absorbable state

_____ 10. J-shaped organ bound at both ends by the cardioesophageal and pyloric sphincters

_____ 11. Fingerlike projections that increase the small intestines' surface area and that house blood and lymph capillaries

_____ 12. The muscular passageway leading from mouth to anus

_____ 13. Rhythmic contractions that mix and propel materials in the GI tract

_____ 14. Stores bile manufactured by the liver

_____ 15. First section of the small intestines

_____ 16. Digestive gland secreting enzymes that break down all categories of digestible foods, including proteins, carbohydrates, and fats

_____ 17. Largest internal organ in the body; carries out more than 500 functions

_____ 18. Longitudinal folds in the stomach's lining that allow expansion

Bibliography

Applegate EJ: *The anatomy and physiology learning system,* ed 2, Philadelphia, 2000, WB Saunders.

Crawley J, Van De Graaff KM: *A photographic atlas for anatomy and physiology,* Englewood, Colo, 2002, Morton.

Crooks R, Stein J: *Psychology: science, behavior, and life,* New York, 1988, Holt, Rinehart, Winston.

Damjanov I: *Pathology for the health-related professions,* Philadelphia, 1996, WB Saunders.

Ford CW: *Where healing waters meet: touching mind and emotions through the body,* Barrytown, NY, 1992, Station Hill Press.

Goldberg S: *Clinical anatomy made ridiculously simple,* Miami, 1984, Medmaster.

Gould BE: Pathophysiology for the health-related professionals, Philadelphia, 1997, WB Saunders.

Haubrich WS: *Medical meanings: a glossary of word origins,* New York, 1984, Harcourt Brace Jovanovich.

Jacob S, Francone C: *Elements of anatomy and physiology,* Philadelphia, 1989, WB Saunders.

Kalat JW: *Biological psychology,* ed 2, Belmont, Calif, 1984, Wadsworth.

Kapit W, Elson LM: *The anatomy coloring book,* ed 3, New York, 2002, Benjamin Cummings.

Kordish M, Dickson S: *Introduction to basic human anatomy,* Lake Charles, La, 1995, McNeese State University.

Marieb EN: *Essentials of human anatomy and physiology,* ed 4, New York, 1994, Benjamin Cummings.

McAleer N: *The body almanac,* Garden City, NY, 1985, Doubleday.

Merck Research Laboratories: *Merck manual,* ed 17, Whitehouse Station, NJ, 1998, Author.

Mosby's medical, nursing, and allied health dictionary, ed 4, St Louis, 1994, Mosby.

Newton D: *Pathology for massage therapists,* ed 2, Portland, Ore, 1995, Simran.

Premkumar K: *Pathology A to Z: a handbook for massage therapists,* Calgary, 1996, VanPub Books.

Solomon EP, Phillips GA: *Understanding human anatomy and physiology,* Philadelphia, 1987, WB Saunders.

Taber's cyclopedic medical dictionary, ed 13, Philadelphia, 1977, FA Davis.

Thibodeau G, Patton K: *Structure and function of the body,* ed 11, St Louis, 2000, Mosby.

Tortora GJ: *Introduction to the human body: the essentials of anatomy and physiology,* ed 3, New York, 1994, HarperCollins.

Tortora GJ, Grabowksi SR: *Principles of anatomy and physiology,* ed 9, New York, 2000, John Wiley.

Werner R: *A massage therapist's guide to pathology,* ed 2, Baltimore, 2002, Lippincott Williams & Wilkins.

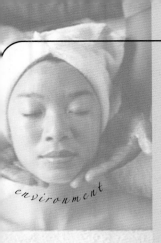

environment

Urinary System

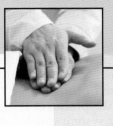

22

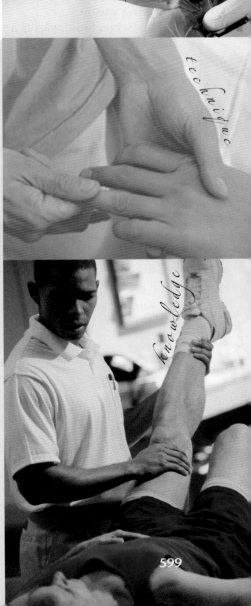

pressure

technique

knowledge

"One doesn't discover new lands without consenting to lose sight of the shore for a very long time."

—Andre Gide

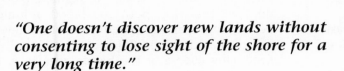

STUDENT OBJECTIVES

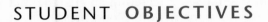

After completing this chapter, the student should be able to:

- Describe functions of the urinary system
- Identify basic structures of the urinary system, and explain their individual functions
- Name parts of the kidney and its nephron
- Trace blood flow through a kidney, including filtration and re-absorption
- Explain the processes of filtration, reabsorption, tubular secretions, and urine production
- Discuss how the antidiuretic hormones renin and aldosterone aid in regulating blood pressure, water balance, and blood volume
- Name types of urinary pathologies, giving characteristics and massage considerations of each

INTRODUCTION

The human body is a complex machine, and as such, it does not perform properly if residues from fuel combustion and other processes are not removed. The cells of the body machine metabolize nutrients, which produce wastes such as carbon dioxide, and heat. The breakdown of proteins produces the nitrogen wastes such as ammonia and urea, which are toxic to the system. Sodium chloride, sodium sulfate, phosphate, and hydrogen molecules and ions also accumulate as a result of metabolic activities. All of these waste materials must be excreted from the body for homeostasis to be maintained and for metabolism to function optimally.

Excretion of waste products is such a large task that no single body system can handle it alone. Several systems contribute to waste elimination.

- **Respiratory.** Waste elimination is done through expiration.
- **Integumentary.** Sweating is a method of eliminating wastes.
- **Digestive.** Solid wastes are eliminated through excretion.
- **Urinary.** Wastes are excreted through urination.

FUNCTIONS

The functions of the urinary system are as follows:
1. **Eliminate metabolic waste.** Cellular metabolism produces waste products that are released in the urine. These waste products include excess potassium ions, carbon dioxide, ammonia, heat, and urea.
2. **Regulate blood pH and its chemical composition.** The kidneys possess specialized cells that monitor the acid-base balance of the blood. Metabolic wastes are laundered from the blood, and substances such as glucose, sodium, vitamins, and minerals are reabsorbed into the blood to adjust its chemical composition. Hydrogen ions are secreted from the blood into the urine as needed to maintain the blood's pH balance.
3. **Regulate blood volume and fluid balance.** The kidneys control the amount of water reabsorbed into the circulatory system to regulate blood volume. In this way, both the blood volume and body's water balance are altered. If fluid levels are not regulated, excess fluids collect in the tissues, producing edema of the hands, feet, face, heart, and other body areas.
4. **Regulate blood pressure.** The kidneys continuously monitor blood pressure and help maintain a normal range by secreting an enzyme that stimulates vasoconstriction. Blood pressure is also kept in balance by the regulation of blood volume. Blood pressure is maintained by interaction of the circulatory, endocrine, and nervous systems.
5. **Maintain homeostasis.** With the removal of metabolic wastes, the body maintains homeostasis by regulating the chemical composition of the blood, by regulating blood volume and maintaining fluid balance and blood pressure. Because of these many functions, the kidneys are the major homeostatic organs of the body. Malfunction of the kidneys causes dangerous changes in blood composition, which often lead to death.

ANATOMY AND RELATED PHYSIOLOGY

The urinary system contains four basic structures: kidneys, ureters, urinary bladder, and urethra (Figure 22-1). The kidneys filter the blood and direct the urine to the ureters, which transfer the urine to the urinary bladder for storage. The bladder is then emptied through the urethra to the outside of the body. The filtered blood is routed back to general circulation.

Kidneys

The **kidneys** are a pair of organs located bilaterally in the upper lumbar region of the spine. They are bean-shaped (convex laterally and concave medially) and are slightly smaller than a fist. The kidneys are located behind the abdominal peritoneum (**retroperitoneal**) and are surrounded by a fibrous renal

Terms and Their Meanings Related to the Urinary System	
Term	**Meaning**
antidiuretic	against or opposed; urine flow
Bowman's capsule	English physician (1816-1892)
calyx	cup
diuretic	urine flow
ducts of Bellini	Italian anatomist (1643-1704)
glomerulus	little ball
hilus or hilum	a trifle
juxtapose	close by, adjacent, side by side
loop of Henle	German anatomist (1809-1885)
macula densa	spot; thick
nephro or nephra	kidney
peritubular	around, about; like a tube
renal	kidney
renin	kidney
retroperitoneal	backward; the peritoneum
trigone	three-cornered figure

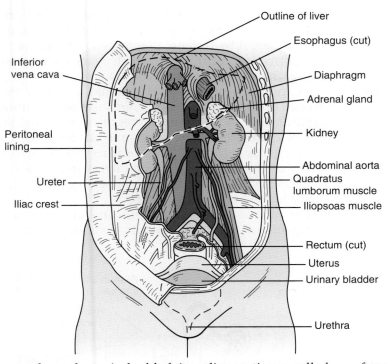

Figure 22-1   General urinary system and important landmarks.

capsule and are imbedded in adipose tissue called perirenal fat; this fat serves as a barrier against trauma and the spread of infection. Because of the presence of the liver, the kidney on the right side of the body is slightly lower than the one on the left.

Because the kidneys do not have the extra protection of the abdominal peritoneal lining or the rib cage, massage tapotement (percussion) is contraindicated over the kidney area in the dorsum of the body. It may be helpful to draw the kidneys on a fellow student with a washable, nontoxic marker to identify the location of these structures.

The **renal hilus** is the indentation located in the medially concave region of the kidney; here is where the renal arteries, renal veins, and the ureters enter and exit. The interior compartment of the renal hilus houses the **renal pelvis**, which is the funnel-shaped origin of the ureters. Each kidney is divided into two major regions: the cortex (outer region) and the medulla (inner region) (Figure 22-2).

The kidneys are composed of millions of minute structures known as **nephrons**, the basic filtering units of the kidney that are responsible for filtering waste products from the blood, which are later excreted. It is possible to lose many nephrons, or even an entire kidney, and maintain good health. The filtration process is accomplished in the nephrons by a vast and intricate network made up of two different routing vessels—one that channels blood through the nephron and one that collects urine from the nephron and routes it to the renal pelvis.

The process begins in the section of the nephron known as the **glomerular capsule** (Figure 22-3).

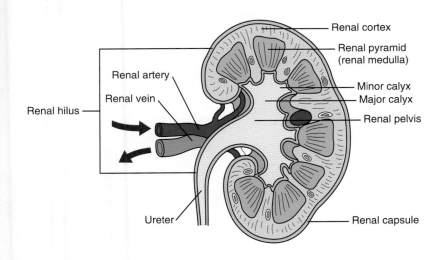

Figure 22-2   The kidney.

The glomerular capsule then becomes the **renal tubule**, a urine routing vessel. Contained within the glomerular capsule are loops of minute blood vessels called **glomeruli**. It is here in the glomerulus that blood plasma crosses over into the glomerular capsule in the first stage of the blood filtration–urine formation process.

A second network of blood vessels branches off before the glomerulus; these vessels are called the **peritubular capillaries**, which are interwoven with corresponding renal tubules. These two structures are interlaced, providing a larger surface area for waste product exchange and water reabsorption. The renal tubules move the urine through the internal portion of the kidney or the medulla to the

ureters. Bundles of renal tubules in the medulla are called **medullary pyramids**. Each kidney, composed of eight to 18 renal pyramids, contains many straight collecting tubules, which gives each pyramid a striated appearance.

At the apex of the renal pyramid, a small, expanded duct, the minor **calyx**, encloses one or more papillae. Four to 13 minor calyces are in the renal sinus of each kidney. Several minor calyces unite to form a major calyx. Only two or three major calyces are in each kidney. The major calyces join to form the renal pelvis, which is the upper region of the ureter located at the renal hilus.

The filtration process depends on blood pressure being higher in the glomeruli than in the renal

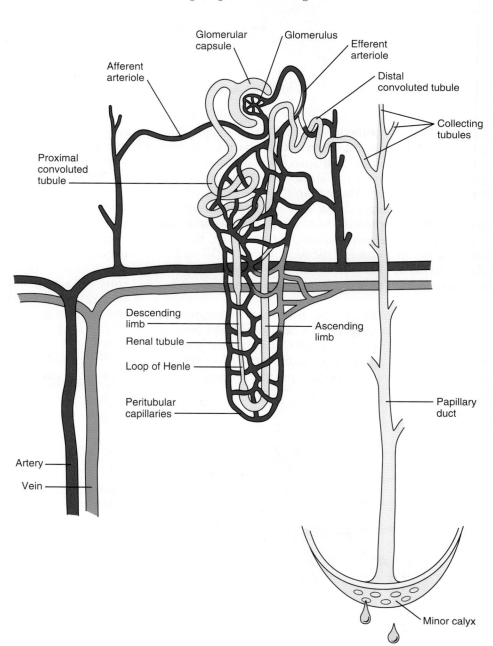

Figure 22-3   Nephron: urine pathway and blood supply.

tubules so that fluid can easily move across the cellular membrane. This process is clearly understood if the path of the blood is traced throughout the kidneys.

Blood Vessels and Blood Flow in the Kidneys

Oxygen-rich blood enters the kidneys by the renal artery where it branches off the abdominal aorta (Figure 22-4). As the renal artery enters the renal hilus, the artery becomes smaller, subdividing and looping through the kidney in two paths, with one consisting of the afferent arterioles and the other consisting of the peritubular capillaries. The afferent arterioles are high-pressure vessels that feed the glomerular capillaries. Here in the glomeruli is where blood plasma, with its dissolved solids, crosses over into the renal tubules. From the glomerular capillaries, the blood flows into the efferent arterioles. This is one of the few places in the body that arterial flow moves through a capillary network and into another artery instead of into a vein.

The second, smaller vascular path feeds directly into the peritubular capillaries, bypassing the glomeruli. The peritubular capillaries surround the renal tubule, where most reabsorption of water occurs. The blood from the efferent arterioles then joins with the flow from the peritubular capillaries, and together, they stream into the venous system. The venous structures grow larger and larger and return the blood directly to the inferior vena cava.

Fluid Movement

Most body fluids move through vessels and across membranes by either hydrostatic pressure and osmosis. Hydrostatic pressure is the pressure exerted on fluids by the weight of the fluid itself, the pressure of muscle contraction, or the pressure on fluids from an external source (massage). Osmosis is the movement of fluids and their particles from an area of low

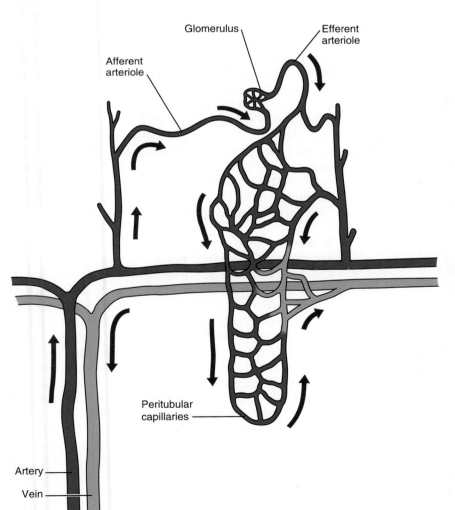

Figure 22-4 Close-up of the blood supply to and from the renal tubule.

concentration (most dilute) to an area of high concentration (least dilute). This action continues until the two concentrations equalize. Osmosis does not depend on pressure but rather on the concentration of dissolved elements that lie in the solutions on each side of a cell membrane or vessel wall. The kidneys use both hydrostatic pressure and osmosis in the process of urine production.

The Filtration Process

Filtration of the blood and formation of urine is a three-step process. First, the watery blood plasma is filtered in the glomeruli; second, water, nutrients, and ions are reabsorbed into the bloodstream from the renal tubules; and third, tubular secretions of unwanted elements are discharged back into the filtrate (Figure 22-5). Urine is then produced.

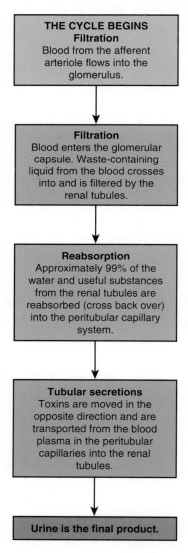

Figure 22-5   Urine formation.

For Your Information

The entire blood supply of the body passes through the kidneys every 3 minutes, during which only about 1% of the blood plasma crosses the glomeruli for waste removal processing by the kidneys. It takes about 5 hours to process all the blood plasma in the human body.

Filtration

In the first step of the filtration process, blood enters the glomerular capsule. Because of hydrostatic pressure, waste-containing liquid from the blood crosses into and is filtered by the renal tubules. The bloodstream retains proteins and formed elements of the blood that are too large to cross the membrane. Toxins, excess free ions, and nonessential substances such as urea, uric acid, ammonia, drug residue, excess minerals and water-soluble vitamins (especially B vitamins; this is why your urine turns bright yellow when taking these supplements) are collected in the renal tubules and allowed to leave the body in the urine, which is a solution of water and dissolved waste. The filtration process is so efficient that about 45 gallons (180 liters [L]) of filtrate are produced in a 24-hour day. Not all of this water is excreted as urine. Most of it is reabsorbed back into the blood.

For the filtration step to occur, the pressure of the blood in the glomeruli is higher than the pressure of the filtrate in the renal tubule. The afferent arteriole feeding the glomerular vessels has a relatively large diameter, whereas the lumen of the efferent arterioles is much narrower. This pressure is approximately 60 mm Hg in the glomerulus as compared with only 18 mm Hg in the renal tubules.

Reabsorption

Approximately 99% of the fluids removed from the blood are reabsorbed. The reabsorption process occurs when water and useful substances from the renal tubules are reabsorbed through the semipermeable membrane into the peritubular capillary system. This happens despite the fact that pressure is greater in the blood vessels than in the renal tubules, and is the result of osmosis. Because most of the water has moved across to the renal tubule, the filtrate is very diluted, and the blood and plasma in the peritubular capillary network are highly saturated with proteins and other solutes. Osmosis causes the reabsorption of water into the bloodstream and continues until the concentrations of the solutions on both sides of the membrane equalize. The majority of the body's water, along with much-needed substances such as glucose and amino acids, are retained and returned to the blood through the process of reabsorption.

Tubular Secretion

In the reabsorption phase, water and necessary nutrients are recovered from the filtrate by crossing back from the renal tubules to the bloodstream. In the final phase of the filtration process, toxins are moved in the opposite direction. These toxins are transported from the blood plasma in the peritubular capillaries into the renal tubules.

Tubular secretion rids the body of toxic elements and controls blood pH. Toxins are secreted back across the cell membrane from the blood to the filtrate. These toxins may include organic compounds and ions. Toxic organic compounds such as creatinine and histamine may occur naturally within the body, or they may be residue from drugs introduced into the body, such as penicillin. Ion levels must be regulated to maintain various bodily functions. The secretion of hydrogen ions is a major factor in the regulation of blood pH. Potassium ion secretion prevents a buildup of ions that would affect heart rhythm.

Urine Flow in the Kidneys

Urine production begins in the renal cortex (urine-manufacturing facility) as the watery portion of the blood plasma exits the glomerulus and then enters the first section of the renal tubule called the *glomerular capsule* (Figure 22-6, *B*). The glomerular capsule is a funnel-shaped pouch that surrounds the glomerulus. Once it crosses from the glomerulus into the glomerular capsule, the filtered fluids are referred to as **filtrate**. This filtrate first flows into the proximal convoluted tubule, the walls of which are lined with microvilli; they create a larger surface area for more efficient fluid exchange. The proximal convoluted tubule feeds into the loop of Henle, which is a hairpin-shaped structure divided into a descending and ascending limb. From here, the filtrate flows into the distal convoluted tubule and then into collecting tubules located in the medulla (urine collecting facility) of the kidney.

These straight collecting tubules route the urine produced in the cortex into large papillary ducts. When the concentrated filtrate of the kidney reaches the calyces, it is then called *urine.*

Encourage your clients to drink lots of water (0.5 oz of water per 1 lb of body weight). Without an adequate water intake, kidneys cannot adequately do their job. Increasing water intake often helps kidneys balance electrolytes; this may reduce muscle cramping. This is also good advice for therapists.

Ureters

The **ureters** are two slender hollow tubes about 10 inches long that transport urine formed by the kidneys to the urinary bladder. Like the kidneys, the ureters are located bilaterally; each kidney has one

ureter. Urine is drained by peristaltic activity from the major and minor calyces, and from the renal pelvis in the kidneys to the urinary bladder. This peristaltic activity continues until urine reaches the urinary bladder. Each ureter enters the urinary bladder through a specialized valve, which prevents backflow of urine as the bladder contracts and empties. When the bladder is empty, the ureters are spaced about 2 cm apart. However, when the bladder expands, the ureters move about 5 cm apart.

Urinary Bladder

Located in the pelvis behind the symphysis pubis, the muscular **urinary bladder** provides a temporary storage reservoir for urine. Within the urinary bladder is a small triangular region called the trigone. The three corners of the trigone are marked at the top by the left and right ureter ducts and at the bottom by the internal urethral orifice. The urinary bladder is often filled with and emptied of urine. The following two types of structures allow expansion of the urinary bladder: (1) folds within the interior lining, or rugae, that allow the urinary bladder to distend and (2) transitional epithelium, which changes shape as pressure is exerted on the epithelial lining. This tissue expansion puts pressure on pressure-sensitive receptors located in the muscular wall, which causes the internal urethral orifice to relax and results in the conscious desire to void (urinate). On demand, the cerebral cortex of the brain sends impulses to the external urethral orifice muscle to relax, and urination, or **micturition**, takes place.

Urethra

The **urethra** is a small tubular structure that transports urine from the urinary bladder out of the body during urination. The internal sphincter muscle closes the proximal end of the urethra, whereas the external sphincter muscles are located in the wall of the urogenital diaphragm. The internal urethral sphincter contains visceral muscle, and the external urethral sphincter contains skeletal muscle and is typically under voluntary control after the age of 15 months.

The length of the urethra differs in males and females. In females, the path of the urethra is located anterior to the vagina and exits between the vaginal opening and clitoris. The female urethra is relatively short (about 1.5 inches). This and the fact that the female urinary orifice is close to the anal opening may account for the much higher incidence of bladder infections in women.

Opening at the distal end, or the glans penis, the male urethra extends from the center of the prostate and passes through the length of the penis (about 8

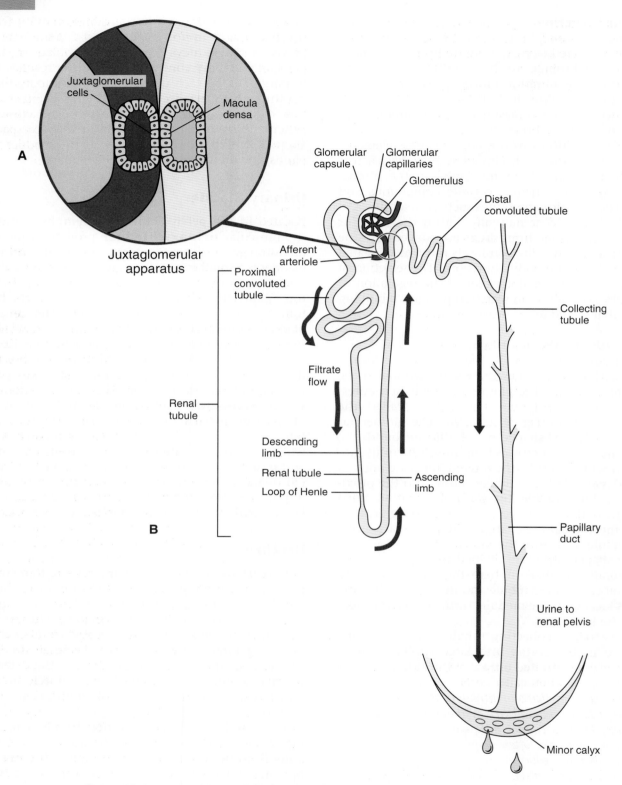

Figure 22-6 **A,** Juxtaglomerular apparatus. **B,** Cutaway view of the nephron focusing on urine pathway.

inches, depending on penile length). Both semen from the testes and urine from the urinary bladder may be transported by the male urethra.

For Your Information

URINE

Urine is concentrated filtrate from the kidneys that is 96% water and 4% dissolved wastes (urea, creatinine, uric acid, sodium chloride, potassium, sulfates, phosphates, and drug residue). Urine tends to be slightly acidic, and a normal amber color. The more concentrated the urine, the darker its color. Abnormal constituents in urine may include albumin, glucose, red blood cells, white blood cells, bilirubin, kidney stones, and bacteria.

The average adult produces anywhere from 1 to 2 quarts (1000 to 2000 ml) of urine per day. Chemical, nervous, and even physical factors can affect the amount of urine produced and excreted by the body. An example of a chemical factor is the consumption of coffee, tea, and many carbonated beverages. Stimulating the production of urine, these drinks have a diuretic effect on the urinary system. A **diuretic** (substance promoting the formation and excretion of urine) can increase urine production by increasing the amount of blood fluid crossing the glomerulus, or it can decrease the amount of water reabsorbed from the renal tubule; both increase urine production. Anxiety often suppresses the body's urge to void. During periods of physical activity, the heart beats more rapidly, moving the blood through the kidney faster and increasing urine production.

Cryotherapy has a diuretic effect on the body. General cold applications cause vasoconstriction of the superficial vessels of the skin, which results in a temporary increase in blood pressure. The raised blood pressure increases the amount of glomerular output and hence urine production.

CONTROLLING THE WATER BALANCE OF THE BODY

The bloodstream is responsible for water transfer to and from all the cells of the body and for oxygen and nutrient exchange. The key to the water balance of the entire body is regulating the fluid balance of the blood. The secretion of antidiuretic hormone (ADH) regulates the control of water balance of the body. If the bloodstream becomes concentrated as a result of the loss of water through sweat or urination, the posterior pituitary gland releases ADH, which stimulates the kidneys to reabsorb more water. If the blood is too dilute, the pituitary reduces the production of ADH, and the kidneys begin to produce more urine. Along with the water, important substances such as glucose are reabsorbed into the bloodstream.

KIDNEYS, BLOOD PRESSURE, AND BLOOD VOLUME

Blood pressure is directly proportional to blood volume. As blood volume increases, blood pressure increases accordingly. The kidneys depend on blood pressure to function properly. As long as systemic blood pressure is sufficient, the kidneys filter the blood and produce urine. However, if arterial blood pressure drops too low, renal pressure becomes inadequate to force substances out of the blood into the tubules, and filtrate formation stops. It makes sense that a mechanism that controls blood pressure and blood volume is located in the kidney.

The mechanism monitoring the blood pressure is known as the **juxtaglomerular apparatus**. It consists of two specialized groups of cells known as the *macula densa* and *juxtaglomerular cells* (Figure 22-6, *A*). The macula densa is located in the ascending limb of Henle's loop. The juxtaglomerular cells are located in the afferent arteriole. The macula densa and the juxtaglomerular cells lie next to each other where the renal tubule touches the afferent arteriole. The juxtaglomerular cells monitor changes in blood pressure in the afferent arteriole, and the macula densa, which functions like a chemoreceptor, monitors the concentration of the filtrate.

When blood pressure or chloride ion concentration of the filtrate drops, the juxtaglomerular apparatus responds by secreting the enzyme **renin** into the bloodstream. Renin reacts with the blood in the lungs, a process that eventually results in a substance called **angiotensin II**, a powerful stimulant that has two major effects. First, it works directly on the blood vessels by causing vasoconstriction, which raises the blood pressure; second, it stimulates the adrenal cortex to release the hormone **aldosterone**. Aldosterone promotes the retention of sodium, which stimulates the reabsorption of more water back into the blood plasma. The plasma volume of the blood increases, and blood pressure rises correspondingly. When blood pressure becomes too high, the renin secretions are decreased, as is blood pressure.

URINARY PATHOLOGIES

Cystitis. Cystitis is an inflammation of the urinary bladder and/or ureters. It occurs more often in women. This condition is often caused by a bacterial infection from neighboring organs such as the kidney or urethra. Cystitis is often characterized by pain, blood in the urine, and by urgency and frequency of urination.

Massage over the abdominal area is contraindicated, although a full body massage may be beneficial. Encourage the client to take the full course of antibiotics and to increase fluid intake.

Glomerulonephritis. Also known as *Bright's disease*, glomerulonephritis is an inflammation of the glomeruli. This disease often follows other infections and is characterized by blood in the urine, edema, and hypertension.

Massage should be very light and soothing and of shorter duration. Do not try to reduce edema with lymphatic massage. Moving the fluid back into the blood may overload the heart.

Gout. Gout is a condition characterized by high levels of uric acid in the blood as a result of high production or an inability of the kidneys to excrete this substance. The uric acid is converted to sodium urate crystals, which are often deposited in joints, kidneys, and other tissues. Gout is more common in men than in women. The great toe is a common site for the accumulation of sodium urate crystals, causing painful swelling. When gout settles in the joints, it is called *gouty arthritis*.

Massage and passive range of motion are contraindicated during an acute phase of gout because of the inflammation and pain. However, cold packs could be beneficial. If the client is not having a flare-up, light massage can be done on the surrounding areas. Range of motion and local massage, however, are contraindicated.

Renal dialysis. Renal dialysis is the process of using an artificial kidney to remove wastes from the blood. This process is accomplished by diffusing previously unfiltered blood across a semipermeable membrane, then the cleansed blood flows back into the body.

A client who is undergoing dialysis may not be a good candidate for massage. Permission from the client's physician is a must. He may be taking anticoagulants. Because deep pressure can cause subcutaneous bleeding, a light massage of short duration is best. The client may have a shunt or catheter. This allows blood to be drawn without resticking. The catheter site should be avoided during the massage.

Renal failure. Renal failure is the inability of the kidneys to perform their essential functions (e.g.,

filtering the blood, collecting and secreting wastes, retaining essential elements). This condition is caused by an impediment to renal blood flow such as hemorrhage, trauma, obstruction of the urinary tract, toxic substances (e.g., mercury), or renal disease (e.g., glomerulonephritis). If a client has progressive renal failure, he may be on hemodialysis.

Permission from the client's physician is a must. A light, soothing massage of short duration is best because the client may bruise easily.

Uremia. Often seen in renal failure and glomerulonephritis, uremia denotes a toxic level of urea and other nitrogenous waste products in the blood. Uremia is the result of a renal insufficiency and abnormal retention of these waste products normally removed by the kidneys.

See Renal Failure.

Urinary incontinence. The inability to control urination is referred to as urinary incontinence. This condition may be the result of an infection or damage to the central or peripheral nervous system or injury to the urinary sphincter or perineal structures, which can occur during childbirth. Urinary incontinence is often precipitated by laughing, coughing and sneezing, late stages of pregnancy, or straining while lifting heavy objects.

Massage is fine. The lower abdomen may be a local contraindication.

Urinary tract infection. Urinary tract infection (UTI) is an infection of one or more structures of the urinary system. Most UTIs are caused by bacteria and are more common in women than in men because women have a short urethra and it is located near the anus. Bacteria from feces can be transported to the urethra as a result of improper toilet habits (i.e., wiping from back to front rather than from front to back). The most common symptoms of UTIs are increased urination, burning and pain during urination, and, if the infection is severe, blood and pus in the urine.

BOX 22-1

Effects of Massage on the Urinary System

- **Increases urine output.** Massage activates dormant capillary beds and recovers lymphatic fluids for filtration by the kidney. This, in turn, increases the frequency of urination and amount of urine produced. Massage is also relaxing. This promotes general homeostasis and increases urine output.
- **Promotes the excretion of nitrogen, inorganic phosphorus, and sodium chloride in urine.** Levels of these metabolic wastes are elevated in urine after massage.

Encourage your client to take the full treatment of the physician-prescribed antibiotics. Also encourage her to drink water each day (½ oz of water per 1 lb of body weight) to flush out microbes. Massage depends on how the client is feeling. If the symptoms are severe, massage may be the last thing the person wants. If the symptoms are less severe, abdominal massage should be avoided, but a general massage would be fine. Keep in mind that the client may need to take frequent trips to the bathroom.

See Box 22-1 for the effects of massage on the urinary system.

SUMMARY

The urinary system maintains homeostasis in the body by accomplishing several functions. This system eliminates metabolic waste; regulates the pH and chemical composition of the blood; and regulates blood volume, fluid volume, and blood pressure. This small system accomplishes these varied functions with only four types of organs: a pair of kidneys, a pair of ureters, a urinary bladder, and a urethra.

The kidney is a highly complex bean-shaped organ located bilaterally in the upper lumbar area. Kidneys have two main divisions—the cortex and the medulla—that are covered with a tough renal capsule. The renal hilus is the point where the artery and vein connect to permit blood circulation through the kidney, and is the origin of the ureters. The cortex carries out the process of urine manufacture, and the medulla houses the urine collecting apparatus. The chief structural and functional unit of the kidney is the nephron, which is responsible for the filtration process. This is accomplished by two interlaced networks of vessels—one carrying blood and the other carrying urine. The blood is carried through some specialized vessels known as *glomeruli* and *peritubular capillaries.* In the glomeruli, the liquid portion of the plasma filters across into the renal tubules, which are urine transport structures. Excess water and certain needed elements are reabsorbed from the renal tubules back into the bloodstream in the peritubular capillaries. The product remaining in the renal tubule is known as *filtrate.* Other toxins are secreted into this filtrate, which is collected and becomes urine.

The urine flows out of the kidneys through a pair of ureters and into the urinary bladder, where the liquid is stored until it can be excreted from the body. When full, the bladder is emptied through a tube to the outside known as the urethra.

MATCHING

Write the letter of the best answer in the space provided.

A. Antidiuretic hormone
B. Renal medulla
C. Glomeruli
D. Juxtaglomerular apparatus
E. Renal cortex
F. Urethra

G. Renal hilus
H. Aldosterone
I. Urinary bladder
J. Retroperitoneal
K. Ureters

L. Nephron
M. Micturition
N. Medullary pyramids
O. Kidneys
P. Urine

_____ 1. The basic filtering unit of the kidney

_____ 2. A small tubular structure that transports urine from the urinary bladder out of the body during urination

_____ 3. Hormone promoting the retention of sodium, which stimulates the reabsorption of more water back into the blood plasma

_____ 4. Two slender hollow tubes transporting urine from the kidneys to the urinary bladder

_____ 5. Concentrated filtrate from the kidneys that is 96% water and 4% dissolved wastes

_____ 6. Inner region of the kidney called the *urine collecting facility*

_____ 7. Bean-shaped pair of organs; the major homeostatic organs of the body

_____ 8. Mechanism monitoring blood pressure consisting of the macula densa and the juxtaglomerular cells

_____ 9. Indentation in the medial concave region of the kidney where arteries, veins, and the ureters enter and exit

_____ 10. Word meaning *urination*

_____ 11. Hormone that stimulates the kidneys to reabsorb more water

_____ 12. Bundles of renal tubules in the medulla

_____ 13. Muscular organ providing a temporary storage reservoir for urine

_____ 14. Outer region of the kidney called the *urine manufacturing facility*

_____ 15. Loops of minute blood vessels in the glomerular capsule

_____ 16. Word meaning *behind the abdominal peritoneum*

Bibliography

Applegate EJ: *The anatomy and physiology learning system,* ed 2, Philadelphia, 2000, WB Saunders.

Crawley J, Van De Graaff KM: *A photographic atlas for anatomy and physiology,* Englewood, Colo, 2002, Morton.

Damjanov I: *Pathophysiology for the health-related professions,* Philadelphia, 1996, WB Saunders.

Gould BE: *Pathophysiology for the health-related professionals,* Philadelphia, 1997, WB Saunders.

Gray H, Pick TP, Howden R: *Gray's anatomy,* ed 29, Philadelphia, 1974, Running Press.

Haubrich WS: *Medical meanings: a glossary of word origins,* New York, 1984, Harcourt Brace Jovanovich.

Jacob S, Francone C: *Elements of anatomy and physiology,* Philadelphia, 1989, WB Saunders.

Kalat JW: *Biological psychology,* ed 2, Belmont, Calif, 1984, Wadsworth.

Kapit W, Elson LM: *The anatomy coloring book,* ed 3, New York, 2002, Benjamin Cummings.

Kordish M, Dickson S: *Introduction to basic human anatomy,* Lake Charles, La, 1995, McNeese State University.

Marieb EN: *Essentials of human anatomy and physiology,* ed 4, New York, 1994, Benjamin Cummings.

McAleer N: *The body almanac,* Garden City, NY, 1985, Doubleday.

Merck Research Laboratories: *Merck manual,* ed 17, Whitehouse Station, NJ, 1998, Author.

Moore KL: *Clinically oriented anatomy,* ed 2, Baltimore, 1985, Williams and Wilkins.

Mosby's medical, nursing, and allied health dictionary, ed 4, St Louis, 1994, Mosby.

Newton D: *Pathology for massage therapists,* ed 2, Portland, Ore, 1995, Simran.

Premkumar K: *Pathology A to Z: a handbook for massage therapists,* Calgary, 1996, VanPub Books.

Solomon EP, Phillips GA: *Understanding human anatomy and physiology,* Philadelphia, 1987, WB Saunders.

Taber's cyclopedic medical dictionary, ed 13, Philadelphia, 1977, FA Davis.

Thibodeau G, Patton K: *Structure and function of the body,* ed 11, St Louis, 2000, Mosby.

Tortora GJ: *Introduction to the human body: the essentials of anatomy and physiology,* ed 3, New York, 1994, HarperCollins.

Tortora GJ, Grabowksi SR: *Principles of anatomy and physiology,* ed 9, New York, 2000, John Wiley.

Werner R: *A massage therapist's guide to pathology,* ed 2, Baltimore, 2002, Lippincott Williams & Wilkins.

UNIT FOUR

A User's Guide to Complementary and Adjunctive Therapies

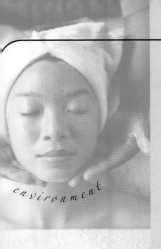

environment

Hydrotherapy and Spa Applications

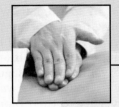

23

pressure

"Nothing on earth is so weak and yielding as water, but for breaking down the firm and strong, it has no equal."

—Lao Tzu

STUDENT OBJECTIVES

technique

After completing this chapter, the student should be able to:

- Define hydrotherapy, spa, cryotherapy, and thermotherapy
- Develop clinical reasoning skills needed for the practice of hydrotherapy
- Select the proper type of hydrotherapy treatment for your client
- Describe the three physical states of water
- List and explain the four factors that contribute to how water affects the body
- Name the benefits and contraindications for cold and heat
- Discuss the hunting response
- List the four sensations felt by the client during an ice treatment
- Outline guidelines to ensure safe application of hydrotherapy and spa methods
- Demonstrate or explain pack, compress, and wrap application methods
- Demonstrate or explain bath and shower applications
- Demonstrate or explain friction applications

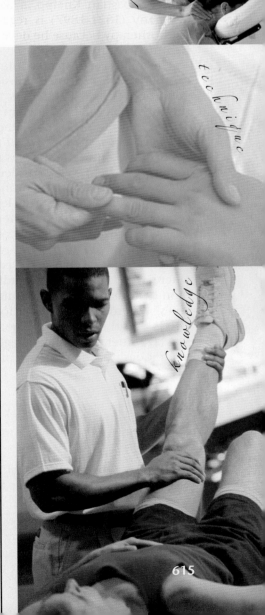

knowledge

INTRODUCTION

Water has always been used to maintain health, manage pain, and treat physical and emotional ailments. The Babylonians, Romans, Greeks, Chinese, Japanese, and Egyptians used and advocated the healing effects of water in the form of various baths, packs, and frictions. Bath temperatures were adjusted to the needs of each individual bather and to affect the intended therapeutic outcome. In Sparta, laws were passed that made frequent bathing mandatory. Water, in its various forms, continues to be employed to enhance the health and well-being of individuals and can be used to add therapeutic value to massage therapy. Hydrotherapy and spa techniques are ways for massage therapists to add diversity to their practice.

Hydrotherapy is the internal and external therapeutic use of water and complementary agents. This chapter addresses external uses only. Water is often heated or cooled for use in specific applications. Father Sebastian Kneipp, a Bavarian monk of West Germany (1821-1897) is regarded as the Father of Hydrotherapy because he developed numerous water treatments still used today.

The inclusion of spa techniques in the study of hydrotherapy is obvious if considering the origin and definition of spa. The letters "S-P-A" were scribbled on the marble walls of ancient public baths of Rome. This coded message, translated from the Latin term *salude per aqua,* meaning *health or healing through water.* In those times the spa was more than just a place to feel good. It was considered a sacred space—a place to experience transformation and healing on both spiritual and physical levels. In the sixteenth century, people traveled to the town of Spa, Belgium, to "take the waters" as a way of rest, retreat, find lost health, preserve vitality, and rejuvenate.

The term **spa** has evolved to describe a place where water therapies are administered. The common denominator for both massage and water therapies, according to international spa expert Robin Zill, is that the "skin is the portal of entry" for both. Massage therapists have begun to add these spa techniques to their menu of services, which can range from simple hot towels to scrubs to steam baths to body wraps. Clients enjoy these additional ways to relax and revive themselves. This chapter offers exposure and training in several methods of spa and hydrotherapy applications to help increase your repertoire of modalities and further your optional career path as a spa technician.

WATER AS A HEALING AGENT

The liquid known as *water* turns into a solid called *ice* at 32° F and into a vapor called *steam* at 212° F. The physical energy that can be added or removed to change the state of water is heat. Adding heat to ice excites the molecules and causes them to move farther apart, changing a block of ice into a puddle of water and a puddle of water into a cloud of water vapor (Figure 23-1). Removing heat from water turns vapor into liquid and liquid into solid. The word *hydrotherapy* finds its roots in the Greek word *hydro,* meaning *water.* Hydro- as a prefix is defined as *fluid* or *liquid.*

To help students comprehend the scope of hydrotherapy, this chapter introduces the student to the factors that contribute to how water effects the body, the effects of hot (thermotherapy) and cold (cryotherapy), and application methods. Often cold and heat are combined in the same treatment to induce a specific therapeutic effect. Soaps, essences, aromatics, minerals, seaweed (thalassotherapy), carbon dioxide, oxygen, and healing agents are often added to the water to enhance its therapeutic value. The indications and contraindications assist you in applying these special baths safely and effectively in your practice of massage.

The body's ability to maintain homeostasis in a changing environment is the key that unlocks the benefits of hydrotherapy. As the nervous system perceives changes in temperature, the body responds as follows with alterations in the flow of blood and lymph:

• Heat applications cause the skin to become hyperemic as a result of dilation of blood vessels; perspiration is produced in an attempt to cool the body.

Figure 23-1 The three physical states of water.

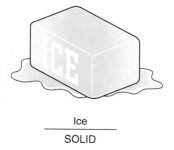

Ice
SOLID

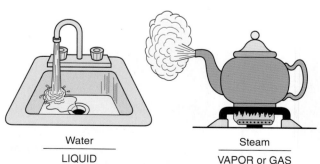

Water
LIQUID

Steam
VAPOR or GAS

617

- Cold applications cause the skin to blanch initially resulting from the vasoconstriction; the skin then becomes hyperemic and a burning sensation may be felt as heat is carried to the application site by the bloodstream in an attempt to warm the area.

By increasing and decreasing blood and lymph flow, hydrotherapy application can assist the body in detoxifying. Water is the universal solvent, and the electrolytes of the body follow the flow of water. By using water (hydrotherapy) externally, the internal flow of water (blood and lymph) can be changed to assist the healing process, move oxygen and nutrients to a desired location, and remove toxins. Other physiological effects are listed later in the chapter.

For Your Information

In 1785, Antoine Lavoisier proved that water is composed of two parts hydrogen and one part oxygen. (Author C.S. Lewis added "one part magic.")

The four major factors that contribute to how water affects the body are *temperature, moisture, mineral content, and mechanical stimuli.*

Temperature

Temperature changes the effect of water on the body. In general, brief cold application causes an initial action of constricting blood vessels and reducing blood flow. Prolonged cold application produces a reaction that stimulates dilation of blood vessels and increases blood flow. This also reduces swelling and decrease inflammation. Hot or warm applications cause an initial action of increasing blood flow whereas prolonged heat application depresses blood flow and increases swelling and inflammation. Both cold and hot application reduces pain and discomfort through the *gate theory* (see Chapter 5). The greater is the difference between the body temperature and water temperature, the greater is the physiological effect. For a more detailed look at the physiological effect of temperature, see Table 23-1. Watsu massage and the LeBoyer method of child birthing use water at near-skin temperature to relax the body. For more information about Watsu, see the biography on its founder, Harold Dull.

Ask for client feedback regarding temperature and comfort, just as you would ask a client if the pressure applied is appropriate during a massage. Adjust the temperature as needed. Extreme hot and cold can harm your client, so the therapist must always be aware of the temperature of the water. Water temperatures below 32° F or above 124° F can cause tissue damage. Although it is helpful to test the water temperature using your fingertips, use caution when placing a hand or foot into water of unknown temperature. For a more accurate reading, use a thermometer (thermometers can be purchased at a pool or spa supply store). Bear in mind when using hot water from a faucet that most water heaters are set at about 140° F (Box 23-1).

BOX 23-1

Temperature Conversion

Fahrenheit to Celsius
Subtract 32, then multiply by $5/9$
$(°F - 32) \times 5/9 = °C$
EXAMPLE: $(212° F - 32) \times 5/9 = 100° C$

Celsius to Fahrenheit
Multiply by $9/5$, then add 32
$(°C \times 9/5) + 32 = °F$
EXAMPLE: $(0° C \times 9/5) + 32 = 32° F$

TABLE 23-1

Temperature Ranges and Effect on the Body

Fahrenheit	Celsius	Description	Effect on the Body
212	100	Boiling point of water	Burn
110+	43+	Painfully hot	Possibly injurious
104-110	40-43	Very hot	Tolerable for short periods
98-104	38-40	Hot	Tolerable, reddens the skin
92-98	33-38	Warm-neutral	Comfortable
80-92	27-33	Tepid	Slightly below skin temperature
65-80	18-27	Cool	Produces goose flesh
55-65	13-18	Cold	Tolerable, but uncomfortable
32-55	0-13	Very cold	Painfully cold
32	0	Freezing point of water	Burn

HAROLD DULL, MA

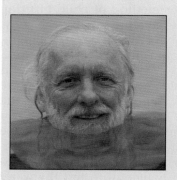

Born: December 18, 1935.

"The body is movement. Breath is life. And the base of our being is the support of others."

No direct path to a career in facilitating health is evident, so it is no surprise that a physics major who decided to become a beatnik poet is the man behind one of the latest forms of hands-on therapy. Watsu is the combination of water and shiatsu. The name was coined by wordsmith and bodyworker Harold Dull. Developed 15 years ago, it is a hybrid of Zen shiatsu, flotation, joint mobilization, and stretching.

The oldest of four boys, Harold Dull was born in Seattle to parents in real estate. He attended the University of Washington with the intention of studying physics, prelaw, or philosophy. He wound up studying poetry instead, became a writer, and was part of the poetry renaissance.

"At age 40 I had never had a massage," Dull says, "but I decided to begin studying Zen shiatsu in San Francisco with Wataru Ohashi and Reuho Yamada." Dull finally traveled to Japan to complete studies with world-renowned master Shizuto Masunaga. When he returned home, he began teaching others the ancient Japanese art and later emphasized how to combine shiatsu with the hot spring therapy he had enjoyed at Harbin Hot Springs Resort in California. In its earlier incarnation, Watsu was dubbed Wassage. Dull used a board set up in a hot tub. In time, however, he began doing his unique form of bodywork in Harbin's hot springs.

In Watsu the water is the medium as is the message. Its buoyancy helps practitioners and clients by supporting body weight, so that small practitioners are able to handle large clients. The water also helps the therapist see, feel, and listen to what's going on with the client's body. As the body rises and falls with each breath, the water helps the practitioner identify areas that need work. The water, maintained at body temperature, also soothes the client, releasing tense muscles, taking the load off joint articulations, and helping increase flexibility and range of motion.

Step into a conventional massage room and you may not feel the result of your massage until after the therapist begins, but immerse yourself in water and you immediately feel different—lighter. As you relax into your breathing pattern, supported by your therapist, you gradually let go as the tickle of the water filling your ears silences a chaotic world and lulls you into a heightened state of relaxation.

One writer describes her experience with Watsu as follows:

The surprise, for me, was just how profound this was. It has become a cliché to say that a therapy works "on many different levels," but that is actually an excellent description of Watsu. Deeply rooted physical tensions and ailments are worked on more easily, while the experience of being safely held and moved through the water also touches profound emotional and spiritual levels.

—From Diana Brueton: "Watsu, flowing free in water," *Kindred Spirit Quarterly.*

Dull notes that it is "the unconditional acceptance that is so powerful. So many injured people are treated as less than what they once were." In addition to its emotional impact, Watsu has reportedly helped headache pain. Muscle spasms disappear, and chronic lower back pain and spine misalignment have been corrected.

Dull's vision is to make the therapeutic value of his work, especially the added benefit of the sense of unconditional acceptance it brings, available to everyone. "From an equipment standpoint, you need a 10-foot diameter pool with about 4 feet of water, which should be maintained at body temperature," he explains, adding that new ways will be discovered to heat water at a lower cost.

Moisture

Moisture content in this context applies to the amount of humidity in the air. Steam baths at 100% humidity help moisten the mucous membranes of the nasal passages and throat and help keep the skin supple. The air naturally does feel heavier, and it may be more difficult to breathe. In saunas, where the humidity ranges from 6% to 20%, the air may be easier to inhale but can also be drying and irritating to the skin and mucous membranes for some people.

Mineral Content

The mineral content of water is another factor that influences the therapeutic on the body. Famous spa resorts are often sought out for the health-giving properties of mineral waters. Three kinds of mineral waters found at spas include saline water containing dissolved salts used for its purgative effects, rust-colored water filled with iron oxide used for its restorative effects, and sulfur water used for its cleansing effects. The effects of natural springs may be duplicated by adding minerals to water, in which the most commonly used are sea salt (sodium chloride), Epsom salt (magnesium sulfate), and baking soda (sodium bicarbonate). These minerals draw out toxins as the body attempts to balance the percentages of saline content between the water and skin. It is a common practice in massage to recommend that a client soak in a tub with salt and baking soda after the massage to enhance the detoxification process and reduce postmassage soreness. The recipe for the bath is 1 part salt and 1 part baking soda (e.g., 1 cup of each) in a tub of warm water and a soaking for 20 minutes. Rinse off after the tub soak.

Mechanical Stimuli

Water, weighing 8.33 lb per gallon, is often used for its mechanical effect. Water may be pressurized during the application, as in a whirlpool or hydrotub, or by using a pressurized hose, as in a shower or spray. Water is valued for its pressure effect and as a means of applying physical energy to the tissues while promoting relaxation and health. Products may be applied to the skin to exfoliate and then rinsed off with cool or warm water. Using forcible water or stimulating the skin during the treatment intensifies the body's response.

> *Everything flows.*
> —Heraclitus

THERMOTHERAPY

Thermotherapy is the external application of heat for therapeutic purposes. The body can only tell whether something is hot or cold in relation to the skin temperature. Heat is transferred into the body only when the temperature of the water is greater than the body temperature. Heat moves into the tissues using one of the following four methods of delivery:

1. **Conduction** involves the exchange of thermal energy while the body's surface is in direct contact with the thermal agent or conductor (e.g., hot packs, immersion baths).
2. **Convection** involves transferring heat energy through circulating currents of liquid or gas (e.g., sauna, steam bath).
3. **Radiation** is the transfer of heat energy in rays (e.g., infrared lamps).
4. **Conversion** involves one energy source changing (or converting) into a heat energy source as it passes into the body (diathermy, ultrasound). This method is generally not used by massage therapist but is within the scope of practice for chiropractic, physical, and occupational therapy.

Effects of Heat Application

In general, short-term applications of heat have a stimulating effect on the body while prolonged applications of heat have a depressing effect on the body. Some physiological effects of heat are as follows:

- Increases sweating so evaporation can create a cooling effect.
- Stimulates vasodilation as excess heat is dissipated through the skin (skin appears hyperemic).
- Increases local blood flow.
- Increases oxygen absorption.
- Increases blood volume by stimulating circulation in dormant capillary beds.
- Increases metabolism.
- Reduces pain.
- Relieves stiffness and soreness.
- Increases relaxation.
- Increases range of motion in joints.
- Increases white blood cell count by producing an artificial fever (heat application must be between 102° F and 104° F).
- Stimulates immune system and inhibits the growth of many bacteria and viruses (heat application must be between 102° F and 104° F).
- Reduces muscle spasms by inhibiting the efferent motor nerve activity and muscle spindle activity.
- Increases extensibility of collagen (scar tissue and tendons).

• Distends and softens superficial fascia. Heat alters the viscoelastic state of fascia, just as the heat created by handling modeling clay makes it more pliable. Massage manipulations are much more effective after the tissues have been prepared by heat.

Contraindications of Heat

Most of the following conditions are contraindicated for thermotherapy because of the effect heat has on the circulation of blood and swelling. Heat may irritate certain conditions. Avoid heat application in the following circumstances:
• Acute injury
• Autoimmune conditions
• Clients with an aversion to heat
• Area over a fresh bruise or any hemorrhaging under the skin
• Recent burns, including sunburn
• Cardiac impairment
• Cerebrovascular accident (CVA) or stroke
• Edematous conditions
• Area directly over the eyes
• Cases of fever
• Hypertension or hypotension
• Immediately after an injury (due to the possibility of internal bleeding)
• Inflammation
• Area over joint prosthetics
• Area over implants
• Malignancy or chronic illness
• Significant obesity
• Open wounds, blisters, or abrasion burns
• Phlebitis
• Area over a pacemaker
• Pregnancy, with the exception of paraffin baths on hands, elbows, knees, and feet
• Rosacea
• Sensory impairments, individuals who cannot report subjective reactions (e.g., infants or elderly people), or when the client has the inability to react appropriately to excessive temperature changes (e.g., infants or elderly people, people with diabetes, clients with mental conditions, clients with multiple sclerosis)
• Skin infections or rashes
• Area directly over a tumor or cyst
• Clients who are weak or debilitated

For Your Information

The unit used for measuring heat energy is the calorie. Specific heat of water is 1. It takes 1 calorie of heat to raise 1 gram of water 1° Celsius.

CRYOTHERAPY

Cryotherapy is the external, therapeutic application of cold. Cold application is the safest, simplest, and most effective method for reducing pain and swelling in injuries and has replaced the use of heat in many rehabilitation clinics. The application of cold has several very distinct physiological effects. During the first 9 to 16 minutes of cold application, the area undergoes a reduction of blood flow through a reflex called *vasoconstriction*. This reduction in the size of the blood vessels causes the skin to appear blanched or pale; local edema is reduced, and hematoma formation is controlled.

If cold application continues, a sudden deep-tissue *vasodilation* occurs. This can last from 4 to 6 minutes. This increase in the diameter of the blood vessels is a thermoregulatory response to restore homeostasis and raises local temperature. After a few minutes, vasoconstriction resumes and the cycle continues. One cycle of vasoconstriction and vasodilation takes about 15 to 30 minutes. This up-and-down cycle is the **hunting response** (Figure 23-2). The alternating action and reaction of the body to cold application brings blood into and out of the area, flushing out tissue debris and bringing in much needed oxygen. This cycling between vasoconstriction and vasodilation creates a vascular pump or vascular gymnastics, which creates an increased deep local circulation, one of the most important effects of cryotherapy.

During the cold treatment, clients experience the following sensations: (1) coldness or cooling, (2) burning, (3) stinging or aching, and (4) numbness. Allow cold application to remain on the body until the fourth and final phase (this may take anywhere from 5 to 20 minutes). Remove the cold application immediately after numbness to prevent tissue damage from excessive cold.

Caution must be used when applying cold. If local or general application is prolonged (more than 20 minutes), tissue damage may result in the form of frostbite and/or hypothermia. Both conditions are harmful to the client. If the client is already chilled before the cryotherapy treatment, do not apply cryotherapy. It may be helpful to administer a hot foot bath to help the client feel more comfortable before proceeding with the cryotherapy.

Effects of Cold Application

Like heat application, short applications of cold have a stimulating effect on the body and prolonged applications of cold have a depressing effect on the body. The following are some other effects that occur:
• Reduces acute inflammation
• Reduces swelling
• Reduces muscle spasm

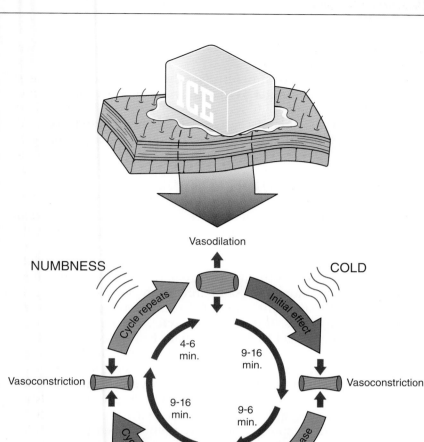

Vasodilation

NUMBNESS

COLD

Cycle repeats

Initial effect

4-6 min.

9-16 min.

Vasoconstriction

Vasoconstriction

9-16 min.

9-6 min.

Cycle repeats

Second phase

STINGING or ACHING

BURNING

Vasodilation

Figure 23-2   The hunting response.

- Reduces pain through reduced nerve conduction velocity
- Reduces muscular spasticity by reducing muscle spindle activity
- Stimulates circulation (prolonged use of cold)
- Stimulates vasodilation (prolonged use of cold)
- Decreases metabolism
- Temporarily decreases local oxygen supply
- Decreases tissue damage
- Reduces blood clot formation
- Increases urine production

Contraindications of Cold

The contraindications for cold application are as follows:
- Arthritis
- Aversion to cold
- CVA (stroke) survivor
- Cold or plastic allergies
- Open wounds
- Hypertension (cold application may cause a transient increase in blood pressure)

- Raynaud's syndrome (ischemia of the extremities of the body caused by cold exposure or emotional stimuli); this is most prominent in the fingers, toes, ears, and nose
- Rheumatoid conditions
- Sensory impairments: individuals who cannot report subjective reactions (e.g., infants or elderly people) or the client cannot react appropriately to excessive temperature changes (e.g., infants, elderly people, people with diabetes, those with mental conditions, clients with multiple sclerosis)
- Skin infections or rashes

MINI-LAB

Arrange a meeting with a local physical or occupational therapist. Ask her how and why she uses ice, heat, and water in rehabilitation. Prepare a summary and present it to the class.

SAFETY AND PROCEDURAL GUIDELINES

Maintain your hydrotherapy equipment in good working order, and clean each item at the beginning or end of each workday. Place a towel on equipment that will be in direct contact with the client, such as stools and benches. Surfaces that come in direct contact with the client and all reservoirs that collect perspiration or exfoliated skin cells must be cleaned after each treatment. If body fluids such as blood come into contact with therapy equipment, a solution of water and chlorine bleach (10 parts water to 1 part chlorine bleach) can be used to disinfect the equipment.

Maintain hot tubs, spas, steam cabinets, and whirlpools in compliance with public and multiple-use standards. Place a nonslip mat on the floor for clients to step on. If water collects on the wet room or bathroom floor, wipe it up immediately to prevent accidents (floor drains are helpful). If hydrotherapy equipment is kept in the massage room, make sure it is not in a high-traffic region of the room. If a client accidentally touches a hot hydrocollator unit, it may burn the skin.

Water is a powerful substance that can damage massage tables, floors, and walls. Preventive measures can be taken such as not splashing water and covering furniture with a protective cloth. The following guidelines can help provide a safe and effective treatment:

- Plan ahead and assemble all necessary articles.
- Make sure the wet room is warm.
- If providing full-body treatments, consider asking the client to bring a swimsuit or providing disposable undergarments.
- Check and monitor the water temperature.
- Check the client's comfort level.
- Use a timer to limit treatment duration. Do not overtreat.
- Ask the client not to eat at least 1 hour before the appointment.
- Before treatment, perform a client consultation.
- Review contraindications (reevaluate for precautions each time the client returns).
- Explain the entire procedure.
- Give clear directions on where to place clothing and personal belongings, how much clothing to remove, and how to lie on the table.
- Avoid use of liniments before treatment.
- Remain with the client or within easy calling distance.
- Do not wait for thirst to kick in; offer water or juice before, after, and during treatment.
- Be available to assist the client on and off the table if treatment is more than 15 minutes because she may feel woozy.
- Instruct client about patting the skin dry after wet treatments.
- After treatment, allow the client to rest for at least 10 minutes so that body temperature can return to normal.
- Document the type of treatment, products used, duration of treatment, and client's reactions.

APPLICATION METHODS

These hydrotherapy treatments can be used exclusively or as part of the massage therapy session. Review the guidelines previously listed before using any application method. Note that the application descriptions that follow are both informational and instructional. Most hydrotherapy applications can be classified into one of three categories: *packs, baths,* and *rubs* (Box 23-2). A **pack** is a bag, sack, or other item used to apply or retain heat or cold. A **bath** is a broad category of hydrotherapy application encompassing partial or full immersion in water, wax, light, heated air, or steam. Hydrotherapeutic **frictions** encompass shampoos; brushing; polishes; scrubs; glows; and frictions with the hands, cloth, brush, sponge, or grainy agent rubbed on the skin's surface. A rinse and quick, vigorous drying are also essential elements.

Pack

A pack is usually a cloth bag used to apply local heat or cold. However, electrically heated mitts, booties, or even stones that have been heated in hot water or

---

BOX 23-2

Hydrotherapeutic Applications at a Glance

Packs	Baths	Frictions
Body wraps	Blitz gus	Body polish
Cold gel pack	Cold immer-	Cold mitten
Cold pack	sion bath	friction
Contrast pack	Contrast bath	Dry brush mas-
Cool compress	Foot bath	sage
Cryokinetics	Hot air bath	Ice massage
Heated mittens	(sauna)	Salt glow
and booties	Hot immersion	Shampoo
Hot compress	bath	
Hot or cold	Paraffin bath	
stones	Plunge	
Hot pack	Scotch hose	
Hydrocollator	Shower	
pack	Sitz bath	
Product pack	Spray	
or mask	Steam bath	

chilled in a freezer can be used. Any product applied to the skin, such as mud or seaweed, is also referred to as a *pack* (e.g., mud pack, clay pack). Heat is often used to enhance penetration of these products. Variations of pack applications are *compresses* and *wraps*. A **compress** is typically a wet cloth that has had water wrung from it and is applied to the skin's surface. Examples are hot compresses, cold compresses, and spinal compresses. A **wrap** is basically a large pack, covering most of the body through the use of large wet or dry sheets or blankets; the most common use is a body wrap.

Hot Compress

A hot compress is a cloth dipped in warm to hot water, wrung out, folded, and placed on the skin. If the compress is uncomfortably hot, lay it inside a dry towel before placing it on the skin. Most often, hot compresses are laid on the forehead, over the spine, or across the back (Figure 23-3). The massage can continue during use, avoiding the treatment area. These packs are used primarily to soothe and relax clients during the massage session. The heat moves quickly to the client's skin, leaving the compress cool, so refresh it often. For a spinal compress, fold a towel lengthwise to achieve a 3- or 4-inch width and place the hot compress inside and along the entire length of the spine (Figure 23-4). The procedure is as follows:

1. Dip a washcloth in warm to hot water; squeeze out any excess water.
2. Layer the cloth by folding it in half and even quarters.
3. Apply to the affected area.
4. Leave the compress on until cool (5 to 10 minutes).
5. Remove or replace with a fresh compress if needed.

Hot Pack

Hot packs are usually commercially manufactured available in a variety of styles. Some are electrical, some must be heated in a microwave, others must be filled with hot water (hot water bottle), and some

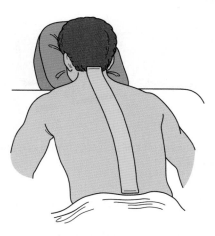

Figure 23-4 Spinal compress.

must be prepared in a heated tank (see the following section on Hydrocollator Pack) or an electric hot towel cabinet. Other names for hot packs are *fomentation packs*. Hot packs are often used by massage therapists in preparing an area for massage because heat softens the fascia and dilates the superficial blood vessels. The liability is that they do block access to and observation of the treatment area, but you may continue to massage adjacent areas. The procedure is as follows:

1. Heat pack before use.
2. Apply to affected area.
3. Leave on for a maximum time of 5 to 20 minutes.

Hydrocollator Pack

A hydrocollator pack is a specialized hot pack consisting of a canvas pouch filled with silicon granules, which hold heat in the pack for about 30 minutes. The packs are kept submerged in a stainless steel kettle that remains at about 165° F (Figure 23-5). The therapist removes the packs from the tank with a pair of tongs or cloth tabs that extend from the pack above the surface of the water. The pack is placed in a special terrycloth wrap or a regular towel folded several times. This pack is placed on top of the client's body and never underneath. One disadvantage of hot pack use is that the packs can burn the skin if left on too long or if insulating material is not placed between the pack and the client's skin. As with hot packs, hydrocollator packs also block the therapist's access and observation of the treatment area, but you may proceed with the massage in other areas. Periodically check the skin under the pack to make sure it does not show signs of irritation or damage. The procedure is as follows:

1. Wrap the hydrocollator pack in up to six layers of terry cloth or Turkish toweling.
2. Place the wrapped pack on the client's skin.
3. To modify the intensity of the heat, add or subtract cloth layers between the pack and the skin.

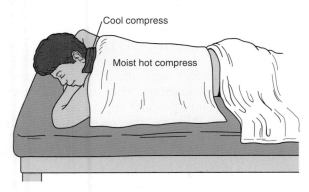

Cool compress

Moist hot compress

Figure 23-3 Back hot compress with cool compress on neck.

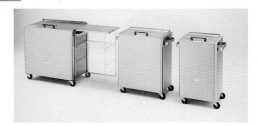

Figure 23-5 Hydrocollator unit. (Courtesy of TouchAmerica, Hillsborough, N.C.)

4. If the client begins to perspire, place a cold compress on the back of the neck.
5. Allow the pack to remain on the treatment area for 20 minutes.

Heated Mittens and Booties

Two types of heated mittens or booties are available for use. The first kinds are filled with buckwheat and warmed in a microwave oven (Figure 23-6). The second are small, electric wraps for the hands and feet. On the electric models, use an extension cord if the cord is not long enough to allow the client to lay down while in use. Sometimes a moisturizing agent such as paraffin wax or an essential oil–enhanced product is applied to soften the skin before these are slipped over the hands or feet. Other services may be performed while these remain on the client. The procedure is as follows:
1. Preheat the mitts or boots.
2. Apply product to the hands or feet

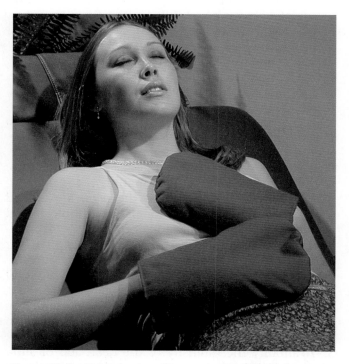

Figure 23-6 Heated mitts. (Courtesy of Golden Ratio, Emigrant, Mont.)

3. Wrap the hands or feet in a plastic bag or surround them with a plastic wrap.
4. Slide the heated mitts or boots on the hand or feet.
5. Slip off after 15 minutes.
6. Remove any excess product.

Hot or Cold Stones

Hot and cold stones have been used by Native Americans for centuries. Teaching application of hot and cold stones began in Arizona by Mary Hannigan and has become a popular spa technique, especially in Ayurvedic treatments. Stones can be used to apply heat and cold to the body's tissues. Basalt is recommended for the "hot" stones, and marble is recommended for the "cold" stones (Figure 23-7). They can be placed directly on the body or over a thin cloth, or held in your hand and used as a massage tool. Exercise caution because the hot stones can burn the skin with improper use. Like a compress, the temperature of stones changes quickly as heat moves into or out of the body, respectively. To properly work with the stones, attend a workshop taught by a qualified instructor. The procedure is as follows:
1. Heat the basalt stones in water 130° to 140° F or chill the marble stones in a freezer or icy water for about 15 to 20 minutes.
2. Apply to desired area.
3. Allow the stones to remain on the skin until the hot stones are cool. Cool stones are simply moved across the affected area several times.
4. Replace with fresh stones as needed.

Product Pack or Mask

Product packs or masks may be used to enhance the skin's health and appearance. Products include moisturizers such as oil, creams, lotions, and natural agents such as moor mud, clay, volcanic ash (fango), charcoal, seaweed, and algae. The amount of product used usually depends on the type of product used and the size of the client. Heat is often used to enhance the product, which adds nutrients into the skin or draws toxins from the skin. Body packs or masks are applied **topically** (on the surface) and are generally used for remineralization, revitalization, and rejuvenation. The procedure is as follows:
1. Apply the product according to the manufacturer's recommendations. This may mean cleaning the skin before product application.
2. Leave on the skin for the recommended time frame.
3. If needed, use a hot compress or heat lamp to enhance the product's healing properties.
4. Remove the product with hot towels or a shower.
5. Apply moisturizer to hydrate the skin.

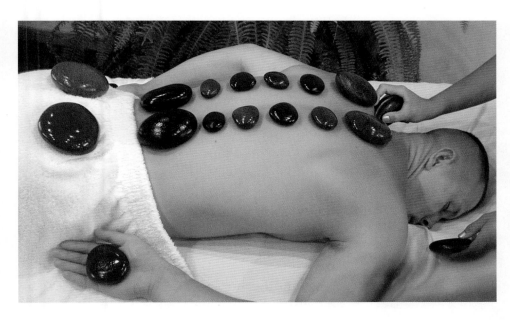

Figure 23-7 Stone layout. (Courtesy of Golden Ratio, Emigrant, Mont.)

Cool Compress

A cool compress is a cloth dipped in cool to cold water, wrung out, folded, and placed on the skin. Most often, cool compresses are laid on the forehead during thermotherapy or over an inflamed area, or are used to soothe an area right after deep massage. As with hot compresses, treatment can continue on other areas, but the compress quickly becomes warm and should be refreshed (Figure 23-8). The procedure is as follows:

1. Dip a washcloth in cool to icy water; squeeze out any excess water.
2. Layer the cloth by folding it in half or even quarters.
3. Apply to the affected area.
4. Leave the compress on until warm (5 to 10 minutes).
5. Remove or replace with a fresh compress if needed.

Cold Gel Pack and Cold Pack

A cold gel pack is a plastic bag filled with a special gel that does not freeze to a solid block mass and retains cold for about 20 minutes (Figure 23-9). Cold packs are either commercial plastic bags filled with icy water or homemade with a zipped plastic bag filled with icy water. Be sure to double-layer the zipped plastic bag to prevent leakage. A solution of two-thirds water and one-third alcohol may be mixed in a zipped plastic bag and kept in the freezer. The alcohol will prevent the water from freezing solid. The main advantage with cold packs over cold gel packs is that the ice quickly melts and the water becomes warm over the course of treatment, reducing the chance of tissue damage. If tissue under the pack is puffy or raised, remove the pack immediately and rewarm the area with a warm compress. Cold packs are often used to decrease inflammation or to reduce the chance of soreness after deep massage. Cold pack use does block the treatment area, but the massage can continue in other areas. Check the skin periodically

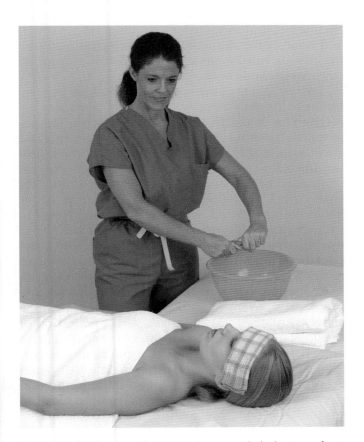

Figure 23-8 Supine client with damp washcloth across forehead while therapist prepares fresh compress.

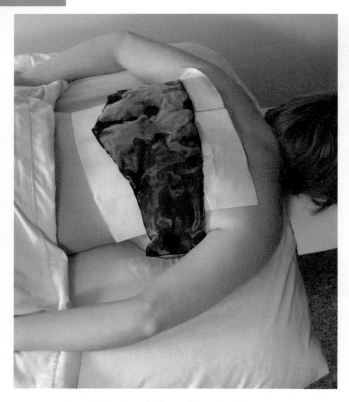

Figure 23-9   Cold gel pack.

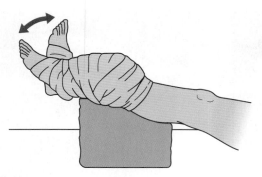

Figure 23-10   Ice applied to an injury while the client is doing active range of motion.

for indications of tissue damage such as mild frostbite. The procedure is as follows:

1. Lay a paper towel or thin cloth such as a pillowcase around the pack. If the cloth is too thick, the cold transfer is reduced.
2. Apply to the affected area.
3. Leave the pack on for a maximum time of 5 to 20 minutes.

Cryokinetics

The application of cold pack followed by full range of motion is **cryokinetics**. The goal of this procedure is full functional use of the affected area. The pain-reducing effects of ice allow the client to push through the discomfort barrier and achieve range of motion faster and easier (Figure 23-10). The resulting movements encourage decongestion of the injured area and free restricted muscles. The procedure is as follows:

1. Apply an ice pack or other method of cold application (cold immersion bath or ice massage) to chill the affected area.
2. Allow the ice to remain on the treatment area until numb (10 to 15 minutes).
3. Ask the client to actively and slowly move the joint by mirroring back to you demonstrated movements. The therapist may elect to resist movement as in an isometric exercise. Never use a motion that causes pain. Maintain communication so that progress can be monitored.

- If the client is unable to actively move the joint, passively move the affected joint.
- Allow the movements to continue until the tissue warms up and feeling is restored (about 3 to 5 minutes).
4. Reapply the ice until the client experiences numbness.
- The area can be re-iced and exercised up to 3 more times.

Body Wrap

A body wrap uses a sheet or bandaging material to wrap the body. As many types of body wraps are available as styles of massage. Some wraps increase circulation, and some reduce swelling; others soften and nourish the skin, and some help eliminate toxins. Wraps can be divided into to two categories; cover wraps and compression wraps.

Cover wraps cover the body with sheets for a predetermined time to increase perspiration, promote relaxation, or detoxify and cleanse the system. The objective is to raise the body temperature, increase circulation, and encourage penetration of a therapeutic substance (e.g., herbal teas, clay, moor mud, or seaweed). The sheets may be applied wet or dry. Wet cover wraps typically use sheets soaked in herbs, hence the name *herbal wrap*. Specific herbs are used to make a tea (decoction or infusion), and the sheets used to wrap the body are soaked in the tea. A **decoction** is a tea made from boiling parts of the plant (e.g., bark, roots, or seeds). An **infusion** is a tea made from steeping the parts of the plant (e.g., stems and leaves). Dry cover wraps are most often used with the above-mentioned product mask. After application of the body mask, dry sheets are used to wrap the client. Time is allowed for penetration of the healing agent.

Compression wraps encase the body in elastic bandages that have been soaked in a solution to increase circulation or detoxify the system. The objective is to contour the body and reduce fluids (temporarily). The therapist must be mindful to not mislead the client into thinking that compression wraps are a method of weight reduction.

The principle behind body wraps is simple. With the body covered in sheets, blankets, and other insulating material, the body temperature rises and the body registers a fever. The physiological sweat response cools the body, eliminating the toxins the body "thinks" is causing the fever. While the pores are open, vital nutrients from the natural agents are absorbed into the skin.

This section outlines cover wraps only. Useful items are hot towel cabinets or a hydrocollator to warm damp towels; covered laundry container; nonbreakable, quart-sized dishes, a body wrap product; toner; mist pump; body lotion or cream; and loofah or natural bristle brush. If you administer a detoxification wrap, the client may feel nauseated after treatment. A cup of cool peppermint tea should help ease the nausea. The procedure is as follows:

1. Prepare the table in the following order:
   - Foam pad or egg crate foam pad
   - Plastic table sheet
   - Cotton thermal blanket
   - Washable wool or fleece blanket
   - Mylar foil or thermal plastic wrap
   - Cotton sheet

   Place a towel folded lengthwise at the tabletop. The towel should be placed between the plastic sheet and the cotton thermal blanket and then folded over the top cotton sheet (Figure 23-11). This towel should be in contact with the client's face and neck once the body is wrapped.

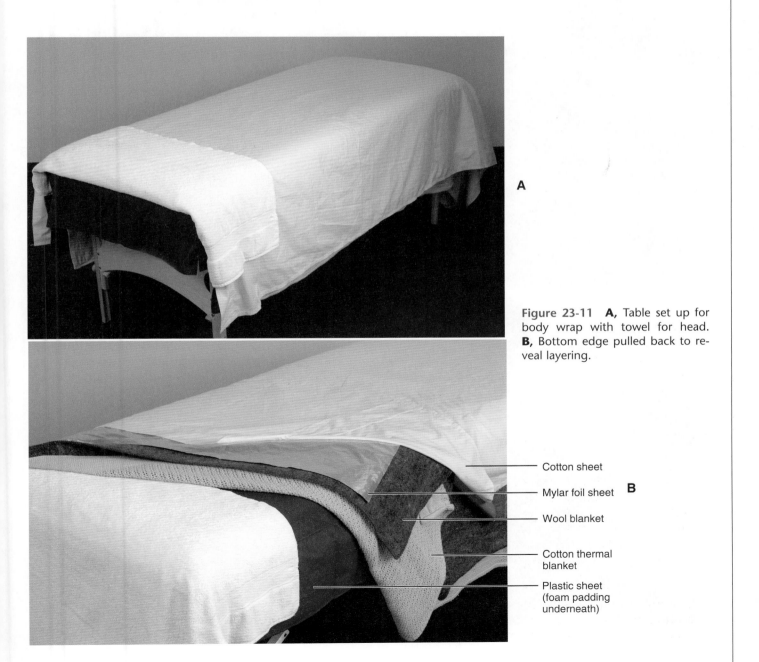

A

B

Cotton sheet

Mylar foil sheet

Wool blanket

Cotton thermal blanket

Plastic sheet (foam padding underneath)

Figure 23-11 **A,** Table set up for body wrap with towel for head. **B,** Bottom edge pulled back to reveal layering.

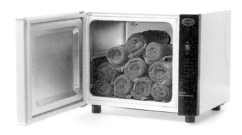

Figure 23-12 Hot towel cabinet. (Courtesy of Touch America, Hillsborough, N.C.)

2. Wet 10 hand towels, wring out excess water, and place them in a hot towel cabinet (Figure 23-12) or other container to become warm (they need time to heat up before spa treatment begins). Use a product that can be wiped off the client with hot towels, *especially if you do not have a shower facility.*
3. Allow the client to shower, soak in tub, or take a steam bath; you can also wipe him down with hot towels to open the pores and prepare the skin.
4. Ask the client to lie on the table. The head should be on the towel. Drape the client to keep him warm.

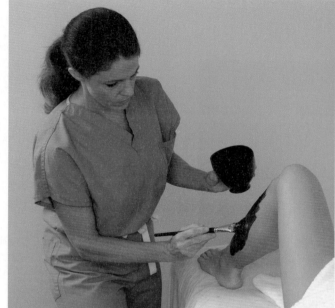

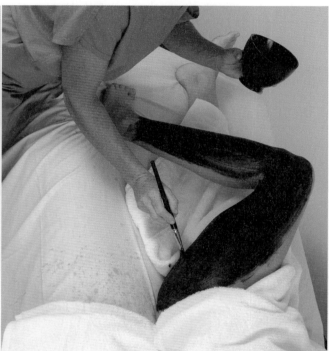

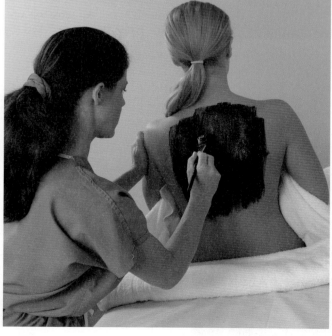

Figure 23-13 A, Therapist applying mud on supine client's leg. **B,** Therapist applying mud on supine client's hip. **C,** Therapist applying mud on seated supine client's back. Note towel covering client's buttocks.

5. Using a dry natural bristle brush or a dry loofah, do a dry brush massage with the client remaining in a supine position. This step is optional (see recommended procedure that follows).

6. Apply product with a disposable-gloved hand or a paintbrush with the client in the supine position only (if possible, warm product first). For the back of the legs, flex the hip and knee (Figure 23-13, *A*); for the hip, internally rotate the hip (Figure 23-13, *B*); for the back, help the client up to a seated position (Figure 23-13, *C*).

7. If using hot linens soaked in herbs or other essences, ask the client to stand briefly, lay the open wet, wrung out sheet or towels on the table, and ask the client to lie back down.

8. Wrap the layers of sheeting around the client snugly. Keep the face exposed. You may finish with one additional winter blanket. Place bolsters under neck and knees. If the client feels claustrophobic, loosen the wrap around the head and neck. If the client is still feeling claustrophobic, allow him to take the arms out or uncover the feet.
   • Allow the client to stay wrapped for up to 30 minutes. Remain nearby.
   • While the client is in the cocoon, you may cover the eyes with an eye rest cushion or cool compress, press into certain spots for a mini-acupressure treatment, or do an aromatherapy scalp massage.

9. Unwrap the client. If the client received an herbal wrap, drape a sheet over him and let him air dry, allowing more time for the herbs to penetrate into the skin. If the client has just received a product mask, escort him to the shower facility.

The running water should already be warm. Showering is optional after an herbal wrap.
   • If wiping off the product (and client is not showering), keep the client warm by unwrapping only the area being wiped. As you wipe off the product with the heated damp towels, place them in the covered laundry container.

10. Using a mist bottle, apply toner or floral water.
11. Apply moisturizer.

Contrast Packs

One of the most potent technique in hydrotherapeutics is to combine heat and cold (Table 23-2). This application technique is known as the *contrast packs* or the **contrast method**. The two variations are *alternate contrast packs* and *simultaneous contrast packs*. The alternate contrast pack is the most commonly used variation. Alternating cold and heat applications intensifies the circulatory effect on the tissues, and the cycles of vasoconstriction and vasodilation that cold and heat create help remove metabolic wastes.

During a simultaneous contrast treatment, a cold pack is placed on the area of complaint and a heat pack is placed at the same time next to the cold pack (Figure 23-14). For example, a painful rotator cuff injury could be treated with the client lying prone with a cold pack under his shoulder and a hot pack on the top of his back covering the shoulder. Not only do the heat impulses interfere with the cold impulses, but the sensation of heat comforts the client and induces relaxation. The alternate method procedure is as follows:

1. Apply a cold pack on the affected area for 10 to 15 minutes.

TABLE 23-2

Comparative Effects of Cold and Heat

Physiological Response	Initial Effect of Cold	Prolonged Effect of Cold	Initial Effect of Heat	Prolonged Effect of Heat
Heart rate	Increases	Decreases	Decreases	Increases
Vascular response	Vasoconstriction	Vasodilation	Vasodilation	Vasoconstriction
Depth of action	Superficial	Deep	Superficial	Superficial
Effect on pain	Reduces	Reduces	Reduces	Reduces
Fascial response	Unchanged	Softens	Softens	Softens
Tissue damage	Decreases	Decreases	Nonapplicable	Nonapplicable
Analgesic	No	Yes	Yes	Yes
Anesthetic	No	Yes	No	No
Inflammatory response	Decreases	Decreases	Increases	Increases
Renal response	Stimulates	Inhibits	Nonapplicable	Nonapplicable
Digestive response	Stimulates	Inhibits	Inhibits	Inhibits
General response	Stimulates	Depresses	Stimulates	Depresses

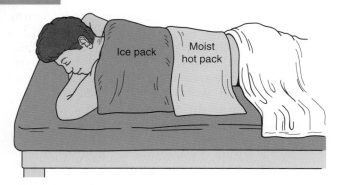

Figure 23-14   The simultaneous contrast method.

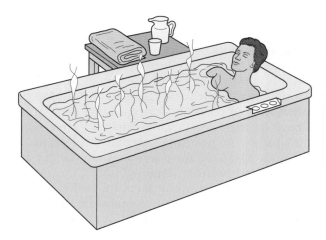

Figure 23-15   Whirlpool immersion.

2. Remove the cold pack and apply a heat pack for 10 minutes.
3. Remove the heat pack and reapply the cold pack another 10- to 15-minute period.
4. Repeat the alternate use of cold and heat for a total of 2 to 3 times.
   The simultaneous method procedure is as follows:
1. Place the hot pack on the affected area and a cold pack underneath the applied area or next to the cold pack.
2. Remove both the cold pack and hot pack after 10 to 15 minutes.

Baths

Baths, or *balneology,* is a broad category of hydrotherapy application encompassing partial or full immersion in water, wax, light, heated air, or steam. Also included in this section are bath techniques such as *showers* and *sprays*. A general rule about bath treatment times is that the greater is the difference between body and water temperatures, the shorter is the treatment time. Baths that are used to generate perspiration, such as steams and saunas, are physically demanding and should be limited to once a week. Make sure you offer your client drinking water after each bath treatment or encourage your client to drink water after each bath treatment.

Hot Immersion Bath

Hot immersion baths include full or partial body immersion with the client sitting in a tub (spa tub, hot tub, hydrotub, or whirlpool tub) (Figure 23-15). Because of the heat and pressure effects on the tissues of the body, both whirlpool baths and spa tubs are also known as *hydromassage* treatments. Whirlpool and spa tubs use agitated water mixed with air propelled by jets positioned on the sides and bottom of the tub. If using the bath soon after an injury, adjust the jets to push water toward the sides of the tank and not on the affected area and use tepid to warm water. The addition of hot water and pressure may exacerbate an in-

jury. By definition, *whirlpool* is a tub for soaking or receiving jets of water against the skin, draining the water after each use (Figure 23-16). A *spa* tub is similar to a whirlpool tub, but the water is treated to remain clean and sanitary for multiple uses. *Hot tubs* are just for soaking without the agitated water.

Hot immersion baths are best used before a massage session because it helps to soften superficial fascia and relax muscles, making them more pliable. Additives may be used to add to the bath's therapeutic value. Epsom salts (named for the mineral springs in Epsom, England) or commercial bath

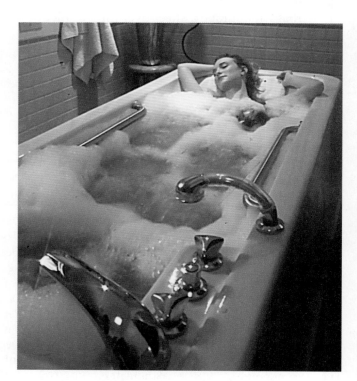

Figure 23-16   Hydrotub. (Courtesy of Golden Ratio, Emigrant, Mont.)

salts such as Batherapy turn the immersion bath into a mineral bath. If the client becomes too warm during treatment, but is not ready to leave the tub, she may lift her arms out of the water, exposing a greater surface area of the skin to allow for evaporative cooling. If the client feels weak or dizzy, stop the bath immediately and assist her out of the bath.

When water immersion is combined with light exercise, a *Hubbard tank* is used. Named after its inventor, Carl Hubbard, this tank is often used in rehabilitation clinics because the buoyancy of the water allows easier movement and produces a soothing sensation. This type of treatment is indicated for individuals with weak or painful muscles or joints.

The procedure for immersion baths is as follows:

1. Ask the client to shower with soap before treatment (the hydrotherapy tub is a soaking, not a cleansing, chamber).
2. Instruct the client on how to enter and exit the tub safely. Assistance may be required.
3. While the client is soaking, offer a cup of cool water in a nonbreakable cup and a cool washcloth for the face. Soaking time ranges from 15 to 20 minutes, depending on the water temperature and client's comfort.
4. After treatment, allow the client to take a 2- to 3-minute tepid shower or use a cool damp cloth to wipe off the skin. Client may also elect to take a cool plunge (discussed later in this chapter).
5. Place the client in a warm, quiet place and allow her to rest and drink water for 10 to 20 minutes. This is a very important part of the bath.

Hot Air Bath or Sauna

A **sauna bath** uses hot-air with temperatures ranging from 170° to 210° F with 10% to 20% humidity. If humidity is too low (below 10%), you run the risk of drying out mucous membranes. A special wooden cabin must be built or purchased to withstand and insulate these intense temperatures. All bathers must be in good health and if the client feels weak or dizzy, discontinue treatment immediately. Novices should take a sauna with temperatures ranging from 170° to 190° F. Experienced bathers can stand temperatures from 185° to 210° F. Sauna baths are often used before a body wrap, massage, or other hydrotherapy treatments. A dry sauna is indicated for general tension and insomnia, but it also increases metabolism and circulation and aids in the removal of toxins. Because of the intense heat and minerals lost during the sweating response, clients must be well hydrated before, during, and after treatment. The procedure is as follows:

1. Ask the client to shower before treatment.
2. Offer a cup of cool water in a nonbreakable cup and a cool washcloth for the face.

3. After the initial sweat, have the client take a tepid shower, or use a wet loofah sponge to rub the skin vigorously to increase the cleansing element. If desired, the client may re-enter the sauna. Treatment time ranges from 20 to 30 minutes, depending on the client's tolerance to dry heat.
4. After treatment, allow the client to take another 2- to 3-minute tepid shower or use a cool damp cloth to wipe off the skin. Client may also elect to take a cool plunge (discussed later in this chapter).
5. Place the client in a warm, quiet place and allow her to rest and drink water for 10 to 20 minutes.

Steam Bath

Steam baths use hot vapors in a confined area to maintain temperatures between 105° and 120° F with 100% humidity. Steam baths, or sweat lodges, are used to decrease stress and assist removal of toxins from the body. The client typically feels relaxed and sedated after the treatment. However, if the client feels weak or dizzy during treatment, discontinue treatment immediately.

A *steam canopy* that fits over a wet table is an inexpensive way to offer clients the benefits of a steam bath. A steam cabinet that allows the head to be exposed is called a *Russian bath* (Figure 23-17). Ensure that plenty of water is in the water reservoir before the client enters and place a towel on the seat or bench. Instruct the client to stay away from direct contact with the steam jet. If the cabinet or room becomes too hot, vent by slightly opening the door.

Steam baths are often used before a body wrap, massage, or other hydrotherapy treatments. You may add essential oils to the water for an aromatherapy steam bath. Add lavender for a sedative effect; rosemary to increase circulation; or eucalyptus for a stimulating effect and to increase respiratory drainage. Dry out the unit daily to prevent mildew. Clean the

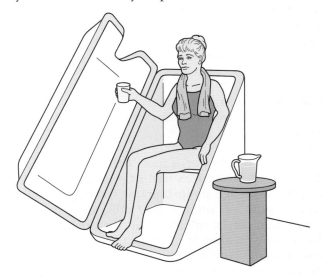

Figure 23-17 Steam cabinet or Russian bath.

unit on a regular basis with a disinfectant. The procedure is as follows:

1. Ask the client to shower before treatment.
2. Offer a cup of cool water in a nonbreakable cup and a cool washcloth for the face.
3. Treatment time ranges from 5 to 20 minutes, depending on client's tolerance to steam.
4. After treatment, allow the client to take a 2- to 3-minute tepid shower or use a cool damp cloth to wipe off the skin. Client may also elect to take a cool plunge.
5. Place the client in a warm, quiet place and allow her to rest and drink water for 10 to 20 minutes.

Paraffin Bath

Paraffin baths are dipped baths using a heated waxy mixture. Paraffin wax treatments are used to apply heat and are particularly useful on angular bony areas such as the hands, wrists, elbows, knees, ankles, and feet. Lotion or alcohol can be applied to the treatment area to help remove hardened wax. The paraffin wax is kept in a thermostatically controlled vessel at 125° to 134° F. The molten wax can be painted on the affected part instead of dipped, but the latter is most widely used. A mixture of volcanic ash (fango) and wax is a treatment mixture called *parafango*. These treatments soften the skin and are used for pain relief. Paraffin baths are indicated for clients who have painful, arthritic joints, sprains, strains, or bursitis. Recalling the contraindications for thermotherapy, do not apply to joints that are hot and swollen. The procedure is as follows:

1. Clean and dry the treatment area thoroughly before the wax dip.
2. Dip the body part into and out of the wax bath quickly.
3. Repeat the process 4 to 6 times or until a thick layer of wax is formed (at least ¼-inch thick). Allow time for the wax to dry between dippings.
4. Wrap the waxed area with a plastic wrap and then with a towel (the towel serves as insulation).
5. Allow the treated area to rest for up to 15 minutes or until the client reports that he can no longer feel heat.
6. Remove the wax covering.
7. Discard the used paraffin wax mixture.

Foot Bath

Typically warm to hot, a foot bath is often used before foot reflexology, as part of a foot treatment, or as part of other hydrotherapy treatments (Figure 23-18). Additives such as goat milk, essential oil, or Epsom salts can be used to create a more luxurious or therapeutic treatment. Commercial foot baths are available that combine vibration with hot soak. Foot baths, or *pedi-baths,* are often given before paraffin dips mentioned above. A dry brush massage or a dry towel rub is also a great addition to a foot bath. The procedure is as follows:

1. Pour heated water in a vessel large enough to accommodate both feet. Products may be added to the water at this time.
2. Place both feet in water for about 10 minutes.
3. Remove feet one at a time and dry with a thick towel.

Sitz Bath

More of a physical therapy modality than spa application, a **sitz** bath is a sitting bath with the water covering the hips and often coming up to the navel. The bath chamber is usually designed so the legs can remain out of the water. The water temperature ranges from 90° to 102° F. If the water is cool for a tonic treatment, the bath is only 3 to 8 minutes long. Warmer water creates a sedating, calming effect with treatment time ranging from 20 to 45 minutes. Healing agents such as salt or alum usually accompany the bath water. As an alternative, the feet may be placed in a tub of water that is warmer than the sitz bath (see Figure 23-18). This provides a contrast that increases circulation. A sitz bath is often indicated for relief of menstruation pain or postchildbirth pain; however, it is contraindicated in cases of pelvic inflammation. The procedure is as follows:

1. Assist the client into the sitz tub filled with water of the desired temperature.
2. Cover the client and tub with a dry sheet for a feeling of comfort and protection.
3. Assist the client out of the tub after the time frame indicated by the water temperature (cool water requires a shorter bath time and warmer water offers clients a longer bath time).

Cold Immersion Bath

Cold immersion baths involve soaking an affected area in a container of icy water. This application method is ideal for injured, inflamed or swollen hands and feet. Because this procedure is often uncomfortable, clients may elect to leave their fingers

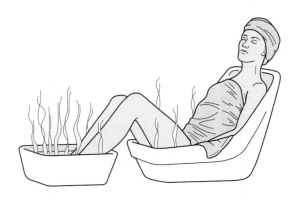

Figure 23-18   Sitz bath and foot bath.

or toes out of the icy water, or they may choose to dip a hand or foot repeatedly into the icy water until they are accustomed to the temperature or the hand or foot is numb. The procedure is as follows:

1. Immerse the affected area in a tub of tepid water.
2. Add plenty of ice—enough to chill the water quickly.
3. Keep the area immersed in icy water for 5 minutes.
4. Once the immersed area is numb, instruct the client to draw pictures or trace the alphabet in the icy water with his fingers or toes.
5. Remove from icy water and dry immediately.

Cold Plunge

A deep-water cool plunge, typically follows a sauna, steam bath, whirlpool, or hot tub. This cold spa option is often found in large spas and resorts. The water is maintained at a chilly 50° to 60° F. The objective of a cold plunge is to rapidly close the skin's pores and blood vessels that have been dilated by a heat treatment; this is a variation of the contrast method. The procedure is as follows:

1. After taking a sauna, an immersion bath, or a steam bath, have the client stand on the edge of the vessel containing the chilly water.
2. Ask the client to jump or step down quickly.
3. Have the client remain in the water from 2 to 30 seconds, or whatever she can bear.
4. Ask the client to step out of the chilly water and dry off immediately.

NOTE: You may follow up with another heated body treatment, but have the client remain in the second treatment about half the amount of time of the first treatment.

Shower

A bath technique where water is sprayed in fine streams from a showerhead under low to medium pressure is a **shower**. The two most popular varieties of spa showers are Swiss showers and Vichy showers. A *Swiss shower* features water jets that spray from overhead and side angles at varying heights while the client stands (Figure 23-19). The water pressure and temperature varies to create a stimulating or invigorating effect. A *Vichy shower* (named for its origin in Vichy, France) is a water shower spraying from multiple overhead-mounted showerheads while the client lies on a table, usually to remove treatment products (Figure 23-20). The needlelike streams alternate with hot and cold water. European Vichy showers use warm water only.

Spray

A type of shower called a *spray,* is a single fine jet of lightly pressurized warm or cool water. The therapist can use a spray attached to a rubber hose to "massage" a client while she is in a hot, whirlpool, or spa

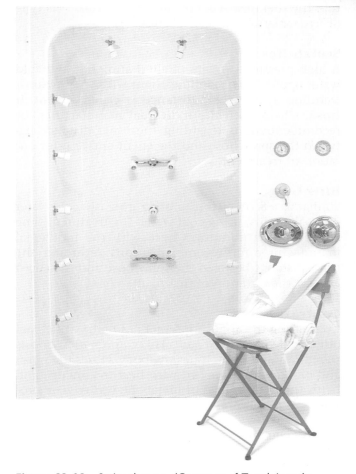

Figure 23-19   Swiss shower. (Courtesy of TouchAmerica, Hillsborough, N.C.)

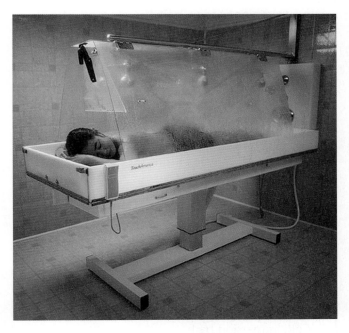

Figure 23-20   Vichy shower. (Courtesy of TouchAmerica, Hillsborough, N.C.).

tub; the therapist remains outside the tub. This type of hydromassage is very relaxing.

Scotch Hose

A high pressured stream of alternating hot and cold water applied to a standing client with the therapist standing at a specific distance is called a **Scotch hose**. Check with the individual manufacturer for recommendations regarding the exact distance between the spray hose and the client and also for duration of treatment.

Blitz Gus

Similar to a Scotch Hose, a **blitz gus** uses cold water only. Naturally, using cold water, the treatment time is only a few minutes. Check with the individual manufacturer for recommendations regarding the exact distance between the spray hose and the client and for the duration of treatment.

Contrast Bath

Combining the application of a hot bath with a cool one is called a *contrast bath*. This combination boosts the immune system, tones the body, closes the pores and blood vessels opened with heat treatments, and helps the body get rid of metabolic wastes. The procedure is as follows:

1. After taking a sauna or immersion or steam bath, have client use a cold plunge, cold shower, or blitz gus for 1 to 2 minutes. Cold plunge is a shorter treatment time.
2. Have the client dry off immediately.

NOTE: You may follow up with another heated body treatment, but have the client remain in the second treatment about half the amount of time of the first treatment.

MINI-LAB

Choose one or all of the following hydrotherapy applications. Administer the treatment to a classmate and write a narrative report.
A. Salt glow
B. Body wrap
C. Body shampoo
D. Hot pack

MINI-LAB

Choose one or all of the following cold applications. Administer the treatment to a classmate and write a narrative report.
A. Cold immersion bath
B. Ice pack
C. Hot immersion bath

Frictions

Friction applications such as shampoos, brushing, polishes, scrubs, glows, and ice massage are treatments given with vigorous rubbing of the hands or a cloth, brush, sponge, or grainy agent rubbed on the skin's surface. Additionally, a rinse and a quick-drying after treatment application is essential. These application methods unclog follicles and pores, refine the skin, remove dulling surface cells and rough, textured skin, increase circulation, and reduce swelling. Once a month is the maximum recommendation time for exfoliation such as polishes, scrubs, and glows. Avoid open wounds, sunburns, sensitive skin or application immediately after shaving or waxing. If a product is used, the amount of product depends on client size. Pressure used during frictions must be monitored and is easily known by directly asking the client. The treatment will feel warm, but if a severe burning sensation occurs, discontinue treatment. If a brush, sponge, or loofah is used during treatment, wash in a sink with hot, soapy water and a disinfectant, or place in the top basket of a dishwasher and run it through a cycle. Allow to air dry.

Shampoo

Body shampoos involve gently scrubbing the body with a brush dipped in warm, soapy water. After working up a generous lather, pour a pail of water over the client's skin. *Swedish shampoos* include a pail of hot water over the client's skin. A *Turkish shampoo*

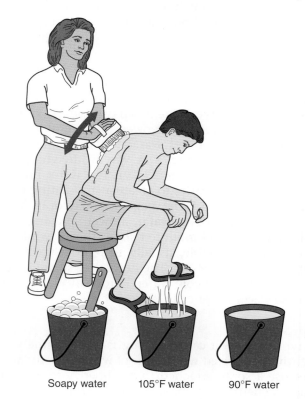

Soapy water   105°F water   90°F water

Figure 23-21   Swedish and Turkish shampoo.

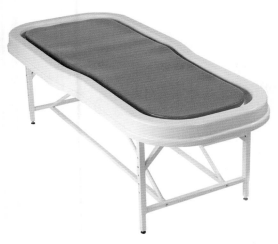

Figure 23-22   Wet table. (Courtesy of Golden Ratio, Emigrant, Mont.)

is the same thing as a Swedish shampoo, with one exception; after the hot pail pour, conclude with a tepid pail pour (Figure 23-21). Another application method is to sit the client on a water-resistant stool in a room that has a floor drain. For variation, try administering Swedish or Turkish shampoos outdoors under a canopy. If no canopy is available, make sure it is a clear and warm day, and choose an area that is quiet and private. The procedure is as follows:

1. Ask the client to sit on a stool or bench, stand, or lie on a wet table (Figure 23-22) or massage table modified for wet treatments (Figure 23-23). The client should be wearing only a towel.
2. Dampen the client's skin.
3. Pour a mild liquid soap on a brush, loofah, or bath pad. Use a circular or linear motion on the skin to work the soap into a lather.
4. After the body (except the face) is covered with lather, pour a pail of water at 105° F over the

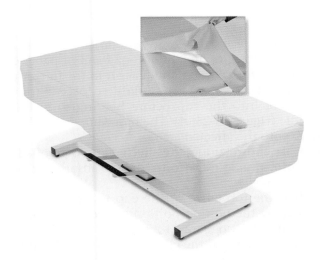

Figure 23-23   Massage table with wet sheet. (Courtesy of Golden Ratio, Emigrant, Mont.)

client's skin (Swedish method). If desired pour a pail of water at 90° F over the client's skin (Turkish method).
5. Follow with a lukewarm shower.
6. Dry the client immediately.

Dry Brush Massage
Highly stimulating to the skin, a dry brush massage uses a dry natural bristle brush or loofah to friction massage the skin. Brushing is usually a short, brisk stroke toward the heart or following lymphatic channels. This treatment is often used before a body wrap or a product mask to mildly exfoliate the skin and stimulate superficial glands so that following treatments work better. The procedure is as follows:
1. Ask the client to sit on a stool or bench, stand, or lie on a massage table. The client should be wearing only a towel.
2. Using a dry brush, scrub the skin using moderate pressure.
   Note: If a burning sensation occurs, reduce pressure and speed or discontinue treatment.

Body Scrub
A body scrub uses a coarse, gritty substance to exfoliate the skin. The products used for scrubs are fairly abrasive, and care must be taken not to rub too hard or fast or allow the product to dry out. Currently, a wide variety of scrubbing agents are available that range from gentle to abrasive. If the client complains of a burning sensation during the application, discontinue the treatment and pour tepid to cool water on the skin. The procedure is as follows:
1. Dampen the client's skin.
2. Take approximately 1 heaping tablespoon of the product and distribute between your palms. Add water if needed. Apply the product. Hold an extremity (arm or leg) in one hand, and use a brisk upward and downward movement with the other while the client holds the extremity stiff.
3. Rinse the product off with a warm pail pour or follow with a warm shower.
4. Dry the client immediately.

Salt Glow
A **salt glow** is a rubbing application of wet salt on the skin (Figure 23-24). Often a mixture of salt and sesame oil is used. Salt glows can be used to exfoliate the skin and are beneficial if the client is undergoing a fast or other self-cleansing regimen. This procedure should not be used on freshly shaven legs, cuts, abrasions, or skin rashes because the salt will burn. Some clients may be allergic to iodine so noniodized salt is recommended. A brisk back-and-forth friction is used to apply the salt; circular friction is used around joints. However, a light friction is indicated if the client has fair, ruddy, or thin skin be-

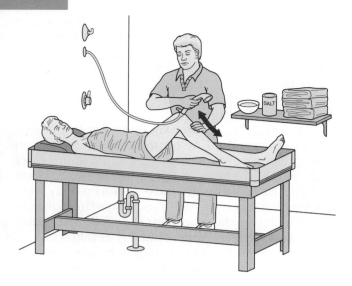

Figure 23-24   Salt glow.

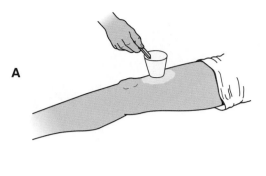

A

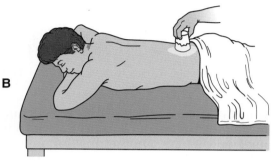

B

Figure 23-25   Ice massage. **A,** Frozen ice cip with handle. **B,** Frozen ice cip with top edges torn.

cause of the possibility of skin irritation. The procedure is as follows:

1. Have the client sit on a stool or bench, stand, or lie on a wet table or massage table modified for wet treatments.
2. Put ½ cup of salt (kosher, table, Epsom, sea, or other natural salt) or salt mixture in an unbreakable quart-size dish. Add just enough water or oil to make the grains stick together but not enough to dissolve the salt. It should be the consistency of slush.
3. After moistening the skin with water, take approximately 1 heaping tablespoon of the moistened salt in the hands, and distribute between your palms. Hold an extremity (arm or leg) in one hand, and use a brisk upward and downward movement with the other while the client holds the extremity stiff. Rinse the area off with warm water and proceed with the salt application and rinsing until the entire body is complete.
4. Follow with a lukewarm shower.
5. Dry the client immediately.

 The cure for anything is salt water—sweat, tears, or the sea.

—Isak Dinesan

Body Polish

The use of a fine grainy substance to gently exfoliate, refine, and buff the skin is called a *body polish.* The products used to polish are not as coarse or abrasive as scrubs and glows. The sensation left on the skin after a polish treatment is very invigorating. This application is often combined with other treatments. It is also more common for localized treatments, a

shampoo, clay pack, toner, and moisturizer for a *back facial.* The procedure is as follows:

1. Dampen the client's skin.
2. Take approximately 1 heaping tablespoon of the product and distribute between your palms. Add water if needed. Apply the product. Hold an extremity (arm or leg) in one hand, and use a brisk upward and downward movement with the other while the client holds the extremity stiff.
3. Rinse the product off with a warm pail pour or follow with a warm shower.
4. Dry the client immediately.

Ice Massage

Ice massage combines the use of ice with circular friction. To begin, fill a 6- or 8-oz foam or paper cup two thirds full of water and place it in the freezer until the water has turned to solid ice. Insert a tongue depressor into the cup before freezing to give it a handle (Figure 23-25, *A*). The procedure is as follows:

1. Expose the affected area.
2. Place a towel under the affected area or a rolled-up towel around the affected area to absorb the melting ice water.
3. Tear the top edges of the cup to expose the ice, leaving the bottom portion of the cup to protect your fingers (Figure 23-25, *B*).
4. Place the ice on the client's skin and move it very quickly in small circular motions.
5. Continue the ice massage over the affected area for 5 to 10 minutes or until numb.

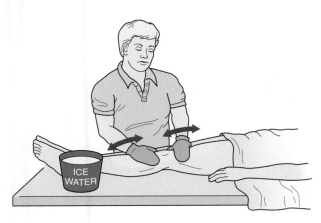

Figure 23-26   Cold mitten friction.

6. Remove the towel.
7. Dry the treatment area.

Cold Mitten Friction

Cold mitten friction is an application of cold with mittens dipped in icy water and friction movements at a force of 5 to 10 lb of pressure. Coarser mitts or a loofah sponge may be used for greater friction effects. This treatment is a tonic treatment because it is thought to aid in the prevention of colds, low energy and endurance, poor resistance to infections, poor circulation, and anemia (Figure 23-26). Ice application through cold mitten friction causes blood vessels to contract and dilate, promotes heat production, and reduces swelling. The procedure is as follows:

1. Place your client on a wet table or a massage table modified for wet treatments.
2. Have the following items nearby:
   • Two or more towels
   • Friction mitts (a washcloth wrapped around the hand with the edge tucked in or mitts made by simply sewing along the sides of a folded washcloth)
   • A pail of icy water 50° to 60° F or less
3. Dip the mitts into the icy water. Arrange the mitts on your hands. Begin at the legs and work up with vigorous back-and-forth friction movements.
4. Dip the mitts again and repeat the process.
5. Quickly remove the mitts.
6. Cover the area with a towel and rub vigorously over the skin until it is thoroughly dry.

SUMMARY

As long as man has known pain, so too has he turned to water for relief from it. Hydrotherapy is the use of water for its healing properties. Each type of application has its own beneficial effects, contraindications, safety issues, and procedures regarding its use. Water can be used for different therapeutic effects by varying its temperature, moisture content, mineral content, and mechanical application. Variations in temperature result in the use of thermotherapy (heat) applications and cryotherapy (cold) applications.

Both thermotherapy and cryotherapy can be applied by means of packs, baths, and frictions. Pack application methods include hot compresses, hot packs, hydrocollator packs, heated mittens and booties, hot or cold stones, product packs or product masks, cool compresses, cold gel packs and cold packs, cryokinetics, body wraps, and contrast packs.

Bath application methods include hot immersion baths, hot air baths, saunas, steam baths, paraffin baths, foot baths, sitz baths, cold immersion baths, cold plunges, showers, sprays, scotch hoses, blitz gus, and contrast baths. Friction application methods include shampoos, dry brush massages, body scrubs, salt glows, body polishes, ice massage, and cold mitten friction.

Today these varied hydrotherapy applications have become known as spa techniques. Spa techniques can be added to the massage therapist's repertoire of modalities to offer a greater variety of services, increase therapeutic effectiveness and client satisfaction, and make the massage therapist more competitive and marketable.

MATCHING I

Write the letter of the best answer in the space provided.

A. Hydrotherapy
B. Thermotherapy
C. Convection
D. Cryotherapy

E. Contrast method
F. Spa
G. Conduction

H. Radiation
I. Cryokinetics
J. Ice massage

_____ 1. Transferring heat energy through circulating currents of liquid or gas

_____ 2. A place where water therapies are administered

_____ 3. The application of ice combined with circular friction

_____ 4. The combination of heat and cold in the same treatment

_____ 5. The exchange of thermal energy while the body's surface is in direct contact with the thermal agent

_____ 6. The application of a cold pack followed by full range of motion of the affected area

_____ 7. The internal and external therapeutic use of water and complementary agents

_____ 8. The transfer of heat energy in rays

_____ 9. The external, therapeutic application of cold

_____ 10. The external application of heat for therapeutic purposes

MATCHING II

Write the letter of the best answer in the space provided.

A. Compress
B. Pack
C. Cold gel pack
D. Compression body wrap

E. Salt glow
F. Wrap
G. Hydrocollator pack

H. Cover body wrap
I. Body shampoo
J. Cold mitten friction

_____ 1. Rubbing application of wet salt on the skin

_____ 2. A plastic bag filled with a special gel that retains cold for about 20 minutes and does not freeze to a solid block mass

_____ 3. An application of cold with mittens dipped in icy water and friction movements at a force of 5 to 10 lb of pressure

_____ 4. A specialized hot pack consisting of a canvas pouch filled with silicon granules, which hold heat for about 30 minutes

_____ 5. A body wrap that covers the body with sheets soaked in herbs and other substances to increase perspiration, promote relaxation, or detoxify the system; the wrap cocoons the body, generating and maintaining heat to encourage penetration of an applied product

_____ 6. Water is wrung from a wet cloth and applied to the skin's surface

_____ 7. Gently scrubbing the body with a brush dipped in warm soapy water; after working up a generous lather, a pail of water is poured over the client's skin

_____ 8. A large pack covering most of the body through the use of large, wet or dry sheets or blankets

_____ 9. A body wrap where the body is covered in elastic bandages that have been soaked in a solution; the objective is to contour the body

_____ 10. A bag, sack, or other item used to apply or retain heat or cold

MATCHING III

Write the letter of the best answer in the space provided.

A. Bath
B. Sauna bath
C. Paraffin bath
D. Cold plunge

E. Swiss shower
F. Scotch hose
G. Immersion bath
H. Steam bath

I. Sitz bath
J. Shower
K. Vichy shower
L. Blitz gus

_____ 1. Hot-air bath with temperatures ranging from 170° to 210° F in 10% to 20% humidity

_____ 2. Full or partial body immersion with the client sitting in a vessel such as whirlpool, spa or hot tub, or a Hubbard tank

_____ 3. Hot vapor bath where the temperature is maintained at 105° to 120° F at 100% humidity

_____ 4. A bath technique where water is sprayed in fine streams from a showerhead under low to medium pressure

_____ 5. A dipped bath of a heated waxy mixture

_____ 6. A broad category of hydrotherapy application encompassing partial or full immersion in water, wax, light, heated air, or steam

_____ 7. A shower with water spraying from overhead needlelike valves at varying heights

_____ 8. A sitting bath with the water covering the hips, often coming up to the navel

_____ 9. A high-pressure stream of _cold water_ applied to a standing client with the therapist standing at a specific distance

_____ 10. A deep-water pool plunge with water temperature maintained at a chilly 50° to 60° F

_____ 11. A high-pressure stream of _alternating hot and cold water_ applied to a standing client with the therapist standing at a specific distance

_____ 12. A shower with water spraying from multiple overhead-mounted showerheads while the client lies on a table; the needlelike streams alternate with hot and cold water

Bibliography

Associated Bodywork and Massage Professionals: *Touch training manual,* Evergreen, Colo, 1998, Author.

Barnes L: Cryotherapy: putting injury on ice, *Physician Sportsmed* 7(6):130-136, 1979.

Capellini S: *The royal treatment,* New York, 1997, Dell.

De Vierville JP: Taking the waters: a historical look at water therapy and spa culture over the ages, *Massage Bodywork: Nurtur Body, Mind, Spirit* pp 12-20, Feb/Mar, 2000.

Drez D: *Therapeutic modalities for sports injuries,* St Louis, 1986, Mosby.

Hannigan MD: *LaStone therapy: the original hot stone massage,* Tucson, Ariz, 1999, Author.

Herriott E: Steam and sauna therapy applications with massage, *Massage Mag* pp 32-35, May/June, 1997.

Klafs D, Arnheim DD: *Modern principles of athletic training,* St Louis, 1981, Mosby.

Knight K: *Cryotherapy: theory, technique and physiology,* Chattanooga, Tenn, 1985, Chattanooga Corporation.

Lawrence DB: *Waterworks,* New York, 1989, Putnam.

Leibold G: *Practical hydrotherapy,* Wellingborough, England, 1980, Thorson.

Marx L: An odyssey through spa therapies, *Massage Mag* pp 45-48, May/June, 1997.

Mellion MB: *Sportsmedicine secrets,* Philadelphia, 1994, Hanley and Belfus.

Minton M: Body and spa, *Massage Mag* pp 89-99, Sept/Oct, 2001.

New Life Systems: *The body book,* Minnetonka, Minn, 2001, Author.

Nikola RJ: *Creatures of water,* Salt Lake City, 1997, Europa Therapeutic.

Tepperman PS, Devilin M: Therapeutic heat and cold: a practitioner's guide, *Postgrad Med* 73(1):69-76, 1983.

Thrash A, Thrash, C: *Home remedies: hydrotherapy, massage, charcoal and other simple treatments,* Seale, Ala, 1981, Yuchi Pines Institute.

Tuckerman B: How to add body wraps to your practice, *Massage Mag* pp 92-96, Nov/Dec, 1999.

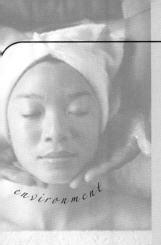

environment

Clinical Application of Massage Therapy

24

Michael A. Breaux, LMT

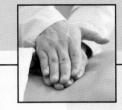

"You can't turn back the clock, but you can wind it up again."

—Bonnie Prudden

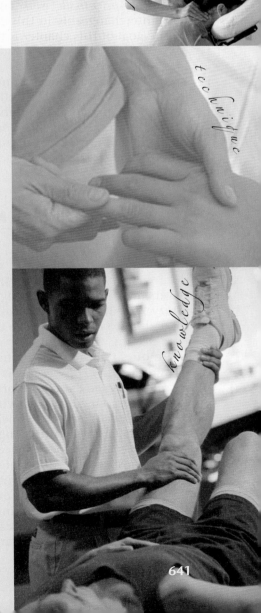

pressure

technique

knowledge

STUDENT OBJECTIVES

After completing this chapter, the student should be able to:

- List typical causes of injury
- List stages of rehabilitation in sequential order
- Name factors that affect recovery time
- Define *trigger points* and describe how to identify them by their symptoms
- Identify several common pathologies and their treatment protocols
- List three important issues of aftercare
- Explain how to avoid the most common mistake of clinical massage
- Demonstrate techniques for gauging pressure and pain
- Discuss common injuries with their clients

INTRODUCTION

Massage was originally used to ease the pain of human ills and conditions. The recent growth of the massage industry has created a proliferation of massage therapists who are better educated and more experienced than in the past. Massage therapists have become licensed health care practitioners. Research has documented the efficacy of massage. Insurance companies are recognizing massage services as being worthy of payment and reimbursement. The need for clinical application of massage is here.

Most injuries and disorders respond well to massage therapy and ancillary modalities, although some are better suited to specific forms of treatment. In general a first-degree tear of the supraspinatus could be treated with relaxation techniques such as Swedish massage or clinical techniques such as ischemic compression, cross-fiber friction, and myofascial release. For purposes of clarity and consistency, the terms *deep-tissue work* and *clinical massage* are used interchangeably in this chapter.

The goal of this chapter is to provide information on a variety of injuries, conditions, tissue pathologies, and recommendations for area-specific treatment that can be used alone in a clinical setting or as a focused segment of a 1-hour session. Information covered in previous chapters is reexamined here, including scope of practice and tissue healing, in addition to defining causes of injury, stages of rehabilitation, aftercare, and common mistakes therapists make.

WHY LEARN CLINICAL MASSAGE?

Choosing and using more aggressive deep-tissue techniques is important for several reasons. When dealing with prescribed treatments and third-party payers, *time* is often a limiting factor. It is often necessary to pursue potent treatment techniques and modalities to rehabilitate the client in a timely manner. Healing time is often swifter with deep-tissue techniques than it is with other techniques.

Additionally, *effectiveness* is key. *Medicine and Science in Sports and Exercise* reported a study where massages were applied with varying degrees of pressure to groups of laboratory rats who had chemically induced Achilles tendonitis. The analysis showed that those subjects receiving applications of deep-pressure massage responded with greater degree of healing (as evidenced by increased fibroblast count) than did those with light or medium pressure on the surgical control group. NOTE: The terms deep-tissue massage and deep-pressure massage can also be used interchangeably in clinical applications.

Another reason is *need.* Some clients are going to request clinical massage techniques or deep-tissue massage. Massage therapists should develop a basic understanding of clinical massage applications. It makes therapists more marketable; they are more likely to be hired to work in a chiropractic, physical therapy, or hospital setting. Even the practitioner who specializes in relaxation techniques periodically encounters clients who have rotator cuff strains, tennis elbow, whiplash, and other injuries. If the therapist is not prepared to meet their needs, these clients are referred to someone who can. Learning other techniques is like cross-training in sports activities—these therapists are prepared for a diverse practice.

LIMITATIONS WITHIN YOUR SCOPE OF PRACTICE

The massage therapist's scope of practice is limited according to state or local law (if applicable). Laws vary, and every massage therapist should familiarize themselves with the laws in their area. Massage can be applied to injuries, conditions, disorders, and/or illnesses. In some areas, massage therapists are specifically prohibited from treating illnesses because treatment of illness constitutes practicing medicine, which violates the law. However, massage therapy can be used to treat the symptoms of an illness. Physicians routinely prescribe massage therapy to relieve the stress, pain, and muscular symptoms of a wide variety of illnesses including cancer.

At no time during treatment should the massage therapist render a diagnosis of disease or a prognosis of care. Massage therapists should never attempt to manipulate joints through the use of high-velocity chiropractic adjustments. Neither should the massage therapist prescribe medications (not even over-the-counter remedies such as aspirin, herbs, or supplements) or procedures that are outside of the massage therapist's scope and training. If legal, massage therapists may commonly recommend the use of hot or cold hydrotherapy, stretching, range of motion, compression bandages, and so on. Although massage therapists cannot diagnose, they can and must assess the client's condition (see Chapter 8). Assessment is vital in the proper formulation of a treatment protocol for the client. When the client's condition is outside of the massage therapist's level of training, experience, or scope, then the therapist should refer the client to a physician for evaluation.

Massage therapists often work in settings such as hospitals, chiropractic clinics, or physical therapy clinics and may be tempted to practice outside their scope. Resist this voice of ego. We are not doctors, nurses, chiropractors, occupational therapists, or physical therapists.

When it comes to muscle work, what we do is statistically safer and often more effective than surgery, medication, injections, and electrostimulation. If you truly want to do more than just massage, then consider a career in medicine, nursing, chiropractic, occupational therapy, or physical therapy. Do not discredit your fellow massage therapists and risk injury to your clients by trying to "play doctor" (see Chapter 2).

INJURY REHABILITATION

Many clients seek out massage services to rehabilitate injuries and the resulting pain and muscular soreness attributed them. These may be due to a variety of reasons including sports injuries, motor vehicle accidents, repetitive motion injuries, surgical treatment, and postural distortions. In treating these conditions, it is important to understand typical causes of injury, stages of rehabilitation, and the principles behind them. These stages of rehabilitation are discussed in the following section and are based on principles of neurological law (see Chapter 17). It is recommended that you review mechanisms of the pain cycle (see Chapter 5) and the physiology of tissue healing (see Chapter 11).

Typical Causes of Injury

No one is a stranger to injury. Activities that cause soreness, pain, or injury include the following:

New activities to which your body is not accustomed. Examples include beginning a new exercise regimen, doing a new task at your current job, or changing jobs. Muscle tenderness is generally temporary, lasting until the body adapts to the new regimen.

Weekend warrior activities that use a completely different set of muscles than you use during the week. Examples include doctors that go hunting, accountants that do National Guard weekends, or teachers that work in the garden on the weekend. Muscle soreness tends to be episodic, recurring each time the weekend activity is repeated.

Body in a particular position for an extended period. Examples are hip or knee pain from sitting on the floor for a long period to wrap presents or neck pain from turning your head to talk to friends behind or beside you while on a long drive. Muscle pain tends to be episodic, occurring once and then going away after treatment (treatment may include a tincture of time).

Repeated movements of any kind. Examples are low-back pain from bending and lifting, elbow pain from scanning groceries as a checkout clerk, or shoulder problems from trying to repeatedly pull-start a lawn mower. These repetitive motion disorders tend to be progressive in nature with muscle pain and inflammation worsening over a period.

Trauma. Examples are major trauma such as automobile accidents, slips and falls, or recovery from surgery and minor traumas such as subluxations, allergies, infestations, psychological, or metabolic disorders (diabetes, and so on). Injuries from trauma tend to be pervasive and activity-limiting. Occasionally, they resolve of their own accord but often require therapy.

Pain and soreness are a normal part of the inflammatory response to injury; they are the body's message for you to slow down. Although massage can be used effectively to speed healing and reduce pain and soreness, some rehabilitative activities have the opposite effect. Muscular pain may increase if an injury is stretched or exercised too soon. Stress and emotional concerns, such as finances and unhealthy personal relationships, may increase the perception of pain. The use of neurostimulants such as amphetamines, caffeine, and sugar may also increase the client's perception of pain.

Healing rates may be retarded by the slowing of the metabolism through excessive alcohol or barbiturate use; decreasing the supply of oxygen through smoking, sleep apnea, or respiratory illness; or depleting bodily resources through disease such as diabetes, autoimmune diseases, or acquired immunodeficiency syndrome (AIDS). To effectively treat injuries, the massage therapist must understand the stages of rehabilitation.

Stages of Rehabilitation

The following are regarded as stages of rehabilitation and, as such, must be addressed in a sequential order. Rearranging the order or omitting one of the stages may hinder the rehabilitation process or exacerbate the condition. For example, stretching a muscle before eliminating the spasm may cause tearing or tissue trauma. NOTE: Stages 4, 5, and 6 may be outside a massage therapist's scope of practice in some states, or the therapist may need to be dually licensed as a physical trainer, athletic trainer, or nutritionist.

Stage 1: Reduce Muscle Spasm
Massage not only reduces spasms but relieves ischemia and trigger points and reduces trigger point formation. Ischemia is relieved by local increase in circulation achieved with massage. Massage relieves neurovascular entrapment by relaxing taut muscles and fascia. Muscles in spasm exert a pull on their attachment sites and sometimes cause certain bones or cartilaginous tissues to be tractioned out of place or increase intrajoint pressure. Massage to the muscles

crossing the affected joints causes muscles to relax and may reduce the intrajoint pressure. Although massage itself cannot correct dislocations or subluxations of joints, it is an important component of the rehabilitation process. To speed recovery time and reduce trauma, massage therapists are now part of the treatment team along with chiropractors, physical and occupational therapists, and orthopedists.

Stage 2: Assess and Correct Faulty Body Mechanics

This can be accomplished through movement therapy and client education. The therapist uses assessment of gait patterns, shoe wear, dysfunctional postures, and inefficient movement habits to help the client make changes in their activities of daily living (ADLs). These changes may be facilitated by teaching the client new postures for sleeping, sitting, or working or by referring them to other specialists for braces, orthotics, or exercise.

Stage 3: Restore Flexibility to Muscles and Joints

Once muscle spasms have been reduced and dysfunctional biomechanical patterns have been identified and corrected, stretching and range of motion can be used to begin to return tissues to their full resting length. Dr. David Simons indicates that stretching is essential to the treatment of a muscle after releasing trigger points to rebalance the tissues surrounding an affected joint. It is important to address all muscle groups associated with the motion of the joint.

Stage 4: Rebuild Muscle Strength

To prevent repeated injury, involved muscles and muscles that cross affected joints must be strengthened. Strengthening can be done with light to moderate weight training and resistance exercises using rubber tubing, small dumbbells, or exercise machines. If the exercise exacerbates the pain or condition, it should be stopped immediately, reassessment should be made, and rehabilitation should resume at the appropriate stage.

Stage 5: Build Endurance

Cardiovascular and aerobic exercise can help build the client's endurance while further building strength. Swimming, walking, running, and biking are all conditioning exercises for building endurance.

Stage 6: Address Diet, Stress Reduction, and Emotional Well-Being

Behavior modification can enhance the health of the client and prevent further episodes of re-injury. Work with your client to get them to adopt a healthy lifestyle that includes a balanced diet, regular exercise program, plenty of fluids, mental/emotional stress reduction, and a massage therapy maintenance plan.

Trauma, Tissue Damage, and Healing

Trauma

Tissue damage results from injury by a physical or mechanical means, chemical irritants, or exposure to extreme temperatures. Injuries resulting from trauma may be acute or chronic, and it is here that the clinical massage therapist can be of the most use. You may often see tissue damage referred to as *lesions,* but a lesion has a much broader definition. A **lesion** is any noticeable or measurable deviation from the normal composition of healthy tissue. A lesion can be a mole, wart, or break in the skin. It can be a tear in the muscle, tumor in the brain, fracture of a bone, or even discoloration of the eye. Once injured, the body's need to regain tissue integrity stimulates a healing process. Damaged tissue is replaced or repaired through several different methods. Which process is stimulated depends on the degree of trauma.

Resolution

At the mild end of the trauma range, reparation of mildly injured tissues occurs by a process known as *resolution.* In this process, tissues/cells are slightly damaged (e.g., a mild sunburn). As long as the cellular membrane is intact, and the nuclear contents are unharmed, the body repairs the damage.

Regeneration

Repair of mild to moderately injured tissue can also occur by the process of regeneration. Regeneration occurs when damaged tissue is replaced with new tissue of the same type. Enough undamaged tissue must be in the area for it to reproduce itself. In a moderate injury such as a skinned knee, the open wound becomes sealed with a scab, and the healthy cells underneath the scab divide until the skin has been reproduced completely; then the scab is sloughed off. No loss of tissue function occurs when an injury is healed through regeneration because the injured tissue has been replaced with the same type of tissue.

Fibrosis

In some cases the injury itself may be geographically too large to be repaired by regeneration or the injury may be moderate to severe in nature and may require a different method of healing. As the trauma or injury becomes greater, the bodily reaction to it is proportional. In these cases the body initiates a repair process known as *fibrosis.* When not enough of the original tissue is left to repair the wound, fibrosis replaces the original tissue with a different kind of tissue. Specialized cells, known as *fibroblasts,* are mobilized to the site of injury to create scar tissue. The fibroblasts secrete collagen fiber strands to bind up the wounded tissue. The collagen fibers laid down in the fibrosis process are formed randomly and are consequently poorly organized. The resulting scar, although strong, may be either bulky and soft or fibrous and tough. In either case, fibrosed scar tissue in muscle, tendon, or ligament causes a loss of the tissue's natural elasticity. In other words, the fibrotic scar creates a strong bond in the tissue, but does not provide the function of the tissue it is replacing.

Remodeling. After fibrosis occurs, some changes must occur within the scar tissue if it is to become pliable and function efficiently after healing. This process is called *remodeling* or the scar maturation phase. During remodeling, the body is continually restructuring the scar tissue by a simultaneous destruction and creation of collagen fibers. Remodeling occurs to tissues that are subjected to longitudinal stress such as the stretching of muscle and tendon tissues. For more information on inflammation and tissue healing, see Chapter 11.

Relative Recovery Times

Before studying the relative recovery times for the various tissues, it must be understood that these recovery times are simply ranges for healing. The following factors affect the relative recovery time or rate of healing:

Age. Children heal faster than adults.

Wound condition. A clean wound heals faster. Wounds that are stitched close the gap that has to be bridged, thereby decreasing the surface area that must be repaired. Stitching also supports the tissue and removes the stress placed on it by the pull of skin, muscle, or other tissues. Foreign objects, infection, bleeding, or disturbances to the wound (e.g., excessive mobility of the tissue) can slow or halt the rate of recovery. In some cases, the wound will just not heal at all. In these cases, recovery stops and the tissue dies (necrosis).

Rehabilitation. Some tissues, such as muscle, may physically repair themselves completely as far as a tear is concerned. However, this process may take an extended period in the absence of rehabilitation. Likewise, the tissue may not regain all of its function, flexibility, or strength without rehabilitation. Clients undergoing rehabilitation (massage, stretching, exercise, and so on) tend to respond faster and perform better than those who recover without assistance.

Health of the patient. Diseases like diabetes can negatively impact the rate of healing.

Nutrition. Good nutrition with an adequate supply of vitamins, minerals, and protein promotes heal-

ing; improper nutrition retards the healing process.

Circulation. For tissue to heal, oxygen delivery and waste product removal are necessary to sustain cellular reproduction. In severe injuries, fibroblast cells must be transported to the site of injury. Because these prerequisites are all provided by the circulatory system, circulation is probably the most important factor in the rate of tissue healing. Additionally, blood supply is different for different tissue types, so time factors for healing and recovery are also different.

The healing rates of these various types of tissues are detailed as follows:

1. **Skin.** Skin has the most abundant blood supply of all the commonly injured tissues and heals the fastest, at about 3 to 7 days. If the damage requires stitching, most sutures are ready to be removed in 5 to 7 days. Mild contusions of the skin heal in about 5 days.
2. **Muscle.** Muscle tissue is the next fastest because of its vascular supply. Muscle soreness usually resolves itself within 24 to 72 hours. Mild (minor) muscular tears may heal as quickly as 3 to 7 days; if exacerbated by further strenuous activity, it may take as long as 3 weeks. Moderate muscle strains take 1 to 6 months for complete rehabilitation (restoration of function, strength, and so on). Some moderate and all severe muscle strains require surgery. Mild contusions can heal within a few days, moderate may take 4 to 6 weeks to heal, and severe contusions may not resolve themselves for 2 to 6 months.
3. **Bone.** Bone tissue is the next fastest healer. Simple fractures that can be cast may heal in about 3 weeks for children or 5 weeks for adults. Fractures that cannot be cast (e.g., clavicle or rib) may take 4 to 5 weeks for children or 6 to 10 weeks for adults. Healing time varies with the configuration of the fracture; type, size, and density of the bone fractured; and age and health of the patient.

For Your Information

The bones of adults have a larger amount of calcified tissue, whereas the bones of children have a greater ratio of living bone tissue and flexible cartilage to calcified tissue. Most bones do not completely calcify until after puberty. The higher amount of living bone tissue provides more raw material for the repair of fractures. Children also have a greater amount of growth hormone in their systems, which stimulates a faster recovery than those of adults. As humans progress through the drying-out process called aging, the bones of adults, especially the elderly, grow more brittle and more susceptible to fracture.

4. **Tendons.** Tendons are relatively avascular collagenous tissues. A mild strain (tear) of the tendon may take 5 to 7 days to heal, a moderate strain requires 7 to 10 days, and a severe strain always requires surgical attention to correct. The tendon may take 3 to 6 weeks to heal after surgery and even longer to be totally rehabilitated. The majority of tendon injuries occur at either the musculotendinous junction or the tenoperiosteal junction. In musculotendinous injuries, the tissue becomes frayed at the junction of the tendon and the muscle. In severe injuries, the two separated ends retract like a severed rubber band. This typically leaves a palpable and sometimes visible bulge or knot under the skin where the ends have rolled up. An injury of this magnitude requires surgery. Sometimes the severed ends can be sutured back together; sometimes the surgical repair is similar to that of the avulsion fracture mentioned later in this section. Most massage therapists in clinical practice are presented with mild to moderate tendon injuries. Trigger points often form in the musculotendinous junction and may refer pain distally. Common musculotendinous junction injury sites may include the following:
   - Soleus for running and jumping (Figure 24-1, *A*)
   - Finger flexors of the forearm for racket sports, weight training, and golf (Figure 24-1, *B*)
   - Finger extensors of the forearm for racket sports, weight training, and golf (Figure 24-1, *C*).

   A severe injury at the tenoperiostial junction is also know as an *avulsion fracture.* In other words, the tendon tears loose where it is rooted to the bone. In severe injuries, the torn tendon often takes a small piece of bone with it. Again, the tendon curls up below the skin, leaving a palpable bump. A pin must be screwed into the bone at the old site of tendon attachment. The tendon tissue must then be sutured to the pin. Healing time after either of the above surgeries is generally 3 to 6 weeks and even longer to reach total rehabilitation. In mild injuries, the tendon may try to reattach itself; sometimes in this process, a bone spur develops as the bone tries to grow out to reach the frayed tendon. This may result in the calcification of part of the tendon. Common tenoperiosteal junction injury sites may include the following:
   - Supraspinatus, infraspinatus, and teres minor for pitching, throwing, tennis, and weight training (Figure 24-2, *A*)
   - Subscapularis for pitching, throwing, and swimming (Figure 24-2, *B*)
   - Finger extensors of the forearm for racket sports, weight training, and golf (Figure 24-3, *A*)
   - Finger flexors of the forearm for racket sports, weight training, and golf (Figure 24-3, *B*)

   Other injuries may involve the entire tendon and may produce inflammation from overuse; this is usually referred to as *tendonitis.* Common tendonitis sites may include the following:
   - Achilles tendonitis: Gastrocnemius for running, basketball, and volleyball (Figure 24-4, *A*)
   - Hamstring tendonitis: Biceps femoris, semitendinosus, and semimembranosus for sprinting and hurtling (Figure 24-4, *B*)
   - Peroneal tendonitis: Peroneus longus and peroneus brevis for lateral ankle sprains (Figure 24-4, *C*)
   - Patellar tendonitis: Quadriceps femoris for basketball, volleyball, and running (Figure 24-4, *D*)

5. **Ligaments.** Ligaments are fairly avascular collagenous tissues. A mild sprain may result in minor tears or stretching of the ligament. Ligaments are under tension but are usually just overstretched in the mild to moderate sprain injury. This stretching may cause joints to become sloppy, hypermobile, or unstable. Mild sprains take about 2 months to heal. Some moderate sprains may resolve themselves within 6 months. Other moderate sprains and all severe sprains require surgical intervention to stabilize the joint. Because ligaments tend to be shorter than tendons, a complete rupture may not leave enough ligamentous material for surgical repair. In these cases, the orthopedic surgeons often "borrow" some tendon from a nearby muscle to replace the ligament. For example, pieces of the iliotibial band may be used to repair the anterior cruciate ligament (ACL) of the knee. Physical healing of the ACL repair is generally 3 to 6 weeks, but complete rehabilitation with a return to full tissue strength may take about 20 weeks. Common ligamentous injury sites for athletes may include the following:
   - Anterior and posterior cruciate ligaments of the knee for basketball, tennis, and football (NOTE: This cannot be accessed for massage) (Figure 24-5, *A*)
   - Lateral and medial collateral ligaments and the anterior and posterior cruciate ligaments of the knee for football, skiing, and soccer (Figure 24-5, *A*)
   - Sacrotuberous ligament of the hip for sprinting, dancing, and distance running (Figure 24-5, *B*)
   - Calcaneofibular ligament and anterior talofibular ligament for football, basketball, and volleyball (Figure 24-5, *C*)

6. **Nerves.** At one time, nerve tissue damage was thought to be permanent but now medical experts believe that only the central nervous system does not experience nerve regeneration. Peripheral nerves do have the ability to heal, but the regeneration rate is extremely slow. The body may compensate for a severed peripheral nerve by

rerouting the nerve signals down an adjacent nerve pathway.

7. **Cartilage.** Cartilages such as the menisci of the knee are avascular and cannot repair themselves. Some clients learn to adapt to minor cartilaginous injuries and live with them. If the injury is severe, it requires surgery to correct (Box 24-1).

CLINICAL MASSAGE: A PRIMER

This section examines techniques, specific tissue pathologies associated with injury, their treatment, and aftercare. Methods for avoiding mistakes; gauging pressure; and focusing on the causes, symptoms,

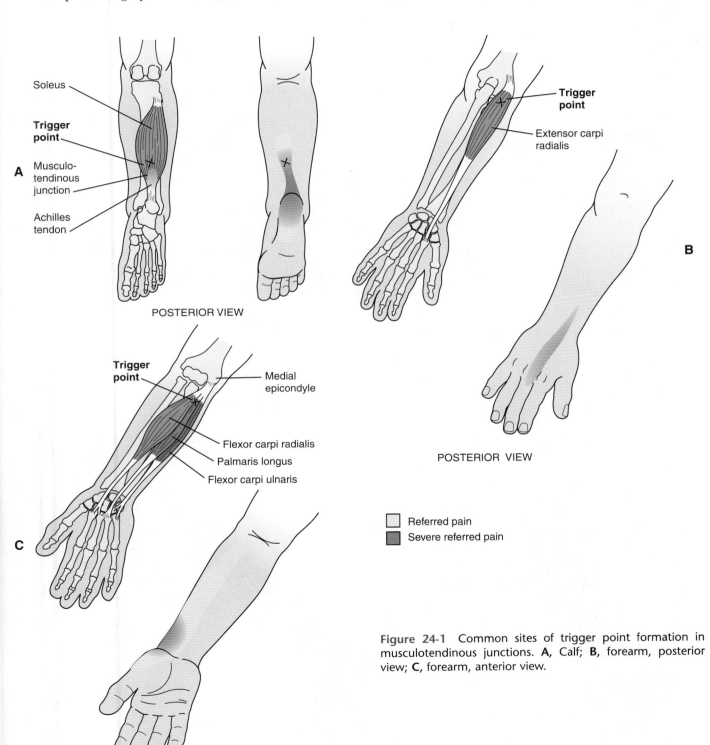

Figure 24-1 Common sites of trigger point formation in musculotendinous junctions. **A**, Calf; **B**, forearm, posterior view; **C**, forearm, anterior view.

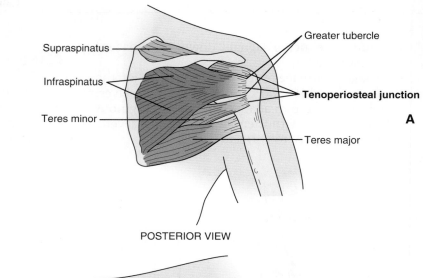

Supraspinatus

Infraspinatus

Teres minor

Greater tubercle

Tenoperiosteal junction

Teres major

POSTERIOR VIEW

A

Figure 24-2 Common tendon injuries at the tenoperiosteal junction for posterior rotator cuff (**A**) and anterior rotator cuff (**B**).

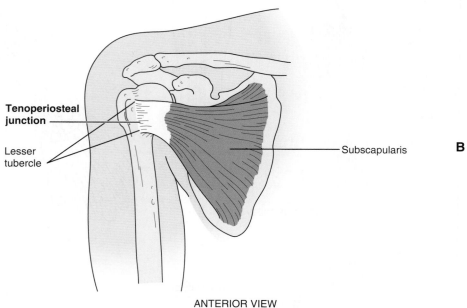

Tenoperiosteal junction

Lesser tubercle

Subscapularis

ANTERIOR VIEW

B

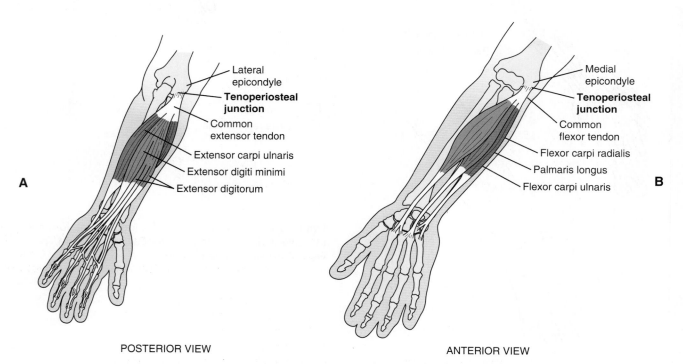

Lateral epicondyle

Tenoperiosteal junction

Common extensor tendon

Extensor carpi ulnaris

Extensor digiti minimi

Extensor digitorum

A

POSTERIOR VIEW

Medial epicondyle

Tenoperiosteal junction

Common flexor tendon

Flexor carpi radialis

Palmaris longus

Flexor carpi ulnaris

B

ANTERIOR VIEW

Figure 24-3 Common tendon injuries at the tenoperiosteal junction for posterior forearm (**A**) and anterior forearm (**B**).

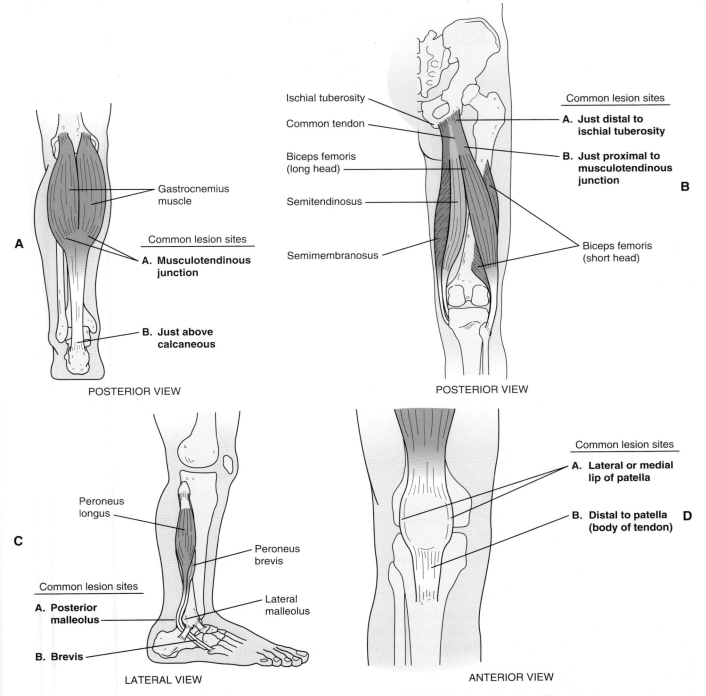

Figure 24-4 Common tendonitis injuries of the calf (**A**), hamstrings (**B**), lateral lower leg (**C**), and knee (**D**).

and treatment strategies of common injuries are also discussed.

Common Techniques Used In Clinical Massage Applications

This section addresses application of specific massage techniques associated with a clinical practice. These techniques are geared to handle tissue pathologies that are discussed in the section that follows. The therapist has the flexibility to use any massage technique at any time, but the following techniques are primarily used:

- Ischemic compression
- Cross-fiber friction
- Myofascial release
- Flushing effleurage
- Joint mobilization and stretching

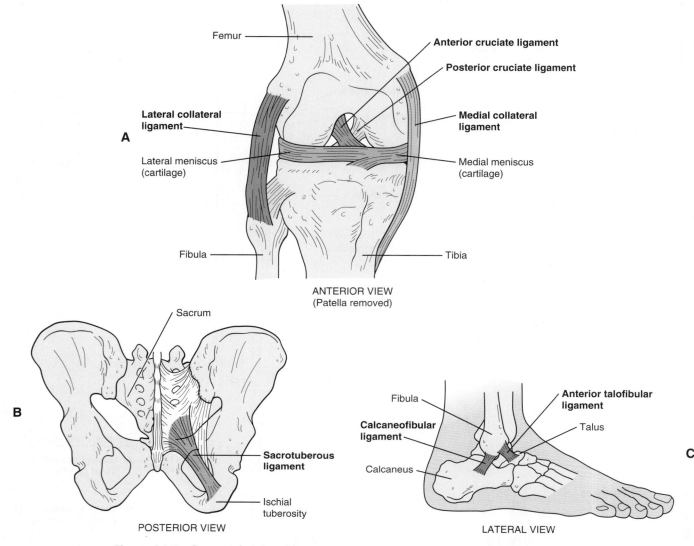

Figure 24-5   Commonly injured ligaments of the knee **(A)**, posterior hip **(B)**, and lateral ankle **(C)**.

To understand these techniques in depth, the general treatment protocol of a clinical massage session should be noted (Figure 24-6). The first step is the *assessment phase*, when the therapist is reviewing the client's intake form and history, checking joint ranges of motion, postural distortions, and other assessments (see Chapter 8). The *preparatory phase* follows, where lubricant is applied to the skin and the therapist begins to warm the tissues. Effleurage, pétrissage, and superficial warming friction are often used to prepare the area for deep-tissue techniques. As the tissues warm up, the therapist precedes directly to the *palpatory phase*, where tissues are explored for pathologies. The decrease in friction offered by the lubricant allows for easier recognition of trigger points, tight fibrous bands, adhesions, and anomalies such as cysts. The therapist may also

check for restriction of movement in the joints before beginning the application of clinical massage.

At this point the therapist enters the *treatment phase* where ischemic compression, cross-fiber friction, myofascial release, joint mobilization, and stretching. After treatment comes an *interval phase* where the therapist moves to an adjacent area for treatment, allowing the original treatment area a chance to rest. In the *retreatment phase*, the therapist returns to the original area of complaint and retreats it, hopefully finding decreased tension and soreness. Next comes the *recovery phase* in which the treated tissues are flushed with a final effleurage to help remove metabolic waste and reduce residual soreness.

After recovery is the *aftercare phase*. The therapist instructs the client in the use of ice, proper hydra-

BOX 24-1

Working With Athletes

Athletes must be handled differently than the average client. Athletes are constantly training their bodies to be stronger and function more effectively. They tend to fuel it with proper nutrition and stretch regularly to maintain elasticity. For these reasons, the metabolism and hence the healing factors of athletes tend to function more efficiently than that of the average client. Athletes snap back faster from muscular soreness and minor muscular injuries, often at about half the time it takes an inactive person to mend. However, it is prudent to remember that damage to ligaments and tendons have a fairly consistent healing time and will heal no faster in athletes than in the average client.

Another factor to remember is that although it is often necessary to ask the average client to reduce physical activities and devote some time to rest while recovering from an injury, this does not always hold true for athletes. Recommending that they stop exercise is counterproductive to their training and interferes with the trust necessary for the therapeutic relationship to function properly. It is generally better to get them to cut back on their training, by either cutting back one third on repetitions, one third on weight, or one third on time spent training.

Another factor to consider with athletes is the sport in which they participate. Each sport has its own set of muscular problems. In other words, marathon runners have different areas of muscular soreness than a golfer; swimmers have trigger points in different muscles than a gymnast.

The following factors may predispose the athlete to injury; review them with your active clients.

Improper Warm-up

Soft tissues must be warm to achieve elasticity. Failure to properly warm up puts the athlete at risk for muscular tears and fascial restrictions that limit performance. Aerobic activity should be used to raise the heart rate and get the blood moving through the muscle groups associated with the competitive activity. A stretching routine should follow. A minimum time frame of 15 to 20 minutes should be spent on warm-up. Warm-up should be increased as the athlete ages to accommodate the natural loss of flexibility associated with the aging process. If competing outdoors, a good rule of thumb is that the cooler the weather, the longer the warm-up should be.

Unsuitable Equipment

Braces, helmets, or pads that do not fit; worn-out shoes; and a bow that is not the right size for the archer are all exam-

ples of unsuitable equipment. Likewise, handlebars and bicycle seats that are not positioned correctly can damage an athlete's form and performance and can predispose him to injury.

Lack of Flexibility

Again, muscles that do not stretch can be overloaded by more powerful opposing muscle groups. Stretching is the answer; every athlete should have a stretching schedule in his or her training routine. Remind them that muscle is like clay; it tends to stretch when warm and break and tear when cold. Stretch after a warm-up and a cool-down.

Inadequate Training

Working too hard or not getting enough rest between sessions can negatively impact health and performance. Look for overtraining symptoms of irritability, fatigue, depression, sleeplessness, weakening of immune system, persistent muscular soreness, and an elevated morning pulse.

Muscle Strength Imbalances

The powerful quadriceps group is often so much stronger than the hamstrings that a sprinter can tear the hamstring with quadriceps contractions. Refer the athlete to an exercise specialist, athletic trainer, or physical therapist for specific muscle testing and weight training to balance strength. The best thing a massage therapist can do for his athletic clients is to study kinesiology.

Miscellaneous Factors

Improper diet and dehydration; competing in abnormal weather conditions such as rain, snow, or extreme temperature and humidity; structural factors such as fallen arches, spinal curvatures, and pelvic distortions; emotional distractions from unhealthy personal relationships; and finances can all contribute to injury.

Remember that regardless of the injury, the body is always seeking to repair itself and return it to normal. Look over the previous information and help your client identify any training-related mistakes. If you are working with an athlete who is in pain and you are unsure about how to help her, refer her to a therapist who has the necessary knowledge and experience or to another health care professional such as an athletic trainer or physical/occupational therapist.

---

tion, and any modifications to ADLs. The following discussion highlights the various techniques of treatment in detail.

Ischemic compression is sustained digital pressure applied to trigger points to relieve pain and discomfort. It is referred to as *ischemic compression* because the skin tends to blanch because of com-

pression of the capillaries and temporary loss of blood flow to the area. Ischemic compression may also be referred to as *trigger point work*. Although ischemic compression is one of the primary clinical massage techniques, it may also be used between the various strokes of a Swedish massage session to address specific trigger points.

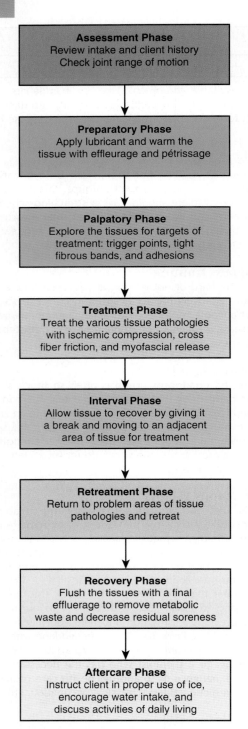

Assessment Phase
Review intake and client history
Check joint range of motion

Preparatory Phase
Apply lubricant and warm the
tissue with effleurage and pétrissage

Palpatory Phase
Explore the tissues for targets of
treatment: trigger points, tight
fibrous bands, and adhesions

Treatment Phase
Treat the various tissue pathologies
with ischemic compression, cross
fiber friction, and myofascial release

Interval Phase
Allow tissue to recover by giving it
a break and moving to an adjacent
area of tissue for treatment

Retreatment Phase
Return to problem areas of tissue
pathologies and retreat

Recovery Phase
Flush the tissues with a final
effluerage to remove metabolic
waste and decrease residual soreness

Aftercare Phase
Instruct client in proper use of ice,
encourage water intake, and
discuss activities of daily living

Figure 24-6 Flowchart for clinical application protocol of massage therapy.

Once the trigger points have been identified, apply direct pressure with thumb, forefinger, knuckle, or elbow. Generally, the pressure is exerted straight down into the trigger point, perpendicular to the body's surface (Figure 24-7). The tissue is compressed between the therapist's hand and the bony structures that support it. For areas that do not have good skele-

tal support, such as the abdomen, and for areas that contraindicate direct pressure to underlying structures, such as the sternocleidomastoid, the muscle may be lifted and a pincer gripped between thumb and forefinger (Figure 24-8). The pressure is held for 8 to 12 seconds or until a softening of the tissue is perceived. Often, the application of ischemic compression to a trigger point results in a local twitch response. When a local twitch response occurs, the ischemic compression may sometimes be held until the spontaneous twitching of the surrounding tissues ceases, even if it exceeds 15 seconds.

For muscles that have a tendency to roll under pressure, such as the biceps brachii and the erector spinae group, the therapist may have to remove some lubricant or stabilize the muscle with the opposite hand to prevent rolling.

Cross-fiber friction, or *deep transverse friction*, is a type of clinical massage developed by Dr. James Cyriax (see the Biography in Chapter 7). Cross-fiber friction is an excellent technique for breaking adhesions between muscle layers and encouraging the healing of strains and scar tissue. It may be applied with one or more fingertips moving perpendicular to the direction of tissue fiber (Figure 24-9).

When the therapist is working in multiple layers of muscle or for areas where it is hard to judge the direction of muscle fiber, it is often necessary to use circular friction or apply the back and forth movement of cross-fiber in multiple directions to make sure the correct area has been addressed (Figure 24-10).

Cross-fiber friction is often uncomfortable, so timing and depth must be carefully judged. Treatment time should be limited to 1 minute on any one injury site. The depth of cross-fiber friction should be performed within the pain tolerance of the client.

Myofascial release is a group of manual techniques used to reduce fascial restrictions. Several technique variations achieve this result, including deep gliding, pin and glide, torquing, and skin rolling.

The preferred myofascial release technique is the deep glide. It consists of slow, deep, controlled glide and is usually performed along the entire length of the muscle fibers. To be effective the excursion of the stroke must be long enough to cause the downward pressure to create a wave effect that separates muscle and fascia layers. This can be done with thumb, index finger, fist, forearm, elbow, knuckles, or the back of the hand without removing lubricant. To achieve a greater depth, the therapist may use both hands; one to direct the glide longitudinally and the other to exert downward pressure on top of the first hand. This technique does require some upper body strength or use of the therapist's weight, but it is fast and efficient.

The pin and glide technique is a variation of the deep glide. One hand anchors the tissue with pres-

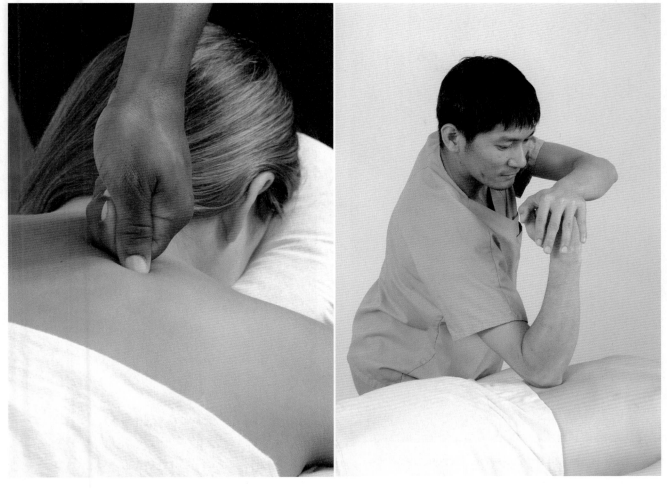

Figure 24-7 **A,** Applying ischemic compression on trigger point with thumb; **B,** using an elbow.

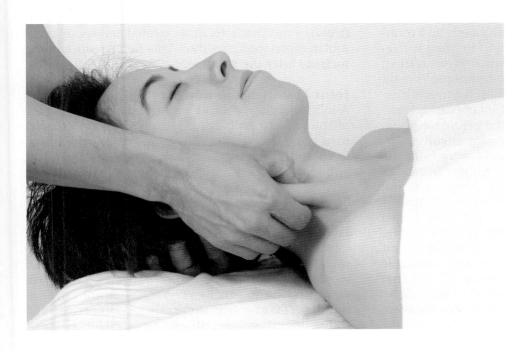

Figure 24-8 Applying ischemic compression on trigger point using a pincer grip on the sternocleidomastoid.

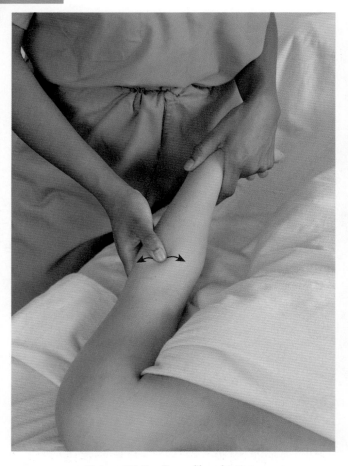

Figure 24-9   Cross-fiber friction.

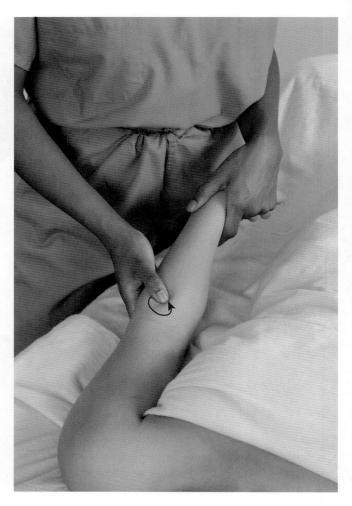

Figure 24-10   Circular friction.

sure as the other glides away from it, stretching and releasing the muscle and fascia (Figure 24-11).

Torquing is generally used for extremities and involves grasping the limb with both hands and rotating the tissues around the bone and holding it (Figure 24-12). As the fascia and muscular layers release, the tissue begins to loosen. This technique is a bit time-consuming but is more practical for treating extremities than other variations of myofascial release. Massage lubricant must be removed before torquing.

Skin rolling, or *Bindegewebsmassage,* involves lifting of the skin and superficial fascia away from the muscle by grasping it between the thumbs and index fingers. This roll of tissues is then compressed and rolled in a wave across the length of the treatment area (Figure 24-13). The movement is then repeated in a perpendicular direction to the original rolling. This technique is highly effective and brings instant hyperemia to the tissues but can be uncomfortable for those clients with fascial restrictions or adhesions. The treatment must be repeated in both directions and massage lubricant must be removed before application.

Flushing Effleurage
After deep-tissue techniques, a series of final effleurages are made to flush treated tissues of accumulated metabolic residue. This helps reduce client soreness after the massage.

Joint Mobilization and Stretching
A joint mobilization can vary from a simple jostling of the joint to progressive stretching of the muscles to a complete range of motion. Jostling mobilizations and progressive stretching reeducate the joint and its associated muscles on how movement can now be performed free of restrictions (Figure 24-14). Taking the associated joint(s) through a therapist-assisted complete range of motion allows the massage therapist to reassess range of motion. Taking the joint to its extremes also serves to lengthen the muscles and fascia by stretching. It is generally better to start with jostling of a joint, move to progressive stretching, and then finally achieve a full range of motion. This may happen in one session or over a series of several sessions, depending on client response.

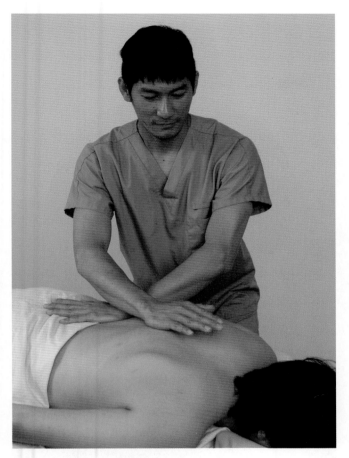

Figure 24-11 Myofascial release techniques of the deep glide or pin and stretch.

Injury Classification, Tissue Pathologies, and Treatment Strategies

Injuries are typically classified according to time of origin or occurrence. An **acute** injury is one of sudden onset and last only a few hours to a few days. They have a recognizable cause such as an auto accident or slipping on ice. Acute injuries generally result in some form of lesion. Although the cause of acute injuries is seldom a mystery; they too can act as a catalyst for the formation of chronic secondary problems, which are covered later in this chapter. Rapid onset injuries may include a whiplash sustained in a motor vehicle accident or a hamstring tear in a sprinter. Acute injuries should generally be treated with rest, ice, compression, and elevation. The therapist should wait 72 hours from the time of injury before beginning treatment.

A **chronic** injury is one that is long-standing, usually weeks, months, or even years. Because of the length of time, the original cause may or may not be known. Chronic injury clients may pursue other types of treatment such as painkillers, steroid injections, and even surgery, before finally arriving at your door. They usually seek out a massage therapist

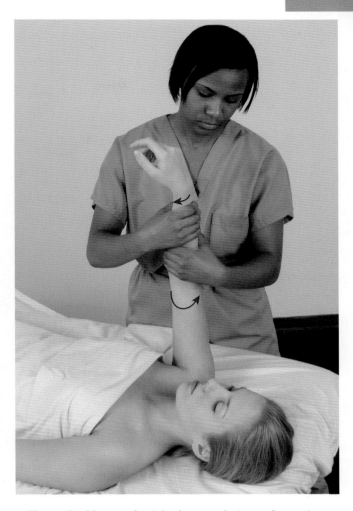

Figure 24-12 Myofascial release technique of torquing.

because of unsatisfactory progress with other options. Over time the original strain in the tissue may have healed, or it may have become chronic and given rise to other tissue pathologies such as trigger points, muscle strains, and scar tissue.

When dealing with the tissue pathologies of injuries and conditions, the question usually is which came first. This is especially true in injuries that have a gradual onset. A prolonged increase of muscular tone may lead to spasm. Sustained periods of spasm, inflammation, and pain often give rise to adhesions. The adhesion of muscles and fascia changes the engineering of movement and creates stress. This stress may produce trigger points, which in turn can restrict movement and lead to the further development of microtears (strains) in the tissues (Figure 24-15).

Trigger Points

Pathology

Trigger points are hypersensitive areas found in muscles, fascia, tendons, ligaments, skin, perios-

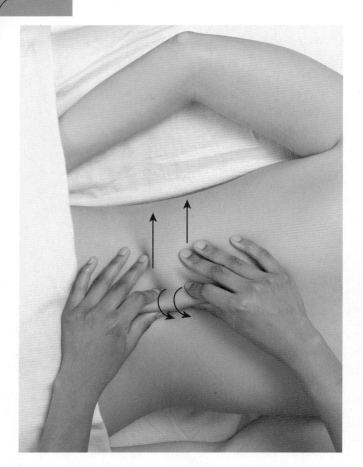

Figure 24-13   Myofascial release technique of skin rolling.

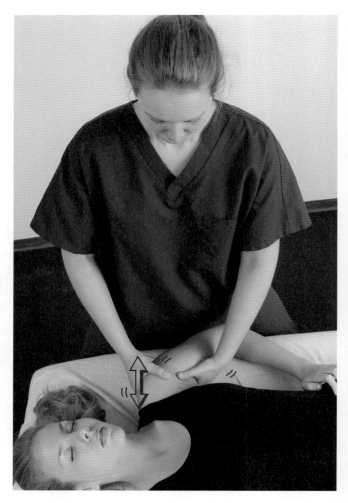

Figure 24-14   Passive range of motion of shoulder on supine client.

teum, and even organs. The term *hypersensitive* indicates that it takes little additional stimulation to cause discomfort. Experts have varying theories regarding the physiological mechanisms of the trigger point. One of these theories is that minute muscular tears, even on the cellular level, can cause a leakage of calcium ions from the sarcoplasmic reticulum. When the controlled flow of calcium through the ion channels occurs after nerve stimulation, muscular contraction is the result. The uncontrolled leakage of calcium from a tear may set up a condition of minute spasm, creating localized nodules surrounding the tear.

When subjected to ischemic compression, these areas elicit local tenderness and may exhibit referred pain phenomena. **Referred pain phenomena** is the tendency of trigger points to produce sensations (e.g., pain, tingling, numbness, itching, aching, heat, cold) distal from that of the trigger point. Occasionally, the pain is produced beneath the trigger point itself. According to Dr. Simons, the pain is referred distally from the site of the trigger point 73% of the time and the pain is produced locally 27% of the time. Often the referred pain sensation is reproduced

when ischemic compression is applied to the trigger point.

Trigger points may be classified as either active or latent. **Active trigger points** are noticeably painful even when no external physical stimulation takes place; they refer pain in specific patterns to other areas of the body. Both the local pain and referred pain of the active trigger point may be either constant or episodic in nature. Treatment may increase the local sensation of discomfort and the referred pain patterns. In general, the farther the referred pain sensation travels, the more active the trigger point. Trigger point location and their corresponding zones of referred pain are typically constant from one person to the next. This phenomena was discovered by Dr. Janet Travell and Dr. Simons while doing research on myofascial pain syndromes (see Dr. Travell's biography in Chapter 18). The consistency of trigger point locations and pain

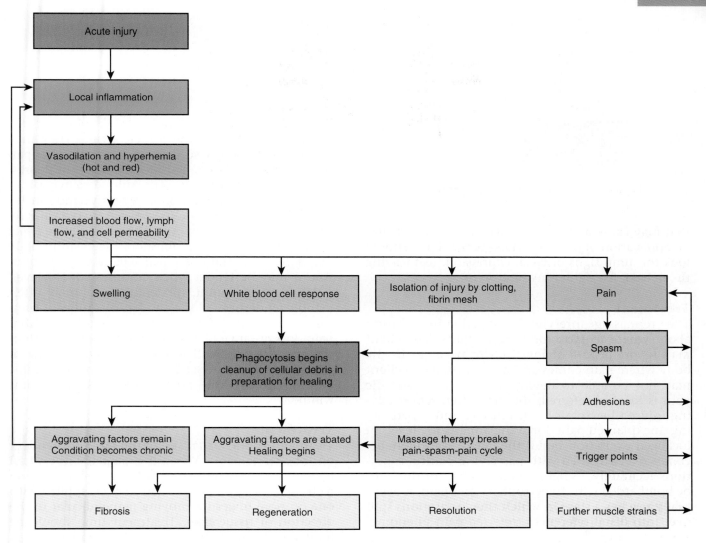

Figure 24-15   Flowchart of injury dynamics.

referral patterns enabled maps to be made of this particular pathology (Figure 24-16).

Latent trigger points are identical to active trigger points with one important exception; they do not hurt all the time. Latent trigger points remain hidden until activated by some stressor such as physical activity, emotional stress, or direct pressure on the muscle; then they are elevated to active status. Latent trigger points may cause muscles to weaken, shorten, or become stiff. Latent trigger points may be even more important to treat than active trigger points because they are so insidious, lying hidden and dormant and then suddenly producing pain unexpectedly. Often latent trigger points are found during palpation. The client may comment, "I didn't even realize it hurt there." Although active trigger points are best managed with periodic, focused, clin-

ical sessions, the management of latent trigger points is best handled with regular massage sessions.

On application of ischemic compression, the massage therapist may notice two other important symptoms of a trigger point: local twitch response and/or jump sign. The **local twitch response** is a reflexive impulse that causes the affected muscle or an adjacent muscle to fire spontaneously. This muscle firing basically results from a summation of sensory nerve information. When the sensation of pressure and discomfort caused by the ischemic compression is added to the existing pain of the trigger point, the total sensory input tends to overload the nerve pathway. The body shunts some of this electrical energy back down the motor nerve that causes a local reflexive contraction of surrounding tissues. The **jump sign** is a spontaneous reaction of pain or discomfort

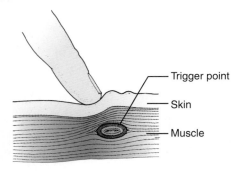

Figure 24-16   Palpation of a trigger point.

that may cause a client to wince, jump, or verbalize on application of pressure. Massage therapists should look for jump signs of facial expression, feet leaving the bolster, fist tightening, and so on.

Treatment

The pre-massage interview helps gather information about where to look for trigger points. The client may report persistent localized pain—areas in the body where pain comes and goes. Although a client may not be able to determine whether a specific pain is local or referred, she may often report having injured her rotator cuff muscles and experiencing unexplained pain down the arm. As the levels of localized excitation build, the client eventually becomes overwhelmed with perceiving painful sensations accurately. As her nervous system continues to be bombarded with hypertonicity and pain, it eventually reaches a state in which these sensations spill over into distal references (referred pain phenomenon).

This referred pain phenomenon can be used as an assessment tool. Look for trigger points that reproduce certain pain patterns. This is especially true for athletes who may experience pain symptoms that are positional in nature during competition. However, they cannot identify the same pain while inactive. In these cases, the therapist may apply pressure to different points until the pain they feel during movement is reproduced.

Trigger points can be palpated in muscle tissue as knots; lesions; or tight, fibrous bands (Figure 24-17). Ischemic compression may be applied to the trigger point for 7 to 15 seconds. If the pressure produces a local twitch response, pressure may be maintained until this muscle firing stops, even if it exceeds the 15-second recommendation. Cross-fiber friction may also be used to treat trigger points, especially when found as tight fibrous bands of muscle or tendon. Failure to properly address trigger points may interfere with muscle flexibility and may result in further muscle strains.

Everyone is ignorant, only in different subjects.

—Will Rogers

Muscle Strains

Pathology

Muscle strains are a pathological or traumatic discontinuity or tear of the muscle tissue. They may occur as microscopic surface tears or noticeably palpable tears that can be felt as separations or depressions in the muscle tissue. The mild tears may occur as a result of overworking or repetitive motion injuries, whereas moderate to severe tears typically result from trauma or sometimes the cumulative effect of long-term muscular abuse. Athletes informally may refer to a strain as a *pull*. Like a trigger point, strains may be tender when compressed. However, unlike a trigger point, moderate strains may often exhibit tenderness at the sudden cessation of pressure. Symptoms of strains may include localized pain, loss of range of motion, and loss of strength in the affected muscle. The more severe the grade of the strain (see the section on grading of strains in Chapter 15), the more severe these symptoms will be.

Treatment

Treatment of the actual site of the tear is dependent on it being palpable. When it is palpable, the strain is predominantly addressed with cross-fiber friction techniques. Cross-fiber friction may be applied with one or more fingertips moving perpendicular to the direction of tissue fiber. Treatment time should be limited to 1 minute to prevent microtrauma of overworking the tissue.

Scar Tissue

Pathology

Scar tissue is the connective tissue formed as a result of the healing process. Scar tissue may form on the skin to close an open wound, it may form in underlying soft tissues that have been torn, or both. An **adhesion** is a scar that occurs when two or more layers of tissue, which normally glide freely over one another, become adhered (often after an injury or surgery). These adhered tissues interfere with the normal glide between the tissue layers, and interrupt normal biomechanics. A **cicatricial** is a scar with considerable contraction resulting from the way it healed naturally (like a burn scar) or the way it was sutured. The contractions may pull nearby structures, like a lip, eyelid, nipple, or navel out of their normal position of symmetry. A **keloid** is a hypertrophic scar, usually containing blood vessels; it is

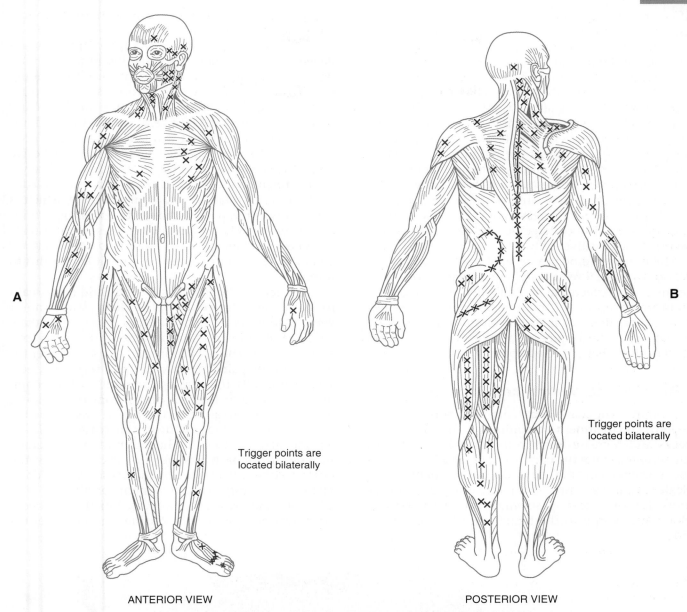

A

B

Trigger points are located bilaterally

Trigger points are located bilaterally

ANTERIOR VIEW

POSTERIOR VIEW

Figure 24-17   Trigger point map, anterior **(A)** and posterior **(B)** views.

often smooth, and either red or pink in color. Scar tissue is a necessary by-product of the healing process, but the formation of excessive or abnormal scar tissue can be counterproductive. Scar tissue may cause a reduction in movement as evidenced by pain, stiffness, weakness, and loss of mobility, which should be addressed with massage.

Treatment

Massage techniques can be used to reduce abnormal scar tissue formation after most types of injuries and surgeries. Cross-fiber friction is generally the technique of choice used to address scar tissue. It can be

applied superficially to the tissues of the skin to improve keloid scar appearance, or it can be done deeply to break up adhesions; reduce fibrosis; and treat scar tissue found in muscles, tendons, and fascia. Chucking, or parallel friction, can be applied to the scar. The depth should be determined by the client's comfort level. Treatment is easier if the scar is over a bony surface such as the knee, sternum, or ilium because the underlying skeletal tissue provides a base to work against.

Superficial scars, however, must sometimes be treated with skin rolling myofascial techniques. If the skin is loose enough, the abdominal scar can be lifted and braced from the back with one hand while the other hand treats the scar with cross-fiber friction. If possible, the scar may be lifted and pincer gripped between thumb and index finger to treat with cross-fiber friction (Figure 24-18). Note, however, that although this works after an appendectomy, it will not work after a tummy tuck; it is counterproductive to try and stretch skin when the purpose of the surgery was to tighten it. In these cases, treat the scar against the abdominal wall. Make sure that you know about any internal staples, pins, wires, or supportive meshes. Do not friction across these structures—it may damage the tissues. Obtain a doctor's release before treating a postinjury or post-surgery scar. Hypoallergenic lotions are recommended for sensitive skin.

The preferred modality of treatment for adhesions is also myofascial release. When myofascial release is applied to an affected area, a palpable and sometimes auditory separation of the tissues occurs. It may feel crunchy or sticky, or it may even make a squeaking sound much like a squeegee being run across glass as the layers are being peeled apart.

Aftercare: Ice, Water, and Education

For clients who have problems with soreness after deep-tissue treatment, recommend the use of ice packs and increase water consumption. Ice numbs the soreness while the pack is in place and minimizes the soreness felt the next day (see Chapter 23). Healthy muscle tissue is well hydrated. Excessive muscular tonus and spasm may restrict the flow of blood and lymph in the tissues. Drinking plenty of water helps flush out the toxins such as lactic acid and reduce residual soreness.

It is also necessary to educate the client receiving deep-tissue work about expectations regarding their pain level after injury and treatment. First, they should be taught that some increase in soreness is quite common and may be expected. This is true for almost any new therapeutic modality (e.g., chiropractic adjustments, electrostimulation, acupuncture, exercise, yoga stretching, and so on), but it is especially applicable when the client has been injured. The body perceives the treatment as increased sensory input, and this adds to the level of total neuromuscular activity, which is commonly felt as pain. Although the occasional "miracle" client feels better after just one session, it usually takes between four and six sessions before the body becomes acclimated to the new treatment and begins to respond.

The client in Box 24-2 is feeling little or no pain for days 1 and 2. On day 3, the client is in a motor vehicle accident, which does not cause immediate pain at the time of injury but does cause some soft-tissue trauma. The next morning, day 4, the client is in significant pain and cannot fully turn the neck. The client calls the massage therapist who recommends waiting at least 72 hours from the accident before starting treatment. On day 7, treatment begins. Some clients experience an increase in pain after the first treatment. These symptoms generally subside within 48 hours, but that is often when the next treatment is given. For this reason it is recommended that deep-tissue treatments be given at least 48 hours apart or every other day. Small peaks occur after treatment, and then declines in pain level be-

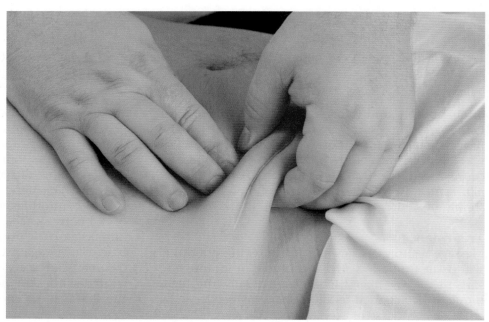

Figure 24-18 Therapist working on scar tissue using the braced-from-behind techniques.

BOX 24-2

Possible Symptoms of Trigger Points

- Pain and referred pain
- Local twitch response
- Palpation as knots; nodules; lesions; or tight, fibrous bands of tissue
- Glandular dysfunction (over- or underproduction of sweat, sebum, and so on)
- Sensations of numbness, coldness, tingling, or itching
- Muscular weakness, muscular tightness, or muscular spasm
- Abnormal skin color (excessively pale or red)
- Visceral dysfunction (halitosis, heartburn, vomiting, constipation, or diarrhea)

gin. Sometime between the fourth and sixth treatment session, the pain level drops below what it was when the client first came to the massage therapist and continues to fall until normalcy is returned. This may take 2 weeks to several months, depending on the severity of the injury and the client's activity level.

No one likes to hear that a client is hurting more after receiving a massage, but educating the client on the dynamics of clinical massage can help improve client morale. Likewise, instructing a client in proper aftercare puts part of the responsibility for recovery on the client. If the client chooses to ignore the aftercare recommendations and soreness results, then the therapist cannot be held liable for the client's posttreatment discomfort. When clients are noncompliant with the recommended aftercare and experience increased pain, a notation should always be made on their treatment record.

For Your Information

Massage therapy itself is a physically demanding profession, but clinical massage is even more so because of the pressures exerted through the hands. Although we were not designed to continuously bear weight with our fingers, hands, wrists, and arms, many of the common injuries associated with long years of massage practice can be prevented or alleviated through a combination of massage therapy and chiropractic care. For example, an intense burning across the heel of the palm could simply be a subluxation of the navicular bone causing impingement of the radial nerve. This condition is often corrected by a single adjustment. Find a chiropractor that practices the Gonstead method of chiropractic care and is proficient at adjusting the joints of the ex-

tremities and the spine. Trigger points in the finger flexors and extensors can be addressed with self-massage or by setting up regular weekly trades with another massage therapist.

The Most Common Mistake: Overworking

Overworking the tissue, especially injured tissue, is the most common mistake novice therapists make. The two types of overworking mistakes that can negatively affect any given treatment area are (1) working too deep and (2) working too long. Experience is the best teacher. Until you progress to a point where you are comfortable judging pressure, tissue density, and tissue resistance, limit your pressure and duration of treatment. For the beginning therapist, the general rules for deep-tissue massage are no more than 15 minutes of deep treatment to any one given region and no more than a total of 3 minutes of ischemic compression or cross-fiber friction on any spot.

Additionally, it is better to treat the area for a short time and then move to another muscle for awhile before returning to the original treatment site. In other words, three 1-minute treatments to the rhomboids are better than one 3-minute treatment.

Clinical massage is, by its very nature, an aggressive form of therapy. As far as depth is concerned, pressure is applied up to the client's level of tolerance. Ask the client to imagine a five-point scale of discomfort where 0 is no pain and 5 is equal to childbirth or having an icepick shoved into the thumbnail. You want to maintain a level of discomfort equivalent to a count of 3 or 4. To learn this scale yourself, see the sections later in this chapter on Gauging Pain and Pressure and the Pain Scale.

The preceding suggestions are basic guidelines for the beginning therapist. With experience, the therapist gains skill and confidence. Using the following four factors, the clinical massage therapist can properly judge how to modify treatment times:

1. **The amount of massage experience the client has had.** Someone who has had weekly massages for the last 10 years is going to be more comfortable receiving clinical massage. An experienced client will be better able to give direction and feedback to the therapist, even if it is their first session together. You can increase treatment time at the request of an experienced massage receiver.
2. **The experience of the therapist.** A therapist with 5 or more years of full-time massage experience can use their own judgment when exceeding the recommended guidelines.
3. **The level of familiarity between the client and the therapist.** If you are just starting to practice clinical massage, but have done 50 to 100 mas-

BONNIE PRUDDEN

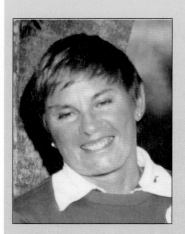

Born: January 29, 1914.

"Seeing ahead is fun. But pushing is very hard work."

The next time your hands grasp a taut trapezius, remember this: a woman, who, if she would have had her way, would have changed our physiological history. At the tender age of 2, your client would have already begun an exercise and strengthening program, supervised by her mother. The body on the table would be flexible, coordinated, and toned—and so would your own.

She is Bonnie Prudden, known in massage circles for her groundbreaking work in myotherapy, but her vision was to change the course of physical education and to develop stronger bodies from the very beginning, rather than provide pain relief for bodies unable to cope with the physical and emotional stress of everyday life.

Why should an individual be so passionate about jumping jacks and push-ups long before fitness became a fad? As a survivor of the Depression, alcoholic and abusive parents, an orphanage, and a stint in Marymount Convent (which she said was like trying "to lock a wild horse in a closet"), Bonnie Prudden found the outlet she so desperately needed in physical training. She was angry, and that anger fed her boundless, but undisciplined, energy. Prudden says she has physical educators to thank for teaching her the lessons of truth and honor. By contrast, Prudden laughs that her longtime assistant recalls learning nothing more from her physical education classes than the rules for 21 games.

Her fight for better bodies began in the early 1940s. Prudden was part of a team that tested the physical fitness level of children all over the world. The conclusions were frightening. American children were some of the weakest and were getting weaker.

"We are regressing physically," she explains. "Children ride the bus to school, sit down for class, ride the bus home, then sit in front of the TV or play video games until it's time to go to bed. We are a dying nation," Prudden claims, "dying from the inside out."

Ironically, Prudden was unable to recruit physical educators to join her crusade for better health and fitness. However, armed with passion and statistics, she did convince President Eisenhower to start the President's Council on Fitness. (Remember those tests you took in junior high to earn your patch from the president and how you yearned to be the fastest one up and down the rope, the longest distance jumper, or the strongest to throw the softball?)

To some, implementation of such a program would have been considered a milestone. To Bonnie Prudden, it was a compromise. She knew children could—and should—be stronger. She responded by publishing book after book on the subject and even introduced the first infant exercises in Sports Illustrated as early as the 1960s.

But it was completely by accident that she came across myotherapy. Through a combination of seeking relief from her own pain after a skiing accident and familiarity with the work of Drs. Hans Kraus, Janet Travell, and Desmond Tivy, myotherapy was born. Travell says it was sheer serendipity.

One morning Prudden woke up for a mountain climb with a neck so stiff it threatened to change her plans. While examining her neck, Dr. Kraus, an associate eager to get on with the climb, grabbed a spot and Prudden said, "I thought my eyeballs might pop out of my head, it hurt so bad." But when he let go, her neck was straight.

During work with Dr. Tivy, Prudden's job was to circle the patient's painful area for the doctor to inject—a method pioneered by Janet Travell—then

BONNIE PRUDDEN—cont'd

show the client how to exercise the area to prevent further problems. During one of these sessions, Prudden "marked the spot," and the pressure itself took care of the pain without injection. These events, coupled with her knowledge of anatomy and physiology, led to the study and development of myotherapy.

At the most basic level, myotherapy (*myo,* meaning *muscle; therapy,* meaning *service to*) involves the application of noninvasive pressure to painful muscular areas or specific prescribed points that may cause pain in another location (referred pain or satellite pain). Pressure is applied to these areas—using the finger, elbow, or a special tool—long enough to cut off or limit the oxygen supply to the area and/or fatigue the muscle, thus effecting change.

These painful areas or trigger points are consistently located irritable spots in a muscle that contribute to pain. This recurring pattern allowed Travell and then Prudden to map these points. (For a more scientific definition of trigger points, see various literature and studies conducted by Dr. Janet Travell. Travell laid much of the groundwork for myotherapy. Therapists and students interested in trigger point therapies can benefit from the excellent illustrations and body mapping found in her text, coauthored with Dr. David Simons, *Myofascial and Pain Dysfunction: The Trigger Point Manual,* volumes 1 and 2 (Williams and Wilkins, 1983 and 1992), as well as the medically oriented approach to, and definitions of, myofascial pain disorders.)

Prudden's textbooks on this subject, unlike Travell's, are written in laypeople's terms. Basically, any number of things can cause trigger points. It could have happened the summer you were 8 and the hay bale came crashing down on your head or just the other day when you lifted the desk to move it a couple of inches away from the wall. It may have even happened during your trip from your mother's womb into your new world. Regardless of the injury or insult to the muscle, trigger points may lie dormant until an emotionally or physically stressful event becomes the proverbial straw that breaks the camel's back. The affected muscle goes into spasm, which splints or guards the area in an attempt to limit usage and prevent further injury. This spasm-pain-spasm cycle shortens the muscle. Myotherapy returns the muscle to its lengthened, relaxed state.

But myotherapy does not stop there. Injured and insulted muscles were probably weak or shortened muscles from the start. That is why exercise, which includes stretching, is as integral to the success of myotherapy as the application of pressure to prescribed trigger points.

Massage therapists across the country are beginning to combine different styles of massage, including myotherapy, to address the special needs of clients. For instance, some massage therapists use traditional Swedish massage strokes to warm up the tissue and locate trigger points during the first half of the massage session. Later in the session, they return to these painful areas to apply deeper work, such as myotherapy, concluding with effleurage to flush out toxins that may have been released during the deeper work.

Prudden's advice for massage therapists? Exercise and stretch religiously. "You can't help people if you're not in good condition yourself," she warns. She also acknowledges the emotional toll of full-time massage therapy work and recommends a creative outlet such as dance, drawing, or sculpting, which she has incorporated into her school curriculum. She adds that it is important for students to get out and teach the community what they have learned about taking care of the body and managing pain.

BONNIE PRUDDEN—cont'd

Today the 89-year-old Prudden takes exercise as seriously as ever, although she has reluctantly heeded her body's message to slow down, which means she does not expect a body with two hip replacements to scale any major mountains. She personally teaches and inspires students at the Bonnie Prudden School for Physical Fitness and Myotherapy in Tucson, Ariz. To learn more about myotherapy, check out Prudden's books on the subject: *Myotherapy, Bonnie Prudden's Complete Guide to Pain-Free Living* (Ballantine Books, 1985) and *Pain Erasure* (M. Evans & Co., 2002).

sages on one certain client, the established rapport and familiarity with the client's body are reason enough to exceed the treatment time for that client.

4. **Physical condition of the client.** Clients who are physically fit, such as professional athletes, are often more "body aware" than the average client.

MINI-LAB

Using a medical dictionary such as *Dorland's Illustrated Medical Dictionary* or a reference book such as Travell and Simons' *Myofascial Pain and Dysfunction*, find and define words that could be used to describe a knot or ropiness, tonus or tension, thickening or swelling, tenderness or discomfort, and numbness. Use these appropriately in the objective portion of your treatment record.

Gauging Pain and Pressure

To be consistent in the application of pressure, develop a reliable system for gauging the subjective experience of pain (Figures 24-19 and 24-20). The following pain scale may be used or modified to suit your practice. Copies of this scale should be available for your clients to use as a reference when explaining their pain to you.

Common Pathologies, Their Symptoms, Causes, and Treatment

The following is a list of common conditions:
- Carpal tunnel syndrome
- Cervical, thoracic, or lumbar strains
- Spinal fusion
- Spinal laminectomy
- Rotator cuff strains
- Sciatica
- Temporomandibular joint dysfunction
- Thoracic outlet syndrome

A discussion of these conditions, including pathology, symptoms, causes, and treatment, follows.

Carpal Tunnel Syndrome

Pathology. Carpal tunnel syndrome is the narrowing or stenosing of the carpal tunnel, which usually results from repetitive motion injury. The carpal tunnel is located at the distal center wrist and proximal palm of the hand and transports the median nerve and finger flexor tendons. As swelling increases, the transverse carpal ligament compresses the median nerve. Compression decreases motor and sensory function of the median nerve and may even entrap the tendons and limit finger movement. As these ten-

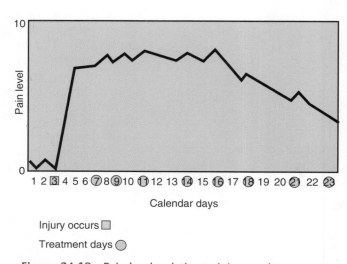

Figure 24-19   Pain levels relative to injury and treatment.

The Pain Scale

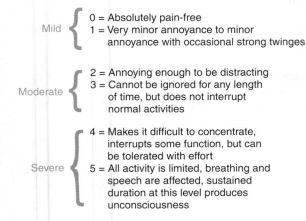

Mild {
0 = Absolutely pain-free
1 = Very minor annoyance to minor annoyance with occasional strong twinges

Moderate {
2 = Annoying enough to be distracting
3 = Cannot be ignored for any length of time, but does not interrupt normal activities

Severe {
4 = Makes it difficult to concentrate, interrupts some function, but can be tolerated with effort
5 = All activity is limited, breathing and speech are affected, sustained duration at this level produces unconsciousness

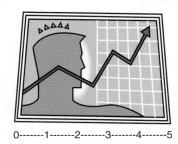

0-------1-------2-------3-------4-------5

Figure 24-20   The pain scale.

dons become irritated, extra synovial fluid is secreted, and extra interstitial fluid causes edema. The accumulated fluid compresses the nerve. Chronic inflammation causes the tendon sheaths to thicken, compounding the problem. Carpal tunnel may also be the by-product of a carpal fracture, arthritis, ligament avulsion, subluxation of the lunate, or generalized fluid retention from pregnancy or a medical condition.

Symptoms. Carpal tunnel syndrome is one of the most overdiagnosed and misdiagnosed ailments today. Sometimes forearm pain is misdiagnosed as carpal tunnel when it is actually just an accumulation of multiple trigger points in the flexors and extensors located in the forearm. In rare cases, thoracic outlet syndrome may produce symptoms that are similar to carpal tunnel and may be misdiagnosed as such.

The symptoms of carpal tunnel syndrome may occur in only one forearm or bilaterally and may include pain or burning, numbness or tingling distal to the wrist, loss of grip strength, and clawing or drawing up of fingers in severe cases.

Causes. Most carpal tunnel syndrome is a result of repetitive motion injuries such as the following:
- Overuse in keyboarding (either computer or piano), lifting and scanning groceries with the same hand
- Weight bearing with hands, along with improper arm-to-wrist angle (chiropractors, massage therapists, and gymnasts)

Treatment. For clients with this syndrome, local massage over the wrist is contraindicated if acute inflammation is present. Use or recommend ice (see Chapter 23.) In chronic conditions, elevating the limb and using effleurage or lymphatic drainage

techniques to move fluid out of the extremity can reduce edema. Penetrating moist heat can help soften and allow stretch of fibrous adhesions. Passive movement of the elbow, wrist, and finger joints maintains range of motion. Ischemic compression, cross-fiber friction, and deep thumb stripping is recommended for the finger flexors and extensors and their tendons crossing the wrist.

Cervical, Thoracic, or Lumbar Strains
Pathology. Muscular strains of the muscles surrounding the spine account for the highest number of injuries today. The most common pathology of spinal-related strains is the microtearing of muscle fiber with localized spasm and pain. Although many of these injuries are well within the scope of the massage therapist, the chance of disc or vertebral involvement is always possible, which necessitates referring the client to their chiropractic or medical physician for further diagnosis.

Symptoms. Characteristics of a back or neck strain may include decrease in neck or back range of motion, spasm, stiffness, pain, limitation of normal activities, and severe cases may cause an interruption of sleep.

Causes. Muscular strains may be the result of any of the following:
- Motor vehicle accident
- Sports injuries
- Slips and falls
- Improper lifting technique or repetitive lifting of heavy loads
- Repetitive motion injuries

Treatment. Depending on the location of the strain, ischemic compression, cross-fiber friction, myofascial release, and deep thumb stripping are recommended for either of the following groups of muscles:

Cervical region
- Cervical paraspinals
- Trapezius
- Splenius capitis and splenius cervicis
- Levator scapulae
- Scalenes
- Sternocleidomastoid

Thoracic region
- Trapezius
- Rhomboids
- Latissimus dorsi
- Intercostals
- Thoracic paraspinals

Lumbar region
- Lumbar paraspinals
- Gluteals
- Quadratus lumborum
- Iliopsoas

Ice is the preferred treatment in all acute injuries and is used posttreatment. Heat can be used to loosen up the area before treatment as long as no swelling or inflammation is present. Clinical massage can be used to manage the pain and restore some lost mobility. Clients with long-standing back pain may elect surgical procedures to address the condition. The section below discusses ramifications of clients with spinal fusions and laminectomies.

Spinal Fusion

Pathology.   When the spine is fused in a surgical procedure, a damaged intervertebral disc is removed and replaced with a fragment of bone harvested from the hip or a cadaver bone bank. Most fusion surgeries are indicated for ruptured or deteriorating disks. The intent is to maintain the space between the two vertebrae to keep them from collapsing and compressing the nerve root. The net result is that the two vertebra are fused into one longer segment; the back loses one joint and so has a slight decrease in mobility. Many patients of successful fusion surgeries have complained that the hip site where bone was harvested experiences more pain than the fusion site itself. Most fusions are performed on either the lumbar or cervical spine; thoracic fusions are rare. If the fusion fails, then nerve compression occurs as the vertebrae collapse back together. Pain is often excruciating and usually limits all activity including sleep.

Symptoms.   Traits of a successful fusion may include loss of mobility, stiffness, and some pain. Characteristics of a failed fusion include the following:
- Excruciating pain
- Debilitating limitation of normal activities
- Interruption of sleep

- Possible loss of muscular control in severe cases (e.g., rubbery knee)
- Failed lumbar fusions may also cause groin pain, rectal pain, and even impotence in men in severe cases

Causes.   Fusion failure may be the result of any of the following:
- Improper healing resulting from lack of local blood supply
- Persistent movement at the site, producing a fibrous union that is unstable
- The body may reject the grafted bone tissue (rare)
- Improper healing may result from infection or surgical error (rare)

Treatment.   Depending on the location of the fusion (cervical or lumbar), ischemic compression, cross-fiber friction, and deep thumb stripping are recommended for either of the following groups of muscles:
- Cervical paraspinals
- Trapezius
- Levator scapulae
- Scalenes
- Sternocleidomastoid

OR
- Lumbar paraspinals
- Quadratus lumborum
- Iliopsoas

Clinical massage can be used to manage the pain and restore some lost mobility. Do not perform ballistic movements, extreme ranges of motion, or stretches unless ordered by the client's physician. Putting the client in an extreme stretch could break the fusion, and possibly paralyze the patient, especially if the fusion is weak. Do not be afraid to use trigger point and cross-fiber techniques around the spinal surgical site after it is completely healed; work within the client's level of comfort.

Spinal Laminectomy

Pathology.   A spinal laminectomy is almost the opposite of a fusion; the surgeon removes a section of bone from the vertebra, a piece of the lamina. A laminectomy is indicated when stenosing or narrowing of the canal that the nerve root passes through puts pressure on the nerve. This may cause numbness, tingling, or excruciating pain. The intent is to enlarge the canal around the nerve root. Unfortunately, in some cases, the space created by the bone removal is filled in with scar tissue that may entrap the nerve.

Symptoms.   Traits of a successful laminectomy may include loss of mobility, stiffness, and some pain. Characteristics of a failed laminectomy include persistence of preoperative symptoms, including moderate to excruciating pain, possible interruption of sleep, and general symptoms of discomfort.

Causes.   Laminectomy failure may be the result of pressure against nerve by soft tissues as scarring develops at surgical site and bone spur growth as the body seeks to rebuild the lamina.

Treatment.   Clinical massage can be used to manage the pain and restore some lost mobility. Depending on the location of the laminectomy (cervical or lumbar), ischemic compression, cross-fiber friction, and deep thumb stripping are recommended for either of the following groups of muscles:
- Cervical paraspinals
- Trapezius
- Levator scapulae
- Scalenes
- Sternocleidomastoid

OR
- Lumbar paraspinals
- Quadratus lumborum
- Iliopsoas

Rotator Cuff Strains

Pathology.   Shoulder injuries are one of the most commonly treated injuries for the clinical application of massage therapy. Most shoulder injuries directly affect one or more of the four rotator cuff muscles—supraspinatus, infraspinatus, teres minor, and subscapularis. These four muscles may become symptomatic as a result of adhesive capsulitis or repetitive strain injuries. Trigger points in these muscles set up referred pain and increased tone in surrounding muscles. Because of the arm pain referrals, infraspinatus and teres minor strains are occasionally confused with carpal tunnel syndrome or thoracic outlet syndrome.

Clinical test for suspected rotator cuff injury. The patient should stand with the arm at the side and elbow flexed to 90 degrees. The patient externally rotates the shoulder (humerus) while the therapist resists the movement. If pain and/or weakness is noted, then the rotator cuff is injured.

Clinical test for severe rotator cuff injury. The therapist should abduct and extend the client's affected arm laterally until it is parallel to the floor. The therapist should release the arm with the client supporting it. The client *slowly* lowers the arm to the side. If the arm drops to his side or it cannot be lowered smoothly, then severe inflammation or a severe tear of the rotator cuff is sus-

pected. These types of injuries should be referred to an orthopedic surgeon for proper diagnosis.

Symptoms.   Injuries to the supraspinatus muscle are evidenced by the following:
- Inability to lift arm above shoulder height and/or limited overhead activity such as painting, pruning, and combing, brushing, or washing hair
- Sharp debilitating pain
- Referred pain to the deltoid and the biceps tendon

Infraspinatus and teres minor strains are characterized by the following:
- Limited behind the back movement such as hooking bras, putting on jackets, or removing a wallet
- Dull and fatiguing pain
- Referred pain to suboccipital region, rhomboids, and most of the affected arm

Subscapularis strains are indicated by the following:
- Limited glenohumeral motion, or frozen shoulder, and adhesive capsulitis
- Deep joint pain
- Referred pain to triceps, wrist, infraspinatus, and pectoralis major

Causes.   Rotator cuff injuries may be the result of repetitive motion activities such as the following:
- Carrying a toddler on one hip
- Jobs with the arms extended in front, such as hair styling, keyboarding, or driving
- Sports activities such as golf, tennis, bowling, pitching, or fly fishing

They can also be caused by muscular overload injuries resulting from the following:
- Slips and falls
- Pull-starting a lawn mower or outboard motor
- Carrying heavy suitcases or a massage table

They can also be the result of nonuse, such as with the following activities:
- Sleeping with the arm over or behind the head
- Inactivity during a long surgery (e.g., heart surgery)
- Inactivity following surgery (e.g., mastectomy)
- Putting the arm in a sling or cast

Treatment.   Ischemic compression, cross-fiber friction, and myofascial release should be directed primarily to the four rotator cuff muscles and secondarily to the following muscles:
- Rhomboids
- Levator scapulae
- Trapezius
- Latissimus dorsi
- Deltoids
- Pectoralis major
- Biceps brachii
- Triceps brachii

Because of its location, the subscapularis presents an access challenge. Begin by bolstering under the shoulder joint in the prone position and flexing the elbow so the wrist is at waist level. Then press the lower humerus toward the table. The scapula should pop up, allowing access to the muscles underneath.

After these treatment protocols, gently provide passive range of motion to the affected arm while in the supine position. While passively mobilizing the arm in any direction, take your cues from the client. The motion should be pain free, and the mobilization should stop at the first symptom of pain. Have the client actively pull the arm back down to his side against your slight resistance and repeat a few times, increasing the range slightly with each subsequent movement. Finish with a closed-fist tapotement over the glenohumeral joint and ice the shoulder thoroughly for 20 minutes, covering the entire scapula, deltoid, upper trapezius, and humeral attachments of the pectoralis major and upper biceps brachii.

Aftercare for the client should include the use of ice and some home range-of-motion therapy such as wall-walking. Have the client stand a little less than arm's length distance from a wall. Starting at waist height, have her touch the wall with the fingers of the affected arm. Using her best "yellow-pages" style, let her fingers "do the walking" up the wall very slowly, until she hits a point of pain. At this point, she should pause, slide her hand back down the wall to the starting position and repeat. This should be done for 10 repetitions at least once a day, according to client comfort. If the shoulder responds positively, then continue treatment for 2 to 4 weeks; if the shoulder becomes exacerbated, refer immediately to an orthopedist. NOTE: exacerbation does not include the 24-hour increase in muscular soreness that sometimes follows a deep-tissue treatment.

Sciatica

Pathology. *Sciatica* refers to a condition of inflammation to the sciatic nerve. This can be brought about by compression of the nerve by vertebra or disks in the lumbar spine or by an injury to nerve distal to its exit from the spine. When a disk is involved, it is sometimes a result of muscular imbalances. For example, tight quadratus lumborum and psoas muscles on one side of the spine can act to compress the lumbar vertebrae together. This pressure can cause the disk to migrate to the opposite side of the spine where it bumps the nerve, firing pain down the hip and leg. Therefore when sciatic pain symptoms are presented on one side of the body, always examine the low back carefully on the opposite side of the involved hip or leg. Sciatic pain is directly affected by stress; an increase in emotional stress may cause muscle tightening that exacerbates pain.

In rare cases, sciatic pain can also be caused by entrapment of the sciatic nerve by the piriformis muscle of the affected side. This condition is sometimes referred to as *piriformis syndrome.* Piriformis syndrome results from an anatomical anomaly where one or both branches of the sciatic nerve penetrate the belly of the piriformis muscle instead of passing underneath it. Statistically, in 80% to 85% of the population, the sciatic nerve passes under the piriformis, but in the other 15% to 20%, the nerve bifurcates the muscle. The net result is that tightness in the piriformis puts a chokehold on the sciatic nerve.

Symptoms. Symptoms of sciatica may occur in one or both legs and can include dull, aching pain in the hip or buttock; burning or coldness; numbness or tingling; and sharp, lightening stabs of pain extending down the leg and into the foot.

Causes. Possible causes for sciatica include the following:
- Anatomical predisposition
- Lordosis, obesity, or late-stage pregnancy
- Sitting for long periods (truck drivers or receptionists) or sitting on a thick wallet
- Leg length discrepancies
- Trauma
- Repetitive motion injuries such as improper lifting or bending

Treatment. Recommended treatment is ischemic compression, cross-fiber friction, and myofascial release to the following muscles:
- Quadratus lumborum
- Gluteus minimus
- Gluteus medius
- Gluteus maximus
- Piriformis

NOTE: Use extreme care when working the piriformis; this muscle is in such close proximity to the sciatic nerve that almost no way is available for applying compression to the muscle without applying pressure to the sciatic nerve itself.

Manual traction to the legs seems to increase effectiveness. Use a towel to traction one leg at a time or a karate belt with loops tied in each end to traction both legs simultaneously (Box 24-3).

Temporomandibular Joint Dysfunction

Temporomandibular joint (TMJ) dysfunction is a common ailment affecting either the jaw joint, its musculature, or both. Its chief symptoms are pain (e.g., jaw pain, toothache, headache, and earache), clicking of the TMJ, and limited range of motion. It is estimated that 60% of the population either clench or grind their teeth, but only 25% are aware of it.

Pathology. TMJ dysfunction is an imbalance and dysfunction of the jaw joint, which is also referred to as the *craniomandibular joint.* The mandible is a unique bone in the human body. It is the only bone in the body that is almost perfectly symmetrical, having mirror images of the same joint at each end. This precision engineering requires that the movement of the jaw also be symmetrical. Dysfunction of the TMJ begins when muscular imbalances occur on one or both sides of the mandible or with postural distortions.

Trigger points form, and tonus increases, often unilaterally, causing a misalignment of the jaw, throwing the bite off. When the body rests, it prefers to have the jaw in a neutral position. If both sets of molars do not touch simultaneously, then the jaw unconsciously hunts for the proper position by clenching or grinding all night long. Clenching and open-mouth strains tend to traumatize the masseter muscles. Grinding (bruxism) tends to traumatize the pterygoids. The temporalis muscles become inflamed because they can be used to bilaterally lock the jaw in place.

Being pain-free is not possible for a client who has active TMJ, so just settle for finding his comfort zone. Pain relief is usually immediate with the majority of clients, achieving a 50% reduction of pain within minutes of treatment. However, the treatment is painful and probably should only be done when the TMJ flares up and the client is at a personal limit on pain tolerance. If done in conjunction with a longer massage session, do this routine first (see treatment that follows). If not treated in a timely manner, muscular TMJ can progress into osseous TMJ. With osseous TMJ the cartilaginous disk is displaced, and the jaw joint itself begins to erode, losing vital bone as the joint degenerates.

Symptoms. TMJ symptoms include some or all of the following:
- Pain, especially jaw pain, toothache, earache, or headache
- Fatigue in the jaw muscles
- Inability to chew gum, nuts, popcorn, granola, or tough meat
- Inability to open mouth to full extension
- Breaking or wearing of tooth enamel or dental work
- Popping, clicking, or grinding in jaw joint

Causes. There are two groups of causes for TMJ. The first is open-mouth strains resulting from the following:
- Trauma from accidents or a blow to the jaw (e.g., whiplash or air bag injury in a motor vehicle accident)
- Normal extension or hyperextension of the jaw for an abnormally long period, as during dentistry or oral surgery

- Hyperextension of the jaw during dentistry or oral surgery
- Muscular imbalance (hyoid muscles injured in a whiplash may become shortened, acting to depress and protract the jaw; this causes the opposing masseter and temporalis muscles to be overworked)

The second group of causes result from repetitive motion injuries, including the following:
- Clenching an ink pen, paintbrush, or car keys in the teeth or chewing fingernails, especially on one side of the mouth only
- Clenching the teeth because of unresolved emotional issues (e.g., anger, fear) while either awake or asleep
- Grinding at new dental work; an asymmetry as small as a grain of sand is noticed, especially if it keeps the molars from touching simultaneously
- Grinding at old dental work that is beginning to deteriorate

Treatment. Ischemic compression and cross-fiber friction should be applied to the masseter, pterygoids, and temporalis. The masseter and lateral pterygoid muscles may be worked externally, or the therapist may glove and insert the index finger carefully into the oral cavity, pincer gripping the masseter and lateral pterygoid through the cheek wall against the thumb (Figure 24-22). NOTE: The use of latex gloves is contraindicated for any client with latex sensitivity, especially in the mouth. See Chapter 4 for more information on safety precautions, latex allergies, and the use of vinyl or latex gloves. Never push the mandible back and do not try to stretch a contracted muscle. If referred pain is a jaw pain in the mandible, focus on the masseter. If the referred pain is an earache, focus on the lateral pterygoid. If the referred pain is a headache, focus on the temporalis.

Thoracic Outlet Syndrome
Pathology. Thoracic outlet syndrome refers to the compression or entrapment of one or more of the structures of the neurovascular bundle located from the neck, upper chest, and axilla. Entrapment is commonly caused by hypertonicity of the pectoralis minor and scalene musculature. Compression may be caused when tightness in these muscles causes a reduction of space between the clavicle and the first rib, reducing the aperture that houses the brachial plexus and related vessels located there. Pain and weakness down the arm are common symptoms. Some clients also experience pain in the chest and neck.

Symptoms. Thoracic outlet syndrome symptoms are diverse and depend on the structure being impinged. Pressure on the sensory branch of the nerve

BOX 24-3

Manual Traction

Leg Traction With Towel

Fold a standard bath-size towel lengthwise in quarters to achieve a long, narrow length of fabric. Standing at the foot of the massage table with the client in the supine position, place the center of the towel underneath the ankle of the affected leg and perpendicular to it. Take the left side of the towel, cross it over the top of the ankle, and let it hang off the foot of the table. Take the right side of the towel, cross it over the top of the ankle, and let it hang off the foot of the table. The towel ends should cross the top of the foot. Now take both towel ends in your hands and lean backward with your body weight, applying static manual traction to the leg. Do not bounce (ballistic moves); just decompress the lumbar spine and hip (Figure 24-21, *A*).

Bilateral Leg Traction With Karate Belt

Take a standard, pleated karate belt and tie a loop in both ends with a double knot. The loop should be large enough to slip over the foot of a large client or even a small shoe. The knot should be securely tied but as flat as possible to be comfortable. Standing at the foot of the massage table with the client in the supine position, slide one loop around the client's right foot. Circle the karate belt behind the therapist's low back and then slide the other loop around the client's left foot. Now slide the karate belt to a comfortable place around your own torso (e.g., around your waist or hips). Lean backward into the belt, exerting a static manual trac-tion on the client's legs as you hold the belt ends just above the knots (Figure 24-21, *B*).

Neck Traction With Towel

Fold a standard bath-size towel lengthwise in quarters to achieve a long, narrow length of fabric. Standing at the head of the massage table with the client in the supine position, place the center of the towel underneath the neck of the client in a perpendicular position. Do not cross the towel across the client's face or throat. Take both towel ends in your hands and lift them straight up toward the ceiling and then superiorly across the client's ears. It may be necessary to experiment with positioning until you are comfortable. NOTE: Earrings should be removed before cervical traction. Lean backward with your body weight, applying static manual traction to the neck. Do not bounce (ballistic moves) and avoid vigorously rotating the towel; just decompress the cervical spine (Figure 24-21, *C*).

• • •

For all three traction procedures, use your weight to exert the traction, being careful not to let the client or sheets slide on the table. Obviously, your weight and the client's weight directly affect how much effort must be used to achieve the traction effect. Traction of this sort should be avoided if the client has had recent fusion, hip replacement, or joint instability. Check with the referring physician before administering this procedure.

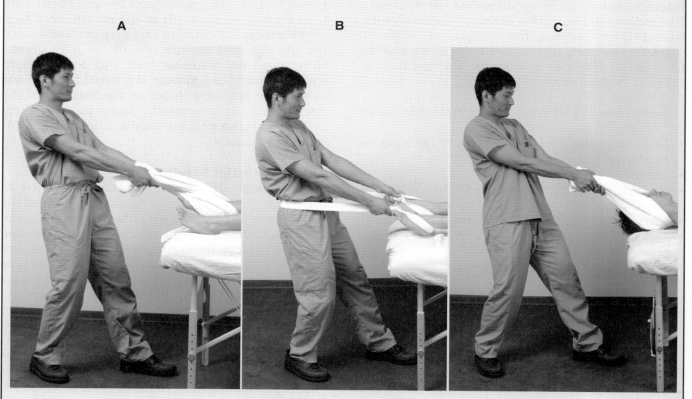

A   B   C

Figure 24-21 **A**, Towel traction on leg; **B**, karate belt traction on legs; **C**, towel traction on neck.

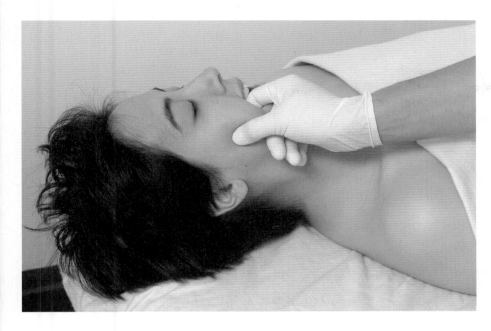

Figure 24-22 Rubber-gloved therapist working inside oral cavity of TMJ client.

may cause pain and numbness or tingling in the arm and chest. Pressure on the motor branch of the nerve may cause arm weakness and loss of grip strength. Pressure on the artery may cause reduction or loss of pulse pain, as well as numbness or tingling down the arm resulting from ischemia. Pressure on the vein may cause edema. This is the result of an increased back-pressure in the vessels creating a surplus of interstitial fluid in the extremity.

Causes. This syndrome can be caused by any of the following:

- Accidents (e.g., slips and falls, whiplash, or seat belt or air bag compression injuries)
- Postsurgical trauma (e.g., mastectomy, lung removal, or breast augmentation)
- Persistent or violent coughing, sneezing, or vomiting

Alternatively, it may be the result of repetitive motion injuries such as playing an instrument, carrying a heavy backpack, or shallow chest breathing that increases the use of accessory breathing muscles.

Treatment. Ischemic compression, cross-fiber friction, and myofascial release should be directed at the scalenes, pectoralis minor, and the anterior and posterior cervical musculature. Manual traction with a towel is also effective in decompressing the cervical spine (see Figure 24-21, *C*).

For Your Information

Use your knowledge of anatomy and kinesiology to locate muscles and their attachments. Have the client perform an isolated contraction of the muscle during palpation to determine correct location. Then have the client relax the muscle for you to locate trigger points and conduct cross-fiber friction.

> *There must be some primal force,*
> *but it is impossible to locate.*
> *I believe it exists, but can not see it.*
> *I see its results.*
> *I can even feel it,*
> *but it has no form.*
> —Zhuangzi, philosopher, 400 BC

SUMMARY

The first section of this chapter reviewed the theory of injury rehabilitation, including causes of injury, stages of rehabilitation, and tissue healing. The second section examined the causes, physiology, and treatment of tissue pathologies, including trigger points, adhesions, increased muscle tone, decreased joint mobility, and scar tissue formation. Additionally, specific deep-tissue clinical techniques for treating these pathologies were covered, including ischemic compression, cross-fiber friction, myofascial release, flushing effleurage, joint mobilizations, and stretching. Also covered in this section were the topics of aftercare, overworking the tissue, gauging pain and pressure. This chapter then explored some common injuries and their causes, symptoms, and treatment strategies. The third section of the chapter consists of an anatomical index that the therapist can use as a reference for specific muscle problems. Using this information, the therapist can now form strategies for area-specific treatment that can be used alone in a short clinical setting or as a focused segment of a 1-hour session.

MATCHING

Write the letter of the best answer in the space provided.

A. Acute
B. Active trigger points
C. Local twitch response
D. Jump sign

E. Myofascial release
F. Chronic
G. Cross-fiber friction
H. Lesion

I. Trigger points
J. Latent trigger points
K. Referred pain phenomena
L. Ischemic compression

_____ 1. Trigger points that do not hurt all the time; they are activated by some stressor such as physical activity, emotional stress, or direct pressure on the muscle

_____ 2. Sustained digital pressure applied to trigger points to relieve pain and discomfort; referred to as *trigger point work*

_____ 3. Another term for *deep transverse friction*

_____ 4. The tendency of trigger points to produce sensations of pain (e.g., pain, tingling, numbness, itching, aching, heat, cold) distal from that of the trigger point

_____ 5. A reflexive impulse that causes the affected muscle or an adjacent muscle to fire spontaneously

_____ 6. An injury of sudden onset

_____ 7. Areas that are noticeably painful even when no external physical stimulation is present; they refer pain in specific patterns

_____ 8. A spontaneous reaction of pain or discomfort that may cause a client to wince or verbalize on application of pressure

_____ 9. An injury that is long-standing; the original cause may not be known

_____ 10. Any noticeable or measurable deviation from the normal composition of healthy tissue

_____ 11. A group of manual techniques used to reduce fascial restrictions; techniques include deep gliding, pin and glide, torquing, and skin rolling

_____ 12. Hypersensitive areas found in muscles, fascia, tendons, ligaments, skin, periosteum, and even organs

Bibliography

Ardion W: *Lecture on temporomandibular joint dysfunction,* Lafayette, La, 1994, Author.

Chaitow L, Walker-DeLany J: *Clinical application of neuromuscular techniques,* vol 1, New York, 2000, Churchill Livingstone.

Chaitow L: *Palpation skills: assessment and diagnosis through touch,* New York, 2000, Churchill Livingstone.

Davies C: *The trigger point therapy workbook: your self-treatment guide for pain relief,* Oakland, Calif, 2001, New Harbinger.

Frazier MS, Drzymkowski JW: *Essentials of human diseases and conditions,* ed 2, Philadelphia, 2000, WB Saunders.

Gehlsen GN, Ganion LR, Helfst R: Fibroblast responses to variation in soft tissue mobilization pressure, *Med Sci Sports Exer* 31:4, 1999.

Gould BE: *Pathophysiology for the health professions,* ed 2, Philadelphia, 2002, WB Saunders.

Hoppenfeld S: *Physical examination of the spine and extremities,* Norwalk, Conn, 1976, Appleton-Century-Crofts.

Klafs C, Arnheim DD: *Modern principles of athletic training,* St Louis, 1981, Mosby.

Lake Charles Memorial Hospital: *Pain scale,* Lake Charles, La, 2002, Author.

Mense S, Simons D, Russell IJ: *Muscle pain: understanding its nature, diagnosis, and treatment,* Baltimore, 2001, Lippincott Williams & Wilkins.

Oviedo Physical Medicine and Rehabilitation: *Pathology for massage therapists,* 1995, Author.

St. John P: *St. John neuromuscular therapy seminars,* manual I, Largo, Fla, 1994, Author.

St. John P: *St. John neuromuscular therapy seminars,* manual II, Largo, Fla, 1994, Author.

Southmayd W, Hoffman M: *SportsHealth: the complete book of athletic injuries,* New York and London, 1981, Quick Fox.

Travell J, Simons D: *Myofascial pain and dysfunction: the trigger point manual,* vol I, Baltimore, 1983, Williams and Wilkins.

Travell J, Simons D: *Myofascial pain and dysfunction: the trigger point manual—the lower extremities,* vol II, Baltimore, 1992, Williams and Wilkins.

Werner R, Benjamin BE: *A massage therapist's guide to pathology,* ed 2, Baltimore, 2002, Lippincott Williams & Wilkins.

Seated Massage

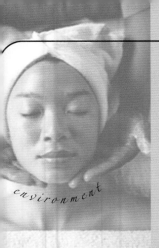

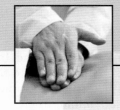

25

Ralph R. Stephens, BSEd

"We can be knowledgeable with another man's knowledge, but we cannot be wise with another man's wisdom."

—Michel De Montaigne

STUDENT OBJECTIVES

After completing this chapter, the student should be able to:

- List major considerations when purchasing a massage chair
- Describe types of seated massage equipment
- State reasons why a massage therapist might choose to massage a client in the seated position
- Explain and demonstrate procedures of sanitation and hygiene
- Properly adjust the massage chair for the client
- Describe proper body mechanics and safety considerations for the massage therapist who uses a massage chair
- Use adaptive professional communication to effectively communicate with the client before and during the massage
- Perform a basic seated massage routine

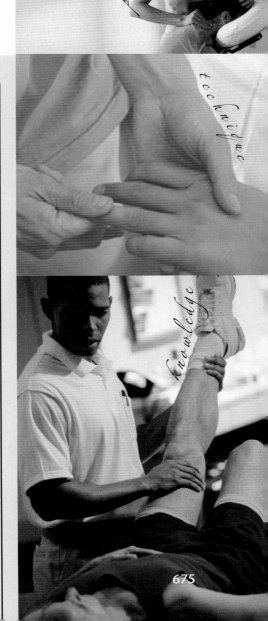

INTRODUCTION

Rubbing a person's shoulders while he or she is sitting in a chair is often instinctive. It is a natural and therapeutic urge. Seated massage is often referred to as *chair massage* and came to prominence through the efforts of David Palmer, whose vision was to make massage therapy safe, convenient, and affordable for anyone, anywhere, anytime. He introduced seated massage in the workplace in the early 1980s. Working at corporations such as Apple, Inc. and Pacific Bell, he developed the idea for a chair to complement the massage. In 1986, he introduced the first special massage chair and coined the term *on-site massage*. Palmer adapted the traditional Japanese system of massage, called *amma,* to create massage routines performed on the client in a special portable chair. Amma routines use acupressure techniques, stretching, and percussion (tapotement).

Seated techniques have made massage more accessible to the mainstream public by making it as convenient and affordable as a haircut. Enterprising therapists have expanded this concept to every imaginable venue. Some of the opportunities to use seated massage are airports, beauty salons, large and small businesses, concerts (public and backstage), chiropractic offices, day spas, numerous events such as fairs and festivals, golf courses, health food stores, hospitals, hospices, institutions, locker rooms, Massage Emergency Response Team (MERT), nursing homes, offices, private practices, retail stores, schools, shopping malls, sporting events, teams, and even street corners.

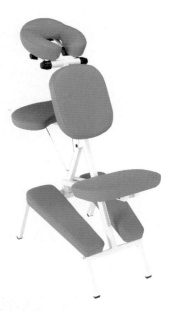

Figure 25-1 A massage chair highlighting the stress points and adjustable joints. (Courtesy of Golden Ratio, Emigrant, Mont.)

For Your Information

The Massage Emergency Response Team (MERT), sponsored by the American Massage Therapy Association, was deployed during the rescue efforts after the Sept. 11, 2001, terrorist attacks on the World Trade Center, Pennsylvania, and the Pentagon. MERT teams primarily used massage chairs to treat rescue workers and others at the disaster sites. The volunteer MERT therapists gave hundreds of seated massages to grateful emergency personnel. Seated massage skills were a vital part of the service rescue workers provided.

Sessions are typically short (5 to 15 minutes), although they can last as long as 30 minutes. The cost is usually $10 to $20, averaging about $1 per minute. Some individuals not familiar with massage find seated massage more acceptable than table massage. There is no need to disrobe. Lubricants are not used. People generally feel less vulnerable seated in a chair

How To Select A Massage Chair

Many different massage chairs are available on the market today. Just as with a massage table, different features appeal to different people. The following are things to keep in mind when purchasing a massage chair:

- The massage chair should be lightweight because you may be moving it from location to location.
- It should be quick and simple to set up and take down.
- It should have enough adjustments to fit a variety of body styles but not so many that you spend a lot of time adjusting the chair. Avoid massage chairs requiring a series of smaller adjustments after making a major adjustment. Simple is better; simple and quick is best.
- It should be sturdy and strong. A creaky or wobbly chair makes the person sitting in it feel insecure and unsafe.
- Be sure the armrest is strong enough to withstand deep compression and deep frictioning techniques performed on the client's arm.
- Face support adjustments on massage chairs should be completely enclosed. Exposed latches and locking mechanisms can pinch therapist's fingers and catch client's hair. Exposed latches and locking mechanisms can also come loose if bumped by the client or therapist and are difficult to keep clean and sanitize.
- The chair manufacturer should offer a trial period during which the chair can be returned for a full refund if the therapist is not completely satisfied. The chair should come with a 5-year or longer warranty.
- It is generally best to buy from a manufacturer that is well established. Such a manufacturer usually provides better customer service, and recognized brands typically have a better resale value should you decide to sell your chair at any time.

than lying on a table, and the time commitment is considerably less, especially when the therapist goes to the client's place of business, or on-site.

Several varieties of seated massage, equipment, and ways to accommodate clients who want a massage in a seated position are known. A massage chair (Figure 25-1) is made by most manufacturers of professional massage tables and offer a desktop face support, which is typically the face support from a massage chair designed to be clamped to or balanced on the edge of a counter, table, or desk. Many of these have chest pads that hang vertically over the edge of the desk. A system of specially designed cushions can hang over the back of an armless chair. These are often the same cushion system used for positioning and support on a massage tabletop. If none of the above-mentioned options are available to you, you can use a stack of pillows on a massage table, a regular table, or chair. As a last resort, the therapist may use a stool or chair, but that option provides no support for the head, upper body, or arms.

REASONS FOR USING THE CHAIR

Reasons for using the massage chair are as follows:
- Massage therapists may use seated massage techniques as their primary modality and source of revenue.
- Massage therapists may use a massage chair as their secondary modality and supplemental source of revenue.
- Seated massage can be used as a promotional tool to introduce the public to massage therapy in a safe, nonthreatening way, thus promoting the therapist's practice in particular and the profession in general.
- Seated massage may be done on-site or in the therapist's office.
- Massage chairs are often used at sporting events.
- Other opportunities include fundraisers, concerts, conventions, airports, beauty salons and spas.
- On-site massage services may be used at professional offices and other workplaces for stress reduction, pain relief, and injury prevention.
- Seated massage is used by therapists in their offices for short treatments of the upper body
- The massage chair is ideal for clients who have difficulty getting on and off a massage table.
- The chair is as versatile as your imagination

Seated massage is most often used for stress reduction and relaxation, as a "stress-buster break"; however, routines can be adapted to address specific complaints such as low back pain, headaches, neck and shoulder tension, and arm and wrist overuse injury. Combining clinical massage techniques with *amma* techniques gives the therapist the option of doing clinical massage in the seated position in either an on-site or private office setting. Individuals are more likely to participate in a program of seated massage if it provides reduction of painful complaints and injuries. Employers are more likely to allow employees to participate if they believe it will prevent injuries, improve morale, and enhance productivity in the workplace.

In research published in 1996, Dr. Tiffany Field of the Touch Research Institute in Miami found that individuals who received a 15-minute seated massage twice a week showed increased cognitive ability, performed better on math tests, and completed problems with increased accuracy and speed. These individuals also experienced a significant decrease in tension compared with individuals who practiced traditional relaxation techniques while seated in a chair without receiving massage. Hence massage does not cost; it pays.

A massage chair takes up less room than a table, making it more adaptable to space limitations. This and the "through-clothes" technique has brought the chair into therapy areas, athletic training rooms, chiropractic offices, and many massage therapists' treatment rooms as an adjunct to their tables for specific work. It is well worth the massage therapist's financial investment and time to acquire a massage chair and learn how to use it effectively.

SANITIZATION AND HYGIENE CONSIDERATIONS

The need for hygiene for the massage therapist and sanitization of the massage chair cannot be overemphasized. The public is aware of the importance of cleanliness, and your clients will notice and appreciate that you keep your equipment sanitary and your work environment clean (see Chapter 4).

When conducting table massage in an office setting, the massage therapist must wash his hands before and after each client. However, with the shorter treatment protocols, it is not economically feasible to take time between clients to wash the hands twice. When working on-site, washroom facilities may be inaccessible. Seated massage therapy procedures must be self-contained, including hygiene.

Seated massage therapists can purchase antimicrobial disposable towelettes from a medical or massage supply business. These disposable towels sanitize your hands, face support, arm rest, and chest pad of the chair between clients. Sanitize the leg rests if the client was wearing shorts or a skirt. These wipes are specially treated to destroy microscopic organisms that can cause diseases, such as staphylococci, streptococci, common cold and influenza viruses, herpes virus, human immunodeficiency virus (HIV), and tuberculosis. As a rule, if a disinfecting agent destroys tuberculosis bacteria, all other microbes are also destroyed. These cleansers help protect the therapist and the client by preventing the spread of contagious pathogens.

It is important to keep your hands clean. The most common way to spread germs is from touching the eyes, ears, and nose. Keep your fingernails short and clean. Using an antimicrobial skin barrier, sometimes called a *skin protectorant,* further protects your hands. These come in creams or foams that when rubbed onto the skin dry to form a barrier. Protect yourself and your clients.

Use a cover on the face cradle to make your clients feel more comfortable and to facilitate keeping the face support cushion clean. These covers help keep makeup off the vinyl. Face cradle covers feel more comfortable on the face than does vinyl fabric. One type of cover is a *nurse bouffant cap,* available through medical or massage supply businesses. Other types of covers are paper towels and specially designed paper covers, with the latter available through massage supply sources.

SAFETY CONSIDERATIONS AND BODY MECHANICS FOR THE SEATED MASSAGE THERAPIST

To prevent repetitive motion injuries, it is essential to use proper body mechanics at all times. Before you set up your massage chair, select an area that allows you to move completely around the chair during the massage. If you use a massage chair carrying case, place it out of the way. Provide a clear, unobstructed pathway for your clients to and from the chair.

Work in the lunge (bow) stance, keeping the feet and body pointed in the direction of the force you are applying. Keep your back straight and your head erect. Your movement and pressure will be generated from the pelvis as you shift your weight from back leg to front leg (Figure 25-2). As you massage, the front knee is flexed and the arms stretched in front, elbows only slightly flexed. For the majority of seated massage techniques, the wrists should not be extended more than 45 degrees.

When using the thumbs, maintain proper thumb alignment by "stacking the bones." This means that the bones of the thumb are in relatively straight alignment with the bones of the wrist and arm. If you look straight down your arm, the thumb is pointing straight ahead. As you use your thumb, the fingers of the working hand may be open or loosely closed. You may also use your fingertips, palm of the hand, or elbow to apply massage techniques. This gives your thumbs a needed break and varies the quality of touch for the client. However, be sure to

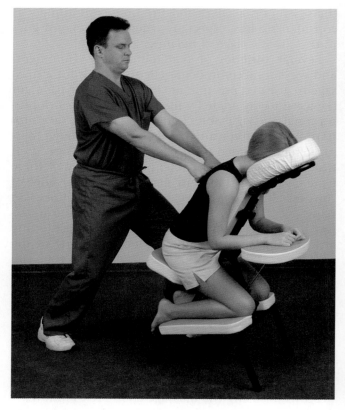

Figure 25-2   Seated massage with therapist in the lunge position.

maintain proper body mechanics at all times. Spread your feet farther apart as you work closer to the floor. Avoid bending the back and neck.

 Ultimately, your only source of funding is satisfied clients.

—Tim Mullen

BEFORE THE SEATED MASSAGE BEGINS

If this is your client's first time to sit in the massage chair, physically demonstrate how to do it properly. As you are sitting in the chair, orally explain what you are doing. For example, "I am sitting in the chair placing my knees and lower legs on these cushions while my forearms rest on this shelf and my face is supported by this crescent-shaped pillow." You will be amazed how many positions your clients will assume without directions. Some sit on the chair backward, whereas others climb onto it as if it were a motorcycle. Although this is entertaining, the client could upset the chair and be injured. Be specific with your directions and actions.

Most massage chairs have adjustments so they can properly support any body size or type (Figure 25-3).

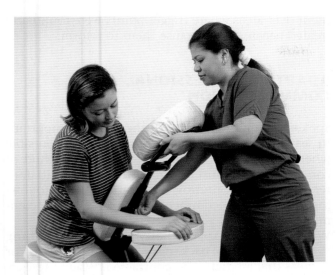

Figure 25-3 Massage therapist making adjustments on chair while client is seated in chair.

Before the seated massage session, adjust the chair to each client; do not expect the client to conform to the chair. The primary adjustments are the seat height, chest pad height, face support height and angle (tilt), and armrest height. A client will typically arch her back or slump if the chair is improperly adjusted to her body. *Be sure the client's back is straight and that the armrest is low enough so that the client's shoulders are not raised.* The proximal end of the forearm is just slightly off the armrest. For most clients the most comfortable position of the face cradle is when the neck is slightly flexed forward. Once the chair is completely adjusted to the client, ask her if any adjustments should be made. Then ask whether the client is comfortable; most clients who do not know how the chair should feel will say yes. However, if given the option to make it better, they will point out any area of discomfort.

Proper Chair Adjustment Per Client

- The client's back is straight and her chest is relatively flat against the chest pad.
- The face cradle is centered around the face and tilted to allow the therapist access to the posterior cervical muscles, without subjecting the client to excessive flexion.
- The armrest is at a height that does not elevate the client's shoulders; the shoulders should be at a natural height with the elbow lightly touching or just a few millimeters above the armrest.
- After asking the client if anything can be adjusted to make the chair more comfortable, ensure that she has no further suggestions or requests.

This simple question takes a few seconds and has a significant impact on the session.

MASSAGE STROKES USED FOR SEATED MASSAGE

Seated massage routines use East Asian and Swedish massage strokes (without oil) and ancillary massage strokes. These strokes include compression, sustained pressure (acupressure), stretching, deep and superficial friction, pétrissage, effleurage, nerve stroke, and tapotement. The strokes used vary according to the training of the therapist.

Compression

Compression is effective on the muscles of the forearm and back. Apply firm pressure primarily from the heel of the hand or loosely clenched fists. During compression of the forearm, face the client with your relaxed fingers pointed toward the client's elbow. Apply pressure straight down while maintaining contact. Instruct the client to exhale as you apply pressure to the back and to inhale as you release. Avoid applying excessive pressure on the floating ribs and the lumbar region due to the kidneys as well as any previous injuries.

Sustained Pressure

Also known as *ischemic compression* or *acupressure*, sustained pressure is usually applied with a finger or thumb, elbow, or a handheld tool. Direct sustained pressure displaces fluids in the tissues being compressed, spreads muscle fibers, and relieves muscle spasms. It is primarily used to relieve trigger and tender points found using palpatory strokes such as deep friction and pétrissage. In East Asian techniques, pressure is applied to points in a pattern to improve or balance energy flow in the meridians.

Deep Friction

Deep friction is applied with the thumb, finger, elbow, loosely clenched fist, palm, or heel of the hand. During friction, engage the skin through the client's clothes and move the skin over the underlying structures. Avoid sliding on the client's skin or clothes. The term *deep* does not denote hard pressure, but the effect of shifting the skin over deeper structures.

Superficial Friction

A warming, stimulating stroke, superficial friction is applied with the palms of one or both hands, in a rapid back and forth movement on the superficial tissues. A variation is to use the ulnar sides of the hands in a sawing motion. This variation is effective for reducing muscular tension around the shoulder joint on either side of the spine and across the top of the upper trapezius.

Pétrissage

Pétrissage involves grasping, lifting, and kneading the tissues or rolling the tissues between the thumb and fingers. This massage movement is used primarily in the neck and upper trapezius (Figure 25-4).

Effleurage

Effleurage, or light stroking, is applied over the client's clothing for relaxation and sedation. Nerve strokes can also be used.

Tapotement

Toward the end of the seated massage, tapotement can be used on the back, head, arms, and hips. Hacking, pounding, and rapping are best for the torso, hips, and arms, whereas tapping and pincement with the fingertips is best on the scalp. Do not use tapote-

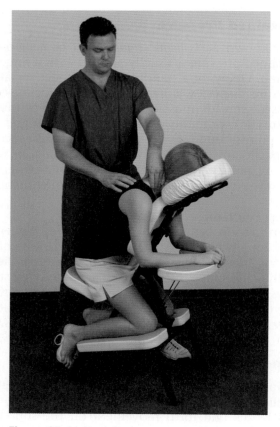

Figure 25-4   Kneading upper trapezius muscles.

ment over areas where trigger points were found and treated because it can cause them to reform.

ADAPTIVE PROFESSIONAL COMMUNICATION

Spoken communication with the client is important in seated massage. Because eye contact is impossible when the client is in the face cradle, a method of communication must be established in the initial interview before beginning the treatment. The following guideline is recommended for establishing communication:

When It Hurts. Explain that you will be examining the tissues of the back, neck, and arms, looking for areas that are tight and contracted. When these areas are located, they will be tender. You should suggest, "Be sure to tell me whenever I find a tender area. Will you do that for me?" Not only does this give the client permission to tell you that something is tender, but she agrees to do so.

When It Gets Better. Continue by saying, "When I find these tender places, I will stop and maintain the pressure. This sustained pressure will cause the nervous system to respond by relaxing the tender area. It may feel to you like I am letting up on the pressure, or it is beginning to feel better. Will you let me know when it gets better?"

If It Refers. You should then add, "When I am examining or maintaining pressure on an area of tissue, you may experience some sensation somewhere else. It could be a pain, tingling, numbness, aching, or some other sensation somewhere besides right where I am massaging. These are trigger points. Will you tell me if you feel any sensation radiating anywhere other than where I am working?"

If It's Too Hard. Say, "If at any time I am working too hard, be sure and tell me right away. Will you do that?" This is important because it gives the client permission to tell you that you are working too hard. Often the client will not tell you this, because she thinks you are the professional and you must be doing it right. She may think it is supposed to hurt. Some clients will endure anything if they believe it may make them better. You can also say, "Let me know if what I am doing feels good or if it hurts, especially if it hurts, because this work should not be painful."

During on-site massage, the massage area may be noisy, making it difficult to hear the client. In this case, ask the client to communicate by raising her hand if she is in pain. If more specific information is needed regarding pain, establish a pain-measuring system on a scale from 1 (no pain) through 5 (excruciating pain). You will know, by the number of

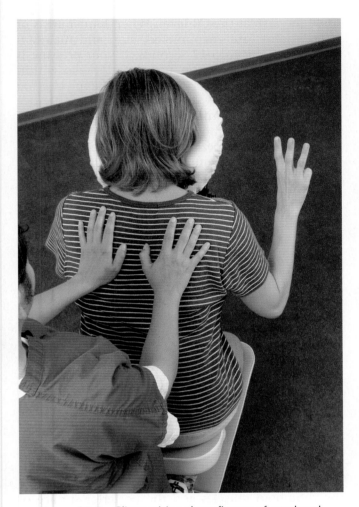

Figure 25-5   Client raising three fingers of one hand.

fingers raised, how she is responding to the pressure (Figure 25-5). This system also may be used in quiet places.

Some people will not tell you that something hurts. They may be accustomed to denying pain. However, the body never lies. You can always tell that you are working too hard when the client begins to pull away from you or unconsciously contracts muscles to limit your access into the tissues. If he is tensing up, squirming, or pulling away, *you are using too much pressure.*

RECORD KEEPING

It is uncommon for seated massage therapists to keep full assessment, plan, implementation, and evaluation (APIE) notes for each client; however, it is prudent to keep a record of each session and to note any unusual findings or observations. Even in seated massage, have your clients fill out an intake form and obtain informed consent. The initial interview

with your client may be brief, but the form should ask questions regarding medications, eye conditions that could be affected by the face cradle (e.g., contacts), and any medical conditions for which they are being treated. Establish your client's primary and secondary complaints.

Clinical seated massage treatments require keeping more detailed notes. Treatment notes document progress and remind the therapist of what procedures were performed and which treatments were helpful. In legal situations, proper documentation is helpful for you and your clients. Also, unless you give each client a receipt, it may not be considered a legal transaction by taxation authorities. To save time, receipts may be prepared in advance with a place to fill in the client's name, date, and amount.

SAMPLE SEATED MASSAGE ROUTINE

The following basic routine is a suggested protocol that you can accomplish in 15 minutes. Use it as a guide but remain creative and intuitive. Accomplish as much as you can for each client within the time allowed. Concentrate the majority of time on the client's primary area of complaint, which is usually the low back, neck, or shoulders. However, in the workplace, forearm, wrist, and hand complaints are quite common. Start with some general strokes to acquaint clients with your touch and to establish their individual sensitivity in receiving; gradually become more specific as you go on. You cannot resolve everything a client has been suffering from for years in one treatment. Even recent injuries usually require multiple treatments (see Chapter 24). One 15-minute session can reduce the main complaint and accomplish some general relaxation, so you have accomplished a great service for the client in that amount of time. Complete the seated massage treatment with general techniques. Work from general to specific, then back to general.

The Upper Back and Neck

Begin the treatment with compression strokes to the paraspinal muscles. Use the heels of the hands or loosely clenched fists. It is important to have the client breathe in rhythm with the compression. Ask your client to take a deep breath and exhale. As he exhales, apply firm pressure to the tissues on either side of the spine (it is ideal if the therapist breathes in the same pattern as the client). Begin between the scapulas and move inferiorly a hand width at a time until the ilium bones are reached. Then move back superiorly a hand width at a time until the starting point is reached. This technique establishes contact with the client, introduces relaxation, and gets him into a regular deep breathing pattern.

You should be standing directly behind the center of the client's back. Keep your arms outstretched with just a slight bend in the elbows, back straight, head erect, moving from the pelvis in a lunge position. If you are using the heels of the hands, the wrists will be significantly extended. If pressure applied with the heels of the hands creates discomfort in your wrists, then switch to a loosely clenched fist. Using a loose fist to apply compression keeps the wrist straight as you apply pressure with the proximal phalanges.

Repeat the above pattern using loosely clenched fists but with a circular deep frictioning stroke. Make four to eight circles with each hand, working simultaneously down and up the sides of the spine. If massaging in circles with both hands at the same time is too difficult or tiresome, you may choose to switch to cross-fiber or chucking friction. Apply four friction strokes medially to laterally over the paraspinal muscles, then four friction strokes superiorly to inferiorly, and then move a hand width and repeat.

Every few minutes, ask the client how he is perceiving the pressure, using the guidelines discussed in the section on Adaptive Professional Communication in this chapter.

Grasp the upper trapezius muscle with both hands, using a pincerlike grip. Begin just lateral to the base of the neck, in about the center of the upper trapezius muscle (Figure 25-6) and pétrissage the muscle between the thumb and fingers. Work laterally to the acromion process, then work medially to the base of the neck, and continue as far superior on the neck as you can while still isolating the trapezius fibers. The trapezius fibers will typically become too small to grasp at the C3 level. When tender areas or trigger points are encountered, stop and maintain the pressure for 8 to 12 seconds. If your pressure is appropriate for the person, he will feel it relax within 12 seconds; if he does not, you are applying too much pressure. Slowly release the pressure and move to another area, returning to the tender area in about 1 minute. It is common for trigger points in the upper fibers of the trapezius to refer to the back of the head and up to the temple area.

You may now move to the side of the client in the chair and grasp and pétrissage the back of his neck in the lamina groove. Work all the way up to the occipital bone and back down to the shoulder. Because the thumb is more sensitive and powerful, you may choose to go to the other side and repeat this step. This decision is based on the sensitivity found in the tissues the first time over them and the client's main complaint. If the main complaint is the neck and shoulders, you will want to be thorough in this area. If the main complaint is in the lower back, less time will be spent in the posterior cervical region.

Tilt the face cradle forward to place the head and neck in 45 degrees of flexion. While standing at the side of the client, use the thumb and second finger of one hand to apply deep frictioning to the tissues between the occiput and C2. Work from lateral to medial and back. These tissues can be tender and ischemic, so be sure to check with the client about appropriate pressures when working this area.

Using the heel of the hand or fingertips, examine the rhomboid muscles and the posterior surface of the scapula with deep circular friction. When massaging the posterior region of the scapula, support

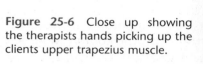

Figure 25-6 Close up showing the therapists hands picking up the clients upper trapezius muscle.

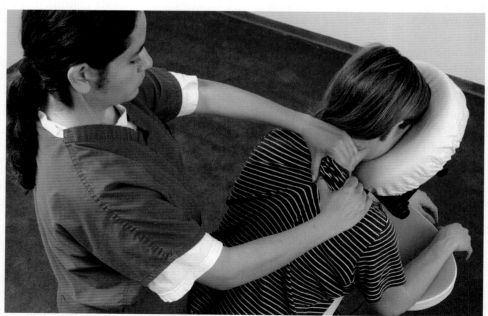

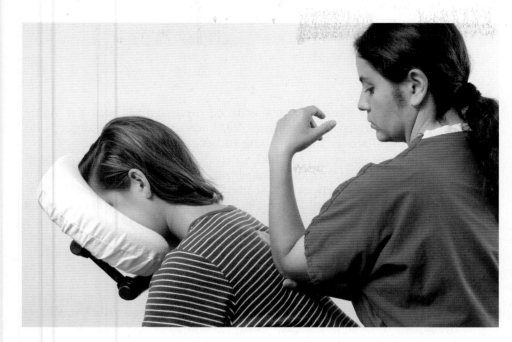

Figure 25-7 Guided elbow technique.

the anterior aspect of the shoulder with the other hand. If this area is the client's primary complaint, a more specific examination of these tissues can be done with the thumbs or a guided elbow (Figure 25-7). When this area is complete, move lateral to the shoulder joint and treat the rotator cuff tendons with circular friction.

Apply circular friction to the area below the scapulas using the heels of the hands, working both sides of the spine at once. This addresses the latissimus dorsi muscle and paraspinal muscles in the midback.

Lower Back

Moving your hand inferiorly, use circular friction to relax the lower back. The quadratus lumborum muscle can be examined and treated effectively in the seated position. This muscle is responsible for many complaints of low back pain. Trigger points in the quadratus lumborum often mimic hip and sciatic nerve pain. Palpate the client's waistline, being careful not to elicit a tickle response. After locating the lateral end of the twelfth rib, apply deep friction with your thumbs in a lateral to medial direction along its inferior surface. As you move medially, you will encounter a hard structure; this is the spine and is often more lateral than expected. Change directions of pressure to 45 degrees medial anterior. Using circular friction, examine the edge of the lumbar spine in the area of the transverse processes. Using deep circular friction, massage this area in thumb-width increments from L1 to the ilium bone. Change the direction of pressure to inferior anterior and treat the su-

perior surface of the ilium laterally to the midline of the body.

The lower portion of the paraspinal muscles can now be examined more thoroughly using fingertips, thumbs, or a guided elbow. Treat one side at a time with deep circular or cross-fiber friction, using sustained pressure on tender areas and trigger points. Apply friction on this area from medial to lateral, allowing the client to rock slightly in the chair. This is effective and relaxing.

Arm

Because no surface is available to compress the biceps and triceps against during seated massage, the therapist is limited to pétrissage, rolling, jostling, nerve strokes, or squeezing the tissues of the upper arm with one or two hands.

Facing the front of the chair, slightly to one side, place the forearm with the palm down on the arm rest to treat the forearm muscles. Apply compression to the extensor muscle group using the heel of the hand, working from wrist to elbow. Repeat this sequence three times, then rotate the arm, palm up, and apply three sets of compression to the flexor muscles.

Roll the hand over, palm down, and instead of compression, repeat this pattern using circular friction applied with the heel of the hand, with your fingers pointed toward the elbow of the client. Work from wrist to elbow in 1- or 2-inch intervals, making five to 10 circles on each spot. Repeat this sequence three times. Rotate the arm, palm up, and repeat the

DAVID PALMER

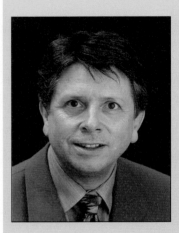

Born: November 27, 1948.

"My vision is to make touch a positive social value in our culture."

The topic of chair massage can hardly be discussed without the name David Palmer surfacing at least once. Read any article on the subject, and you will soon discover that he is the Father of chair massage.

His career in massage began in 1980. Considering his previous profession of 10 years as an administrator of social service programs for nonprofit agencies in Chicago and San Francisco, it seemed only natural that he would focus on a field in which he could have a great effect on the mental well-being of people through the art of touch. He first encountered massage in his early 20s during a Rolfing session. He had been experiencing chronic shoulder pain, and the Rolfing combined with tai chi and stretching gave him a feeling of being back inside his body. It was this experience that led him to explore massage.

After he received a massage in a spa in San Francisco, a series of events over a 3-year period led to his position as director of a massage institute specializing in the Japanese art of *amma*. After only a short period of teaching, he realized that a serious gap existed between the people who wanted to give and receive professional massage. After a little investigating, he came to the conclusion that a significant packaging problem existed in the massage industry.

"The package that the mainstream massage community was selling to the general public was a package that the general public was not interested in buying," he says. It was hard to convince most people to accept an idea that required going into a private room, removing clothing, lying on a table, and being rubbed with oils by a stranger for a costly fee on a regular basis. The whole idea was just too frightening for the average individual. It was then that he gave massage a hard look from a marketing point of view. He says, "They [mainstream massage community] were selling a graduate-level understanding of the field of touch to a population who had not even begun kindergarten regarding touch."

Palmer's solution to this problem was to make massage less frightening and more affordable. The result was his legacy of the seated chair massage. Although this type of massage had been done for thousands of years, as can been seen in ancient Japanese and Chinese woodcuts, Palmer's contribution was to revive its visibility and identity. It would be more difficult to perceive as strange if the massage is given with the client fully clothed on an open sidewalk in a chair.

At the time, the chair massage was being done on a drummer's stool, but in 1983, he decided to create a special chair. He had seen one of the Scandinavian computer chairs called *Balance* with slanted leg rests and thought it would be perfect, if only it had some sort of head rest and chest support. He hired a French cabinetmaker named Serge Bouyssou to be his design partner, and after 2 years the chair was introduced to the national market. The year was 1986, and chair massage was now viewed as being significant enough to have its own physical product.

Vision has clearly been an important factor in David Palmer's career. From the beginning, he saw a challenge and immediately acted on it. Chair massage has given so many people the opportunity to experience the wonderful benefits of massage. It allows the client to safely experience the much needed sense of touch. "We're so touch phobic that you can't grow up in this culture without having some serious issues about touch," says Palmer. "Parents are afraid to touch their kids; teachers can't touch their students; it's crazy out there. My feeling is that we need to shift that around, and massage is a vehicle

DAVID PALMER—cont'd

for doing that because it provides structured touch." Although he fully appreciates the many wonderful benefits of massage, it is not his main interest. He states, "My vision is to make touch a positive social value in our culture." He admits that this is what primarily motivates his professional life.

The most important thing he feels that students can do in their massage therapy program is first learn how to touch and how to be touched. He confesses, "I'm one of those unreformed 1960s brats who thinks it's still possible to change the world." If his previous record is any reflection on his future, he just might succeed.

circular friction moves on the flexor muscles of the forearm (Figure 25-8).

Using the thumbs, apply circular friction to all sides of the wrist. Grasp the client's hand, shake out the arm, and return it to the armrest. Repeat this sequence on the other arm.

Face and Scalp

Facial and scalp massage feels great while in a chair; however, many people do not want their hair or makeup messed up, so always ask first. Apply circular friction to the temples, jaw, face, and forehead (Figure 25-9). During scalp massage, the tissue can be shifted back and forth across the cranium using deep friction in any direction. Gentle tapping or pincement tapotement also works well on the scalp, espe-

cially as part of the general finishing strokes. Tapotement on the cranium is not appropriate if someone has a headache.

Stretches

Stretches are useful in seated massage. Because most individuals spend much of their time in a flexed position, the anterior cervical region and pectoral re-

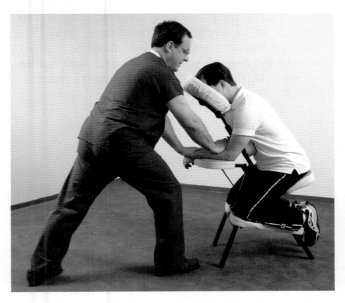

Figure 25-8   Therapist using heel of hand to apply deep circular friction to forearm musculature.

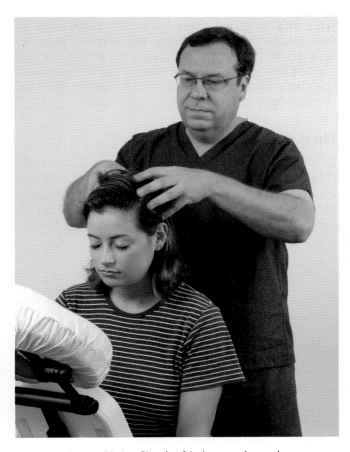

Figure 25-9   Circular friction on the scalp.

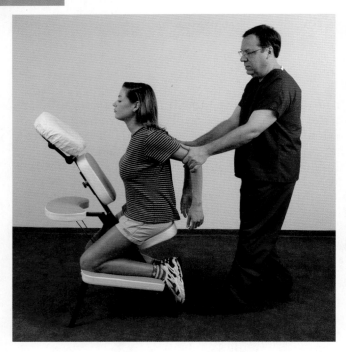

Figure 25-10 Therapist actively assisting client in stretch by pulling elbows back.

gions of the body are typically contracted. Most clients also have chronically internally rotated shoulders. Passive and active assisted stretches can relax and lengthen these habitually contracted tissues (Figure 25-10). Massage therapists should use only those systems of stretching in which they are trained and must always be careful not to overstretch the client's soft tissue and to avoid bouncy (ballistic) or prolonged stretching.

Final Procedure

As the seated massage session draws to a close, the therapist returns to general strokes. If the goal is to leave the client relaxed and sedated, finish with some effleurage and slow downward nerve strokes on the back and shoulders. If the client is returning to work and needs to be more alert, finish with tapotement, superficial (palmar) friction, and faster nerve strokes. Tapping or pincement tapotement on the head, hacking or quacking on the shoulders and back, and pounding or rapping on the hips is a more stimulating way to finish the massage (see Figure 25-10).

When the treatment is complete, tell the client and ask her to get off the chair slowly. Remain close by because many people, especially the elderly, may feel unsteady for a few moments. Some people actually doze off during the seated massage and may need time to become fully oriented. Be prepared to assist your client as needed.

Always have your appointment calendar handy to reschedule appointments and business cards to distribute. As you collect your fee from the client or just thank them and say good-bye, suggest that the client book another appointment. It is also appropriate to mention that if he liked your work, he should recommend it to others.

On completion of all transactions with the client, clean your hands, disinfect the chair, write your case notes, take a few deep breaths, and get ready for the next client.

SUMMARY

Seated massage is an important specialty area in the profession of massage therapy. It allows the therapist to reach a different group of clients who may not be available for traditional table massage. Usually done in a special portable chair, seated techniques can be used on-site at the client's location or the therapist's office. Seated massage sessions tend to be shorter, ranging from 5 to 30 minutes. The work is done through the clothes without lubricants. Seated massage is used for promoting the therapist's private practice or as a complete practice in itself. The portable massage chair has made massage as accessible to the general public as a haircut and has become a valuable adjunct to any therapist's practice.

MATCHING

List the letter of the answer next to the term or phrase that best describes it.

A. Amma
B. Lunge position
C. Explain and demonstrate how to sit in the chair properly
D. Client begins to pull away from you or tense up
E. Massage lubricants
F. David Palmer
G. Lubricated effleurage

H. Select an area allowing the therapist to move around the chair during the massage
I. If you could change anything, what would it be?
J. Raise a hand
K. Antimicrobial disposable towelettes
L. An alternative method of communication

_____ 1. The Father of seated massage

_____ 2. The traditional Japanese system of massage from which Palmer's techniques were derived

_____ 3. Massage media not used in seated massage

_____ 4. At on-site massage locations, this item replaces traditional handwashing

_____ 5. What the massage therapist must do before setting up the massage chair

_____ 6. The position most commonly used by therapists performing seated massage

_____ 7. What must be established with the client because eye contact is not possible

_____ 8. Observation made by the therapist to determine whether he is working too hard or too deep

_____ 9. Request verbalized to the client once the chair is completely adjusted to fit

_____ 10. Activities done if the client is experiencing seated massage for the first time

_____ 11. Method for obtaining the therapist's attention in a noisy treatment area

_____ 12. The stroke not used in seated massage

Bibliography

Field T: Massage therapy reduces anxiety and enhances EEG pattern of alertness and math computations, *Int J Neurosci* 86:197-205, 1996.

Ironson G et al: Massage therapy is associated with enhancement of the immune system's cytotoxic capacity, *Int J Neurosci* 84:205-218, 1996.

Mattes A: *Active isolated stretching,* Sarasota, Fla, 1995, Author.

Palmer D: *How to market on site massage,* Santa Rosa, Calif, 1986, Living Earth Crafts.

Palmer D: *The bodywork entrepreneur,* San Francisco, Calif, 1990, Thumb Press.

Stephens R: *Seated therapeutic massage video seminars,* vol I-III, Cedar Rapids, Iowa, 1996.

Travell JG, Simons DG: *Myofascial pain and dysfunction: the trigger point manual,* vol I-II, Baltimore, 1983, Williams and Wilkins.

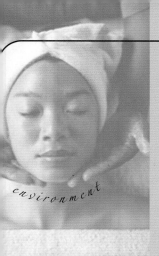

Asian Bodywork Therapy: Shiatsu

26

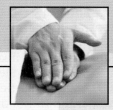

Debra C. Howard, Dipl. ABT (NCCAOM)

"Experience is the hardest kind of teacher. It gives you the test first and the lesson afterward."

—Anonymous

STUDENT OBJECTIVES

After completing this chapter, the student should be able to:

- Define Asian bodywork therapy
- Define shiatsu
- Locate the 12 primary meridians, the Governing Vessel, and the Conception Vessel
- Identify differences in eastern and western approaches to health and medicine
- Describe Yin/Yang theory and major correspondences
- Describe the Five Element theory and major correspondences
- Apply appropriate techniques of varying direction, degree, and intensity to meridians and acupoints during a full-body session
- Define and apply appropriate techniques according to Qi (Ki) deficiency and/or excess conditions in the meridians, while using proper body mechanics

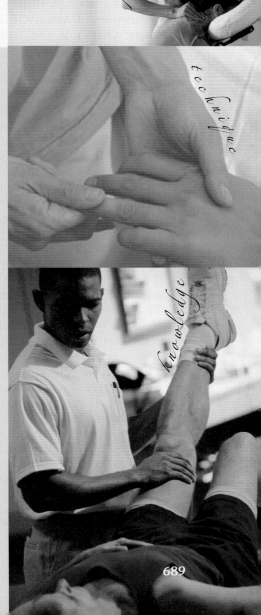

INTRODUCTION

This chapter is designed to give the student a basic introduction to Asian Bodywork Therapy in general and shiatsu in particular. Although this is by no means meant as a complete course of study, this chapter gives the beginning student a provocative glimpse into the world of ancient Chinese theories and techniques that continue to thrive today.

Included in this chapter are sections defining Asian bodywork therapy and shiatsu with a brief history, some basics of Chinese medicine, differences in eastern and western approaches to health and medicine, Yin/Yang theory, Qi (Ki), Five Elements theory, meridians, acupoints, Hara, and dantien, shiatsu theory, shiatsu techniques, and a full-body routine.

WHAT IS ASIAN BODYWORK THERAPY?

According to the American Organization for Bodywork Therapies of Asia (AOBTA), **Asian Bodywork Therapy (ABT)** is the treatment of the human body, mind, and spirit through pressure and/or manipulation. This includes the electromagnetic or energetic field that surrounds, infuses, and brings the body to life. Asian bodywork is based on traditional Chinese medical principles. Traditional Asian techniques and treatment strategies are used to affect and balance the body's energetic systems, combining treatment of the human body, emotions, mind, energy fields, and spirit for the promotion, maintenance, and restoration of health. Many Asian modalities exist, including acupressure, amma, amma therapy, anma, chi nei tsang, jin shin do, jin shin jyutsu, nuad bo rarn (traditional Thai massage), several forms of shiatsu, and tuina. Although many others are also available, this chapter focuses on shiatsu.

All forms of Asian bodywork use a variety of techniques, but their philosophical and theoretical roots are in ancient Chinese medicine (see Chapter 1). Some Asian bodywork techniques predate Chinese medicine. Others were derived from the Chinese medical model. Modalities from both eras spread from China, throughout Asia, and eventually to the rest of the world. Some elements of Swedish massage were developed from Chinese medicine texts translated by the French. Most modern modalities have their roots in Chinese medicine. Most schools that specialize in Asian bodywork therapy teach Chinese medicine as its foundation.

For these reasons, Asian bodywork therapy is considered a distinct profession; to practice Asian bodywork therapy is to practice an important branch of Chinese medicine.

CHINESE MEDICINE

This section gives the student an introduction to the basics of the Chinese medical model; the sections hereafter add more depth to this basic information.

When studying Chinese medicine, it is important to remember that it is a functional medical model. In assessment, energetic qualities of Qi and the other Vital Substances in the body are the focus. Function is the natural by-product of energy. It is said that when the Qi is flowing smoothly, no illness occurs. Signs and symptoms of limited function or dysfunction are clues that energy is not moving, is moving too slowly or quickly, is being overstimulated or drained, or is not being properly nourished. Symptoms also arise from pathological influences.

The Zang/Fu, or Organ Systems in Chinese medicine, are named for the internal organs and include all functions dedicated to that particular organ. Function occurs on all human levels, including emotional, mental, spiritual and physical. These levels are not separate from each other; the Organ System includes these levels in its functions. The **Zang** are the Yin organs; the **Fu** are the Yang organs. The related Vital Substances, meridians, connections to other meridians, elemental relationships, and correspondences are all a part of a particular Organ System. For this reason, names of Organ Systems (e.g., Heart) are capitalized in most texts; names of anatomical organs (heart) are not.

From a Chinese medical point of view, Yin and Yang continuously interact to build and move the Vital Substances through the meridians and vessels to the Zang/Fu. The Zang/Fu interact continuously with each other, the Vital Substances, Yin/Yang, meridians and vessels, and the outside world (food, breath, environmental factors, lifestyle factors, emotional and mental stresses, and so on). The facilitation of the smooth flow of these various energies can restore, maintain, and promote health.

For assessment purposes, client information is gathered through the following **Four Examinations**:
1. Looking
2. Listening/smelling
3. Asking
4. Palpating

In *looking at the client,* the practitioner observes the overall demeanor and mobility, posture, and facial and body characteristics of the client, including color, shape, distinguishing marks, scars, fingernails and even the ears. The tongue is a major source of information and tells much about the interior condition of the client. For example, a yellow coating on the tongue indicates *heat* in the body.

Listening to the client includes not only hearing what he is saying but also listening to what he is not saying. Listening includes paying attention to the sound of the voice, breath, and emotion emanating from each person. Each Element also has an associated sense or sense organ (see the section on The Five Elements). A burnt smell is associated with the Fire Element and is often present in the breath when heat is in the Heart.

Asking refers to the use of the Ten Questions, which are classic inquiries into the state of the body's systems including the client's feelings about heat and cold, appetite and eating habits, sleep patterns, and other daily energy-level highs and lows. Questions regarding digestive, urinary, and eliminative habits; pain; sweat; and menstrual and family medical history are included. Although a paper intake form is helpful, the asking of verbal questions can give the practitioner greater insight into the client's condition and a route to establish rapport with the client.

Palpating is the last of the Four Examinations. Palpation includes feeling for certain qualities in the radial pulses at the wrists (the three locations on each wrist, three depths at each position, and 28 pulse qualities). The abdomen is palpated to check the quality of the Organ Systems' energy at designated areas. The meridians, muscles, and skin are palpated. Some **acupoints**, especially the Shu points (named Yu points in Japan) on the back of the body and the Mu points (named Bo points in Japan) on the front of the body, are used as assessment and treatment points (Figure 26-1). Source points, near the ankles and wrists, are also assessment sites. The practitioner is feeling for the quality of the energy, temperature, moisture levels of the skin, pain, lack of tonicity or hypertonicity of the tissues, areas of stagnation, and any other outstanding features. It can take years of study and practice to perfect one's ability to palpate.

Once the client information has been gathered, the information must be interpreted through Chinese medicine assessment parameters. Specific methods help arrive at an assessment of the body's condition. A basic paradigm (pattern) used is the **Eight Principles**:

- **Yin/Yang:** General principles used to categorize diseases
- **Cold/Hot:** The thermal quality of the disease
- **Interior/Exterior:** The location and process of the disease
- **Empty/Full:** The conditions of the body's protective systems and the pathogenic factors (causes of disease) in the body

These pathogenic factors are divided into Internal and External categories and are described as follows:

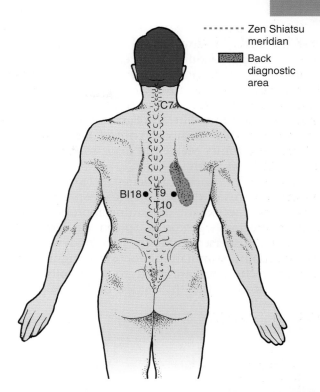

Figure 26-1   Back diagnostic area and Yu points of the liver. (From Beresford-Cooke C: *Shiatsu theory and practice,* Edinburgh, 1999, Churchill Livingstone.)

- **Internal causes of disease:** The emotions: fear and fright, anger, excess joy, pensiveness, grief, and sadness
- **External causes of disease:** The environmental factors: wind, cold, heat and fire, dampness, dryness, and summerheat
- **Other causes of disease:** Poisons, parasites, environmental toxins, plagues, constitutional factors, lifestyle factors, diet, and unforeseen events

Another useful paradigm in Chinese medicine is the Five Element Theory (see the section on The Five Elements). The Five Elements are used to determine a client's constitution, genetic inheritance, and personal story, and also to identify strengths and weaknesses for the life of the individual. Each person is their own particular synthesis of the Five Elements, and a Chinese medicine practitioner uses constitutional determination to educate the person about practical ways to enhance their health. For example, if the Spleen-Pancreas Organ System is constitutionally weak, the person would do well to sing daily, eat plenty of healthy soups, and be mindful of their intake of sweets.

 In the beginner's mind there are many possibilities, but in the expert's mind there are only a few.

—Shunryu Suzuki

The Five Element theory can also be used to assess past processes of disease and possible future processes. When someone has a weakness in Earth, it is unable to fully feed Metal or fully control Water. Wood tends to overcontrol Earth when it is weak.

The Five Element theory also shows the treatment strategy; first, tonify Fire and Earth to begin nourishing Earth so that Earth can control Water and feed Metal. Next, tonify Metal and disperse Wood to take the pressure off Earth.

The art of Chinese medicine is to identify the client's patterns of disharmony (e.g., Spleen Qi deficiency, Earth weak) and determine appropriate treatment strategies (e.g., tonify Spleen Qi, Fire, Earth, and Metal; disperse Wood). In Asian bodywork therapy, acupoint stimulation and differing meridian therapy techniques are used to accomplish these therapeutic goals (see the section on Shiatsu Theory and Techniques).

Traditional Chinese medicine treatment techniques include dietary and lifestyle changes, meditation, exercise, herbal medicines, bodywork, and acupuncture. Other techniques include moxibustion (burning the herb mugwort, an external warming technique); cupping (the use of glass cups as suction over areas of stagnation); gua sha (the art of scraping the surface of the skin); and compresses, liniments, baths, and poultices.

DIFFERENCES BETWEEN EASTERN AND WESTERN APPROACHES TO HEALTH AND MEDICINE

There are many differences in eastern and western approaches to health and medicine. Both have their strengths and weaknesses, successes, and limitations (Table 26-1).

TABLE 26-1

Eastern and Western Approaches to Health and Medicine

Eastern	Western
The body is a garden whose landscape embodies primal forces of nature (Earth, Fire, Wood, Metal, Water) that are connected to all life.	The body is a machine with working parts that are removable, repairable, interchangeable and, in some cases, unnecessary.
Humans are a microcosm of nature.	Humans are autonomous in nature.
A holistic view is taken, addressing the body, mind, and spirit as a whole.	A reductionist view is taken, separating and reducing matter.
Health is based on integrity, adaptability, and continuity.	Health is regarded as the absence of disease, functioning within limits (homeostasis).
A functional model is used, viewing the body, mind, and spirit as interacting systems.	A structural model is used, seeking answers from the body structures (cells and tissues).
The approach is based on energy awareness, assessment, and treatment.	The approach has no regard for body energy.
The approach focuses on health maintenance and prevention.	The approach focuses on curing disease.
Health is cultivated by a partnership between doctor and patient to improve ecological conditions.	Outlook of medicine is a war on disease with doctor as general, disease as enemy, and patient as occupied territory.
Goal of medicine is enhancement of self-healing capacity.	Goal of medicine is to eradicate symptoms and maximize performance.
Eastern (Chinese) medicine was taken to the masses by *barefoot doctors* as a medicine by and for the people, to be learned, taught and practiced by the people whenever possible.	Western medicine is more specialized, technologically based, impractical, and even illegal for the average person to practice.
Training addresses the body/mind as a whole.	Training is centered around a specific body system with intricate knowledge of that system.
Physicians train the people to care for themselves; the patient takes some responsibility for their condition.	Physicians are the authority and take responsibility for the patient's condition.
Herbal medicines are used that have little or no side effects and can be tailored to the individual.	Chemical synthesized drugs are used, with many side effects and dosages based on statistics.

Ancient medicines do not have the capability to eradicate all disease or treat every condition. Modern medicines also do not have all the answers to human ills. Although neither have all the answers, they seem to complement each other well.

For Your Information

Chinese herbal formulas are designed to be a balanced treatment. Few formulas contain a single herb, Radix Polygoni Multiflori (He Shou Wu or Fo ti) and Tienchi, (or Tienchi Ginseng) are examples. When you take other single Chinese herbal remedies, you risk hurting yourself. Always seek a trained professional for assistance.

YIN/YANG THEORY

The Yin/Yang theory is the foundation of the Chinese medical model and therefore Asian bodywork therapy. The familiar black and white icon, the **Tai Ji** (Figure 26-2), symbolizes the observable, continuous movement and interaction of the two main forces of life: energy and matter in the universe. Yin and Yang are complementary opposites—the order that came from the chaos that was before. These ideas stem from ancient Taoist traditions. At the root of Chinese medicine is the concept that the mind, body, spirit, and the entire universe are interconnected, inseparable, and must be treated as such.

According to Lao Tsu's ancient text, *Tao te Ching*, the continuous interaction between Yin and Yang keeps all things creating, moving, and changing in the universe. Although they are seen as two, in reality, they are three. From Chaos came the One: the Tao. From the One came the Two: now the Yin and Yang. From the Two came the Three: Yin and Yang together, or the Tai Ji. From the Three came the 10,000 things: all the things identified in the universe. The following is a list of the few guiding principles about Yin/Yang theory:

- Mutually creating one another
- Mutually controlling one another

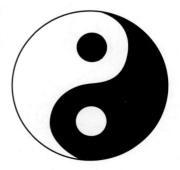

Figure 26-2   Yin/yang symbol.

- Being relative to each other
- Being interdependent
- Not existing without one another
- Eventually becoming one another
- Subdividing infinitely

References to *Yin* and *Yang* relative correspondences are used to categorize and define all things in the universe (Table 26-2). In Asian bodywork therapy, Yin and Yang can be used to define the client's condition and determine appropriate treatment protocol.

In China the energy of the body, mind, and spirit is called **Qi** (Ch'i), which translates as Life Force or Vital Energy. In Japan, it is called **Ki**. Qi is in and around the body, affecting all the senses, tissues, and thoughts. Reciprocally, the body also affects Qi. This concept is one of the foundations of the Chinese medical model and is the therapeutic focus for Asian bodywork therapists.

Qi is not something that can be seen with the average human eye nor even a microscope. If you

TABLE 26-2

Some Relative Correspondences of Yin/Yang

Yin	Yang
Feminine	Masculine
Dark	Light
Cold (numb)	Hot (inflamed)
Moist	Dry
Interior	Exterior
Chronic	Acute
Anterior	Posterior
Medial	Lateral
Inferior	Superior
Community	Competition
Earth	Heaven
Water	Fire
Moon	Sun
Slow (still, lethargic)	Fast (restless, energetic)
Static, storing, conserving	Transforming, changing
Substantial	Nonsubstantial
Matter	Energy
Soft, mushy tissue	Hard, congested tissue
Concave	Convex
Passive (inhibited)	Active (excited)
Pale tongue	Red tongue
Thin pulse	Full pulse
Contraction	Expansion
Deficiency	Excess
Pain is dull, achy, stiff	Pain is sharp or moving
Deep	Shallow (on the surface)
Client says "Mm-mm-mm."	Client says "OW!"

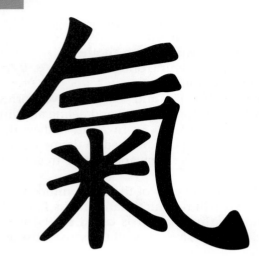

Figure 26-3   Symbol for Qi.

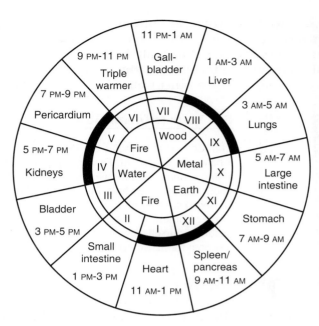

Figure 26-4   Meridian Cycle wheel chart. (Modified from Hass EM: *Staying healthy with the seasons,* Millbrae, Calif, 1981, Celestial Arts.)

dissect the body, it cannot be found. Just like the wind in the trees, Qi is seen by seeing its effects. All living things are infused with Qi (Figure 26-3). Qi is felt by palpating acupoints, abdomen, and skin and muscles or by feeling the auric field, or the energy field surrounding the body. All energy is vibrational and can be palpated when one is attuned to it.

The following are important functions for Qi in the body:

- Heats and protects the body
- Serves as the source of all movement and goes along with all movement
- Governs smooth and harmonious transformations
- Keeps the body's vital substances and organs in place

For Your Information

The Vital Substances in Chinese medicine are Qi, essence (jing), blood (xue), body fluids (jin-ye), and spirit (shen).

Qi has three sources: (1) it is gathered from parents to offspring at birth and represents a person's inherited constitution, (2) it is obtained from the food eaten, and (3) it is extracted from the air breathed.

Qi flows through the 12 primary meridians in a specific order every 24 hours, based on Sun time. This cycle is known as the *meridian cycle,* the Law of Midday/Midnight, or sometimes, the Chinese clock (Figure 26-4). Although Qi is in each channel at all times, a tide flows through every day. The tide peaks in a different meridian every 2 hours; at its opposite time of day is its ebb, the lowest tide. For example, the Lung meridian's high tide is from 3 AM to 5 AM, so its lowest tide is 3 PM to 5 PM.

THE FIVE ELEMENTS

The **Five Elements** show us, through correspondences and relationships, how life processes and relationships work. These theories were deduced over centuries of careful observation of natural phenomena. The Five Elements are the ingredients necessary for life on Earth: (1) Water, (2) Wood, (3) Fire, (4) Earth, and (5) Metal.

Each Element has its fundamental influence, strengths, and weaknesses (Figure 26-5). Each Element has its relationship to all the other Elements

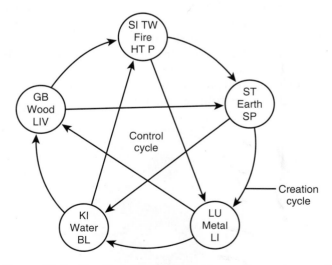

Figure 26-5   Five Element symbol with creation and control cycles and associated meridians.

TABLE 26-3

Five Element Correspondences

Element	Organ Systems	Season	Color	Sense Organ	Joints of the Body	Emotion
Fire	Ht/SI P/TW	Summer	Red	Tongue	Elbows	Excess joy
Earth	SP/ST	Late summer	Yellow	Mouth	Hips	Overthinking
Metal	Lu/LI	Autumn	White	Nose	Wrists	Grief
Water	K/BL	Winter	Black/navy	Ears	Knees, ankles	Fear
Wood	Liv/GB	Spring	Green	Eyes	Shoulders	Anger

Ht/SI, Heart, small intestine; *P/TW,* pericardium, triple warmer; *SP/ST,* spleen-pancreas, stomach; *Lu/LI,* lung, large intestine; *K/BL,* Kidney, bladder; *Liv/GB,* liver, gallbladder.

and they are constantly interacting to keep energy flowing in a series of cycles, described as follows:

- The Creation Cycle is a nourishing cycle; each Element feeds the next in line.
- The Control Cycle is a system of checks and balances, each exerting control over another.
- The Overacting Cycle is a stronger version of the Control Cycle; an Element's control gets excessive and weakens the Element being controlled.
- The Counteracting Cycle attacks backward along the Control Cycle.

The Five Elements are another division of Yin and Yang; each Element holds a Yin/Yang pair of Organ Systems. The Fire Element is associated with four Organs, or two pairs. Many other correspondences are also associated, including seasons of the year, colors, sense organs, joints of the body, emotions, and so on (Table 26-3). These correspondences help us understand associations and relationships of life while helping us understand ourselves.

For Your Information

It is helpful to regard the Five Elements as the Five Transformations or Phases because these concepts do more justice to their meaning. In English, Element is a word that makes one think of separate objects. Transformation or Phase is an entirely different concept (you can see how some confusion over translations occurs). The transformations are not separate; they are connected through relationships and interact continuously. Unfortunately, Element is the word most often used and thus most often recognized; hence, its usage here.

SHIATSU

Shiatsu, which in Japanese means finger (shi) pressure (atsu), is the application of direct, perpendicular pressure applied along meridian lines and tsubos (acupoints and other reactive points on the body) to assist Qi flow in the body, mind, and spirit. Active and passive exercises, rhythmic or steady palm pressure, direct pressure to specific tsubos, and meridian stretching may be part of the protocol (Figure 26-6). A qualified practitioner may recommend dietary and lifestyle changes. Keeping the Qi flowing smoothly is necessary for continued health. Shiatsu is excellent therapy for health maintenance and disease prevention, which directly relates to smoothly flowing Qi.

Shiatsu has been practiced in Japan for at least 2000 years and became systemized during the twentieth century. Tokujiro Namikoshi and Shizuto Masunaga are generally regarded as the fathers of the systemization. Although they were classmates in their early studies, they took shiatsu in different directions. Namikoshi took a more western approach, applying shiatsu to muscles and muscle groups. Masunaga took a more eastern approach, developing Zen shiatsu, which focuses on the body's energy and incorporates ancient extended meridians. Interestingly, both approaches are effective. Shiatsu has been officially recognized as medical therapy in Japan since the mid-1950s.

During a shiatsu session, the client remains fully clothed in loose, comfortable clothing and may receive treatment on a futon mat, massage table, or chair. The practitioner uses thumbs, fingers, hands, elbows, or sometimes feet to apply pressure, bringing balance to Qi flowing through the meridians in the body.

One goal of the shiatsu session is to assist the client in discovering blockages or weaknesses. Other goals may be to facilitate the release of blockages, strengthen weaknesses, calm hyperactivity, and advise the client of postural, lifestyle, or dietary changes that may be helpful. Each session is tailored to the individual and based on their individual goals.

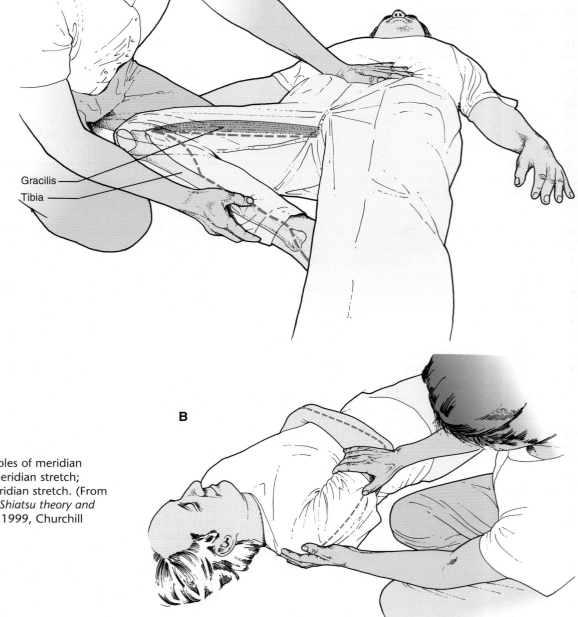

A

Gracilis

Tibia

B

Figure 26-6   Examples of meridian stretches. **A,** Liver meridian stretch; **B,** triple warmer meridian stretch. (From Beresford-Cooke C: *Shiatsu theory and practice,* Edinburgh, 1999, Churchill Livingstone.)

Shiatsu is practiced in many areas of the world and continues to be developed, studied, researched, and enjoyed. Shiatsu is experiencing a movement into the mainstream of health maintenance routines. The AOBTA offers the following definitions for six forms of shiatsu currently available: Five Element shiatsu, Integrative Eclectic shiatsu, Japanese shiatsu, macrobiotic shiatsu (barefoot shiatsu), shiatsu anma therapy, and Zen Shiatsu. Each form has distinguishing characteristics and varying requirements.

Five Element Shiatsu

The emphasis of Five Element shiatsu is to identify patterns of disharmony through use of the four examinations and to harmonize these patterns using an appropriate treatment plan. Hands-on techniques and preferences for assessment vary with the practitioner, depending on their individual background and training. The radial pulse usually provides the most critical and detailed information. Palpation of the back and/or abdomen and a detailed verbal

SHIZUKO YAMAMOTO

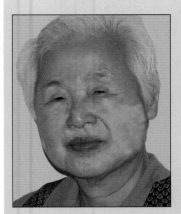

Born: June 1, 1924.

"Carefully observe your activities of thinking, breathing, movement, diet, sex, and sleep, for these are the six fundamentals of health. Within this realm lies success or failure in your physical health and emotional happiness."

Shizuko Yamamoto is a bodyworker, author, and founder of the International Macrobiotic Shiatsu Society. What she believes, teaches, and practices is at once simple and sublime. In a nutshell, she advises us to return to nature as a means to promote health and well-being. Of course this is not a new idea. Around 400 BC, Hippocrates taught that violating nature's laws brought disharmony in the form of physical or emotional sickness. The cure was to recreate balance so that the patient could cure herself.

Centuries after Hippocrates, Chinese medicine made its way to Japan and with it came the art of massage. However, unlike the full spectrum of treatment practiced in Chinese medicine, massage soon became viewed as a pleasurable indulgence for the wealthy, much like the way massage has been viewed for generations. Of course, various practitioners always stuck to the old, more holistic ways of healing. A segment of this group branched out and named their form of massage shiatsu.

Shiatsu is finger, forearm, elbow, or foot pressure and stimulation to certain points on the body and includes rotation and stretching of joints. This pressure frees any blockage in what is the normal route of energy as it moves from organ to organ throughout the body and balances the Qi (Ki), which means Life Force in Japanese.

Macrobiotic is an ancient term that describes healthy people who live a long life. Macrobiotic shiatsu is a blend of hand and barefoot shiatsu, diet, exercise, breathing, stretching, postural rebalancing, and use of medicinal plants to create balance and thus health in individuals. Basic macrobiotic principles are as follows:

1. Health is the natural condition of human beings. It is our birthright.
2. Illness and unhappiness are unnatural conditions.
3. Health or sickness is not an accident or something inexplicable.
4. Sickness arises from how we live as a result of our own actions and thoughts.
5. Food is one of the important factors in determining sickness.
6. We should eat seasonal foods that grow in our own environment.

Illness is not so much shrouded in mystery as it is a function of how you think, breath, move, and sleep; your diet; and your relationships with others. To a certain degree, you can influence your own health, even though it may not be as easy as clicking your heels together three times.

Shizuko Yamamoto was born in Tokyo, the youngest of three brothers and one sister. Her father owned his own company; her mother was a homemaker. After World War II a generous cousin made it possible for her to be trained in yoga, shiatsu, aikido, and Chinese acupuncture, but it was a bout with ill health that changed her life. She had leukemia, lost her eyesight, and had absolutely no energy. She was counseled to eat only fresh, organic foods and whole grains, animal products with no by-products, and no sugar. She began walking for exercise and doing corrective breathing exercises. One month later she felt much better, something that 12 operations had not accomplished. Now she shares her experience and expertise with others worldwide.

"We are nature's creation. Our bodies should be organic. We need clean water and a good environment. We are not just existing as ourselves; we are part of the planet, otherwise we cannot survive."

She travels all over the world and teaches and counsels at a pace that might be grueling for someone half her age. At a mere 5 feet 3 inches, she is sturdy

SHIZUKO YAMAMOTO—cont'd

and exudes energy and warmth. She has worked on many people who were much larger than her when she started her practice in the states. Her clients were not just bigger; they were also less flexible, which she attributes to a higher consumption of animal fats and protein. She has worked on so many people for so many years, her hands sometimes cannot move. To compensate for her size difference and to continue a strong practice for years to come, she developed barefoot shiatsu, a simple yet effective routine wherein the client lies on the floor and the practitioner stands and primarily uses the feet to deliver the treatment.

Yamamoto outlines her advice to beginning massage therapists: "I don't think about money. I concentrate on how I can help." She also recommends being sensitive to clients' needs, maintaining good health, and using good judgment. "Increase your knowledge of your craft; then practice, practice, practice. Maintain a healthy balance in your life."

history serve to confirm the assessment. Also considered during assessment are the client's lifestyle and emotional and psychological factors. Although this approach uses the paradigm of the Five Elements to tonify, sedate, or control patterns of disharmony, practitioners of this style also consider hot or cold; internal or external signs and symptoms. Cindy Banker is one of the major developers of Five Element shiatsu.

Integrative Eclectic Shiatsu

Integrative Eclectic shiatsu, developed by Toshiko Phipps, combines the use of Japanese shiatsu techniques, traditional Chinese medical theory, and Western methods of soft-tissue manipulation. Dietary changes and herbal remedies are also used to create a comprehensive, integrated treatment approach.

Japanese Shiatsu

Shiatsu is pressure applied along meridian lines, usually with the thumbs. Extensive uses of Hara and the Yu/Shu point assessments are also characteristic of shiatsu. The emphasis of shiatsu is the treatment of the entire meridian; however, tsubos are also used. The therapist assesses the condition of the patient's body as treatment progresses; thus assessment and treatment are one continuous process.

Macrobiotic Shiatsu (Barefoot Shiatsu)

Founded by Shizuko Yamamoto and based on George Ohsawa's philosophy that each individual is an integral part of nature, macrobiotic shiatsu sup-

ports a natural lifestyle and heightened instincts for improving health. Assessments are made visually, verbally, and through touch (including pulses) and using the Five Elements. Treatment involves touch, pressure using both hands and bare feet, and stretches to facilitate Qi flow. Dietary guidance, medicinal plants, breathing techniques, and home remedies are also emphasized. Corrective exercises, postural rebalancing, palm healing, self-shiatsu, and Qigong are all integral components of Macrobiotic Shiatsu.

Shiatsu Anma Therapy

Shiatsu anma therapy uses a blend of the two most popular Asian bodywork forms practiced in Japan, shiatsu and anma. Dr. Tsuneo Kaneko introduced traditional Anma Massage Therapy based on the energetic system of traditional Chinese medicine in long form and contemporary pressure therapy based on neuromusculoskeletal system in short form. Ampuku, abdominal massage therapy, is another foundation of anma massage therapy.

Zen Shiatsu

Developed by Shizuto Masunaga, Zen shiatsu is based on the theory of Kyo-Jitsu, as well as the application of Kyo-Jitsu to abdominal diagnosis. Zen shiatsu theory uses extended meridian systems that combine traditional acupuncture meridians with an additional set of expanded meridians. A practitioner of Zen shiatsu uses meridian lines rather than specific tsubos. In addition, Zen shiatsu does not adhere to a fixed sequence, applying this sequence to all clients, but rather seeks and applies a unique sequence on each individual.

For Your Information

When Masunaga included the ancient extended meridian system, it doubled the 12 Primary meridians to 24, with the extended meridians mirroring each other in opposite parts of the body across the transverse plane. For example, in Zen Shiatsu there is a Stomach meridian in the arm as well as the leg.

Ohashiatsu

Developed by Wataru Ohashi, Ohashiatsu is taught at the Ohashi Institutes in New York and Chicago.

Quantum Shiatsu

Pauline Sasaki, who is currently developing Quantum Shiatsu, describes it as a "system of shiatsu where everything is defined in terms of energy as one continuous whole; where time is defined as a sensory experience that is used to make possible the appearance and existence of things, rather than as a reality comprised of irreversible events from birth to death. It is a system that respects life in all its forms, where shiatsu acts as the organizer, not the manipulator."*

Tao Shiatsu

Tao Shiatsu, the manual form of oriental medicine, expresses the Way of Unification, which includes all beings and the Universal Spirit. Master Ryokyu Endo founded this system of health care and healing as a way to promote harmony both within the individual, in their relationship to society and ultimately to the source of all existence: the Tao. The practitioner works with her hands, forearms, and sometimes knees or feet. Continuous steady pressure is applied while synchronizing with the patient's Ki (energy). This enhances the Ki circulation through the network of energy channels or meridians. Each treatment is a combination of deep rhythmic movements, assisted stretches and attention to specific release points. A Tao shiatsu treatment stimulates the internal healing power of the individual and promotes the release of stagnated energy, restoring the unification of body, mind, and spirit.

Watsu

Watsu is a hybrid technique that is conducted in warm water pools. Harold Dull based this system on Zen shiatsu and other techniques. His biography and an explanation of Watsu is available in Chapter 23.

*Sasaki P: Personal communication, 2002.

The level and quality of training varies widely from program to program and person to person. The requirements in the United States are generally a minimum of 500 documented hours of approved curricula for entry-level practitioner status. This is also the minimum number of hours required to sit for the national certification examination for Diplomate of Asian Bodywork Therapy, provided by the National Certification Commission for Acupuncture and Oriental Medicine (NCCAOM).

 First you learn your instrument, then you wail.

—Charlie "Bird" Parker

For Your Information

A *cun* is the body inch in Chinese medicine, used to measure distance on the body. Each cun is measured by the width of the client's own thumb knuckle. The width of four finger knuckles together is 3 cun, two finger knuckles is 1.5 cun, and four fingertips together are 3 cun (Figure 26-7).

MERIDIANS

In Chinese medicine, **meridians** (also called *channels* or *pathways*) are the conduits through which Qi flows. Meridians are a considerable part of the focus when doing Asian bodywork. The 12 primary meridians flow bilaterally in superficial layers of the body, joining internally with other meridians and additional connecting channels, and pass through the internal organs for which they are named. Meridians are an integral part of the Organ Systems of Chinese medicine and join to other areas of the body through acupoints and additional connecting channels. These systemic energetic connections establish links that carry the energy from our food and breath to the rest of the body.

Of the 12 primary meridians, six are Yin and six are Yang meridians. Six meridians nourish each arm

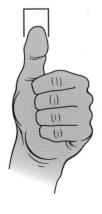

Figure 26-7 Cun illustration.

and connect to the head, back, and torso; six meridians nourish each leg and connect to the head, back, and torso. The anatomical position in the Chinese medical model is a person standing with the hands raised and palms forward, showing the directions of Qi flow.

The Yin meridians are located on the anterior and medial aspects of the body, flow up, and are associated with the solid body Organs that function in storage and nourishment. The Yin meridians are as follows:

- Liver meridian (Liv) (Figure 26-8)
- Spleen-pancreas meridian (SP, usually called *Spleen*) (Figure 26-9)
- Lung meridian (Lu) (Figure 26-10)
- Kidney meridian (K or KI) (Figure 26-11)
- Pericardium meridian (P) (Figure 26-12)
- Heart meridian (Ht) (Figure 26-13)

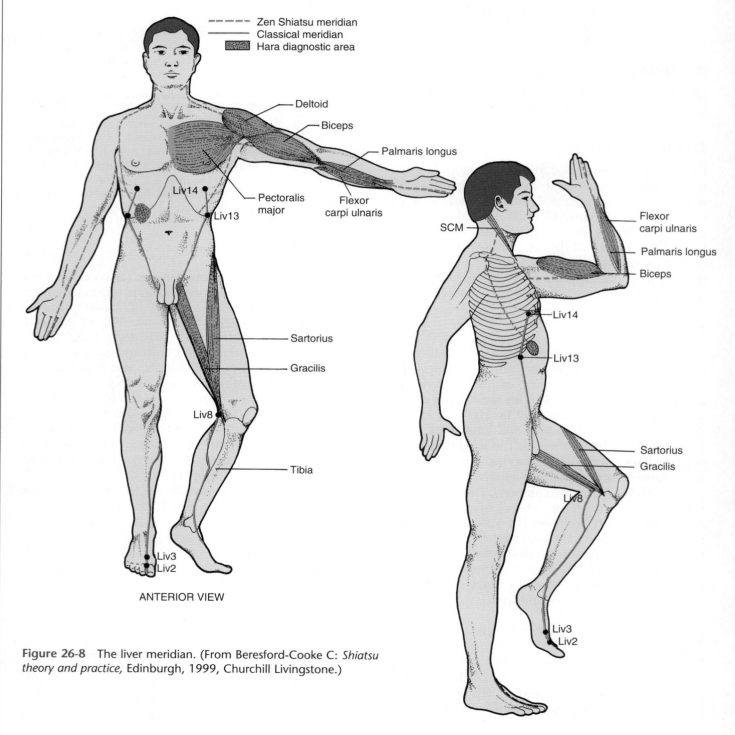

ANTERIOR VIEW

LATERAL VIEW

Figure 26-8 The liver meridian. (From Beresford-Cooke C: *Shiatsu theory and practice,* Edinburgh, 1999, Churchill Livingstone.)

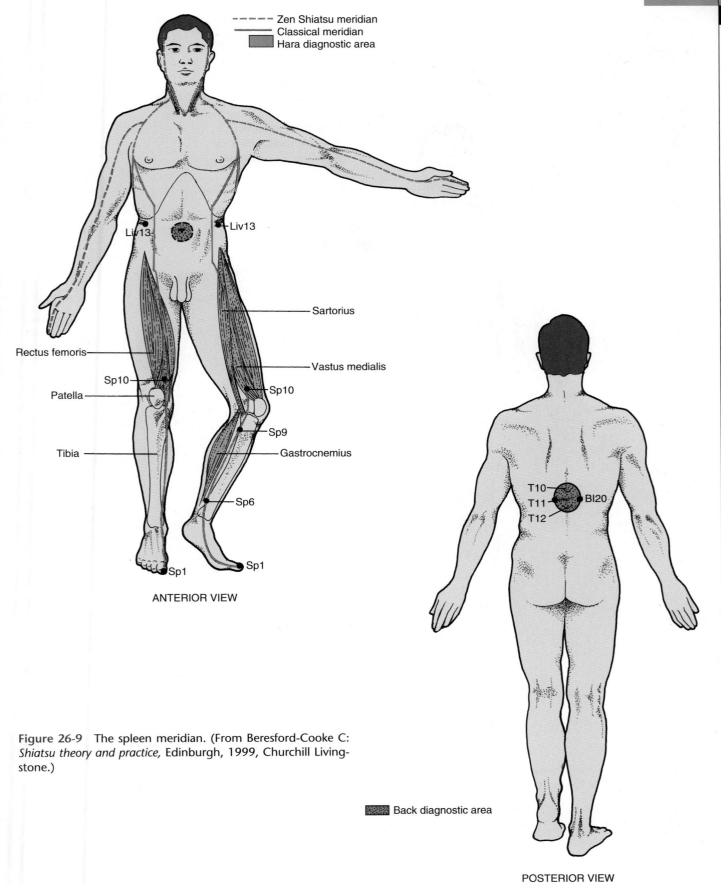

Figure 26-9 The spleen meridian. (From Beresford-Cooke C: *Shiatsu theory and practice,* Edinburgh, 1999, Churchill Livingstone.)

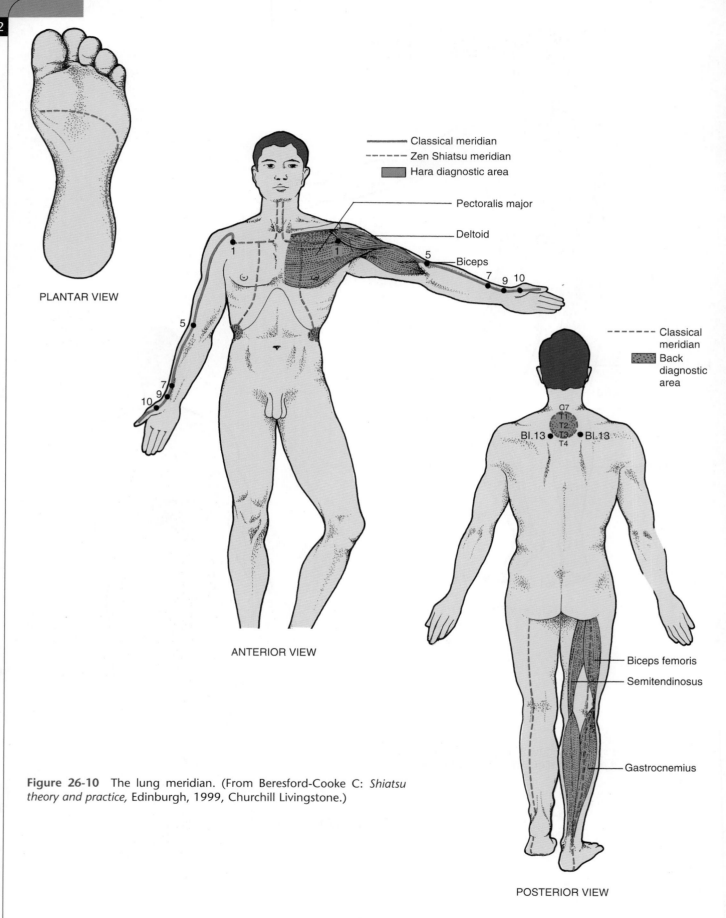

Classical meridian
Zen Shiatsu meridian
Hara diagnostic area

Pectoralis major

Deltoid

Biceps

Classical
meridian

Back
diagnostic
area

Bl.13   Bl.13

PLANTAR VIEW

ANTERIOR VIEW

Biceps femoris

Semitendinosus

Gastrocnemius

POSTERIOR VIEW

Figure 26-10   The lung meridian. (From Beresford-Cooke C: *Shiatsu theory and practice,* Edinburgh, 1999, Churchill Livingstone.)

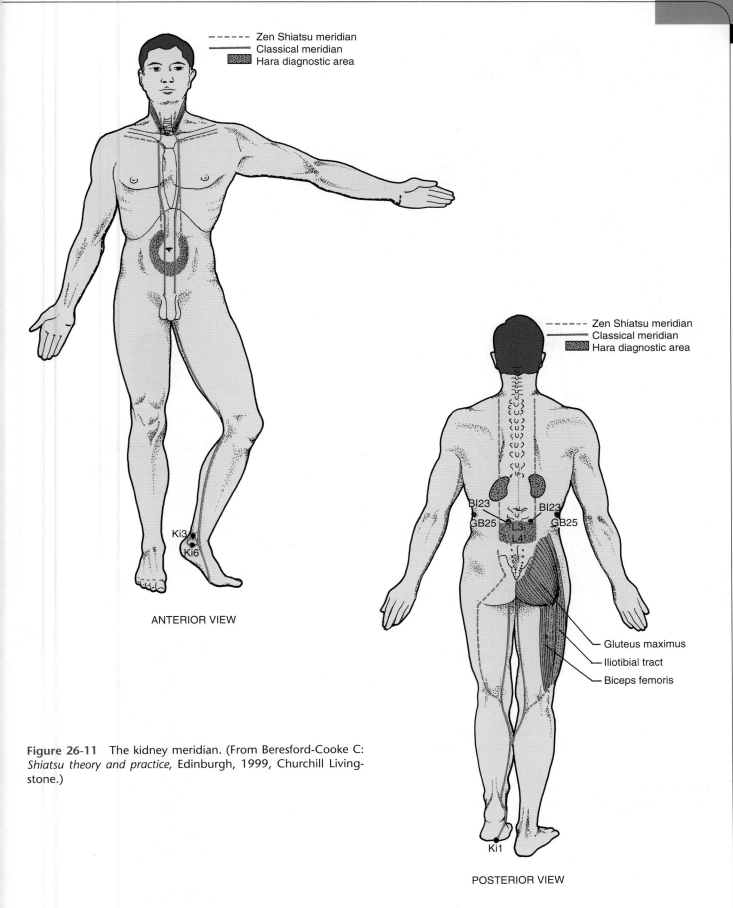

Zen Shiatsu meridian
Classical meridian
Hara diagnostic area

Ki3
Ki6

ANTERIOR VIEW

Zen Shiatsu meridian
Classical meridian
Hara diagnostic area

Bl23   Bl23
GB25   GB25
L3
L4

Gluteus maximus
Iliotibial tract
Biceps femoris

Ki1

POSTERIOR VIEW

Figure 26-11   The kidney meridian. (From Beresford-Cooke C: *Shiatsu theory and practice,* Edinburgh, 1999, Churchill Livingstone.)

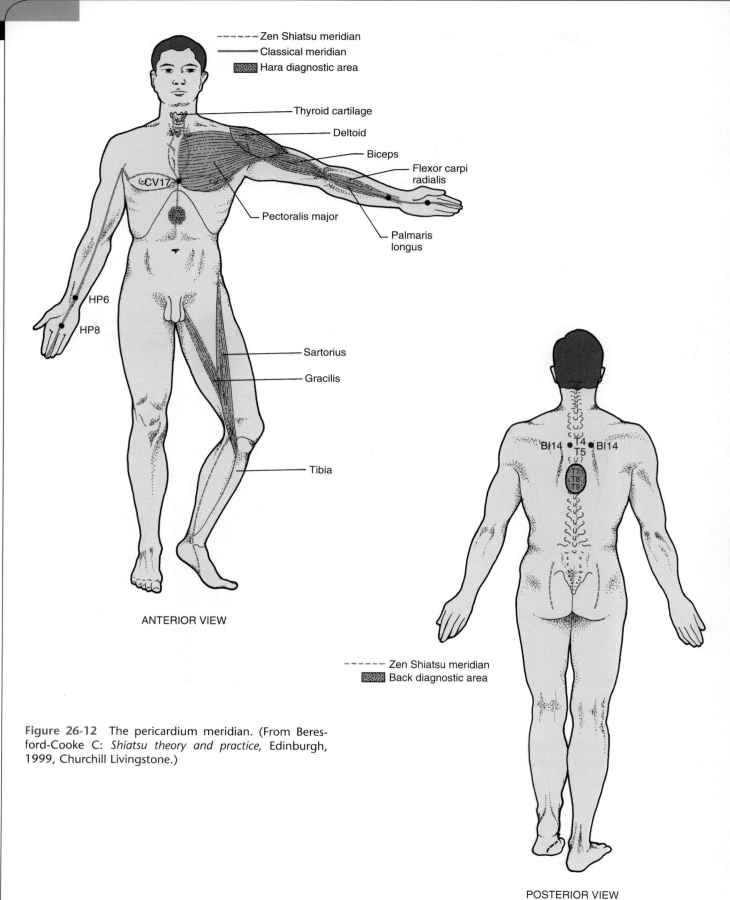

------ Zen Shiatsu meridian
—— Classical meridian
▨ Hara diagnostic area

Thyroid cartilage

Deltoid

Biceps

Flexor carpi radialis

CV17

Pectoralis major

Palmaris longus

HP6

HP8

Sartorius

Gracilis

Tibia

ANTERIOR VIEW

Bl14 T4 Bl14
T5
T7
T8
T9

------ Zen Shiatsu meridian
▨ Back diagnostic area

POSTERIOR VIEW

Figure 26-12   The pericardium meridian. (From Beresford-Cooke C: *Shiatsu theory and practice,* Edinburgh, 1999, Churchill Livingstone.)

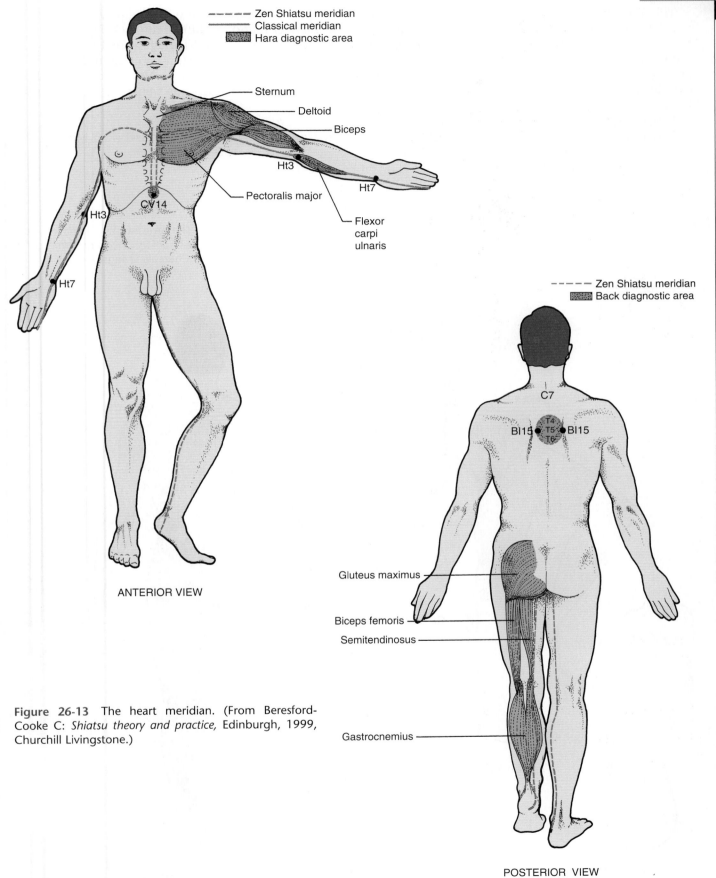

Zen Shiatsu meridian
Classical meridian
Hara diagnostic area

Sternum
Deltoid
Biceps
Ht3
Ht7
Pectoralis major
CV14
Flexor
carpi
ulnaris
Ht3
Ht7

ANTERIOR VIEW

Zen Shiatsu meridian
Back diagnostic area

C7
T4
T5
T6
Bl15
Bl15

Gluteus maximus

Biceps femoris

Semitendinosus

Gastrocnemius

POSTERIOR VIEW

Figure 26-13 The heart meridian. (From Beresford-Cooke C: *Shiatsu theory and practice,* Edinburgh, 1999, Churchill Livingstone.)

The Yang meridians are located on the posterior and lateral aspects of the body, begin or end in the head, flow down, and are associated with hollow body Organs. These Organs' functions are to digest and excrete food and fluid and to communicate with exterior body orifices. The Yang meridians are as follows:

- Large intestine meridian (LI) (Figure 26-14)
- Small intestine meridian (SI) (Figure 26-15)
- Gallbladder meridian (GB) (Figure 26-16)
- Bladder meridian (BL) (Figure 26-17)
- Stomach meridian (ST) (Figure 26-18)
- Triple warmer meridian (TW) (Figure 26-19)

The Eight Extraordinary Vessels are considered deep reservoirs of the body's energies and are as follows:

1. Governing Vessel (Du Mai)
2. Conception or Directing Vessel (Ren Mai)

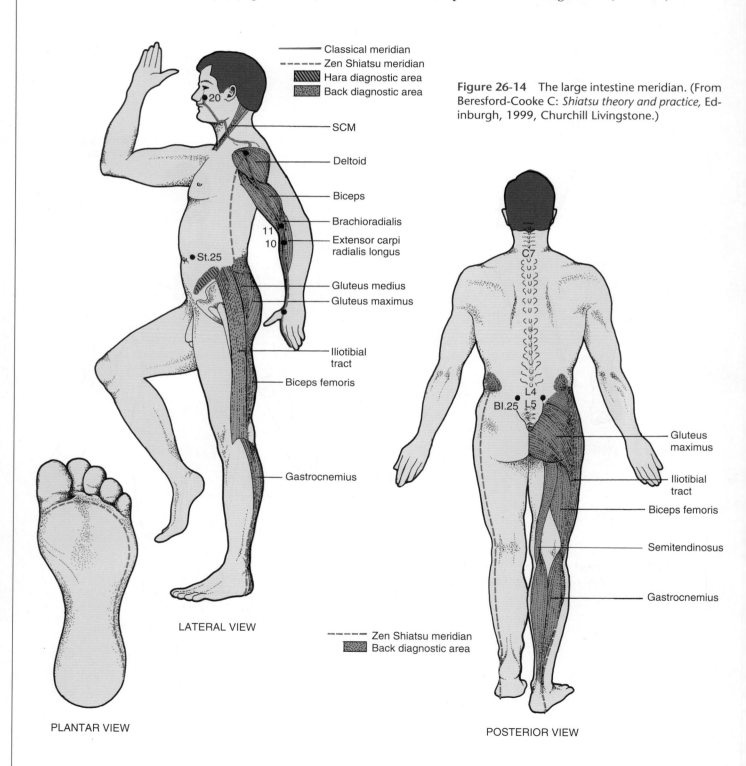

Figure 26-14   The large intestine meridian. (From Beresford-Cooke C: *Shiatsu theory and practice,* Edinburgh, 1999, Churchill Livingstone.)

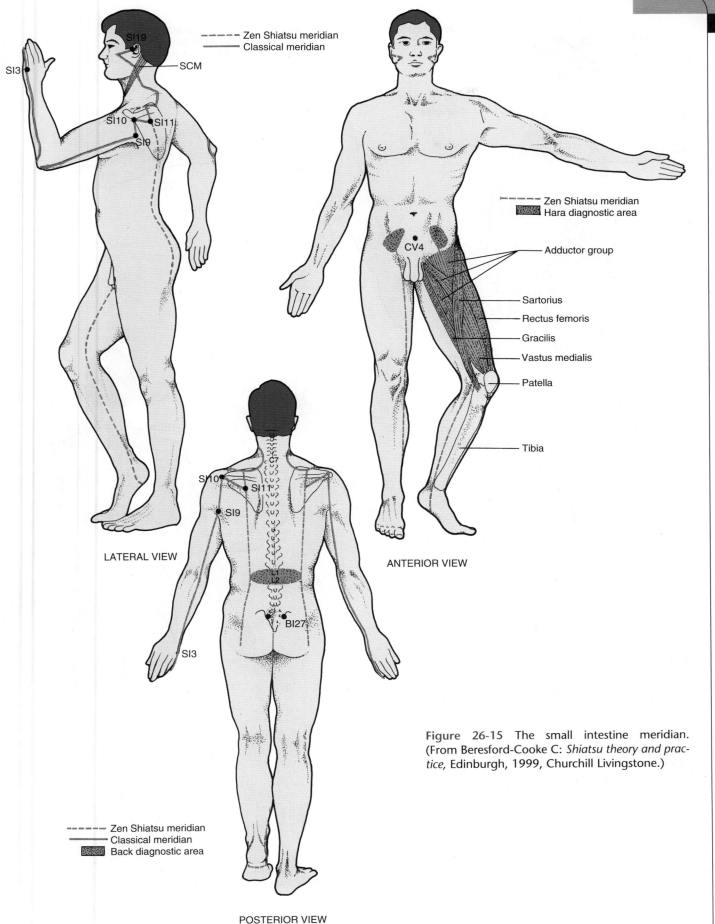

SI19
SCM
SI3
SI10   SI11
SI9

------ Zen Shiatsu meridian
—— Classical meridian

LATERAL VIEW

------ Zen Shiatsu meridian
Hara diagnostic area

Adductor group

Sartorius
Rectus femoris
Gracilis
Vastus medialis
Patella

Tibia

CV4

ANTERIOR VIEW

C7
SI10
SI11
SI9

L1
L2

BI27

SI3

------ Zen Shiatsu meridian
—— Classical meridian
Back diagnostic area

POSTERIOR VIEW

Figure 26-15 The small intestine meridian. (From Beresford-Cooke C: *Shiatsu theory and practice*, Edinburgh, 1999, Churchill Livingstone.)

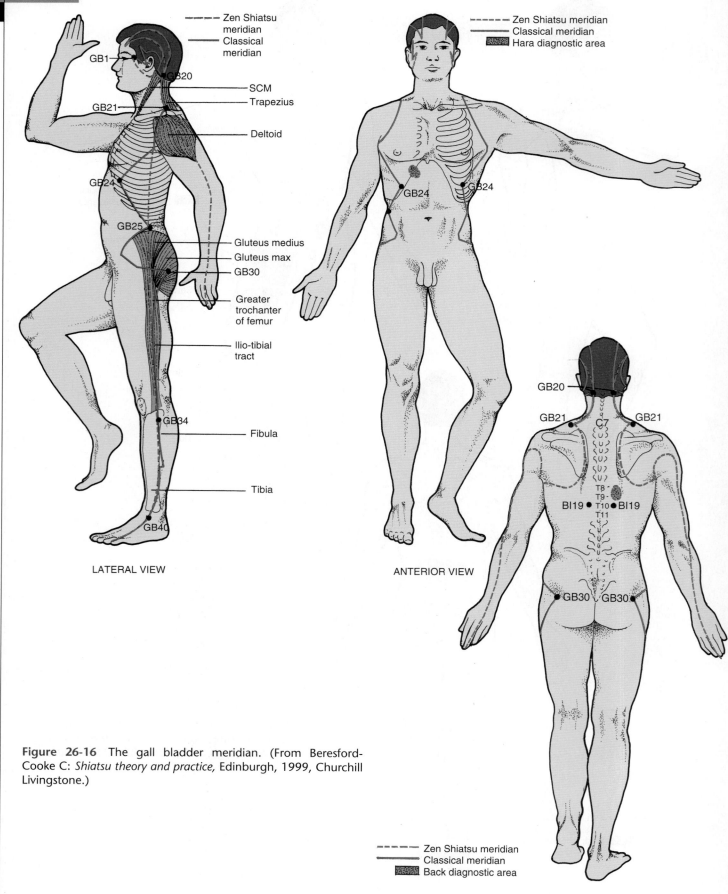

Figure 26-16 The gall bladder meridian. (From Beresford-Cooke C: *Shiatsu theory and practice,* Edinburgh, 1999, Churchill Livingstone.)

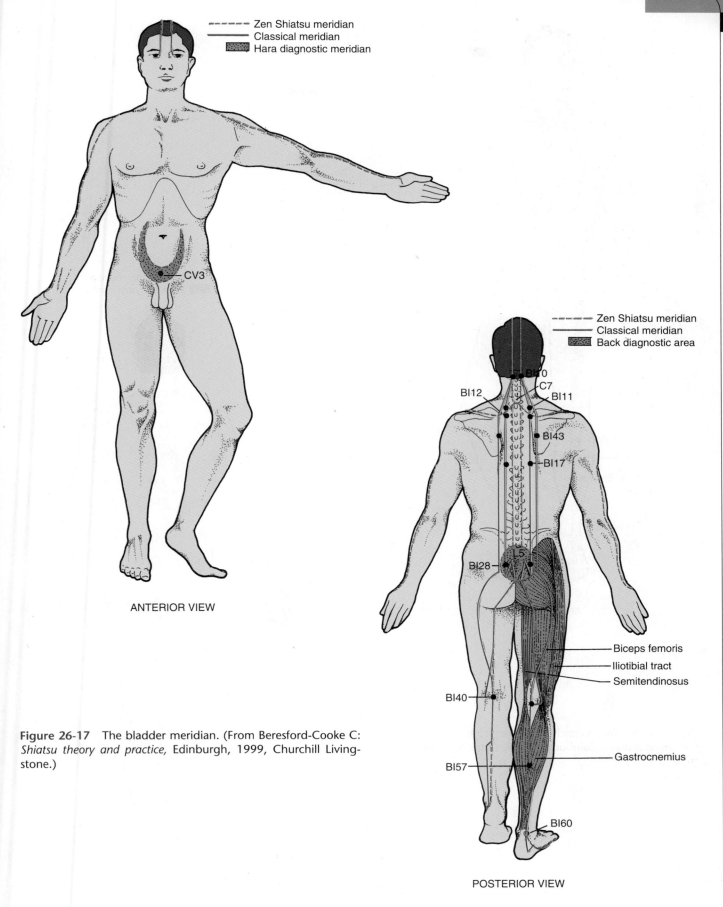

ANTERIOR VIEW

POSTERIOR VIEW

Figure 26-17   The bladder meridian. (From Beresford-Cooke C: *Shiatsu theory and practice,* Edinburgh, 1999, Churchill Livingstone.)

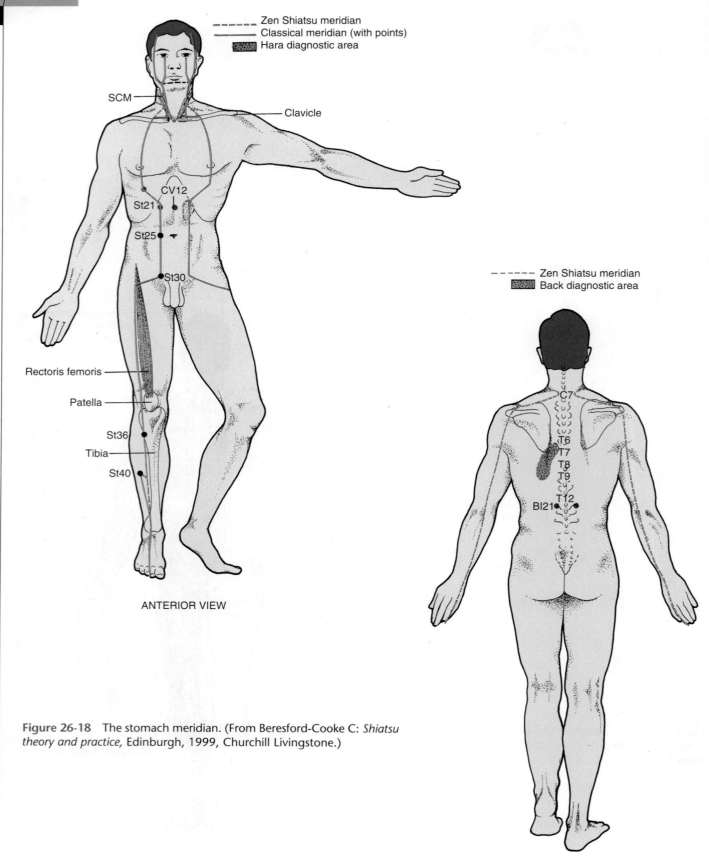

Figure 26-18 The stomach meridian. (From Beresford-Cooke C: *Shiatsu theory and practice,* Edinburgh, 1999, Churchill Livingstone.)

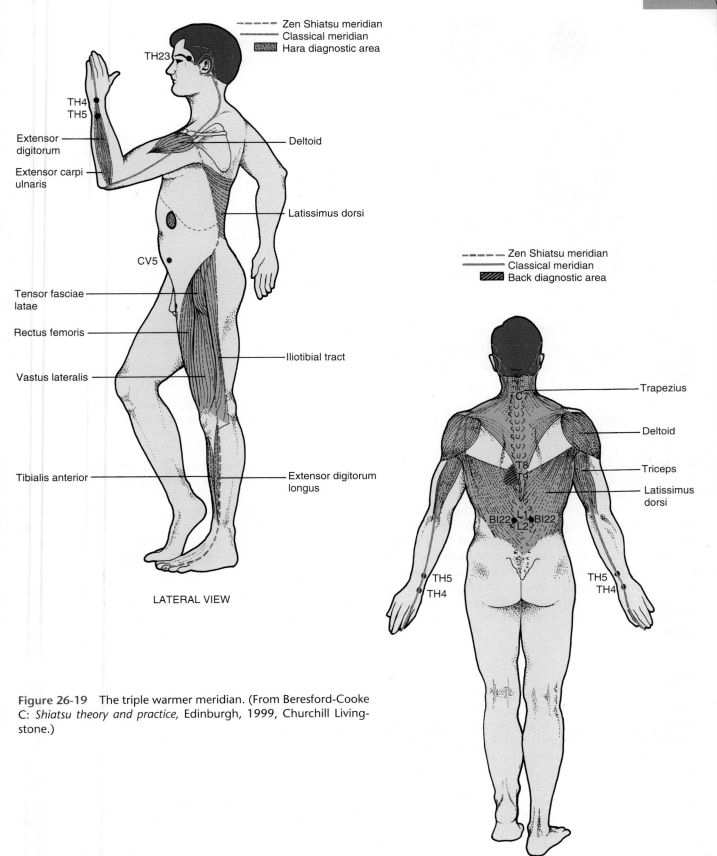

LATERAL VIEW

POSTERIOR VIEW

Figure 26-19   The triple warmer meridian. (From Beresford-Cooke C: *Shiatsu theory and practice,* Edinburgh, 1999, Churchill Livingstone.)

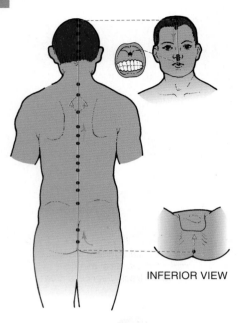

INFERIOR VIEW

POSTERIOR VIEW

Figure 26-20 The Governing Vessel. (From Maciocia M: *The foundations of Chinese medicine,* Edinburgh, 1989, Churchill Livingstone.)

3. Yin Linking Vessel (Yin Wei Mai)
4. Yang Linking Vessel (Yang Wei Mai)
5. Yin Heel Vessel (Yin Qiao Mai)
6. Yang Heel Vessel (Yang Qiao Mai)
7. Penetrating Vessel (Chong Mai)
8. Belt or Girdle Vessel (Dai Mai)

The Governing Vessel and the Conception Vessel are the two extraordinary vessels with their own acupoints. The Governing Vessel begins at the tip of the coccyx and moves up the spinal column, over the midline of the head, down the center of the face, and into the mouth (Figure 26-20). The Conception Vessel begins at the perineum and ascends the midline of the anterior torso and neck to also end in the mouth (Figure 26-21).

ACUPOINTS

Acupoints are points on the body that influence and are influenced by body energy. These specific points have been mapped out for many centuries. Acupoints in Chinese medicine all have names that pertain to their function and/or location. Bubbling Spring or Gushing Spring is the name of an acupoint located on the bottom of the foot and pays homage to that point's function as a source of nourishment flowing upward. Acupoints are also named according to the meridian on which they are located and the direction of Qi flow. For example, Bubbling Spring is known as K1. The Qi flow of the Kidney meridian begins at K1, flows up the anterior and medial aspects

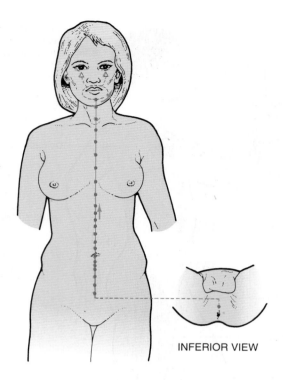

INFERIOR VIEW

ANTERIOR VIEW

Figure 26-21 The Conception Vessel. (From Maciocia M: *The foundations of Chinese medicine,* Edinburgh, 1989, Churchill Livingstone.)

of the body, and ends at K27, under the sternoclavicular joint. The twenty-seventh point of the Kidney meridian is the last point of that meridian.

Acupoints are used in assessment and treatment of the body's energy imbalances. These points are energetic intersections on the highways of the body's energy and the places Qi tends to collect (Figure 26-22).

In Chinese medicine, other points on the body that get a reaction from the client when touched are called **ashi points**. *Ashi* means "that's it!", the typical reaction from the client. Also known as reactive points, ashi points may or may not be on a map of acupoints, but it does not mean they are not important or effective to work with.

Tsubo is the Japanese term used to describe acupoints and other ashi, or reactive points. The tsubo is likened to a vase or jar, or container in which Qi can pool.

HARA

The **Hara**, in Japanese therapies, is the belly—the geographical center of gravity and the energetic center in the body. In China, three of these energy centers are known as dantien; the lower dantien (lower belly), the middle dantien (in the center of the chest) and upper dantien (just above and between the eyes, the third eye).

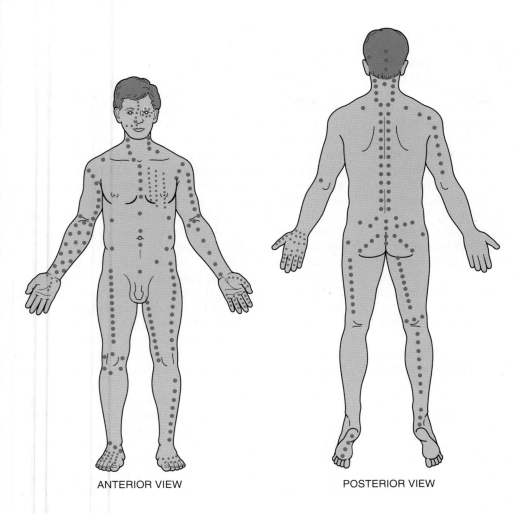

ANTERIOR VIEW   POSTERIOR VIEW

Figure 26-22 Acupoints, anterior and posterior views.

SHIATSU THEORY AND TECHNIQUE

The Hara is located in the central/lower abdomen, the center of which is about 2 finger-widths below the navel. When coming from the hara, a practitioner is being biomechanically efficient by using body weight and structure rather than upper body strength and muscle.

A healthy Hara is expressed by good health, balanced energy, and honorable interaction with the world. Many exercises and meditations are used in Qigong and Tai Chi to strengthen the Hara. Focused intention in an area of the body that provides more balance helps us stay more centered. A strong Hara serves to strengthen the entire body on every level: energetically, physically, mentally, emotionally, and spiritually.

When practicing Asian bodywork therapy, the Hara is the central pivot point while leaning into the client with body weight and not pushing or straining (see Chapter 6). Staying relaxed and centered encourages the client to seek and hopefully find this same state. Both client and practitioner benefit from this reciprocal exchange.

Shiatsu theory is simplistic on the surface; locate the energy imbalances in the body, then take appropriate steps to facilitate balance. If the Qi is weak, build it up. If the Qi is excessive, tone it down. If the Qi is stuck, help it move. Shiatsu connects, balances, and rejuvenates harmony with all life.

Qi imbalances may be almost any shape or size, with some smaller than a fingertip, larger than the palm of your hand, localized, or systemic. Some imbalances affect the entire meridian and its connecting meridians. An imbalance in an Organ System affects the associated meridian and an imbalance in the meridian eventually affects the associated Organ. The benefits of regular treatment are made clear when this relationship is understood and honored.

This section is about identifying and treating deficiencies and excesses of Qi in a meridian, a basic and important part of Asian bodywork therapy. Shiatsu and other Asian bodywork sessions are often a continuous process of assessment and treatment.

Sensing Qi imbalances is a good way to begin learning to feel the meridian and its Qi flow.

As mentioned earlier, a meridian is like a pathway. A number of noticeable, palpable effects are located along the pathway. It is helpful to think of the pathway as a place for water to flow, like a stream (although Qi is not water, the flowing process is similar). Along the stream may be rocks and stones that block the flow. Holes where the water collects into pools may be found. When palpating a meridian, it is important to remember the pathway is one continuous flow—when it is visualized this way, one can notice the blockages and pools more easily.

When a deficiency of Qi is in a meridian, the practitioner notices signs that are more Yin in nature. A few signs of Qi deficiency areas that are cooler or cold to the touch, excessive moisture on the skin, weak musculature that feels loose and soft, complaints of vague and achy pain, deep and empty areas that feel like holes or valleys on the pathway, and the presentation of chronic conditions.

When a deficiency of Qi is determined, the therapist responds by using tonifying techniques that strengthen, build, awaken, and fill the meridian with Life Force. This is done using gentle, invigorating techniques. Several techniques accomplish this, such as perpendicular pressure and quick, light movements in a clockwise motion. Warming and strengthening techniques are also tonifying, such as isometric contractions (proprioceptive neuromuscular facilitation), hot packs and compresses, holding and baking techniques (using the palms of the hands opposite each other on the body part to generate heat), working in the direction of Qi flow, and encouraging empty areas to fill with Qi. A general rule of thumb is to tonify deficiencies first, thus building the person's foundational energy (Table 26-4).

When there is excess of Qi in a meridian, the practitioner notices signs that are more Yang in nature. These signs may include areas that are warm or hot to the touch, dry skin, hypertonic muscle tissue, specific, acute pain at or near the surface, areas that feel stuck, swollen, and/or hardened to the touch, and presentation of acute conditions.

When an excess of Qi is determined, dispersing/sedating techniques are used to move stuck Qi, untie knots, calm hyperactivity, and spread Qi around. The practitioner realizes that excessive Qi can be painful and works in a gentle, careful, yet deliberate, manner. Dispersing techniques include nonperpendicular pressure, counterclockwise circles and motions, broader pressure using the palm or foot, cold packs, range-of-motion techniques with the breath, rocking and jostling, working against the direction of Qi flow and encouraging the extra energy to move about throughout the rest of the meridian.

The shiatsu therapist uses his body weight to lean into the client's body (Figure 26-23); perpendicular pressure is the goal. Angle the pressure toward the center of the body part. Ideally, the pressure is perpendicular to the body area/part, not the floor. While doing shiatsu, keep the Hara toward and near the area you are going to be working while leaning into the client's body. Keep the Hara up off the ground to lean. Transfer the weight from the Hara into your hand(s), elbow, foot, and so on, keeping the shoulders down and the rest of the body loose and open (Figure 26-24).

When doing bodywork, meridian knowledge guides the practitioner through the body landscape. Work each meridian with gentle, relaxed, rhythmic, and direct pressure, covering the entire area and following the flow of the meridian's Qi (Figure 26-25). Always keep both hands on the client, even if one hand is stationary. The stationary hand is referred to as the *mother hand;* it is comforting and reassuring and diverts attention from the working or moving hand. Begin with light palm pressure, gathering information with each pass over the meridian. As you gain more knowledge of the meridian's condition, reassess and modify pressure, using tonifying or dispersing techniques as needed. Use enough pressure to "meet the Qi"—that is, enough so that you can feel the resistance in the tissue but not so much that you cause discomfort. Follow the meridian as many times as it takes to open the flow of Qi. Spend extra time in areas that house Qi deficiencies and excesses (Figure 26-26).

TABLE 26-4

Opposing Symptoms to Ascertain Imbalances With Corresponding Treatment Plans

Qi Imbalance	Qi Deficiency	Qi Excess
Looks and feels like	Cold, moist, tired, achy pain, weak, chronic	Hot, dry, excitable, specific pain, strong, acute
Treatment plan	Tonifying	Dispersing/sedating
Techniques used	Perpendicular pressure, light and vigorous clockwise motions, warming and strengthening techniques	Nonperpendicular pressure, broader, slower and firmer; counterclockwise motions, cooling techniques

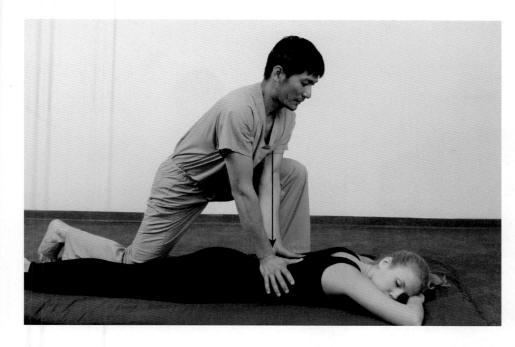

Figure 26-23 Leaning into the back.

When using the thumbs and fingertips, note the pressure used (Figure 26-27). Too much pressure may not only cause the client discomfort, but it also impedes the practitioner's ability to feel Qi flow. Qi flow may feel like a pulsing under the skin or like electrical charges under the fingers.

MINI-LAB

To begin to palpate Qi, look over a meridian chart and try this exercise. Find two acupoints on one meridian of a classmate or friend. Place a fingertip gently on each one. To make it more interesting, choose points that are relatively distant from each other. Add enough pressure to feel the points resist your touch. Maintain pressure; ask your friend to verify pressure comfort. Still maintaining pressure, close your eyes and focus your awareness in your fingertips. Movement under each fingertip may occur; the movement may be subtle, or it may be obvious—from an electrical sensation or a pulsing sensation to actual movements of the tissues. Alternately hold and stimulate the points with small, circular motions. Do these points feel connected? Do the sensations feel balanced or steady? Do both points vibrate alternately or simultaneously? Be patient with yourself; palpating Qi may take some time. It is advisable, however, to spend not more than 3 minutes on any two points. Be ready to remove your hands should the client request it. Ask your friend to pay attention and to share the experience. Both giver and receiver can benefit from the exchange.

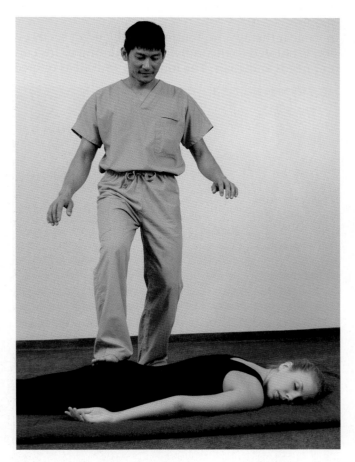

Figure 26-24 Therapist using foot, leaning in with bent knee while keeping the rest of the body loose and open.

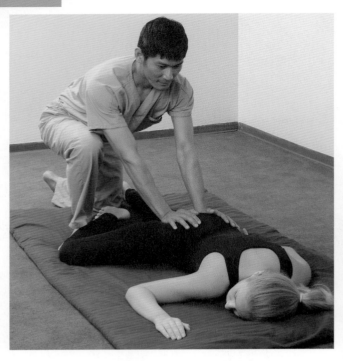

Figure 26-25   Frogging the leg.

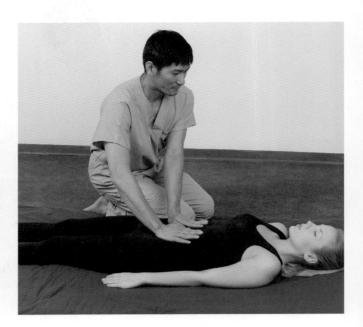

Figure 26-26   Hara work.

A ROUTINE TO PRACTICE

In shiatsu therapy, no routine is really used; each session is tailored to the individual according to his current needs and goals. The following routine is offered for the practice of technique and body mechanics, with the understanding that it is only an outline for early training.

Please review the entire section before proceeding with practice. This routine is designed to work the channels in each body area, rather than following

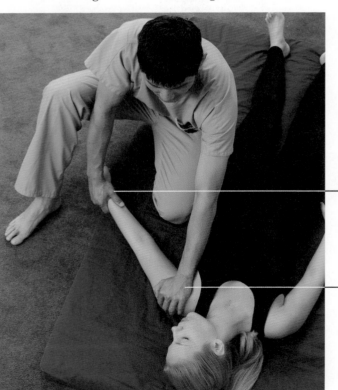

Working
hand

Mother
hand

Figure 26-27   Thumbing the arm.

the channels from beginning to end. This routine is designed to be read aloud, with students simultaneously practicing the techniques after an instructor demonstration. Remember the following:

- Lean; do not press.
- Use perpendicular pressure (for the most part, as required).
- Stay relaxed, centered, and focused.
- Let your own Qi flow.
- Tonify deficiencies.
- Disperse excesses.

NOTE: As with any bodywork, do not invade the client's privacy, physically or energetically.

The Beginning

Ask the client to lie down in a supine position. Support her with bolsters as needed. Students must ground and center themselves and focus in their own Hara.

Make the first contact with both hands (choose the shoulders, ankles, or feet), resting there a moment to get energetically connected with the client. Gently rock the client, moving each portion of the body until you have moved the entire body as you make your way up/down/around. No need to rock the head, it will move along with the spine. If the client is rocked in her own timing, the practitioner feels no effort, and the client experiences relaxation. Use some gentle range-of-motion techniques now; this is an opportunity for the client's body to reintegrate into a whole being at the beginning of your time together. Use your body weight to facilitate range-of-motion techniques.

Make your way to the head and spend a few moments working on the head and face with perpendicular, direct pressure; this helps calm the client's mind and immediately enhances relaxation. It does not take long, and the routine brings you back here later. Hence, do not overdo it. Work the ears; more than 100 acupoints are in each ear that reflex to the entire body. Gently squeeze the outer ear between your thumb and index finger, moving from lobe to top.

Before a client falls asleep, ask him to turn to a prone position; use bolsters as needed. If your client has trouble lying on a mat with his head turned to one side, use a small bolster under the anterior portion of the shoulder they are facing.

Back and Lateral Meridians: Bladder and Gallbladder

Straddle the client (only when prone) so that you are centered over the back (Figure 26-28). Stand up or try a one-knee-down stance; change the stance often so that you can stay comfortable, even if this means resting on both knees. Use your legs more than your

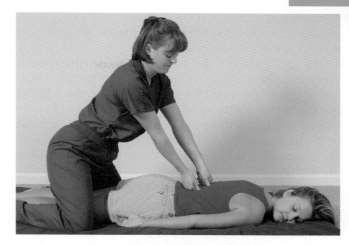

Figure 26-28 Working the back while straddling the prone client.

back. Gently rock and loosen the entire back of the body, making your way from the shoulders to the feet and back again. Use your thumbs along either side of the spine.

Next, begin *cat-walking* (Figure 26-29), alternating pressure from hand to hand as you work in a rhythmic pattern down the BL meridian, on either side of the spine from the upper back to the sacrum. This movement twists the spine and helps loosen tight muscle attachments. Use perpendicular pressure. Come back to the upper back and work from the medial borders of the scapulae for the outer BL channel and follow it to the ischial tuberosities.

Continue in the same manner by leaning into the back with simultaneous pressure in both hands, beginning at the upper back, following the client's exhalation. Never force the client to exhale but follow the breath to the bottom, backing out as he inhales again. Move another palm width down the back and lean in again as he exhales. Make your way down the

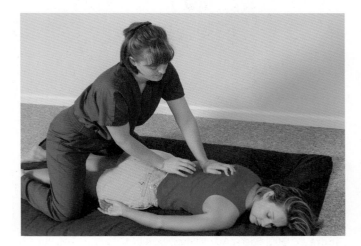

Figure 26-29 Cat-walking on the Bladder meridian.

BL meridian, inner portion first and then outer, until you have worked to the ischial tuberosities again. Be sure to cover the entire area.

The last pass on the BL channel is with specific pressure using thumbs or fingertips. Locate the intercostal spaces between T3 and T4, just at the edge of the transverse processes of the vertebra. You will be on the outer edge of the paraspinal muscles, 1.5 **cun** out from the spinous processes (see FYI, p. 699). Lean into these specific acupoints as the client exhales, continuing along the BL meridian (inner and outer portions), until you reach the ischial tuberosities again.

Next, place both hands, one over the other, crosswise over the sacrum. Roll your weight around on the outside of your hands with pressure to the client's comfort. This is to move the sacrum, not the skin.

Now sit on the floor to one side of your client with his arm out to the side and your body between the arm and the hips. Begin *see-saw walking* (Figure 26-30). Using your foot, gently lean into the side of the body by extending your leg from a bent position, adding pressure from your foot to the body. Begin under the arm and continue in a pattern down the side of the body, a portion of the GB meridian. Be sure to monitor your foot position; do not pinch the breast tissue between your foot and the mat. As you lean out, bring the arm with you so that the client is rocking back and forth as you make your way down

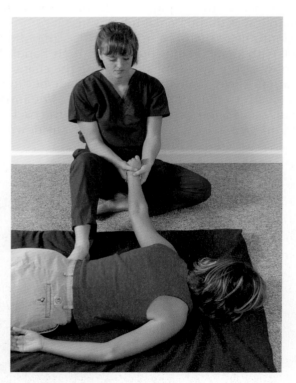

Figure 26-30 See-saw walking, working a portion of the GB meridian.

the side. Be careful in the area of the eleventh and twelfth ribs and kidneys. Always begin with gentle pressure; you can add more. Turn your foot so the outer edge is in the space between the ribs and the iliac crest and lean in. Work down the side and leg as far as you can comfortably reach with your foot, switching to your other foot as needed.

Posterior and Lateral Shoulder and Arm Meridians: Large Intestine, Triple Warmer, and Small Intestine

The next area to work is the shoulder and arm (remain beside the one to which you are closest). Begin work on each limb with joint mobilization techniques. Start with the shoulder and then the elbow, wrist, and hand. Opening the joints first often relieves minor imbalances before more specific work (See Chapter 7.)

After you have opened the joints, work the hand well. Reposition the arm so that the elbow and the shoulder are extended and the hand is palm down. Proceed with perpendicular pressure to the three meridians in the posterior arm from the wrist to the shoulder. These are the LI, TW, and SI meridians, and they all continue to the face. Generally, the channels are worked three times: once with light palm pressure, again with heavier palm pressure, and finished with more specific pressure using thumbs and/or fingertips (i.e., palm- palm-thumb).

When you complete the arm, transition to the other side and begin see-saw walking to the other side. Work that arm as above, place it in a comfortable position; restraddle the back.

Cat-walk down the back one more time and all the way to the sacrum. Work the buttocks well, one side at a time, using feet, loose fists, and/or elbows. When using the foot into the buttocks, be sure to lean your weight into your foot and bend the knee as you lean in. Using the heel of the foot would be specific, so be careful. Try different foot positions and pressures. Get feedback from your client. If you wish to continue down the hamstrings using the foot, stay more than a foot's width away from the popliteal fossa. Using the foot behind and on the iliotibial band can be effective when applied with firm, yet gentle, pressure.

Posterior Leg Meridians: Lateral, Bladder and Gallbladder; Medial, Kidney

Continue by taking one leg in your hands and again begin with joint mobilizations. Mobilize the joints of the hip, knee, ankle, and foot. Then, using palm-palm-thumb pressure, work the BL channel from the ischial tuberosity to the little toe. Use light pressure in the popliteal fossa.

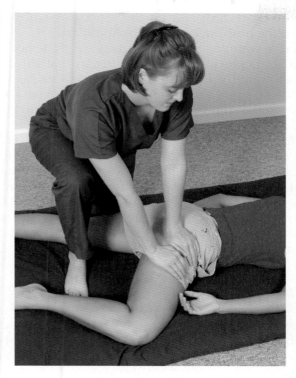

Figure 26-31 Working the client's Gallbladder meridian.

Next, frog the leg out to the side (always mind your client's comfort) and work down the GB to the fourth toe (Figure 26-31). The iliotibial band is usually tight in the upper leg, so work gently at first and try some dispersing techniques. The peroneus longus can usually handle a lot of pressure. When you bring the leg back to a neutral position, raise the hip slightly off the ground to allow it to re-center when the leg is not frogged.

Work the foot well and then begin moving up the K meridian from under the ball of the foot and up the inside of the back of the leg (i.e., palm-palm-thumb). Most people need the K channel tonified so apply tonification techniques. Transition to the other leg and repeat as above.

Anterior Leg Meridians: Medial, Spleen-Pancreas and Liver; Lateral, Stomach

Ask your client to please roll over and use bolsters as necessary. Work the feet again. Use perpendicular pressure to open the areas between the metatarsals.

Proceed with joint mobilizations to the client's left leg. Next, reposition the leg so that the SP channel can be worked. Her foot is at the opposite ankle; support her knee with your knee or a bolster (palm-palm-thumb). The SP meridian is often sensitive, so be careful.

Next, move the leg so her foot is toward the opposite knee to work the Liv channel. Continue

supporting their knee (palm-palm-thumb). Proceed by placing the leg back in a straight position to work the ST meridian down the leg to the middle toes. Transition to the right leg and repeat.

The Hara and Chest

Now on the client's right side, rock the hips side to side and lean into the anterior superior iliac spine with your palms and cat-walk. Settle yourself into a comfortable position next to the Hara and gently place both hands on the center of the abdomen. Let your hands rest there a moment and then begin with gentle perpendicular pressure using flat fingers, one hand over the other (Figure 26-32). Begin at the base of the ascending colon and follow peristalsis around in a spiraling pattern toward the center of the Hara. Do not put direct pressure into the solar plexus or the navel. When you reach the central point, 2 cun below the navel, lightly rest one hand over the area and reach under the low back with the other hand. Bake the Hara by generating heat between the palms of your hands. Leave the heat there when you remove your hands.

Continue next by working directly up and on both sides of the sternum with perpendicular pressure until you reach the sternoclavicular joints. Try using the outside edges of your hands and/or fingertips here. At the upper chest, turn your hands into loose fists (or use fingertips) and work out toward the anterior shoulder under the clavicles. Lean into both shoulder joints simultaneously as your client exhales.

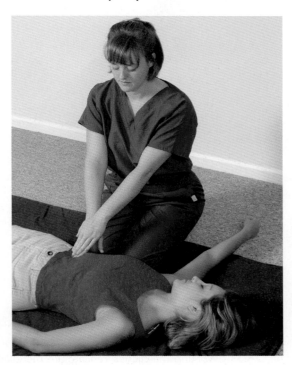

Figure 26-32 Gently pressing the client's Hara.

Anterior Arm Meridians: Lung, Pericardium, Heart

Take the right arm and start joint mobilizations. To work the Lu channel, bring the arm down at a 45-degree angle from the shoulder with the palm up and palm-palm-thumb the meridian. For the P meridian, bring the arm directly out to the side at a 90-degree angle; do not put heavy, direct pressure onto the bicep. For the Ht channel, bring the arm up from the shoulder at a 45-degree angle (Figure 26-33). Transition to the other arm and repeat.

The Neck, Head, and Face

Sit above the client's head and get comfortable. Cat-walk into the tops of the shoulders, changing the angle of pressure to cover the entire area, using palm-palm-thumb. Do some gentle neck joint mobilizations, never forcing it in any way. Place both hands under the neck and rest there a moment. Begin with perpendicular pressure on either side of the cervical spine using the fingertips, working from the base of the occiput to the intercostal space between T2 and T3. Repeat several times.

Turn the head gently to one side and support if necessary. Work with perpendicular and circular pressure into the scalp, using as much pressure as is comfortable for the client. Work the entire side and back of the head; turn and do the other side and back. Place the head back in a neutral position.

Place your fingertips under the base of the occiput and apply pressure simultaneously so that the chin rises toward the ceiling as the client exhales. Ask him to inhale again and as he exhales, flex the neck forward so the chin is near the top of the sternum. Place the head down gently.

To work the face, use perpendicular pressure. Gliding strokes are not comfortable to the client without a lubricant. Use thumbs and/or fingertips and make your way from forehead to chin, using both hands and working from the midline of the face toward the outside. Squeeze the tissue on the top of the chin and jaw around to the ears and work the ears. Thank the client and cordially end the session.

SUMMARY

Asian bodywork therapy, as one of the major branches of ancient Chinese Medicine, has evolved over the centuries into many different modalities, including shiatsu. Shiatsu is the application of direct pressure of varying direction, degree, and intensity to the body. Shiatsu therapy includes but is not limited to simultaneous assessment and treatment, range-of-motion techniques, meridian stretches, and direct pressure.

Eastern and western approaches to health and medicine differ in several ways and offer different treatment plans. Both have successes and challenges, although they complement each other well.

Yin/Yang theory shows us the basic components of all things and how they interact. Qi is the Life Force and the Vital Energy in all living things. The Five Element theory can figure prominently in shiatsu therapy. The Five Elements are an expanded system of functional relationships that apply to all aspects of life and the universe. All of these systems of thought were developed after careful observation of natural phenomena and can assist in assessment and treatment of the client.

Shiatsu theory includes but is not limited to factors to determine Qi deficiency and excess and associated techniques to address each imbalance. The body mechanics, attention, and focus of the practitioner are important factors.

Shiatsu is practiced today in many different countries with varying degrees of training and curricula. In the United States, a national certification examination is often taken. Research is being conducted now in the United States and other countries. Shiatsu was officially recognized as medical therapy in Japan in the mid-1950s.

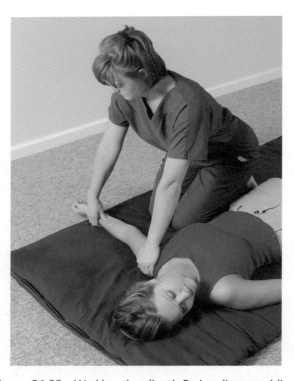

Figure 26-33   Working the client's Pericardium meridian.

MATCHING

List the letter of the answer next to the term or phrase that best describes it.

A. Cupping   F. Gua sha   K. Tsubo
B. Asian bodywork therapy   G. Hara   L. Tai Ji
C. Qi   H. Ashi points   M. Dantien
D. Meridians   I. Moxibustion   N. Cun
E. Ki   J. Acupoints   O. Shiatsu

__E__ 1. In Japan, the energy of the body, mind, and spirit

__H__ 2. In Chinese medicine, these are points on the body that get a reaction from the client when touched; means "that's it!"

__B__ 3. The treatment of the human body, mind, and spirit by pressure and/or manipulation; this includes the electromagnetic or energetic field, which surrounds, infuses, and brings the body to life

__D__ 4. In Chinese medicine, these are the channels or pathways through which Qi flows

__F__ 5. The art of scraping the surface of the skin

__N__ 6. The body inch in Chinese medicine; the width of the client's own thumb knuckle

__A__ 7. The use of glass cups as suction over areas of stagnation

__C__ 8. In China, the energy of the body, mind, and spirit

__J__ 9. The Chinese term used to describe specific points on the body that influence and are influenced by body energy

__G__ 10. In Japan, the geographical center of gravity, and the energetic center in the body

__M__ 11. In China, the geographical centers of gravity and the energetic centers in the body

__I__ 12. An external warming technique by burning the herb mugwort

__K__ 13. The Japanese term used to describe acupoints and ashi points

__L__ 14. The familiar black and white icon, which symbolizes the interaction of Yin and Yang

__O__ 15. Means finger pressure in Japanese; the application of direct, perpendicular pressure to assist Qi flow in the body, mind, and spirit

Bibliography

Beinfeld H, Korngold E: *Between heaven and earth: a guide to Chinese medicine,* Ballantine Books, 1991, New York.

Beresford-Cooke C: *Shiatsu theory and practice,* Edinburgh, 1996, Churchill Livingstone.

Dubitsky C: *Bodywork shiatsu: bringing the art of finger pressure to the massage table,* Rochester, Vt, 1997, Healing Arts Press.

Ferguson P: *Take five: the five elements guide to health and harmony,* Lithia Springs, Ga, 2000, Newleaf.

Holland A: *Voices of Qi: an introductory guide to traditional Chinese medicine,* Seattle, 1997, Northwest Institute of Acupuncture and Oriental Medicine.

Kaptchuk T: *The web that has no weaver: understanding Chinese medicine,* Chicago, 1983, Congden and Weed.

Maciocia G: *The foundations of Chinese medicine,* Edinburgh, 1989, Churchill Livingstone.

Tsu L: *Tao te ching* (translated by GF Feng, J English), New York, 1972, Vintage Books.

Xinnong C, editor: *Chinese acupuncture and moxibustion,* Beijing, 1987, Foreign Languages Press Beijing.

UNIT FIVE

Business Practices

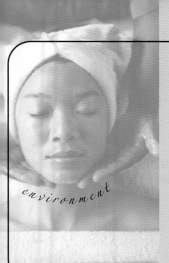

environment

The Business of Massage

27

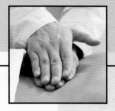

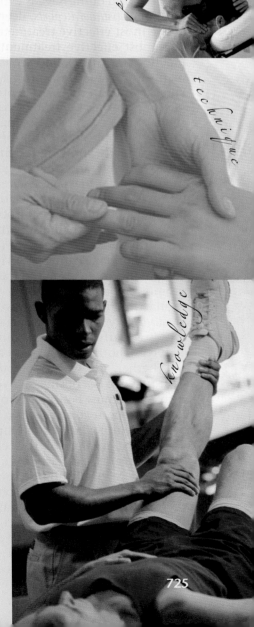

pressure

technique

knowledge

"To accomplish great things we must not only act, but also dream; not only plan, but also believe."

—Anonymous

STUDENT OBJECTIVES

After completing this chapter, the student should be able to:

- Identify your primary values
- Write a vision and a mission statement
- Develop a business plan
- Create a curriculum vitae
- Describe various promotional activities
- Design a business logo, letterhead, business card, and promotional flyer
- Write three sample business advertisements
- List five business resources
- Describe how you will grow and evolve in the field of massage therapy
- Create a plan for avoiding burnout
- Make a commitment for investing toward retirement

INTRODUCTION

Achieving gratification from a career in massage therapy can happen in two ways: through monetary compensation and personal satisfaction. Many students enter this profession because they felt "drawn" or "called" to become a massage therapist. For some, the attraction is simply a matter of the personal success achieved as a massage *client.* What does a career in massage mean to you?

- The financial reward of a full-time job
- The supplemental income of a part-time job
- More free time without loss of income
- Personal recognition
- Travel opportunities
- Being your own boss
- The personal fulfillment of helping others
- Flexible hours
- A retirement career

The world of massage is evolving. In the May 2000 issue of *Consumer Reports,* deep massage was reported as the most effective treatment for fibromyalgia, second most effective treatment for back pain (chiropractic care is first), and second most effective treatment for headaches (prescription drugs are first). Furthermore, in the 1994 September/October issue of *Money Magazine,* being a massage therapist is listed as the Best Business for Enjoying Life While You Work.

Many people go into business for themselves without ever really knowing the first thing about it. They love their craft, and they are good at it, but being able to give a great massage is rarely the cause of a failed business. It is rather the lack of business acumen and insufficient capital. The purpose of this chapter is to provide the new therapist with basic business knowledge to build a prosperous practice, from surveying the site and laying the foundation (planning and development) to erecting the framework (employment, promotion, and support) to the finishing touches, regular maintenance, and eventual remodeling (diversifying your income, tracking your finances, avoiding burnout and planning for retirement). This chapter is both a tool kit and a survival kit.

Whether you work for yourself or someone else, your practice is a business. If your practice is going to thrive, you must become a proficient businessperson. However, perseverance often makes the difference between employed and unemployed.

The first section of this chapter identifies your hopes, dreams, and aspirations. You will map your approach by beginning a business plan, followed by acquiring business permits, obtaining the proper insurance, and determining startup costs. Once these essential elements have been established, you need to market yourself and your services, advertise and promote your business, write contracts and proposals, locate resources, plan career advancement, diver-sify your income, and return something to the community through volunteering. Finally, you will learn how to manage discouragement, avoid burnout, and plan for retirement.

SURVEYING THE SITE AND LAYING THE FOUNDATION: BUSINESS PLANNING AND DEVELOPMENT

Massage therapists have two main choices of employment: they can work for someone else or they can become self-employed. The majority of therapists, even those that start out working for someone else, eventually become self-employed. Starting your own business may seem like a daunting project but if you break it down into steps and take one step at time, it can be accomplished by anyone.

Why do businesses fail? Dun and Bradstreet, the world's largest business database manager, claims that 90% of all businesses fail because lack of business planning and not lack of professional skills. This section assists the student therapist in business planning and development. You will first conduct a survey of your personal values by listing your dreams and desires and stating the purpose of your business. The practice you are building requires a vision, mission, and working plan. Having a vision, mission, and business plan helps you keep your attention and business focused. This will become your map because it shows you how to get where you want your business to go. After developing a business plan, we will then explore business entities, obtaining the necessary licenses and insurance to lay the foundation of your practice.

What Do You Value?

Your massage practice will reflect who you are. Who you are (your character) and how you behave (your personality) naturally come from your needs, desires, attitudes, and beliefs about life. A big part of your success is, and will be, embedded in your personal, business, and spiritual philosophies. If your work is not an extension of your self—that is, if your inner and outer life are not congruent—you will experience a mental and emotional tug of war.

Identifying what you value is often difficult because values themselves are abstract concepts. However, as experience teaches us and scientific research tells us, we spend time and energy on things we value or on acquiring things we value. Using a backdoor approach, the following activity may help you identify important elements about yourself.

On a sheet of paper, list 15 to 20 things you like or want to do. These can range from cooking to hiking to reading to your kids to watching television or to getting *or* receiving massages. After reading over your list, write a *value* to the right of each activity. For example, cooking may be linked to spending time with family, creative expression, or nurturing. This evaluation may take some time, but the underlying motivation of each activity should emerge. During this exercise, you will be shifting the focus from things you like or want to do to things you value.

Next, create a new list from the values you have identified in the previous section. From the most important to the least important, number each value. Although it may feel like soul searching, this exercise is often liberating because it helps you identify your most important values, making it easier to make decisions involving your energy and your time—two of your most valuable assets! This list will change to reflect your changing needs.

Copy the new list on several sheets of paper, and tape it where you can see it, such as on the bathroom mirror, on the refrigerator door, on the dashboard of your car. This is also a beneficial activity to teach clients for stress reduction. If your clients feel overwhelmed, ask them to go through this process and help them identify what is important to them.

 Things which matter most must never be at the mercy of the things which matter least.

—Goethe

Vision Statement

Every business follows a path. Several signs indicate what type of path you will take or are currently taking. Some indicators are profit (or loss), décor, services offered, clientele, referral base, and your own level of satisfaction. Any type of business should be guided by a vision instead of the therapist's worries, anxieties, or fears. The harsh truth is that if you do not consciously design your business vision, circumstances will. Unless you give thought to it and create your vision, you will be trying to navigate your business without an idea about where you are and where you are headed.

A vision statement embraces what you want—the desires for your business. Built from your value list, your business vision should both create excitement and energize you. This vision is not necessarily a preview of the future but a glimpse of how things could be if certain obstacles were removed (e.g., time, money, training, experience, confidence and so on). Embark on a "vision quest" and describe on paper what you see. Wake up the following morning and move about as if you are living this vision—a vision of how busy you are, the kind of work environment in which you are located, the kind of modalities you are practicing, and so forth. Continue building this vision until it is complete. When talking about your business with others, speak of it affectionately and not with impatience. As you create your vision, no-

tice how it makes you feel. If it does not feel right, alter the vision till it makes you smile and stirs you into action. Note if you must make any changes within yourself to fulfill your business vision. Once your vision is clear, move on to writing your mission statement and then on to the business plan. The business plan will help you turn your dreams into a reality.

 Argue for your limitations and they're yours.

—Richard Bach

Mission Statement

A mission statement, or statement of purpose, briefly and succinctly defines your type of business and its objective. Mission statements give businesses direction. The U.S. Constitution can be viewed as a mission statement. When writing your mission statement, you might say that you are in the massage industry and your mission is to help people relax or feel better. This textbook has a mission too; its mission is to assist in the educational process of individuals who wish to become knowledgeable, well-informed, and competent massage therapists.

A few guidelines are available for writing a mission statement. First, it must be short. If not, you are probably not going to remember it or read it often; it is a good idea to be able to recite it by memory. Next, it must focus on meeting the needs of other people while not conflicting with your own. Every successful massage therapist will tell you the same thing; when your focus is serving humanity, opportunities are never in short supply. Last, your mission statement must be totally compatible with your most important values; it will evolve as you evolve, so it must be flexible and revised as needed. Your birthday or New Year's Day may be a good time to reevaluate it on an annual basis.

 A true definition of an entrepreneur comes closer to: a poet, visionary, or packager of social change.

—Robert Schwartz

Business Evaluation and Planning

Once you have gotten to know more about your values, dreams, and mission, it is time for evaluation and planning. The following is a list of questions; it is the beginning of your business map. Remember, there is no single "right way" to construct a successful business; the trick is to find your own way—one that fits who you are and what your business represents.

Answering the following questions to the best of your ability will help you (1) identify your business parameters and (2) develop a better understanding of what areas need attention. It is better to begin responding to the questions now. Put them down on paper and go back to them after graduation for completion, refinement, and implementation. The components of basic business and marketing plans are personal information, general description of your business, services, fees and pricing, competition, your location and operations, and your management and personnel. Sections of the business plan appear throughout the chapter as boxes. Read or answer these questions as you go along. A complete list of questions for the business plan is located at the end of the chapter.

Business Plan: Personal Information

- What is my experience in this business, if any?
- What do I love about my work?
- What are my weaknesses and shortcomings?
- What are my strengths and talents?
- What is special and distinct about me as a massage therapist? Why will these appeal to clients?
- What are my values?
- What have I learned about this business from fellow therapists, teachers, trade journals, and trade suppliers?

Business Plan: General Description of Business

- What is my vision statement?
- What is my mission statement?
- What services do I or will I offer? Describe these services and the benefits of these services.
- For what purpose will people buy my services?
- Am I willing to change what I offer, to some extent, to meet my client's changing needs?

The only place where success comes before work is in the dictionary.

—Vidal Sassoon

Choice of Business Entity

Business enterprises may take many forms. Common choices in for-profit entities include *proprietorships, limited liability companies, partnerships,* and *corporations.* The choice of format has compliance, tax, and liability consequences that call for consultation with lawyers, accountants, and other experts; however, some insight into these matters can make these consultations more efficient and beneficial.

Proprietorship

Proprietorship, or *sole proprietorship,* has a single owner. It is the simplest and least expensive to open. The owner provides all the capital and receives all the profits. Legally, there is no distinction between the business and owner. Creditors of the proprietorship may look to both the owner's personal assets and business assets to satisfy their claims. Also, people injured by an employee of the proprietorship during the course of employment may pursue a claim against the owner of the proprietorship. In the case of a proprietorship that uses a different name than that of the owner, the proprietor often must make a filing under local statutes to protect the use of the assumed name, which is referred to as a *doing business as* (DBA). The profits or losses of the business are reported on the owner's personal tax return, which in most cases is on schedule C of a 1040 federal individual tax return. A sole proprietorship is recommended for the small-business person who is just getting started. Other benefits of sole proprietorship are that the owner has complete control and that the business may be easily terminated.

Advantages
- It is easy to start.
- You own it, and you control it.
- Profit and loss is reported on a schedule C on your individual 1040 tax return.

Disadvantages
- You are personally liable; any court judgment may affect your personal assets.
- If you decide to expand, locating financial resources (loan or credit) depends on your personal credit history and net worth.

What You Will Need To Do
- Obtain an occupational license, which is issued by the city and/or county/parish in which you operate.
- Acquire liability insurance.

Limited Liability Company

Limited liability company (LLC) has appeared fairly recently as an organizational choice. As a consequence of the check-the-box regulations, the owner of a single-member company can treat the business as a corporation for tax purposes or report any income and expense on the owner's schedule C 1040. An LLC with two or more members may elect corporate or partnership taxation. Members can generally limit their liability to their equity in the company. However, as a practical matter, banks, landlords and other significant creditors may require the members to personally guarantee some of the company's obligations. LLCs contrast with limited partnerships in that a member can retain protection against the company's general creditors while actively participating in the business. The laws of most jurisdictions permit the owners of limited liability companies to conduct most of their affairs in private.

Advantages

- It is easy to start.
- It is the same as proprietorship or partnership (LLC can be either).
- Members retain protection against the company's creditors while actively participating in business activities.

Disadvantages

- Banks, landlords, and other significant creditors may require the members to personally guarantee some of the company's financial obligations
- If more than one member exists, each member is required to file a separate tax return
- If you decide to expand, locating financial resources (loan or credit) may depend on the personal credit history and net worth of the LLC members

What You Will Need To Do

- Contact an attorney to discuss creating an LLC.
- Obtain an occupational license, which is issued by the city and/or county/parish in which you operate.
- If the LLC has more than one member, acquire federal and state identification employee numbers.
- Acquire liability insurance.

Parnerships

Partnerships have a flow-through taxation. Each partner files his or her own individual tax return (1040) and the partnership accounts for its income and losses on tax form 1065. Business partnerships are similar to domestic partnerships in that both parties agree to share both the responsibilities and rewards of the business. Like domestic partnerships, it helps if business partners have good personal chemistry (similar to domestic partnerships, business partnerships have about a 50% mortality rate). Additionally, like domestic partners who choose not to formally marry, two people can enter the business relationship without a formal written agreement. However, it is advisable to have a written agreement drawn up and reviewed by an attorney. Investment expense is usually shared among the partners, while authority is divided. Partnerships can have *general partners* who have shared responsibility for decisions, share in the profits, and share in personal liability. *Limited partners,* referred to as *silent partners,* do not actively participate in the management of the partnership but still receive a profit and are only liable up to the amount of their personal investment. Most small business partnerships are general partnerships that have no limited partners.

Advantages

- It is easy to start.
- Startup costs are divided between two or more people.
- Provides a broader base of skills and interest (two heads or better than one).

Disadvantages

- Decision making must be shared with partner(s).
- If one partner dies, the other is left with the business debts.
- As with sole proprietorship, the partners are liable for business-related mistakes.
- Unlike a sole proprietorship, this means you can be personally liable for suits against your partner (the exception to this would be a limited liability partnership, which is a separate legal structure with limiting liability).
- Although a partnership is only a tax-reporting rather than a tax-paying entity, it must still file a tax return.
- Think carefully about entering into a partnership with your best friend; many business partnerships end in dispute.

What You Will Need To Do

- Obtain an occupational license, which is issued by the city or county/parish in which you operate.
- Acquire liability insurance.
- Consider drawing up a partnership agreement.
- Acquire federal and state identification employee numbers.

Corporations

For Internal Revenue Service (IRS) purposes, a small business may either be an S corporation or a C corporation. A C corporation pays federal taxes on its taxable income. Subject to exceptions, the income or loss of an S corporation flows to its shareholders in proportion to share ownership. A properly organized and operated corporation of either type limits the owner's liability. Limiting liability is the principal reason most small-business owners organize in the corporate format. After the corporation is organized by the articles of incorporation with the secretary of state or other appropriate states (and, if applicable, local) officers, shares of stock are issued to the stockholders. The shareholders must elect a board of directors annually, which oversees business operations. Corporate officers who run the daily affairs of the company can be elected or appointed by the board. Apart from filing tax returns, corporations must pay fees annually and give certain notices to state government periodically. Questions that organizers may wish to discuss with their attorneys include the following: (1) What happens if the shareholders disagree on a fundamental issue? (2) If a death or divorce changes share ownership, will the remaining shareholders have a right to purchase and, if so, at what price? (3) What happens if a shareholder working in the business becomes disabled?

Advantages

- You are not liable to third parties.
- Your personal assets cannot be attached in a lawsuit against the business.
- The practice can continue in the event an owner leaves or dies.
- Because of its limited liability and accounting requirements, the corporate structure is attractive to a broader range of financial resources; over time, a profitable corporation is a more attractive risk to banks and investors.
- Your financial risk is generally limited to the amount you pay for your stock.

Disadvantages

- A corporation is the most legally complicated business structure, and creating a corporate entity requires the assistance of an attorney.
- C corporations pay taxes separately from its shareholders (Form 1120); if the corporation pays dividends to its shareholders, such payments are not tax deductible to the corporation, but the shareholders are required to pay tax on the dividend distribution.
- Most states charge a corporate franchise tax each year.

What You Will Need To Do

- Employ an attorney to help draw up articles of incorporation.
- File the articles of incorporation with the state where you wish to be incorporated (usually the secretary of state); you may ask the attorney you hire to take care of this.
- Obtain an occupational license, which is issued by the city or county/parish in which you operate.
- Acquire federal and state employee tax identification numbers.
- Acquire liability insurance

Licenses, Permits, and Registrations

The following is a list of licenses and permits that may be required before starting your massage therapy business. Each state, county/parish, and municipality is different in how these licenses and permits are issued. Please contact your local city hall for the proper procedure. The local Small Business Administration (SBA) also may be of assistance.

If you do not know whether your state has a massage licensing board, contact your state attorney's office or the secretary of state. If no massage board or a state licensing program is available for massage, contact the National Certification Board for Therapeutic Massage and Bodywork (NCBTMB) at (800) 296-0664 and request an application for certification. Al-

though not required, you may want to do this anyway, for the recognition of being nationally certified.

If your state does have a licensing board, request by mail or telephone an information packet, application, and list of upcoming testing dates. Carefully read the state requirements, and ensure that the educational program you choose meets or exceeds the state standards. Preparation for certification may include successfully completing an approved course of study and an internship program. Some states require not only a minimum number of hours but also a number of hours in specific subject areas. It may also be helpful to get a copy of your state's massage therapy laws. Many massage therapy boards will not provide them for you, so you may have to check at your local library or download the laws off the Internet.

Provisional License

In most states a massage therapist must obtain a state license before she is allowed to practice. However, because of lag time between graduation and state testing, many states grant a provisional license to therapists who have completed their pre-licensing coursework. Although not mandatory, it allows the therapist to legally practice for a specified period. This time frame may be for a fixed period such as 1 month, or it may be flexible, being valid until the next scheduled state testing date. The provisional license assumes that the therapist is fully trained and will be able to pass the state examination. In some states the required provision may be that a licensed therapist must be willing to supervise the unlicensed therapist. In other words the provisionally licensed therapist must not do any massages unless the supervising therapist is on the premises. In this way, if problem situation arises, the provisional therapist can ask for advice from the licensed therapist. Other restrictions are also made, such as with advertising. Some states may require that provisionally licensed therapists state in all advertisements that they are provisionally licensed and that they must list the name and license number of their supervising therapist. Check with your own state or regional law for specifics. An extra form and fee often must be submitted to the state to apply for a provisional license.

State License

Once you have graduated from a massage therapy program, it is time to take the state examination or become nationally certified. Obtain an application form from the state or national board and fill it out completely; an incomplete application may delay or void your testing date and may cost you a resubmission fee. If your application is approved, you may be able to apply for a provisional or temporary license while you are waiting for the examination date and your test scores. If not, do not practice massage for compensation until you have received verification that you have successfully passed your state examination. In some states, you may have passed your examination but you cannot legally practice until you receive your state license. This procedure varies from state to state so obtain specific licensing instructions from your state board.

Your state board of massage therapy exists to protect the public. It is not its responsibility to inform you of proposed or current changes in the law. It is up to each massage therapist to keep abreast of changes in the state law by attending open board meetings or local massage therapy association meetings.

Occupational License

In most cities, you must acquire a business (occupational) license to operate any kind of business. Contact the clerk of court, city planning department, or appropriate public office in your area. Typically, part of the procedure of obtaining your business license is to have your business location approved through the city zoning department and the fire marshal. This process includes a home, or "cottage," business. All business licenses and permits should be displayed in a public place.

Sales Tax Permit

If you sell any product to a client, you may be required to obtain a sales tax permit through state or county/parish taxing authorities. You will receive a tax payer identification number and instructions on how to pay your sales tax, which usually involves monthly, quarterly, or twice yearly tax payments. You are usually allowed to choose a payment schedule when you apply for your sales tax number. Some municipalities tax services such as massage, whereas others do not.

Registration of a Business Name

If you have a business name (other than your name), you must register it with the city, county, or parish clerk's office. Also known as a *trade name,* or a *doing business as (DBA)* name, the statement filed with the clerk's office protects you from other businesses using your name and ensures that you are not using a name currently registered by someone else in your area.

Federal Tax Identification Number

Also known as an *employer identification number* (EIN), a federal tax identification number is issued to a business if you have employees or are incorporated. If your business falls into either of these categories, apply for an EIN by filling out form SS-4, available at

Business Plan: Operating Procedures

- What type of licenses are required for me to operate my business?
- What will be the opening date of my business? What hours of the day and days of the week will I be in operation?
- What will my office policies be for late clients, cancellations, out-of-date gift certificate redemption, insufficient funds checks, and credit card sales?

Business Plan: Management and Personnel

- What is my management experience?
- What do I predict my legal structure will be?
- Who will be the other key figures in my business? Include an organizational chart, list of duties/backgrounds of key individuals, outside consultants/advisers, and board of directors.
- How will services be provided? Will I do all the work or will I use employees or contract labor?
- Describe the types of support my business may require, including child care, janitorial service, lawn and garden care, bookkeeping, and accounting.
- Describe the wages and benefits I can offer each type of employee and support person.

your local IRS office. Your EIN will usually begin with the prefix 72-. All other business can operate using an individual social security number.

Insurance Needs

What types of insurance do you have? What types of insurance will you need to operate your business? Insurance needs vary from person to person and time to time. Find out which type of insurance is required by law for your business to operate. Additionally, an insurance agent should be contacted to discuss your individual insurance needs. Some of your commercial and personal insurance needs can be obtained through professional massage organizations. The following sections help you understand the different types of insurance that affect your business.

Professional Liability

Also referred to as *malpractice insurance* and *errors and omission insurance,* professional liability covers liability costs rising from your professional activities. Massage therapists are accountable for their actions and may be held liable for any mistakes made while performing their service, such as soft-tissue damage. Most affordable professional liability policies are available through the major massage and bodywork professional associations. This type of insurance can also be purchased while you are a student. If you operate a home-based practice, your homeowner's policy does not cover your professional activities. Professional liability is required in most states.

General Liability

Also referred to as *premise liability*, general liability takes care of liability costs that are a result of bodily injury, property damage, and personal injury incurred when the client is on your premises. An example would be if your client slips and falls on your property or if a tree limb falls and damages a client's parked car.

Business Personal Property

This type of insurance covers the cost of business property such as a desk, massage table, chairs, and stereo equipment in your business location. Again, your homeowner's policy probably does not cover the costs of your business property if you operate a home-based business. An inexpensive rider can usually be purchased under your homeowner's policy to cover these costs in the event of flood, fire, or theft.

Automobile Insurance

Some states require that you have an automobile policy that is rated for business use if you travel to and from a client's home or office.

Health Insurance

Expenses such as doctor visits and hospitalization are covered with health insurance. If you are self-employed, this type of insurance can be purchased through the *National Association for the Self-Employed* (NASE).

Life Insurance

If you have dependents, this type of insurance provides your loved ones with financial support in the event of your death. *Term life* is the least expensive choice and is the insurance policy most frequently purchased.

Business Plan: Insurance Needs

- What are your insurance needs? These may include professional and general liability; business personal property; automotive, life, and health insurance; and disability insurance.
- Have you contacted an agent to discuss what types of policies they offer and the cost and benefit of each?

Disability Insurance

If you need income protection, you may want to obtain disability insurance. This type of insurance provides you with disability income in the event that you cannot work as a result of a disability such as an illness or injury.

Determining Startup Cost

Startup costs vary from person to person and one geographical region to the next. Take a realistic look at how much money you will need to open your doors. This section assumes that you will be working for yourself. Once you have made your initial calculations, you can make adjustments before purchases are made if you find that the figures are high. For example, you may decide that it will be more advantageous financially to ask another therapist to share certain expenses with you. High overhead and an office are risky when you are just starting out and do not have any clients. Some of these items, such as advertising and printing costs, must eventually be repeated. Box 27-1 is a worksheet that helps clarify startup costs.

THE FRAMEWORK: EMPLOYMENT, PROMOTIONAL STRATEGIES, AND SUPPORT

Great diversity exists within the categories of the self-employed and employee massage therapist. This section explores various employment opportunities and strategies for promoting massage through the use of advertising, marketing, business cards, brochures, and Internet websites. It focuses on the importance of a curriculum vitae (CV) and how to develop contracts and proposals, get publicity, and write press releases. Lastly, this section examines the advantages of support services that can be gained by networking with other therapists, business owners, and health care professionals.

Employment Opportunities

A career in massage therapy offers many employment opportunities for working with people in the health and fitness industry, beauty and spa industry, travel and recreation industry, and health care industry. A variety of settings are available for massage therapists including the following:
Acupuncturists
Airports
Athletic teams and dance companies
Casinos
Chiropractic clinics
Corporate wellness programs
Cruise lines

BOX 27-1

Determining Startup Costs

Opening a business checking account _____
Equipment and machinery (massage tables, stereo, phone) _____
Room furnishings and fixtures (shelves, lamp, chair) _____
Office rent (first and last month's rent plus security deposit) _____
Telephone deposit and installation costs _____
Utility deposits and installation costs _____
Legal and professional services (accountant, attorney) _____
Personnel _____
Insurance (auto, general liability, malpractice, property, prepayments) _____
Professional society membership (often regarded as insurance payment) _____
Initial licenses and permits _____
Remodeling _____
Initial office supplies (appointment book, stapler, pens) _____
Initial massage supplies (linens, massage lubricant) _____
Advertising and promotion _____
Printing cost (business cards, gift certificates, stationery, forms) _____
Petty cash _____
Miscellaneous _____
TOTAL _____

Day spas
Facial, nail, and beauty salons
Golf, tennis, and country clubs
Gyms and health clubs
Hospitals
Hotels
Nursing homes
Onsite massage in offices
Pain management clinics
Physical therapy and sports medicine clinics
Private practice (in office or out-call)
Psychiatric treatment centers
Resorts
Shopping malls
Upscale grocery stores
Veterinarians and race tracks (animal massage)

Marketing

Marketing involves moving your goods and services from the provider to the consumer. This process involves promoting your business with image, purpose, and direction. Ideas include the following:
- Paid advertising and publicity
- Passing out business cards at a local country club
- Giving gift certificates to potential referral sources
- Sending a proposal to a hospital for massage services
- Setting up a booth at a local heath fair
- Sending a resume to a prospective employer

In developing a marketing strategy, consider your competition. Asking yourself direct questions and answering honestly about your competitors helps you develop and evaluate marketing ideas. Consider the following discussion when building your marketing strategy.

Advertising

Making your business noticeable to the public by purchasing print or broadcast media is advertising. Airtime or space can be purchased from the media. **Media** are systems of mass communication. Massage therapists often use media in the form of yellow page advertising, newspaper and newsletter advertising (display or classified), radio or television commercials, direct mailing, or even the Internet by setting up a website. Most media sell advertising and offer prospective customers a media kit. Media kits include things such as the coverage area and market information including total population statistics by groups (women, men, teens and children); information about households with televisions, cable, and videocassette recorders; and demographics about household income, education levels and occupation. Also included is a price sheet. This lays out the deadlines and pricing structure; history of the company; its mission statement, owners, and stock listing; and any advantages regarding buying this

Business Plan: Marketing and Competititon

- What do I want my business identity to be? Describe the image you want to project. *You never get a second chance to make a first impression.*
- What do I want people to say to others about my services?
- Who is my target market? Who will want to buy my services? Identify important characteristics such as age, gender, occupation, income, and so on.
- Who else provides a similar service? In order of their strength in the market, list my five closest competitors by name and address. Next, describe each competitor's strengths and weaknesses. What have I learned from my competitors' operations and their advertising?
- What will my fee schedule look like? How have I determined these fees? Will this price cover material costs, labor costs, and overhead?
- What are my competitors charging?
- How am I different from my competitors in ways that matter to potential clients? Refer to the previous business plan section on personal information.

particular media over other media. Lastly, it should include a Web address so that people can go online to learn more about the company or business or obtain a telephone number, address, and contact person. Polish up on your telephone skills before such calls come in (Chapter 10).

When choosing the right advertising for your business, consider not only the price but also the amount of return, its target audience, circulation, and when it is released. For example, more people read Sunday papers, but only a certain sector of the population read the travel section of the newspaper. People who are working most likely not watch soap operas, and only about 5% of people who get your direct-mail piece actually read it, with even fewer actually calling for an appointment. Advertising also influences your business image in the client's mind. The appearance of the advertisement is just as important as when it comes out and what it says (Figure 27-1). It helps to solicit the help of advertising specialists. Some therapists employ an advertising agency, which helps make decisions about how, when, and where to advertise.

Advertising lets people know who you are and what services you provide. *General advertising* announces or reminds the current or potential clients about your business. *Specific advertising* targets an objective such as gift certificate sales or increasing the purchase of a new or existent service (e.g., body wraps or reflexology). By determining your target group, you can decide what advertising and promotional strategies are

most effective because the most effective advertisements target a specific population. Keep in mind that a lag time always exists between action and results, and you cannot always predict the results.

Business plan: Advertising, Promotion, and Location

- How can I get the attention of the people I want to reach? Which advertising media are appropriate for my business and targeted clients?
- What other channel(s) will I use to reach clients such as networking, referrals, and publicity?
- How can I discover which promotion is working?
- Plan an advertising budget for 6 months. Include specific media you will use and the cost of each.
- What type of location does my business require? Describe the type of building your business needs, including office and studio space, parking, exterior lighting, security needs, and proximity to other businesses for added exposure.
- Where do I plan to locate my business? Is this location right for my business and me?
- Describe the geographical area my business will serve. Are sufficient numbers of potential clients located there?
- What type of layout is needed for my business? Include layout for reception area, restroom, hydrotherapy and spa room (if applicable), retail and inventory areas, and gift certificate sales.

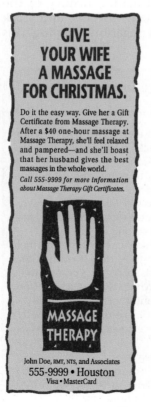

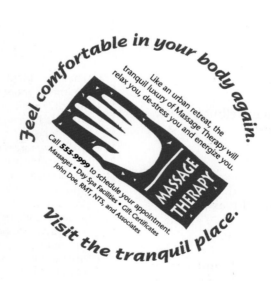

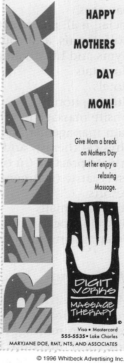

Figure 27-1   Various ways to advertise in display ad for a massage therapy practice.

Business Cards

Business cards should let people know who you are, what services you provide, and how to contact you while projecting a favorable image. Your card should be well-spaced and not crowded with words or graphics; beauty lies in simplicity. If you have a logo, use it on your business card and on every other piece of printed material. Make sure the type style or font is clear and easy to read and the telephone number with area code is easily located by a larger and bolder type. If you have an office in your home, you may choose to specify your geographical area (e.g., the Garden District) but not your home address. Be sure to proofread all information before it goes to print.

Be generous and hand your business cards out often. They serve no purpose in a box on the shelf. As you give them to people, introduce yourself and tell them about your line of work. Business cards may also be used for appointment cards. You may even use your business card as part of an incentive program by writing something on the back like "$10 off next massage." Be creative and have fun, but remember, this is your "face."

MINI-LAB

Design your own business card, letting it reflect your area of specialty.

Brochures

The purpose of a brochure is to explain to prospective clients in some detail about you and your services. Professionally printed brochures are more expensive than business cards, but because of space, they can be very effective in promoting your business. If you have an adequate computer, printer, and computer program, you can print your own. The most popular format is a trifold, which is printed double-sided on an 8.5" × 11" sheet of paper. This size can also be used as a mailer.

Begin your brochure with an attention grabber that conveys some benefit of massage, such as "Feel comfortable in your body again." Then describe the benefits people often experience (in your clients' words). Next, describe what you actually do and give a brief autobiography. In your autobiography, state a brief description of your qualifications and, if appropriate, your years of experience. Your telephone number should be large and readable at the end of the brochure. Close with a statement that may provoke action, such as, "Call now." Use vivid language, appealing to vision, hearing, and emotion (e.g., "One part therapy, one part luxury," or "Visit the tranquil place"). Note that you do not have to say things directly, as with "Feel comfortable in your body again" or "Must be experienced to be fully understood." What are the mental images that come to mind when you read those words? A brochure reads more easily if you use bullets and attractive graphics instead of paragraphs of text.

If you include your fees and menu of services, print them on a separate sheet of paper that slips into your brochure as an insert. Avoid dating your flyer; put "practicing since 1994" instead of "10 years of experience." Use fax machines and electronic mail to send out your brochure when someone calls you with an inquiry.

Once you have a rough draft, give it to three trusted friends and ask for feedback. Revise it as often as needed. Ensure that after reading your brochure, a potential client then knows what needs you fulfill and how you are different from others providing a similar service.

Internet Websites

Although radio and television advertising are occasionally cost prohibitive for those with small practices, an Internet website can be an inexpensive way to reach large numbers of clients. The exposure can range from a free listing on established massage sites to creating and publishing your own website.

Curriculum Vitae

A curriculum vitae (CV), also known as a *résumé,* is an autobiographical sketch that documents all your achievements, including occupational, avocational, academic, and personal information that you wish to disclose to a prospective employer or business contact. Even if you are self-employed, your CV can help you in business meetings, with developing business relationships, and in acquiring a referral base. A well-written CV lets your business contacts know who you are and what you can offer their employers, members, clients, or patients. A well-written and properly distributed CV can help you advance your practice.

Before you sit down to write your CV, take time to reflect on your life. What accomplishments are you proud of? What are the things that have brought you the most joy? Your list of accomplishments may include acting in a community play or assisting with a political campaign. Now, study the list. You might notice a pattern of personal strengths or interests emerging. You may find that you are a natural leader or that you work best with groups of people. This information can help you write your personal data section.

Begin organizing and writing your CV. The most widely used format is the *reverse chronological format,* which emphasizes your education and work experience from most to least recent. Begin by posting your name, address, and telephone number at the top center of the page at a larger font the rest of the text. Use the headings of the next few sections to organize your CV or the format provided in Figure 27-2.

Résumé of
James Michael Brown

■ **James Michael Brown**
555 Seoul Drive
Middleton, LA 77777
315.555.1212

Massage Therapy Work Experience

■ **Owner and Operator** of The Body Shoppe-Massage Therapy by James Michael Brown and Associates, 1987-Present.
Gulf Coast Physical Therapy, **Primary Massage Therapist,** 1987-1989.
Middleton Hospital, **Outpatient Massage Therapist,** 1989-1990.
Gulf Coast Chiropractic Clinic, **Primary Massage Therapist,** 1989-1994.

Education

■ **Gulf Coast Academy of Massage Therapy,** Middleton, LA, 1987.
Gulf Coast State University, Middleton, LA, Associate Degree in History, 1989.

Massage Therapy Certification Credentials

■ Gulf Coast Academy of Massage Therapy, **Certified Massage Therapist,** 1987.
Texas Department of Health and Hospitals, **Registered Massage Therapist,** 1990.
Louisiana Board of Massage Therapy, **Licensed Massage Therapist,** 1992.
National Certification Board for Therapeutic Massage and Bodywork, **National Certification,** 1993.
Infant Massage Instructor Certification, **Certified Instructor,** 1990.
Neuromuscular Guild of America, **Neuromuscular Therapy Certification,** 1995.

Continuing Education Credentials

■ Aromatherapy for Massage, Gulf Coast Academy of Massage Therapy, 1988.
Massage for the Expectant Mother, IMICA, 1989.
Infant Massage Instructor Certification, IMICA, 1990.
Sportsmassage I, Connecticut College of Massage, 1991.
Sportsmassage II, Connecticut College of Massage, 1992.
Anatomy Refresher for Massage Therapists, Gulf Coast Academy of Massage Therapy, 1993.
The Cadaver Dissection Experience, Connecticut College of Massage, 1994.
Insurance Billing and the Massage Professional, Connecticut College of Massage, 1996.
Advanced Hydrotherapy Workshop, Gulf Coast Academy of Massage Therapy, 1996.

Professional Activities

■ Member, American Association of Massage Practitioners, 1987-Present.
Member, AAMP's National Sports Massage Team, 1987-Present.
Captain, AAMP's National Sports Massage Team, 1992.
Assistant Convention Coordinator, Texas Chapter of the AAMP, 1991.
Member, AAMP's Texas Sports Massage Team, 1992-Present.
Leisure Learning Program, Middleton, LA, 1988-Present.

Awards and Achievements

■ Eagle Award for Small Business Achievement, 1996.
Olympic Games, Sportsmassage Therapist, Gymnastic Venue, Atlanta, GA, 1996.

Publications

■ "Massage and Sports Injuries," *Sportsguide Magazine* Fall 1990.
"Ice and Tennis Elbow," *Sportsguide Magazine* Winter 1990.
"The Runner's Survival Kit-Massage Included," *Sportsguide Magazine* Spring 1991.
"Not for Humans Only-Massaging Your Horse" *Sportsguide Magazine* Summer 1991.
"When Hamstrings Hurt...," *Sportsguide Magazine* Fall 1991.
"The Shoulder Injuries of Duck Season," *Sportsguide Magazine* Winter 1991.
"And you Don't Even Need a Prescription...," *Sportsguide Magazine* Sprint 1992.
The Relaxation Vacation: a Guide to Massage When Traveling, Lifetime Publishing, Middleton, LA, 1995.

Hobbies and Interests

■ Big Brothers/Big Sisters of the Gulf Coast, Volunteer Big Brother
Travel
Singing

Figure 27-2   A sample résumé.

Education. List all your academic achievements in reverse chronological order. If you did not attend college, list your high school; if you did attend college, omit your high school in this section. Your education section should include the name of the educational institution, any college degrees, postgraduate degrees, certificates, or any awards or honors. Also include the schools you attended and any major and minor courses that have helped you as a massage therapist (e.g., psychology, anatomy and physiology, or kinesiology). If you have attended any postgraduate workshops, list them after your formal educational achievements.

Work Experience. Starting with the most recent, list all the jobs held within the past 10 years. Include the names of your employers, titles or positions held, job descriptions, and starting and termination dates. Focus on your field experience while you were at school. Did you provide sports massage for athletes? Did you massage residents in a nursing home? Select the activities that enhance your qualifications, such as hobbies, sports, and professional affiliations.

Personal Data. Although not necessary, this section is your opportunity for the reader to know about you. List your marital status, number and ages of your children, your general health status, and whether you are a nonsmoker. Use only the personal information what will help you project the positive image that you began to formulate in the preceding sections. You might even mention that you like to coach baseball or that you enjoy playing chess. This may create a pleasant image to the reader.

Once your CV is organized, type it on 8.5" × 11" white bond paper. Keep your writing style simple. After you have proofread it once, let three other people proofread it for you. This is a good system for reducing grammar and spelling errors. Typos in a professional CV are taboo.

If you have a specific employer in mind, send him your CV along with a well-written cover letter addressed to a specific person in the company or organization. Avoid phrases such as "Dear Madam," "Dear Sir" or "To Whom It May Concern." Spell his or her full name correctly. If you are invited to an interview or a business meeting, call the day before to confirm. Arrive 15 minutes before the meeting begins. Within a week, send him a thank-you note and mention how much you enjoyed the opportunity to share ideas.

Contracts and Proposals

When embarking on a new business venture, you may be asked to write a business contract or a proposal. Writing down these ideas and formal agreements does many things. It outlines and details your ideas, helps avoid communication problems, states specifically how problems will be handled and who will handle them when they do arise, and helps keep both parties focused.

A contract is a written agreement between two or more parties that communicates expectations, duties, and responsibilities. A signed and dated contract is enforceable by law. Ideally, all parties should draw up an informal contract, or draft, outlining what they perceive as a reasonable agreement. Make sure your draft (1) clarifies the business relationship of each party (e.g., lessor, lessee, employer, employee, partner, independent contractor, and so on), (2) states the duration of the contract (e.g., 6 months, 1 year, or more), and (3) predetermines on what grounds the contract can be terminated, if before the previously agreed time. Write down any other ideas you have concerning the proposed business arrangement. Regardless of which party prepares the final draft of the contract, have your attorney look over it to point out possible problems. Everything is negotiable, but do negotiate *before* signing.

A proposal is a written idea put forward for consideration, discussion, or adoption. Many massage therapists entering the field have the opportunity to approach businesses that do not offer massage therapy and to create a position for themselves or for other therapists. The following sections are elements that should be included when writing a proposal to a sports group, nursing home, or any other business endeavor where you wish to be hired or volunteer your services.

Cover Letter. The cover letter of the proposal is actually your *letter of introduction* and should include your name (or name of person submitting the proposal), title, and all contact information such as your mailing address, e-mail address, telephone number, cellular phone number, and pager number. This page should also include the title of the project and a 25-word summary introducing your concept of the proposed massage therapy services.

Objective. This broad statement should embody the aim and/or expected results of the project, for example, "by providing stress reduction services to the employees of said corporation and to enhance employee productivity and reduce absenteeism." Next, the objective describes whom the project will serve and the geographic location. Then, discuss the significance and need for this project; compare your project with other projects in the same field and/or geographic locations (when applicable). Lastly, state the anticipated outcomes and a method of evaluating and reporting these outcomes.

Logistics.   Logistics are the managing details of the operation—that is, the what, when, and where section of the proposal. If you are familiar with the facility, you may recommend a specific location where massage services will be provided. Briefly discuss physical arrangements such as room dimensions, bathroom location, lighting, equipment, and supplies. Mention which of these items you are willing to provide. Are you proposing full-time or part-time work? Will massage services be available during the day, evenings, or weekends? One idea is to propose a part-time availability and to increase your hours as demand increases. Within what time frame would you conduct the proposed massage services? What hours of the day will massage services be offered, and who will pay for them? Also include who should be contacted as ideas are developed and problems arise. State which person in the company will be responsible for managing the project, and define your organization's contact person, if different from the person negotiating the proposal. Specify how you can be reached. Also include a mutually agreed on mediator (or third party) to help settle disputes if irreconcilable problems arise.

Qualifications.   This section introduces you as a health care professional. Include a brief CV of your training and experience. If you do not have postgraduate experience, focus on the field experience you acquired while you were in school. Introduce other people (e.g., staff or volunteers) who are key to the project and provide their backgrounds. Mention any professional affiliations such as the American Massage Therapy Association (AMTA), National Certification Board for Therapeutic Massage and Bodywork (NCBTMB), Associated Bodywork & Massage Professionals (ABMP), and if the participating massage therapists are insured.

Funding.   This important section outlines the projected budget for the project and includes the amount you are contributing, if any; the names and amounts of funds received from other participants; and the amount you are requesting from the agency or corporation. If needed, suggest plans for additional fund-raising. The budget should include both expenses and revenues for the entire proposed project. If revenue is to be generated by this project, outline who will benefit financially. This section should also include payment schedules and payment method.

Summary.   Your summary, or closing remarks, should recap your proposal and convey a sense of warmth, camaraderie, confidence, and willingness to be of service in this project. It is helpful to include a brief synopsis on a separate sheet of paper listing or bulleting all the elements in your proposal, outlining

their contents, which can be used during the meeting in which your proposal is presented before the board members. Do not use complete sentences but rather a rough description of what each element entails. This is similar to using note cards for a speech; it will keep you on track and allow others to follow your presentation easily.

MINI-LAB

Using the guidelines outlined in this chapter, write a proposal and a contract.

Publicity

Publicity is free media exposure. You can attract attention for your business in many ways. One way is to *become the expert.* After you have some initial experience in massage therapy, write a column for a local paper or magazine. Write about anything with which you are experienced and tie it back into massage. Stress and stress reduction are always good topics. If you like sports, write about ways to manage common sports injuries. Submit this information for publication to newspapers, magazines, or newsletters as an article. Contact them ahead of time and request a copy of their writers' guidelines. Use this information when preparing your final draft. If accepted, you may even be paid for your work. Take advantage of the release date and run a display advertisement in the same publication, or if you have the time and resources, publish your own newsletter.

Use this same information and dispense it by speaking publicly; give talks, speeches, or lectures. You may be asked to appear on a television or radio show. You can also begin teaching classes or workshops in massage or a related topic. Promoting massage instead of your practice is an effective way of increasing clientele. This is called a *soft sell.* Tell people about massage and teach them how to use it to take care of themselves. Pass out informational material that includes your name and contact information. They can contact you if they have any questions or need to schedule an appointment.

Another way to use publicity is to participate in *community service* or to *volunteer.* A volunteer is someone who renders aid or performs a service without direct monetary gain. It is done of your own free will, usually with a sense of charity, but virtually every known religion or philosophy is concerned with some form of volunteerism or charity. Volunteerism is also a way to give back to the community that supports your practice. Through donations of time and talent, massage can touch lives. There are many ideas for volunteering such as doing postevent sports massage at local athletic events or donating gift certificates to civic and church groups as door prizes or auction items for fundraisers. Get a group of therapists together, and support your local police and fire departments by offering free foot rubs or massages to each officer or firefighter. Donate time at retirement homes or with hospice programs. When donating time, wear professional attire with a nametag or monogrammed shirt. Not only will you be promoting massage, personal recognition will come as more and more people recognize your name. Donate gift certificates to schools for teacher appreciation week. The possibilities are limited only by your imagination.

Press Releases. Part of your promotional strategy might include publicity writing and submitting press releases to newspapers as a way of letting people know what you are doing. Each workshop you attend, each office you hold, and each lecture you give should be announced in the newspaper as a noteworthy event. This provides a subtle reminder of who you are and gives the message that you are active in your community and your profession (Figure 27-3). A press release is not an advertisement. If yours sounds like an advertisement, the editor of the newspaper will not print it.

Begin your press release with something that a newspaper normally considers interesting and newsworthy. Keep it simple and use a writing style that is direct and delivers a clear, concise message.

MINI-LAB

Using the guidelines outlined in this chapter, write a press release.

When writing your press release, use short words, sentences, and paragraphs and write in the present tense as much as possible. Make sure your press release answers the who, what, where, when, why, and how of your event. Use inverted pyramid style of journalistic writing—that is, place the most important information in the beginning of the press release and less important information in each subsequent paragraph. This way, if the editor has to cut the size of the release, important information located at the beginning of it will not be eliminated (most editors cut from the bottom of the release). Lastly, and most importantly, proofread your work and ask at least three other objective people to proofread it. The following guidelines are helpful in putting together you press release:
- Type on 8.5" × 11" white bond paper.
- Leave a 2" margin on the top and bottom of the press release; side margins are 1.5".
- Date it and identify it as a press release by typing the words PRESS RELEASE at the top center of the

page, followed by the phrase *For Immediate Release.* A specific date can be substituted if the release should be delayed.
- At the upper left-hand corner of the page, identify yourself (or the appropriate person) as the *Contact Person* and include an address and daytime telephone number.
- Type only the lead sentence in capital letters; it should be action-oriented.
- Double-space the text if the press release is for print and triple space the release if it is for broadcast. Confine the release to one page (if possible) and type on only one side of the paper. If the press release is more than one page, write MORE at the bottom of the first page. End the press release with either -30- or consecutive number symbols (#) tabbed consecutively across the page.

Preceptors, Resources, and Networking

Building a support structure is vital for the health of any business. This involves reaching out to others and asking for help. Several methods are available for accomplishing this. First, locate an established therapist and ask her to become your preceptor. These meetings often can be arranged by your massage instructor. Participating in a preceptorship can be rewarding for both the novice and the preceptor. During class time, instructors are available to teach you the knowledge and skills of your trade. A *preceptor* is someone who guides you during your postgraduate clinical practice; this is similar to a mentor. She may be physically on premises while you engage in your professional activities, or she may be available to be contacted as you have questions about how to handle certain situations. This person may be one of your instructors but most often is a veteran massage therapist who has agreed to help you get started. Someone who was once a massage student and new graduate herself can better understand your concerns.

You can also locate a business coach, which is a cross between a consultant and a teacher and not necessarily in the massage business. This person helps you bridge the gap between where you are and where you want to be. They may offer honest, direct feedback and professional advice. Your business coach may be a chiropractor, physical/occupational therapist, banker, or experienced self-employed person. Do not be afraid to approach people from whom you would like to learn (Figure 27-4). These individuals are often flattered that you are asking them for their guidance and can act as a sounding board if you need help in making decisions. The following is a list of keys to finding and keeping a business coach relationship:
1. Find someone you admire.
2. Find someone who is successful.
3. Find someone who is willing to be a coach.

PRESS RELEASE

Contact Person: James M. Brown

Release Date: February 28, 2003

Phone: (318) 555-1212

TRIATHLETES RECEIVE MASSAGES: February brought to Metropolis the Tenth Annual Super-Man Triathlon.

The morning was surprisingly cold and windy. One would think the only people bold enough to brave the weather would be the triathletes…well, think again.

At 6:45 AM, a group of people started transporting massage tables and equipment to the race site. These dedicated individuals were staff and students of the Gulf Coast Academy of Massage Therapy in nearby Middleton. School owners Ann and Barry McDonald coordinated the event in association with the Greater Metropolitan Runners Association and the Orthopedic Clinic of Dr. Cary Ellender, the event sponsor. The massage students and faculty volunteered their time to assist athletes before and after the event. The 22 massage tables were never vacant. Of the 230 entrants in the event, approximately 178 received complimentary sportsmassage. "I give the massage therapists an A+," commented the winner of this year's event, William Saunders.

"The massage is what I look forward to after the race," said another participant. Many people received their first massage during the event and expressed their desire to incorporate massage into their fitness and training routine.

Gulf Coast Academy of Massage Therapy students traveled from all over Louisiana and Texas to participate in this year's event. The students participating included Laura Ardoin, Connie Bertrand, James Brown, Sehoya Butterworth, Geoffrey Curtis, Jamie Dubus, Charlie Duhon, Robbie Byrd, Charmaine Clement, Edward Griffin, Lanette Hidalgo, Clark Kent, Jill Maggiore, Faye Morvant, Debra O'Sonnier, Sam Parker, Martin Sheila, Jackie Short, Bo Scroggins, Sara Smith, Moxie Sporl, and Gert Verrett. Ernie Ogg, Susan Cormier, Cheryl Lavergne, Ann Gott, Tony Chapman, and Ken Duhon, school alumni, also donated their time and expertise for the event.

For additional information about sportsmassage or the Gulf Coast Academy of Massage Therapy, call (318) 555-1212.

#   #   #   #   #   #   #   #   #   #   #

Figure 27-3   A sample press release.

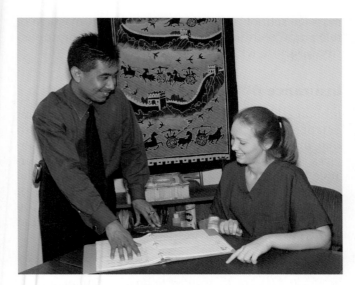

Figure 27-4 Massage therapist meeting with business coach.

It isn't what you know when you start, but what you learn when you get out there.

—Carol Kresge

4. Be willing to learn from his mistakes.
5. Give something back to him. Money is probably not appropriate in this circumstance, but find a service that he needs such as cooking or baby-sitting or give a gift such as flowers, a book, or even a massage. Show him how much he is appreciated.
6. Remember that regardless of what advice is offered the decision and responsibility are ultimately your own.

Another important aspect of support is using established business resources. These include a variety of business and civic organizations such as your public library, the Small Business Association (SBA), and the Service Corps of Retired Executives (SCORE). Most major hospitals have medical librarians who can help you locate important information. Often your secretary of state's office can put you in touch with these resource organizations. Membership in a professional bodywork organization is also am important resource tool. Belonging to a massage association helps you keep up with current trends, exchange ideas with the only people who truly understand your problems, and actively support your industry as a whole. Attend massage conferences and conventions often. There is nothing quite as inspiring as thousands of people gathered together who share a common experience.

If you are fortunate to live in the vicinity of a college or university, most colleges and universities have a business and marketing department. Volunteer your business as a project for graduate students who must analyze and prepare business proposals. The college library, which typically has more scientific resources available, is also a wealth of information and generally includes large periodical indexes such as *Index Medicus*.

The next support method involves networking, which is essentially a referral system. During this process, you are reaching out and developing business relationships with vast groups of people who are looking for the same thing you are—promoting their businesses. You may network informally by referring your clients to people you know or with whom you do business. Formal networking involves joining a networking group, local Chamber of Commerce, or other civic or social group to begin meeting people. When you meet someone that is a potential networking associate, exchange business cards and clearly state your line of work. People often remember what you do rather than your name, which is why business cards are important. At your next opportunity, write down where and when you met them and who introduced you. Keep track of all the business cards you collect in a rotary file, a computer program, or a special card folder.

As your base of support widens, you will have a number of people you can call when you have a question, need guidance, or want a sounding board for your concerns. At the same time, it is also a reciprocal process; be there for your network friends. So much of this business comes by word of mouth; it makes sense to network.

FINISHED TOUCHES, REGULAR MAINTENANCE, AND REMODELING: HOW TO STAY IN BUSINESS

Now that your business is started and you have learned some ways to nurture and promote it, it is important to know the long-term strategies for *staying* in business. The economics of private practice move in a spiral, not linear, pattern. This section explores ideas for diversifying your income, adding insurance billing and reimbursement to your practice, and monitoring the pulse of your business through basic accounting and financial reports. This section also discusses taxes and tax deductions, hiring employees and independent contractors, handling insufficient funds checks, preventing professional burnout, and investing in your future.

Diversifying Your Income

The business world is a jungle, and the law of the jungle is survival of the fittest. One way for massage therapists to survive in the ever-changing business environment is by diversifying their income.

Diversification helps minimize the effects of fluctuation in the market (the consumer or stock market); diversification helps take off financial stress while you are building a clientele. The idea of diversity follows the same idea as in financial investments: do not put all your eggs in one basket. It is easier to find 10 places to scrape up $1000 each year than to find one place that provides $10,000. Diversify your income by using different strategies for producing revenue. Here are a few ideas to protect you from extinction.

Retail sales can bring in extra money. Clients may choose to buy individual containers of massage cream; massage tools; relaxation music on cassette tapes or compact discs; aromatherapy oils, candles, or bath salts; and eye, neck, and back pillows. If you are going to sell retail goods, make sure that you have the proper license requirements. You must also collect and pay sales tax regularly. The following should be considered when engaging in retail sales:

- Make sure that the items you sell are affordable. Many clients will buy a $5 item, but only a few will buy a $100 item.
- Have a significant markup. Common markups are between 50% and 100%.
- The items should be related to massage or relaxation. Do not sell candy and cigarettes.
- Do not tie up your money in a large inventory.
- Sell what you use yourself or what you would recommend.

Expand your services by offering clients a variety of treatment options. Some therapists offer whirlpool baths, steam rooms, saunas, salt scrubs, facials, and other services. Make sure that the services offered do not take away from the atmosphere of the massage environment. The sound of hair dryers and the smell of nail polish and acetone are usually not conducive to relaxation.

Specialized training is a good way to attract new business and expand your client base. Most states and the NCBTMB require massage therapists to earn continuing education units (CEUs) each year. It may be worthwhile to take additional training for developing a new area of expertise. Learn an approach or technique that is unique to your community—something that will fill a gap in the existing market. For example, if you practice relaxation massage, attend a workshop in hydrotherapy, get some experience in the field, and develop a day spa facility.

Work in more than one location. This is especially true if you are self-employed. Locate part-time work a couple of afternoons a week for a chiropractor. Offer chair massage at the local health food store, a busy office building, or anywhere else with high traffic. Practice foot reflexology treatments at shoeshine booths and split the proceeds with the owner. Take a new technique you learned and teach it at the local massage school. Offer a low-cost class in massage or relaxation techniques at your local college or university for those who want to learn massage.

Insurance Billing and Reimbursement

Insurance billing is another aspect of expanding your practice and increasing your income. As clients learn that insurance coverage is available for massage services, therapists will be contacted regarding insurance billing and reimbursements. During the initial intake, it might be a good idea to ask your client if they have been involved in an accident recently. You may begin to see a client, only to find out later that he was involved in an accident.

 If I had really wanted to do all this damned secretarial work, I'd have gone to secretarial school.

—S. Devillier

Furthermore, because massage has been proven effective in treating musculoskeletal and myofascial pain, more doctors are referring to massage therapists. Physical therapists are hiring massage therapists to work in their offices. When the time-consuming work of massage is handled by massage therapists, the physical therapist becomes free to perform the more technically demanding tasks of evaluations, assign exercise protocols, and so on. Chiropractors also are taking advantage of the success of massage therapy by employing therapists within their practices and billing insurance for massage services.

All insurers use medical codes to process claims. A claim is a formal request for payment or reimbursement. The two important codes used by the medical community are ICD-9-CM and CPT. *ICD-9-CM* diagnostic codes are found in the *International Classification of Disease, Ninth Edition: Clinical Modifications*. All diagnosticians use this book of codes when identifying and prescribing treatment and therapy for their patients. The *Physicians' Current Procedural Terminology* (CPT) codes define services and procedures offered by health care providers. Massage and hydrotherapy treatment all fall under the physical medicine codes that are numbered in the 97000 series. As of 2002, codes that massage therapists can use are as follows:

97010—Hot and Cold Packs
97124—Massage
97140—Manual Therapy
97139—Unlisted Modality

Avoid using codes written for physical and occupational therapist, such as 97001 (Physical Therapy Evaluation) and 97002 (Physical Therapy

Re-Evaluation). Check with your state licensing board or related agency about which codes massage therapist are legally able to use. The codes do change periodically. For updated treatment codes, check with local chiropractors, physical therapists, other massage therapists who file claims for clients, insurance billing companies, and trade journals.

Most states require that massage therapists chart daily to develop and evaluate the effectiveness of a treatment plan for each client (see Chapter 8). The therapist should be meticulous with the charting of insurance claims because patient records are often subpoenaed by attorneys for use in court. Never release your patient records unless the request is accompanied by a release signed by the patient. You may bill a copying fee of 25 cents per page; do not send original documents. You may be called to testify in a mediation or hearing. You should charge the attorney hired by your client a rate of 2 to 4 times your normal hourly fee for court appearances.

The two main types of insurance claims are *major medical* and *personal injury.* Major medical claims are often referred to as *third-party claims* (the third party is the medical or health insurance company). Each insurance company has its own rules and regulations regarding coverage, and each insurance company writes numerous policies with each policy having its own guidelines. Verify (in writing if possible) each policy's specific requirements, allowances, and limits. It is often better to call the company on the phone to verify coverage, deductible, and so on. Unfortunately, prior verification does not always guarantee payment. Some clients may know this information, but you should always verify it before treatment.

A prescription from a medical or chiropractic physician is necessary for filing third-party claims. Most major medical policies carry a deductible, which is a way of making the client share in the coverage. A deductible must be paid out of the client's pocket before the insurance company makes any payment. Deductible amounts vary and may be $200 to $1000 or more per year per person. Once the deductible has been met, then the client must still pay a co-payment, which is a fixed rate or a percentage of the bill. Some policies require a fixed co-pay for all office visits; the client pays the first $25 and the insurance is billed for the rest. Some policies require that the client pay a percentage such as 20% of the bill, and then the insurance company will pick up the rest. Most third-party payers will not make payment on injuries that are someone else's fault; they will insist that the liable party's insurance be filed against.

Personal injury claims can be divided into three general categories: workers' compensation, motor vehicle accidents, and miscellaneous injury.

Workers' compensation is a state-operated benefits program for workers who are injured while on the job. Contact the workers' compensation board in your state and obtain approval and a health care provider number before beginning treatment. Most states also require a physician's referral before claims can be considered for payment. No deductible or co-payment is involved with workers' compensation; 100% of all reasonable and customary costs are paid. To calculate these costs, insurance companies use a scale based on average charges for a geographic region. Regions with greater population densities usually support larger fees. The workers' compensation pay scale is often used as the standard for setting the rates for the third-party payers. An attorney is involved in some workers' compensation cases, and some clients choose to handle the negotiations themselves.

Motor vehicle accident claims fall into two main categories: auto liability and AutoMed. Auto liability claims are claims filed for injuries sustained to passengers of one car who were injured through the fault of another car. The insurance claim is filed through the insurance company of the person at fault. Most states require a minimum level of auto liability insurance, such as $10,000. Even if the auto insurer does not require a prescription for treatment, it is generally better to have one. No deductible or co-payment is involved with auto liability; 100% of all reasonable and customary costs are paid. An AutoMed claim covers injuries to the client or her passengers if she is at fault for the accident. The limits on this policy may be low ($1000) and used up quickly, especially if other professionals are billing to it besides you. An attorney is involved in some auto accident cases, and some clients choose to handle the negotiations themselves.

Miscellaneous injury claims may include slips and falls, injuries from pet attacks, and so on. If the injury occurred at a business or residence, then the claim is filed against the business liability or homeowner's insurance. Attorneys are often involved with these types of personal injuries. No deductible or co-payment is involved with these miscellaneous personal injury liability claims; they pay 100% of all costs. You must have a physician's referral before the treatment bill can be considered for payment.

Prioritizing Insurance Claims

The first rule of insurance filing is to *never compromise your cash flow.* In other words, do not take insurance cases over cash-paying clients. Insurance cases should be used to fill in the dead time in your practice. Realize that insurance clients may be seen as often as three times a week, so one client will take up a lot of your time. The second rule is to *avoid cases that involve attorneys whenever possible.* These are the most risky insurance claims regarding payment. By the very nature of litigation, it slows down the payment process. Occasionally, a case is lost, so in such an instance, you will not be paid. When an attorney is not involved, the therapist can often bill the insurance company weekly or monthly for long treatment periods. With an attorney involved, you may not get payment until the case is settled, which can sometimes take years. If an attorney is involved, request that the attorney or the client pay your bill (or at least 50% of it) during treatment to increase your cash flow or, in the event that your client's attorney loses the case, to protect yourself from a significant loss. If the attorney is unwilling to negotiate, you do have the right to refuse to accept the case. Paperwork for insurance claims is time consuming and runs up costs because it takes away from time with your regular clientele (Figure 27-5). You can also hire a medical billing company to take care of treatment authorization and filing for you.

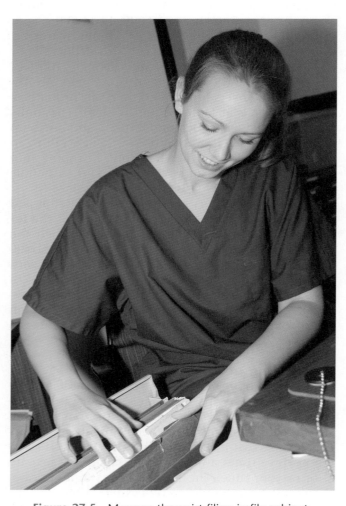

Figure 27-5 Massage therapist filing in file cabinet.

Accounting

Accounting can be defined as the art of interpreting, measuring and describing economic activity. Whether you are preparing a household budget, balancing a checkbook, preparing an income tax return, or running your massage practice or a major corporation, you are working with accounting concepts (Box 27-2). Accounting has often been called the *language of business*. Begin by opening up a business checking account. Use this account when depositing all money earned as a result of your business and paying business expenses. If possible, use checks to pay for all business-

---

BOX 27-2

Accounting Terminology

Accounting: The art of interpreting, measuring and describing economic activity.

Accounts payable: Money you owe to suppliers.

Accounts receivable: Money owed to you.

Accrual-basis accounting: Charging the income and expense to the period in which they were incurred or recognized.

Assets: Things that offer value to the company. Current assets are cash on hand; fixed assets are hard goods such as machines, equipment, furniture, vehicles, property, and buildings that are owned by the company.

Balance sheets: A summary of the company's *assets, liabilities,* and owner's *equity* at an exact point in time.

Cash-based accounting: Record transactions, both monies collected and expenses, at the time they are received or paid.

Cash flow: The amounts and sources of money coming into and going out of the company.

Credits: Entries made on the *right side* of an account. Credits reduce assets and expense accounts and increase liability, capital, and income accounts.

Debits: Entries made on the *left side* of an account. Debits increase assets and expense accounts and reduce liability, capital, and income accounts.

Depreciation: The process of spreading out the deduction for the cost of an asset over time.

Equity: The difference between total assets and liabilities; also called *net worth.*

Gross income: The money earned or accumulated before deductions.

Inventory: Unsold retail items on hand.

Liabilities: What the business owes, both current and long-term liabilities.

Net income: The money left after expenses.

Petty cash: Cash used to pay for incidental expenses. Usually set up and treated like a separate account.

Profit and loss statement: A statement of income that outlines revenues and expenses over a fixed period, indicating whether your business made a *profit* or a *loss.*

related expenses because this provides the best documentation of payment. If you are sharing expenses with another therapist, avoid co-mingling funds to maintain your separate business entity.

Establish a petty-cash account by writing yourself a check and cashing it. Keep this money in a separate envelope or small lock box. This fund is for small incidental business expenses you pay in cash. Do not put cash received from clients in this account. Write *petty cash* on any receipts and file them in the lock box. When the fund is running low, total the receipts and write another check to cash for the amount of the receipts. This will replenish the fund to its original balance. Most businesses keep $100 to $200 in this fund. At any given time, you should be able to count the money and receipts and balance back to the originally established total.

Acquiring an accountant or a bookkeeper can help you with record keeping, financial statements, and preparation of tax forms. A good accountant can help you save money and evaluate tax consequences of tax deductions and major purchases. Software packages can be purchased for less than $200 that help with all your accounting needs. If you have an accountant or plan on getting one, ask her which software program she recommends because you will be giving her copies of files on disks periodically throughout the year. Your records should outline some basic information such as *cash flow, inventory and purchases, payroll* (if applicable), *assets,* and some financial reports such as *cash flow statements, profit and loss statements,* and *balance sheets.*

Cash Flow

Record all monies received from clients and collected from other sources such as retail sales. Deposit this money in the proper account and balance this account when your statement arrives in the mail. The two ways to track cash flow are cash-based and accrual-based. Cash-based accounting requires you to record the transaction, both monies collected and expenses, at the time they are received or paid. Accrual-based accounting involves charging the income and expense to the period in which they were incurred or recognized. For example, if you gave a massage last month and you will not be collecting payment until this month, record the transaction in last month's financial statement with an accounts receivable for the money due this month.

Inventory and Purchases

Document all your purchases of business supplies. If you are involved with the retail sales of massage products such as lubricants, music, or books and periodicals, record when these items were purchased, how much you paid for them, and how much they

sold. Your inventory is the unsold retail items you have on hand.

Payroll

If you have employees, keep track of their federal wages, taxes, and social security taxes withheld, as well as any taxes and social security paid to local and state governments.

Assets

Keep a record of your fixed assets such as equipment, machines, furniture, computer and computer peripherals, vehicles, and other business-related property. The value of these items will be depreciated at tax time. Depreciation is the process of spreading out the deduction for the cost of an asset over time. Some fixed assets can be deducted in one fiscal year. Check with your accountant to see whether it is more tax-advantageous for you to take the deduction in one or multiple years.

Financial Reports

All of the financial information you gather (cash flow, inventory, purchases, payroll, and assets) are vital in preparing three key financial reports. The accuracy of these financial reports reflect the accuracy of the financial information you collect and record throughout the year. These reports will help you to track business and financial trends and spot potential problem areas that may need attention. If you are trying to get a business loan or have another financial need, you will probably need to produce these reports.

Cash Flow Statements. These statements provide an overview of the amounts and sources of money coming into and going out of the company. Because cash flow is regarded as the *life-giving blood of a business,* keeping track of these amounts and having the opportunity to regulate these amounts may make the difference between whether your business thrives.

Profit and Loss Statements. Profit and loss (P & L) statements are essentially statements of income that outline revenues and expenses over a fixed period, indicating whether your business made a *profit* or a *loss.* Most businesses prepare these statements monthly, quarterly, or annually.

Balance Sheets. Balance sheets summarizes all of the company's *assets* and *liabilities* and the owner's *equity* at an exact point in time, usually at the end of a quarter or a fiscal year.

Assets. Business assets are things that offer value to the company. Assets are divided into current and fixed assets. *Current assets* are cash on hand, including petty cash; money in checking and savings accounts; accounts receivable (money owed to you); prepaid expenses such as deposits on rent, utilities, and insurance, and the value of your inventory. *Fixed assets* include machinery, equipment, and furniture such as a massage table, computer, telephone, answering machine, wet room spa, and steam cabinet. Vehicles, property, and buildings that are owned by the company are also considered fixed assets.

Liabilities.   What the business owes are its liabilities, which can be classified as current and long-term liabilities. Examples of *current liabilities* are accounts payable (what you owe to suppliers); payments you owe on business loans within 1 year; accrued expenses such as salaries, wages, and commissions that you owe but have not yet paid; and taxes that you owe but have not paid. Examples of taxes are payroll, sales, income, property, and self-employment taxes. *Long-term liabilities* are mortgage payments for your business location and promissory notes taken out on the business' behalf for major purchases. Long-term liabilities are expenses that extend beyond one calendar year.

Equity.   Also called *net worth,* equity is the difference between your total assets and your liabilities.

Taxes

All businesses and individuals pay tax on their income. *Gross income* is the money one earns or accumulates before deductions. What you have left or the money you pocket after deductions is your *net income.* Taxes, which are an unavoidable part of running and keeping a business, include sales tax, income tax, and self-employment tax. Not all of these

will apply to your situation, but it is always a good idea to have some understanding of what each type of business tax entails. Tax laws change periodically; consult with your accountant about current tax information.

Sales Tax
If you sell any product to a client, you may be required to collect sales tax. These collected taxes are paid to state and local governments on a regular basis, usually once a month. Some municipalities tax services, whereas others do not. You will also need a sales tax number. Contact your local department of revenue and taxation for more information.

Income Tax
Federal and state taxes must be paid on profits gained by your business operations. These profits are derived from your revenues minus your expenses. The percentage paid to the federal government relates to the amount of your bottom line (how much you actually made). The amount paid to state and local governments vary from region to region. Contact your state and local department of revenue for more information. Track throughout the year how much profit (or loss) you are generating. If you notice a large profit during the year, begin preparing for a sizable income tax payment by saving money or by making quarterly estimated tax payments.

Self-Employment Tax
Most self-employed people pay a quarterly self-employment tax of 15.3% (both the employer's and the employee's portion of Social Security and Medicare taxes), in addition to income tax, to the federal government on their business net income. You may also be required to pay an amount to your state and local governments on a quarterly basis. Ask your accountant or contact the Department of Revenue and Taxation for more information. Some localities also tax equipment used in business. Your local city hall is a good place to check for information as this percentage changes.

Tax Deductions
For tax purposes, keep all your business receipts, past income tax returns, and documents related to your tax returns for 7 years. Anyone who is regarded as self-employed (files Schedule C on Form 1040) or operates as a corporate business can deduct business-related expenses. The IRS says that you may deduct any ordinary and necessary items from your business, so you may deduct needed items that may not be common in other businesses but that make your business function more efficiently. Be sure to consult with your accountant to help you make timely decisions when purchasing assets (from a tax

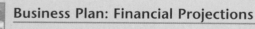

Business Plan: Financial Projections

- How much money do I have to begin this business?
- What are my capital equipment, supply list, and other startup costs?
- If money is to be borrowed, do I have a bank and loan officer in mind?
- How will my business be profitable? Produce an income projection (P & L statement), balance sheet, cash flow statement, and breakeven analysis. The projection should cover 3 years—the first year projected monthly, and the next 2 years projected quarterly.
- Based on these documents, how much money will I need to make to stay in business?
- What are the growth opportunities?

liability perspective). Examples of tax deductions are as follows:

- Accounting and bookkeeping fees
- Accounting courses (may be deductible as continuing education)
- Advertising and promotion
- Bank service charges and card merchant fees
- Books and periodicals
- Business-related insurance
- Continuing education and professional development
- Conventions and conferences of business and trade organizations
- Computer courses to help your organize data or run your business effectively
- Depreciation on major purchases
- Gifts to and entertaining current or prospective clients (IRS limits apply)
- Health Insurance (70% in 2002 and 100% in 2003)
- Interest on business and investment loans; business bank card interest and annual fees incurred
- Laundry and cleaning services
- Legal, consulting, and professional services
- License fees
- Mileage (cents per mile or deduct a percentage of actual cost); excluding travel to and from work; keep a mileage log
- Office supplies (including lubricants)
- Postage and shipping
- Printing and duplication
- Rent (home office; use a ratio of office space to total square footage)
- Repairs to office or equipment
- Uniforms and protective clothing
- Utilities and phone (home office; use a percentage of utilities; should be the same percentage used to determine rent amount; cannot deduct personal phone line but can deduct business-related long distance calls or get a separate business line)

Employees and Independent Contractors

When your business has grown to the point where you are turning down clients because of already heavy workload, it may be time to recruit another therapist. Massage therapists often associate with each other and other businesses as common law employees or independent contractors. These classifications have extensive legal and tax consequences.

An employer usually sets the hours and place for employee massage services. Employers generally provide employees with the tools and materials required to perform the work and exercise at least a measure of control and supervision over how the employees go about their tasks. The employment relationship typically involves a single employer and continues for an indefinite period (i.e., term of employment).

Independent contractors, in most cases, receive a fee based on completion of the task. They usually have special skills, training, or licensure that allows operation without detailed supervision by others. Independent contractors may even provide their own tools and equipment. They generally determine the precise time for performing services and work for more than one party.

Contracting parties occasionally attempt to characterize employees as independent contractors. This temptation may arise from an employer's responsibility to withhold income taxes on wages, contribute to social security, pay unemployment compensation insurance, and obtain workers' compensation coverage. These are significant compliance and financial burdens, particularly when the employer lacks bookkeepers and other associates adept at handling the necessary paperwork.

However, a mischaracterization can expose an employer to interest and penalties for missing tax payments. A common law employee treated as an independent contractor may take legal action for gaps in social security and unemployment compensation coverage. Even worse, if the employee has failed to pay income taxes due, the employer may have to pay the employee's taxes to the extent of the tax-withholding shortfall. A massage therapist considering an independent contractor relationship should obtain tax advice from a lawyer or accountant to confirm that a proper characterization of the relationship exists.

MINI-LAB

In your own words, define success and security.

Insufficient Funds Checks

When you receive a insufficient funds check, call the client and politely explain the situation. Tell him that you are mailing him a letter to serve as official notification and ask him for a specific time and date when he can deliver or mail payment. Write this information down. It is best to receive payment in a certified check, cash, or money order. Be sure to collect any insufficient funds check fees. Send two copies of the letter: one by certified mail with return receipt requested and one by regular mail.

If you have not received payment within 10 days after receiving verification that the certified letter was claimed, or if your certified letter was not picked up or refused, contact your local district attorney's office. Do not open the certified letter if it is returned to you. The district attorney's office may require a copy of the certified letter, your returned receipt card, or the unopened returned certified letter before collection can be pursued.

If you accepted a postdated check and it was returned, you have accepted a check knowing the person did not have money in her bank account. In this case, the district attorney's office may not be able to help you.

In any case, be pleasant, patient, understanding, and persistent. See Box 27-3 for a sample letter to be used in these circumstances.

How to Prevent Burnout

Burnout is the condition of being tired of or unhappy with one's work. It does not discriminate against any race, gender, religion, or age and is not specific to one type of profession. It affects everyone from teachers to neurosurgeons. Symptoms of burnout can include simple disinterest in the job, dreading your next client, boredom, restlessness, inability to remain focused, fatigue, and outright hatred of a job or associates. It can include depression, lack of productivity, increased tardiness, increased absenteeism, decline of social skills, workaholism, and a decline in professional boundaries. The added stress can also affect your health.

Burnout affects people for different reasons. Many massage therapists are entrepreneurs and are highly motivated, hardworking people. Many self-employed people have difficulty setting limits on their professional time. Because it is hard to delineate a 40-hour week, self-employed people may overwork.

Not setting and maintaining limits for yourself or your time is maintaining poor boundaries and over scheduling, which may lead to early burnout. If burnout is the result of overwork, it is possible that the therapist is mad at herself for not maintaining good boundaries. The inherent danger with this type of burnout is that at times this anger can manifest toward the client. The strategies for dealing with it are varied and depend on the type of problem. A few suggestions for managing burnout follow:

Nurture yourself. Eat right, get enough rest, and exercise. Spend time with people you enjoy, read a book, or take a photography class. Rediscover things you like to do or try new things that you might enjoy. Write down 10 things you currently like to do and how long it has been since you have done them. This activity may be quite revealing. List each activity on a separate strip of paper and place the strips in a jar. When you feel excessively stressed or on the verge of burnout, pick one of the activities from the jar and do it. This is also a great stress-reduction activity for your clients.

Sojourn. It is extremely important that massage professionals schedule a certain amount of time off for themselves *every week*. Be flexible; if your massage days are Monday through Friday, take off Saturday and Sunday, or if everyone wants Saturday massages, take off Sunday and Monday. Remember that you cannot give away what you do not have and that it is necessary to recharge your own batteries. It is important for a therapist to book some time off for himself on a *daily* basis. For example, if you know that you do not function well without food, schedule a lunch and a snack break every day. Do not forget to take a vacation at least once a year. Get away from the office, especially if you work out of your home. Better yet, get out of town. If you feel the need, take a break from massage altogether. Shift gears and take a sabbatical. Use this time to not only recharge your batteries but also to reevaluate important decision or situations.

BOX 27-3

Sample Letter to Client Regarding Insufficient Funds

NOTE: Personalize the terms in bold type to fit your specific situation.

YOUR LETTERHEAD WITH NAME, LOGO, ADDRESS, AND TELEPHONE AND FAX NUMBERS HERE

Name
Address
City, State, Zip
Date
Dear **Name**,

The check we received from you in the amount of **fifty dollars ($50.00)** dated **August 15, 2003**, was returned.

We understand that occasionally these mishaps occur as a result of mathematical errors, mistakes on the bank's behalf, or a deposit not being credited to your account. These situations are often embarrassing, but please be assured that we are willing to work with you.

Please bring the above-mentioned amount plus a **twenty-dollar ($20.00)** insufficient funds check charge for a total amount of **seventy dollars ($70.00)** to our offices as soon as possible. This payment must be made in cash, money order, or certified check. If you cannot come by our office, you have 10 days from receipt of this letter to mail your payment to us at the above address. Please do not send cash through the mail.

We are happy to provide you with massage therapy services and try to keep all collection attempts inside our office. Please note the following office policies:

1. Payment is due at the time of service.
2. Should a check or credit card fail to clear, a notice (this letter) is sent to the client.
3. Failure to comply with making payment of the original amount plus insufficient funds fees within the designated time frame will result in filing collections with the district attorney's office.
4. We reserve the right to place any client whose check or credit card has failed to clear on a cash-only basis.

Please contact us so that we can take care of this matter.

Sincerely,

Terry White, L.M.T.
cc: certified mail, regular mail, file

Stimulate yourself. Some therapists burn out from the boredom of repetitive routines and not being challenged. Use CEUs for this purpose. Take a class in something interesting and outrageous, not just massage technique and anatomy. Workshops also bring you together with your colleagues.

Relax. Get massages yourself! Regular massages are a necessity because of the tremendous physical requirements of this job. The recommended minimum is one massage per month. There is no maximum number of massages you can receive; just make sure you can afford the time and the money, or just trade off massages with your colleagues (Figure 27-6).

> " *I am indeed rich, since my income is superior to my expense, and my expense is equal to my wishes.*
>
> —Edward Gibson

Building a Cash Reserve and Investing in Your Future

Putting away money for a rainy day is more important for massage therapists because of the influx of clients, so cash flow fluctuates from day to day. You

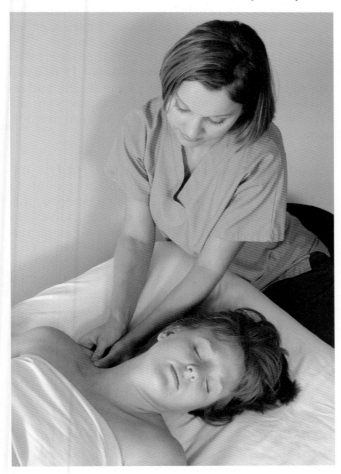

Figure 27-6 Get massages yourself.

need to build a cash reserve to get you through tough times when more money is going out than coming in, you are unemployed, or any other financial disaster occurs. Because you will always have bills to pay, do not wait till you have extra money to begin saving. Instead, consider yourself a creditor. Once a month, pay yourself 10% of what you gross. Put this money in a liquid account (e.g., savings account or an interest-bearing checking account) so you can access it quickly and easily. When you have enough money saved to pay for 1 to 6 months of living expenses, you have reached your goal of an adequate cash reserve to be used in emergencies, and you are ready to begin your next financial goal, investing.

Do not wait until you have a goal (college for children, retirement) to start investing in your future. Continue with the 10% rule (pay yourself 10% of your gross income). This money will be invested so it can grow over time. If you work for a company that makes regular contributions to a retirement account or offers incentive for you to put money in a retirement account, you are among the few. Most therapists are self-employed or work for small companies that do not participate in employee retirement plans; therefore massage therapists must become motivated and disciplined enough to invest for themselves to meet future financial goals. The following investment guidelines can help you with market investing:

Invest for the long term. The market does not move in one direction all year, but historically the stock market moves up over time, even with relatively sharp downturns. Investing for the long term allows you to weather the inevitable storms. This strategy is not unlike a marriage commitment. However, if you cannot sleep at night worrying about your investments, you probably should not be investing in the market or you are in the wrong area of the market.

Invest systematically. It is almost impossible to buy stocks when they are at their lowest (unless you have a crystal ball). If you invest the same dollar amount and buy the same stock or fund regularly and systematically, you will naturally buy it at different prices. Over time, your average cost will be lower than the average price of the stock or fund. This strategy is called *dollar cost averaging.*

Diversify. Do not put all your eggs in one basket. If you allocate your money among several different types of securities (stocks, bonds, funds), your portfolio performs better. A financial portfolio is all of the various investments held by an individual investor. What you choose to buy will depend on your need for income and your personality (whether you can handle it when the stock, bond, or fund price fluctuates), and risk tolerance. Many investors use the *diversity by five* strategy, which is to carefully select five quality stocks (names you know such as Coca Cola, Wal-Mart, or Exxon Mobil). Odds are that three of these will perform well, one will offer a stellar performance, and one will be disappointing.

Use professional advice. Finding a good financial advisor is tricky. Brokers make their living whether you make money or not; they get a commission if you buy or sell. Many horror stories have been told about unscrupulous financial advisors who recommend purchasing something for an exorbitant fee that only later you discover was never performed even though you were charged. Ask around for someone who gives you the pros and cons of an investment and lets you make the decision. It is important that you like him and trust him. Ask him for references too.

Securities

Securities are the vehicles in which you put your money to optimize your return. Types of securities are stocks and bonds. A fund contains many types of securities. The securities listed in the following sections will help you decide where to invest. Unless your money is invested in a retirement account or other tax shelter, you will owe tax on your investment income.

Stocks. Buying stock establishes your proportionate ownership in that company represented by shares. As a stockholder, you reap rewards of the company's profits and also suffer the company's losses. The two types of stock are common stock and preferred stock. Most stocks pay their stockholders dividends. A dividend is part of a company's earnings that is distributed at regular intervals to its shareholders; dividends can be reinvested to buy more shares or can be paid to you in cash.

Bonds. A bond is basically a loan. Examples of bonds are corporate bonds (loan to a corporation), municipal bonds (loan to a municipality or revenue district), and government bonds and types of government bonds called treasury bills (loan to Uncle Sam). When you purchase a bond, most agencies you loan money to pay you interest on a biannual basis. Interest on municipal and government bonds is usually tax-free. When the bond matures (ranges from 1 to 40 years), the agency returns your initial investment. Most people who buy bonds need to receive a regular income from their investments, such as individuals already retired.

Funds. A mutual fund is established by an investment company that pools money from its shareholders and invests it in a variety of securities. Each individual mutual fund has varying degrees of its investment objectives and accompanying risks. Some

mutual funds charge a fee to join and to withdraw; other funds are no-load, which means no fee is charged when shares are bought or sold. Index funds are unmanaged mutual funds that seek to replicate the performance of established market indices. Some well-known indexes include the Dow Jones Industrial Average, Standard & Poor's 500 Index, the NASDAQ Composite Index, Russell 2000, and the Consumer Price Index.

Retirement Accounts

The federal government wants you to save for your own retirement too. In fact, they help you out by allowing you to treat contributions to your retirement account like a tax deduction. Some restrictions include how much you can claim as a deduction ($3000 or a percentage of your gross).

If you withdraw funds from a retirement account, you have 90 days to replace it or you may pay income tax on the amount withdrawn plus a 10% penalty. The income you earn from your investment is tax-deferred, so taxes are not due till you begin withdrawing the money at retirement. At this future time, you will probably be in a lower tax bracket (the exception is the Roth IRA). You can borrow against retirement accounts, so it can be regarded as an asset and therefore loan collateral. The most common retirement accounts are an Individual Retirement Account (IRA), Simplified Employee Pension Plan (SEP), Savings Incentive Match Plan for Employees (SIMPLES), and Annuities. You have till April 15 to make contributions for the previous year and rules and restrictions change annually. Please consult your accountant or your financial advisor for current information.

Individual Retirement Account (IRA). Traditional IRAs are tax-deferred retirement accounts in which some or all contributions may be deductible from current taxes, depending on the individual's adjusted gross income and coverage by an employer-sponsored retirement plan. Through 2007, the maximum deductible contribution is $4000. It will increase to $5000 in 2008 and be subject to annual adjustments thereafter. Under these conditions, you are taxed on the distribution, but not penalized. You can invest the money in a wide variety of ways (CDs, stocks, bonds, or funds). A Roth IRA, which was created through the Taxpayer Relief Act of 1997, does not allow you to write off contributions, but income derived as a result of distributions during retirement are tax-free.

Simplified Employee Pension Plan (SEP). In many ways, they are similar to an IRA, except SEPP allows an employer to make tax-deductible contributions to the employees retirement account while they are also contributing.

Savings Incentive Match Plan for Employees (SIMPLE).
A SIMPLE IRA is a company-sponsored retirement plan that allows employees to contribute through deductions from their paycheck. The company must match the employee contribution or contribute 2% of the employee's annual gross income to any employee who earns more than $5000 or more during the year.

Annuities.
Often used as a retirement account, an annuity is a type of investment in which the policy holder makes a lump sum or installment payments to an insurance company. The income is tax-deferred and distributions are made at retirement. This type of account is expensive to open and maintain because of many hidden costs.

SUMMARY

Basic business consists of three phases: preparatory work, actual business operation, and long-term strategies for the future operation of your business. The preparatory work includes the development of a business plan (Box 27-4), which should be built around your personal values, goals, visions, and professional mission. Your business plan will include details of all phases of your future business, such as services offered, hours, fees, marketing, insurance needs, startup costs, and necessary licenses and permits. Once this is accomplished, you can open your doors.

It has been said that anyone can open a business, but keeping it open is the hard part. Business growth depends on how we relate to the public, both individually as clients and collectively as a target market for our advertising and promotional strategies. This applies to the use of media and networking with other professionals.

Finally, proof of true business success is defined in terms of longevity. You can go the distance by diversifying your income, managing your finances with basic accounting and financial reports, planning tax strategies, avoiding professional burnout, and investing wisely for retirement.

If you find all this business thinking helpful, realize that this is just the tip of the iceberg. You can learn more about business in many ways. Your public library is a wealth of books about promotion, publicity, advertising, marketing, and selling. Your local massage schools, universities, and many professional organizations also offer continuing education courses in business.

BOX 27-4

Business Plan

Introduction
- Cover letter
- Table of contents

Personal Information
1. What is my experience in this business, if any?
2. What do I love about my work?
3. What are my weaknesses and shortcomings?
4. What are my strengths and talents?
5. What is special and distinct about me as a massage therapist? Why will these appeal to clients?
6. What are my values?
7. What have I learned about this business from fellow therapists, teachers, trade journals, and trade suppliers?

General Description of Business
1. What is my vision statement?
2. What is my mission statement?
3. What services do I or will I offer? Describe these services and the benefits of these services.
4. For what purpose will people buy my services?
5. Am I willing to change what I offer, to some extent, to meet my client's changing needs?

Operating Procedures
1. What types of licenses are required for me to operate my business?
2. What will be the opening date of my business? What hours of the day and days of the week will I be in operation?
3. What will my office policies be for late clients, cancellations, out-of-date gift certificate redemption, insufficient funds checks, and credit card sales?

Management and Personnel
1. What is my management experience?
2. What do I predict my legal structure will be?
3. Who will be the other key figures in my business? Include an organizational chart, list of duties/backgrounds of key individuals, outside consultants/advisers, and board of directors.
4. How will services be provided? Will I do all the work, or will I use employees or contract labor?
5. Describe the types of support my business may require, including child care, janitorial service, lawn and garden care, and bookkeeping and accounting.

Continued

BOX 27-4

Business Plan—cont'd

6. Describe the wages and benefits I can offer each type of employee and support person.

Insurance Needs

1. What are my insurance needs? These may include professional and general liability, business personal property, automotive, life and health insurance, and disability insurance.
2. Have I contacted an agent to discuss what types of policies they offer and the cost and benefit of each?

Marketing and Competition

1. What do I want my business identity to be? Describe the image you want to project. *You never get a second chance to make a first impression.*
2. What do I want people to say to others about my services?
3. Who is my target market? Who will want to buy my services? Identify important characteristics such as age, gender, occupation, income, and so on.
4. Who else provides a similar service? In order of their strength in the market, list my five closest competitors by name and address. Next, describe each competitor's strengths and weaknesses. What have I learned from my competitors operations and from their advertising?
5. What will my fee schedule look like? How have I determined these fees? Will this price cover my material costs, labor costs, and overhead?
6. What are my competitors charging?
7. How am I different from my competitors in ways that matter to potential clients? Refer to the previous business plan section on personal information.

Advertising, Promotion, and Location

1. How can I get the attention of the people I want to reach? Which advertising media are appropriate for my business and targeted clients?
2. What other channel(s) such as networking, referrals, and publicity will I use to reach clients?

3. How can I discover whether a promotion is working?
4. Plan an advertising budget for 6 months. Include specific media you will use and the cost of each.
5. What type of location does my business require? Describe the type of building your business needs, including office and studio space, parking, exterior lighting, security needs, and proximity to other businesses for added exposure.
6. Where do I plan to locate my business? Is this location right for my business and me?
7. Describe the geographic area my business will serve. Are sufficient numbers of potential clients located there?
8. What type of physical layout is needed for my business? Include layout for reception area, restroom, hydrotherapy and spa room (if applicable), retail and inventory areas, and gift certificate sales.

Financial Projections

1. How much money do I have to begin this business?
2. What is my capital equipment, supply list, and other startup costs?
3. If money is to be borrowed, do I have a bank and loan officer in mind?
4. How will my business be profitable? Produce an income projection (profit and loss statements), balance sheet, cash flow statement, and break-even analysis. The projection should cover 3 years—that is, the first year projects monthly and the next 2 years project quarterly.
5. Based on these documents, how much money will I need to make to stay in business?
6. What are the growth opportunities?

Supporting Documents

- Tax returns for the last 3 years
- Personal financial statements
- Copy of proposed lease for building space
- Copy of licenses and other legal documents
- Copy of your curriculum vitae

MATCHING I

Write the letter of the best answer in the space provided.

A. Sole proprietorship
B. Media
C. Curriculum vitae
D. Publicity

E. Marketing
F. Contract
G. Preceptor

H. Professional liability
I. Advertising
J. Mission statement

_____ 1. Making your business noticeable to the public by purchasing print or broadcast media

_____ 2. Systems of mass communication

_____ 3. Promoting your business with image, purpose, and direction

_____ 4. A written agreement between two or more parties that communicates expectations, duties, and responsibilities; this agreement is enforceable by law

_____ 5. Business of a single owner

_____ 6. Free media exposure

_____ 7. Malpractice insurance

_____ 8. Someone who guides you during your post-graduate clinical practice

_____ 9. An autobiographical sketch that documents all your achievements: occupational, avocational, and academic

_____ 10. Statement of purpose

MATCHING II

Write the letter of the best answer in the space provided. Some will be used more than once.

A. Inventory
B. Dividend
C. Equity or net worth
D. Cash-based accounting

E. Balance sheet
F. Securities
G. Profit and loss statement
H. Individual retirement account

I. Gross income
J. Accounts receivable
K. Portfolio
L. Depreciation

_____ 1. Unsold retail items you have on hand

_____ 2. Money owed to you or your business

_____ 3. All the various investments held by an individual investor

_____ 4. The process of spreading out the deduction for the cost of an asset over time

_____ 5. Statement of income that outline revenues and expenses over a fixed period, indicating whether your business earned a profit or a loss

_____ 6. Tax-deferred retirement account in which some or all contributions may be deductible from current taxes, depending on the individual's adjusted gross income and coverage by an employer sponsored retirement plan

_____ 7. The difference between your total assets and your liabilities

_____ 8. Part of a company's earnings distributed at regular intervals to its shareholders

_____ 9. The money one earns or accumulates before deductions

_____ 10. Vehicles you put your money in to optimize your return

_____ 11. A financial statement that summarizes all of the company's assets, liabilities, and owner's equity at an exact point in time, usually at the end of a quarter or a fiscal year

_____ 12. Accounting method where you record the transaction, monies collected, and expenses at the time they are received or paid

Bibliography

Ashley M: *Massage: a career at your fingertips,* ed 2, Mahopac Falls, NY, 1995, Enterprise.

Associated Bodywork and Massage Professionals: *Successful business handbook,* Evergreen, Colo, 2001, ABMP.

Barnhart T: *The five rituals of wealth: proven strategies for turning the little you have into more than enough,* New York, 1996, HarperCollins,.

Beck MF: *Theory and practice of therapeutic massage,* ed 2, Albany, NY, 1994, Milady.

Boldt LG: *Zen and the art of making a living: a practical guide to creative career design,* New York, 1993, Penguin Books USA.

Charles Schwab: *Investment choices.* Available at http://www. schwab.com, February 10, 2002.

Consumer Reports: *The mainstreaming of alternative medicine,* pp 17-25, May 2000.

Denning E: Massage therapy medical codes for 2002, *Massage Bodywork: Nurtur Body, Mind, Spirit* pp 144-145, Feb/Mar 2002.

Downes J, Goodman JE: *Barron's dictionary of finance and investment terms,* ed 5, Hauppauge, NY, 1995, Barron's Educational Services.

Edward Jones: *Approaching retirement.* Available at http://www.edwardjones.com, February 10, 2002.

Fritz D: *Fundamentals of therapeutic massage,* St Louis, 1995, Mosby.

Gaedeke R, Tootelian D: *Small business management,* ed 3, Needham Heights, Mass, 1991, Simon and Schuster.

Grodzki L: *Building your ideal private practice: how to love what you do and be highly profitable too!* New York, 2000, WW Norton.

Harrison BJ: *Business practices: a guide to starting your massage therapy practice in New Mexico,* Albuquerque, 1994, Author.

Meigs WB, Roberts F: *Accounting: the Basis for business decisions,* ed 7, New York, 1987, McGraw-Hill.

Money Magazine: p 56, Sept/Oct 1994.

Palmer DA: *The bodywork entrepreneur,* San Francisco, Calif, 1990, Thumb Press.

Sohnen-Moe C: *Business mastery: a guide for creating a fulfilling, thriving business and keeping it successful,* ed 3, Tucson, Ariz, 1997, Sohnen-Moe Associates.

Reflexology

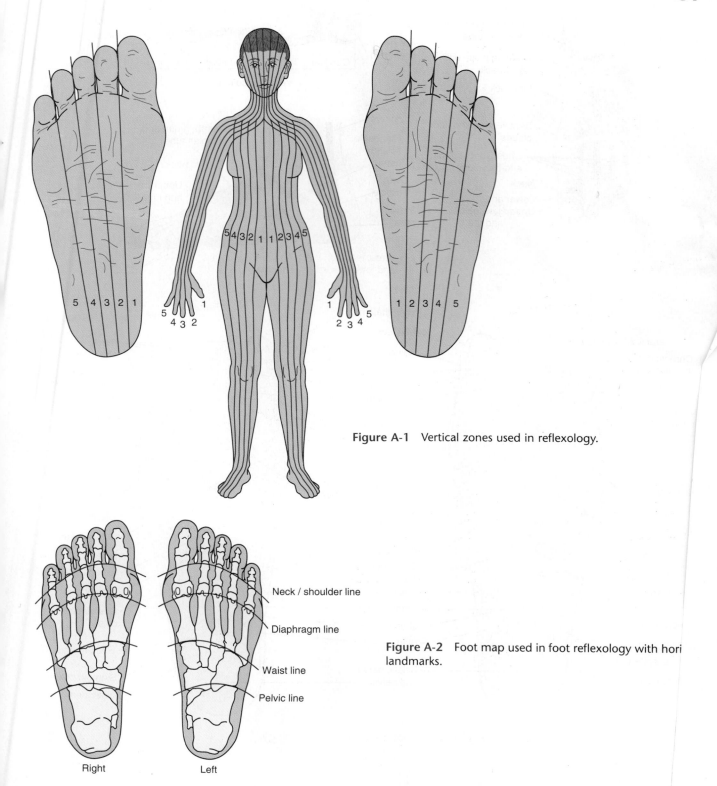

Figure A-1 Vertical zones used in reflexology.

Neck / shoulder line

Diaphragm line

Waist line

Pelvic line

Figure A-2 Foot map used in foot reflexology with hori landmarks.

Right   Left

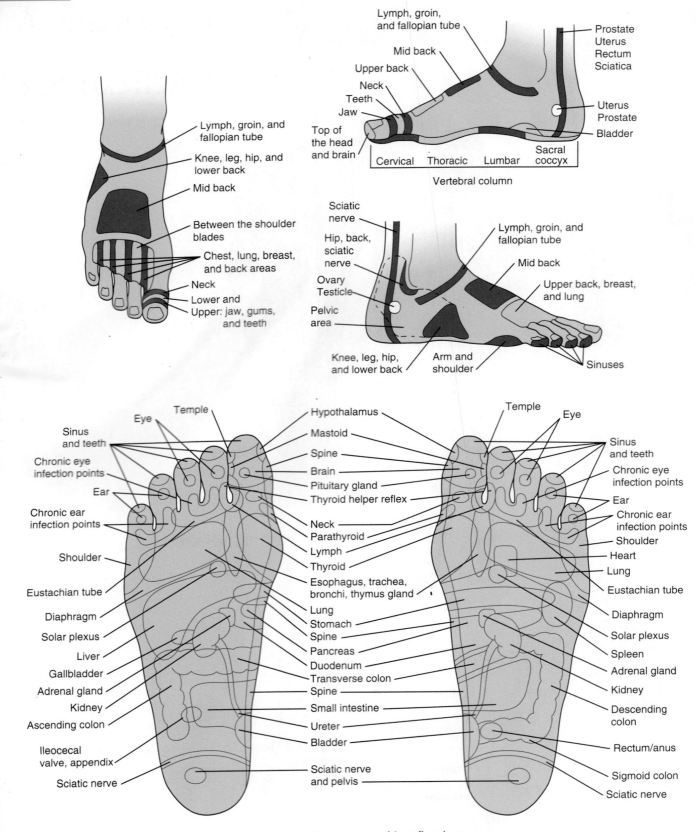

Figure A-3   Foot map used in reflexology.

Major Chakra Centers

Chakra	No.	Element	Color	Endocrine Gland	Musical Note	Physiological Function	Psychological Function
Crown	7	Nonapplicable	Silvery white	Pineal	B	Biorhythms (circadian and diurnal rhythms)	Spirituality, connection with the universe, oneness
Brow (third eye)	6	Nonapplicable	Purple/indigo	Pituitary	A	The senses	Meditation, vision, insight, creativity, realization
Throat	5	Ether	Blue	Thyroid	G	Vocal communications	Self-image, self-love, self-expression
Heart	4	Air	Green	Thymus	F	Respiratory, cardiovascular, lymphatic/immune functions	Love of others, compassion, harmony
Solar plexus	3	Fire	Yellow	Pancreas	E	Digestion, enzymatic functions	Personal power, life force, emotions, pleasure, mental capacity, ambition
Sacral	2	Water	Orange	Gonads	D	Reproduction, colon	Relationships, sexual energy, purification
Root	1	Earth	Red	Adrenals	C	Elimination, movement	Survival, security, transmutation

Business Forms

Daily Income Log for: Month _____ Year _____										Page ___ of ___

					Payment Method (check one)					
No.	Date	Client Name	Fees Paid	Tips Paid	Cash	Check	Charge	Gift Cert	Comp	Comments
1										
2										
3										
4										
5										
6										
7										
8										
9										
10										
11										
12										
13										
14										
15										
16										
17										
18										
19										
20										
21										
22										
23										
24										
25										
26										
27										

Total no. of clients seen this period ⟶

Total Fees for this page ⟶

Total Income for this page (fees + tips) ⟶

⟵ Total Tips for this page

⟵ Cumulative Gross Monthly Income

Copyright © 2003 by W.B. Saunders Company. All rights reserved.

Figure A-4 Daily income log. (Permission is hereby granted to reproduce this form in its entirety, including the copyright notice, for commercial or instructional use but not for resale.)

Yearly Business Expenses by Quarter for the _____ Calendar Year

Category	First Quarter		Second Quarter		Third Quarter		Fourth Quarter	
Advertising								
Auto expense								
Bank service charges								
Books and periodicals								
Childcare								
Continuing education								
Donations								
Entertainment and gifts								
Furniture and fixtures								
Insurance								
License fees								
Miscellaneous								
Office supplies								
Postage and shipping								
Printing and duplicating								
Prof. asso. memberships								
Prof. services (legal, acct.)								
Refunds								
Rent								
Repairs								
Retail merchandise								
Taxes								
Telephone								
Travel								
Utilities								
Wages—contract labor								
Wages—salary								
Wages—owner's draw								
Totals								
Grand Total								

Figure A-5   Yearly business expenses by quarter. (Permission is hereby granted to reproduce this form in its entirety, including the copyright notice, for commercial or instructional use but not for resale.)

Gift Certificate Sales Log for: Month _____ Year _____

Page _____ of _____

No.	Date Issued	Certificate Number	Client Name on Certificate	Name of Purchaser	Purchaser's Telephone	Certificate Value	Method of Payment	Date Redeemed
Ex.	01/02/02	1000	John Jacobs	Sherrie Jacobs	555-1212	$45.00	check	01/23/02
1								
2								
3								
4								
5								
6								
7								
8								
9								
10								
11								
12								
13								
14								
15								
16								
17								
18								
19								
20								
21								
22								
23								
24								
25								
26								
27								
28								
29								
30								

Figure A-6 Gift certificate sales log. (Permission is hereby granted to reproduce this form in its entirety, including the copyright notice, for commercial or instructional use but not for resale.)

Glossary

Abdominal Anterior trunk.

Abduction Movement away from the median plane. *Horizontal abduction* refers to the direction of abduction.

Absolute contraindication Condition in which massage is inappropriate, is not advised, and may be harmful.

Absorption The processes by which the products of digestion move into the bloodstream or lymph vessels and then into the body's cells.

Acetylcholine A chemical stored in vesicles at the axon terminal located at the end of the motor neuron. It mediates nerve activity to the skeletal muscles.

Acetylcholinesterase An enzyme secreted into the synaptic cleft to clean up any residual acetylcholine.

Acne An infection of the sebaceous glands and hair follicles caused by bacteria.

Acquired immunity Diverse but specific responses to invaders involving lymphocytes.

Acquired immunodeficiency syndrome (AIDS) AIDS is a disease caused by the human immunodeficiency virus (HIV).

Acupoints Points on the body that influence and are influenced by body energy.

Acromegaly Caused by the overproduction of growth hormone characterized by an elongation and enlargement of the bones of the extremities, face, and jaw.

Acromial The area on the top of the shoulder.

Actin A thin myofilament. Actin is pulled over myosin filaments to produce muscular contraction.

Action potential A measurement of electrical difference between the charge inside and the charge outside a neural cell membrane; sometimes referred to as the electrical impulse.

Active movement Involves the therapist describing or demonstrating the movement while the client actively performs the movement.

Active-assisted movement Performed by the client while the therapist assists throughout the range of motion.

Active-resisted movement Involves the therapist applying gentle resistance while the client is actively engaged in the movement.

Active transport The movement of important atoms and molecules such as ions against the concentration gradient from low levels to high levels to maintain such vital processes as nerve conduction.

Active trigger points Trigger points that are noticeably painful even when there is no external physical stimulation; they can refer pain in specific patterns to other areas of the body.

Acute Refers to those conditions that last for a short time, usually a few days to a few weeks; typically these conditions have a sudden onset and run a severe course.

Adaptation A decrease in sensitivity to a prolonged stimulus.

Addison's disease Caused by partial or complete failure of adrenal functions, often resulting from an autoimmune disease, local or general infection, or adrenal hemorrhage.

Adduction Movement toward the median plane. *Horizontal adduction* refers to the direction of adduction.

Adhesion A scar that occurs when two or more layers of tissue, which normally glide freely over one another, become adhered (often after an injury or surgery). These adhered tissues interfere with the normal glide between the tissue layers and interrupt normal biomechanics.

Adipose tissue A type of loose connective tissue, specialized for fat storage. This connective tissue insulates the body against heat loss, provides fuel reserves for energy, and provides a cushion around certain structures (e.g., heart, kidneys, and some joints).

Adrenal glands (suprarenals) These important glands are located superior to each kidney and are among the most vascular organs in the body. They are divided into two regions (cortex and medulla), each producing different hormones.

Adrenocorticotropic hormone A pituitary hormone that regulates the endocrine activity of the adrenal cortex, especially cortisol secretion.

Age spots Also referred to as *senile lentigo* or *liver spots,* age spots are tan or brown patches found on the skin of older people, especially those who have had excessive exposure to the sun.

Agonist The muscle that is most responsible for causing desired joint action.

Aldosterone A hormone produced by the adrenal cortex. This hormone causes the kidneys to retain sodium, which stimulates the reabsorption of more water back into the blood plasma. The plasma volume of the blood increases, and blood pressure rises correspondingly.

Alimentary canal A mostly coiled, muscular passageway leading from mouth to anus.

Allergies Hypersensitivity and overreaction to otherwise harmless agents.

All-or-none response Each individual muscle fiber, when sufficiently stimulated, will contract to its fullest extent. Likewise, in the absence of sufficient stimuli, each muscle fiber relaxes to its full resting length. This refers to nerve impulses as well.

Alveolar sacs Two or more alveoli that share a common opening.

Alveolus Tiny sacs attached to the bronchioles. They are made of a single layer of epithelial tissue blended with elastic tissue.

Amino acids The building blocks of protein. There are 22 identified amino acids vital for proper growth, development, and maintenance of health.

Amma (Amno) A Chinese style of massage; regarded as the precursor to all other therapies, manual and energetic.

Amphiarthrotic These joints are slightly movable (only a few millimeters).

Anal canal The final portion of the colon located between the rectum and the anus.

Anatomical position A standard body position; the body is erect and facing forward, the arms are at the side, the palms are facing forward with the thumbs to the side, and the feet are slightly apart with toes pointing forward.

Anatomy The study of the structures and shape of the human body and their positional relationship to one another.

Androgens A group of adrenal hormones that maintain male sexual characteristics.

Anemia A condition in which the oxygen-carrying capacity of the blood is decreased because of a decrease in red blood cells or a decrease in the amount of functional hemoglobin in the blood.

Aneurysm A weakness and dilation in the wall of a blood vessel.

Angina pectoris Often felt as chest pain, angina pectoris is frequently caused by constriction of coronary arteries and myocardial anoxia (lack of oxygen in the heart muscle).

Angiotensin II A powerful stimulant that has two major effects. First, it works directly on the blood vessels by causing vasoconstriction, which raises the blood pressure; second, it stimulates the adrenal cortex to release aldosterone.

Ankylosing spondylitis This is an inflammatory disease leading to calcification and fusion of the joints between the vertebrae and the sacroiliac joint.

Anorexia nervosa The prolonged avoidance of eating.

Anothomia Work written by Mondino dei Luzzi in 1316. Considered to be the first modern treatise on human anatomy.

Antagonist The opposing muscle that must resist or yield to the joint motion initiated by the agonist.

Antebrachial Pertains to the forearm; between the wrist and elbow.

Antecubital Space in front of the elbow or at the bend of the elbow.

Anterior (ventral) Pertaining more to the front of a structure.

Antidiuretic hormone (vasopressin) Decreases urine output by stimulating the kidneys to reabsorb water into the blood.

Anus The terminal end of the anal canal.

Aortic semilunar valve The semilunar valve between the left ventricle and the aorta.

Apnea A temporary cessation or absence of spontaneous respiration, typically 15 seconds in duration.

Aponeurosis A broad, flat tendon that attaches skeletal muscle to bone, to another muscle, or to the skin.

Appendicitis An inflammation of the vermiform appendix often detected by acute pain in the lower right quadrant of the abdomen, vomiting, fever, and elevated white blood cell count.

Arachnoid The middle layer of the meninges possessing many threadlike strands, giving it a cobwebbed appearance.

Areolar connective tissue One of the most widely distributed types of connective tissue. It has several types of cells: macrophages, fibroblasts, mast cells, plasma cells, adipocytes, and a few white blood cells.

Arndt-Schultz law Weak stimuli excite physiological activity, moderately strong ones favor it, strong ones retard it, and very strong ones arrest it.

Aromatherapy The use of scents for therapeutic purposes.

Arrector pili The muscle of the hair that allows it to stand upright.

Arrhythmia Any deviation from a normal heart rate pattern.

Arterial pulse The expansion effect that occurs when the left ventricle contracts, producing a wave of blood that surges through and expands the arterial walls.

Arteries Blood vessels that move blood away from the heart.

Arterioles Smaller, thinner branches of arteries.

Arthritis Several chronic diseases characterized by inflammation, swelling, and pain in the joints.

Articular cartilage The hyaline cartilage associated with joints that covers the epiphysis.

Articulations Where bones meet; joints.

Asclepiades Founder of the group of ancient Greek physicians known as the Methodists.

Ashi points In Chinese medicine, points on the body that get a reaction from the client when touched.

Asian Bodywork Therapy (ABT) The treatment of the human body, mind, and spirit by pressure and/or manipulation. This includes the electromagnetic or energetic field, which surrounds, infuses, and brings the body to life.

Asthma A chronic, inflammatory disorder in which the smooth muscles in the walls of the smaller bronchi and bronchioles spasm to close or partially close the respiratory passageways.

Atherosclerosis An arterial disorder associated with a buildup of plaque (made of lipids) in the blood vessels.

Athlete's foot A superficial fungal infection of the foot characterized by discoloration of the skin and a ridge of red tissue.

Atrioventricular bundle (bundle of His) A bundle of conducting fibers arising from the distal portion of the atrioventricular (AV) node; it quickly branches into a right and left bundle, which run in the interventricular septum to the right and left ventricle.

Atrioventricular node The node in the interventricular septum that is designed to work at a slower rate than the sinoatrial node to give the atria plenty of time to empty of blood.

Atrioventricular valves The heart valves separating the atria from the ventricles.

Atrium The superior heart chambers that receive blood from the body through large veins.

Atrophy A decrease in the size of muscle fibers or a wasting away of muscles from poor nutrition, lack of use, motor unit dysfunction, or lack of motor nerve impulses.

Aulus Celsus Ancient Roman writer, considered to be the first important medical historian.

Autoimmune disease Part of a large group of diseases characterized by an alteration of immune functions. These disorders result from an attack by the body's own immune system.

Autonomic nervous system Involuntary system supplying impulses to smooth muscle, cardiac muscle, and glands.

Avicenna (980-1037) Name by which Persian physician Abu-Ali al-Husayn ibn-Sina was known in the West. He authored over 100 books that compiled all the theoretical and practical medical knowledge of his time and was thus greatly influenced by the works of Galen of Pergamon.

Axillary Armpit region.

Axillary nodes Lymph nodes located in the axillary region.

Axon A single cylindrical extension of a neuron that transmits impulses away from the cell body.

Axon terminal Fine filament-like terminal extension of the axon.

Ayur-Veda Part of Hindu tradition, regarded as a sacred practice.

Æculapius (Asclepius) A legendary physician who became the Greek god of medicine and healing.

Bacteria Unicellular microorganisms, most of which are not pathogenic and do not require living tissue for survival.

Ball-and-socket joint Also referred to as a *triaxial joint*, this type of joint permits all movements and offers the greatest range of motion; examples are the hip and shoulder joints.

Baroreceptor Pressure-sensitive receptor cells that affect blood pressure by sending impulses to the cardiac and vasomotor centers in the medulla oblongata.

Basal cell carcinoma A slow-growing skin cancer characterized by lesions that begin as small raised nodules that ulcerate.

Basilar membrane A membrane within the cochlea, containing sensory cells.

Bath(s) A broad category of hydrotherapy application encompassing partial or full immersion in water, wax, light, heated air, or steam.

Bell's palsy Unilateral facial paralysis of sudden onset due to inflammation of the facial nerve.

Belly (gaster) of a muscle The central portion or bulk of a muscle.

Benign A condition that is not cancerous or life threatening.

Biarticular Muscle that crosses two joints, acting on both joints.

Bicuspid (mitral) valve The left atrioventricular valve containing two flaps or cusps.

Bile Produced from the hemoglobin in worn-out red blood cells, bile is not an enzyme but an *emulsifier*. It physically breaks apart large fat globules in the gastrointestinal (GI) tract into smaller ones and provides a larger surface area for fat-digesting enzymes to work.

Biogenic amines These are the simplest hormone molecules and are derived from amino acids; examples are peptide hormones. These substances regulate blood pressure, elimination of waste, body temperature, and many other functions.

Blisters A collection of fluid below the epidermis sometimes caused by pressure or friction.

Blitz gus A high-pressure stream of cold water applied to a standing client standing at a specific distance.

Blood Red liquid connective tissue.

Blood pressure The pressure exerted by blood on an arterial wall during contraction of the left ventricle.

Blood-brain barrier A very selective semipermeable membrane that controls which substances are allowed into the brain.

Body mechanics Also known as *biomechanics;* the proper use of postural techniques to deliver massage therapy with the utmost efficiency and with minimum trauma to the practitioner.

Body shampoo   Gently scrubbing the body with a brush dipped in warm soapy water. After working up a generous lather, water is poured over the client's skin.

Bolus   A ball-like, masticated lump of swallowed food.

Bone   The hardest and most solid of all connective tissue, bone consists of compact and spongy bone, collagenous fibers, and mineral salts.

Bone marrow   Tissue located in the medullary cavity of bones.

Bony markings   Markings located on the exterior surface of bones where muscles, tendons, and ligaments attach and where nerve and blood vessels pass. These exterior marks are also called *surface markings.*

Borelli, Giovanni Alfonso (1608-1679)   Italian anatomist who carried out extensive anatomical dissections and analyzed the phenomenon of muscular contraction.

Boundaries   The limits we establish between ourselves and others regarding various aspects of our lives.

Bow stance   Also known as the *archer stance* or *lunge position,* the bow stance is used when applying any stroke in which the therapist proceeds from one point to the next along the client's body; the feet are placed on the floor in a 30- to 50-degree angle, one pointing straight forward (lead foot) and one pointing off toward the side (trailing foot). The lead foot points in the direction of movement.

Brachial   Refers to the upper arm.

Bradycardia   Slow heart rate (less than 50 to 60 beats per minute).

Brain   One of the largest organs in the body, containing an estimated 9 to 15 billion neurons. The brain is divided into four major regions: *cerebrum, diencephalon, cerebellum,* and *brain stem.*

Brain stem   The inferior part of the brain that contains three main structures: *midbrain, pons,* and *medulla oblongata.*

Breathing (pulmonary ventilation)   The mechanical process required to move air in and out of the lungs. The two phases of breathing are inspiration and expiration.

Bright, Timothy (c. 1551-1615)   British Renaissance–era physician who taught and published on the use of baths, exercise, and massage to restore health.

Bronchi   The large air-conduction passageways leading to each lung. Each tubelike structure is reinforced with hyaline cartilage to keep it open.

Bronchioles   Smaller divisions of the bronchi.

Bronchitis   An inflammation of the bronchial mucosa causing the bronchial tubes to swell and extra mucus to be produced.

Bronchogenic carcinoma   Also known as *lung cancer,* this condition is caused by a long-term irritant such as air pollution, cigarette smoke, asbestos, or coal dust.

Bruise   Also known as a *contusion,* a bruise is an injury that does not break the skin. It is caused by a blow and is characterized by swelling, discoloration, and pain.

Brunner's (duodenal) glands   Intestinal glands that secrete alkaline mucus.

Buccal   Pertaining to the cheek area.

Bulimia   Characterized by overeating (bingeing) and self-induced vomiting (purging).

Bunion   Abnormal medial tilting and enlargement of the joint between the first metatarsal of the great toe and the associated proximal phalanx.

Burn   When the skin is damaged by heat, radiation, electricity, or chemical agents.

Bursae   A collapsed saclike structure with a synovial membrane that contains synovial fluid.

Bursitis   Acute or chronic inflammation of the bursae. It is caused by infection, trauma, disease, or excessive friction or pressure in the joint.

Calcitonin   Thyroid hormone that decreases blood calcium and phosphorus levels by stimulating osteoblasts (bone-forming cells) to make bone matrix. This causes calcium and phosphorus to be deposited in the bones.

Calf (sural)   Pertaining to the calf area of the lower leg.

Calyx   A small expanded duct located at the apex of the renal pyramid. Note that there are *minor* and *major calyces.*

Cancerous disease   Disease characterized by the uncontrollable growth of abnormal cells that invade surrounding tissue and metastasize. Cancer is not contagious, but it can spread internally.

Capillaries   Blood vessels with thin, permeable membranes.

Capillary exchange   The process by which nutrients and oxygen are provided to tissues and waste from cells is removed.

Carbohydrates   Also known as starches and sugars, carbohydrates are classified according to molecular structure as mono-, di-, and polysaccharides.

Carbon monoxide poisoning   A toxic, often lethal condition that is caused by the absorption of carbon monoxide through inhalation.

Carcinogen   Cancer-causing agent.

Cardiac arrest   The sudden and complete cessation of the heartbeat, stopping all cardiac output, including pulmonary and systemic circulation.

Cardiac cycle   The cycle of events occurring with each alternating contraction and relaxation of the heart muscle, coordinated by the conducting system.

Cardioesophageal sphincter The superior sphincter, found at the junction between the esophagus and the stomach.

Carpal Pertaining to the wrist.

Carpal tunnel syndrome A painful repetitive strain injury of the hand and wrist caused by compression of the median nerve.

Cartilage An avascular, tough, protective tissue capable of withstanding repeated stress. Cartilage is the slowest tissue to heal because it has no direct blood supply.

Cauda equina The ends of the spinal cord, which fan out like a horse's tail.

Caudal (inferior) Situated below or toward the tail end.

Cecum The first section of the colon that is a small saclike structure located in the right lower quadrant of the abdomen.

Cell The fundamental unit of all living organisms and the simplest form of life that can exist as an independent self-sustaining unit. Cells are the building blocks of the human body.

Cell body (cyton) Part of the neuron that contains the nucleus and other standard equipment (i.e., organelles) of the cell.

Cell membrane Separates the cytoplasm from the surrounding external environment.

Central (deep) Pertaining to or situated at a center of the body.

Central nervous system Part of the nervous system that occupies a central or medial position in the body. It is primarily concerned with interpreting incoming sensory information and with issuing instructions in the form of motor response. The major components of the central nervous system include the brain (cerebrum, cerebellum, diencephalon, brain stem), meninges, cerebrospinal fluid, and spinal cord.

Centripetally Toward the center.

Cephalic (superior, cranial) Situated above or toward the head.

Cerebellar cortex The thin outer layer of the cerebellum.

Cerebellum A cauliflower-shaped structure located posterior and inferior to the cerebrum. The cerebellum is concerned with muscle tone, coordinates skeletal muscles and balance (posture integration and equilibrium), and controls fine and gross motor movements.

Cerebral cortex A thin gray layer covering the outer portion of the cerebrum.

Cerebral palsy A group of motor disorders resulting in muscular incoordination and loss of muscle control.

Cerebrospinal fluid A clear, colorless fluid circulating around the brain and spinal cord; it func-

tions as a shock absorber and provides a medium for nutrient exchange and waste removal.

Cerebrum The largest part of the brain that governs all higher functions (i.e., language, memory, reasoning, and some aspects of personality).

Cervical Pertaining to the neck area.

Cervical nodes Lymph nodes located at the cervical region.

Chemoreceptor Sensory receptor activated by chemical stimuli that detect smells, tastes, and chemistry changes in the blood.

Chen-chiu ta-ch'eng Sixteenth-century Chinese work, written by Yang Chi-chou, that contains a discussion about pediatric massage.

Chief cell Another type of exocrine cell in the stomach that produces the gastric enzyme pepsinogen, which is a precursor of pepsin.

Chronic Refers to conditions that have a long duration—in some cases a lifetime.

Chronic fatigue syndrome A condition characterized by the onset of disabling fatigue, sometimes due to a viral infection.

Chronic illness A condition of the body for which there is no known cure.

Chyme A thin viscous fluid that is formed as food is blended with digestive enzymes.

Cicatricial A scar with considerable contraction due to the way it healed naturally (e.g., a burn scar) or the way it was sutured.

Cilia Projections on the outer surfaces of certain cells that can produce movement of particles or fluids.

Circumduction Occurs when the distal end moves in a circle and the proximal end is relatively fixed; it can be described as cone-shaped range of motion but is actually a combination of several movements such as flexion, extension, adduction, and abduction.

Cirrhosis A chronic degenerative disease of the liver in which the hepatic cells are destroyed and replaced with fibrous connective tissue, giving the liver a yellow-orange color.

Client abuse Physical or emotional harm sustained by the client due to *deliberate* acts of the therapist. An abusive therapist is one who makes a conscious decision to take advantage of a client physically, sexually, financially, or emotionally.

Client neglect Physical or emotional harm sustained by the client due to lack of knowledge or insensitivity on the therapist's behalf.

Coagulation The ability of blood to clot.

Cochlea A coiled, fluid-filled cavity of the inner ear.

Coccygeal Inferior region of the spine.

Code of ethics A set of guiding moral principles that governs one's course of action.

Colitis An inflammation of the mucosa of the large intestine and rectum characterized by weight loss, intestinal ulcerations, diarrhea, and bleeding of the colon wall.

Colon The final path of intestines undigested and unabsorbed food takes before it is eliminated by the body.

Compress In hydrotherapy, a wet cloth that has had the water wrung from it and is applied to the skin's surface.

Concentric contraction A type of isotonic contraction occurring as the muscle shortens, pulling on a bone to produce movement.

Conduction The exchange of thermal energy while the body's surface is in direct contact with the thermal agent or conductor (e.g., hot packs, immersion baths).

Cone Photoreceptor of color vision. Cones have short, blunt projections.

Confidentiality The nondisclosure of privileged information; that is, it may not be divulged to a third party without the client's permission.

Congestive heart failure In congestive heart failure the heart is a failing pump. Causes include coronary artery disease, long-term hypertension, and myocardial infarct (areas of dead heart tissue from a previous heart attack).

Connective tissue The most abundant and ubiquitous tissue of the body. Some connective tissue types serve as nutrient transport systems, some defend the body against disease, some possess clotting mechanisms, and some act as a supportive framework and provide protection for vital organs.

Constipation Infrequent or difficult passing of stools.

Contamination A process that occurs when an infectious, or causative, agent enters an organism (e.g., airborne, fluid-borne, direct contact). Once the organism is contaminated, the next phase is infection.

Continuity In massage, it is the uninterrupted flow of strokes and to the unbroken transition from one stroke to the next.

Contracture An abnormal, usually permanent condition of a joint in which it is fixed in a flexed position.

Contraindications Conditions in which massage is not indicated. Types are *absolute* and *local contraindications*.

Contralateral Related to opposite sides of the body.

Contrast method In hydrotherapy, the combined use of cold and heat.

Convection Transference of heat energy through circulating currents of liquid or gas (e.g., sauna, steam bath).

Conversion One energy source changing into a heat energy source as it passes into the body.

Corns Thickened cone-shaped skin resulting from repeated friction or pressure. Corns occur primarily over toe joints and between the toes.

Coronary artery disease In coronary artery disease the coronary arteries are narrowed so that there is a reduced blood flow to the heart. The three main causes are atherosclerosis, coronary artery spasm, and blood clots.

Corpus callosum Large fibrous bundles of transverse fibers that provide a communicative pathway for impulses to move from one hemisphere to another.

Corpus Hippocraticum Collection of ancient Greek works that summarized much that was known about disease and medicine in the ancient world. Compiled by Hippocrates and his followers.

Cortisol Adrenal hormone that affects carbohydrate, protein, and fat metabolism and when needed produces an antiinflammatory response.

Costal Referring to the ribs.

Coulter, John S. American physician who, in 1926, became the first full-time academic physician in the field of physical medicine, which became known as physiatry.

Countertransference An emotional reaction of the therapist that reflects the therapist's own inner needs and conflicts; a reaction to the client's behavior of transference.

Coxal Regarding the hip region.

Cranial nerves Nerves exiting the brain.

Cranial (superior, cephalic) Situated above or toward the head.

Craniosacral outflow (parasympathetic nervous system) An anabolic system that conserves the body's energy resources.

Crepitus A noise produced by the body.

Cretinism A congenital deficiency of the thyroid hormones characterized by a lack of physical and mental development.

Crohn's disease A progressive inflammatory disease of the colon and/or ileum.

Cross-contamination The passing of microorganisms from one person to another.

Crural Regarding the entire leg.

Cryokinetics The application of cryotherapy followed by full range of motion of the affected area.

Cryotherapy The external, therapeutic application of cold.

Cubital Pertains to the elbow.

Cushing's disease Classified as a metabolic disorder caused by an overproduction of adrenocortical steroids.

Cyanosis The presentation of bluish or dark purplish skin due to reduced blood flow, oxygen deficiency, and an increase in carbon dioxide.

Cystic fibrosis A genetic disorder involving the overproduction of all exocrine glands, especially the pancreas, and the mucosa of the respiratory system.

Cystitis An inflammation of the urinary bladder and/or ureters caused by a bacterial infection from a neighboring organ such as the kidney, prostate, or urethra.

Cytoplasm The gel-like intracellular fluid within the boundaries of the cell membrane.

Dantein An ancient Chinese "center of gravity"; a topographical/meditative point of reference and the center of physical and spiritual balance.

Davis' law If muscle ends are brought closer together, then the pull of tonus is increased, thereby shortening the muscle, which may even cause hypertrophy. If muscle ends are separated beyond normal, then tonus is lessened or lost, thereby weakening the muscle.

De Arte Gymnastica Work written by Girolamo Mercuriale (1569) that is considered to be the first book written in the field of sports medicine.

Deep (central) Pertaining to or situated at a center of the body.

De Humani Corporis Fabrica Written by Andreas Vesalius in 1543, the work is considered one of the most important studies in the history of medicine.

De Medicina Medical text written by Aulus Celsus that bridged the gap between the Roman medical writers and the earlier Greek *Corpus Hippocraticum*.

Decoction A liquid, such as a tea, made from boiling plant products, usually bark, roots, or seeds.

Decompression sickness (bends) The unusual absorption of nitrogen, carbon dioxide, and oxygen in the body's tissues that impairs normal tissue oxygenation.

Decubitus ulcers Ulcers caused by constant deficiency of blood to tissues that have been subjected to prolonged pressure.

Defecation The process of eliminating indigestible or unabsorbed material from the body.

Deficiency disease Caused by a lack of an essential vitamin or nutrient. Typically interferes with the body's growth and development or helps to establish metabolic diseases. Examples include *scurvy* (deficiency of ascorbic acid or vitamin C), *rickets* (deficiency of vitamin D), and *beriberi* (deficiency of thiamine, or vitamin B_1).

Deglutition Swallowing.

Deltoid Curve of the shoulder and upper arm formed by the large deltoid muscle.

Dendrite Typically short, narrow, and highly branched neural extensions that receive and transmit stimuli toward the cell body.

Dense connective tissue Densely packed, strong collagenous fibers with fewer cells than loose connective tissue.

Dense irregular connective tissue Possesses collagen fibers that are ordinarily irregularly arranged. It can resist pulling forces in several directions.

Dense regular connective tissue Possesses bundles of collagen fibers in an orderly parallel arrangement that gives great strength and can resist pulling forces in two directions.

Depression Lowering or dropping a body part.

Depth In massage, the distance traveled into the body's tissues achieved through pressure application.

Dermatome An area of skin that a specific sensory nerve root serves.

Dermis Region of skin under the epidermis containing adipose tissue, many blood vessels, and nerve endings.

Diabetes A family of metabolic disorders that alter the fluid balance of the body, characterized by *polyuria*, an excessive excretion of urine, and *polydipsia*, or excessive thirst.

Diabetes insipidus Caused by a posterior pituitary gland dysfunction that results in deficient production of antidiuretic hormone.

Diabetes mellitus A group of disorders that lead to elevated blood glucose levels (hyperglycemia).

Diagnosis Identifying a disease or illness by scientific evaluation from a qualified health care practitioner.

Diaphysis The shaft of a long bone.

Diarrhea Frequent passing of unformed, loose, watery stools.

Diarthrotic joints Also known as *synovial joints*, these are freely movable joints, allowing movement in one, two, or three dimensions.

Diastole The static pressure against the arterial wall during the rest or pause phase between ventricular contractions.

Diencephalon Located approximately in the center of the brain; houses two primary structures: *thalamus* and *hypothalamus*.

Diffusion The movement of molecules, or other particles, from an area of high concentration to a area of low concentration.

Digestion The mechanical and chemical processes that occur as food is mixed with digestive enzymes and converted into an absorbable state.

Digital Pertaining to digits; fingers or toes.

Disassociation A coping mechanism to deal with traumatic events in which the person "leaves the body," does not feel, or believes that the abuse is happening to someone else.

Disinfection The process of removal of pathogenic microorganisms or their toxins from surfaces by chemical or mechanical agents.

Dislocation Occurs when bones are forced out of their normal position in the joint cavity.

Distal Farther from the point of reference, usually away from the midline.

Diuretic Any substance that promotes the formation and excretion of urine.

Diverticulosis Pouchlike herniations of the colon wall where the muscle has become weak.

Dorsal cavity Located on the back, or posterior, aspect of the body; it is further divided into the cranial cavity (containing the brain) and the spinal, or vertebral, cavity (containing the spinal cord).

Dorsal (posterior) Pertaining more to the back of a structure.

Dorsiflexion Flexing the foot dorsally so that the toes are moving toward the shin.

Dorsum Regarding the top of the foot.

Draping Covering the body with cloth.

Duodenum The first section in the small intestine. It is between 10 and 12 inches long.

Dura mater The outermost meningeal layer, which is thick, durable, and lies up against the bone.

Eccentric contraction A type of isotonic contraction when the muscle lengthens during a contraction.

Ectoderm The outermost of the three cell layers that gives rise to the structures of the nervous system, the mucosa of the mouth and anus, and the epidermal tissues.

Eczema An acute or chronic superficial inflammation characterized by redness, watery discharge, crusting, scaling, itching, and burning.

Effleurage The application of unbroken gliding movements that are repeated and follow the contour of the client's body.

Eicosanoids Also called *local* or *tissue hormones,* eicosanoids are produced by almost every cell in the body. They work on the cells that produce them or on nearby cells.

Eight Principles According to traditional Chinese medicine, these are Yin/Yang (general principles used to categorize diseases), Cold/Hot (the thermal quality of the disease), Interior/Exterior (the location and process of the disease), and Empty/Full (the conditions of the body's protective systems and the causes of disease in the body).

Elastic cartilage Cartilage that is soft and more pliable than hyaline or fibrocartilage and gives shape to the external nose and ears and to internal structures, such as the epiglottis and the auditory tubes.

Elastic connective tissue Has an abundance of elastic fibers. It can be stretched and restored to its natural shape. It is found in ligaments connecting adjacent vertebrae, in the trachea, and in the bronchi.

Electrocardiogram A graphic tracing of the variations in electrical potential caused by the excitation of the heart muscle and detected at the body surface.

Elevation Raising or lifting a body part.

Ellipsoidal joints Also referred to as *biaxial joints,* ellipsoidal joints are essentially a reduced ball-and-socket joint. Ellipsoidal joints allow flexion, extension, abduction, and adduction, but rotation is not permitted (e.g., radiocarpal joints).

Embolus A blood clot, bubble of air, or any piece of debris transported by the bloodstream.

Emphysema Destruction of the alveoli, producing abnormally large air spaces that remain filled with air during expiration.

Encephalitis Inflammation of the brain typically transmitted by the bite of an infected mosquito.

Endangerment site Area on the body containing superficial delicate anatomical structures that are unprotected by bone or muscle and are therefore prone to injury.

Endocardium The thin, inner lining of the heart that is continuous with the endothelial lining of the heart chambers and blood vessels, as well as with the valves of the heart.

Endocrine glands Glands with cells that produce secretions called *hormones* that diffuse directly into the bloodstream. Also known as "ductless glands." The bloodstream carries the hormones to the sites of action.

Endocytosis A process that moves large particles across the cell membrane into the cell. The two main types of endocytosis are *phagocytosis* and *pinocytosis.*

Endoderm The innermost cell layer that gives rise to the lining of the alimentary canal, lining of the respiratory passages, and all tissues of the organs and glands.

Endomysium The protective covering that encloses each muscle fiber.

Endoneurium The connective tissue covering that surrounds each nerve fiber.

Endoplasmic reticulum A complex network of membranous channels within the cytoplasm.

Enzyme A catalyst that accelerates chemical reactions.

Epicardium The thin outer layer of serous membrane surrounding the heart. This protective layer possesses adipose tissue and the blood vessels that nourish the heart.

Epidermis The superficial region of the skin that consists of four or five layers. Composed solely of epithelial tissue, the epidermis is relatively avascular. Oxygen and all nutrients reach the epidermal cells by diffusion of tissue fluids from the underlying dermis.

Epiglottis　One of the single laryngeal cartilages that closes the trachea during swallowing, preventing food from entering the inferior respiratory passageways.

Epilepsy　The presence of abnormal and irregular discharges of cerebral electrical activity.

Epimysium　The tough and thick fascial layer that wraps the entire muscle.

Epinephrine (adrenaline)　An adrenal hormone that increases blood pressure by stimulating vasoconstriction rather than by affecting cardiac output.

Epineurium　Connective tissue wrapping around nerves.

Epiphyseal plate　A flat plate of hyaline cartilage between the diaphysis and epiphysis of growing bones.

Epiphysis　The ends of a long bone.

Epithelial tissue　Tissue that lines or covers the internal and the external organs of the body; lines blood vessels and body cavities; and lines the digestive, respiratory, urinary, and reproductive tracts. The functions of this tissue include protection, absorption, filtration, secretion, excretion, and diffusion.

Eponychium (cuticle)　The tough ridge of epidermis that grows out over the nail from the proximal nail fold.

Erb's palsy　Often caused by birth injury to the upper brachial plexus, causing paralysis in the arm.

Ergonomics　The scientific study of anatomy, physiology, and psychology relating to humans' work; adjusting the environment and equipment to support the alignment and balance of the body in its activities.

Erythrocytes　Red blood cells, or red corpuscles.

Esophagus　The muscular tube that connects the pharynx to the stomach. The esophageal lining secretes mucus to aid in the transport of food.

Estrogen　Promotes the development of secondary sex characteristics in females. It is also known as the "feminizing" hormone because it is responsible for female secondary sex characteristics. During the menstrual cycle, estrogen triggers the preparation of the female genital tract for fertilization and implantation of the early embryo and helps keep calcium in bones.

Eversion　Elevation of the lateral edge of the foot so that the sole is turned outward.

Exhalation　See expiration.

Exocrine glands　Glands containing cells that produce glandular secretions and use ducts to transport their products to the site of action.

Expiration (exhalation)　A process that occurs when the diaphragm relaxes and ascends back up toward the thoracic cavity. Air is forced out of the lungs.

Extension　Straightening or increasing the angle of a joint. *Hyperextension* is a continuation of extension beyond the anatomical position, as in bending the head backward, and may or may not be used by some textbook authors.

External　Nearest the outside of a body cavity.

External (pulmonary) respiration　Gas exchange in the lungs between blood and air in the alveoli that came from the external environment.

Exteroceptors　Sensory nerve endings located in the skin, mucous membranes, and sense organs, responding to stimuli originating from outside of the body, such as touch, pressure, or sound.

Facial　Regarding the face.

Fascia　Connective tissue that varies in thickness and density; types are superficial *fascia* and *deep fascia*.

Fasciculi　Bundles of muscle fibers bound by perimysium.

Fast twitch A (pink muscle)　Type of fatigue-resistant fiber that is intermediate in diameter. It contains large amounts of myoglobin, many mitochondria, and numerous capillaries but breaks down ATP quickly.

Fast twitch B (white muscle)　Rapidly fatigable fibers. They possess the largest diameter and have the smallest amount of myoglobin, few mitochondria, and few capillaries.

Fats　Fats are composed of lipids or fatty acids and can range in consistency from a solid to a liquid.

Femoral　Pertaining to the femur or the thigh area; area between the hip and the knee.

Fibrinogen　One of the solutes in plasma that functions in blood clotting. When necessary, fibrinogen is converted to an insoluble fibrin, forming the foundations of a blood clot.

Fibrocartilage　It has the greatest tensile strength of all cartilage types. Fibrocartilage is found in the intervertebral disks, in the meniscus of the knee joint, and between the pubic bones (pubic symphysis).

Fibromyalgia　A chronic inflammatory disease that affects muscle and related connective tissues.

Fibrosis　A process in which the original tissue type is replaced with a different kind of tissue. Fibrosis occurs when the damage is so severe that there are not enough healthy cells to reproduce the tissue required or when the damaged tissue does not have the ability to readily reproduce itself. The scar tissue formed by fibrosis is usually stronger than the original tissue.

Filtrate　The term used to refer to filtered fluids once they have crossed from the glomerulus into the glomerular capsule.

Filtration   The movement of particles across the cellular membrane due to pressure.

Filum terminale   The threadlike lower end of the spinal cord.

Five Elements   In oriental medicine, the ingredients necessary for life, which are water, wood, fire, earth, and metal.

Fixators (stabilizers)   Specialized synergists that stabilize the joint over which the prime mover exerts its action. This allows the prime mover to perform a motion more efficiently.

Flaccid   Muscles lacking normal tone that appear flattened rather than rounded.

Flexion   Bending or decreasing the angle of a joint. *Lateral flexion* refers to the direction of flexion.

Follicle-stimulating hormone   Stimulates oogenesis, or egg development, in the ovaries. It also stimulates estrogen production by the ovaries. In men, follicle-stimulating hormone stimulates sperm production, or spermatogenesis, in the testes.

Fomite   An inanimate object.

Four Examinations   According to traditional Chinese medicine, these include looking, listening/smelling, asking, and palpating.

Fracture   A fracture is a break, chip, crack, or rupture in a bone.

Free nail edge   The most distal portion of the nail; what we trim because of nail growth.

Free nerve endings (nociceptors)   Bare nerve endings that detect pain.

Friction   In massage, compressing tissues in several directions.

Friction(s)   In hydrotherapy, frictions encompass shampoos, brushing, polishes, scrubs, glows, and frictions with the hands, a cloth, a brush, a sponge, or grainy agent rubbed on the skin's surface. A rinse and a quick, vigorous drying are essential elements.

Frontal   Regarding the forehead

Frontal (coronal) plane   The plane passing through the body from side to side to create anterior (ventral) and posterior (dorsal) sections.

Fu   The Yang organs, according to traditional Chinese medicine.

Fungus   A microorganism that requires an external carbon source; multicellular fungi reproduce by spore formation. Fungal agents include molds and yeast, and their growth is promoted by warm, moist environments. Only a few fungal varieties are pathogenic.

Furuncle   A boil or an abscess caused by the staphylococcal bacteria resulting in necrosis (death) of a hair follicle.

G cells   Endocrine glands located in the gastric mucosa that secrete the hormone *gastrin,* which initiates the production and secretion of gastric juice and stimulates bile and pancreatic enzyme emission into the small intestines.

Gait   A person's walking pattern.

Galen of Pergamon (c. 130-200)   Roman physician who synthesized and unified Greek medical knowledge. His works dominated Western medicine for over 1500 years.

Gallbladder   A pear-shaped sac located in a depression on the inferior surface of the liver that stores bile manufactured by the liver.

Gallstones   The result from the fusion of cholesterol crystals in bile.

Ganglion   A cluster of nerve cell bodies located in the peripheral nervous system.

Gastroesophageal reflex disease (GERD)   Failure of the cardioesophageal sphincter to close normally after food has entered the stomach.

Genetic disease   Caused by an imperfect genetic code in the chromosomes (structures found in the nucleus of every cell of the body). Examples of genetic diseases are Down syndrome, cystic fibrosis, sickle cell anemia, and hemophilia. These genetic disorders are not contagious, but may be passed down from generation to generation.

Geriatric   Refers to clients who are 70 years of age and older.

Gestational diabetes mellitus   May occur in women in the second and third trimesters of pregnancy. Hormones secreted by the placenta disturb the function of insulin, causing expectant mothers to become glucose intolerant.

Gliding joints   Also referred to as *triaxial joints,* these joints permit movements limited to gliding in flexion, extension, abduction, and adduction (e.g., intercarpal and intertarsal joints).

Glomerular capsule   The section of the nephron where urine formation begins.

Glomerulonephritis   Also known as *Bright's disease,* glomerulonephritis is an inflammation of the glomeruli and is often characterized by blood in the urine, edema, and hypertension.

Glomerulus   Loops of minute blood vessels contained within the glomerular capsule.

Glucagon   Secreted by the alpha cells of the pancreatic islets of Langerhans, glucagon increases blood glucose levels, producing hyperglycemic effects.

Gluteal   Curve of the buttocks formed by the large gluteal muscles.

Goblet cells   Cells that produce mucus in the nasal cavity, which moistens the air and traps incoming foreign particles.

Goiter   An enlarged thyroid gland associated with hyperthyroidism, hypothyroidism, inflammation, infection, or lack of iodine in the diet.

Golgi apparatus   A series of four to six horizontal membranous sacs typically located near the nucleus and attached to the endoplasmic reticulum for the purpose of altering proteins and lipids.

Golgi tendon organ Receptor that is stimulated by both tension and excessive stretch, located at the musculotendinous junction. This protective mechanism helps to ensure that muscles do not become excessively stretched or do not contract too strongly and damage their tendons.

Gout Characterized by high levels of uric acid in the blood due a high production or an inability of the kidneys to excrete this substance. When gout settles in the joints, it is called *gouty arthritis.*

Gouty arthritis A condition characterized by high levels of uric acid; gout settles in the joints.

Graham, Douglas O. American physician and Swedish massage practitioner who authored several works on the history of massage.

Graves' disease Caused by hyperthyroidism and characterized by related anxiety, fatigue, tremors of the hands, loss of appetite, and increased metabolic rate. An enlarged thyroid (goiter) and enlarged lymph nodes, as well as an unusual protrusion of the eyeballs, often accompany this condition.

Greater omentum A double-layered structure that attaches from the greater curvature of the stomach and the duodenum, draping down over the coils of the small intestine, to the transverse colon.

Groin (inguinal) Area where the thigh meets the abdomen.

Gustatory organ The chemoreceptor nestled in spherical pockets on the superior and lateral surfaces of the tongue that detect primary tastes of sweet, sour, bitter, and salty.

Gyri Elevations of the cerebral cortex.

Hair follicle Pouchlike depressions in the skin that enclose the hair shaft.

Hair-follicle receptors Nerve receptors that respond briefly to hair movement; also known as *hair root plexuses.*

Hara The Japanese ancient "center of gravity"; a topographical/meditative point of reference and the center of physical and spiritual balance.

Harvey, William (1578-1657) British anatomist who demonstrated that blood circulation in animals is caused by the beat of the heart.

Haustra A series of pouches created as "gathers" or "tucks" along the length of the colon.

Haversian canals Minute vascular canals found in osseous tissue that run longitudinally through the bone.

Heart A hollow organ, located in the mediastinal region of the thoracic cavity, that pumps blood.

Hemoglobin A red respiratory pigment in erythrocytes.

Hemophilia A genetically determined condition in which a clotting factor is missing in the blood, making it difficult or impossible for the blood to clot.

Hemopoiesis The formation of blood cells.

Hemorrhage Excessive bleeding, either internally (from blood vessels into tissues) or externally (from blood vessels directly to the surface of the body).

Hemorrhoids Hemorrhoids, or *piles,* are varicosities of the rectal veins.

Hepatic portal system A pathway of blood that starts and ends with veins; it collects blood and nutrients from the digestive organs (stomach, intestines, gallbladder, spleen, and pancreas), delivering them to the liver for storage.

Hepatitis Inflammation of the liver.

Hernia A protrusion of an organ or part of an organ through its surrounding connective tissue membranes or cavity wall.

Herniated disk Protrusion of the nucleus pulposus from the annulus fibrosus of an intervertebral disk.

Herpes simplex A viral infection that has the ability to lie dormant for extended periods without expressing any signs or symptoms of disease.

Hilton's law A nerve trunk that supplies a joint also supplies the muscles of the joint and the skin over the insertions of such muscles.

Hinge joints Also referred to as *monaxial joints,* movements are limited to flexion and extension (e.g., elbow, knee, and interphalangeal joints).

Hippocrates of Cos (c. 460-375 BC) Greek physician; generally considered the "father of modern Western medicine."

Histamine A compound, found in all cells, that is released in allergic, inflammatory reactions, causing dilation of capillaries, decreased blood pressure, and constriction of smooth muscles of the bronchi.

Hodgkin's disease Cancer of the lymph nodes.

Homeostasis A relatively stable condition of the body's internal environment within a very limited range.

Homolateral (ipsilateral) Related to the same side of the body.

Hormonal control system A system whereby hormones themselves can stimulate or inhibit the release of other hormones in the endocrine system.

Hormone Internal secretions that are the "chemical messengers" of the endocrine system. They act as catalysts in biochemical reactions and regulate the physiological activity of other cells in the body.

Human growth hormone (somatotropin) Pituitary hormone that stimulates protein synthesis for maintenance of muscle and bone growth. It also plays a role in metabolism.

Hunting response An up-and-down cycle of vasoconstriction and vasodilation that occurs if an initial ice application continues more than 9 to 16 minutes. One cycle of vasoconstriction and vasodilation may take from 15 to 30 minutes.

Hyaline cartilage An elastic, rubbery, smooth type of cartilage that covers the ends of bones (epiphysis), connects the ribs to the sternum (costal cartilage), is part of the larynx and the nose, and forms the C-shaped rings of the trachea.

Hydrotherapy The internal and external therapeutic use of water and complementary agents.

Hygiene The collective principles of health preservation.

Hyperemia The observable reddened and warmed skin that results from increased blood flow.

Hyperesthesia Increased hypersensitivity to touch often perceived as a painful sensation. The irritation to touch may be caused by emotional stress, chronic pain, shingles, or nerve compression.

Hypertension A common, often asymptomatic disorder of elevated blood pressure; 140/90 mmHg is regarded as the threshold of hypertension, and 160/95 is classified as serious hypertension.

Hyperthyroidism Condition characterized by an enlarged thyroid, nervousness and tremor, heat intolerance, increased appetite with weight loss, rapid forceful pulse, and increased respiration rate.

Hypertrophy An increase in the size and diameter of muscle fibers without cell division.

Hypodermis (subcutaneous layer, superficial fascia) A layer of tissue under the dermis.

Hypoglycemia An excessive loss in blood glucose levels that can result in a variety of symptoms including weakness, lightheadedness, headaches, excessive hunger, visual disturbances, anxiety, and sudden changes in personality.

Hypothalamus Governs many important homeostatic functions such as regulating the autonomic nervous and the endocrine systems by governing the pituitary gland, which controlls hunger, thirst, temperature, anger, aggression, release of hormones, sexual behavior, sleep patterns, and consciousness.

Hypothyroidism A deficiency of thyroid activity, hypothyroidism is marked by fatigue and lethargy; weight gain; slowed mental processes; skin dryness and slow digestive, heart, and respiration rates. More common in women, this condition may lead to cretinism.

Hypoxia A decrease in the amount of oxygen in the blood.

Ice massage The use of ice with circular friction.

Ileocecal sphincter (valve) Sphincter located between the ileum of the small intestine and the cecum of the large intestine.

Ileum The final division of the small intestine; it is approximately 9 feet long.

Immunity An anatomical and physiological defense reaction to invading microorganisms.

Impetigo An inflammatory skin infection caused by staphylococcal or streptococcal bacteria.

Infectious disease Highly contagious diseases caused by a biological agent, such as a virus or a bacterium. Examples are pneumonia, measles, and tuberculosis.

Inferior (caudal) Situated below or toward the tail end.

Inflammation The body's reaction to soft-tissue injury. Inflammation is a protective mechanism, and its purpose is to stabilize and prepare the damaged tissue for repair. The primary symptoms of inflammation are local heat, swelling, redness, pain, and decreased function or range of motion.

Informed consent Client's authorization for professional services based on adequate information provided by the attending therapist. This information includes modalities used, expectations, potential benefits, possible undesirable effects, and professional and ethical responsibility.

Infusion A liquid, usually a tea, made from steeping plant products, typically stems and leaves.

Ingestion The process of orally taking materials into the body.

Inguinal nodes Lymph nodes located in the inguinal region.

Inhalation See inspiration.

Insertion The insertion, usually located laterally or distally, is the muscle attachment located on the more movable bone and undergoing the greatest movement.

Inspiration (inhalation) The flow of air into the lungs that occurs when the diaphragm contracts and descends into the abdominal cavity and when the external intercostal muscles contract to raise the ribs.

Insulin Secreted by pancreatic beta cells, insulin decreases blood glucose levels by enhancing the uptake of glucose into the cells.

Integrity The condition of being whole and undivided; the firm adherence to a code of moral or artistic values.

Intention A consciously sought out goal or a desired end based on a plan of action.

Internal Nearer the inside of a body cavity; within.

Internal (tissue) respiration The gas exchange between blood and the body's tissues.

Interneurons (association neurons) These neurons connect sensory neurons to motor neurons.

Interoceptors Receptors located in the viscera that respond to stimuli originating from within the body regarding the function of the internal organs, such as digestion, excretion, and blood pressure.

Interosseous ligament (membrane)   A tough membrane that interconnects select bones (e.g., ulna and radius) by attaching to their periosteum.

Interstitial cells of Leydig   Within the testis these groups of specialized cells produce and secrete androgens, namely testosterone.

Intimacy   A sensual bond to another in which choice, mutuality, reciprocity, trust, and delight exist.

Inversion   Elevation of the medial edge of the foot so that the sole is turned inward.

Ipsilateral (homolateral)   Related to the same side of the body.

Irritable bowel syndrome   A condition of the large intestine characterized by abnormal muscular contraction and excessive mucus in stools.

Ischemia   A reduction of oxygenated blood to a body organ or part, often marked by pain and tissue dysfunction.

Ischemic compression   Sustained digital pressure applied to trigger and tender points to relieve pain and discomfort.

Islets of Langerhans (pancreatic islets)   Groups of specialized cells within the pancreas. The pancreas contains over 1 million islets, each consisting of alpha cells and beta cells.

Isometric contractions   Contractions in which the muscle increases in tension but does not change its length or the angle of the joint.

Isotonic contractions   Contractions in which the muscle changes length against resistance and movement occurs.

Jejunum   The intermediate portion of the small intestine that joins the duodenum with the ileum; it is approximately 6 feet long.

Joint capsule   A sleevelike continuation of the periosteum of the bones involved in the joint.

Joint cavity   The enclosed space between the bones of the joint filled with synovial fluid.

Joint mobilization   Moving a joint through its normal range of motion.

Jump sign   A spontaneous reaction of pain or discomfort that may cause a client to wince, jump, or verbalize upon application of pressure.

Juxtaglomerular apparatus   A mechanism monitoring blood pressure consisting of two specialized groups of cells: the *macula densa* and *juxtaglomerular cells*.

Kellogg, John Harvey (1852-1943)   American popularizer of health concerns. Kellogg wrote numerous articles and books on massage that brought the issue to the general populace.

Keloid   A hypertrophic scar usually containing blood vessels; it is often smooth and either red or pink in color.

Keratin   A cordlike protein that provides protection by waterproofing the skin's surface (it is insoluble in water).

Ki (Qi)   Japanese term used to describe the concept of energy.

Kidneys   Paired organs located bilaterally in the upper lumbar region of the spine. They are bean-shaped, (convex laterally and concave medially, like a kidney bean) and are slightly smaller than a fist.

Kinesiology   The study of human motion.

Krause end bulbs   Although the operating mechanism of Krause end bulbs is not exactly known, they are believed to be stimulated by lowering temperatures.

Kupffer's cells   Phagocytic cells that line the sinusoids of the liver and filter bacteria and other foreign material out of the blood before sending it through the hepatic vein.

Kyphosis   Often called *hunchback* or *hyperkyphosis*, kyphosis is an exaggeration of the normal posterior thoracic curve.

Lacteals   The lymph capillaries in the villi of the small intestines that assist in the absorption of fat.

Large intestine (colon)   The final path undigested and unabsorbed food takes before it is eliminated by the body.

Laryngitis   Inflammation of the larynx that often results in loss of voice, commonly caused by respiratory infections or irritants such as cigarette smoke.

Larynx   Formed by three single and three paired pieces of cartilage; voicebox.

Latent trigger points   Identical to active trigger points with one important exception: they do not hurt all the time. Latent trigger points remain hidden until activated by some stressor such as physical activity, emotional stress, or direct pressure, and then they are elevated to active status.

Lateral   Oriented farther away from the midline of the body.

Lateral nail folds   The sides of the nail where they meet the skin.

Law of facilitation   When an impulse has passed once through a certain set of neurons to the exclusion of others, it will tend to take the same course on future occasions, and each time it traverses this path the resistance will be less.

Lesion   Any noticeable or measurable deviation from the normal composition of a healthy tissue. Examples of lesions include a mole, a wart, or a break in the skin.

Lesser omentum   A fatty, membranous extension of the peritoneum that attaches from the right side of the stomach and first section of the duodenum to the liver.

Leukemia   Also called "cancer of the blood," leukemia is a cancer of white blood cells.

Leukocytes   White blood cells or white corpuscles.

Lice   Parasitic insects that are highly contagious. Lice are diagnosed with the presence of egg sacs on the hair shaft.

Ligament   Connective tissue that connects bone to bone. Functionally, ligaments are an extension of the bone to allow lightness, flexibility, and added strength.

Ling, Pehr Henrik (1776-1839)   Swedish physiologist and gymnastics instructor. Ling is considered the "father of Swedish massage." He developed his own system of medical gymnastics and exercise, known by several different names—the Ling System, Swedish Movements, and the Swedish Movement Cure. An important part of the Ling System was a particular style of massage, known today as Swedish massage.

Liquid connective tissue   Vascular tissue consisting of blood, lymph, or interstitial fluid.

Liver   The largest internal organ in the body, located in the upper right quadrant of the abdominal cavity.

Lobe   Region of the cerebrum named for the bone each lies beneath: the frontal, parietal, temporal, and occipital lobes.

Local contraindication   Condition in which massage can be administered while avoiding the infected area or area in question; local contraindications merit caution and adaptive measures to ensure that the massage is safely administered.

Local twitch response   An involuntary firing or twitching in a muscle (a reflex motor output) in response to the sensory stimulation (pressure) on a trigger point.

Loose connective tissue   Regarded as the packing material of the body, it attaches the skin to underlying structures, serves to wrap and support the body cells, fills in the spaces between structures (i.e., organs, muscles), and helps to keep them in their proper place.

Lordosis   Often regarded as hyperlordosis, lordosis, or *swayback,* is an exaggeration of the anterior curvature of the lumbar concavity.

Lucas-Championniere, Just (1843-1913)   French physician who advocated the use of massage and passive-motion exercises after certain injuries.

Lumbar   Pertaining to the low back between the ribs and the hips.

Lumen   The open space within a vessel.

Lungs   The spongy, highly elastic, paired organs of respiration.

Lunula   The whitish half-moon shape at the base of the nail.

Lupus   An autoimmune, inflammatory disease of connective tissue that occurs mostly in young women.

Luteinizing hormone   In women stimulates ovulation and the production of estrogen and progesterone by the ovaries; in men stimulates testosterone secretion by the testes.

Lyme disease   A recurrent form of arthritis caused by the bacterium *Borrelia burgdorferi,* which is transmitted via tick bite.

Lymph   The fluid of the lymph system.

Lymph capillaries   Lymph vessels that are larger, more irregular, and more permeable than blood vessels.

Lymph nodes   Bean-shaped structures located along lymph vessels that collect and filter lymph. These are powerful defense stations that help to protect the body from unwanted invaders.

Lymphatic trunks   Large vessels in the lymphatic system. These trunks join to form one of two lymphatic ducts.

Lymphedema   An accumulation of interstitial fluid (swelling) in the soft tissues due to local or general inflammation, obstruction, or removal of lymph vessels.

Lymphocyte   A type of white blood cell comprising about 25% of the total white blood cell count, increasing in number in response to infection. Two forms occur: B cells and T cells.

Lysosome   Membrane-bound organelle containing various digestive enzymes.

Macula   Special receptor in the wall of the inner ear that help determine orientation with respect to gravity. Each macula contains a membrane with groups of modified hair cells, or cilia, that are attached to sensory nerves.

Major duodenal papilla   A dilation that is formed by the juncture of the pancreatic and bile ducts as they open into the small intestines.

Malignant   A condition that worsens and causes death if not treated.

Malignant melanoma   Cancer of the melanocytes in the skin, which begins as a raised dark lesion with irregular borders and appears uneven in color.

Manav Dharma Shastra   Ancient Hindu work (c. 300 BC) that mentions the use of therapeutic massage.

Mandibular   Region of the lower jaw.

Massage   The systematic and scientific manipulation of the soft tissues of the body for the purpose of improving and maintaining health; it can also be defined as organized, intentional touch.

Mastication   Chewing.

Meatus   Creaselike passageways that subdivide the three nasal conchae.

Mechanical response   A physiological response of the body brought on by force or pressure; tissues being pulled, lifted, rubbed, compressed, and manipulated.

Mechanoreceptors   Sensory receptors that respond to mechanical stimuli and are located in the skin, ears, muscles, tendons, joints, and fascia. They detect sensations such as touch, pressure, blood pressure, vibration, stretching, muscular contraction, proprioception, sound, and equilibrium.

Media   Systems of mass communication.

Medial   Oriented more toward or near the midline of the body.

Mediastinal   A portion of the thoracic cavity occupying the area between the lungs.

Medulla oblongata   The most inferior portion of the brain stem that is often considered the most vital part of the brain; it contains the respiratory center, the cardiac center, and the vasomotor center. The medulla also controls gastric secretions and reflexes, such as sweating, sneezing, swallowing, and vomiting.

Medullary cavity   The hollow space in the bone's center containing the bone marrow.

Medullary pyramids   The bundles of renal tubules in the renal medulla. Each kidney, composed of 8 to 18 renal pyramids, contains many straight collecting tubules, which gives each pyramid a striated appearance.

Meissner corpuscle   Receptor for light touch, responding to both the actual movement and the length of the movement across the skin.

Melanin   Skin pigment that contributes to the color of the skin but is also found in the hair and in the iris of the eye. Melanin granules serve to protect the underlying cells from ultraviolet radiation.

Melanocyte-stimulating hormone   Stimulates the distribution of melanin granules, thereby increasing skin pigmentation.

Melatonin   A pineal hormone that may be involved in the control of circadian rhythms (occurring daily, such as sleeping and eating) and in the growth and development of sexual organs. When injected into the body, melatonin produces drowsiness.

Membrane   Thin, soft, pliable sheet of tissue that covers the body, lines tubes or body cavities, covers organs, and separates one part of a cavity from another.

Meninges   Special connective tissue membranes that envelop the entire central nervous system (brain and spinal cord); they contain three layers: the pia mater, the arachnoid, and the dura mater.

Meningitis   An infection or inflammation of the meninges often characterized by a sudden severe headache, vertigo, stiff neck, and severe irritability.

Mercuriale, Girolamo (1530-1606)   Italian Renaissance–era physician who synthesized ancient medical writings. He wrote *De Arte Gymnastica*, considered to be the first book written in the field of sports medicine.

Meridians   In traditional Chinese medicine, meridians (also called *channels* or *pathways*) are the conduits through which Qi flows.

Merkel disk   Receptor that responds to superficial pressure and skin displacement.

Mesentery   A large, fan-shaped section of the peritoneum, connecting the small intestine to the posterior abdominal wall.

Mesoderm   The midlayer of the three germ layers that becomes the muscles and connective tissues of the body, as well as vascular and lymphatic tissue.

Metabolic disease   Disease that involves abnormal activities of cells and/or tissues such as diabetes, cardiovascular conditions, and jaundice. Metabolic diseases are not contagious but may originate from a contagious disease such as hepatitis, which can lead to jaundice or vice versa.

Metabolism   The total of all the physical and chemical processes that occur in a given organism (i.e., those that are considered to be signs of life).

Metaphysis   In mature bone, this is where the diaphysis and the epiphysis meet.

Metastasis   The process of cancerous cells spreading to distant parts of the body, usually through the bloodstream or the lymphatic circulation.

Methodists   A group of ancient Greek physicians who supported a simplistic view of healing and generally restricted their treatments to bathing, diet, massage, and a few drugs.

Mezger, Johann (1839-1909)   Dutch physician who is generally given credit for making massage a fundamental component of physical rehabilitation. He is also credited for the introduction of French terminology into the massage profession.

Micturition (voiding)   Also known as urination, micturition is the act of emptying the bladder by passing urine out of the body through the urethra.

Midbrain   The most superior structure of the brain stem that houses voluntary motor tracts descending from the cerebral cortex to the spinal cord.

Midsagittal (median) plane   A plane that runs longitudinally, or vertically, down the body, anterior to posterior, dividing the organism into right and left sections. This plane creates a right lateral and a left lateral portion of the body.

Migraine headaches   Also called *vascular headaches*, migraines are caused by dilation of cranial blood vessels.

Minerals   Essential nonorganic compounds found in nature that are needed by the body to build bone, control muscle activity, support various organs, and transport oxygen and carbon dioxide in the body.

Mitochondrion   An oval-shaped organelle lying within the cytoplasm; considered the cell's "power plant" because it is a site for cellular respiration, which provides most of a cell's adenosine triphosphate supply.

Modality   A general term used to denote any technique, procedure, or product used to produce a positive response for the client.

Mole   A collection of melanocytes. Most moles are present a birth (often referred to as a birth mark) and some can become cancerous if visible changes occur.

Mononucleosis   An acute viral infection caused by the Epstein-Barr virus (EBV).

Motor end plate   An expansion at the end of some motor nerves.

Motor neurons   Neurons responsible for carrying messages of contraction (or in some cases, inhibiting contraction) to a muscle or gland.

Motor unit   A single motor neuron and all of its associated skeletal muscle fibers. A single muscle is composed of many motor units.

Mucosal associated lymphoid tissue (MALT)   Lymphoid cells in the mucosa or submucosa of the alimentary canal. These are tonsils, Peyer's patches, and the appendix.

Mucous membranes (mucosae)   Membranes that line openings to the outside of the body. This type of membrane is found in the respiratory, digestive, reproductive, and urinary tracts. Mucous membranes secrete a viscous, slippery fluid called mucus.

Multiarticular   Muscle crossing more than two joints.

Multidimensional relationships   Relationships that exist in addition to the therapeutic relationship.

Multiple sclerosis   The progressive destruction of myelin sheaths in the central nervous system.

Mumps   An acute viral disease caused by a Paramyxovirus (an airborne member of the herpes family).

Muscle cramp   See muscle spasm.

Muscle fatigue   The inability of a muscle to contract even though it is still being stimulated.

Muscle (neuromuscular) spindle   Stretch-sensitive receptor that wraps around intrafusal muscle fibers (striated muscle fiber within a muscle spindle) and monitors change in the length of a muscle and the rate of that change.

Muscle spasm   An increase in muscle tension with or without shortening due to excessive motor nerve activity.

Muscle strains   A pathological or traumatic discontinuity or tear of the muscle tissue.

Muscle tissue   Extremely elastic, muscle tissue is very vascular and has the unique ability to shorten (contract) and to elongate to produce movement.

Muscular dystrophy   A collection of genetically transmitted diseases, muscular dystrophy is characterized by the progressive atrophy of skeletal muscles without any indication of neural degeneration or damage.

Myasthenia gravis   A weakness in the muscles characterized by chronic fatigability.

Myelin sheath   A fatty material around most axons that electrically insulates the neuron and increases the speed of nerve impulse conduction.

Myocardial infarction   A heart attack followed by death (necrosis) of myocardial tissue due to an interrupted coronary blood supply.

Myocardium   The thick muscular layer that makes up the bulk of the heart wall.

Myofascial   The skeletal muscles and related fascia.

Myofascial release   Refers to a group of manual techniques used to reduce fascial restrictions.

Myofilaments   Bundles of smaller structures called actin and myosin that comprise a myofibril.

Myoglobin   A chemical similar to the hemoglobin molecule present in red blood cells.

Myosin   The thicker myofilament.

Myosin heads   Ball-like structures on myosin filaments.

Nail bed   The skin beneath the nail; it appears through the clear nail, oftentimes as a series of longitudinal ridges.

Nail body   The main visible part of the nail.

Nail root   Where nail production takes place.

Nails   The thin hard plates found on the distal surfaces of the fingers and toes.

Nasal   Regarding the nose region.

Nasal conchae   The superior, middle, and inferior nasal conchae are the ridges that extend out of each lateral wall of the nasal cavity.

Natural immunity   Nonspecific responses to invading pathogens.

Necessary care   Care or therapy that is appropriate and relates to the client regaining function and the ability to perform activities of daily living.

Negative feedback system   A process of the endocrine system that triggers the negative, or opposite, response; this process may or may not involve the nervous system.

Nei Ching   Chinese medical text that serves as the classic on traditional Chinese medicine. The work contains descriptions of therapeutic touch procedures and their uses. Written sometime around 2600 BC.

Nephrogenic diabetes insipidus   Much the same as diabetes insipidus, except that the cause is kidney dysfunction, often a result of disease or damage.

Nephron   The basic filtering unit of the kidney responsible for filtering waste products from the blood.

Nerve A collection of impulse-carrying nerve fibers.

Nerve compression Also known as *nerve impingement,* nerve compression is similar to a nerve entrapment except that the pressure against the nerve is due to contact with hard tissues such as bone or cartilage.

Nerve entrapment Also known as *entrapment neuropathy,* nerve entrapment refers to dysfunction of a nerve as a result of pressure against it by adjacent soft tissues such as muscle, tendon, fascia, and ligaments.

Nervous tissue Oddly shaped cells that can pick up and transmit electrical signals by converting stimuli into nerve impulses. Located in the brain, spinal cord, and peripheral nerves, nervous tissue possesses characteristics of excitability and conductibility.

Neural control system Hormones secreted because of direct nerve stimulation.

Neuroglia (glial) cells Connective tissues that support, nourish, protect, insulate, and organize the neurons.

Neurology The study of the functions and disorders of the nervous system.

Neuromuscular junction A fluid-filled space between nerve endings and muscle fibers.

Neuron The basic nerve cell possessing two major properties: excitability and conductibility.

Neuropathy Decrease or change in sensation.

Neurotransmitters A collective term for a vast range of chemicals that facilitate, arouse, or inhibit the transmission of nerve impulses between synapses.

Nissen, Hartvig Prominent early practitioner of Swedish massage (created by Pehr Ling) in the United States. He helped popularize Ling's methods with his numerous publications.

Nociceptor Receptor for detecting pain.

Nodes of Ranvier Gaps located at certain intervals along an axon; during neural activity, impulses jump from one node to another, resulting in an increased rate of conduction.

Nonverbal communication Involves the transmission of messages by means other than the spoken word.

Norepinephrine (noradrenaline) Hormones that help the body to maintain the stress response. The effects of norepinephrine are increased heart rate, blood pressure, and blood glucose levels and dilation of the small passageways of the lungs.

Nuchal Regarding the posterior neck region.

Nucleus The largest organelle in the cytoplasm; the control center of the cell.

Obesity Abnormal increase in subcutaneous fat tissue, primarily in visceral regions of the body.

Objective data Information that is measurable and quantitative, such as the size and shape of a mole, whether the right shoulder is higher than the left, or if the left knee is swollen (larger) and by how many centimeters more than the right.

Occipital Posterior inferior surface of the head.

Olfaction Refers to the sense of smell.

Oral Pertaining to the mouth.

Oral cavity Also known as the *mouth,* the oral cavity contains the tongue, teeth, gums, and openings from the salivary ducts. Digestion begins in the oral cavity.

Orbital (ophthalmic) Pertaining to the eye area.

Organelles Small cellular structures that provide special functions such as reproduction, storage, and metabolism. Types of organelles are the nucleus, ribosomes, endoplasmic reticulum, Golgi apparatus, mitochondria, and lysosomes.

Origin The tendinous attachment of the muscle on the less movable bone or attachment during the muscle's action.

Osmosis The movement of a pure solvent, such as water, from an area of low concentration (most dilute) to an area of high concentration (least dilute). This action continues until the two concentrations equalize.

Ossification The process by which bone develops.

Osteoarthritis Progressive erosion of articular cartilage due to chronic inflammation of the joints.

Osteoblasts Bone-forming cells found in the periosteum.

Osteoclasts Bone-destroying cells that help maintain homeostasis and repair bone.

Osteocytes Mature osteoblasts that soon become embedded in bone matrix.

Osteoporosis Decreased bone mass; this increases the susceptibility to fractures.

Otoliths Calcium carbonate particles floating above the macula of the ear that shift position as the body moves; when this occurs, the cilia are disturbed, which initiates a nerve impulse.

Outcome The client's response to therapy and progress toward short- or long-term goals.

Oval window The ear membrane that covers the opening of the cochlea.

Ovaries Functioning both as endocrine and exocrine glands, the ovaries are located in the abdominopelvic region of the female body.

Oxytocin Hormone involved in milk expression from the mammary glands and uterine muscular contraction.

Pacinian (laminated) corpuscle Pressure-sensitive receptor that responds to skin displacement and high-frequency vibration, adapting quickly to external stimuli.

Pack In the field of hydrotherapy, a pack is a bag, sack, or other item used to apply or retain heat or cold.

Palliative care Care or therapy that eases or reduces pain.

Palmar Refers to the anterior surface or palm of the hand.

Palpation Assessment through touching with purpose and intent.

Palsy An abnormal condition characterized by paralysis. The three most common forms are Bell's palsy, cerebral palsy, and Erb's palsy.

Pancreas Both an endocrine and an exocrine gland, the pancreas is a carrot-shaped organ located inferior and posterior to the greater curvature of the stomach.

Pancreatic islets (islets of Langerhans) Groups of specialized cells within the pancreas. The pancreas contains over 1 million islets, each consisting of both alpha and beta cells.

Pancreatitis An inflammation of the pancreas, usually the result of trauma, alcohol abuse, infection, or certain medications.

Papillae Projections on the tongue.

Papule A small, round, firm, elevated area in the skin, varying in size from a pinpoint to that of a small pea.

Paracelsus (1493-1541) Name by which Philippus Aureolus Theophrastus Bombastus von Hohenheim was generally known. Paracelsus was a Swiss physician and chemist who promoted chemically prepared medicines instead of herbal remedies.

Paraffin bath Dipped bath with a heated waxy mixture.

Paralysis Loss of muscle function and/or sensation.

Parasympathetic nervous system (craniosacral outflow) An anabolic system that conserves the body's energy resources.

Parathyroid glands Tiny glands, usually numbering four, located on the posterolateral surface of the thyroid lobes.

Parathyroid hormone Increases blood calcium levels by stimulating osteoclast (bone-destroying cells) activity and breaks down bone tissue. The liberated calcium is released in the bloodstream, and blood calcium levels increase. Parathyroid hormone also increases calcium reabsorption from urine and the intestines back into the blood.

Paré, Ambroise (c. 1510-1590) French military surgeon. In addition to inventing several surgical instruments, he was among the earliest modern physicians to discuss the therapeutic effects of massage, especially in orthopedic surgery cases.

Parietal cell One type of exocrine cell in the stomach. These cells produce intrinsic factor, a substance required for the absorption of vitamin B_{12} from the small intestine to the bloodstream. They also produce hydrochloric acid, a component of gastric juice, which breaks down protein and activates many gastric enzymes.

Parkinson's disease A progressive, degenerative neurological disorder marked by the destruction of certain areas of the brain (specifically, dopamine-producing neurons) and depletion of the neurotransmitter dopamine.

Passive movements Applied by the therapist while the client remains relaxed (or passive).

Patellar Region of the knee cap.

Pathogen A living biological agent capable of causing disease.

Paul of Aegina (625-690) Greek physician who was one of the most important medical men of his time and one of the last of the Greek compilers.

Pectoral Pertaining to the upper anterior thorax or chest area.

Pedal Referring to the foot.

Pediatric Young people between 3 and 18 years of age.

Pelvic Inferior region of the abdominopelvic cavity.

Peptide hormones Peptide, or protein, hormones are derivatives of amino acid chains. These hormones are water soluble. They attach to the cell membrane and introduce a series of chemical reactions to alter the cell's metabolism.

Pericarditis An inflammation of the parietal pericardium that may be due to trauma or infectious disease.

Pericardium The tissue layers surrounding the heart.

Perimysium A fascial layer within the muscle that binds together fasciculi.

Perineal Region between the anus and the genitals; inferior pelvic cavity.

Perineurium Connective tissue covering around each nerve fascicle.

Periosteum Fibrous, dense, vascular connective tissue sheath around the bone that penetrates the bone like nails, anchoring itself to the bone.

Peripheral nervous system Part of the nervous system composed of the nerves exiting the central nervous system.

Peripheral (superficial) Pertaining to the outside surface, periphery, or surrounding external area of a structure.

Peripheral vascular disease An abnormal condition that decreases circulation in the hands and feet; involves the flow of blood and lymph.

Peristalsis Wavelike involuntary contractions that mix and propel materials in the gastrointestinal tract.

Peritoneum The largest serous membrane in the body that envelops the entire abdominal wall. Sections of the peritoneum include the mesenteries, the parietal and visceral peritoneum, and the greater and lesser omentum.

Peritonitis An acute inflammation of the peritoneum produced by bacteria or irritating substances that gain access to the abdominal cavity.

Peritubular capillaries A second network of blood vessels branching off before the glomerulus that is interwoven with corresponding renal tubules.

Pétrissage A cycle of rhythmic lifting, squeezing, and releasing of tissue.

Peyer's patches Groups of lymphatic nodules found in the mucous membrane of the small intestine that combat pathogens ingested.

Pfluger's law of generalization When the irritation becomes very intense, it is propagated in the medulla oblongata, which becomes a focus from which stimuli radiate to all parts of the cord, causing a general increase of tonus in all muscles of the body.

Pfluger's law of intensity Reflex movements are usually more intense on the side of irritation; at times the movements of the opposite side equal them in intensity, but they are usually less pronounced.

Pfluger's law of radiation If the excitation continues to increase, it is propagated upward, and reactions take place through centrifugal nerves coming from the cord segments higher up.

Pfluger's law of symmetry If the stimulation is sufficiently increased, motor reaction is manifested, not only by the irritated side but also in similar muscles on the opposite side of the body.

Pfluger's law of unilaterality If a mild irritation is applied to one or more sensory nerves, the movement will take place usually on one side only, the side that is irritated.

Phagocytosis Phagocytosis, or "cell eating," is the process by which specialized cells engulf harmful microorganisms and cellular debris, break them down, and expel the harmless remains back into the body.

Pharynx Also called the throat, the pharynx is the tubular structure that transports food, liquid, and air to their respective destinations.

Phlebitis An inflammation of the veins, often accompanied by a thrombus (blood clot).

Photoreceptor Sensory receptor that is sensitive to light stimuli. There are two types: rods and cones.

Physiology The study of how the whole body and its individual parts function in normal body processes.

Physiopathological reflex arc An abnormal reflex arc caused by increased stimuli entering the spinal cord.

Pia mater The innermost meningeal layer, which is thin, vascular, and lies close to the brain.

Pineal gland The pineal gland, or epiphysis cerebri, is a pinecone-shaped structure in the brain, attached to the roof of the third ventricle and inferior to the corpus callosum. Although its function is not clear, the pineal gland produces and secretes the hormone melatonin.

Pinocytosis Pinocytosis, or "cell drinking," is almost identical to phagocytosis except that the targeted object is liquid.

Pitch The quality of a tone or sound, which is dependent on the relative rapidity of the vibrations.

Pitting edema Prolonged existence of pits produced by applying pressure to the skin.

Pituitary gland The bilobed pituitary gland is located in the sella turcica of the sphenoid bone and extends from the hypothalamus by a stalklike structure known as the infundibulum.

Pivot joints Also known as *monaxial joints,* these joints allow movements that are limited to rotation (e.g., atlantoaxial and proximal radioulnar joints).

Plantar Pertaining to the bottom surface of the foot.

Plantar fasciitis Inflammation of the plantar fascia at the calcaneus, medial aspect of the foot, and insertions of tibialis posterior.

Plantar flexion Extension of the ankle so that the toes are pointing downward, increasing the ankle angle anteriorly.

Plasma A straw-colored liquid that helps transport blood cells.

Platelet plug The process by which platelets enlarge, become sticky, and clump together, forming a plug, which helps to seal the damaged vessel.

Platelet (thrombocyte) Fragmented cells that help to repair leaks in the blood vessels through various clotting mechanisms.

Pleurisy Inflammation and/or adhesion of the pleural membranes characterized by stabbing pain during breathing.

Plexus A network of intersecting nerves.

Plicae circulares Circular folds in the lumen of the small intestine.

Pneumonia An infection or inflammation of the alveoli due primarily to the bacterium *Streptococcus pneumoniae;* however, other infectious agents such as bacteria, protozoans, viruses, and fungi may be responsible.

Poliomyelitis Poliomyelitis, or *polio,* is an infectious disease transmitted through fecal contamination or nasal secretions. It is caused by one of the three polioviruses and can range in severity from relatively asymptomatic to severe paralysis.

Pons The large rounded area below the midbrain that relays messages from the cerebral cortex to the spinal cord.

Popliteal   Area located on the posterior aspect of the knee.

Posterior (dorsal)   Pertaining more to the back of a structure.

Posture   The position of the body in space, such as standing, sitting, or lying down.

Prescription   A written order by a physician or nurse practitioner authorizing massage therapy treatment.

Pressure   The application of force applied to the client's body.

Progesterone   Hormone that prepares the endometrium for pregnancy and helps to maintain the corpus luteum once conception and implantation occur. One cause of spontaneous abortion (miscarriage) is a drop in progesterone levels.

Prolactin   Hormone that stimulates the mammary glands to create milk production in women.

Pronation   Medial (inward) rotation of the forearm; the palm is turned down.

Prone   Lying face or belly down in a horizontal, recumbent position.

Proprioception   A kinesthetic sense that helps us consciously orient our body in space without the use of vision.

Proprioceptor   A special type of mechanoreceptor detecting stimuli within the body itself. Examples of proprioceptors are muscle spindles, Golgi tendon organs, and baroreceptors.

Proteins   Naturally occurring organic compounds that contain large combinations of amino acids.

Protozoa   These single-celled organisms are considered the lowest form of animal life; pathogenic protozoa can only survive in a living subject and are commonly transmitted through contaminated food, water, and feces.

Protraction   Movement forward.

Proximal   Nearer to the point of reference, usually toward the trunk of the body.

Pruritus   Severe itching of the skin caused by dryness, sweat retention on the skin, kidney failure, allergic reactions, fungi, or parasitic agents such as scabies or body lice.

Psoriasis   Distinct, red, flaky skin elevations marked by periods of remission and exacerbation.

Pubic   Pertaining to the region of the pubic symphysis or the genital area.

Pulmonary circuit   The pathway of blood from the heart to the lungs and back.

Pulmonary edema   A condition involving an excessive amount of blood and interstitial fluid in the lungs.

Pulmonary respiration   See external respiration.

Pulmonary semilunar valve   The semilunar valve between the right ventricle and the pulmonary trunk.

Pulse   See arterial pulse.

Purkinje (conducting) fibers   Conducting fibers from the bundle of His that spread an impulse throughout the myocardium, causing the ventricles to simultaneously contract and expelling blood from the ventricles to the arteries.

Pustule   A small raised elevation of the skin, often with a "head" containing lymph or pus.

Pyloric sphincter   The sphincter located between the stomach and the small intestine.

Qi (Ki)   Chinese term used to describe the concept of energy.

Radiation   The transfer of heat energy in rays (e.g., infrared lamps).

Range of motion   A measure of possible joint movement from the least to the greatest by a particular joint.

Raynaud's syndrome   Periodic attacks of vasospasm of blood vessels in the body's extremities, especially the most distal parts, such as the toes, fingers, ears, and nose.

Recidivism   Relapse into the previous condition, such as substance abuse.

Reciprocal inhibition (Sherrington's law)   When a muscle receives a nerve impulse to contract, its antagonist receives simultaneously an impulse to relax.

Recruitment   The process of motor unit activation based on need of strength.

Rectum   The lower end of the colon that usually contains three circular folds that overlap when empty and grow in size as the rectum fills with "ready to excrete" wastes. The main function of the rectum is storage.

Referral forms   Forms generally produced by the provider and given to and filled out by a physician or nurse practitioner authorizing massage therapy treatment.

Referred pain phenomena   The tendency of trigger points to produce sensations (pain, tingling, numbness, itching, aching, heat, cold) distal from that of the trigger point.

Regeneration   Tissue healing that occurs when damaged tissue is replaced with new tissue of the same type. There must be enough undamaged tissue in the area to reproduce itself.

Reflex   An instantaneous, involuntary response to a stimulus originating from either inside or outside the body.

Reflex arc   The smallest, simplest portion of the nervous system capable of receiving stimuli and yielding a response; the functional unit of the nervous system.

Reflex sympathetic dystrophy   A complex disorder or group of disorders affecting the muscles and nerves of limbs that may develop as a result of trauma (e.g., accident, repetitive motion, or surgery).

Reflexive response A physiological response of the body due to reaction of a stimulus, often mechanical stimulation of nerve receptors.

Relaxin Hormone that softens the connective tissue in the body of a pregnant woman, which is helpful for loosening up ligaments in the pelvis for fetal delivery. It also helps to dilate the cervix during labor and delivery.

Remodeling (scar maturation phase) The process by which collagen fibers in the scar tissue are formed randomly following fibrosis.

Renaissance The intellectual and artistic movement (a "rebirth") beginning in northern Italy in the fourteenth century and extending throughout much of Europe by the seventeenth century.

Renal dialysis (hemodialysis) The process of using a mechanical kidney to remove substances from the blood in an attempt to restore its electrolyte and acid-base balance.

Renal failure The inability of the kidneys to perform essential functions (i.e., filtering the blood, collecting and secreting wastes, retaining essential elements).

Renal hilus The indentation located in the medial concave region of the kidney; where the renal arteries, renal veins, and the ureters attach.

Renal pelvis The funnel-shaped origin of the ureters located in the interior compartment of the renal hilus.

Renal tubules A urine-routing vessel.

Renin An enzyme secreted by the juxtaglomerular apparatus in response to a drop in blood pressure and a drop in the chloride ion concentration of the filtrate. This enzyme serves as a catalyst to change inactive angiotensin into active angiotensin II.

Repetitive motion injuries Also known as *repetitive strain injuries,* repetitive motion injuries are self-inflicted injuries related to inefficient biomechanics including general posture, sporting movements, and work habits.

Resolution Tissue healing involving tissue replacement. This occurs as long as cellular membranes are intact and nuclear contents are present.

Respiratory diaphragm A dome-shaped muscular partition that separates the thoracic cavity from the abdominal cavity; the main muscle of respiration.

Respiratory distress syndrome An acute infantile lung disease characterized by inelastic lungs, respiration rate of more than 60 per minute, and nasal flaring.

Reticular connective tissue A type of loose connective tissue; forms the framework of certain organs and provides support.

Retina A delicate nervous tissue membrane of the eye that is continuous with the optic nerve.

Retinaculum Bandagelike retaining band of connective tissue found at the ankles and wrists to keep tendons and tendon sheaths in place.

Retraction Movement backward.

Retroperitoneal Refers to structures located behind the peritoneum.

Rh factor The presence or absence of the Rh protein on the erythrocyte membrane. There are two types: Rh positive (about 85% of the population) and Rh negative (about 15% of the population).

Rhazes (c. 850-932) Name by which Persian physician Abu Bakr Muhammad ibn-Zakariya al-Razi was known in the West. He was a noted physician of his time and the first important Arab medical writer.

Rheumatoid arthritis Systemic arthritis that destroys the synovial membranes of joints characterized by flare-ups and remissions.

Rhythm In massage, rhythm is the repetition or regularity of massage movements.

Ribosomes Small granules of ribonucleic acid (RNA) and protein in the cytoplasm of cells.

Right lymphatic duct One of the two main lymphatic ducts that move lymph from the right arm, right side of the head, and right half of the thorax and enter the right subclavian vein.

Ringworm A group of fungal diseases characterized by itching, scaling, and sometimes painful lesions manifested as a raised red-ringed patch.

Rod Type of photoreceptor that is a thin cellular structure with slender rodlike projection very sensitive to dim light (night vision) and to shades of black, white, and gray.

Rosacea A chronic form of acne usually involving the middle third of the face, rosacea is characterized by persistent redness and swelling.

Rotation Circular movement when a bone moves around its own central axis. *Lateral* and *medial rotation* refer to direction of rotation. *Upward* and *downward rotation* are terms reserved for the scapula.

Ruffini end organs These receptors alert us when the skin comes into contact with deep or continuous pressure. Some references indicate that Ruffini end organs detect the sensation of heat.

Rugae Longitudinal folds in the stomach, urinary bladder, and vagina to permit expansion.

Sacral Pertaining to the sacrum of the spinal column.

Sacroiliac Between the sacrum and the ilium bone.

Saddle joints Also known as *biaxial joints,* saddle joints allow all movements, but rotation is limited (e.g., carpometacarpal of the thumb).

Sagittal plane A plane that passes through the body parallel to the midsagittal or median plane.

Saliva A clear, nondigestible, viscous fluid secreted by the salivary glands in the mouth.

Salt glow   A rubbing application of wet salt on the skin.

Sanitation   The application of measures to promote a healthful, disease-free environment.

San-tsai-tou-hoei   Japanese publication (c. 1610) that mentions both passive and active massage procedures.

Sarcolemma   The cell membrane that envelopes each individual muscle fiber.

Sarcomere   The muscle's contractile unit.

Sarcoplasm   The cellular fluid that is contained in each skeletal muscle fiber.

Sarcoplasmic reticulum   Fluid-filled system of cavities encircling each sarcomere that stores and releases calcium ions.

Sauna bath   A hot-air bath with temperatures ranging from 170° to 210° F in 10% to 20% humidity.

Scabies   Highly contagious infection caused by parasitic mites that crawl under the skin's surface and cannot be seen by the naked eye. The female mite excretes a material that causes intense itching (typically at night).

Scapular   Referring to the shoulder blade.

Scoliosis   Lateral deviation or curvature in the normally straight vertical line of the vertebral column, usually in the thoracic region.

Scotch hose   A high-pressured stream of alternating hot and cold water applied to a standing client.

Sciatica   Inflammation of the sciatic nerve often experienced as a dull pain and tenderness in the buttock region with sharper radiating pain or numbness down the leg.

Scleroderma   An autoimmune disorder affecting blood vessels and connective tissues.

Scope of practice   The working parameters of a particular profession according to training, education, and licensure.

Sebaceous (oil) glands   Glands that possess ducts (exocrine) and are attached to the hair follicle. Sebaceous glands secrete sebum.

Seborrhea   A topical disease of the sebaceous glands, marked by an increase in the amount of oily secretions.

Sebum   A mixture of fats, cholesterol, proteins, and inorganic salts secreted by sebaceous glands; it is mildly antibacterial, antifungal, and lubricates both the hair and the skin.

Self-disclosure   Honest and open sharing of thoughts, feelings, ideas, and insights.

Semilunar valves   Heart valves between both ventricles and their adjacent arteries.

Sensory neurons   Neurons carrying impulses from nerve receptors to the brain or spinal cord.

Separation   Injury in which the joint structure is simply pulled and stretched; the bone is not displaced out of the joint capsule.

Serous membranes   Membranes that line closed body cavities that do not open to the outside of the body. These membranes consist of two layers, parietal and visceral, and secrete a thin, serous fluid between these layers, which lubricates organs and reduces friction between the organs in the thoracic or abdominopelvic cavities.

Sherrington's law (reciprocal inhibition)   When a muscle receives a nerve impulse to contract, its antagonist receives simultaneously an impulse to relax.

Shiatsu   Japanese term that means finger (shi) pressure (atsu); the application of direct, perpendicular pressure applied along meridian lines and tsubos (acupoints and other reactive points on the body) to assist Qi flow in the body, mind, and spirit.

Shingles   An acute infection of the peripheral nervous system caused by the reactivation of the latent herpes zoster (chickenpox) virus.

Shin splints   Strain of either the anterior or posterior tibial muscles, marked by pain along the shin bone.

Shower   A bath technique in which water is sprayed in fine streams from a shower head under low to medium pressure.

Sickle cell disease   An inherited type of severe, chronic anemia in which red blood cells are "sickled." This shape greatly reduces the amount of oxygen that can be supplied to the tissues.

Sinoatrial node   The node that lies within the right atrium and initiates the cardiac impulse, stimulating both the right and left atria to contract.

Sinusitis   Inflammation of the paranasal sinuses.

Sinusoids   Specialized venous channels located in the liver.

Sitz bath   A sitting bath with the water covering the hips and often coming up to the navel. The bath chamber is usually designed so that the legs can remain out of the water.

Skin pallor   This term refers to an unnatural paleness or lack of skin color.

Skin tags   Tiny flaps of skin.

Sliding filament theory   The theory that discusses how muscle filaments slide past each other to change muscle length.

Slow twitch (red muscle)   Fatigue-resistant fibers that are small in diameter and have copious amounts of a red respiratory pigment called myoglobin.

Small intestines   The longest section of the alimentary canal situated in the central abdomen and framed by the large intestine. This muscular tube is bound at both ends by the pyloric sphincter (at the stomach) and the ileocecal sphincter (at the large intestine).

Sodium-potassium pump   A mechanism that actively transports ions (sodium and potassium) across a cell membrane against an opposing concentration gradient.

Somatic nervous system   Voluntary system governing impulses from the central nervous system to the skeletal muscles.

Somatic reflexes   Reflexes responsible for the contraction of skeletal muscle, such as when the doctor taps the patellar tendon with a rubber hammer (knee-jerk or patellar reflex).

Spa   A place where water therapies are administered.

Spasticity   Increased muscle tone and stiffness associated with an increase in tendon reflexes.

Sphincter   A ring of muscle fibers that regulates movement of materials from one compartment of the gastrointestinal tract to another.

Sphincter of Oddi   Regulates the flow of secretions from the pancreas, liver, and gallbladder.

Sphygmomanometer   The instrument used to measure blood pressure, most often in the brachial artery.

Spina bifida   A congenital defect characterized by a lack of osseous development in the lamina (posterior vertebral arch).

Spinal cord   Located in the vertebral canal of the vertebral column, the spinal cord is an extension of the brain stem from the foramen magnum to the region of L2.

Spinal nerves   Nerves exiting the spinal cord.

Spleen   A lymphatic organ; functions appear to be defense (destroys bacteria), hemocytopoiesis, destruction of red blood cells and platelets, storage of these destroyed and worn-out blood cells, and returning these blood cells to the liver for bile production.

Spondylolisthesis   An anteriorly displaced vertebra, usually the fifth lumbar vertebra over the first sacral vertebra.

Spondylosis   A general term for degeneration of the spine due to osteoarthritis; often called "arthritis of the spine."

Sprain   Joint trauma that stretches or tears ligamentous attachments, causing pain and possible temporary disability.

Squamous cell carcinoma   A type of skin cancer that arises from the epidermis, beginning as a scaly pigmented area that may develop into an ulcerated crater.

Standards of practice   A list of standards to assist professionals in making good decisions while conducting day-to-day responsibilities with their scope of practice.

State-dependent memory   Type of memory triggered by duplicating the original position of a client, location or amount of pressure, body move-ments, and emotions at the time an abusive or traumatic event occurred.

Steam baths   Hot vapor baths where temperatures are maintained at 105° to 120° F at 100% humidity.

Sterilization   A technique for destroying microorganisms using heat, water, chemicals, and/or gases.

Steroid hormones   Steroid hormones are derived from cholesterol and alter a cell's activity by turning genes on or off.

Stimuli   Any change in the internal or external environment.

Stomach   The stomach is a J-shaped organ that is essentially an enlargement of the gastrointestinal tract bound at both ends by sphincters.

Strain   A muscle or tendon injury due to a violent contraction, forced stretching, or synergistic failure.

Stratum corneum   The outermost layer of the skin.

Stratum germinativum   Also known as the *basal layer,* this is the innermost or matrix layer of the epidermis. The stratum germinativum undergoes continuous cell division and produces all other layers.

Stratum granulosum   A layer of cells containing an accumulation of keratohyalin granules, distinguishing it from other skin layers under a microscope. This layer is three to five cells deep, depending on the thickness of the skin.

Stratum lucidum   The translucent layer between the stratum corneum and the stratum granulosum. In thin skin, the stratum lucidum is absent.

Stratum spinosum   The stratum spinosum, or "prickly layer," is a bonding and transitional layer between the stratum granulosum and the stratum germinativum because it possesses cells of both these layers.

Stretch marks   Also called *striae,* stretch marks are silvery to white marks characterized by linear scars. These streaks often result from extreme stretching of the skin.

Stretching   Drawing out a single muscle (and its synergist) to its fullest length.

Stroke   Also known as a *cerebrovascular accident (CVA),* a stroke is an occlusion (blockage) of cerebral blood vessels by an embolus, thrombus, or cerebrovascular hemorrhage.

Stroke volume   The amount of blood ejected from the left ventricle during each contraction of the heart.

Subcutaneous layer   See Hypodermis.

Subjective data   Any information you gain from the client.

Sudoriferous (sweat) glands   Exocrine glands located in the dermis that secrete sweat, or perspiration. The primary functions of sudoriferous glands are to regulate body temperature and to eliminate waste products.

Sulci Grooves or depressions of the cerebral cortex.

Summation The amount of stimuli needed (both in frequency and number of fibers stimulated) to create a nerve impulse.

Superficial fascia See Hypodermis.

Superficial (peripheral) Pertaining to the outside surface; the external area of a structure.

Superior (cranial, cephalic) Situated above or toward the head.

Supination Lateral (outward) rotation of the forearm; the palm is turned up.

Supine Lying face up or belly up in a horizontal, recumbent position.

Surfactants Phospholipids made by the cells forming the alveoli that assist in exchange of gas, reduce surface tension, and contribute to the elasticity of pulmonary tissue.

Swedish gymnastics Movements to reduce pain, to restore mobility, and to maintain heath; these stretches and joint mobilizations can be applied passively, actively, or actively with assistance or resistance.

Swedish massage A systematic and scientific manipulation of the soft tissues of the body for the purpose of establishing or maintaining good health.

Sydenham, Thomas (1624-1689) English physician who emphasized clinical observation rather than theory.

Sympathetic nervous system (thoracolumbar outflow) A catabolic system that is involved with spending body resources and with preparing the body for emergency situations.

Symptom Anything the client subjectively notices as unusual or uncomfortable.

Synapse A junction between two neurons, or between a neuron and a muscle or gland, where they connect to transmit information.

Synaptic cleft See Synapse.

Synaptic end bulbs Bulblike structures at the end of axon terminals.

Synaptic transmission The electrochemical method by which the nerve impulse from one neuron bridges the synaptic cleft to convey nerve impulses to the next neuron. This is a one-way conduction from the axon of one cell to the dendrite of another.

Synaptic vesicles Sacs storing chemicals called neurotransmitters, located at synaptic end bulbs.

Synarthrotic A type of joint in which movement is absent or extremely limited.

Synergists Muscles that aid the prime movers by causing the same movement.

Synovial fluid Also known as *synovia*, this viscous fluid is found in joints, bursae, and synovial sheaths; a viscous liquid that provides nutrition and lubrication to the joint so that it can move freely without friction.

Synovial membranes Lines the joint cavities of freely moving joints (e.g., shoulder, hip, knee). Synovial membranes secrete synovial fluid.

Synovial sheaths Synovial sheaths are similar to bursae but are tubular instead of flat.

Systemic circuit The pathway blood from the left ventricle of the heart through numerous arteries into the capillaries, then through the veins to the right atrium of the heart.

Systole The pressure exerted on the arterial wall during active ventricular contraction.

Table mechanics Includes client positioning (prone, supine, side-lying, or seated), positioning equipment (bolsters and pillows), and draping.

Tachycardia Rapid heart rate (more than 100 beats per minute).

Taenia coli Thick, longitudinal bands located in the tunica muscularis of the large intestine that resemble thread gathering fabric.

Tai Ji The black and white icon representing Yin/Yang, or the supreme ultimate.

Tapotement Repetitive staccato striking movements of the hands, moving either simultaneously or alternately.

Target cell Cell that contains receptor sites, which are chemically compatible and join with their corresponding hormone.

Tarsal Regarding the ankle.

Taylor, Charles Fayette American physician who, along with his brother, George Henry Taylor, introduced the Swedish movement system (created by Pehr Ling) into the United States; helped popularize Ling's methods with his publications.

Taylor, George Henry American physician who, along with his brother, Charles Fayette Taylor, introduced the Swedish movement system (created by Pehr Ling) into the United States; helped popularize Ling's methods with his publications.

Techne Iatriche Term used to refer to the ancient Greek knowledge that comprised their philosophy of a "healing science."

Temporomandibular joint dysfunction A common ailment afflicting either the jaw joint, its musculature, or both.

Tendinitis Inflammation of the tendon, accompanied by pain and swelling.

Tendon A cord of tough fibrous connective tissue that anchors the ends of muscle to bone, fascia, or other connective tissue structures.

Tendon sheaths Tubular structures found where tendons cross multiple joints (e.g., hands and feet) and lined with synovial membrane.

Testes The reproductive glands located in the male scrotum that function both as endocrine and exocrine glands.

Testosterone An androgenic hormone that promotes secondary male sex characteristics, libido (sex drive), and sperm production.

Thalamus A relay station and interpretation center of the brain for all sensory impulses except olfaction.

Thermoreceptor Receptor sensitive to temperature changes, located immediately under the skin.

Thermotherapy The external application of heat for therapeutic purposes.

Thixotropy The ability of fascia to change the ground substance in its matrix from a gel to a sol state, and vice versa.

Thoracic Region between the neck and the respiratory diaphragm.

Thoracic duct The lymphatic duct that drains lymph from parts of the body not drained by the right lymphatic duct.

Thoracic outlet syndrome One of the repetitive strain injuries affecting the hand and wrist; caused by compression of the median nerve by the transverse carpal ligament.

Thoracolumbar outflow (sympathetic nervous system) A catabolic system that is involved with spending body resources and preparing the body for emergency situations.

Thrombocyte (platelet) Blood cell fragments that help repair leaks in the blood vessels through various clotting mechanisms.

Thrombosis An abnormal vascular condition characterized by thrombus (blood clot) formation in an unbroken blood vessel.

Thymopoietin Both thymosin and thymopoietin are immunological hormones that play a role in the body's growth, development, and sexual maturation and in the growth and maturation of antibodies, namely T cells.

Thymosin See thymopoietin.

Thymus gland A bilobed gland posterior to the sternum in the mediastinal region of the thorax. It is large in infants, reaches its maximum size at puberty, then atrophies and is replaced by adipose tissue in adults.

Thyroid gland Located at the base of the neck, posterior and inferior to the larynx. The butterfly-shaped thyroid gland is a bilobed gland connected in the center by a mass of tissue known as the *isthmus.*

Thyroid-stimulating hormone Stimulates the thyroid gland to produce and secrete triiodothyronine (T_3) and thyroxine (T_4).

Thyroxine (T_4) Both triiodothyronine (T_3) and thyroxine regulate growth and development and influence mental, physical, and metabolic activities. These hormones consist of a small peptide molecule bound to iodine.

Tissot, Simon André (1728-1797) French hygienist who was an important figure in physical therapy. He published several works on gymnastics and massage.

Tissue A group of similar cells that act together to perform a specific function.

Tissue respiration See internal respiration.

Tonsils A group of large specialized lymph tissues embedded in the mucous membranes in the throat.

Tonus A state of continuous, partial muscle contraction.

Topical Pertaining to the surface.

Torticollis Torticollis, or wryneck, involves spasms of the sternocleidomastoid muscles. The scalenes, trapezius, and the splenius muscles may also be involved.

Trachea A tube from the larynx to the upper chest. Located anterior to the esophagus, it measures about 5 inches long and consists of 16 to 20 half-ring hyaline cartilages.

Tract A bundle of nerve fibers running down the spinal cord in columns.

Transference The unconscious tendency to assign to others feelings and attitudes associated with significant persons in one's early life, especially the client's transfer to the therapist of feelings associated with a parent.

Transient ischemic attack An event of temporary cerebral dysfunction caused by ischemia or reduced blood circulation.

Transverse (horizontal) plane The plane that passes through the body and creates superior (cephalic or cranial) and inferior (caudal) sections.

Transverse (T tubules) Extensions in the sarcolemma within a muscle.

Treatment record Documentation obtained by information gained subjectively from the client; objectively through assessments; and the actual treatment notes, evaluation methods, and outcomes.

Tricuspid valve The right atrioventricular valve containing three flaps or cusps.

Trigger points Hypersensitive areas found in muscles, fascia, tendons, ligaments, skin, periosteum, and even organs.

Triiodothyronine (T_3) See Thyroxine.

Tropomyosin See Troponin.

Troponin Both troponin and tropomyosin are protein molecules present on actin molecules. These protein molecules mark the sites of attachment of the myosin filament during contraction.

Tsubo Japanese term used to describe acupoints.

Tuberculosis A chronic lung infection caused by the bacterium *Mycobacterium tuberculosis.*

Tunica externa The outermost layer of arteries and veins.

Tunica interna The innermost layer of arteries and veins.

Tunica media The middle layer of arteries and veins.

Tunics The layers of the alimentary canal: the mucosa, the submucosa, the muscularis, and the serosa.

Tympanic membrane The eardrum, which separates the outer ear from the middle ear.

Ulcer A lesion in a membrane, usually in parts of the digestive tract exposed to acidic gastric juice.

Umbilical Referring to the area of the midabdomen or navel.

Uniarticular Muscle that crosses one joint.

Universal donor A person with type O blood. Type O blood does not react to the other blood types.

Universal precautions A system of preserving health that may include any combination of the following: mandatory handwashing, vinyl gloves, protective eyewear, nose-face masks, protective clothing, laundering of linens and uniforms, cleaning of disinfecting equipment, and proper methods for disposing of used medical supplies and biological material.

Universal recipient A person with type AB blood. These persons can receive all other blood types.

Uremia A toxic level of urea and other nitrogenous waste products in the blood due to a renal insufficiency and abnormal retention of these waste products normally removed by the kidneys.

Ureters Two slender hollow tubes that transport urine formed by the kidneys to the urinary bladder. The ureters are located bilaterally—one ureter for each kidney.

Urethra A small tubular structure that transports urine from the urinary bladder out of the body during micturition (urination).

Urinary bladder A hollow muscular organ located in the pelvis behind the symphysis pubis that provides temporary storage for urine.

Urinary incontinence The inability to control micturition.

Urinary tract infection An infection of one or more structures of the urinary system often caused by bacteria.

Urine A solution of water and dissolved waste.

Varicose veins Dilated veins possessing incompetent valves.

Vascular spasm Occurs when the smooth muscle in the broken blood vessel begins to spasm; this may reduce blood flow for up to 30 minutes.

Vasoconstriction When the diameter of a blood vessel narrows.

Vasodilation When the diameter of a blood vessel enlarges.

Veins Blood vessels that drain the tissues and organs and return blood back to the heart and lungs.

Venous pump The one-way valve system to prevent backflow, together with the pumping action of muscular contraction in the limbs.

Ventral (anterior) Pertaining more to the front of a structure.

Ventral cavity Located anteriorly to the dorsal cavity, the ventral cavity is further divided into the thoracic and abdominopelvic cavities.

Ventricle The inferior heart chamber that pumps blood to the body's organs and tissues.

Venules Smaller, thin branches of veins.

Vermiform appendix A worm-shaped lymph gland, 3 to 6 inches in length, suspended from the inferior portion of the cecum.

Vertebrae Bones of the vertebral column.

Vertebral Pertaining to the spinal (vertebral) column.

Vesalius, Andreas (1514-1564) Flemish physician. His *De Humani Corporis Fabrica* (1543) is considered one of the most important studies in the history of medicine.

Vibration Rapid shaking, quivering, trembling, or rocking movement applied with the fingertips, the full hand, or an appliance.

Villi Fingerlike projections housing blood and lymph capillaries located in the lining of the small intestines.

Virus Considered to be a nonliving entity because it does not carry out independent metabolic activities. A virus can only replicate itself within the cell nucleus of a living plant or animal host.

Visceral (autonomic) reflexes Homeostatic reflexes such as coughing; sneezing; blinking; and corrections to heart rate, respiratory rate, and blood pressure.

Vital capacity The total amount that can be forcibly inspired and expired from the lungs in one breath.

Vitamins Organic compounds that are essential for normal physiological and metabolic functioning of the body.

Vocal cords Bands of elastic ligaments that are attached to the rigid cartilage of the larynx by skeletal muscle. A space exists between the folds and when air passes over them they vibrate and produce sound. The tighter the skeletal muscles pull the vocal folds, the higher the pitch of the voice.

Volkmann's canals Osseous canals that vertically connect Haversian canals.

Volume The loudness of sound.

Volunteer Someone who renders aid or performs a service without monetary gain. The service is performed of his or her own free will, usually with a sense of charity.

Warrior stance Also known as the *horse stance,* the warrior stance is used to perform massage strokes that traverse relatively short distances and to reach over to the far side of the body. Both feet are placed on the floor a little more than hip distance apart with toes pointing forward.

Wart Also known as a *verruca,* a wart is a mass of cutaneous elevations caused by a contagious virus, papillomavirus. Most warts are not cancerous, although some can be.

Weber-Fechner law The least noticeable increase in the intensity of a human sensation is always brought about by a constant proportional increase in the previous stimulus. To increase the intensity of a sensation in arithmetical progression, it is necessary to increase the intensity of the stimulus in geometrical progression.

Whiplash A sprain/strain of the cervical spine and the spinal cord at the junction of the fourth and fifth cervical vertebrae, occurring as the result of rapid acceleration (causing extension) or deceleration (causing flexion) of the body.

Wrap In hydrotherapy, a large pack covering most of the body through the use of large wet or dry sheets or blankets; the most common use is a body wrap.

Zang The Yin organs, according to traditional Chinese medicine.

Index